Handbook of
Self and Identity

Handbook of
Self and Identity

Edited by

Mark R. Leary
June Price Tangney

THE GUILFORD PRESS
New York   London

2003

© 2003 The Guilford Press
A Division of Guilford Publications, Inc.
72 Spring Street, New York, NY 10012
www.guilford.com

Printed in the United States of America

This book is printed on acid-free paper.

Last digit is print number: 9 8 7 6 5 4 3 2 1

Library of Congress Cataloging-in-Publication Data

Handbook of self and identity / edited by Mark R. Leary and June Price Tangney.
    p. cm.
  Includes bibliographical references and index.
  ISBN 1-57230-798-6
  1. Self. 2. Identity (Psychology) I. Leary, Mark R. II. Tangney, June Price.
  BF697 .H345 2003
  155.2—dc21   2002005520

About the Editors

Mark R. Leary, PhD, is Professor of Psychology at Wake Forest University. His research interests focus on social motivation and emotion, particularly processes involving the self. Dr. Leary has written or edited several previous books, including *Social Psychology and Dysfunctional Behavior* (1986, Springer-Verlag), *Self-Presentation: Impression Management and Interpersonal Behavior* (1995, Brown & Benchmark), *Social Anxiety* (with R. M. Kowalski; 1995, Guilford Press), *Interpersonal Rejection* (2001, Oxford University Press), and *Selfhood: Identity, Esteem, Regulation* (1999, Westview). He is also Editor of the journal *Self and Identity.*

June Price Tangney, PhD, is Professor of Psychology at George Mason University. She is coauthor (with Ronda Dearing) of *Shame and Guilt* (2002, Guilford Press) and coeditor (with Kurt Fischer) of *Self-Conscious Emotions: The Psychology of Shame, Guilt, Embarrassment, and Pride* (1995, Guilford Press). Dr. Tangney is currently Associate Editor of *Self and Identity* and Consulting Editor of *Journal of Personality and Social Psychology, Personality and Social Psychology Bulletin, Psychological Assessment, Journal of Social and Clinical Psychology,* and *Journal of Personality.* Her research has been funded by the National Institute on Drug Abuse, the National Institute of Child Health and Human Development, and the John Templeton Foundation.

Contributors

Arthur Aron, PhD, Department of Psychology, State University of New York at Stony Brook, Stony Brook, New York

Mahzarin R. Banaji, PhD, Department of Psychology, Harvard University, Cambridge, Massachusetts

Roy F. Baumeister, PhD, Department of Psychology, Case Western Reserve University, Cleveland, Ohio

Jennifer S. Beer, BA, Department of Psychology, University of California, Berkeley, California

Marilynn B. Brewer, PhD, Department of Psychology, Ohio State University, Columbus, Ohio

Peter J. Burke, PhD, Department of Sociology, University of California, Riverside, California

Charles S. Carver, PhD, Department of Psychology, University of Miami, Coral Gables, Florida

Jennifer Crocker, PhD, Department of Psychology, University of Michigan, Ann Arbor, Michigan

Susan E. Cross, PhD, Department of Psychology, Iowa State University, Ames, Iowa

Edward L. Deci, PhD, Department of Clinical and Social Sciences in Psychology, University of Rochester, Rochester, New York

Thierry Devos, PhD, Department of Psychology, San Diego State University, San Diego, California

David Dunning, PhD, Department of Psychology, Cornell University, Ithaca, New York

Carol S. Dweck, PhD, Department of Psychology, Columbia University, New York, New York

Jamie L. Goldenberg, PhD, Department of Psychology, Boise State University, Boise, Idaho

Brian M. Goldman, MS, Department of Psychology, University of Georgia, Athens, Georgia

Jonathan S. Gore, MS, Department of Psychology, Iowa State University, Ames, Iowa

Jennifer T. Gosselin, MA, Department of Psychology, George Mason University, Fairfax, Virginia

Heidi Grant-Pillow, PhD, Department of Psychology, New York University, New York, New York

Jeff Greenberg, PhD, Department of Psychology, University of Arizona, Tucson, Arizona

Jennifer S. Guinn, BS, Department of Psychology, University of Texas at Austin, Austin, Texas

Susan Harter, PhD, Department of Psychology, University of Denver, Denver, Colorado

Amy Kegley Heim, PhD, Department of Psychology, Boston University, Boston, Massachusetts

E. Tory Higgins, PhD, Department of Psychology, Columbia University, New York, New York

Michael A. Hogg, PhD, Center for Research on Group Processes, School of Psychology, University of Queensland, Brisbane, Queensland, Australia

Michael H. Kernis, PhD, Department of Psychology and Institute of Behavioral Research, University of Georgia, Athens, Georgia

John F. Kihlstrom, PhD, Department of Psychology, University of California, Berkeley, California

Stanley B. Klein, PhD, Department of Psychology, University of California, Santa Barbara, California

Mark R. Leary, PhD, Department of Psychology, Wake Forest University, Winston-Salem, North Carolina

Geoff MacDonald, PhD, School of Psychology, University of Queensland, Brisbane, Queensland, Australia

James E. Maddux, PhD, Department of Psychology, George Mason University, Fairfax, Virginia

Walter Mischel, PhD, Department of Psychology, Columbia University, New York, New York

Robert W. Mitchell, PhD, Department of Psychology, Eastern Kentucky University, Richmond, Kentucky

Carolyn C. Morf, PhD, Behavioral Science Research Branch, National Institute of Mental Health, Bethesda, Maryland

Lora E. Park, BS, Department of Psychology, University of Michigan, Ann Arbor, Michigan

Tom Pyszczynski, PhD, Department of Psychology, University of Colorado, Colorado Springs, Colorado

Peter J. Rentfrow, BA, Department of Psychology, University of Texas at Austin, Austin, Texas

Frederick Rhodewalt, PhD, Department of Psychology, University of Utah, Salt Lake City, Utah

Richard M. Ryan, PhD, Department of Clinical and Social Sciences in Psychology, University of Rochester, Rochester, New York

Barry R. Schlenker, PhD, Department of Psychology, University of Florida, Gainesville, Florida

Constantine Sedikides, PhD, Department of Psychology, University of Southhampton, Southhampton, United Kingdom

Carolin J. Showers, PhD, Department of Psychology, University of Oklahoma, Norman, Oklahoma

John J. Skowronski, PhD, Department of Psychology, Northern Illinois University, Dekalb, Illinois

Deborah L. Sorrow, BA, Department of Psychology, University of Utah, Salt Lake City, Utah

Jan E. Stets, PhD, Department of Sociology, University of California, Riverside, California

William B. Swann, Jr., PhD, Department of Psychology, University of Texas at Austin, Austin, Texas

June Price Tangney, PhD, Department of Psychology, George Mason University, Fairfax, Virginia

Abraham Tesser, PhD, Institute of Behavioral Research, University of Georgia, Athens, Georgia

Dianne M. Tice, PhD, Department of Psychology, Case Western Reserve University, Cleveland, Ohio

Kathleen D. Vohs, PhD, Department of Psychology, Case Western Reserve University, Cleveland, Ohio

Harry M. Wallace, PhD, Department of Psychology, Case Western Reserve University, Cleveland, Ohio

Drew Westen, PhD, Departments of Psychology and Psychiatry, Emory University, Atlanta, Georgia

Anne E. Wilson, PhD, Department of Psychology, Wilfred Laurier University, Waterloo, Ontario, Canada

Joanne V. Wood, PhD, Department of Psychology, University of Waterloo, Waterloo, Ontario, Canada

Virgil Zeigler-Hill, MA, Department of Psychology, University of Oklahoma, Norman, Oklahoma

Preface

In retrospect, it is difficult to understand why behaviorism dominated academic psychology so completely throughout much of the 20th century. The notion that we might be able to explain the complexities of human behavior without any consideration of what people might be *thinking and feeling* now seems absurd. In overlooking important aspects of human experience and important antecedents of human behavior, behaviorism stymied for decades many areas of research that involved cognitive or mentalistic concepts.

One of the fatalities of the behaviorist monopoly was the self. Building on millennia of thought in philosophy, William James had given the self a prominent place in his groundbreaking 1890 text. Reading James's chapter "The Consciousness of Self," many turn-of-the-century psychologists and sociologists could not escape the sense that people's thoughts and feelings about themselves were important determinants of their behavior. No doubt, James influenced many early theorists—most prominently Baldwin, Cooley, and Mead—who shared and elaborated upon this view, but mentalistic concepts such as the self were all but banished from mainline behavioral and social science once behaviorism took hold.

Now, a century later, the self has reappeared with a vengeance. One cannot make much progress through most areas of human psychology without encountering constructs involving the self, and contemporary sociology is replete with self-related research as well. Even animal researchers have come full circle to an appreciation of the fact that at least some nonhuman animals have the capacity to self-reflect and that this ability has implications for understanding their behavior. In addition to the hundreds of thousands of scholarly articles and chapters that have been published about the self in the past 30 years, there now exists a thriving international, interdisciplinary society for scholars who study self and identity, as well as a new journal called *Self and Identity* that started publication in 2002.

Given the tremendous advances in theory and research on the self over the past few decades, the time seemed ripe to assimilate the work in this burgeoning area within a *Handbook of Self and Identity*. From the start, we faced massive challenges in terms of deciding which lines of work should be covered in such a volume and the scientists who would be invited to contribute to it. There is far more important, influential work on the topic than can be glimpsed in a single volume, as well as more noted scholars who have contributed important work than could contribute chapters.

Looking at the literatures on self and identity as a whole, we concluded that the study of self and identity has emerged in five overlapping domains and so organized this volume along those lines. Following two introductory chapters in Part I that provide a broad historical and conceptual perspective on self and identity, the chapters are organized into five sections. Part II examines the *content, structure, and organization* of the self. A great deal of theory and research has been devoted to cognitive aspects of the self—not only the content of people's thoughts about themselves but how this self-relevant information is organized, stored, and retrieved. The chapters in Part II cover topics such as identity, self-concept, self-memory, self-organization, the implicit self, and the stability of self-thought.

Perhaps the greatest benefit of the human capacity for self-awareness is that it allows people to control their own behavior in ways that are not possible for animals that do not possess a self. The chapters in Part III—dealing with *agency, regulation, and control*—focus on the processes by which people regulate themselves—processes involving self-awareness, self-control, the use of self-standards, and self-efficacy. Although researchers still do not understand precisely how people turn self-generated intentions into deliberate self-directed behavior, the chapters in Part III show how far our understanding has progressed in the past 20 years.

The topics covered in Parts II and III involve largely "cold" self-processes, focusing on how people develop, process, store, and use information about themselves. The chapters in Part IV, in contrast, deal with "hot" processes that involve motivation and emotion. A great deal of research has studied self-motives such as self-enhancement and self-verification, as well as how self-thought and self-evaluation are related to emotions such as pride, shame, and guilt. The chapters in this section share a common focus on self-processes involving *evaluation, motivation, and emotion*.

One criticism that has been leveled at some research on self and identity is that it has treated the self in a disembodied, decontextualized manner, thereby losing much of its inherently interpersonal nature. The chapters in Part V redress this complaint as they focus on *interpersonal aspects of the self*. Clearly, much of what happens when people interact—in relationships, groups, or casual interactions—is influenced by how the individuals construe themselves. In turn, those self-construals are greatly affected by interpersonal and cultural factors.

The chapters in Part VI deal with the *development of the self*—among nonhuman animals, over evolutionary time, and during childhood and adolescence. Most psychologists would agree that newborn babies, like most nonhuman animals, have at most a rudimentary bodily or ecological self but no capacity for true self-awareness or self-relevant thought. Chapters in this section address many interesting questions about the selves of other animals, how the human self evolved from presumably self-less hominids, ways in which self-thoughts and self-evaluations change with age, and why the development of the self sometimes goes awry, resulting in emotional and behavioral problems.

One of the most notable things about human beings that distinguishes them from all other animals is their ability to self-reflect, to form images and ideas of what they are like, to ponder important questions about themselves, to seek outcomes that are congenial to their sense of self, to exert deliberate control over themselves, and to engage in other acts of selfhood. Although our understanding of these processes will undoubtedly advance in the coming years, researchers and theorists have made enormous strides in illuminating these quintessential human processes related to the self. This volume represents an attempt to integrate and summarize state-of-the-art knowledge about self and identity in a single, comprehensive volume. In the closing chapter in Part VII, we reflect on common themes that have emerged across the five areas of self-functioning and speculate on what the future holds for the next generation of research on the self.

MARK R. LEARY
JUNE PRICE TANGNEY

Reference

James, W. (1890). *The principles of psychology*. New York: Holt.

Contents

PART VI. PHYLOGENETIC AND ONTOLOGICAL DEVELOPMENT

PART VII. EPILOGUE

PART I

INTRODUCTION

1

The Self as an Organizing Construct in the Behavioral and Social Sciences

MARK R. LEARY
JUNE PRICE TANGNEY

Major advances in science often occur when the work of a large number of researchers begins to converge on a single unifying construct. Within psychology, for example, "learning" dominated the psychological landscape of the 1950s, "attitude" served as a rallying point in the 1960s, "attribution" was pervasive during the 1970s, and "cognition" was ubiquitous during the 1980s. Even when the specific topics studied under a particular conceptual umbrella vary widely, the overlapping and complementary findings of many researchers often lead to a rapid, synergistic accumulation of knowledge. In retrospect, periods in which a large number of researchers rally around the same maypole may appear somewhat faddish. Nonetheless, progress on a particular topic is often rapid when researchers invest a good deal of time and effort in it.

Since the 1970s, one such unifying construct within psychology, sociology, and other social and behavioral sciences has been the self, as tens of thousands of articles, chapters, and books have been devoted to self-related phenomena. The various topics that have fallen under the umbrella of the self have been quite diffuse—self-awareness, self-esteem, self-control, identity, self-verification, self-affirmation, self-conscious emotions, self-discrepancy, self-evaluation, self-monitoring, and so on—leading Baumeister (1998) to conclude that "self is not really a single topic at all, but rather an aggregate of loosely related subtopics" (p. 681). In one sense, this is undoubtedly true. Yet virtually all of these phenomena involve, in one way or another, the capacity for self-reflection that lies at the heart of the self.

Although a great deal of behavior occurs automatically and nonconsciously (Bargh & Chartrand, 1999), many complex human behaviors involve some degree of self-reflection. Some phenomena—such as long-term planning, choking under pressure, self-conscious emotions (e.g., shame and guilt), self-verification, and deliberate self-presentation—simply cannot occur in animals that are unable to self-reflect. Other phenomena—such as interpersonal communication, conformity, cooperation, mating, and nonsocial emotions such as sadness and fear—do not necessarily require self-reflection yet are drastically modified when people think about themselves. It seems impossible to understand the complexities of human behavior without reference to the human capacity to think about oneself. Indeed, reflexive consciousness may be the most important psychological characteristic that distinguishes human beings from most, if not all, other animals.

In light of the obvious importance of self-reflection to understanding human behavior, it is curious that behavioral and social scientists took so long to move the study of the self to a prominent position, particularly given that its importance was recognized millennia ago. The beginnings of intellectual discussions of the self are often traced to Plato (circa 428–347 B.C.E.), but we find Eastern writers wrestling with the problem of the self even earlier. The *Upanishads,* written in India as early as 600 B.C.E., the *Tao te Ching* in China (circa 500 B.C.E.), and the philosophy of Gautama Buddha (circa 563–483 B.C.E.) dealt extensively with questions about self, reflexive consciousness, and identity that still interest researchers today. In fact, many of the insights of these early philosophers were surprisingly astute, foreshadowing recent "discoveries" in behavioral and social science.

For nearly two millennia afterward, most discussions of the self appeared in religious and theological contexts, as writers analyzed the evils of egotism, pride, and selfishness and pondered ways to help people escape the self-centeredness that the writers believed interferes with spiritual insight and leads to immoral behavior. During the Enlightenment, most major philosophers tackled the problem of the self, including Descartes, Locke, Hume, Leibnitz, Berkeley, and Kant. The first detailed psychological discussion of the self did not appear until William James (1890) devoted a chapter of his *Principles of Psychology* to "The Consciousness of Self." James not only laid a strong conceptual foundation for the study of the self but also touted the importance of the self for understanding human behavior and set a strong precedent for regarding the self as a legitimate topic of scholarly investigation.

Oddly, however, behavioral scientists did not pick up where James left off for many years, due in large measure to the domination of psychological thought by behaviorism on one hand and psychoanalysis on the other. Most academic researchers were persuaded by behaviorism's admonition to avoid mention of invisible internal entities such as the self, and those enamored by psychoanalysis couched investigations of psychological processes in Freudian terms. Although Freud posited the existence of an executive ego that struggled to manage the individual's intrapsychic affairs, his conceptualization was too far removed from prevailing constructs in academic psychology to promote widespread adoption among behavioral scientists.

Even so, several influential theorists emphasized the importance of the self for understanding human behavior, and society more generally, during the early and mid-20th century. Charles Horton Cooley (1902) was particularly instrumental in bringing the self to the attention of sociologists, and George Herbert Mead (1934) extended and refined Cooley's ideas with a psychological twist. Likewise, Ellsworth Faris (1937) and Herbert Blumer (1937) further promoted the study of the self in sociology, leading to the development of what became known as "symbolic interactionism." A little later, Erving Goffman's (1959) seminal work on self-presentation stimulated another wave of interest in the self. Although Goffman himself dismissed psychology's view of an inner self, the researchers who imported the study of self-presentation into psychology assumed that the self was intimately involved in self-presentation (E. Jones, 1964; Schlenker, 1980).

At about the same time, the neo-Freudians began to offer perspectives on the self that not only differed markedly from Freud's notion of the ego but that also tied the self to interpersonal processes. Alfred Adler, Karen Horney, and Harry Stack Sullivan, for example, all provided views of the self that were more palatable to many academic psychologists than the original incarnation of psychoanalysis had been (Ansbacher & Ansbacher, 1964; Horney, 1950; Sullivan, 1953). Over time, these ideas evolved into the clinical perspectives known as ego psychology, self psychology, and object relations theory (Kurzweil, 1989).

By the mid-1950s, Gordon Allport (1955, p. 37) observed:

Perhaps without being fully aware of the historical situation, many psychologists have commenced to embrace what two decades ago would have been considered a heresy. They have re-introduced self and ego unashamedly and, as if to make up for lost time, have employed ancillary concepts such as self-image, self-actualization, self-affirmation, phenomenal ego, ego-involvement, ego-striving, and many other hyphenated elaborations which to experimental positivism still have a slight flavor of scientific obscenity.

Much of this work within psychology had a humanistic bent, as exemplified by Carl Rogers's (1959) theories of personality and psychotherapy and Abraham Maslow's (1954) work on fully functioning (i.e., self-actualized) individuals. However, although they provided many new ideas, the efforts of the neo-Freudians, humanists, and symbolic interactionists led to little systematic empirical research on the self.

Three developments converged to increase the attention given to the self by academic psychologists and sociologists in the second half of the 20th century. The first concerted empirical interest in the self arose in the context of self-esteem in the 1950s and 1960s (Berger, 1952; Coopersmith, 1967; Janis & Field, 1959; Rosenberg, 1965). Not only did these writers demonstrate the importance of self-esteem as a psychological construct, but they also provided self-report measures that stimulated a good deal of research. This early work on the predictors and concomitants of self-esteem then led to an interest in how people maintain their self-esteem in the face of various threats to their identity. Beginning in the 1960s, theorists began to use self-esteem motivation to explain a variety of phenomena, including conformity, self-serving attributions, reactions to self-relevant feedback, attitude change, prosocial behavior, and group behavior (e.g., Aronson, 1969; Bradley, 1978; Gergen, 1971; Greenwald, 1980; Jones, 1973).

The second development, the cognitive revolution in psychology, legitimized the study of thoughts and internal control processes. Armed with new models of how people attend to and process information—many of them rooted in computer metaphors—researchers began to conceptualize the self in terms of attention and cognitive

processes (Markus, 1977). Self-awareness theory (Duval & Wicklund, 1972) was particularly instrumental in changing how psychologists viewed the self, and led to control and cybernetic approaches to self-regulation (Carver & Scheier, 1981; Hull & Levy, 1979). Studying self from a cognitive framework also led to an expansion of interest in identity, which, although long a popular topic within sociology (Burke & Tully, 1977; McCall & Simmons, 1966; Rosenberg, 1965; Stryker, 1980), attracted more attention after identity and self-concept were explicitly cognitivized (Epstein, 1973; Markus, 1980).

Third, the publication of several measures of dispositional attributes related to the self also prompted a surge of interest in self-related topics in the 1960s and 1970s. In addition to the measures of trait self-esteem mentioned earlier (Coopersmith, 1967; Janis & Field, 1959; Rosenberg, 1965), measures of self-monitoring (Snyder, 1974), self-consciousness (Fenigstein, Scheier, & Buss, 1975), and self-concept (Wylie, 1974) fueled a great deal of theoretical and empirical attention to the self. The ease with which research could be conducted using self-report measures of these characteristics was both a blessing (in that it generated a proliferation of research interest) and a curse (because it led to a large number of hastily designed studies). By the 1980s, the self had emerged as a vibrant and central topic of investigation, and, by a decade later, interest in the self dominated many areas of psychology and sociology. Progress on each of these topics did not always inform the others as much as one might have liked (see Mischel & Morf, Chapter 2, this volume), but the fact that so many researchers were studying related constructs pushed our understanding of self and identity forward at a fast clip.

The Meanings of "Self"

In one sense, it is surprising that psychologists and sociologists took so long to embrace the relevance of the self for understanding human behavior. Not only had its importance been discussed in philosophical circles for nearly 3,000 years, but also influential early figures such as James, Cooley, and Mead had stressed its utility as an explanatory construct. In another sense, however, it is perhaps surprising that progress in understanding self and identity has been as rapid as it has. From the beginning, the topic has been bogged down in a conceptual quagmire as muddy as any in the social and behavioral sciences. Although psychologists and sociologists often have had difficulty agreeing how to define and conceptualize their constructs, "self" has been particularly troublesome. Not only have we lacked a single, universally accepted definition of "self," but also many definitions clearly refer to distinctly different phenomena, and some uses of the term are difficult to grasp no matter what definition one applies.

To see that this is the case, consider what the term "self" refers to in each of the following phrases, each of which has received attention by self researchers: self-awareness, false self, turning against the self, expanding the self, self-talk, honoring the self, vulnerability of the self, loss of self, self-disclosure, the border between self and others, social self, self-schema, traumatized self, sense of self, lack of time for the self, possible self, self-actualization. At best, inspection of these and other self terms suggests that "self" does not mean the same thing in all of these constructions; at worst, one begins to wonder what the term "self" actually means in any of them. To complicate matters, different writers have used precisely the same terms differently, and sometimes individual writers have used "self" in more than one way within a single paper.

Semantic debates in science are often unproductive. Magee (1985, p. 49) warned that "the amount of worthwhile knowledge that comes out of any field of inquiry . . . tends to be in inverse proportion to the amount of discussion about the meaning of words that goes into it. Such discussion, far from being necessary to clear thinking and precise knowledge, obscures both, and is bound to lead to endless argument about words instead of matters of substance." Despite Magee's warning, however, we feel compelled to spend a few pages grappling with the definition of self and self-related constructs. At minimum, we hope to alert researchers to the ways in which "self" is used and to urge them to choose their words with care.

Disparate Uses of "Self"

We have identified five distinct ways in which behavioral and social scientists commonly use the word "self" and its compounds (e.g., "self-esteem," "self-regulation," "self-verification"). (Olson, 1999, discussed eight uses of "self" among philosophers, some of which overlap with ours.)

Self as the Total Person

First, writers sometimes use the word "self" as more or less synonymous with "person," which also seems to be common in everyday language. In this usage, one's "self" is just that person, him- or herself. The compound "self-mutilation" relies on this meaning (the individual mutilates his or her own person), as do "self-monitoring" (the person monitors him- or herself as a person) and "self-defeating behavior" (the person is undermining his or her personal well-being). Similarly, writers sometimes use "self" to refer to the person him- or herself when "oneself" or "themselves" would be clearer (as in a study that found that "lack of time for self" was a common complaint among respondents).

Although this is obviously a perfectly acceptable use of "self" in everyday writing, uses that equate the self with the person do not refer to the psychological entity that is actually of interest to self researchers. From a psychological standpoint, most people (social and behavioral scientists included) do not seem to think that a person *is* a self but rather that each person *has* a self (Olson, 1999). If this is so, using "self" as a synonym for person in psychological writing is unnecessary and potentially confusing. When one means the person him- or herself, using "person" or reflexive pronouns, such as "oneself," will avoid confusion.

Self as Personality

Other writers have used "self" to refer to all or part of an individual's personality. For example, Wicklund and Eckert (1992) equated self with one's "behavioral potentials" (p. 3), and Tesser (2002, p. 185) suggested that the self is "a collection of abilities, temperament, goals, values, and preferences that distinguish one individual from another. . . ." Similarly, when Maslow (1954) wrote about "self-actualization," he was referring to actualization of a person's *personality*—a personality that was integrated, nondefensive, and optimally functioning. Again, using "self" as a rough synonym for personality appears to be acceptable in everyday discourse. Even so, using "self" to refer to a person's personality or the totality of aspects of a person that make him or her psychologically unique also breeds confusion. If a person's self is that person's personality, does that mean that all personality researchers are studying the self? In our view, the term "personality" captures this meaning far better than "self" does (although the self is obviously relevant to understanding aspects of personality).

Self as Experiencing Subject

James (1890) introduced a distinction, subsequently adopted by generations of theorists and researchers, between two intertwined aspects of the self—the self as subject and the self as object. The self-as-subject, or "I," is the psychological process that is responsible for self-awareness and self-knowledge; many writers have called this entity the "self-as-knower" to distinguish it from the "self-as-known." Thus many writers use "self" to refer to the inner psychological entity that is the center or subject of a person's experience.

This use of "self" is reflected in the phenomenology of selfhood. Most people have the sense that there is an experiencing "thing" inside their heads that registers their experiences, thinks their thoughts, and feels their feelings. Further, many people report that this mental presence is at the core of who they really or most essentially are (Olson, 1999). The fact that there is no specific neurophysiological structure underlying this experience of self does not undermine the subjective sense that there is a conscious entity—a self—"in there" somewhere.

Self as Beliefs about Oneself

James contrasted the "self-as-knower" (the *I-self*) with the "self-as-known" (the *Me-*

self). Many uses of "self" refer to perceptions, thoughts, and feelings about oneself—the various answers that a person might give to questions such as "Who am I?" and "What am I like?" Thus, when we speak of a "fragmented sense of self," we presumably mean that an individual's beliefs about him- or herself do not form a coherent whole. Likewise, when people "enhance the self," they are inflating the positivity of their beliefs about themselves, and when they "self-disclose," they are sharing the information they have about themselves with other people. Processes such as "self-verification" and "self-affirmation" also involve people's perceptions of and beliefs about themselves.

In our view, it seems important to distinguish clearly between a person's "self" per se and the person's knowledge or beliefs about him- or herself. It does not seem useful to regard the self as nothing more than a person's beliefs about himself or herself as a person (cf. Epstein, 1973). Fortunately, most writers have used terms such as "self-concept," "self-image," "self-schema," or "self-beliefs" to refer specifically to people's conceptualizations of or beliefs about themselves.

Self as Executive Agent

A fifth usage regards the self as a decision maker and doer, as the agentic "ghost in the machine" that regulates people's behavior. As Hamachek (1971) noted, one aspect of the self involves "the personality structure that represents the core of decision-making, planning, and defensiveness" (p. 6). Baumeister's (1999) discussion of the "executive function" of the self nicely captures this usage. Far from the problematic homunculus or psychodynamic ego that befuddled researchers of earlier generations, the executive self is often conceptualized as a cybernetic, self-control process (Carver & Scheier, 1981). When we speak of processes involving "self-control" and "self-regulation," we are referring to this executive feature of the self.

A Conceptual Morass

As we have shown, various writers have used "self" to refer to the person him- or herself, to the person's personality, to the seat of a person's self-awareness, to a person's knowledge about him- or herself, and to the source of agency and volition. A reader for whom "self" connotes any one of these definitions of self may easily misinterpret writers who use other definitions. For example, when we say that infants and most nonhuman animals do not possess a self, do we mean that they fail to meet the criteria for being a person, have no personality, lack subjectivity, do not have a concept of who or what they are, or can not exercise deliberate self-control? In one sense, we may mean all of these things, but in another sense, we may mean none of them. Similarly, the prefix "self-" refers to a quite different construct in terms such as self-observation, self-actualization, self-talk, self-schema, and self-regulation.

A Plea for Clarity

Our intention is not to offer the final word on the meaning of "self" but rather to alert writers to the widespread semantic confusion that exists, to urge them to consider their uses of "self" carefully, and to offer a few suggestions. First, we think that there are good reasons to avoid using "self" as a synonym for both "person" and "personality" in scholarly writing. Not only do clearer and more precise words than "self" exist for these constructs, but also most work in the social and behavioral sciences that focuses on the self deals with something other than the total person or the personality.

Each of the other three uses of "self" described earlier has some merit. The self is, in fact, somehow involved in (1) people's experience of themselves (though a self is not needed for consciousness per se), (2) their perceptions, thoughts, and feelings about themselves, and (3) their deliberate efforts to regulate their own behavior. However, none of these three specific uses of "self" captures the nature of the self in a way that encompasses all of the others. Thus we must either concede that "self" has at least three very different meanings (not a desirable state of affairs if we desire precision and clarity) or else arrive at a definition that encompasses all three of these uses.

If we dig down to the fundamental, essential quality that underlies all three of these uses of the term "self," we arrive at the hu-

man capacity for reflexive thinking—the ability to take oneself as the object of one's attention and thought. Virtually all scholarly interest in the self involves, in one way or another, phenomena that involve this capacity for reflexive consciousness. At its root, then, we think it is useful to regard the self as the psychological apparatus that allows organisms to think consciously about themselves. The self is a mental capacity that allows an animal to take itself as the object of its own attention and to think consciously about itself.

This definition of self accommodates the three preceding connotations. The special psychological apparatus that permits self-reflection affects the nature of conscious experience (because people can think about the self-relevancy of what they experience), underlies all perceptions, beliefs, and feelings about oneself (because self-conceptualization requires the ability to self-reflect), and allows people to deliberately regulate their own behavior (because self-regulation requires thinking about personal goals and how to meet them). Furthermore, with a few exceptions (such as "self-mutilation"), most hyphenated psychological constructs that have "self-" as a prefix—such as self-efficacy, self-deception, self-schema, self-presentation, and self-control—all refer to constructs, processes, or phenomena that, at their base, involve the ability to think reflexively about oneself.

Whether or not others agree with our basic definition of self, one way to avoid confusion is to use precise terms in place of the ambiguous "self." All of those hyphenated "self" terms serve us well in this regard. For example, if the focus is on the self as object, terms that denote thoughts about the self should be used as appropriate, such as "self-schema," "self-concept," "self-belief," or others. In our experience, a clearer, more precise term than "self" can almost always be found except when referring to the cognitive mechanism that allows reflexive self-thinking to take place, for which "self" is the only designation.

Carving Up the Self Pie

Starting with the idea that the self is the mental apparatus that underlies self-reflection, we can begin to bring order to the vast array of phenomena that self researchers have studied by considering the self-processes that have been of greatest interest to investigators. At the risk of oversimplifying, most of the psychological phenomena that have been studied with regard to the self involves one of three basic psychological processes—attention, cognition, and regulation. These three processes are inextricably related, and it is rare for one to occur without one or both of the others. For example, focusing attention on oneself often results in self-relevant cognitions and allows the possibility of regulation, thinking about oneself requires self-attention, self-regulation requires both self-attention and self-cognition, and so on. Even so, these seem to be distinct psychological processes that have different consequences and that are probably controlled by different regions of the brain.

Attentional Processes

At the most basic level, possession of a self allows people to direct their conscious attention to themselves, either spontaneously or purposefully. (In the case of deliberate self-attention, the regulatory function described subsequently is also involved.) Only a few other animals appear to possess a self that has a rudimentary capacity for self-attention, namely chimpanzees, orangutans, and possibly dolphins (Gallup & Suarez, 1986; Mitchell, Chapter 28, this volume). As considerable work on self-attention has shown, simply focusing attention on oneself has important effects on thought, emotion, and behavior (Carver & Scheier, 1981; Duval & Wicklund, 1972), and self-awareness is required for most other self-related processes.

Cognitive Processes

Possession of a self allows people to think consciously about themselves. Some of these self-thoughts involve one's current state and situation, others involve one's enduring attributes and roles, and others involve memories and imaginings, such as of oneself in the past or future. The capacity for self-relevant thought underlies the construction of a self-concept and identity, as well as the development of the various standards that

guide people's actions and influence their emotions, such as standards involving what they should do or be (Higgins, 1987). Among other things, self-relevant cognitions provide the link between the social world and the individual.

Executive Processes

The ability to attend to and think about oneself, both now and in the future, allows the possibility for human beings to regulate themselves. Unlike other animals, people can decide to control how they think, feel, and behave, then set about to do so. Of course, people's efforts at self-control are met with mixed success, but the possession of a self at least allows the possibility that one can occasionally escape the influence of one's environment, history, and internal state to act in autonomous, self-directed ways.

Theorists have found it a challenge to conceptualize the executive aspect of the self in a way that avoids positing something like a homunculus. If a person controls his or her responses through volition, who or what is doing the controlling? Cybernetic, computer, and neural-network models have all helped in this regard, explaining how interconnected elements of a physical system can allow the system to autoregulate in complex ways. However, none of these models can easily account for precisely how people make conscious, deliberate, intentional choices. Our sense is that this problem will not be addressed adequately until the larger problem of consciousness is solved. Once we understand how consciousness can arise from biological matter, we ought to be in a better position to talk about how it is that consciousness can focus on itself, allowing an organism to think about its own thoughts and direct the responses of the body in which it resides.

What about Motivation and Emotion?

Beyond capacities for self-relevant attention, cognition, and regulation, many writers have also imbued the self with motivational and emotional qualities, positing special self-motives (such as motives for self-enhancement and self-verification) and self-relevant emotions (such as pride, shame, and embarrassment). However, the relationship between the self and motivation and emotion is indirect and complex, and we do not think that the evidence at present is sufficient to conclude that the self possesses motivational or emotional qualities of its own.

The difficulty in addressing this question is that self is not essential for either emotion or motivation in the same way that it is required for self-attention, self-thought, and self-regulation. An organism absolutely must have a self in order to attend to, think about, and regulate itself. On the contrary, self-less animals experience emotions and have motives, and human beings also demonstrate automatic, nonconscious motives and affective reactions that do not involve self-reflection (Bargh & Chartrand, 1999). Put simply, many emotional and motivational processes do not require a self. Even so, possessing a self clearly extends people's range of motivational and emotional experiences far beyond those of other animals, and the self appears to underlie several motivational and emotional phenomena that appear to be unique to human beings.

The Self and Emotion

Having a self changes the nature of emotional experience by allowing people to create emotions in themselves by imagining self-relevant events, reacting emotionally to symbolic images of themselves in their own minds, consciously contemplating the causes of their reactions, and deliberately regulating their emotional experiences (Leary, in press). By being able to think about themselves, people can create subjective events that elicit emotional reactions. These emotions are not part of the self per se but are rather the consequences of certain self-thoughts and other appraisals.

However, one special category of emotions does appear to require a self. The "self-conscious emotions"—such as embarrassment, shame, guilt, and pride—occur only when people either judge themselves relative to their personal standards or imagine how they are being regarded by other people (Miller, 1996; Tangney & Dearing, 2002; Tangney & Fischer, 1995). Most theorists concur that self-reflection is necessary

in order for people to experience these emotions and that neither nonhuman animals who lack a self nor human infants before the ages of 18–24 months appear to experience these emotions (Buss, 1980; Lewis, 1992; Lewis & Brooks-Gunn, 1979; Lewis, Sullivan, Stanger, & Weiss, 1989).

It is unclear at present whether these self-conscious emotions should be considered part of the self (inasmuch as they cannot occur without it) or whether they are best regarded as the output of an integrated cognitive–affective system that is linked to the self. Given that the underpinnings of many of the self-conscious motives may be found in nonhuman animals (particularly in encounters among conspecifics involving dominance and submission; Gilbert & Trower, 1990), it may be best to regard them for now as emotions that have been appropriated by the self. Clearly, the precise nature of the link between the self and emotion deserves concerted research attention (Leary, in press).

Self-Motives

Likewise, possession of a self opens the possibility of motivated actions that are not possible without one. Writers have postulated several self-related motives, including self-esteem maintenance (or ego defense), self-verification, self-appraisal, self-actualization, self-affirmation, and self-expansion. What is not clear, however, is whether it is best to attribute these motives to the self per se (as if the self *wants* certain things for itself) or to view them as self-mediated ways to satisfy other, more basic motives and needs. We do not question that people behave in ways that make it appear as if they are inherently motivated to preserve their self-esteem, to maintain a consistent view of themselves, to seek accurate information about themselves, and so on, nor that self-reflection is often involved in these processes. Yet, rather than reflecting freestanding self-motives that are especially dedicated to fostering some quality of the self (such as a positive evaluation, consistency, integrity, or expansion), these pervasive proclivities may emerge from more general and fundamental motives, such as to minimize unpleasant affect or reduce uncertainty.

Put differently, having a self gives people additional ways of dealing with negative feelings and uncertainty that are not available to other, self-less animals. Other animals must take behavioral action to change their emotions (such as fleeing a predator) or to reduce uncertainty (such as exploring a novel stimulus). Armed with a self, however, people may influence their feelings simply by thinking about themselves and their worlds in certain ways. So, for example, people can engage in self-deception or self-affirmation to make themselves feel better, can overestimate the amount of control that they have over events to reduce anxiety, can construe themselves in ways that give them a consistent and, thus, more useful self-image, or can decide that more certainty exists than is, in fact, the case. In each instance, they are cognitively manipulating information in ways that achieve certain psychological outcomes, in a sense "cheating" the system by reaping the subjective effects of events that they experience only in their minds. Viewed in this way, these phenomena seem to emerge from self-mediated efforts to satisfy other motives rather than from freestanding motives of the self, although the jury is obviously still out on this issue.

Thus it may be more parsimonious to conclude that emotional and motivational systems are intimately linked to the self but are not an inherent part of it. Thus, for example, emotion and motivation may be affected when people compare themselves with their standards or with their past selves (Carver & Scheier, 1981; Higgins, 1987), contemplate their failures, shortcomings, and moral lapses (Tangney & Dearing, in press), think about how other people perceive them (Leary & Kowalski, 1995), ponder their goals and how to achieve them (Cantor & Zirkel, 1990), or assess their ability to perform certain tasks (Maddux, 1999). In each case, reflexive consciousness, along with self-generated affect, may energize and direct behavior, but the emotional and motivational systems themselves are independent of the mechanism that is responsible for self-reflection (i.e., the self). People's thoughts about themselves (which do involve the activity of the self) influence their emotion and motivation in much the

same way that thoughts about many things in the world can affect what they feel and desire at any particular time.

Self-Constructs, Self-Processes, and Self-Phenomena

Table 1.1 lists, in alphabetical order, a number of constructs, processes, and phenomena that, in one way or another, deal explicitly with the self. Although the list is by no means exhaustive, it provides a flavor for the variety of phenomena that have been studied under the rubric of the self. Importantly, as suggested earlier, the "self-" prefix means something different in different terms. So, for example, the "self" in "self-destructive behavior" seems to refer to something different from the "self" in "self-awareness." (Terms that do not refer to the psychological self in any way, such as "self-fulfilling prophecy," are not included.)

The first thing one notices is the sheer number of "self"-related terms. Just out of curiosity, we looked to see how many hyphenated "self" terms appeared in the abstracts in the *PsycInfo* computerized database through June of 2001. Eliminating the term "self-report," we found over 150,000 abstracts that contained a hyphenated "self" term, and this did not include such other central "self" terms as ego and identity! The most frequent ones included "self-concept" and "self-esteem" (with more than 20,000 references each), "self-control" and "self-disclosure" (with approximately 5,000 references each), and "self-actualization," "self-monitoring," "self-confidence," and "self-awareness" (each with more than 2,000 references).

Inspection of Table 1.1 also shows how splintered research on the self is at present. Very little effort has been devoted into exploring how each of the constructs, processes, and phenomena relate to other entries in Table 1.1. A smattering of work has examined the relationships among different constructs (such as Tesser, Crepaz, Beach, Cornell, and Collins's [2000] efforts to show the substitutability of various processes that involve self-esteem maintenance), but such efforts have been sparse. Researchers may wish to give additional attention to how

Table 1.1. Self-Related Constructs, Processes, and Phenomena

Desired/undesired self	Self-blame	Self-handicapping
Ego	Self-care	Self-help
Ego defense	Self-categorization	Self-identification
Ego extension	Self-completion	Self-identity
Ego ideal	Self-complexity	Self-image
Ego identity	Self-concept	Self-management
Ego integrity	Self-confidence	Self-monitoring
Ego strength	Self-conscious emotions	Self-organization
Ego threat	Self-consciousness	Self-perception
Feared self	Self-control	Self-preservation
Future/past self	Self-criticism	Self-presentation
Ideal self	Self-deception	Self-protection
Identity	Self-defeating behavior	Self-reference
Identity orientation	Self-definition	Self-regard
Ought/should self	Self-development	Self-regulation
Possible selves	Self-disclosure	Self-reliance
Self-acceptance	Self-discrepancy	Self-schema
Self-actualization	Self-doubt	Self-silencing
Self-affirmation	Self-efficacy	Self-talk
Self-appraisal	Self-enhancement	Self-trust
Self-assessment	Self-esteem	Self-verification
Self-awareness	Self-evaluation	Self-worth

their particular topic of interest relates to other self-processes more generally. Our current microtheories of specific self-related phenomena will take us only so far in understanding the self as a whole.

When we first designed Table 1.1, we planned to indicate beside each construct whether the term refers primarily to an attentional, cognitive, or executive feature of the self or to an emotional–motivational phenomenon in which the self is inherently involved. However, we quickly despaired of making these designations. Virtually every construct on the list involves at least two— and often three or four—of these features. For example, "self-awareness" is clearly an attentional phenomenon at heart, yet it is tied intimately to self-cognition, self-regulation, and self-relevant motivation and emotion (Carver & Scheier, 1981), and researchers who have studied self-awareness have often been interested in its cognitive, regulatory, motivational, or emotional concomitants rather than in self-attention per se. Likewise, "self-efficacy" is a cognitive phenomenon that relates directly to regulatory, motivational, and emotional processes (Maddux, 1999), and "self-conscious emotions" are emotional phenomena that necessarily involve self-attention and self-cogni-

tion and that have regulatory implications (Tangney & Fischer, 1995). Our inability to unequivocally categorize any of the constructs in Table 1.1 is instructive because it shows that the attentional, cognitive, and regulatory aspects of the self are intimately interconnected, with pervasive links to emotion and motivation.

Conclusion

It seems virtually impossible to develop a full understanding of human behavior without taking into account the fact that human beings can attend to, think about, and act on themselves in ways that are not possible for any other animal. Major strides have been made in understanding the self over the past century (Hoyle, Kernis, Leary, & Baldwin, 1999), and, now that self research is no longer stigmatized as it once was, progress should continue at a fast pace.

Although we are optimistic about the state of self theory and research, our optimism is tempered slightly by the fact that the field is composed of a large number of pockets of self-contained research literatures that have yet to be adequately integrated. With a few exceptions, behavioral and social scientists, perhaps with good reason, have avoided large-scale theorizing in favor of limited-domain theories, leaving the big picture to philosophers of mind. Although the philosophers have contributed many useful ideas and theoretical perspectives on the self (see Gallagher & Shear, 1999), they have generally not tied those ideas to the extensive empirical literature in psychology and sociology. As a result, social and behavioral scientists have not rushed to embrace those perspectives, to use them to interpret their own findings, or to base their research on them. The future of self research will depend in large measure on how successfully broad theoretical advances are able to link together specific bodies of research that deal with self and identity.

References

Allport, G. W. (1955). *Becoming*. New Haven, CT: Yale University Press.

Ansbacher, H. L., & Ansbacher, R. R. (Eds.). (1964). *Superiority and social interest: A collection of later writings by Alfred Adler*. Evanston, IL: Northwestern University Press.

Aronson, E. (1969). Dissonance theory: Progress and problems. In R. P. Abelson, E. Aronson, W. J. McGuire, T. M. Newcomb, M. J. Rosenberg, & P. H. Tannenbaum (Eds.), *Cognitive consistency theories: A sourcebook* (pp. 5–27). Skokie, IL: Rand McNally.

Bargh, J. A., & Chartrand, T. L. (1999). The unbearable automaticity of being. *American Psychologist, 54,* 462–479.

Baumeister, R. F. (1998). The self. In D. Gilbert, S. T. Fiske, & G. Lindzey (Eds.), *The handbook of social psychology* (pp. 680–740). New York: Oxford University Press.

Berger, E. M. (1952). The relation between expressed acceptance of self and expressed acceptance of others. *Journal of Abnormal and Social Psychology, 47,* 778–782.

Blumer, H. (1937). Social psychology. In E. P. Schmidt (Ed.), *Man and society* (pp. 144–198). New York: Prentice-Hall.

Bradley, G. W. (1978). Self-serving biases in the attribution process: A reexamination of the fact or fiction question. *Journal of Personality and Social Psychology, 36,* 56–71.

Burke, P. J., & Tully, J. (1977). The measurement of role/identity. *Social Forces, 55,* 881–897.

Buss, A. H. (1980). *Self-consciousness and social anxiety*. San Francisco: Freeman.

Cantor, N., & Zirkel, S. (1990). Personality, cognition, and purposive behavior. In L. A. Pervin (Ed.), *Handbook of personality: Theory and research* (pp. 135–164). New York: Guilford Press.

Carver, C. S., & Scheier, M. F. (1981). *Attention and self-regulation: A control-theory approach to human behavior*. New York: Springer-Verlag.

Cooley, C. H. (1902). *Human nature and the social order*. New York: Scribner's.

Coopersmith, S. (1967). *The antecedents of self-esteem*. San Francisco: Freeman.

Duval, S., & Wicklund, R. A. (1972). *A theory of objective self-awareness*. New York: Academic Press.

Epstein, S. (1973). The self-concept revisited: Or a theory of a theory. *American Psychologist, 28,* 404–416.

Faris, E. (1937). *The nature of human nature*. New York: McGraw-Hill.

Fenigstein, A., Scheier, M. F., & Buss, A. H. (1975). Public and private self-consciousness: Assessment and theory. *Journal of Consulting and Clinical Psychology, 43,* 522–528.

Gallagher, S., & Shear, J. (Eds.). (1999). *Models of the self*. Thorverton, UK: Imprint Academic.

Gallup, G. G., Jr., & Suarez, S. D. (1986). Self-awareness and the emergence of mind in humans and other primates. In J. Suls & A. G. Greenwald (Eds.), *Psychological perspectives on the self* (Vol. 3, pp. 3–26). Hillsdale, NJ: Erlbaum.

Gergen, K. J. (1971). *The concept of self*. New York: Holt, Rinehart & Winston.

Gilbert, P., & Trower, P. (1990). The evolution and manifestation of social anxiety. In W. R. Crozier (Ed.), *Shyness and embarrassment* (pp. 144–177). New York: Cambridge University Press.

Goffman, E. (1959). *The presentation of self in everyday life*. Garden City, NY: Doubleday Anchor.

Greenwald, A. G. (1980). The totalitarian ego: Fabrication and revision of personal history. *American Psychologist, 35,* 603–613.

Hamachek, D. E. (1971). *Encounters with the self*. New York: Holt, Rinehart, & Winston.

Higgins, E. T. (1987). Self-discrepancy: A theory relating self and affect. *Psychological Review, 94,* 319–340.

Horney, K. (1950). *Neurosis and human growth*. New York: Norton.

Hoyle, R. H., Kernis, M. H., Leary, M. R., & Baldwin, M. W. (1999). *Selfhood: Identity, esteem, regulation*. Boulder, CO: Westview Press.

Hull, J. G., & Levy, A. S. (1979). The organizational functions of the self: An alternative to the Duval and Wicklund model of self-awareness. *Journal of Personality and Social Psychology, 37,* 756–768.

James, W. (1890). *The principles of psychology*. New York: Holt.

Janis, I. L., & Field, P. B. (1959). A behavioral assessment of persuasibility: Consistency of individual differences. In C. I. Hovland & I. L. Janis (Eds.), *Personality and persuasibility* (pp. 55–68). New Haven, CT: Yale University Press.

Jones, E. E. (1964). *Ingratiation*. New York: Appleton-Century-Crofts.

Jones, S. R. (1973). Self- and interpersonal evaluations: Esteem theories versus consistency theories. *Psychological Bulletin, 79,* 185–199.

Kurzweil, E. (1989). *The Freudians: A comparative perspective*. New Haven, CT: Yale University Press.

Leary, M. R. (in press). The self and emotion. In R. J.

Davidson, K. R. Scherer, & H. H. Goldsmith (Eds.), *Handbook of affective sciences*. New York: Oxford University Press.

Leary, M.R., & Kowalski, R.M. (1995). *Social anxiety.* New York: Guilford Press.

Lewis, M., & Brooks-Gunn, J. (1979). *Social cognition and the acquisition of self.* New York: Plenum Press.

Maddux, J. E. (1999). Personal efficacy. In V. J. Derlega, B. A. Winstead, & W. H. Jones (Eds.), *Personality: Contemporary theory and research* (2nd ed., pp. 229–256). Chicago: Nelson-Hall.

Magee, B. (1985). *Philosophy and the real world: An introduction to Karl Popper.* LaSalle, IL: Open Court.

Markus, H. (1977). Self-schemata and processing information about the self. *Journal of Personality and Social Psychology, 35,* 63–78.

Markus, H. (1980). The self in thought and memory. In D. M. Wegner & R. R. Vallacher (Eds.), *The self in social psychology* (pp. 102–130). New York: Oxford University Press.

Maslow, A. H. (1954). *Motivation and behavior.* New York: Harper & Row.

McCall, G., & Simmons, J. L. (1966). *Identities and interactions: An examination of human association in everyday life.* New York: Free Press.

Mead, G. H. (1934). *Mind, self, and society.* Chicago: University of Chicago Press.

Miller, R. S. (1996). *Embarrassment: Poise and peril in everyday life.* New York: Guilford Press.

Olson, E. T. (1999). There is no problem of the self. In S. Gallagher & J. Shear (Eds.), *Models of the self* (pp. 49–61). Thorverton, UK: Imprint Academic.

Rogers, C. (1959). A theory of therapy, personality, and interpersonal relationships, as developed in the client-centered framework. In S. Koch (Ed.), *Psychology: A study of a science* (Vol. 3, pp. 184–256). New York: McGraw-Hill.

Rosenberg, M. (1965). *Society and the adolescent self image.* Princeton, NJ: Princeton University Press.

Schlenker, B. R. (1980). *Impression management.* Monterey, CA: Brooks/Cole.

Snyder, M. (1974). Self-monitoring of expressive behavior. *Journal of Personality and Social Psychology, 30,* 526–537.

Stryker, S. (1980). *Symbolic interactionism: A social structural version.* Menlo Park, CA: Benjamin/Cummings.

Sullivan, H. S. (1953). *The interpersonal theory of psychiatry.* New York: Norton.

Tangney, J. P., & Dearing, R. L. (2002). *Shame and guilt.* New York: Guilford Press.

Tangney, J. P., & Fischer, K. W. (Eds). (1995). *The self-conscious emotions: The psychology of shame, guilt, embarrassment, and pride.* New York: Guilford Press.

Tesser, A. (2002). Constructing a niche for the self: A biosocial, PDP approach to understanding lives. *Self and Identity, 1,* 185–190.

Tesser, A., Crepaz, N., Beach, S. R. H., Cornell, D., & Collins, J. C. (2000). Confluence of self-esteem regulation mechanisms: On integrating the self-zoo. *Personality and Social Psychology Bulletin, 26,* 1476–1489.

Wicklund, R. A., & Eckert, M. (1992). *The self-knower: A hero under control.* New York: Plenum.

Wylie, R. (1974). *The self-concept* (Vol. 1). Lincoln: University of Nebraska Press.

2

The Self as a Psycho-Social Dynamic Processing System: A Meta-Perspective on a Century of the Self in Psychology

WALTER MISCHEL
CAROLYN C. MORF

In spite of many historical vicissitudes, the concept of "self" has been central in psychology from James at the start of the last century, to Rogers in its middle years, to the contemporary explosion of work on this topic, as reflected in the chapters in this volume. During the same hundred years this now highly popular construct also has been condemned as a gratuitous fiction that merely re-names the dreaded homunculus that sits inside the person and is made its causal agent. That specter could be avoided easily if the self is treated just as a set of concepts about the self—individual, relational, and collective—as it was in its early resurgence in psychology in the 1970s, concurrent with the beginnings of the cognitive revolution after a long lull during decades of behaviorism. However, in a rapidly accelerating trajectory, self research and theory soon grew greatly beyond those beginnings in new directions to raise again issues concerning the self's agency and associated motivations and emotions. This field now is bursting with important findings, creating fresh challenges, and offering exciting prospects, while at the same time still struggling with classic problems.

In this chapter, we have two goals. First, we seek to provide a perspective on the current state of the science of the self. In our view, this state is robust and vibrant but it also is complex and diffuse, with relevant work scattered across diverse sub-fields and disciplines that often operate in remarkable isolation, impervious to developments just across the boundaries. As a result, integration and the growth of a cumulative science of self is exceedingly difficult, making it extremely important to cross those boundaries if we are to construct a more unifying framework for understanding the self. At present, the disparate self-relevant strands include work in areas beyond social cognition and social psychology that range from personality and clinical psychology and psychiatry, to developmental psychology, to cognitive science, sociology, philosophy, and more. Although the breadth of this work makes even a comprehensive overview an unrealistic goal, we discuss in the first major section some of the shifting boundaries and expansions of the concept of self over the last century. We also examine some of the particularly difficult challenges with which self research has struggled throughout much of its history and that still confront it currently. Because of their importance, we then focus in depth on the homunculus problem and its current state, and examine the fuzzy and often confusing entangled relations between the self and personality.

Despite the dispersed literature and research on the self, there seems to be a growing consensus about the essentials that "selfhood" encompasses. We begin the second major section by presenting our reading of these consensus statements about the nature of the self. Most important, we see a clear recognition emerging from this consensus that the self needs to be conceptualized as an organized coherent system. Many promising indications of the outlines for such a system are beginning to appear and seem virtually waiting to be articulated, and many of the sub-processes and sub-systems already have been specified in depth, again documented in this volume. Our second goal in this chapter is to draw and build on these developments to discuss a potentially integrative approach—a preliminary model—toward a comprehensive self-system that seems to be emerging from many converging lines of theory and research. We do not see this system as "ours," but rather as an effort to integrate diverse already existing contributions—it is a system that rests on, and is intended to reflect, decades of cumulative contributions from our science.

In this system the self and its directly relevant processes (e.g., self-evaluation, self-regulation, self-construction) may be conceptualized fruitfully as a coherent *organization* of mental–emotional representations, interacting within a system of constraints that characterize a person (or a type) distinctively. In its complex organization and processing dynamics, it draws as a metaphor on current connectionist theory. But it also is a motivated, proactive knowing, thinking, feeling action system that is constructed, enacted, enhanced, and maintained primarily in interpersonal contexts in the social world within which it develops. Through this organized system the person experiences the social, interpersonal world and interacts with it, in characteristic self-guided ways, in a process of continuous self-construction and adaptation.

In the second section we formulate this model with the hope that it offers a unifying perspective for viewing the relations among diverse lines of previous and current work on the self, while also having heuristic value for future research and theory. Then in the third and final major section, we examine the implications for further theory and research, and consider the prospects for the future in efforts to build a cumulative science of the self.

Perspectives on a Century of Self Research: The Locus of the Expanding Self in Psychology

Expansion of the Self Construct and Its Implications

The long and fascinating history of the psychology of self and selfhood lies outside the scope of this chapter, and has been comprehensively reviewed elsewhere (see Baldwin, 1905; Baumeister, 1987). We therefore begin only with a selective thumbnail sketch of the recurrent issues and some of the more recent major trends insofar as they can inform the understanding of where the field is now and where it might go next. But while we bypass the history of the self in any detail, one can hardly proceed without noting that the self for many centuries played a key part in the work of philosophers concerned with the problem of human consciousness from Descartes (1637/1970) on, just as it still engages contemporary philosophy. Its modern account in psychology generally is seen as beginning with William James (1890, 1892), who foreshadowed much of how we conceive of the self today. James notes and analyzes the flux of consciousness co-existing with the sense of continuity in the stream of thought, the importance of habit (or what now is called automaticity), and the selectivity of consciousness, of attention, and of all the workings of the human mind. In his famous chapter on the self he elucidates most of the topics that still define much of the agenda of contemporary self research. These include the feelings and emotions of self, the diverse aspects of self, self-esteem, the self-as-knower, the I and the Me and how the former appropriates the latter—to name just a few.

The recognition that the self is essentially a *social* phenomenon that arises out of social experiences has regained popularity in contemporary views on the self. It was evident already in the writings of John Dewey (1890), C. H. Cooley (1902), George Herbert Mead (1934), and other symbolic interactionists, and within clinical psychology, psychiatry, and personality (e.g., in the interpersonal theory of H. S. Sullivan). The implications of this social nature of the self for the development of a comprehensive model of the self-system will be one of the major themes of this chapter. A second enduring theme, recognized since the first half of the last century, is the importance for adaptation and coping of the "executive functions" (e.g., self-regulation, self-defense) of the self, emphasized first by the "ego psychologists", stemming originally from the psychodynamic Freudian tradition (see Mischel, 1998, for an overview). This is evident, for example, in Anna Freud's focus on ego defenses and in the theories and clinical practice of Alfred Adler and Carl Jung. Furthermore, in the second half of the last century the self-evaluative functions of the self, as in self-esteem, as well as the importance of the concept of identity, became central in the "object relations" theories of clinicians like Melanie Klein and, more recently, Heinz Kohut (1971) and Otto Kernberg (1976, 1984).

Guardians of the self construct during the reign of behaviorism. Through these developments, the clinical–personality area turned out to be the guardians of the self construct during the concurrent period of behaviorism that dominated mainstream American academic psychology from the 1930s to the 1960s. In this time frame, behaviorism virtually killed the self as a legitimate topic for psychological inquiry in mainstream academic research, and banned it as outside of what was then defined as the boundaries of the science. Thus, although the psychology of self and selfhood began at least at a theoretical level with the start of psychology, its modern impact on the development of the science was not felt widely for many years.

Within clinical psychology, interest in the self resurfaced as the core of a humanistic protest movement in the 1950s. The protest was against the then-dominant influences of American behaviorism, as well as against psychoanalytic theory coming from Europe, and its strongest spokesperson was Carl Rogers. The essence of the protest was directed on the one side against the unconscious id-based (sex and aggression) motivational determinism of Freudian theories. On the other side, it was directed equally at the mechanistic push–pull determinism of behaviorism, as seen in Skinner's regnant position on the powers of "stimulus control." In refreshing contrast, it was Rogers who articulated the view that "behavior is basically the goal-directed attempt of the organism to satisfy its needs in the field as perceived" (1951, p. 491). In his words, "there is one central source of energy in the human organism ... a tendency toward fulfillment, toward actualization, toward the maintenance and enhancement of the organism," and it was the self and the experiences of the self that played a central role in this process. This then-rebellious viewpoint created great interest, especially among humanistically oriented psychologists and clinicians. However, it also soon ran into challenges, most notably that the self was a homunculus—a "little man in the head" that performed all sorts of feats—that worried many thoughtful psychologists when dealing with a self like this one hypothesized by Carl Rogers: "when the self is free from any threat of attack, then it is possible for the self to consider these hitherto rejected perceptions, to make new differentiations, and to reintegrate the self in such a way as to include them" (1947, p. 365).

The concern of course was that for Rogers the self seemed to take on a life of its own beyond the "me" or "I" distinct from the whole person and from what he or she does—it is even a self that can "reintegrate the self." Unwilling to give the self such extraordinary causal powers, Gordon Allport—one of the construct's early defenders even at the height of behaviorism—noted then: "To say that the self does this or that, wants this or that, wills this or that, is to beg a series of difficult questions. The psychologist does not like to pass the buck to a self-agent. ... It is unwise to assign our problems to an inner agent who pulls the strings" (1961, pp. 129–130).

Sharing Allport's concerns, personality psychologists refrained for many years from dealing with the motivated self and turned instead to more static alternatives such as broad trait descriptions of "what people are like" and to individual differences in those qualities. In that spirit, in the 1950s and 1960s, research was done on individual differences in global self-esteem. But beyond that, the self received little empirical attention and remained excluded until the cognitive revolution in the 1970s rapidly transformed psychology itself.

The cognitive revolution: self as a knowledge structure. At that time, social psychologists, in an effort to avoid the homunculus problem and influenced by the cognitive revolution, turned to examining the self as an essentially "cool" cognitive, unmotivated knowledge structure—an information-processing machine based on computer analogs of the 1970s (as reviewed in Linville & Carlston, 1994). The resurgence of interest in the self, indeed its virtual explosion, during the 1970s returned the self-concept to the realm of legitimate study for empirical psychologists, mostly housed within the domain of social cognition (Markus & Zajonc, 1985). The research work during this time dealt primarily with "self as known" or as object, and significant advances were made, especially in understanding the self's structure (e.g., Greenwald & Pratkanis, 1984; Linville & Carlston, 1994). Use of the computer metaphor, and advances in cognitive psychology, such as the distinction between declarative and procedural knowledge, facilitated conceptualization of many complex features of the self, such as the diverse, multiple forms of its expressions, and the seemingly paradoxical co-existence of its stability and malleability. The same period of the cognitive revolution also contributed an arsenal of new methods—from rediscovering the diverse uses of reaction time, to priming procedures, to innovative recall and recognition measures that have become essential quotidian tools for social psychologists.

But soon the self-construct and research about it expanded dramatically as self researchers began to look beyond the self as object to consider its functions as a "doer," thereby re-infusing the self with agentic qualities. Thus in the 1980s the self construct continued to expand and acquired personal agency and such basic processing dynamics as self-evaluation, self-enhancement, self-defense, self-regulation, and self-control. This enrichment and expansion of the self-construct further vitalized the area. For example, knowledge structures have been extended to include outcome expectations, action-evaluation, and affective information and even to prescribe goals and desires (as discussed by Hoyle, Kernis, Leary, & Baldwin, 1999). But this also raised again classic problems about the self as a causal agent: clearly these processes of the self involve not only "cool" mental representations or knowledge structures about the self but also imply motivation. Furthermore, they link to evaluative and emotional reactions and ultimately to behavioral outcomes that can be of profound significance for the person, ranging from failed New Year's resolutions to destructive relationships to suicide. An attempt to address these processes thus has to be able to speak to such questions as *why* an individual who seems to seek intimacy also experiences and enacts relationships in ways that undo them. Likewise, one needs to understand *why* the diabetic for whom dieting is a central self-relevant goal and who resolved to skip dessert failed to forgo the chocolate pastry on the tray when it was presented by the waiter. In short, it is difficult if not impossible to understand agentic processes such as self-regulation and self-control without invoking explanatory mechanisms. Hence the self soon became motivated, driven by goals and a wide range of motives, expectations, beliefs, values, and so on (e.g., Cantor, 1990; Cantor & Kihlstrom, 1987; Emmons, 1991, on goals; Gollwitzer & Bargh, 1996; Mischel, 1973; Pervin, 1982, 1989). And of course the more agentic and autonomous the self became, the more the homunculus threat returned, and again faced contemporary research and theory building on the phenomena of self and selfhood.

Avoiding the Homunculus in an Agentic Self: Gains and Risks of the Motivated Self

The explosion of interest in the motivated self in recent years has both re-vitalized research in the area and re-introduced fundamental challenges for generating satisfying models that can account for those diverse and basic self-relevant activities. Emboldened by the current popularity of hypothesized motives as mediating units, homunculus fears receded, and students of the self again have been hypothesizing increasingly numerous self-motives which are invoked to try to explain the phenomena that led to their creation. As Prentice (2001) noted in a perceptive commentary on the state of contemporary self research—echoing Allport's (1961) concerns forty years later—the current proliferation of self motives, while generative, also has its down side. In her view, such motives as a " need for self-expansion" are being created with reasoning that "comes perilously close to circularity: The motive provides an explanation of the data at the same time that the data provide evidence of the motive. Clearly the hazards inherent in motivational theorizing have not gone away simply because self researchers have become less concerned about them" (Prentice, 2001, p. 324).

One is reminded of Henry Murray's long lists of motives that covered the alphabet virtually from A to Z (e.g., need for abasement, need for atonement) 70 years ago. As one critic of the history of our field has quipped, one begins to wonder if it is in danger of becoming another case of "déjà vu all over again." The challenge is how to conceptualize the agentic functions of the self as a "doer" while avoiding the homunculus threat that buried the self during 30 years of behaviorism, or that kept it "cool" during the era of social cognition. That requires a model for understanding the self and its diverse processes with increasing depth while side-stepping the traps of pseudo-explanations into which the concept of a self as causal agent can quickly lead.

Fortunately, while the homunculus is difficult to bury, there now are abundant illustrations of motivational analyses that avoid circularity and that illuminate the underlying processes that help make sense of the phenomena that need to be explained. For example, promising first steps toward building a processing framework at least for the self's regulatory functions have been taken with concepts like feedback loops and self-regulation theories (e.g., Carver & Scheier, 1981; Gollwitzer & Bargh, 1996; Higgins

& Kruglanski, 1996), and many such efforts are represented in this volume. The distinguishing feature of these approaches as efforts to control the homunculus problem is that they go much beyond post-hoc naming of motives. They focus on the specifics of the processes that generate the phenomena of interest by explaining, for example, the ways in which self-regulation becomes possible through the use of cognitive reframing strategies (e.g., Kuhl, 1985; Mischel, Cantor, & Feldman, 1996). These process analyses, as seen in this volume, illuminate the multi-faceted aspects of the self and its functions. However, while they address in depth diverse component part-processes, the need for a coherent explanatory model of the functioning self-system as a whole has remained largely unmet, although some initial steps toward that goal are available (e.g., Cantor & Kihlstrom, 1987; Hoyle et al., 1999; Linville & Carlston, 1994). The needed next step now is to contextualize these part-processes within a coherent, comprehensive self-system that functions as an organized whole and allows their interconnections and dynamics to be seen as they work within a person, not just as isolated components.

Toward that goal, further advances in theory now seem possible as a result of recent developments in fields from social cognition and personality through cognitive psychology and neuroscience, for example, through neural networks and connectionist modeling (e.g., Read & Miller, 1998; Rumelhart & McClelland, 1986; Shoda & Mischel, 1998). These developments may make it possible to conceptualize the individual as an actor with agency or agentic power who self-regulates, plans, exerts self-control, and pursues goals proactively. If appropriately applied and extended, they may enable a conception that captures the person as a thinking, feeling being who self-reflects and self-evaluates, while also taking account both of the impact of the social context and of automatic implicit processing.

The Self and Personality: An Entangled Relationship

Given that the self seems key in virtually all psycho-social processes of central importance to the person, it is unsurprising that as research and theory on the self evolved in recent decades, the boundaries between self processes and structures and personality processes and structures have become particularly fuzzy. If, as Tesser (2002) noted, the self now is "*a collection of abilities, temperament, goals, values, preferences that distinguish one individual from another* . . ." it becomes close to the conception of what are commonly thought of as key aspects of personality (e.g., Cantor & Kihlstrom, 1987; Cervone & Shoda, 1999; Higgins & Kruglanski, 1996; Mischel, 1973; Mischel & Shoda, 1995; Pervin, 1989, 1994). Yet historically the self and personality have been split apart as constructs and as fields of study in American academic psychology.

The Self in Relation to the Two Traditions of Personality Psychology

The nature of the relation between self and personality of course depends crucially on how each construct and area is defined. On close examination, those definitions and the cuts they produce in how the phenomena of interest are identified, partitioned, and pursued are highly consequential—and have become increasingly confusing over the years, with serious consequences for the research agendas, theories, and training programs in both fields. The confusion that developed is understandable because the cuts made evolved more from historical accident and arbitrary disciplinary boundaries and old traditions than by design or in response to the phenomena discovered in a century of research on self and self-relevant processes. Such historical "accidents" have made the self more or less in the province of social psychology and particularly social cognition, whereas the person became the province of personality psychology.

An unfortunate consequence is that in practice, both self researchers and personality researchers frequently lack awareness of the relevant literature just across the boundary. Both areas are trying to understand such critically self-relevant phenomena as self-control, self-regulation, self-evaluation, perceived self-discrepancies, self-standards, goal-setting, reactions to success and failure, self-affirmation, self-defense processes, conflict, and the like. Given the overlap in their interests and subject matter, they nevertheless inevitably—albeit often unknowingly—develop parallel concepts, measures, and findings, thus shadowing each other rather than building on each other in complementary ways that would enhance the growth of a more cumulative science. Yet, much of the prolific theory and research about the self in psychology has not been linked to the dynamics of the personality processing system with which the self—no matter how conceptualized—is necessarily closely related and indeed entangled. On the other side, much of the work in the last 20 years of personality psychology has ignored self-relevant processes and focused on stable traits conceptualized as broad behavioral tendencies or dispositions, as in the so-called "Big Five" (e.g., Hogan, Johnson, & Briggs, 1997).

Consequently, mainstream personality psychology has devoted relatively less attention to the role of self-relevant processes in the cognitive and affective processing dynamics that characterize different individuals and types, and the adaptations and interpersonal constructions that characterize so much of their lives. Conversely, by examining self-processes in isolation from a dynamic personality system, it has become difficult to understand how people can engage in apparently self-defeating or paradoxical self-regulatory behaviors and goal pursuits. Moreover, it has been impossible to address how such self-processes might develop in the first place.

The fuzziness and confusion of the boundaries between self and personality is further complicated by the fact that personality psychology itself has two distinct traditions, each with its own conception and definition of the nature of personality, and often these two approaches have themselves been in conflict. Hence, to address the basic links between self psychology and personality psychology, one has to begin by being clear about the kind of personality psychology one has in mind.

Personality as Traits. In one mainstream tradition, personality psychology deals primarily with —and is virtually synonymous with—individual differences in basic traits. In this tradition, currently represented by the "Big Five," individual differences are conceptualized in terms of behavioral dispositions, or traits, that predispose individuals to engage in relevant behaviors (e.g., McCrae & Costa, 1999). In this vein, dispositions and their behavioral expressions are assumed by definition to correspond directly: the more a person has a trait of conscientiousness, for example, the more conscientious the person's behavior is expected to be. The basic assumption is that these traits are essentially stable and played out in the life course in characteristic ways. The focus is on identification and description of the broad traits that people "have" enduringly. The aim is to identify individual differences in these basic traits, and these traits are used as explanations of why people differ in the important ways that they do. If personality is equated with traits that are stable predispositions of this sort, it may "predispose" the self and its vicissitudes in particular directions, but it is quite distinct from the self and its construction over the life course. In contrast, many contemporary self-researchers have focused more on what goes on inside the person's head, that is, how the way people "think" about things affects their behavior.

Another reason for a lack of overlap between the two traditions is that self researchers have been more interested in understanding *general* processes, common to all people. They have been interested in individual differences only insofar as people differ in their levels of isolated self-processes (e.g., high/low self-monitoring, or high/low self-handicapping), but these do not lead to characterizations of differences in entire personality types or categories. Trait psychologists, on the other hand, have always been concerned with these more molar typologies (e.g., extraversion, neuroticism, etc.)

However, the personality-equals-traits equation is by no means universally shared, and does not seem one that self researchers would want to accept because it excludes the very processes of greatest relevance to the self, such as the person's core goals, motivations, and conflicts. In 1981, in a prescient although rarely cited paper, Athay and Darley (1981, p. 291) emphasized that in more than a half century of research the construct of personality disposition "has been burdened by psychologists with more than its share of misleading connotations." The effect, they said, is that "it has become difficult not to think of the term as a syn-

onym for 'personality trait,'" resulting in an "extremely unfortunate equation" that by now has become virtually automatic. In this conclusion they sounded a theme voiced previously (e.g., Mischel, 1973), and reiterated more recently (e.g., Cervone & Shoda, 1999; Mischel, Shoda, & Mendoza-Denton, 2002; Pervin, 1994), as considered next.

Personality as a Dynamic Processing System. Rejecting the traits-equals-personality equation, an alternative and fundamentally different, second conception of personality also has evolved throughout the history of the field, and it is has much closer affinity to theory and research on the self. In this tradition, personality is construed as a system of mediating processes and structures, conscious and unconscious. The focus is on how these mediating processes can explain how and why people think and feel as they do, and on their interactions with the social world throughout the life cycle (e.g., Mischel & Shoda, 1995, 1998). Freud's theory, of course, was only the first and boldest of personality process theories in what by now has become a long tradition whose pioneers include such figures as Alfred Adler, Harry Stack Sullivan, Henry Murray, Kurt Lewin, and George Kelly. In contemporary personality and social psychology, mediating process models have had a substantial resurgence during the social cognition era in the last two decades (see Cervone & Shoda, 1999; Gollwitzer & Bargh, 1996; Higgins & Kruglanski, 1996; Pervin & John, 1999).

As part of this same era, much of the work in this second tradition of personality currently is essentially "social cognitive–affective" in its focus (e.g., Cervone & Shoda,1999; Derryberry, 2002; Higgins, 1996b; Higgins & Kruglanski, 1996; Mischel & Shoda, 1995; 1998; Morf & Rhodewalt, 2001a, 2001b.). But while most of these efforts seem to be predominantly "social cognitive" in their preferred theoretical language, encompassing the role of automatic and unconscious processing (e.g., Bargh, 1997; Kihlstrom, 1987, 1990), this approach now also is concerned with the goals and motivations that underlie behavior central to self and self-regulation (e.g., Gollwitzer & Bargh, 1996; Read & Miller, 1989, 1998). However, unlike work on isolated self-processes, this tradition tries to capture and account for "personality-like" types or individual differences at the person level.

It does so by addressing the internal cognitive–affective–motivational states and "processing dynamics" of the person and their interpersonal as well as intra-personal expressions as the person adapts to and shapes the social environment. This approach is exemplified in the Cognitive Affective Personality System (CAPS) model (Mischel & Shoda, 1995) and is directly relevant to—and overlaps with—current self theory and research. Nevertheless, much of this work is located in areas often defined as personality and developmental psychology, or at their outer edges and hyphenated inter-faces, and is cast in terms in which the self is not the focus. Consequently, it is easily perceived as outside the disciplinary boundaries of traditional research on the self and irrelevant, although it may be substantively central.

Costs of Splitting the Self from its Personality System

Regardless of disciplinary boundaries and conventions, there is an intrinsic natural connection between the self and the personality system. Thus splitting the self from its personality system would be manifestly dysfunctional for self theory. It would leave the self disconnected from the individual's motivations and life pursuits, including self-evaluation and self-assessments, planning and control processes, and so forth—the list is long—as well as from its development. The costs of splitting self from personality are equally (or even more) severe for personality theory. They leave the personality without a self, split from its most central driving motivations and organizing processes (such as self-regulation, self-enhancement, self-construction, self-protection), in danger of being little more than a static list of traits or factors. It reflects not a natural division dictated by differences in the phenomena relevant to understanding the self and personality but rather unfortunate disciplinary divisions and historical accidents that may carve nature at just the wrong joints.

In short, research on the self on the one side, and on personality processes on the other, represents two different traditions of theory, research strategies, and findings that have been asking closely related questions about people from two different but overlapping vantage points for many years. As a result there now are two literatures from two different starting points and vantage points that address aspects of the self: they are seeming to converge and virtually screaming for an integration. The next part of this chapter we hope will facilitate such an integration within a unifying conceptual framework.

Summary and Preview

To recapitulate, concurrent with the onset of the cognitive revolution and the decline of behaviorism, explosive growth has characterized the study of the self and the role given to it within psychology, as the chapters in this volume attest. This expansion, which endows the self with diverse agentic functions and emotional as well as cognitive aspects, brings self research and theory to the intersection of a host of other closely related areas, most notably process approaches to personality, social cognition, and motivation-emotion. The question then becomes, What kinds of mechanisms and processing model are needed to deal with the motivated self as a "doer" as well as "thinker" and "feeler," and the frequently perplexing vicissitudes of the self?

In the next part of this chapter, we address those mechanisms, and consider an emerging framework—preliminary, tentative, and open to progressive revision—of the self-system and the self-construction process. The outlines for such a framework are already visible and are being articulated with increasing convergence (e.g., Baumeister, 1998; Hoyle et al., 1999). Perhaps we are at one of those special moments in the history of a profoundly complex problem in which a consensus is forming, at least about the general conceptual framework needed to catch up with the cumulative findings from diverse areas after a century of prolific research.

Toward a Pscho-Social Dynamic Processing Model of the Self

Consensus on the Characteristics of the Self

In the attempt to outline a comprehensive self-system, the first question to ask is,

What phenomena must such a system explain? One then can proceed to map out the essential characteristics that such a system must have to explain those phenomena. Fortunately, at this juncture a broad cumulative agreement regarding the features of the self and "selfhood" is seen in recent integrative summaries that capture the essence of the current consensus view (e.g., Baumeister, 1998; Hoyle et al., 1999). From these reviews it quickly becomes clear that the self is stable *and* variable, consistent *and* inconsistent, rational *and* irrational, planful *and* automatic, agentic *and* routinized. Further, the self in contemporary psychology is not just a knowledge structure and thus "known," but is also a "doer" and indeed a "feeler," as much driven by affect as guided by cognition. Moreover, a unique, central feature of the self is self-awareness and conscious self-thinking that allows the person to reflect on experiences and to monitor and evaluate his or her reactions. Nevertheless, some of the experiences of the self and its expressions also may be at implicit levels outside awareness. While this is all merely descriptive, in our reading a consensus is also emerging regarding two core features of the self that provide a basis for developing an explanatory approach that can account for these complexities and seeming inconsistencies: (1) the self is an organized dynamic cognitive–affective–action system, and (2) the self is an interpersonal self-construction system.

With regard to the first feature, the widely shared desire in the field to conceptualize the self as a system can be seen in examples such as, "The self is a dynamic psychological system, a tapestry of thoughts, feelings and motives that define and direct—even destroy—us" (Hoyle et al., 1999, p. 1). Likewise, Dweck, Higgins, and Grant-Pillow (Chapter 12, this volume) emphasize the need to view the self as a system, and suggest that it is goals that give the self-system "real life and important meaning." This view of the self as a system recognizes that the diverse aspects and functions of the self are not isolated components or unconnected part processes and knowledge structures but rather interacting facets of a coherent system that operates at multiple levels concurrently. It suggests that the self may be usefully conceptualized *not* simply

as a *collection* of attributes, as in Tesser's (2002) definition mentioned earlier, but rather as a coherent organization of mental–emotional (cognitive–affective) representations. Further, it portrays the self as a motivated, dynamic, action system. It is dynamic in that the system continuously accommodates and assimilates to information from the social world within which it is contextualized, and it is an action system insofar as it generates behavior. These actions are motivated, and the meanings and goals that inform and guide them are largely constructed interpersonally in the social world.

While the view that the self is essentially a social product is far from new, for many years its significance was unappreciated. In recent years, however, it has again become evident that it may be difficult, if not impossible, to understand the self detached from its social context (e.g., Athay & Darley, 1981; Baldwin & Holmes, 1987; Hoyle et al., 1999; Markus & Cross, 1990). Consequently, to understand the self requires studying individuals with regard to their interpersonal behavior, much of which may consist of efforts to get others to respond in ways that are consistent with one's goals or projects. These efforts reflect the motivated and agentic qualities of the self-system, which importantly include ways of behaving and thinking "aimed at asserting, protecting, or repairing identity or self-esteem" (Hoyle et al., 1999, p. 20). To capture "who someone is," then, one needs to understand the person's identity goals through their expression in social interaction: it is within those interactions that the individual's self-theory is constructed, validated, and revealed.

In the consensus view, the self is not simply passively reactive to the social world: it is, rather, a motivated, goal-directed self-regulatory system that is proactive and agentic. This requires that the self-system also subsume such executive functions as planning, interpreting, and monitoring behavior and selectively processing information about both the self and the social world. And essential to performing such functions is the self-system's "capacity for reasoned self-reflection" (e.g., Baumeister, 1998; Hoyle et al., 1999, p.2). Indeed, perhaps the most distinguishing feature of the self-system is that it deals with how people construct self-relevant meanings by reflecting on themselves, their past, and their possible futures. In the present view, however, while the meaning system of the self requires as its sine qua non self-awareness and conscious self-thinking, it is not necessarily always either conscious or self-aware, and often operates automatically and nonverbally (e.g., Bargh, 1997). In short, absent self-awareness and consciousness, one cannot imagine a self system; but a self without implicit processes and indirect manifestations would be insufficient to capture the complexities and diverse, often conflicted aspects of the self system, which operates concurrently at multiple levels of awareness.

Our goal in the sections that follow is to sketch a framework for viewing the self as a Psycho-Social Dynamic Processing System that we believe captures the essence of the discussed consensus regarding the key aspects and functions of the self, and that helps to account for them systematically. We do so in an attempt to respond to what we see as the main theoretical challenge that now faces the field. Namely, there is a need to collectively articulate the kind of processing self-system that enables the self to perform the core functions summarized in the consensus—a system that we hope will have heuristic value for future research and theory-building.

We share the increasing recognition that connectionist models and parallel distributed processing systems may have some of the necessary general processing characteristics for such a self-system. They therefore may be especially relevant at least as metaphors (e.g., Graziano & Tobin, 2001; Morf & Rhodewalt, 2001b; Nowak, Vallacher, Tesser, & Borkowski, 2000). In the proposed self-system that follows we draw on this metaphor and borrow from these connectionist contributions; therefore, we begin with a brief summary of the basic processing characteristics of connectionist models.

Connectionist Models as Metaphors for a Self-System

Neurally inspired connectionist and parallel distributed processing (PDP) models that deal with knowledge and memory seem promising because they can take account of multiple simultaneous processes without invoking a single central control. They offer a metaphor for a self-system that may help us to understand the phenomena of selfhood, while minimizing the homunculus threat discussed earlier. Briefly, in a connectionist model a concept (or object) is represented by a *distributed representation,* where each representation is a different pattern of activation across a large number of simple processing units (Rumelhart & McClelland, 1986). These interconnected units send activation to each other over weighted links (which can be either excitatory or inhibitory) and these weights get updated (or adjusted) every time as activation flows through the system.

It is important to understand that concepts are not stored as discrete units, but rather are represented by different patterns of activation across many units. Therefore, concepts or memories represented by different patterns of activation across many units are never retrieved "as is," but rather reconstructed each time there is activation in the system. Furthermore, because the whole system is connected and each unit can be involved in the representation of many different concepts, whenever one part is activated or "worked on," other parts are affected also and possibly changed (via the weight adjustments). The implication is that any "reconstruction" will be imperfect and affected by the person's other knowledge. Learning and development occur through subtle changes in the weights over time.

Especially relevant for the self's functions, connectionist models can account for a system that is "biased," as the self-system surely is, because patterns of activation are constrained and guided by the existing network, because patterns of activation are generated to satisfy mutual constraints across the excitatory or inhibitory links. Thus connections are activated and updated in nonrandom, predictable ways. For example, if threat to a particular person's self-esteem in certain types of situations (e.g., threats of abandonment by partner, of being outperformed by another person) tends to activate rage which in turn activates behavior that derogates the source of the threat, such a pattern may be seen predictably in future similar situations (e.g., Ayduk, Downey, Testa, Yen, & Shoda, 1999; Morf & Rhodewalt, 1993).

Because such networks can perform highly sophisticated information processing that is essential for complex higher level functions, these new processing approaches indeed seem potentially central for work on the self. More than a promissory note, such connectionist models or systems have been shown repeatedly to produce meaningful, coherent, and adaptive patterns of complex behavior that reflect the dynamic interplay among multiple processes (Kashima & Kerekes, 1994; Kunda & Thagard, 1996; Read & Miller, 1998; Shoda & Mischel, 1998; Smith & DeCoster, 1998). One major distinct advantage of these systems, to reiterate, is that they do not require a central control plan. They are able to generate exceedingly complex patterns of behavior as a function of the network of *relationships* among the units that make up the system. These models thus provide an appealing route for conceptualizing the self and its processes in network terms while avoiding the homunculus problem: the agency is in the organization of the network, and no internal controller needs to be invoked, as was the case in the earlier information processing models of the 1970s.

Furthermore, the conception that memories and concepts, including about the self, personality, and other people, are constructed rather than retrieved speaks directly to the nature of the self-construction process. All concepts are freshly generated or reconstructed within the constraints of the system but also in dynamic interaction within a particular context that activates and updates the system. This allows a view of self-construction as a process of adaptation in which, consistent with Piaget, actors accommodate available, familiar thought and action patterns to deal with the continuously changing specifics of the immediate situation. It is a view of the mind and brain's plasticity that brings potential rigor and formal modeling methods to bear, at least by analogy, on studies of the construction of the self.

In the sections that follow, we consider the essential aspects and functions of the self in the framework of the proposed Psycho-Social Dynamic Processing System. The discussion of this model is organized around the two key consensus features of the self, as noted above: (1) The self is an organized, dynamic cognitive–affective–action system and (2) the self is an interpersonal self-construction system.

The Self as an Organized Cognitive–Affective–Action System

General Processing Characteristics, Units, and Dynamics of the Self-System

Conceptualizing the self-system as an organized, dynamic, cognitive–affective (knowing–feeling) action system requires that one address the nature of the units in the system, the relationship and organization among these units, and their dynamic functioning. Following an essentially connectionist, network-like metaphor, we begin with the assumption that in this type of processing system the mental representations consist of cognitions and affects (emotional states) that interact and interconnect within a stable network that guides and constrains their activation. These characteristics are similar to those of the Cognitive Affective Processing System (CAPS), which provides an integrative social–cognitive–affective framework for personality processes and dynamics (Mischel & Shoda, 1995; Shoda & Mischel, 1998). When applied to the self-system, however, there is a necessary shift in focus to identify the types of cognitive–affective units or representations needed in a self-system, if it is to perform its diverse functions.

The types of cognitive–affective units in the self-system may be thought of as mapping onto diverse psychological variables and constructs found to be important for understanding self-relevant processes. These include representations of self-knowledge and self-concepts (e.g., self-esteem), self-relevant goals, beliefs–expectancies (e.g., self-efficacy) about the self, the person's theories about the self, self-relevant affects (e.g., anxiety, shame, pride, eagerness), and values central for the self. Also encompassed are self-regulatory and self-evaluative standards, and self-construction competencies and mental representations of strategies and scripts for generating diverse types of social behavior. In positing cognitive–affective units at this high level of abstraction, we depart from the connectionist metaphor in which the units, strictly speaking, have no meaning. We do so as a short-cut to enable conceptual links to the large research literature on the importance of these variables in research on the self. In connectionist terms, our constructs and units are themselves composed of activation patterns among much lower-level units (as also discussed in Shoda & Mischel, 1998). Cognitive–affective units operate both at automatic and volitional levels, and are basic for self-regulation and effective pursuit of goals central to the self (Gollwitzer & Bargh, 1996; Mendoza-Denton, Ayduk, Mischel, Shoda, & Testa, 2001; Mischel, 1973).

These self-units are organized into distinctive networks for each person. The distinctive organization of the interrelations among the units is the result of an individual's genetic endowment, and biological history (e.g., temperament), as well as his or her social learning and developmental history within the particular culture and subculture. These factors underlie the organization of the system, and it is this organization that determines which units become activated together in the system's interactions with the social environment. Thus the organization and structure of the system consists of the relatively stable links and connections formed among the units, as well as the strength of their associations. Consistent with a connectionist model, then, patterns of activation are what create and "run" the self-system.

This activation can have various sources. First, it can occur in response to social stimuli during interpersonal interactions that are encountered or self-initiated. Activation, however, can also be generated internally, as in self-reflection and rumination. For example, in thinking about particular aspects of the self, associated affective reactions (anxiety, shame, guilt, pride, eagerness, fears) may be activated, and further activate a cascade of other cognitive, emotional, and behavioral reactions (e.g., efficacy expectations, self-doubts, defensive denials). These activations quite literally involve an active contextualized construction or reconstruction process *in situ* rather than a retrieval or enactment of pre-existing entities from storage.

However, because the pattern of activation must satisfy, at least locally, the constraints represented in the network connection weights, each person is characterized by a relatively stable activation network among the units within the self-system. The *processing dynamics* of the self-system, thus, refer to the system's characteristic patterns of activation among the cognitive–affective units within it, in relation to different features of the social environment. Individual differences, then, are the result of differences in the chronic accessibility of the units (e.g., Higgins, 1996a) and, equally important, in the distinctive organization of the interrelations among them (Mischel & Shoda, 1995). Differential accessibility and organization also contribute to enduring individual differences in the types of features of situations that people select and to which they are particularly responsive. Change in the system occurs slowly as a result of subtle adjustments of association strengths among the units as different parts of the system are activated and reconstructed in particular contexts.

Multiple Levels of Functioning and Sub-Systems

The self-system functions at multiple levels and subsumes a number of sub-systems that operate concurrently and in parallel; therefore it can be useful to conceptualize subsystems for in-depth analyses of various self-relevant processes at different levels of abstraction. While several of the chapters in this volume illustrate in detail the utility of such subsystem analysis, here we wish only to underline that sub-systems and particular self-relevant processes do not operate in isolation, but rather are played out and exert their influence in their specific interactions and inter-dependent functioning within the total self-system. Further, within an organized, coherent self-system, not all subprocesses are necessarily equal: they likely are organized into super-ordinate and subordinate hierarchies in terms of their importance and priorities for the functioning and maintenance of the system as a whole. One of the reasons for postulating an organized self-system is that it calls attention to the issue of the nature of the hierarchies and interactions that characterize the system—an issue easy to bypass when the focus is restricted to sub-systems. At least implicitly in self research, constructs like the self-concept and identity play an important role in guiding and constraining such organization by providing the super-ordinate goals within that organization. The existence of such organization and of coherence within the system of course does not imply that it is conflict-free. On the contrary, conflicting goals and behavior tendencies in different contexts and domains can be understood in terms of the concurrent operation of different goals and different motives in parallel and at different levels of the system exerting their reciprocal influences in tandem (e.g., Emmons & King, 1988; Graziano & Tobin, 2001). Furthermore, the nature of the organization among self components with regard to such issues as their integration, fragmentation, and compartmentalization also needs to be addressed (e.g., Donahue, Robins, Roverts, & John, 1993; Linville, 1987; Showers, 1992).

The operations of the self-system, and the interactions among sub-systems, are illustrated in such core processes as self-regulation and self-control in the course of goal pursuit. Although these processes to a large degree involve automaticity (e.g., Bargh, 1997), effortful, sometimes self-conscious, interruptions of the automatic flow also occur and are fundamental for effectiveness of the self-system. Effortful control is particularly important for diverse self-regulatory and self-control functions that require overriding more accessible, automatic, and impulsive response tendencies (e.g., fight or flight) with effortful, more adaptive but less easily accessible interventions in the service of goals important to the self.

To be effective, sustained effortful control requires a variety of strategies that include planning, rehearsing, self-monitoring, and strategic attention control to overcome highly accessible but potentially dysfunctional impulsive tendencies with more appropriate, thoughtfully mediated action scripts (Gollwitzer & Moskowitz, 1996; Mischel, Cantor, & Feldman, 1996). To be maintained over time, these control efforts have to be converted from conscious and effortful to automatic and spontaneous control. In this sense, the enactment of "willpower" to allow continued goal pursuit depends on the automatic interaction between these more automatic and more effortful sub-systems. We elaborate on the interactions between these two sub-systems

here because they are particularly key for self-regulation. However, while illustrative of subsystem interactions in general, this by no means captures the full complexity of the relations among subsystems, nor even between cognition and emotion, that underlie such emotions as sadness, anger, contempt, love, and interest—all of which are self-relevant and important ingredients within the self-system and for the experienced self.

Hot/Cool or Implicit/Explicit Sub-Systems in Self-Regulation

Several theorists have postulated similar frameworks of two such orthogonal, though potentially continuously interacting, processing systems, each of which is responsive to different input features, and operates by its own processing rules and characteristics (e.g., Epstein, 1994; Metcalfe & Mischel, 1999). While the terms employed by each theory are somewhat different, in essence one system tends to be more affect-based or "hot" and thus more automatic, impulsive, and faster to respond. The other system is based more on logic and reason and is "cool," thus involving slower, more mediated and effortful cognitive processing. In the self-system, such processes as the encoding or knowledge representations of the self and of the situation, and the self-relevant goals-values, expectations, plans, and attention control strategies that become activated within the particular context are activities of the "cool" or "know" system. However, to the degree that these activations are not merely isolated "cool" cognitions or "know" structures when relevant to the self, but also are intimately interconnected with emotions and affect-laden representations, they operate in continuous interaction with the "hot" system. Likewise, although each system has its biological basis in different brain systems, these also continuously interact (Ledoux, 1996; Metcalfe & Mischel, 1999; Posner & Rothbart, 2000).

Self-relevant behavior is the product of the joint operation of the two systems. Their relative dominance/balance is determined by individual differences in self-regulation, and situational variables that either prime rational formal analysis or induce emotional arousal. For example, the presence of high stress or negative arousal (either acutely within the situation or chronically within the person) increases hot activation and attenuates the operations of the cool system. Interactions among these two systems become particularly important as the person inevitably runs into barriers, frustrations, and temptations that activate hot, impulsive responding in the course of pursuing long-term goals. Persistence and adaptation in the face of these barriers in pursuit of goals central for the self depend on purposeful self-regulation and mental control. In these control processes, the hot representations of events are transformed in ways that strategically cool them, for example, through ideation (e.g., thinking of a marshmallow as a cloud instead of as soft, chewy and yummy), and/or self-distraction (Mischel et al., 1996). Individuals who have such self-regulatory competencies highly accessible can more adaptively and automatically use their attention control skills and meta-cognitive knowledge of effective ways to self-control in the service of effective long-term pursuit of goals central to the self.

Thus far we have described the self-system's basic units, processing characteristics and some of its self-regulatory operations in motivated goal-pursuit. But we have been mute about the origins and nature of those motivations and goals, and equally silent about the evolution of the system itself. To do so requires contextualizing the general cognitive–affective self-system explicitly within the interpersonal world in which it develops its distinctiveness and, as it were, constructs itself. We therefore turn next to the interpersonal self-construction process through which self-relevant goals and the meaning structures within the system are acquired and maintained.

The Interpersonal Self-Construction Process

The self-system described above emerges not spontaneously but through a process of self-construction in which there is continuous reciprocal interaction between the dynamics of the system and the demands and affordances of the particular situation and contexts (e.g., Athay & Darley, 1981; Tesser, 2002; Vygotsky, 1978). This emphasis on the interpersonal nature of the self departs from the traditions in personality and self psychology that for much of the last century focused on self-contained inner, intra-psychic processes and dynamics, e.g., as exemplified in Freud's theories of the internal warfare among the sub-systems of personality. In sharp contrast to the traditional exclusive inner-system focus, we share the view of many other contemporary self theorists that the self is fundamentally interpersonal. Moreover, the self-construction process is intrinsically rooted within, and dependent upon, interpersonal processes that unfold in the social world (e.g., Baldwin & Holmes, 1987; Hoyle et al., 1999; Markus & Cross, 1990). And these interpersonal processes and "situations" involve not only significant other individuals but also relevant social groups that ultimately become part of one's "collective self" (e.g., Sedikides & Brewer, 2001). Indeed, interpersonal processes may precede changes in intra-personal processes, and the latter may be adapted subsequently to take the interpersonal into account. The social experiences and processes are seamlessly connected to the intra-individual dynamics that they reflect and that in part create them and they become an inextricable component of the experiential self (as illustrated in Morf & Rhodewalt, 2001a, 2001b).

Role of Pre-dispositions

The construction of the self does not begin with a blank slate. Biological and genetic history, as well as social learning history, developmental processes, and cultural–social influences, interact dynamically and continuously in the developing self system (e.g., Tesser, 2002). It is by now a truism that individuals differ in multiple biochemical–genetic-somatic factors. These may be conceptualized as *pre*-dispositions, with emphasis on the "pre" to make clear that they are biological precursors that may manifest indirectly as well as directly at the other levels of analysis in diverse and complex forms (Mischel & Shoda, 1999).

These pre-dispositions ultimately influence such personality and self-relevant qualities as sensory and psychomotor sensitivities and vulnerabilities, skills and competencies, temperament (including activity level and emotionality), chronic mood, and affective states (e.g., Plomin, DeFries, McClearn, & Rutter, 1997). In turn these all interact with social cognitive, social learning and cultural-societal influences, mediated by, and conjointly further interacting reciprocally with, the self-system that becomes constructed over time. Consequently, these pre-dispositions influence the organization of the self-system, the self-construction process, and the behavioral-signatures that ultimately characterize the person (Mischel & Shoda, 1995). Self-construction is thus born out of the interactions between these pre-dispositions and the evolving self-system in its dynamic transactions with the social interpersonal world in which it is contextualized.

Development of the Meaning System

In the process of constructing the self-system, as the person interacts with the social world, social stimuli acquire their personal cognitive and affective meanings. They are a result both of the person's more automatic, nonreflective reactions and interpretations of social events, as well as of his or her more deliberate reflections and evaluations. The self-system thus is a *motivated meaning system* insofar as the self-relevant meanings and values that are acquired in the course of its development (or self-construction) inform, constrain, and guide the interpretations of experience, goal pursuits, self-regulatory efforts, and interpersonal strategies. In this life-long self-construction process, identity, self-esteem, and self-relevant goals, values, and life projects are built, maintained, promoted, and protected. Through the self-construction process the self-system takes shape and, in turn, affects, as well as being influenced by, the social contexts and networks that constitute its social world. In this sense, self-construction is a developmental process in which the self-system that emerges is in part its product and in part its architect. It begins with relations to caretakers, and it continues throughout the life course.

The nature of care-giving beginning in early life has an immense impact on the self-system, self-evaluations, and the types of attachment and social relationships that develop (e.g., Crittenden, 1990; Harter, 1999). To illustrate, consider briefly Gunnar's (2001) studies on the social–emotional significance of dyadic processes in infancy. She shows the crucial role of mother–child relationships as

regulators of the physiology of stress, which in turn dramatically influences the development of self-regulatory competencies and well-being in later self development. For example, such maternal qualities as focused attention and sensitive care-giving in the first year of life seem to be key for building an "outer ring" of support. This interpersonal outer ring helps to buffer the intra-personal "inner ring of support" essential to reduce the otherwise elevated cortisol levels in stress reactions that, in turn, have potentially negative effects on further adaptation and constructive self development.

These early attachment experiences affect the types of mental `working models' that are constructed: working models serve like templates through which subsequent relationship experiences may be selected, filtered and interpreted (e.g., Andersen, Chen, & Miranda, 2002; Baldwin, 1992; Hazan & Shaver, 1987). The formation and expression of these attachment relationships already points to the proactive and interactive (rather than reactive–passive) nature of the self-construction process in early life. One sees this, for example, in the toddler's ways of dealing with the separation situation, or with the intrusive demands of an over-controlling mother. The impact of the caretaker in these situations depends on the self-regulatory strategies the toddler uses to deal with the experienced stressors (e.g. Sethi, Mischel, Aber, Shoda, & Rodriguez, 2000)— although those strategies themselves were influenced by the nature of the earlier care-giving. The picture is one of dynamic reciprocal interactionism rather than of one-way influences, either from mother to child or in the opposite direction. The strategies that evolve in these interactions begin to be visible early in life and appear to have significant stability and long-term implications for the types of self-construction and competencies that develop and that in turn impact on the efficacy of goal pursuit and self-esteem (Ayduk et al., 2000; Mischel, Shoda, & Rodriguez, 1989; Sethi et al., 2000).

Processes in Self-Construction: A Pro-Active, Motivated System

As the person acquires strategies for dealing with different types of interpersonal situations during the life course, he or she develops a preferred theory of the self. This self-theory at first may be rudimentary, but it becomes elaborated and increasingly complex over time as the person seeks to test and validate it in the social world (Epstein, 1973). To be clear, we do not assume that people are highly cognizant about their self-theories. Even when increasingly multi-faceted and enriched, self-theories likely remain largely implicit, although they also have diverse explicit expressions.

Much still remains to be learned about just how self-theories influence the operations of the self-system, but it is clear that they do so, significantly affecting the directions that self-construction takes (e.g., Harter, 1999; Hoyle et al., 1999; Sedikides & Brewer, 2001). Moreover, extensive research already documents their importance in guiding the acquisition of goals/values, self-evaluations, motivations, and regulatory competencies; in selecting the life tasks and projects that are pursued; and in proactively constructing the particular types of interpersonal situations and relationships that become the person's interpersonal world (Cantor et al., 1991; Emmons, 1989, 1991; Little, Lecci, & Watkinson, 1992; Mischel et al., 1996; Pervin, 1989; Zirkel & Cantor, 1990). Thus actions in the service of self-construction are biased in the selection and interpretation of social feedback and performance outcomes, motivated at least in part by the desire to build, affirm, and protect identity and self-esteem in line with the person's self theory (e.g., Hoyle et al. 1999; Morf & Rhodewalt, 2001a). In developing and testing these theories, the person is "first of all an actor rather than a thinker or a theorist" (Athay & Darley, 1981, p. 283)."

People, however, are not unlimited in the self-theory or identity they can construct, but rather do so within the limits—and opportunities—of the evolving self-system (e.g., Bolger & Zuckerman, 1995; Buss, 1997; Emmons, Diener, & Larsen, 1986). Adjustment and change in self-theories and in the system are possible, but not without boundaries: in terms of the connectionist metaphor, it is constrained by the connections and "weights" already formed in the system. These weights reflect the talents, skills, and abilities, as well as the goals and construction competencies, of the self-sys-

tem. The self-construction process provides and modifies progressively the weights in the system's development as the individual learns new skills and/or different social stimuli and experiences acquire their cognitive–affective meanings and value and become "reinforcing."

In short, the self-system, as it were, constructs its niches (Tesser, 2002) in a developmental process of accommodation and assimilation, in part shaping its own social environments as much as it is shaped by them. In turn, the self-system reacts in characteristic ways to those situations, cognitively, affectively, and behaviorally. Self-construction is an intrinsically interactionist process: the theories of self are based on and modified by the experiences in the interpersonal world, just as the latter are influenced by and in part created by those theories. In time, over the life course these interactions progressively generate the unique trajectories and defining experiences and relationships of the self.

Expressions of the Self-System

The essentials of the self-system were described above in terms of its two key features: it is an organized, knowing–thinking–feeling–action system, and it is an interpersonal system that is constructed and re-reconstructed in social contexts and relationships throughout its development, maintenance, and transformations over the life course. Personally, we experience the self-system and its phenomenological realities subjectively, and these experiences and self-reflections are themselves consequential. As observers in our scientist roles, we know the self-system through its behavioral expressions—from the actions observed in the social world, the inferences made about inner states, or the measurements taken—from self-reports to brain scans. It is through these expressions that we see the consistency and variability of the self, discern its characteristic behavioral signatures, and come to understand its underlying goals and dynamics. And it is through these expressions that we begin to perceive the depths and uniqueness of each person's self-system. Some of these expressions are considered next.

Consistency and Variability in the Self-System and Its Expression

The self-system is responsive to contexts but is itself relatively stable in its organization and processing dynamics—in this sense the self is both "stable and variable." The *states* within the system refer to the activation levels of the cognitions and affects at a given time (Shoda & Mischel, 1998). These states, which vary across different situations (e.g., with mother, with partner) in stable patterns, in part reflect the external situations encountered, and the past experiences of the person, and encompass what is commonly referred to as the "working self-concept." When the current situations change, these states vary readily and over time form a continuous stream, reflecting the history of the situations encountered, as well as the distinctive organization of the self-system contextualized in its interpersonal world.

Whereas the cognitions and affects that are activated at a given time in the self-system may change as the situation does, *how* they change, and the *relations* among them, are assumed to reflect the relatively stable structure and organization of the self-system. For example, whenever a person encounters an individual with a certain configuration of features relevant to the self, the kinds of thoughts and feelings that are activated follow a particular predictable pattern. It is within this organized system, and the stream of thoughts and feelings generated by it, that the phenomenological self experiences the social world.

The Signatures of the Self-System

If one traces the changes in the variable "states of the self"—the thoughts and feelings activated, and the behaviors generated—and plots them as a function of psychologically salient features of situations, as the person goes from one situation to another a profile with a characteristic elevation and shape should emerge theoretically. Consistent with the theory, it has been shown to do so empirically as well as through formal modeling (Shoda & Mischel, 1998; Shoda & Tiernan, 2002; Zayas, Shoda, & Ayduk, 2001). This profile constitutes the individual's characteristic IF–THEN personality signature (Mischel & Shoda, 1995). When

these IF–THEN relations are self-relevant, for example in interpersonal contexts in which aspects of the relational self with significant others become activated in stable predictable patterns, they may be thought of as *signatures of the self* and of the self-system, as illustrated in work on transference (Andersen et al., 2002) and narcissism (Morf & Rhodewalt, 2001a, 2001b).

The novel point here is that the stable characteristics of the processing system are reflected and seen not just in consistencies across situations. Importantly, they are seen also, and unexpectedly, in the way a person's thoughts, feelings, and behavior *vary* as a function of specific features of situations in predictable, stable IF–THEN patterns (she does, feels A when X but B when Y). These signatures of the self can provide a window into their underlying meanings and the nature of the self-system. Consider, for example, two colleagues who display the same amount of overall "sociability." One, however, is always exceptionally warm and friendly with his students but not with his senior colleagues, while the other consistently shows the opposite pattern. Such stable patterns of IF–THEN relationships seem to provide at least a glimpse into the motivations and goals that may underlie them (Cervone & Shoda, 1999; Shoda, 1999a, 1999b), and a route for studying them systematically.

Predictable Patterns of Variation

This analysis captures two key features of the self that often have appeared to be paradoxical. As Hoyle and colleagues (1999, p. 23) noted, these two "(apparently) contradictory features of the self are that at one level the self system is ever-changing; at another it is stable over time. In short, the self is both responsive to social contexts but also stable in the face of highly variable social inputs. In this sense, as they also note, the self is both variable and fixed.

The present analysis in terms of variable states of a system that is responsive to contexts but that is itself stable in its organization (Mischel & Shoda, 1995; Shoda & Mischel, 1998) converges with the views and findings of self researchers. Their account of the seeming paradox of variability and consistency in the self is given in terms of the distinction between working self concepts that are engaged in particular situations combined with a relatively stable constellation of working self-concepts (e.g., Hoyle et al., 1999; Markus & Kunda, 1986). The present analysis, however, tries to go a step beyond viewing the self as containing both the working concept of the moment and the collection of other available working self-concepts. It does so by addressing the nature of the processing system that intrinsically generates both enduring overall levels of behavior, as reflected in overall stable levels of self-esteem and types of characteristic social behavior (sociability, conscientiousness), and also in stable, potentially predictable *patterns of variability* across different situations. This analysis allows a fresh perspective for understanding and unpacking many seemingly paradoxical, self-defeating, and bizarre behaviors and conflicts within the self-system (Morf & Rhodewalt, 2001b).

Individual Differences in Self-Systems

Individual differences in self-systems at the most basic levels are conceptualized both in terms of differences in the chronic accessibility of particular cognitive–affective units and of the distinctive organization of interrelationships among them, that is, in their processing dynamics. For example, a person may be characterized by having academic competence as a central goal for the self, and also by becoming easily anxious about it. Thus both the goal and the anxiety are at a high chronic accessibility level. In addition, when that goal is activated, it may be connected to the anxiety activation, which in turn may trigger a stable pattern of self-defense. These dynamics may unfold in a stable pattern of cognitive–affective internal reactions, as well as manifested with distinctive coping reactions in interpersonal relations (reflecting the organization of interconnections in the system).

Given the interpersonal nature of the self, and therefore the need to construct adaptive coping mechanisms and strategies for optimizing those relationships, both empathy and role-taking and role-playing ability may be especially important aspects of individual differences. Likewise, the ability to make subtle discriminations between different types of social situations so that behavior can be appropriately monitored and adapted to the specific affordances and constraints appears to have functional value and to enhance favorable outcomes (Chiu, Hong, Mischel, & Shoda, 1995). To the degree that individuals share similar goals, interpersonal competencies, and processing dynamics in the self-construction process, they can be studied together as constituting particular *self-construction types* (as is discussed in more detail in Part III of this volume). Research on these types needs to specify the distinctive nature of their processing dynamics and characteristic strategies, and to connect them to the self-signatures that they generate. Those signatures and the underlying processing dynamics in turn become the focus of assessment in the study of self-construction types.

Summary

To recapitulate, the self-system posited, consistent with the connectionist metaphor, is an organized meaning system, guided and constrained by the organization of relationships among the person's self-relevant cognitions and affects. These units operate concurrently at different levels and the specific interactions of these levels (e.g., hot, affective automatic processes with cool, cognitive processes) underlie the self-regulatory and self-control efforts made in goal pursuit. The characteristic processing dynamics of the system are activated in relation to perceived self-relevant features of situations, and played out primarily in interpersonal contexts and relationships. Through the interactions of the system with the interpersonal world, different social stimuli and experiences acquire their value and cognitive–affective meanings, and in the course of development the weights in the system are progressively modified.

The expressions of the self-system may be seen in particular predictable, characteristic patterns of stable IF–THEN relationships (she does A when X, but B when Y)—the distinctive self-signatures of the person. Thus, consistent with the consensus view regarding the defining characteristics of the self, the psychosocial dynamic processing system captures a self that is both variable across different types of situations, but relatively stable within them. It is an agentic do-ing system, an organized cognitive–affective (knowing, thinking, feeling) system, and it is an interpersonal system.

Implications, Applications, Prospects

In this concluding section we consider some of the implications that follow for theory and research from the type of Psycho-Social Dynamic Processing System for the self proposed above. We also discuss some of the challenges and prospects for the future that seem to us to follow. We begin by examining whether such a system is in fact really needed, and just what might be gained from it.

Why a Systems Approach is Needed: Potential Gains

Much concern has been expressed by contemporary researchers that the self is suffering from a rapidly spreading prefix disease. In this disease, the self and a hyphen seem to be becoming the prefix for virtually every psychological process, from self-enhancement and self-regulation to self-control and self-reflection to self-awareness and self-monitoring to self-everything, ad infinitum. The same wry but distressing sentiment is expressed in phrases like Abraham Tesser's (1996) "self-zoo"—a heterogeneous, ever-growing collection of assorted concepts, hypothesized selves, self-constructs, and self-relevant processes. These concerns have led to a growing belief that to get over the "zoo problem" the self needs to be conceptualized as a coherent, organized system (e.g., Hoyle et al., 1999). Nevertheless, with Occam's razor and parsimony in mind, one still may ask whether positing such a system is mostly a bow in a currently fashionable "modeling" direction that creates unnecessary complexities. Or does it really have advantages for the study of the self with significant implications for the research agenda of the future?

In our view, the field may benefit from the type of self-system described here for many reasons. First, it would indeed facilitate going beyond studies of the diverse aspects and sub-processes of the self as a proliferating collection of unconnected aspects

and variables or isolated part processes (see also, Smith, 1996). That is necessary because self-relevant processes do not operate in isolation and independently but concurrently in parallel and at multiple levels. Most important, recall that in a processing system that is in line with the connectionist metaphor, the whole system is connected so that when one "part" is activated the others also may be affected and potentially changed (through adjustment in their "weights"). Hence the components cannot be properly understood alone because it is their organization within the system that constrains and guides their interactions and determines how they work.

The agentic, doing aspects, previously characterized as different motives, are now inherent qualities of the larger interacting system that operates at many levels concurrently that are manifested in different expressions or forms. In this "organic" dynamic system, apparently paradoxical behavior can be understood as the result of the parallel operations of the system at these multiple levels, for example more automatic versus more controlled, implicit and explicit, affective and cognitive, and so forth. Thus a systems approach makes it easier to avoid having to invoke a panoply of different motives for each diverse manifestation and function of the system, hopefully reducing the homunculus threat.

Conceptualized within the connectionist metaphor, the particular expressions of the system that are (re-) constructed and manifested at a given moment depend on the particular aspects of the system that are expressed in the specific context and situation observed. In a sense, it is the system's "momentary local solution" for satisfying the mutual constraints inherent within its network of links, as expressed in that instant. Psychologically, the specific context can be quite different for the individual than it is for an outside observer, because its meaning for the individual, which is often based on enduring concerns, may not be apparent to the observer. These distinctive subjective meanings of the salient features of the situation constitute its psychological *active ingredients* (Higgins, 1996a; Lewin, 1931; Shoda, Mischel, & Wright, 1994). This is to say that different features of the self-system might be activated and acted upon than the onlooker might have expected from observing more "objectively" (or normatively) salient features of a situation (Bargh & Ferguson, 2000). When the psychological features of the situation that are salient for the particular individual are understood, his or her seemingly paradoxical behaviors can be seen as the non-mysterious and indeed potentially predictable reflections of the state of the system within that context (Shoda et al., 1994). The type of self-system posited also is needed to address the phenomena of the self as they are experienced and unfold within a particular person over the course of time—a goal to which self theorists beginning with William James have been committed, but with little progress in a century. To study the continuous stream of experience and behavior requires attention to the *variability* intrinsic to such experience and their dynamics. It thus requires a systems approach that takes account of the variability of the states of mind and consciousness that James long ago noted, and the interactions between these states and the events that prime them. In this regard, the type of interactionist self-system described may provide a route for the more rigorous idiographic study of the flow of these experiences of the self and facilitate finding the stability and consistencies within them (e.g., Brown & Moskowitz, 1998; Eizenman, Nesselroade, Featherman, & Rhoda, 1997; Fleeson, 2001; Shoda & Tiernan, 2002). Such research should be facilitated by the concept of the stable self-signatures of IF–THEN intra-individual variability that the interactionist system described has been shown to generate.

In this conceptualization, the intra-personal processes within the system are in continuous seamless interaction with the interpersonal relationships within which the system is contextualized. Consequently, the links between the intra-personal dynamics and the interpersonal signatures and strategies of the self are the locus in which the meaning of each can be more fully understood. It therefore should be fruitful to examine them conjointly, rather than partitioning them—sometimes even into different sub-disciplines, as seen in the current tripartite division within the field's flagship research outlet, the *Journal of Personality and Social Psychology*.

Identifying Common Self-Signatures and Self-Construction Types

Although self-signatures are necessarily idiographic, they lend themselves equally to the nomothetic study of the signatures shared by a *self-construction type*. A self-construction type consists of people who have a common organization of relations among mediating units in the processing of certain self-relevant situation features. To identify these individuals, assessments are directed at finding their common self-signatures—that is, the IF–THEN patterns of behavior variation that they share (e.g., Mischel & Shoda, 1995). These patterns in turn provide clues to the common self-construction goals and dynamics that underlie and generate the signatures. Conversely, identifying similarities among persons in their underlying processing dynamics should allow prediction of their shared self-signatures as they are manifested in the self-construction process.

An Example: The Narcissistic Prototype

The concept of self-construction types invites construct validity research to explore the characteristic self-systems and signatures that distinguish different types of self-construction, as illustrated, for example, in research on the narcissistic type (Morf & Rhodewalt, 2001a, 2001b; Rhodewalt & Sorrow, Chapter 26, this volume). The most striking feature of narcissists is that while they engage in virtually relentless efforts of self-affirmation and self-esteem enhancement, these efforts seem to be undone and destroyed as rapidly as they are built up. That happens because in the attempt to self-affirm they employ interpersonal strategies that ultimately destroy the very relationships upon which they are dependent. One can begin to make sense of this paradoxical self-signature by taking account of parallel processes working at different levels within the underlying system that generates the signature for this type distinctively. In the case of narcissism, this seems to involve the conjoint operation of two key features that are paradoxically juxtaposed: grandiosity and vulnerability.

The grandiosity aspect of their self-system is evident at direct and explicit levels in the narcissist's chronic vigilance for situational opportunities in which their grandiose self-concepts can be affirmed and bolstered, reflecting the centrally important self-affirmation goal of narcissists (Morf, Ansara, & Shia, 2001; Morf, Weir, & Davidov, 2000; Rhodewalt & Eddings, 2002). They latch on to these opportunities to promote the self and expend much effort toward providing evidence for their superiority. Simultaneously, narcissists have cynical and unempathic views of others and seem insensitive to others' concerns and situational constraints. Thus, they promote their grandiosity unbounded: they self-report superiority, beyond what is socially acceptable, they engage in self-aggrandizing behaviors, even in situations that call for modesty, derogating others who outperform them, and self-handicapping prior to performance—even when the long-term costs are self-defeating and relationship-destructive. Furthermore, they provide post-hoc interpretations of experiences that ingeniously amplify the positive feedback to them while discounting the negative (documented in Morf & Rhodewalt, 2001a, 2001b).

At other, less directly accessible levels, and perhaps requiring more indirect and implicit assessments, however, the same individuals may be seen to be easily threatened and exceptionally vulnerable in their self-esteem, changing the meaning of their total self-signature (Morf & Rhodewalt, 2001a). The narcissist's vulnerability is much less directly expressed, and thus more difficult to capture. Mostly, it is inferred from their excessive responses and often inappropriate interpersonal behaviors in response to self-esteem threat. It seems reasonable to conclude from these responses that narcissists, while highly sensitive to self-aggrandizing opportunities, are simultaneously, chronically alert to, indeed scanning for, threat and "danger"—a pattern reflecting the second defining feature of their signature, namely, their vulnerability.

When their vulnerability is experienced, however, it does not stay visible long, given that narcissists are experts at counteracting or defensively denying it. In this dynamic, experiences such as being outperformed by a competitor (and they may perceive many people that way) may trigger hot, automatic, emotional activation of feelings like "I am a worthless person" (Morf & Rhode-

walt, 2001b). Concurrently, at an explicit level it may elicit, "unless I can show that I am better than he is—which of course I can, because I am superior," which in turn would quickly replace anxiety or even shame by active other-derogation to reassert the self as superior. The sad aspect of this dynamic is that the derogator never quite seems to persuade himself of his own self-worth, and the labor to affirm self-esteem becomes a ceaseless burden, an endless climb out of quicksand. In short, the narcissistic paradox begins to make sense when one sees that its key features, the juxtaposition of grandiosity and vulnerability, are generated concurrently by a self-system in which each operates in parallel, albeit at different levels, and is expressed behaviorally in different forms.

The Need for Mid-Level Types

As in this example, note that the self-construction prototypes that best lend themselves to such analyses are likely to be cast at middle levels of abstraction, rather than at more superordinate, abstract levels (Cantor, 1990; Cantor & Mischel, 1979; Emmons, 1989; Morf & Rhodewalt, 2001a). It is at this middle level that trait prototypes involve specific, contextualized representations of the self and of others. For example, defensive-pessimists may be defined by a pattern of coping with high experienced anticipatory performance anxiety through mentally rehearsing and working through all the bad outcomes that they can imagine. Concurrently, they also self-protectively set low expectations. They then mobilize themselves by searching for and finding ways to improve performance by increasing their effort and scanning for possible obstacles (Norem & Cantor, 1986).

Likewise, dependency in adults is widely assumed to be linked to a broad disposition of passivity-submissiveness, but nevertheless fine-grained analyses indicate that within some situations it is in fact related to high levels of activity and assertiveness. Specifically, while dependent individuals who are focused on getting along with a peer will self-denigrate, they will self-promote when concerned mostly with pleasing an authority figure (Bornstein, Riggs, Hill, & Calabrese, 1996).

These mid-level prototypes are characterized by particular kinds of cognitive and affective representations of self and others, visible in distinctive patterns of beliefs, values, emotional reactions, self-regulatory processes, and goal-driven interpersonal styles and scripts for social behavior (e.g., Cantor, 1990; Cantor, Mischel, & Schwartz, 1982; Morf & Rhodewalt, 2001a). Global traits like extraversion, in contrast, are cast at super-ordinate levels of abstraction, with insufficient specificity in terms of defining self-regulatory goals, interaction patterns, and cognitive–affective organization. For example, while the self-affirmation goals found in extraversion are a feature of narcissism, they also are seen in other personality types defined by different motivational concerns. What is true for extraversion likewise seems to apply to such broad personality dimensions as aggression (e.g., Crick & Dodge, 1994; Dodge & Somberg, 1987). For example, in an extensive observational study of interpersonal behavior over time in a summer camp, some children were substantially and reliably more aggressive than others when disciplined by an adult. However, and most interesting, the same children also were significantly and consistently less aggressive than others when teased by a peer, while still others were marked distinctively by becoming most aggressive when approached *positively* by others (Mischel & Shoda, 1995). Thus the behavior of these individuals took the form of stable but specific IF–THEN patterns or profiles.

This is to say, in order to be meaningful, that is, to allow predictions of future behavior in particular situations, these broad personality dimensions need to be analyzed to the levels of such profiles. At this level, they may be seen to be expressions of different types of self-construction to the degree that they reflect different types of goals or self-theories. An exciting challenge for future research is to determine more precisely to what degree, and in what ways, a behavioral disposition needs to be contextualized in order to constitute a meaningful self-construction type.

Assessment/Measurement Implications

Both theoretically and empirically, even if two people are similar in their overall levels on a dimension such as "sociability and interpersonal warmth," for example, they will display distinctive, predictable, and meaningful patterns of behavioral variability in their self-signatures. That is, they will differ reliably and meaningfully in terms of when and with whom they are relatively more and less sociable than others, even if they are alike in their total overall degree of sociability (Mischel & Shoda, 1995). Narcissists, for example, will self-enhance on agentic but not on communal qualities (Campbell et al., 2002). Although these IF–THEN patterns are deliberately bypassed in traditional assessment, it is these patterns that provide clues to the individual's goals, values, and the underlying organization of the self-system. IF–THEN self-signatures require IF–THEN assessments: they call for measures that capture the predictable variability of the contextualized self, not just its overall levels. Therefore, they need to be central in assessments designed to do justice to the complexities and diverse manifestations of the self-system in different contexts and relationships, and at different levels. The development of models and methods to identify these signatures and their underlying organization with increasing precision provides an agenda and a host of research challenges. It will be important for future assessments of the self-system to take context and the specifics of the interpersonal situation fully into account if the goal is to capture the richness and depth of different types of self-construction.

To illustrate with another type, consider individuals whose self-construction centers around their anxieties about interpersonal rejection (Downey, Feldman, & Ayduk, 2000). Their "rejection sensitivity" is seen first in intimate relationships when they encounter what could be construed as uncaring behavior (e.g., partner is attentive to someone else), which is likely to lead them to experience thoughts like "she doesn't love me." These cognitions in turn tend to trigger expectations of rejection, abandonment, feelings of anger and resentment, and anxiety and rage at the prospect of abandonment. Coercive and controlling behaviors then become activated, but typically are blamed on the partner's behavior. However, although their defining self-signature includes being more prone than others to anger, disapproval, and coercive behaviors in certain types of intimate situations, it also includes being more supportive, caring, and romantic than most people, for example, in initial encounters with potential partners.

The systems approach to assessment of self-construction types, such as rejection sensitivity illustrated here contrasts in significant ways with current mainstream assessment practices. The latter typically approach the assessment of individual differences guided by the traits=personality model described earlier in this chapter. Therefore global, relatively context-free self-report measures, for example, scales from the Big Five, are usually employed to tap broad factors such as Extraversion or Neuroticism. In contrast, in the systems approach the assessment focus is not limited to broad overall average characteristics, although they can, of course, be included. The focus is on the IF–THEN patterns that characterize the self-signatures of the type, and it seeks to assess these at multiple levels of analysis and measurement, not just with direct, explicit uncontextualized assessments. That also may call for indirect, implicit assessments, such as response latency to "hot" trigger stimuli that activate the vulnerability (e.g. rejection scenes or words), or other indirect tests (e.g., Ayduk et al., 1999, 2001; Greenwald et al., 2002).

To study these signatures systematically requires assessing the individual's thoughts, feelings, and action tendencies (the THEN) in relation to changes in the IF that is activated, internally or externally (Ayduk et al., 1999; Baldwin & Meunier, 1999). Given that at least some of these IF–THEN relations are themselves stable in ways characteristic of the person (Shoda et al., 1994), they also may allow an in-depth analysis of the stream of experience that goes much beyond uncontextualized introspective reports or global assessments. They can even lead to experimental paradigms that identify the important IF trigger stimuli that are linked predictably to changes in the person's cognitive–affective states and behavioral reactions (e.g., Shoda & Tiernan, 2002).

Development of Different Types of Self-Construction

When the self is conceptualized as an organized system, and different people are seen in terms of their different types of self-constructions and organizations, a cascade of new questions invite exploration. While self researchers have made much progress in understanding how self-construction systems are maintained, enhanced, and reconstructed within social interactions, how these self-systems develop in the first place and are linked to long-term social relationships is a topic largely untouched thus far by self researchers. One notable exception is in Susan Harter's (1999) work on development as a self-construction process. She sees the path of self-development as one in which the cognitive-developmental structures that emerge pave the way for more mature self-structures but also represent "a veritable minefield" (p. 11) of potential vulnerabilities for the self-system that can lead to many negative consequences and life outcomes. As one example, she notes that the development of the ability to differentiate self and others as independent agents can greatly deflate the sense of omnipotence, with a consequent increase in frustration and distress, as the caregiver behaves in ways that may not fit the toddler's goals.

The interactions between the young child and his/her significant others as they deal with these stresses and developmental opportunities are the early stage on which self-construction evolves and possible selves begin to take their shapes. Although it is the stage for the development of potential vulnerabilities, it also can lead to increased freedom and opportunities for "self-actualization" and not just to self-defense and safety concerns, using Maslow's (1957) distinction. The challenge for self research is to identify the conditions under which such opportunities for enhanced self-actualization can be optimized, and under which the potential vulnerabilities for the self can be appropriately buffered.

A focus on the development of self-construction types also makes explicit the close connections between self research and diverse research findings and theories that already exist, but often within other sub-disciplines on the fuzzy boundaries of self research—boundaries that need to be readily crossed in research on self-systems. Relevant topics on these boundaries to which new research on the self could be directed include, for example, the development of the person's relational selves and identities (Chen & Andersen, 1999; Harter, 1999) and the development of the person's theory of self and of the possibilities for changes in the self (e.g, Dweck, 1991; Dweck et al., Chapter 12, this volume). In other, related directions is work on the role of the person's theory of mind for explaining self-relevant behavior about oneself and about others (e.g., Malle, 1999), the effects of meta-cognitive understanding (e.g. Mischel & Mischel, 1983) on the experienced self, the nature and consequences of different types of self-perception, and the perception and understanding of significant others who are close to the self (e.g. Chen-Idson & Mischel, 2001).

Prospects for the Future of Self Research: Situating the Self as a Psycho-Social Dynamic Processing System within the Field

Fields and sub-disciplines within psychology, like selves, undergo evolutions and redefine themselves. This was seen in the 1970s when in response to the cognitive revolution much of social psychology quickly metamorphosed into social cognition. An analogous transformation may be under way in the relationship between the study of the self and of personality in academic psychology. As the view of the self is expanding to encompass diverse executive and motivational functions, as was seen throughout this chapter—functions that traditionally have been at the heart of the basic processes and dynamics of personality—the boundaries between the two domains are becoming increasingly fuzzy and potentially dissolving.

Implications of the Expanded Self

In this sense, the psychology of self is becoming the contemporary form of what used to be "ego and object relations" psychology, but now informed by decades of relevant new research and theory-building. At first glance, this kind of shift may seem to be consistent with the view of "personality as antecedents to the self" (Hoyle et al., 1999, p. 17), and of the self as a "mediator between personality and adjustment" (Graziano, Jensen-Campbell, & Finch, 1997). In that view (Roberts & Robins, 2000), personality becomes the attributes a person *has,* and the self-system becomes the dynamic cognitive–affective–action system that deals with what the motivated person *does* and experiences (Mischel, 1973, 1984; Mischel & Shoda, 1999).

In the present view, however, an adequate conception of what the person "has" at the outset of life, and its subsequent developmental course needs to capture the fundamental plasticity of the human brain and of the pre-dispositions that initially reflect the individual's biological inheritance. A close look at human development, as seen, for example, in the self-construction process, suggests not a one-way influence process but a dynamic reciprocal interactionism, exemplified in the two-way influence process between mother and child in early life. And similar continuous two-way influence processes seem to characterize virtually all aspects of bio-psycho-social adaptation, accommodation, and assimilation in its many diverse forms, including in the development and functioning of the brain (e.g., Sutton, 2002).

Self theory and research now seem well-positioned to address the large empty conceptual space between whatever temperamental, affective, and cognitive pre-tuning or pre-wiring the newborn brings to the world and the exquisitely complex patterns of adaptation and self-construction that evolve in the life-long subsequent interactions with the social world. One substantive advantage of casting the processing dynamics that underlie self-construction in a framework of "selfhood" (rather than of personality) is that it bypasses many of the classic century-old assumptions about personality dynamics (e.g., about the nature of unconscious motivational determinism à la Freud, the focus on pathology, the belief that "personality can't change"). Many of these assumptions do not fit the currently emerging view of mind, brain, and their plasticity in interaction with the contexts within which they function. Such plasticity and adaptiveness, however, seems highly compatible with a view of the self that allows the potential for multiple selves and alternative possible selves all organized within a larger interacting self-system. (Note, in contrast, that unlike the possibility of "multiple selves," the concept of "multiple personalities" makes sense only in terms of an illness.) In short, a dynamic self-system may facilitate a more "positive" and optimistic approach to the human potential and the opportunities for self-directed freedom and constructive change (e.g., Aspinwall & Staudinger, in press).

The Self Located at the Intersection of Diverse Disciplines

In light of the expansion of the self as a construct and as a system, the study of the self now seems perched at the intersection—indeed the hub—of areas that include personality processes and dynamics, social cognition, emotion-motivation, developmental psychology, interpersonal behavior, clinical-health psychology-behavioral medicine, and cultural psychology. The recognition of this new position at the hub can influence the journals we read, the conferences we attend, the training we give our students, and, most important, our vision of how to proceed with the most-needed research and theory-building in the study of selfhood. It influences how the science of the self organizes itself, trains its students, and shapes its research projects. A curriculum for the training of the "complete self researcher" ideally now may need to span virtually every area of our science. Indeed, the ideal researcher on the self may have to be one of the endangered species of "generalists" remaining within psychology. Perhaps most important—and the focus of this chapter—it impacts on the type of conceptual framework needed to capture the complexities and scope of self-relevant phenomena and processes with the depth they deserve.

The Psycho-Social Dynamic Processing system for the self outlined in this chapter has tried to build a conceptual bridge that takes account of relevant developments in diverse areas, focusing particularly on both research cast in the language of the self and parallel work on the cognitive–affective processing dynamics of personality. The two lines of research and theory on personality dynamics and on self-construction seem to overlap substantially in the phenomena they seek to understand, and in the principles and procedures that guide their common search. Our hope is that their closer integration in future work will help to build a more cumulative science of both selfhood and personality—or perhaps the two will ultimately converge toward "personhood."

Author Notes

The views expressed in this chapter are those of the authors and do not necessarily reflect official views of the National Institute of Mental Health, the National Institutes of Health, or any other branch of the U.S. Department of Health and Human Services. Preparation of this chapter was supported in part by National Institute of Mental Health Grant MH 39349 to Walter Mischel. Thanks are due to Ozlem Ayduk, Daniel Cervone, Rodolfo Mendoza-Denton, Fred Rhodewalt , Yuichi Shoda , Eliot Smith, Charlene Weir, and Vivian Zayas for many helpful comments on earlier drafts.

Correspondence concerning this chapter and requests for reprints should be addressed to Walter Mischel, Department of Psychology, Columbia University, New York, NY 10027, or Carolyn C. Morf, National Institute of Mental Health, 6001 Executive Blvd., Room 7216, MSC 9651, Bethesda, MD 20892–9651.

References

Allport, G. W. (1961). *Pattern and growth in personality.* New York: Holt, Rinehart and Winston.

Andersen, S. M., Chen, S., & Miranda, R. (2002). Significant others and the self. *Self and Identity, 1,* 159–168.

Aspinwall, L. G., & Staudinger, A. U. (2002). *A psychology of human strengths: Perspectives on an emerging field.* Washington, DC: American Psychological Association.

Athay, M., & Darley, J. M. (1981). Toward an interaction-centered theory of personality. In N. Cantor & J. F. Kihlstrom (Eds.), *Personality, cognition, and social interaction* (pp. 281–308). Hillsdale, NJ: Erlbaum.

Ayduk, O., Downey, G., Testa, A., Yen, Y., & Shoda, Y. (1999). Does rejection elicit hostility in rejection sensitive women? *Social Cognition, 17,* 245–271.

Ayduk, O., Mendoza-Denton, R., Mischel, W., Downey, G., Peake, P., & Rodriguez, M. (2000). Regulating the interpersonal self: Strategic self-regulation for coping with rejection sensitivity. *Journal of Personality and Social Psychology, 79,* 776–792.

Baldwin, M. J. (1905). Sketch of the history of psychology. *Psychological Review, 12,* 144–165.

Baldwin, M. W. (1992). Relational schemas and the processing of social information. *Psychological Bulletin, 112,* 461–484.

Baldwin, M. W., & Holmes, J. G. (1987). Salient private audiences and awareness of the self. *Journal of Personality and Social Psychology, 52,* 1087–1098.

Baldwin, M. W., & Meunier, J. (1999). The cued activation of attachment relational schemas. *Social Cognition, 171,* 209–227.

Bargh, J. A. (1997). Reply to commentaries. In R. S. Wyer, Jr. (Ed.), *The automaticity of everyday life: Advances in social cognition* (Vol. 10, pp. 231–246). Mahwah, NJ: Erlbaum.

Bargh, J. A., & Ferguson, M. J. (2000). Beyond behaviorism: On the automaticity of higher mental processes. *Psychological Bulletin, 126,* 925–945.

Baumeister, R. F. (1987). How the self became a problem: A psychological review of historical research. *Journal of Personality and Social Psychology, 52,* 163–176.

Baumeister R. F. (1998). The self. In D. T. Gilbert (Ed.), *The handbook of social psychology* (pp. 680–740) Boston: McGraw-Hill.

Bolger, N., & Zuckerman, A. (1995). A framework for studying personality in the stress process. *Journal of Personality and Social Psychology, 69,* 890–902.

Bornstein, R. F., Riggs, J. M., Hill, E. L., & Calabrese, C. (1996). Activity, passivity, self-denigration, and self-promotion: Toward an interactionist model of interpersonal dependency. *Journal of Personality, 64,* 637–673.

Brown, K. W., & Moskowitz, D. S. (1998). Dynamic stability of behavior: The rhythms of our interpersonal lives. *Journal of Personality, 66,* 105–134.

Buss, D. M. (1997). Evolutionary foundations of personality. In R. Hogan, J. A. Johnson, & S. R. Briggs (Eds.), *Handbook of personality psychology* (pp. 317–344). San Diego, CA: Academic Press.

Campbell, W. K. (2002). Narcissism and commitment in romantic relationships: An investment model analysis. *Personality and Social Psychology Bulletin, 28,* 358–368.

Cantor, N. (1990). From thought to behavior: "Having" and "doing" in the study of personality and cognition. *American Psychologist, 45,* 735–750.

Cantor, N., & Kihlstrom, J. F. (1987). *Personality and social intelligence.* Englewood Cliffs, NJ: Prentice-Hall.

Cantor, N., & Mischel, W. (1979). Prototypes in person perception. In L. Berkowitz (Ed.), *Advances in experimental social psychology* (Vol. 12, pp. 3–52). New York: Academic Press.

Cantor, N., Mischel, W., & Schwartz, J. C. (1982). A prototype analysis of psychological situations. *Cognitive Psychology, 14,* 45–77.

Cantor, N., Norem, J., Langston, C., Zirkel, S., Fleeson W., & Cook-Flannagan, C. (1991). Life tasks and daily life experience. *Journal of Personality, 59,* 425–451.

Carver, C. S., & Scheier, M. F. (1981). *Attention and self-regulation: A control theory approach to human behavior.* New York: Springer-Verlag.

Cervone, D., & Shoda, Y. (Eds.). (1999). *The coherence of personality: Social-cognitive bases of consistency, variability, and organization.* New York: Guilford Press.

Chen, S., & Andersen, S. M. (1999). Relationships from the past in the present: Significant-other representations and transference in interpersonal life. In M. P. Zanna (Ed.), *Advances in experimental social psychology* (Vol. 31, pp. 123–190). San Diego, CA: Academic Press.

Chen-Idson, L., & Mischel, W. (2001). The personality of familiar and significant people: The lay perceiver as a social cognitive theorist. *Journal of Personality and Social Psychology, 80,* 585–596.

Chiu, C.Y., Hong, Y., Mischel, W., & Shoda, Y. (1995). Discriminative facility in social competence: Conditional versus dispositional encoding and monitoring-blunting of information. *Social Cognition, 13,* 49–70.

Cooley, C. H. (1902). *Human nature and the social order.* New York: Scribner's.

Crick, N. R., & Dodge, K. A. (1994). A review and reformulation of social information-processing mechanisms in children's social adjustment. *Psychological Bulletin, 115,* 74–101.

Crittenden, P. S. (1990) Internal representational models of attachment relationships. *Infant Mental Health Journal, 11,* 259–277.

Derryberry, D. (2002). Attention and voluntary self-control. *Self and Identity, 1*(2), 105–111.

Descartes, R. (1970). *The philosophical works of Descartes* (Vol. 1, p. 101; E. S. Haldane & G. R. T. Ross, Trans.). New York: Cambridge University Press. (Original work published 1637)

Dewey, J. (1890). On some current conceptions of the term "self." *Mind, 15,* 58–74.

Dodge, K. A., & Somberg, D. R. (1987). Hostile attributional biases among aggressive boys are exacerbated under conditions of threats to the self. *Child Development, 58,* 213–224.

Donahue, E. M., Robins, R. W., Roverts, B. W., & John, O. P. (1993). The divided self: Concurrent and longitudinal effects of psychological adjustment and social roles on self-concept differentiation. *Journal of Personality and Social Psychology, 64,* 834–846.

Downey, G., Feldman, S., & Ayduk, O. (2000). Rejection sensitivity and male violence in romantic relationships. *Personal Relationships, 7,* 45–61.

Eizenman, D. R., Nesselroade, J. R., Featherman, D. L., & Rowe, J. W. (1997). Intraindividual variability in perceived control in an older sample: The MacArthur successful aging studies. *Psychology and Aging, 12,* 489–502.

Emmons, R. A. (1989). Exploring the relations between motives and traits: The case of narcissism. In D. M. Buss & N. Cantor (Eds.), *Personality psychology: Recent trends and emerging directions* (pp. 32–44). New York: Springer-Verlag.

Emmons, R. A. (1991). Personal strivings, daily life events, and psychological and physical well-being. *Journal of Personality, 59,* 453–472.

Emmons, R. A., Diener, E., & Larsen, R. J. (1986). Choice and avoidance of everyday situations and affect congruence: Two models of reciprocal interactionism. *Journal of Personality and Social Psychology, 51,* 815–826.

Emmons, R. A., & King, L. A. (1988). Conflict among personal strivings: Immediate and long-term implications for psychological and physical well-being. *Journal of Personality and Social Psychology, 54,* 1040–1048.

Epstein, S. (1973). The self-concept revisited or a theory of a theory. *American Psychologist, 28,* 405–416.

Epstein, S. (1994). Integration of the cognitive and the psychodynamic unconscious. *American Psychologist, 49,* 709–724.

Fleeson, W. (2001). Toward a structure- and process-integrated view of personality: Traits as density distributions of states. *Journal of Personality and Social Psychology. 80,* 1011–1027.

Gollwitzer, P. M., & Bargh, J. A. (1996). *The psychology of action: Linking cognition and motivation to behavior.* New York: Guilford Press.

Gollwitzer, P. M., & Moskowitz, G. B. (1996). Goal effects on action and cognition. In E. T. Higgins & A. W. Kruglanski (Eds.), *Social psychology: Handbook of basic principles* (pp. 361–399). New York: Guilford Press.

Graziano, W. G., Jensen-Campbell, L. A., & Finch, J. F. (1997). The self as a mediator between personality and adjustment. *Journal of Personality and Social Psychology, 73,* 392–404.

Graziano W. G., & Tobin, R. M. (2001). The distributed processing of narcissist: Paradox lost? *Psychological Inquiry, 12*(4), 219–222.

Greenwald, A. G., Banaji, M. R., Rudman, L. A., Farnham, S. D., Nosek, B. A., & Mellott, D. S. (2002). A unified theory of implicit attitudes, stereotypes, self-esteem, and self-concept. *Psychological Review, 109*(1), 3–25.

Greenwald, A. G., & Pratkanis, A. R. (1984). The self. In S. Wyer & T. K. Srull (Eds.), *Handbook of social cognition* (pp. 129–178). Hillsdale, NJ: Erlbaum.

Gunnar, M. (2001, April). Relationships as a central context of early childhood. In D. A. Philips & J. P. Shonkoff (Chairs), *From neurons to neighborhoods: The science of early child development.* Symposium conducted at the meeting of the Society for Research and Child Development, Minneapolis, MN.

Harter, S. (1999). *The construction of the self: A developmental perspective.* New York: Guilford Press.

Hazan, C., & Shaver, P. (1987). Romantic love conceptualized as an attachment process. *Journal of Personality and Social Psychology, 52,* 511–524.

Higgins, E. T. (1996a). Ideals, oughts, and regulatory focus: Affect and motivation from distinct pains and pleasures. In P. M. Gollwitzer & J. A. Bargh (Eds.), *The psychology of action: Linking cognition and motivation to behavior* (pp. 91–114). New York: Guilford Press.

Higgins, E. T. (1996b). Knowledge activation: Accessibility, applicability, and salience. In E. T. Higgins & A. W. Kruglanski (Eds.), *Social psychology: Handbook of basic principles* (pp. 133–168). New York: Guilford Press.

Higgins, E. T., & Kruglanski, A. W. (Eds.). (1996). *Social psychology: Handbook of basic principles.* New York: Guilford Press.

Hogan, R., Johnson, J. A., & Briggs, S. R. (Eds.). (1997). *Handbook of personality psychology.* San Diego, CA: Academic Press.

Hoyle, R. H., Kernis, M. H., Leary, M. R., & Baldwin, M. W. (1999). *Selfhood: Identity, esteem, regulation.* Boulder, CO: Westview Press

James, W. (1890). *The principles of psychology* (Vols. 1 & 2). New York: Holt.

James, W. (1892). *Psychology: Briefer course.* New York: Holt.

Kashima Y., & Kerekes, A. R. Z. (1994). A distributed memory model of averaging phenomena in personal impression formation. *Journal of Experimental Social Psychology, 30,* 407–455.

Kernberg, O. (1976). *Object relations theory and clinical psychoanalysis.* New York: Jason Aronson.

Kernberg, O. (1984). *Severe personality disorders.* New Haven, CT: Yale University Press.

Kihlstrom, J. F. (1987). The cognitive unconscious. *Science, 237,* 1445–1452.

Kihlstrom, J. F. (1990). The psychological unconscious. In L. A. Pervin (Ed.) *Handbook of personality: Theory and research* (pp. 445–464). New York: Guilford Press.

Kohut, H. (1971). *The analysis of the self.* New York: International Universities Press.

Kuhl, J. (1985). From cognition to behavior: Perspectives for future research on action control. In J. Kuhl & J.

Beckmann (Eds.), *Action control from cognition to behavior* (pp. 267–276). New York: Springer-Verlag.

Kunda, Z., & Thagard, P. (1996). Forming impressions from stereotypes, traits, and behaviors: A parallel–constraint–satisfaction theory. *Psychological Review, 103,* 284–308.

Ledoux, J. (1996). *The emotional brain.* New York: Simon & Schuster.

Lewin, K. (1931). The conflict between Aristotelian and Galileian modes of thought in contemporary psychology. *Journal of General Psychology, 5,* 141–177.

Linville, P. W. (1987). Self-complexity as a cognitive buffer against stress-related depression and illness. *Journal of Personality and Social Psychology, 52,* 663–676.

Linville, P. W., & Carlston, D. E. (1994). Social cognition of the self. In P. G. Devine, D. C. Hamilton, & T. M. Ostrom (Eds.), *Social cognition: Impact on social psychology* (pp. 143–193). New York: Academic Press.

Little, B. R., Lecci, L., & Watkinson, B. (1992). Personality and personal projects: Linking the big five and PAC units of analysis. *Journal of Personality, 60,* 501–525.

Malle, B. F. (1999). How people explain behavior: A new theoretical framework. *Personality and Social Psychology Review, 3,* 23–48.

Markus, H., & Cross, S. (1990). The interpersonal self. In L. A. Pervin (Ed.), *Handbook of personality: Theory and research* (pp. 576–608). New York: Guilford Press.

Markus, H., & Kunda, Z. (1986). Stability and malleability of the self-concept. *Journal of Personality and Social Psychology, 51,* 858–866.

Markus, H., & Zajonc, R. B. (1985). The cognitive perspective in social psychology. In G. Lindzey & E. Aronson (Eds.), *The handbook of social psychology* (3rd ed., Vol. 1, pp. 137–230). New York: Random House.

Maslow, A. H. (1957). Some basic propositions of a growth and self-actualization psychology. In G. Lyndzey & C. Hall (Eds.), *Theories of personality: Primary sources and research* (pp. 307–316). New York: Wiley.

McCrae, R. R., & Costa, P. T. (1999). A five-factor theory of personality. In L. A. Pervin & O. P. John (Eds.), *Handbook of personality: Theory and research* (2nd ed., pp. 139–153). New York: Guilford Press.

Mead, G. H. (1934). *Mind, self and society: From the standpoint of a social behaviorist.* Chicago: University of Chicago Press.

Mendoza-Denton, R., Ayduk, O., Mischel, W., Shoda, Y., & Testa, A. (2001). Person × situation interactionism in self-encoding (I am . . . when . . .): Implications for affect regulation and social information processing. *Journal of Personality and Social Psychology, 80,* 533–544.

Metcalfe, J., & Mischel, W. (1999). A hot/cool system analysis of delay of gratification: Dynamics of willpower. *Psychological Review, 106,* 3–19.

Mischel, H. N., & Mischel, W. (1983). The development of children's knowledge of self-control strategies. *Child Development, 54,* 603–619.

Mischel, W. (1973). Toward a cognitive social learning reconceptualization of personality. *Psychological Review, 80,* 252–283.

Mischel, W. (1984). On the predictability of behavior and the structure of personality. In R. A. Zucker, J. Aronoff, & A. I. Rabin (Eds.), *Personality and the prediction of behavior* (pp. 269–305). New York: Academic Press.

Mischel, W. (1998). Metacognition at the hyphen of social-cognitive psychology. *Personality and Social Psychology Review, 2,* 84–86.

Mischel, W., Cantor, N., & Feldman, S. (1996). Principles of self-regulation: The nature of willpower and self-control. In E. T. Higgins & A. W. Kruglanski (Eds.), *Social psychology: Handbook of basic principles* (pp. 329–360). New York: Guilford Press.

Mischel, W., & Shoda, Y. (1995). A cognitive–affective system theory of personality: Reconceptualizing situations, dispositions, dynamics, and invariance in personality structure. *Psychological Review, 102,* 246–268.

Mischel, W., & Shoda, Y. (1998). Reconciling processing dynamics and personality dispositions. *Annual Review of Psychology, 49,* 229–258.

Mischel, W., & Shoda, Y. (1999). Integrating dispositions and processing dynamics within a unified theory of personality: The cognitive affective personality system (CAPS). In L. Pervin & O. P. John (Eds.), *Handbook of personality: Theory and research* (pp. 197–218). New York: Guilford Press.

Mischel, W., Shoda, Y., & Mendoza-Denton, R. (2002). Situation-behavior profiles as a locus of consistency in personality. *Current Directions in Psychological Science, 11*(2), 50–54.

Mischel, W., Shoda, Y., & Rodriguez, M. L. (1989). Delay of gratification in children. *Science, 44,* 933–938.

Morf, C. C., Ansara, D., & Shia, T. (2001). *The effects of audience characteristics on narcissistic self-presentation.* Manuscript in preparation, University of Toronto.

Morf, C. C., & Rhodewalt, F. (1993). Narcissism and self-evaluation maintenance: Explorations in object relations. *Personality and Social Psychology Bulletin, 19,* 668–676.

Morf, C. C., & Rhodewalt, F. (2001a). Expanding the dynamic self-regulatory processing model of narcissism: Research directions for the future. *Psychological Inquiry, 12,* 243–251.

Morf, C. C., & Rhodewalt, F. (2001b). Unraveling the paradoxes of narcissism: A dynamic self-regulatory processing model. *Psychological Inquiry, 12,* 177–196.

Morf, C. C., Weir, C. R., & Davidov, M. (2000). Narcissism and intrinsic motivation: The role of goal congruence. *Journal of Experimental Social Psychology, 36,* 424–438.

Norem, J. K., & Cantor, N. (1986). Anticipatory and post hoc cushioning strategies: Optimism and defensive pessimism in "risky" situations. *Cognitive Therapy and Research, 10,* 347–362.

Nowak, A., Vallacher, R. R., Tesser, A., & Borkowski, W. (2000). Society of self: The emergence of collective properties in self-structure. *Psychological Review, 107,* 39–61.

Pervin, L. A. (1982). The stasis and flow of behavior: Toward a theory of goals. In *Nebraska Symposium on Motivation* (pp. 1–53). Lincoln: University of Nebraska Press.

Pervin, L. A. (1989). *Goal concepts in personality and social psychology.* Hillsdale, NJ: Erlbaum.

Pervin, L. A. (1994). A critical analysis of trait theory. *Psychological Inquiry, 5,* 103–113.

Pervin, L. A., & John, O. P. (1999). *Handbook of personality: Theory and research* (2nd ed.). New York: Guilford Press.

Plomin, R., DeFries, J. C., McClearn, G. E., & Rutter, M. (1997). *Behavioral genetics* (3rd ed.). New York: Freeman.

Posner, M., & Rothbart, M. K. (2000). Developing mechanisms of self-regulation. *Development and Psychopathology, 12,* 427–441.

Prentice, D. A. (2001). The individual self, relational self, and collective self: A commentary. In C. Sedikides & M. B. Brewer (Eds.), *Individual self, relational self, collective self* (pp. 315–326). Philadelphia: Psychology Press/Taylor & Francis.

Read, S. J., & Miller, L. C. (1989). The importance of goals in personality: Toward a coherent model of persons. In R. S. Wyer, Jr., & T. K. Srull (Eds.), *Advances in social cognition: Vol. 2. Social intelligence and cognitive assessments of personality* (pp. 163–174). Hillsdale, NJ: Erlbaum.

Read, S. J., & Miller, L. C. (1998). *Connectionist models of social reasoning and social behavior.* Mahwah, NJ: Erlbaum.

Rhodewalt, F., & Eddings, S. K. (2002). Narcissism reflects: Memory distortion in response to ego-relevant feedback among high- and low-narcissistic men. *Journal of Research in Personality, 36,* 97–116.

Roberts, B. W., & Robins, R. W. (2000). Broad dispositions, broad aspirations: The intersections of personality traits and major life goals. *Personality and Social Psychology Bulletin, 26,* 1284–1296.

Rogers, C. R. (1947). Some observations on the organization of personality. *American Psychologist, 2,* 358–368.

Rogers, C. R. (1951). *Client-centered therapy: Its current practice, implications and theory.* Boston: Houghton Mifflin.

Rothbart, M. K., Derryberry, D., & Posner, M. I. (1994). A psychobiological approach to the development of temperament. In J. E. Bates & T. D. Wachs (Eds.), *Temperament: Individual differences at the interface of biology and behavior* (pp. 83–116). Washington, DC: American Psychological Association.

Rumelhart, D. E., & McClelland, J. L. (1986). *Parallel distributed processing: Explorations in the microstructure of cognition: Vol. 1. Foundations.* Cambridge, MA: MIT Press/Bradford Books.

Sedikides, C., & Brewer M. B. (Eds.). (2001). *Individual self, relational self, collective self.* Philadelphia: Psychology Press/Taylor & Francis.

Sethi, A., Mischel, W., Aber, L., Shoda, Y., & Rodriguez, M. (2000). The relationship between strategic attention deployment and self-regulation: Predicting preschooler's delay of gratification form mother–toddler interactions. *Developmental Psychology, 6,* 767–777.

Shoda, Y. (1999a). Behavioral expressions of a personality system: Generation and perception of behavioral signatures. In D. Cervone & Y. Shoda (Eds.), *The coherence of personality: Social-cognitive bases of consistency, variability, and organization* (pp. 155–181). New York: Guilford Press.

Shoda, Y. (1999b). A unified framework for the study of behavioral consistency: Bridging person × situation interaction and the consistency paradox. *European Journal of Personality, 13,* 361–387.

Shoda, Y., & Mischel, W. (1998). Personality as a stable cognitive–affective activation network: Characteristic patterns of behavior variation emerge from a stable personality structure. In S. Read & L. C. Miller (Eds.), *Con-*

nectionist models of social reasoning and social behavior (pp. 175–208). Mahwah, NJ: Erlbaum.

Shoda, Y., Mischel, W., & Wright J. C. (1994). Intraindividual stability in the organization and patterning of behavior: Incorporating psychological situations into the idiographic analysis of personality. *Journal of Personality and Social Psychology, 67,* 674–687.

Shoda, Y., & Tiernen, S. L. (2002). What remains invariant?: Finding order within a person's thoughts, feelings and behaviors across situations. In D. Cervone & W. Mischel (Eds.), *Advances in personality science* (pp. 241–270). New York: Guilford Press.

Showers, C. (1992). Compartmentalization of positive and negative self-knowledge: Keeping bad apples out of the bunch. *Journal of Personality and Social Psychology, 62,* 1036–1049.

Smith, E. R. (1996). What do connectionism and social psychology offer each other? *Journal of Personality and Social Psychology, 70,* 893–912.

Smith, E. R., & DeCoster, J. (1998). Knowledge acquisition, accessibility, and use in person perception and stereotyping: Simulation with a recurrent connectionist network. *Journal of Personality and Social Psychology, 74,* 21–35.

Sutton, S. K. (2002). Incentive and threat reactivity: Relations with anterior cortical activity. In D. Cervone & W. Mischel (Eds.), *Advances in personality science* (pp. 127–150). New York: Guilford Press.

Tesser, A. (2002). Constructing a niche for the self: A biosocial, PDP approach to understanding lives. *Self and Identity, 1*(2), 185–190.

Tesser, A., Martin, L. L., & Cornell, D. P. (1996). On the substitutability of self-protective mechanisms. In P. M. Gollwitzer & Bargh, J. A. (Eds.), *The psychology of action: Linking cognition and motivation to behavior* (pp. 48–68). New York: Guilford Press

Tice, D. M., & Baumeister, R. F. (2001). The primacy of the interpersonal self. In C. Sedikides & M. B. Brewer (Eds.), *Individual self, relational self, collective self* (pp. 71–88). Philadelphia: Psychology Press/Taylor & Francis.

Vygotsky, L. S. (1978). *Mind in society.* Cambridge, MA: Harvard University Press.

Zayas, V., Shoda, Y., & Ayduk, O. (in press). Personality in context: An interpersonal systems perspective. *Journal of Personality.*

Zirkel, S., & Cantor, N. (1990). Personal construal of life tasks: Those who struggle for independence. *Journal of Personality and Social Psychology, 58,* 172–185

PART II

CONTENT, STRUCTURE, AND ORGANIZATION OF THE SELF

3

Organization of Self-Knowledge: Features, Functions, and Flexibility

CAROLIN J. SHOWERS
VIRGIL ZEIGLER-HILL

From a lay perspective, an expert on self-organization might be expected to provide insight on the sorts of questions that trouble individuals who are prone to introspection and self-awareness. These include the "Who am I?" questions of identity: What are my characteristics, which attributes describe me and which attributes do not? Related to this are questions of self-determination: What is my potential, where should I go, and how should I get there? Surely, people with well-organized selves know what they are striving for, have realistic goals for self-improvement and self-change, and feel confident that they can make choices to further these goals. As laypersons, we also hope that experts on self-organization can help us become more comfortable with our selves. That is, they can show us how to handle our moments of self-doubt and how to manage those aspects of self that we wish to ignore or deny. From the lay perspective, people with well-organized selves should know who they are, where they are going, and how to handle unwanted aspects of self and feelings of self-doubt or uncertainty.

From a technical perspective, the empha-

sis of research on self-organization is less on the character of the well-organized self than on organizational processes—the dimensions people use to organize self-beliefs, how these dimensions of self-organization function, and the potential consequences of each. If there is an especially adaptive type of self-organization, it will most likely be one that matches the motivational and emotional context of the individual rather than one that applies across the board. Nonetheless, whether by intention or accident, the literature on self-organization does speak to the layperson's issues of identity, self-determination, and self-doubt. This chapter reviews a variety of approaches to self-organization that have clear implications for identity and adjustment. We consider how these approaches address the layperson's queries and the related issues they raise.

Organization of Self-Knowledge: Features and Functions

At first glance, the issues addressed by studies of self-organization seem less existential

47

and less enticing than those that laypersons raise. The term "self-organization" typically invokes an information processing model in which organization refers to how items of self-knowledge are organized into categories. Such category structures can be viewed more broadly as associative networks of self-relevant beliefs in which the interconnections or associative links between specific self-beliefs are of paramount importance (Cantor & Kihlstrom, 1987).

The basic assumption of this model is that the amount of self-relevant information in memory is vast, so some form of organization is needed to guide the retrieval of relevant self-beliefs in any information processing context. The subset of beliefs retrieved is called the working self-concept and contains the information that will be brought to bear in that context (Cantor, Markus, Niedenthal, & Nurius, 1986; Markus & Nurius, 1986). Thus the question of self-organization boils down to a question of accessibility. Organizational factors determine which self-beliefs from the vast repertoire will be brought to bear on the information processing task at hand. In this way, organizational factors may allow people to override the content of their self-concepts (Showers, 2000). Whereas traditional information processing models suggested that the sheer number of positive and negative self-beliefs determined a person's global self-evaluation, the present view is that organizational factors may moderate these effects. For instance, even though a great many negative self-beliefs may be available in the total self-repertoire, if the self is organized so that this information does not become accessible as part of the working self-concept, its impact will be minimal. Organizational factors can make specific items of knowledge about the self more or less accessible, altering their impact. In this way, self-organization goes beyond the content of a person's self-beliefs in determining how the self functions (Showers, 2000).

An early approach that generated interest in the organization of self-knowledge was self-schema theory (Markus, 1977; Rogers, Kuiper, & Kirker, 1977). Studies of negative self-schemas, for example, supported the hypothesis that negative information is both available and highly accessible for depressed

individuals (Bargh & Tota, 1988; Gotlib & McCann, 1984; Williams & Broadbent, 1986; Williams & Nulty, 1986). Some studies (e.g., those using a Stroop task with priming) did test specific interconnections between self-relevant beliefs (e.g., Gotlib & Cane, 1987; Segal, Hood, Shaw, & Higgins, 1988; Segal & Vella, 1990). However, that approach did not directly assess the underlying structure of the schemata (Segal, 1988). These studies supported the idea that, for depressed persons, negative information about the self is highly organized.

The working self-concept, as well as the underlying memory structure or associative network from which it is drawn, is most likely continually being reconstructed online (Markus & Nurius, 1986). Connectionist models of the self explicitly represent this on-line process (Smith, Coats, & Walling, 1999). Stability of the interconnections or category structure of that network, then, corresponds to stability in an individual's strategies for accessing that structure. In this view, an individual may have favorite strategies for constructing and updating the working self-concept that are more or less stable across contexts (Cantor & Kihlstrom, 1987). These strategies need not be conscious nor intentional but may simply evolve over time as effective responses in a wide range of situations. To the extent that the individual employs the same organizational strategy over and over, the structures and interconnections will appear stable. However, because the structure is continually reconstructed on-line and because the individual's strategies may vary with context, there is likely to be considerable flexibility in this system as well. Thus a college professor may actively construct her "nutty professor" self-image on the way to a large lecture class (whether she is aware of this process or not), except just prior to an exam, when she recruits the "stern professor" self-image instead.

Reconstructive strategies and the knowledge structures that result from them will be influenced by motivational, emotional, and cognitive processes within the individual, as well as by context. The most fundamental cognitive process involved is categorization, based on a perceiver's judgments of similarity among relevant beliefs. Thus one student may see failure on a history test as similar and related to failure on the racquetball court ("failure" category), whereas another student may see failure at history as similar to success in calculus ("school" category). Emotional processes may influence the accessibility of similarly valenced beliefs, as well as categorization processes (Bower, 1981; DeSteno & Salovey, 1997). For example, Niedenthal and colleagues have shown that people in emotional states are more likely to use emotional features as a basis for categorization (i.e., happy or sad people would be more likely to use the "failure" category; Halberstadt & Niedenthal, 1997; Niedenthal, Halberstadt, & Innes-Ker, 1999).

Finally, a person's motivational state will influence the type of self-knowledge that is relevant and useful (Singer & Salovey, 1988; Woike, Gershkovitz, Piorkowski, & Polo, 1999). For example, a person motivated to feel better (i.e., to self-enhance) may activate the belief "good at calculus" ("school" category) as a form of self-affirmation; a person motivated toward accuracy and problem solving might look for commonalities among a set of failure experiences ("failure" category; cf. Trope, 1986). Taylor and Gollwitzer (1995) suggest that a deliberative mind-set (in which people are considering their options) should encourage realistic thinking and the activation of both positive and negative beliefs, whereas an implemental mind-set (in which people are carrying out the actions they have decided on) is associated with activation primarily of positive beliefs. The very basic motivational distinction between promotion focus (striving to attain good outcomes such as advancement and gain) and prevention focus (trying to avoid bad outcomes such as danger and loss) has been associated with differential accessibility of episodic memories consistent with the goal (Higgins, Roney, Crowe, & Hymes, 1994; Higgins & Tykocinski, 1992). Individuals with a promotion focus recall events that further a goal (e.g., waking up early for class, attempting to catch a movie), whereas individuals with a prevention focus recall experiences that involve avoiding an undesired end state (e.g., not scheduling a class conflict, trying to avoid getting stuck on the subway). Presumably, each of these motivational states involves a reorganization of memory to make goal-relevant experiences more accessible.

Once a working self-concept is constructed and self-knowledge relevant to the current context is accessible, that information influences subsequent behavior. The active self-knowledge can alter interpretations of the current situation, guide behavior, and regulate emotions. In turn, each life experience alters self-structure by building new associations and interconnections among self-beliefs that, in turn, affect future constructed selves. However, when it comes to understanding how the self-concept functions in specific contexts, researchers typically set aside this view of a working self actively constructed on-line and shift their focus to relatively stable features of self-organization.

Multiple Selves: Benefits and Costs

For theoretical and empirical purposes, a person's overall self-concept is typically represented as a set of basic-level categories or self-aspects (cf. Cantor, Mischel, & Schwartz, 1982; Linville, 1985; Rosch, 1978). These categories may be idiographically defined, and each represents a distinct self or persona (Markus & Wurf, 1987). The basis for these multiple self-concept categories may vary from person to person, or even within the person, but they typically correspond to distinct roles, contexts, relationships, activities, traits, states, and the like. The elements of each category are the specific items of self-knowledge associated with that self-aspect. These elements include attributes experienced in that self-aspect, emotional states, behaviors, and episodic memories of past experience (Cantor & Kihlstrom, 1987; Linville, 1985).

Two types of measures assess multiple self-concept categories. One type of measure emphasizes the structure of the elements across self-concept categories. An example is the self-descriptive card-sorting task developed by Linville (1985, 1987) to assess self-complexity (cf. also Niedenthal, Setterlund, & Wherry, 1992; Showers, 1992a). Participants are given a stack of 40 cards, each of which contains a potentially self-descriptive attribute. Participants sort the cards into groups so that each group represents an aspect of themselves or their lives. They may use the cards more than once, or, if an attribute does not describe them, they may set that card aside. The self-concept categories are generated idiographically (e.g., "me at school," "me with my friends," "me when I'm in a bad mood"; Table 3.1).

The second type of measure focuses on a person's tendency to differentiate among multiple self-concepts at the category level. An example is the Self-Attributes Questionnaire (SAQ; Pelham & Swann, 1989; cf. Marsh, Barnes, & Hocevar, 1985; Table 3.2). In this measure, the set of self-aspect domains (e.g., sports, math, language, music, social activity) is chosen by the researcher. The participants provide self-evaluations in each of these domains and other ratings (such as the perceived importance of that domain, the certainty of their self-evaluation, or a description of their ideal self). For both types of measures, the ability to differentiate among different domains or categories of the self is associated with psychological adjustment (e.g., mood) or self-esteem.

Such representations are clearly oversimplified in several ways. First, the amount of self-knowledge represented is a mere fraction of what is available in memory stores. More important, the measures do not capture any interconnections between self-categories. Such interconnections represent the tendency for one aspect of self (e.g., student) to activate another (e.g., racquetball player) and imply that the self has a higher order hierarchical structure (Rosenberg, 1988; Rosenberg & Gara, 1985). This feature of self-structure is not addressed by the measures discussed here.

Most theoretical perspectives suggest that the experience of multiple selves is an inherent part of existence and contributes to psychological well-being (e.g., Gergen, 1972). Multiple selves should be the natural outgrowth of people's ability to discriminate the different features of different situations and the different attributes, attitudes, and behaviors appropriate in each (Mischel, 1973; Snyder, 1974). The notion of multiple selves also follows directly from the idea that people construct working self-concepts

---

TABLE 3.1. Sample Self-Descriptive Card Sort (Self-Complexity = 3.99; Maximum Value = 5.32)

Helpful	Not always "perfect"	Funny	Responsible	Lovable	Looking at the good in everyone
Giving	– Indecisive	Intelligent	Mature	Lovable	Optimistic
Friendly	– Lazy	Happy	Independent	Needed	Giving
Capable	– Isolated	Energetic	Organized	Friendly	Interested
Hardworking	– Weary	Outgoing	Interested		
	– Sad and blue	Fun and entertaining	Hardworking		
	– Insecure	Communicative			

Good work ethic	Making decisions	Taking disappointment hard	Good student	Talented	
Hardworking	– Indecisive	– Sad and blue	Intelligent	Successful	
Capable	– Uncomfortable	– Insecure	Interested	Capable	
Intelligent	– Tense	– Like a failure	Organized	Confident	
Interested	– Insecure	– Hopeless	Hardworking	Fun and	
Successful		– Inferior		entertaining	
Confident		– Isolated			
Mature		– Incompetent			
Independent					
Organized					
Energetic					

Note. Minus sign (–) indicates negative attributes for the purpose of computing compartmentalization (Showers, 1992a). This sort is perfectly compartmentalized (phi = 1.0). From Showers, Abramson, and Hogan (1998). Copyright 1998 by the American Psychological Association. Reprinted by permission.

TABLE 3.2. Self-Attributes Questionnaire

This questionnaire has to do with your attitudes about some of your activities and abilities. For the first ten items below, you should rate yourself relative to *other college students* your own age by using the following scale:

A	B	C	D	E	F	G	H	I	J
bottom 5%	lower 10%	lower 20%	lower 30%	lower 50%	upper 50%	upper 30%	upper 20%	upper 10%	top 5%

An example of the way the scale works is as follows: if one of the traits that follows were "height," a woman who is just below average in height would choose "E" for this question, whereas a woman who is taller than 80% (but not taller than 90%) of her female classmates would mark "H", indicating that she is in the top 20% on this dimension.

1. intellectual/academic ability
2. social skills/social competence
3. artistic and/or musical ability
4. athletic ability
5. physical attractiveness
6. leadership ability
7. common sense
8. emotional stability
9. sense of humor
10. discipline

Now rate how *certain* you are of your standing on each of the above traits (you may choose any letter):

A	B	C	D	E	F	G	H	I
not at all certain				moderately certain				extremely certain

11–20. (same as items 1–10)

Now rate how *important* each of these domains is to you:

A	B	C	D	E	F	G	H	I
not at all important to me				moderately important to me				extremely important to me

21–30. (same as items 1–10)

Now rate yourself relative to your "ideal" self—the person you would be if you were exactly the way you would like to be:

A	B	C	D	E	F	G	H	I
very short of my ideal self				somewhat like and somewhat unlike my ideal self				very much like my ideal self

31–40. (same as items 1–10)

Note. From Pelham and Swann (1989). Copyright 1989 by the American Psychological Association. Reprinted by permission.

in each situation to guide their behavior (Markus & Nurius, 1986). The principal advantage of multiple selves is that they afford flexibility in response. For example, a person with multiple "tennis selves" can respond appropriately in each type of match. He can be his "win-at-all-costs" self when playing a tournament against an opposing team, but his "good sport" self when practicing with a team member (Markus & Wurf, 1987). In extreme circumstances, multiple selves may provide resilience against traumatic events. When the "good scholar" self experiences a crushing rejection from a top journal, the "good parent" self provides a source of self-affirmation (Steele, 1988).

What evidence is there that multiple selves contribute to psychological well-being? Linville (1985, 1987) assessed a feature of multiple self-concept categories known as self-complexity. A person's self-representation is said to be more complex to the extent that, in describing the self, a person identifies a greater number of self categories that are highly elaborated (i.e., represented by many traits or attributes) and that do not overlap (i.e., do not share sets of attributes; cf. Rafaeli-Mor, Gotlib, & Revelle, 1999). Thus each self category should have a unique set of attributes or self-knowledge associated with it. To the extent that multiple selves share many attributes, they are not so distinct, and that reduces the complexity of the self-representation.

The self-complexity–affective-extremity model predicts the associations observed among self-complexity, life stress, and psychological well-being (Linville, 1987). This model suggests that self-complexity minimizes the amount of the self implicated by any external event, and so a complex self buffers the impact of stress, restricting its impact to a small part of the self. As predicted, high self-complexity has been associated with less negative mood in college students under conditions of high life stress (Cohen, Pane, & Smith, 1997; Linville, 1987; see also Dixon & Baumeister, 1991).

Despite the theoretical appeal of multiple selves, an alternative view is that multiple selves create a sense of self-fragmentation (Block, 1961; Donahue, Robins, Roberts, & John, 1993). People with multiple selves may lack a core self, that is, a single self-concept category with a consistent set of attributes that could potentially guide thoughts, feelings, and behavior in a wide range of situations. A person with a core self presumably has resolved conflicting attributes, identified the most central features or domains of self, and integrated them into a whole (James, 1890/1963; Rogers, 1959). One advantage to having a core self is simplicity (Ross & Nisbett, 1991). New working self-concepts do not have to be constructed in each situation, and it is easy to

choose appropriate behaviors that one can do well. Also it is easy to choose which situations to enter, because one's attributes and preferences are consistent (cf. Campbell, 1990; Setterlund & Niedenthal, 1993). Finally, having only a few distinct self-categories may be less taxing than maintaining multiple selves (Donahue et al., 1993; Lecky, 1945). It may be stressful to switch from an ambitious, competitive self in the workplace to a nurturing, expressive self at home. Such shifts among multiple selves may also contribute to the experience of role conflict (Oyserman & Markus, 1993, 1998). In Gergen's (1991) view, the need to accommodate new experiences, new information, or new role models may "saturate" the self, causing us to lose touch with our moral core. Moreover, it is not clear that nonoverlapping selves offer the best buffer for stress. Consider an individual who strives to be nurturing both in the workplace and at home. If the sense of self as a nurturing boss is threatened by an employee's failure, the sense of self as a nurturing parent could potentially stabilize self-perceptions. Thus the argument that overlap among self-aspects tends to augment threats to the self may be misguided. As long as a threat is restricted to one domain, a simple structure of self-attributes could actually provide resilience to threat.

Donahue and colleagues (1993) found empirical support for the benefits of the core self in a pair of studies that used an attribute-focused measure of multiple selves. The task was similar to the self-descriptive card sort in that participants rated the self-descriptiveness of a set of attributes across multiple social roles. However, the task was different from the card sort in that the self-aspect categories (social roles) were provided by the researcher (e.g., student, friend, employee, son or daughter, and romantic partner). Individuals whose self-descriptions across social roles were more differentiated (i.e., more distinct) scored lower on measures of psychological adjustment. Greater self-concept differentiation (SCD) was also associated with more role transitions (e.g., divorce, job changes) over the life span.

The apparent inconsistency between the findings for self-complexity and for self-concept differentiation is resolved in part by Linville's (1985, 1987) model. Under conditions of low stress, a less complex self implicates more of the total self in one's life experiences (presumably, these are positive experiences if stress is low). If participants in the SCD studies typically were experiencing low stress over their lifetimes, then the two lines of research are consistent—both show a negative correlation between the existence of nonoverlapping selves (high self-complexity, high SCD) and psychological well-being when stress is low.[1]

Another possible interpretation is that self-complexity and SCD are unrelated features of self-organization. Perhaps a complex representation of oneself across multiple situations can coincide with a clear representation of a well-integrated core self, producing an exceptionally healthy combination of stability and flexibility. For example, if an individual identified himself, with equal importance, as being nurturing in his parenting role and competitive in his professional role, there could still be a core self ("superdad") that drives behavior when the multiple selves are in conflict and provides a sense of clarity and consistency for the self.

Multiple Selves: A Source of Motivation

We have already indicated how the on-line construction of working selves is influenced by motivational states. However, multiple selves are often a source of motivation in themselves. One dimension along which multiple selves are differentiated is the dimension of time. People easily articulate past, current, and future or possible selves (Cross & Markus, 1991, 1994; Markus & Nurius, 1986). Distinct possible selves (concepts of the self in the future) are the representation of a person's goals. They embody significant hopes, dreams, or fears. They provide motivational anchors, such as the selves that one desires to avoid. Typically, they combine the representation of directions to approach or avoid with expectations of success for those goals. When positive expected selves are balanced by matching feared possible selves, motivational resources are high. The positive expected selves provide direction and the negative feared selves provide energy and persistence, thereby preventing people from drifting from their goals (Oyserman & Markus,

1990). Possible selves also help to defend the current self by providing a context for one's current self-view. Thus, if the present is not going well, a positive possible self may create hope for the future. As the current self changes, possible selves may be adjusted to create discrepancies that are optimal for motivation and well-being (Cross & Markus, 1991).

In the most complex representation of future or possible selves, a person's concept of the self in the future is represented by its own set of multiple selves, corresponding to specific roles, situations, relationships, states, traits, and the like. The complexity of this set of future self-concept categories moderates a person's affective responses to feedback relevant to long-term goals (Niedenthal et al., 1992). Thus the existence of multiple selves, differentiated with respect to time, instantiates motivation by providing representations of goals, defining directions for effort, creating optimal self-discrepancies, and helping to regulate emotional responses.

Some hypothetical selves correspond to specific classes of motivations, such as the promotion focus (ideal self) or the prevention focus (ought self; Higgins, 1987; Higgins, Bond, Klein, & Strauman, 1986; Higgins, Shah, & Friedman, 1997). According to self-discrepancy theory, a structural comparison of these self-guides to the current actual self influences motivation and emotion. Discrepancies between one's ideal self and one's actual self are associated with dejection-related emotions (e.g., disappointment, dissatisfaction, and sadness) presumably because one has failed to reach one's hopes or ideals (i.e., absence of positive outcomes). The discrepancy between the actual self and the self one thinks one ought to be has been linked to agitation-related emotions (e.g., fear, anxiety, and worry), presumably because one has failed to meet obligations or responsibilities (i.e., presence of negative outcomes; Higgins et al., 1986; cf. Tangney, Niedenthal, Covert, & Barlow, 1998). A discrepancy between the actual and the "can" self may create high levels of motivation (Higgins, Vookles, & Tykocinski, 1992). In contrast to the theory of possible selves (according to which discrepancies between actual and possible selves may be adjusted to create optimal levels of motivation and emotion), ideal and ought discrepancies are thought to be relatively stable. These discrepancies may represent repeated experiences with self–other contingencies, especially those involving parents and other caregivers (Strauman, 1996).[2]

Interestingly, none of the empirical studies reviewed here speaks directly to the question of behavioral flexibility, which is probably the strongest argument for the benefits of multiple selves. Multiple selves should allow us to respond flexibly, expressing different attributes in different contexts (cf. Mendoza-Denton, Ayduk, Mischel, Shoda, & Testa, 2001; Mischel & Shoda, 1995). Evidence that such flexibility is associated with the activation of distinct selves or is facilitated by individual differences in self-structures remains elusive.

Multiple Selves: Differentiation by Importance and Self-Evaluation

Another important function of the differentiation of multiple selves is to regulate a person's self-evaluations or, more specifically, their emotional reactions to their self-beliefs. In other words, the differentiation of the self-concept into multiple selves may facilitate (or inhibit) self-enhancement. We review three features of self-organization that contribute to this process: importance differentiation; compartmentalization and integration; and self-concept clarity. Fundamentally, all of these areas of the literature address the issue of how a person deals with negative self-knowledge.

Importance Differentiation

In children, the ability to differentiate among multiple selves emerges around age 8 (Fischer, 1980; Harter, 1999). Prior to this, children are thought to experience themselves as all good or all bad, but in middle childhood, children begin to articulate that they are good in math and poor in sports, for example. Along with this, an additional organizational feature emerges, namely the differentiation of these multiple selves according to their importance. Children who report that their excellent math skills are important and their poor sports performance is unimportant have higher self-esteem than children for whom positive domains are not the impor-

tant ones (Harter, 1999).

In adults, importance differentiation (DI) as measured by the SAQ is correlated with higher self-esteem (Pelham & Swann, 1989). The DI measure is the correlation of a person's self-evaluations across a nomothetic set of life domains with his or her ratings of the perceived importance of each domain. Using a similar measure, Marsh (1993) has argued that correlating domain-specific self-evaluations with nomothetic ratings of importance provides an equally good indicator of a person's psychological adjustment. In either case, there is consistent evidence that differentiation of self-evaluations across multiple domains is linked to global self-evaluations. These findings raise the possibility that people may be able to use self-differentiation in a strategic fashion, adjusting either their self-perceptions (in important domains) or their perceptions of importance (in extremely positive or extremely negative domains) to maintain or enhance self-esteem (cf. Tesser, 2000).[3]

Compartmentalization and Integration

The impact of negative self-beliefs may also be moderated by the evaluative organization of the self, namely, the structure of positive and negative beliefs within self-aspect categories. Showers's (1992a, 2000) model identifies two types of self-organization: In *evaluatively compartmentalized* organization, positive and negative beliefs about the self are separated into distinct self-aspects, so that each self-aspect contains primarily positive or primarily negative information; in *evaluatively integrative* organization, self-aspect categories contain a mixture of positive and negative beliefs. Examples are shown in Table 3.3.

The evaluative organization of self-knowledge may influence the accessibility of positive and negative self-beliefs (Showers, 1995). When an event activates a compartmentalized self-aspect that contains purely positive self-beliefs, a person is flooded with positive self-knowledge and is likely to feel quite good. However, if that person's self-concept were organized in an evaluatively integrative fashion, the same event would activate self-aspect(s) that contained a mixture of positive and negative beliefs. With both positive and negative beliefs about the self in mind, the person with integrative or-

TABLE 3.3. Examples of Compartmentalized Organization ("Harry") and Integrative Organization ("Sally") for Identical Items of Information about Self as Student

"Harry": Compartmentalized organization		"Sally": Integrative organization	
Renaissance scholar (+)	Taking tests, grades (−)	Humanities classes (+/−)	Science classes (+/−)
+ Curious	− Worrying	+ Creative	+ Disciplined
+ Disciplined	− Tense	− Insecure	+ Analytical
+ Motivated	− Distracted	+ Motivated	− Competitive
+ Creative	− Insecure	− Distracted	− Worrying
+ Analytical	− Competitive	+ Expressive	+ Curious
+ Expressive	− Moody	− Moody	− Tense

Note. A positive or negative valence is indicated for each category and each item. The symbol (+/−) denotes a mixed-valence category. Adapted from Showers (1992a). Copyright 1992 by the American Psychological Association. Reprinted by permission.

ganization should have a less positive (and possibly emotionally conflicted) reaction to the event than would the person with compartmentalized organization.

Of course, if an event primed a purely negative compartment, then the compartmentalized individual would be flooded with negative self-beliefs and feel much worse than an individual with integrative organization who experienced the same event. The cumulative impact of compartmentalized organization depends on the frequency with which purely positive or purely negative self-aspects are activated. In other words, there are two types of compartmentalized organization, described as "positive compartmentalized" and "negative compartmentalized" to indicate whether the purely positive or purely negative self-aspects are most important (i.e., most frequently accessed or most central to the self). As long as most experiences activate positive self-aspects, then compartmentalized organization should be preferable to integrative organization. However, when negative self-aspects are activated quite frequently, then integrative organization may be advantageous because it facilitates access to whatever positive self-beliefs exist and thereby minimizes the impact of negative attributes and beliefs.

Findings consistent with this model have been obtained in numerous studies, most of which rely on a self-descriptive card-sorting task to assess self-structure (e.g., Rhodewalt, Madrian, & Cheney, 1998; Showers, 1992a; Showers, Abramson, & Hogan,

1998; Showers & Kling, 1996). In the card-sorting task, participants sort 40 attributes (20 positive and 20 negative) into groups to represent the different aspects of themselves (i.e., their multiple selves). Participants also provide ratings of the positivity, negativity, and importance of these self-aspect categories that indicate whether a person is positive or negative compartmentalized or positive or negative integrative. Feelings about the self are assessed by conventional measures of mood (e.g., Beck Depression Inventory; Beck, Ward, Mendelson, Mock, & Erbaugh, 1961) or self-esteem (Rosenberg, 1965). The predictions of the model of compartmentalization are tested by regressing a measure of mood or self-esteem onto the measures of self-structure and negativity obtained from the card-sorting task.

Results consistent with the model have also been obtained using a self-descriptive listing task (Showers, 1992b, Studies 1 and 2), a self-descriptive paragraph task (Showers, 1992b, Study 2), and the variation of self-evaluations across life domains (Showers & Ryff, 1996). The model has also been applied to the structure of a person's beliefs about a romantic partner or "partner-structure" (Showers & Kevlyn, 1999).

Self-Concept Clarity

For many people, negative self-knowledge may create low self-concept clarity. That is, rather than being incorporated into the self-structure as self-beliefs held with high certainty (cf. Pelham & Swann, 1989), negative self-beliefs may actually coexist with opposite or conflicting beliefs, creating confusion as to one's self-definition. Self-concept clarity, or the tendency to report self-beliefs that are clear and confidently defined, as well as stable and internally consistent, has been established as an individual-difference variable (Campbell et al., 1996, 2000). Individuals with low self-concept clarity have clouded notions of who they are and what traits they possess. Low self-clarity is associated with neuroticism, low agreeableness, low self-esteem, low internal state awareness, chronic self-analysis, and a ruminative form of self-focused attention. Low self-clarity affects decision-making strategies, shifting people away from using similar others as a model for their behavior (Setterlund & Niedenthal, 1993).

The association between low self-clarity and low self-esteem makes sense if people with low self-clarity are endorsing both positive traits and their opposites. Low self-esteem in college students may be characterized by a mixture of positive and negative traits, whereas high self-esteem is characterized by primarily positive traits (Campbell, 1990). Thus low self-esteem in college students may correspond to self-uncertainty rather than to an unambiguously negative view of the self.

So far, no associations between self-concept clarity and measures of self-differentiation have been observed (Campbell et al., 2000). One possibility is that low self-clarity involves self-differentiation gone awry. That is, differentiated or opposite attributes are observed, perhaps without an overarching or integrative structure. If opposite or conflicting attributes are endorsed without being tied to specific contexts or being understood as fitting together in a meaningful way, then confusion rather than a well-integrated self will emerge. Thus low self-clarity may imply a disorganized, unintegrated self, whereas structural parameters such as self-complexity, differentiation, or evaluative integration typically imply a high degree of self-organization.

Self-Organization: A Strategic View

Each dimension or feature of self-organization that we have discussed so far corre-

sponds to a different self-strategy. Structural features such as possible selves or self-discrepancies correspond to motivational strategies that people use to achieve their goals. Structural features such as importance differentiation, compartmentalization, or self-clarity are most likely linked to strategies for emotional self-regulation. On one hand, these structures may reflect a person's favorite strategies, ones to which the person has become accustomed (e.g., whereas one person may use integration to handle negative self-beliefs, another may use importance differentiation). On the other hand, once these structural features are in place, the structures themselves may facilitate the choice of certain strategies. Favorite strategies may evolve because they fit the contexts a person encounters. This process of matching strategy and structure to context is described in the next section.

Dynamics of Self-Organization

Given the view that the working self-concept is continually being reconstructed on-line, the organized self is likely to be a flexible and dynamic system. The dynamics of organizational dimensions can take two forms: short-term flexibility and long-term change.

Short-Term Flexibility

By "short-term flexibility," we mean the matching of the organizational structure to the current context. Because some types of organization are more useful in some contexts than in others, a well-adapted person may shift type of self-organization to fit the context. Taking this process one step further, individual differences in organizational styles may result in idiographic matchings of organization and context, analogous to the behavior–situation profiles documented by Mischel and Shoda (1995) and Mendoza-Denton and colleagues (2001). For example, because both compartmentalization and integration are effective strategies for handling negative self-beliefs, some individuals may rely on increased integration in times of stress, whereas others may become increasingly compartmentalized. In some cases, it may be necessary to know the individual's preferred strategies or styles to predict patterns of change across contexts.

Short-term flexibility has been demonstrated for several of the organizational dimensions described. One striking example involves differential importance in a longitudinal study of college students (Showers et al., 1998). These student participants had been selected for either high or low cognitive vulnerability to depression, as indicated by their scores on measures of attributional style and dysfunctional attitudes (Alloy & Abramson, 1999). Participants' self-organization was assessed at two times when they were experiencing either high or low levels of major negative life events. Those low in cognitive vulnerability to depression showed remarkable resilience when they were experiencing high levels of major negative life events. Although the content of their self-descriptions became more negative under stress, their ratings of the perceived importance of those negative attributes decreased. They perceived the negative attributes they experienced in times of stress to be less important than those they experienced in calmer times. In other words, the structural measure of differential importance changed in an adaptive direction in times of stress, in a way that should reflect good coping.

In the same study, compartmentalization was greater for these resilient individuals when stress was high than when stress was low. Subsequent analyses showed that compartmentalization under conditions of stress was correlated with less depressed mood, even when the effect of differential importance was taken into account. Thus these resilient individuals were able to shift their styles of organization in a way that seemed to be an adaptive response to stress.[4]

In a clever experiment, Margolin and Niedenthal (2000) demonstrated short-term flexibility in self-complexity using a cognitive-tuning manipulation. Some participants expected to receive personality feedback from a psychologist, whereas others expected to transmit personality information to her. Receivers showed greater self-complexity than transmitters. Perhaps receivers were preparing to accommodate the new information, whereas transmitters were trying to focus on a simplified self-representation. Baseline differences notwithstanding, we

may adjust the complexity of our self-representations to fit the task at hand (cf. Zajonc, 1960).

Self-discrepancies also indicate short-term flexibility because of the ease with which they are primed. For example, Higgins and colleagues (1986) selected individuals who possessed both actual-ideal and actual-ought self-discrepancies and randomly primed one or the other. Although it is easy to imagine real-life events priming one discrepancy or the other in a similar way, true flexibility would entail an individual's strategic use of one discrepancy or the other. That is, the ultimate form of flexibility would involve the ability to conjure up the preferred discrepancy (either consciously or nonconsciously) to help guide behavior.

Long-Term Change

Long-term change in self-organization involves either the development of organizational strategies that are new to the individual or the application of previously known strategies to a different class of situations. One of the first organizational dimensions to develop in children is the internal–external dimension, as they increasingly associate their behaviors with stable self-characteristics rather than external influences (Mohr, 1978). Harter and colleagues have documented children's development of the ability to differentiate the importance of multiple-self domains as they mature (Harter, Bresnick, Bouchey, & Whitesell, 1997). A more extreme version of self-differentiation in children is the phenomenon of splitting the self into the "good me" and the "bad me" (Kernberg, 1975). This differentiation, or splitting, is a primitive way of coping with undesired attributes, behaviors, or affect. The good self does not have to acknowledge the bad self. In normal children these selves are increasingly integrated with age, perhaps because children learn to associate their good and bad selves with specific contexts or to differentiate them according to their importance. Thus the roots of organizational features such as self-complexity, compartmentalization, possible selves, and self-certainty have been examined in children. However, with the exception of importance differentiation and, to some extent, self-complexity (Jordan & Cole,

1996), developmental change in these features of self-organization has not been explicitly addressed.

Long-term change in self-organization during the course of adulthood fits many of the models discussed so far, but few concrete data exist. Given the short-term flexibility of differential importance in young adults, it seems possible that people whose self-esteem suffers from a failure of importance differentiation could learn this strategy for enhancing their self-views. The acquisition of this strategy could simply increase flexibility in stressful situations, or, if the strategy of differential importance is applied more broadly, baseline levels of importance differentiation could change.

The theoretical models associated with two dimensions of self-organization—self-complexity and compartmentalization—lend themselves directly to the notion that long-term self-change might occur. First, in Linville's (1985, 1987) self-complexity model, the effectiveness of high self-complexity for dealing with stressful situations raises the possibility that individuals who are exposed to stressful events and manage to cope well will begin to develop greater complexity in their self-views (cf. Fiske & Linville, 1980; Jordan & Cole, 1996; Pelham, 1993). Similarly, in the case of evaluative organization, exposure to certain kinds of stressors or to individuals who model either compartmentalized or integrative thinking may alter a person's preferred strategies for handling specific types of events. Indeed, the finding that compartmentalization increases with stress in low-vulnerability individuals goes against the basic hypothesis that integrative thinking should be most advantageous when negative attributes are salient (Showers, 2002; Showers et al., 1998). However, the stressful experiences of college students may be especially easy to compartmentalize. Perhaps chronic stresses later in life (e.g., a prolonged divorce, career setbacks) are difficult to compartmentalize and require integrative thinking, gradually shifting people who experience such stressors toward that type of organization.

A complete dynamic model of self-organization should take into account both short-term flexibility and the possibility of long-term change in organizational styles. As an example, the dynamic model of compartmentalization accounts for both types of self-change (Showers, 2002). In this model, the likelihood of self-change is related to the occurrence of stress (which activates negative self-beliefs), the organizational alternatives that a person "knows," and the fit between an organizational strategy and features of the current stress. A central feature of the dynamics of this structural system is the relative ease or difficulty of maintaining a compartmentalized or integrative style of thinking.

Of the two types of evaluative organization, compartmentalization seems easy and efficient. The use of the evaluative dimension as a basis for categorization is well established (e.g., Bower, 1981; Osgood, 1969; Niedenthal et al., 1999), whereas integrative structures require a person to override a natural tendency to associate beliefs of the same valence. Moreover, when an integrative person thinks, "I'm insecure, but also creative," that person may have to suppress a negative emotional response to feeling insecure in order to bring the positive belief about creativity to mind. This process most likely requires effort, attention, and other cognitive resources (Showers & Kling, 1996). If integration requires high effort and resources, then people may tend to rely on compartmentalized structures whenever they can, shifting only to integrative ones when the extra effort is warranted. Consistent with this view, nondisordered individuals who were positive compartmentalized in their overall self-structures showed the ability to shift to an integrative style of thinking when they were asked to focus on a specific negative attribute (McMahon, Showers, Rieder, Abramson, & Hogan, in press).[5]

Given the prevalence of compartmentalized self-structures under stress, the effort and attention that integration may require, and the ability of compartmentalized individuals to shift to integrative thinking when they focus on a negative attribute, it seems that integrative structures may be transient and may emerge primarily when individuals are focusing a great deal of attention on negative attributes. Because maintaining integrative structures may be difficult, many people may eventually revert to a compartmentalized style of organization. This dynamic view of self-structure is diagrammed in Figure 3.1.

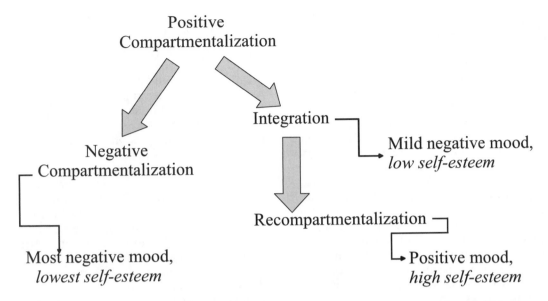

FIGURE 3.1. Dynamic model: How the self-structure may change in response to stressful life events. From Showers (2002). Copyright 2002 by The Guilford Press. Reprinted by permission.

At the top of Figure 3.1, positive compartmentalization is depicted as the baseline style of organization for most individuals. The assumption is that most individuals construct self-concepts that are basically positive and construct their lives to maintain relatively low levels of stress. Under these conditions, they take advantage of the effectiveness and efficiency of a compartmentalized self-structure. From the top, moving down either side of the diagram, Figure 3.1 depicts how self-structures may change when negative attributes become salient (e.g., when stressful events occur).

The left side of the diagram shows the hypothesized shift in self-structure for individuals who are not handling their stress or salient negative attributes especially well. These individuals may shift to a negatively compartmentalized style of organization. The leftmost line indicates that such a shift should be associated with extremely low self-esteem and the most negative mood. The right side of the diagram shows the pattern of change hypothesized for individuals who are coping relatively well with stress or salient negative beliefs. When negative attributes become salient, these individuals may tend to focus attention on them and engage in an integrative thinking process in an attempt to minimize the impact of these at-

tributes. Eventually, however, this effort becomes too much, and many individuals may revert to a compartmentalized style of organization. This process may involve compartmentalizing the stresses or negative attributes that they have experienced; in other words, it may correspond to a recompartmentalization of one's life. People who succeed in recompartmentalizing their self-concepts should be the happiest and experience the highest self-esteem and the greatest psychological well-being.

For example, a person who typically compartmentalizes positive and negative attributes may, at the time of a divorce, expend a great deal of effort to think integratively about his or her negative attributes until that thought process becomes exhausting (or any relevant concerns are resolved). At that point, recompartmentalization would allow the person to focus on primarily positive attributes again. This recompartmentalization may be facilitated by external circumstances. For instance, during child custody negotiations, a person may have many integrative thoughts about his or her failings as a parent, yet find that those negative self-beliefs are more easily recompartmentalized once custody issues are resolved.

As the model suggests, however, there

may be some individuals who remain committed to integrative styles of thinking. These individuals (1) may actually prefer integrative thinking (i.e., are more practiced and find it less effortful than do others); or (2) may have negative attributes (or negative experiences) that are especially difficult to compartmentalize. For example, the loss of a child or parent or a difficult divorce may make it difficult to segregate attributes of self associated with these events from more positive self-domains. In these cases, integration may be a "best-they-can-do" strategy. The upper line on the right in Figure 3.1 indicates that individuals who remain integrative will experience some degree of residual negative mood or lower self-esteem as a result of the focus on negative attributes that this style of organization implies. Integrative structures avoid the strong focus on negative attributes associated with negative compartmentalization, but over the long term integration may never create the strong positive feelings about the self that positive compartmentalization can.

Even though long-term change in self-organization may sometimes occur, it is likely to be the exception rather than the rule. In the case of integration–compartmentalization or self-complexity, self-organization is likely to change gradually as a cumulative response to life stress or in response to rare traumatic events. Similarly, psychological treatment may bring about a one-time change. However, the rule is likely to be substantial stability in the dimensions of self-organization. Even the kinds of short-term flexibility described here are likely to be context-specific deviations from some baseline. Good stability has already been shown for several dimensions of self-organization over periods of several years. Over a 3-year period, for self-discrepancies (actual–ideal and actual–ought combined), $r(45)$ = .56 (Strauman, 1996). In their 2-year study of individuals high and low in cognitive vulnerability to depression (average time elapsed = 22 months, $N = 79$), Showers and colleagues (1998) found the following test–retest stabilities for dimensions of self-organization: compartmentalization, r = .56; self-complexity, r = .46; differential importance, r = .07[6]; proportion of negative self-descriptors, r = .71.

Just as an understanding of the development of self in children actually focuses on organizational features rather than content, so too perhaps the literature on self-change in adulthood should mirror this perspective. A particularly interesting context for studying self-change should be the change that occurs in psychological treatment. Cognitive therapy techniques often claim to focus on changing self-beliefs. However, a closer look suggests that organizational features are involved—changes in self-discrepancies, in goals, and in goal discrepancies. In many cases, changes in organizational features may precede changes in self-beliefs or obviate such change. For example, compartmentalization of negative attributes may be the precursor to excluding those attributes from the self. In some cases, perceptions of unwanted attributes or memories of past behaviors may be quite accurate. Here, organizational factors may minimize the impact of negative knowledge that is unlikely to change. Despite the prevalence and effectiveness of positive illusions (Taylor & Brown, 1994), some individuals face problems that do not lend themselves to illusory strategies, for example, problems of regret and forgiveness for behaviors that are undeniably true. Perhaps by focusing on reorganization, treatment may provide an alternative to constructing positive illusions in situations in which that strategy would be too risky or difficult.

Self-Organization and Stability

Looking beyond short-term and long-term change in self-organization, a third area of self-dynamics is strongly linked to organizational factors. Specifically, organizational features (viewed here as a relatively stable characteristic) may be differentially associated with the likelihood of self-change, either as a cumulative process over time, as a response to specific traumatic life events, or as a minute-by-minute process. For example, a particular configuration of organizational features may be associated with variability in self-evaluations or self-esteem from day to day. Rhodewalt and colleagues (1998) found this to be the case for compartmentalized individuals with narcissistic tendencies (cf. also Campbell et al., 1991; Showers & Kling, 1996; Kernis & Goldman, Chapter 6, this volume). Techniques such as daily diary studies, the mouse task, and dynamic systems models are being used to document changes in self-evaluations (Nowak & Vallacher, 1998; Vallacher, Nowak, & Kaufman, 1994). Nowak, Vallacher, Tesser, and Borkowski's (2000) dynamic systems technique lends itself to a computer model of the evolution of compartmentalized and integrative self-structures over time. Representing the self-concept as a grid of positive and negative elements (self-beliefs), they show how adjacent elements of oppositely valenced information may become integrated to form higher order positive and negative compartments of the self. This approach differs from Showers's (1992a, 2001) view of integration because it allows the valence of the basic elements to change. Nonetheless, it provides a viable model of how information is represented in memory with a focus on the possibilities for and process of self-change.

Future Directions

Specification of Process

Studies of self-structure advance literature at the interface of affect, cognition, and motivation because they are inherently process oriented. For each structural variable, there is an associated process model that specifies how access to specific self-beliefs affects motivational and emotional outcomes. However, very few studies have actually tested the mechanics of those processes to demonstrate that individuals with different self-structures activate different self-beliefs in a given context. Future research will need to develop new methods for observing these processes and probably more diagnostic measures of self-structure as well. For example, studies of self-complexity need to document the spillover process (or lack thereof) and assess the amount of self-knowledge activated by a specific positive or negative event. Similarly, studies of compartmentalization need to assess directly the interconnectedness of similarly and oppositely valenced attributes and the accompanying thought processes. An array of cognitive techniques (e.g., priming, response

latencies, word completion) are available to help document these processes.

Additional Features of Self-Structure

A lingering question from this exploration of self-structure is whether the limited empirical evidence for the existence of a core self can be reconciled with the notion of multiple selves, their inevitability, and their advantages. One possibility is that the core self exists as a separate structure, with many features that are automatically activated. It may vary across individuals in its complexity and in the perceived certainty of its attributes. Uncertainty and too much complexity may be a liability here, causing stress and indecisiveness as the individual struggles to choose appropriate situations and behaviors that are well suited to the core self. At the same time, each person may have a set of multiple selves that represent the working self-concepts commonly constructed in familiar contexts. Each self represents an effective way of behaving in each context, one that has been tested over time. Here, multiple selves may be an asset, facilitating responsiveness to different contexts and affording the opportunity to express a variety of attributes.

A related area that has not been well explored is the hierarchical structure of the self (S. Rosenberg, 1988; S. Rosenberg & Gara, 1985). For example, in one branch of the hierarchical structure, a person could have a complete set of working self-concepts that permits good functioning in those situations likely to be encountered at times of high stress. These selves might facilitate efficiency, satisficing, prioritization, and achieving closure. On another branch of the hierarchical self-structure, a complete set of working self-concepts might be available for times at which stress is low. These selves might facilitate exploration, nurturance, creativity, and attention to detail. Other dimensions, such as mood or energy level, could correspond to distinct sets (branches) of selves. Although throughout this chapter, we have focused on the knowledge structures that compose the personal self, the social selves (i.e, relational and collective identities) may be represented as distinct branches of the hierarchy (Brewer & Gardner, 1996).

A related question has to do with whether some selves are more closely connected than others. To what extent is the self-as-worker likely to activate the self-as-parent, thereby creating either role conflict or a stress buffer? Most likely the strength of such interconnections is an individual difference that goes beyond the question of overlapping attributes (cf. Linville, 1987).

Finally, consider how individuals may differ in the location of the core self within the hierarchy of selves. For some individuals, this core self may be at the top of the hierarchy, consistent with the idea of automatic activation. For others, the core self may be a parallel self, one of the multiple selves that may or may not be activated in any given context.

Additional Dimensions of Self-Differentiation

There has been little exploration of the basic dimensions of self-differentiation. The evaluative dimension is highlighted in work on compartmentalization–integration. However, the tendency for individuals to categorize their self-aspects according to roles, situations, social relationships, traits, states, emotion/affect, or other specific dimensions has not been documented.

Given the burgeoning interest in the distinction between independent and interdependent selves (Heine, Lehman, Markus, & Kitayama, 1999; Markus & Kitayama, 1991), a particularly interesting question is how the structures of these selves differ. Could social relationships displace the evaluative dimension as a basis for categorization of self-knowledge (Cross, Bacon, & Morris, 2000; Cross & Madson, 1997)? Do individuals with interdependent selves define their self-attributes in interrelated rather than in isolated terms (Niedenthal & Beike, 1997)? Do they more easily incorporate the attributes of others into the self? Does interrelatedness foster self-complexity? How does it affect the experience of a core self?

Further Explorations of Flexibility and Self-Change

If research on self-structure is to have much practical application, say for helping people develop more adaptive structures and styles

of thinking, then the area of greatest emphasis should be the area of flexibility in self-organization and long-term change. The practical applications of this work are in helping people change. The literature has established that at least some flexibility exists. The future goal is to be more specific in being able to identify those contexts in which one type of organization or another is adaptive. To do this, two methodological advances are needed. First, we need on-line measures of self-organization, so as to be better able to assess the type of organization being used in any context. Second, we need to develop causal manipulations of organizational features, so that we can clearly assess their effects. In the case of long-term self-change, the greatest need is for longitudinal studies.

The features of self-organization reviewed here can be viewed as a set of organizational tools that individuals can use for the purposes of guiding their behavior, regulating the demands on their cognitive capacities, and regulating their emotional reactions or self-evaluations. Focusing for a moment on the self-evaluative function, people have a wide array of organizational strategies that they can use to maintain or enhance their overall feelings about the self. They can use importance differentiation to minimize the impact of negative self-aspects, they can compartmentalize negative attributes, or they can exert more effort and use evaluative integration. Perhaps they can adjust their self-discrepancies or shrink or expand the self (Aron & Aron, 1986). The greatest challenge for this literature is to understand why one individual chooses a particular style of organization when other equally effective approaches are available. These may be true alternatives that are selected only by the individual's choice. Similar challenges are facing researchers in the area of self-esteem regulation, because they are attempting to sort out whether various self-esteem maintenance mechanisms (e.g., self-affirmation, cognitive dissonance, and social comparison) are substitutable for each other (Tesser, 2000).

Applications to Other Knowledge Structures

The self is but one of the knowledge structures that people use to organize memory and guide behavior. Research on self-organization has important applications to knowledge in other domains. For example, there is a long history of studying the organization of beliefs about stereotyped groups (Wittenbrink, Judd, & Park, 2001) or about attitude objects in general (Judd, Drake, Downing, & Krosnick, 1991). The self is a particularly interesting attitude object because most people have an elaborate, well-organized structure and because elements of self-knowledge have strong evaluative tags with powerful implications for future behavior and emotional response. Currently, interest in close relationships suggests the utility of examining how people organize beliefs about a relationship partner. The ongoing interest in stereotypes and prejudice calls for a reexamination of knowledge structures as a function of motivation to reduce prejudice and the automaticity of stereotyped beliefs (Fazio, Jackson, Dunton, & Williams, 1995; Fazio, Sanbonmatsu, Powell, & Kardes, 1986). Literature on attitude conflict and ambivalence may suggest new ways of looking at evaluatively laden self-beliefs (Cacioppo & Bernston, 1994; Lavine, Thomsen, Zanna, & Borgida, 1998; Priester & Petty, 2001).

Conclusion

This chapter takes the point of view that the organization of self-knowledge is a dynamic process that reflects an individual's current strategy for constructing the self. It addresses four basic issues: (1) the comparative advantages of maintaining a set of context-specific multiple selves versus a single, well-defined core self; (2) the ways in which multiple selves (especially discrepancies between current and future selves) contribute to motivation; (3) how the organization of positive and negative attributes within the self-structure affects mood, self-esteem, and self-clarity; and (4) the possibilities for self-change, both short-term flexibility in response to specific situations and long-term development and change. Future directions include the specification of underlying cognitive processes, including the activation of specific elements within the self-structure; examination of nonevaluative dimensions of self-categorization; and applications of

work on self-organization to a broader range of psychological phenomena.

Returning to the lay perspective, we may consider the extent to which literature on self-organization has addressed the layperson's concerns. First of all, this literature suggests that questions of identity will be answered in terms of both multiple selves and the possibility of a higher order core self. Second, questions of self-determination ("Where should I go?") will be addressed by representations of future and possible selves that embody a person's goals. Third, people may learn to handle self-doubt by reorganizing positive and negative self-beliefs in order to minimize negative impact. Most important, an understanding of self-organization may foster avenues for self-change.

Notes

1. At the same time, most studies of baseline relationships between self-complexity and other personality characteristics suggest that high self-complexity is associated with positive adjustment. Whereas low self-complexity is characteristic of individuals with borderline personality disorder (Gardner, 1997), an anxious–ambivalent attachment style (Mikulincer, 1995), and possibly narcissism (Rhodewalt & Morf, 1995), high self-complexity characterizes individuals who score high on both sociotropy (interpersonal investment) and autonomy (valuing independence; Solomon & Haaga, 1993) and also traumatized individuals who are not experiencing psychological distress (Morgan & Janoff-Bulman, 1994). Both positive, negative, and nonsignificant correlations between self-complexity and self-esteem have been reported (Campbell, Assanand, & Di Paula, 2000; Campbell, Chew, & Scratchley, 1991; Woolfolk, Novalany, Gara, Allen, & Polino, 1995). The mixed findings concerning the relationship between self-complexity and self-esteem may be influenced by past negative events. If self-complexity is a good way to cope with stress, then it is likely to be more prevalent in those individuals who have experienced more negative events. In addition, individuals with low self-esteem are likely to have experienced more negative past events.

2. Self-discrepancy theory (Higgins, 1987; Strauman, 1989) articulates an elaborate structure of multiple selves, for example, by positing that each self-guide (e.g., actual, ideal, ought,

and can) is represented from multiple perspectives (i.e., own and other).

3. Most researchers have weighted self-evaluations by perceived importance to generate an index of psychological adjustment (e.g., Marsh, 1993) rather than using the correlational measures preferred by Pelham (e.g., Pelham & Swann, 1989). These indices necessarily confound positivity and perceived importance. The advantage of the differential importance measures described herein is that they disentangle positivity and importance and generate an index of importance differentiation that is independent of the mean level of a person's self-evaluations. This independence suggests that importance differentiation can be used as a strategy to minimize the impact of negative self-beliefs or maximize the impact of positive ones without changing the content of those beliefs.

4. Similarly, in romantic relationships, most individuals who reported high levels of relationship stress tended to become more compartmentalized in their perceptions of their partner over the course of one year (Showers, 2002).

5. Recall that positive-compartmentalization refers to people with compartmentalized self-structures in which positive self-aspect categories are either more salient or more important than negative self-aspect categories.

6. This measure of differential importance is based on ratings of self-aspects generated in the card-sorting task rather than on responses to the SAQ (Pelham & Swann, 1989).

References

Alloy, L. B., & Abramson, L. Y. (1999). The Temple–Wisconsin Cognitive Vulnerability to Depression Project: Conceptual background, design, and methods. *Journal of Cognitive Psychotherapy, 13,* 227–262.

Aron, A., & Aron, E. N. (1986). *Love and expansion of the self: Understanding attraction and satisfaction.* New York: Hemisphere.

Bargh, J. A., & Tota, M. E. (1988). Context-dependent automatic processing in depression: Accessibility of negative constructs with regard to self but not others. *Journal of Personality and Social Psychology, 54,* 925–939.

Beck, A. T., Ward, C. H., Mendelson, M., Mock, J., & Erbaugh, J. (1961). An inventory for measuring depression. *Archives of General Psychiatry, 4,* 561–571.

Block, J. (1961). Ego-identity, role variability, and adjustment. *Journal of Consulting and Clinical Psychology, 25,* 392–397.

Bower, G. H. (1981). Mood and memory. *American Psychologist, 36,* 129–148.

Brewer, M. B., & Gardner, W. (1996). Who is this "we"? Levels of collective identity and self representations. *Journal of Personality and Social Psychology, 71,* 83–93.

Cacioppo, J. T., & Bernston, G. G. (1994). Relationship between attitudes and evaluative space: A critical review, with emphasis on the separability of positive and negative substrates. *Psychological Bulletin, 115,* 401–423.

Campbell, J. D. (1990). Self-esteem and clarity of the self-concept. *Journal of Personality and Social Psychology, 59,* 538–549.

Campbell, J. D., Assanand, S., & Di Paula, A. (2000). Structural features of the self-concept and adjustment. In A. Tesser, R. B. Felson, & J. M. Suls (Eds.), *Psychological perspectives on self and identity* (pp. 67–87). Washington, DC: American Psychological Association.

Campbell, J. D., Chew, B., & Scratchley, L. S. (1991). Cognitive and emotional reactions to daily events: The effects of self-esteem and self-complexity. *Journal of Personality, 59,* 473–505.

Campbell, J. D., Trapnell, P. D., Heine, S. J., Katz, I. M., Lavallee, L. F., & Lehman, D. R. (1996). Self-concept clarity: Measurement, personality correlates, and cultural boundaries. *Journal of Personality and Social Psychology, 70,* 141–156.

Cantor, N., & Kihlstrom, J. F. (1987). *Personality and social intelligence.* Englewood Cliffs, NJ: Prentice-Hall.

Cantor, N., Markus, H., Niedenthal, P., & Nurius, P. (1986). On motivation and the self-concept. In R. M. Sorrentino & E. T. Higgins (Eds.), *Handbook of motivation and cognition: Foundations of social behavior* (pp. 96–121). New York: Guilford Press.

Cantor, N., Mischel, W., & Schwartz, J. C. (1982). A prototype analysis of psychological situations. *Cognitive Psychology, 14,* 45–77.

Cohen, L. H., Pane, N., & Smith, H. S. (1997). Complexity of the interpersonal self and affective reactions to interpersonal stressors in life and in the laboratory. *Cognitive Therapy and Research, 21,* 387–407.

Cross, S., & Markus, H. (1991). Possible selves across the life span. *Human Development, 34,* 230–255.

Cross, S. E., Bacon, P. L., & Morris, M. L. (2000). The relational-interdependent self-construal and relationships. *Journal of Personality and Social Psychology, 78,* 191–208.

Cross, S. E., & Madson, L. (1997). Models of the self: Self-construals and gender. *Psychological Bulletin, 122,* 5–37.

Cross, S. E., & Markus, H. R. (1994). Self-schemas, possible selves, and competent performance. *Journal of Educational Psychology, 86,* 423–438.

DeSteno, D. A., & Salovey, P. (1997). The effects of mood on the structure of the self-concept. *Cognition and Emotion, 11,* 351–372.

Dixon, T. M., & Baumeister, R. F. (1991). Escaping the self: The moderating effect of self-complexity. *Personality and Social Psychology Bulletin, 17,* 363–368.

Donahue, E. M., Robins, R. W., Roberts, B. W., & John, O. P. (1993). The divided self: Concurrent and longitudinal effects of psychological adjustment and social roles on self-concept differentiation. *Journal of Personality and Social Psychology, 64,* 834–846.

Fazio, R. H., Jackson, J. R., Dunton, B. C., & Williams, C. J. (1995). Variability in automatic activation as an unobtrusive measure of racial attitudes: A bona fide pipeling? *Journal of Personality and Social Psychology, 69,* 1013–1027.

Fazio, R. H., Sanbonmatsu, D. M., Powell, M. C., &

Kardes, F. R. (1986). On the automatic activation of attitudes. *Journal of Personality and Social Psychology, 50,* 229–238.

Fischer, K. W. (1980). A theory of cognitive development: The control and construction of hierarchies of skills. *Psychological Review, 87,* 477–531.

Fiske, S., & Linville, P. (1980). What does the schema concept buy us? *Personality and Social Psychology Bulletin, 6,* 543–557.

Gardner, J. A. (1997). Borderline personality disorder and self-complexity: Application of Linville's self-complexity–affective-extremity hypothesis (Doctoral dissertation, Purdue University, 1998). *Dissertation Abstracts International, 59,* B0416.

Gergen, K. J. (1972). Multiple identity: The healthy, happy human being wears many masks. *Psychology Today, 5,* 31–35, 64–66.

Gergen, K. J. (1991). *The saturated self: Dilemmas of identity in contemporary life.* New York: Basic Books.

Gotlib, I. H., & Cane, D. B. (1987). Construct accessibility and clinical depression: A longitudinal investigation. *Journal of Abnormal Psychology, 96,* 199–204.

Gotlib, I. H., & McCann, C. D. (1984). Construct accessibility and depression: An examination of cognitive and affective factors. *Journal of Personality and Social Psychology, 47,* 427–439.

Halberstadt, J. B., & Niedenthal, P. M. (1997). Emotional state and the use of stimulus dimensions in judgment. *Journal of Personality and Social Psychology, 72,* 1017–1033.

Harter, S. (1999). *The construction of the self: A developmental perspective.* New York: Guilford Press.

Harter, S., Bresnick, S., Bouchey, H. A., & Whitesell, N. R. (1997). The development of multiple role-related selves during adolescence. *Development and Psychopathology, 9,* 835–853.

Heine, S. H., Lehman, D. R., Markus, H. R., & Kitayama, S. (1999). Is there a universal need for positive self-regard? *Psychological Review, 106,* 766–794.

Higgins, E. T. (1987). Self-discrepancy: A theory relating self and affect. *Psychological Review, 94,* 319–340.

Higgins, E. T., Bond, R. N., Klein, R., & Strauman, T. (1986). Self-discrepancies and emotional vulnerability: How magnitude, accessibility, and type of discrepancy influence affect. *Journal of Personality and Social Psychology, 51,* 5–15.

Higgins, E. T., Roney, C., Crowe, E., & Hymes, C. (1994). Ideal versus ought predilections for approach and avoidance: Distinct self-regulatory systems. *Journal of Personality and Social Psychology, 66,* 276–286.

Higgins, E. T., Shah, J., & Friedman, R. (1997). Emotional responses to goal attainment: Strength of regulatory focus as moderator. *Journal of Personality and Social Psychology, 72,* 515–525.

Higgins, E. T., & Tykocinski, O. (1992). Self-discrepancies and biographical memory: Personality and cognition at the level of psychological situation. *Personality and Social Psychology Bulletin, 18,* 527–535.

Higgins, E. T., Vookles, J., & Tykocinski, O. (1992). Self and health: How "patterns" of self-beliefs predict types of emotional and physical problems. *Social Cognition, 10,* 125–150.

James, W. (1963). *The principles of psychology.* New York: Holt. (Original work published 1890)

Jordan, A., & Cole, D. A. (1996). Relation of symptoms to the structure of self-knowledge in childhood. *Journal of Abnormal Psychology, 105,* 530–540.

Judd, C. M., Drake, R. A., Downing, J. W., & Krosnick, J. A. (1991). Some dynamic properties of attitude structures: Context-induced response facilitation and polarization. *Journal of Personality and Social Psychology, 60,* 193–202.

Kernberg, O. (1975). *Borderline conditions and pathological narcissism.* New York: Aronson.

Lavine, H., Thomsen, C. J., Zanna, M. P., & Borgida, E. (1998). On the primacy of affect in the determination of attitudes and behavior: The moderating role of affective–cognitive ambivalence. *Journal of Experimental Social Psychology, 34,* 398–421.

Lecky, P. (1945). *Self-consistency: A theory of personality.* New York: Anchor Books.

Linville, P. W. (1985). Self-complexity and affective extremity: Don't put all of your eggs in one cognitive basket. *Social Cognition, 3,* 94–120.

Linville, P. W. (1987). Self-complexity as a cognitive buffer against stress-related illness and depression. *Journal of Personality and Social Psychology, 52,* 663–676.

Margolin, J., & Niedenthal, P. M. (2000). Manipulating self-complexity with communication role assignment: Evidence of the flexibility of self-concept structure. *Journal of Research in Personality, 34,* 424–444.

Markus, H. (1977). Self-schemata and processing information about the self. *Journal of Personality and Social Psychology, 35,* 63–78.

Markus, H. R., & Kitayama, S. (1991). Culture and the self: Implications for cognition, emotion, and motivation. *Psychological Review, 98,* 224–253.

Markus, H., & Nurius, P. (1986). Possible selves. *American Psychologist, 41,* 954–969.

Markus, H., & Wurf, E. (1987). The dynamic self-concept: A social psychological perspective. *Annual Review of Psychology, 38,* 299–337.

Marsh, H. W. (1993). Relations between global and specific domains of self: The importance of individual importance, certainty, and ideals. *Journal of Personality and Social Psychology, 65,* 975–992.

Marsh, H. W., Barnes, J., & Hocevar, D. (1985). Self–other agreement on multidimensional self-concept ratings: Factor analysis and multitrait–multimethod analysis. *Journal of Personality and Social Psychology, 49,* 1360–1377.

McMahon, P. D., Showers, C. J., Rieder, S. L., Abramson, L. Y., & Hogan, M. E. (in press). Integrative thinking and flexibility in the organization of self-knowledge. *Cognitive Therapy and Research.*

Mendoza-Denton, R., Ayduk, O., Mischel, W., Shoda, Y., & Testa, A. (2001). Person × situation interactionism in self-encoding (I am . . . when . . .): Implications for affect regulation and social information processing. *Journal of Personality and Social Psychology, 80,* 533–544.

Mikulincer, M. (1995). Attachment style and the mental representation of the self. *Journal of Personality and Social Psychology, 69,* 1203–1215.

Mischel, W. (1973). Toward a cognitive social learning reconceptualization of personality. *Psychological Review, 80,* 252–283.

Mischel, W., & Shoda, Y. (1995). A cognitive–affective system theory of personality: Reconceptualizing situations, dispositions, dynamics, and invariance in personality structure. *Psychological Review, 102,* 246–268.

Mohr, D. M. (1978). Development of attributes of personal identity. *Developmental Psychology, 14,* 427–428.

Morgan, H. J., & Janoff-Bulman, R. (1994). Positive and negative self-complexity: Patterns of adjustment following traumatic versus non-traumatic life experiences. *Journal of Social and Clinical Psychology, 13,* 63–85.

Niedenthal, P. M., & Beike, D. R. (1997). Interrelated and isolated self-concepts. *Personality and Social Psychology Review, 1,* 106–128.

Niedenthal, P. M., Halberstadt, J. B., & Innes-Ker, A. H. (1999). Emotional response categorization. *Psychological Review, 106,* 337–361.

Niedenthal, P. M., Setterlund, M. B., & Wherry, M. B. (1992). Possible self-complexity and affective reactions to goal-relevant evaluation. *Journal of Personality and Social Psychology, 63,* 5–16.

Nowak, A., & Vallacher, R. R. (1998). *Dynamical social psychology.* New York: Guilford Press.

Nowak, A., Vallacher, R. R., Tesser, A., & Borkowski, W. (2000). Society of self: The emergence of collective properties in self-structure. *Psychological Review, 107,* 39–61.

Osgood, C. E. (1969). On the whys and wherefores of E, P, and A. *Journal of Personality and Social Psychology, 12,* 194–199.

Oyserman, D., & Markus, H. R. (1990). Possible selves and delinquency. *Journal of Personality and Social Psychology, 59,* 112–125.

Oyserman, D., & Markus, H. R. (1993). The sociocultural self. In J. M. Suls (Ed.), *The self in social perspective* (pp. 187–220). Hillsdale, NJ: Erlbaum.

Oyserman, D., & Markus, H. R. (1998). Self as social representation. In U. Flick (Ed.), *The psychology of the social* (pp. 107–125). New York: Cambridge University Press.

Pelham, B. W. (1993). The idiographic nature of human personality: Examples of the idiographic self-concept. *Journal of Personality and Social Psychology, 64,* 665–677.

Pelham, B. W., & Swann, W. B. (1989). From self-conceptions to self-worth: On the sources and structure of global self-esteem. *Journal of Personality and Social Psychology, 57,* 672–680.

Priester, J. R., & Petty, R. E. (2001). Extending the bases of subjective attitudinal ambivalence: Interpersonal and intrapersonal antecedents of evaluative tension. *Journal of Personality and Social Psychology, 80,* 19–34.

Rafaeli-Mor, E., Gotlib, I. H., & Revelle, W. (1999). The meaning and measurement of self-complexity. *Personality and Individual Differences, 27,* 341–356.

Rhodewalt, F., Madrian, J. C., & Cheney, S. (1998). Narcissism, self-knowledge organization, and emotional reactivity: The effect of daily experiences on self-esteem and affect. *Personality and Social Psychology Bulletin, 24,* 75–87.

Rhodewalt, F., & Morf, C. C. (1995). Self and interpersonal correlates of the Narcissistic Personality Inventory: A review and new findings. *Journal of Research in Personality, 29,* 1–23.

Rogers, C. R. (1959). The essence of psychotherapy: A client-centered view. *Annals of Psychotherapy, 1,* 51–57.

Rogers, T. B., Kuiper, N. A., & Kirker, W. S. (1977). Self-reference and the encoding of personal information. *Journal of Personality and Social Psychology, 35,* 677–688.

Rosch, E. (1978). Principles of categorization. In E. Rosch & B. B. Loyd (Eds.), *Cognition and categorization* (pp. 27–48). Hillsdale, NJ: Erlbaum.

Rosenberg, M. (1965). *Society and the adolescent self-image.* Princeton, NJ: Princeton University Press.

Rosenberg, S. (1988). Self and others: Studies in social personality and autobiography. *Advances in experimental social psychology* (Vol. 21, pp. 57–95). New York: Academic Press.

Rosenberg, S., & Gara, M. A. (1985). The multiplicity of personal identity. In P. Shaver (Ed.), *Review of personality and social psychology* (Vol. 6, pp. 87–113). Beverly Hills, CA: Sage.

Ross, L., & Nisbett, R. E. (1991). *The person and the situation: Perspectives of social psychology.* New York: McGraw-Hill.

Segal, Z. V. (1988). Appraisal of the self-schema construct in cognitive models of depression. *Psychological Bulletin, 103,* 147–162.

Segal, Z. V., Hood, J. E., Shaw, B. F., & Higgins, E. T. (1988). A structural analysis of the self-schema construct in major depression. *Cognitive Therapy and Research, 12,* 417–485.

Segal, Z. V., & Vella, D. D. (1990). Self-schema in major depression: Replication and extension of a priming methodology. *Cognitive Therapy and Research, 14,* 161–176.

Setterlund, M. B., & Niedenthal, P. M. (1993). "Who am I? Why am I here?": Self-esteem, self-clarity, and prototype matching. *Journal of Personality and Social Psychology, 65,* 769–780.

Showers, C. J. (1992a). Compartmentalization of positive and negative self-knowledge: Keeping bad apples out of the bunch. *Journal of Personality and Social Psychology, 62,* 1036–1049.

Showers, C. J. (1992b). Evaluatively integrative thinking about characteristics of the self. *Personality and Social Psychology Bulletin, 18,* 719–729.

Showers, C. J. (1995). The evaluative organization of self-knowledge: Origins, processes, and implications for self-esteem. In M. H. Kernis (Ed.), *Efficacy, agency, and self-esteem* (pp. 101–120). New York: Plenum Press.

Showers, C. J. (2000). Self-organization in emotional contexts. In J. P. Forgas (Ed.), *Feeling and thinking: The role of affect in social cognition* (pp. 283–307). Paris: Cambridge University Press.

Showers, C. J. (2002). Integration and compartmentalization: A model of self-structure and self-change. In D. Cervone & W. Mischel (Eds.), *Advances in personality science* (pp. 271–291). New York: Guilford Press.

Showers, C. J., Abramson, L. Y., & Hogan, M. E. (1998). The dynamic self: How the content and structure of the self-concept change with mood. *Journal of Personality and Social Psychology, 75,* 478–493.

Showers, C. J., & Kevlyn, S. B. (1999). Organization of knowledge about a relationship partner: Implications for liking and loving. *Journal of Personality and Social Psychology, 76,* 958–971.

Showers, C. J., & Kling, K. C. (1996). Organization of self-knowledge: Implications for recovery from sad mood. *Journal of Personality and Social Psychology, 70,* 578–590.

Showers, C. J., & Ryff, C. D. (1996). Self-differentiation and well-being in a life transition. *Personality and Social Psychology Bulletin, 22,* 448–460.

Singer, J. A. & Salovey, P. (1988). Mood and memory: Evaluating the network theory of affect. *Clinical Psychology Review, 8,* 211–251.

Smith, E. R., Coats, S., & Walling, D. (1999). Overlapping mental representations of self, in-group, and partner: Further response time evidence and a connectionist model. *Personality and Social Psychology Bulletin, 25,* 873–882.

Snyder, M. (1974). Self-monitoring of expressive behavior. *Journal of Personality and Social Psychology, 30,* 526–537.

Solomon, A., & Haaga, D. A. F. (1993). Sociotropy, autonomy, and self-complexity. *Journal of Social Behavior and Personality, 8,* 743–748.

Steele, C. M. (1988). The psychology of self-affirmation: Sustaining the integrity of the self. In L. Berkowitz (Ed.), *Advances in experimental social psychology* (Vol. 21, pp. 261–302). New York: Academic Press.

Strauman, T. J. (1989). Self-discrepancies in clinical depression and social phobia: Cognitive structures that underlie emotional disorders? *Journal of Abnormal Psychology, 98,* 14–22.

Strauman, T. J. (1996). Stability within the self: A longitudinal study of the structural implications of self-discrepancy theory. *Journal of Personality and Social Psychology, 71,* 1142–1153.

Tangney, J. P., Niedenthal, P. M., Covert, M. V., & Barlow, D. H. (1998). Are shame and guilt related to distinct self-discrepancies? A test of Higgins's (1987) hypotheses. *Journal of Personality and Social Psychology, 75,* 256–268.

Taylor, S. E., & Brown, J. D. (1994). Positive illusions and well-being revisited: Separating fact from fiction. *Psychological Bulletin, 116,* 21–27.

Taylor, S. E., & Gollwitzer, P. M. (1995). Effects of mindset on positive illusions. *Journal of Personality and Social Psychology, 69,* 213–226.

Tesser, A. (2000). On the confluence of self-esteem maintenance mechanisms. *Personality and Social Psychology Review, 4,* 290–299.

Trope, Y. (1986). Self-enhancement and self-assessment in achievement behavior. In R. M. Sorrentino & E. T. Higgins (Eds.), *Handbook of motivation and cognition: Foundations of social behavior* (pp. 350–378). New York: Guilford Press.

Vallacher, R. R., Nowak, A., & Kaufman, J. (1994). Intrinsic dynamics of social judgment. *Journal of Personality and Social Psychology, 67,* 20–34.

Williams, J. M. G., & Broadbent, K. (1986). Autobiographical memory in suicide attempters. *Journal of Abnormal Psychology, 95,* 144–149.

Williams, J. M. G., & Nulty, D. D. (1986). Construct accessibility, depression and the emotional Stroop task: Transient mood or stable structure. *Personality and Individual Differences, 7,* 485–491.

Wittenbrink, B., Judd, C. M., & Park, B. (2001). Evaluative versus conceptual judgments in automatic stereotyping and prejudice. *Journal of Experimental Social Psychology, 37,* 244–252.

Woike, B., Gershkovich, I., Piorkowski, R., & Polo, M. (1999). The role of motives in the content and structure of autobiographical memory. *Journal of Personality and Social Psychology, 76,* 600–612.

Woolfolk, R. L., Novalany, J., Gara, M. A., Allen, L. A., & Polino, M. (1995). Self-complexity, self-evaluation, and depression: An examination of form and content within the self-schema. *Journal of Personality and Social Psychology, 68,* 1108–1120.

Zajonc, R. B. (1960). The process of cognitive tuning in communication. *Journal of Abnormal and Social Psychology, 61,* 159–167.

4

Self and Identity as Memory

JOHN F. KIHLSTROM
JENNIFER S. BEER
STANLEY B. KLEIN

Modern thought literally begins with the self. René Descartes, beginning his *Meditations* of 1641 from a stance of methodical doubt, quickly discovered that there was one thing he couldn't doubt: that he himself existed. This conclusion, in turn, was based on his experience of himself as a conscious being—hence, "*Cogito, ergo sum*" and "*Sum res cogitans.*" More recently, the editors of the *New York Times Magazine,* in one of six special issues celebrating the year 2000, dubbed the previous 1,000 years "The Me Millennium":

A thousand years ago, when the earth was reassuringly flat and the universe revolved around it, the ordinary person had no last name, let alone any claim to individualism. The self was subordinated to church and king. Then came the Renaissance explosion of scientific discovery and humanist insight and, as both cause and effect, the rise of individual self-consciousness. All at once, it seemed, Man had replaced God at the center of earthly life. And perhaps more than any great war or invention or feat of navigation, this upheaval marked the beginning of our modern era. There are now 20 times as many people in the world as there were in the

year 1000. Most have last names, and many of us have a personal identity or a reasonable expectation of acquiring one. ("The Me Millennium," 1999, p. 20)

This sense of self is critical to our status as persons. In fact, philosophers often use the terms "self" and "person" interchangeably: A capacity for self-awareness is necessary for full personhood. One has a sense of self if one is able to entertain first-person thoughts and if one possesses first-person knowledge. The eye cannot see itself, but the self somehow knows itself: The simultaneous status of self as subject and object of awareness is one of the enduring problems of philosophy. For human beings, at least, and perhaps for some other animals as well, cognition is not simply directed at the external environment. Our minds also turn inward, permitting us to acquire, store, retrieve, and use knowledge about ourselves—which raises a further issue, stated eloquently by Gordon Allport:

This puzzling problem arises when we ask, "Who is the I that knows the bodily me, who has an image of myself and a sense of identity over time, who knows that I have propriate strivings?" I know all these things, and what is more, I know that I know them. But who is it who has this perspectival grasp? . . . It is much easier to *feel* the self than to *define* the self. (1961, p. 128)

Although the self is a thorny metaphysical problem for philosophers, raising questions about mind and body, the homunculus, and whether teleporters can replicate subjective identity, as well as material existence (Gallagher, 2000; Gallagher & Shear, 1999), cognitive psychology offers a simple answer to Allport's question: The self is a mental representation of oneself, including all that one knows about oneself (Kihlstrom & Cantor, 1984; Kihlstrom et al., 1988). The *I* who knows the *me* is the same *I* who knows everything else, and the mental representation of this knowledge is no different, except perhaps in intimacy and richness, than is the mental representation of anything else I know. The solution is perhaps too simple, but it was the solution offered by William James (1890/1980), and it is a start.

What Kind of Knowledge Is Self-Knowledge?

In general, psychology and cognitive science distinguish between two forms of knowledge representation (J. R. Anderson, 1995; Paivio, 1971; see also Paivio, 1986): *perception-based* knowledge representations take the form of *mental images* representing in analog form the physical appearance of objects and the configuration of objects and features in space, whereas *meaning-based* knowledge representations store propositional knowledge about the semantic relations among objects, features, and events. A person's self-knowledge can be construed in similar terms. In fact, the technical distinction between perception-based and meaning-based self-knowledge is anticipated in ordinary language when we refer to the *self-concept* and the *self-image*. Taking the folk-psychological notions of self-concept and self-image literally has yielded a substantial body of research and theory on the self (e.g., Kihlstrom & Klein, 1994).

The Self as Concept

A concept is a mental representation of a category—a set of objects that share some features in common, somehow distinct from objects in other categories. In the classical Aristotelian view, concepts are proper sets, defined by a list of features that are both singly necessary and jointly sufficient to identify an object as an instance of a category. Every instance of a concept has every defining feature, and any object that possesses the entire set of defining features is an instance of the concept.

From the classical point of view, then, the self-concept is identified by a set of features that are singly necessary and jointly sufficient to identify oneself as different from all other persons. This list of features could be utterly trivial: One of the authors (J. K.) of this chapter is the only person who ever lived who was born on October 24, 1948, in Norwich, New York, to Harriet Foster and Waldo Helge Kihlstrom. If he had an identical twin brother, that sibling would (at least) have been born at a slightly different time. In more substantive terms, however, Allport's ideographic view of personality supposes that there is a unique set of psychological features—he called them *central traits*—that distinguish every individual person from every other individual person (Allport, 1937). Assuming that we ourselves are aware of our traits, in Allport's view these psychological characteristics then become the defining features of the self-concept.

Along the same lines, Hazel Markus and her colleagues have suggested that the *self-schema* incorporates those features that are important to one's self-concept, not merely those that are descriptive of the self (e.g., Markus, 1977). In her research, subjects are classified as "self-schematic" for a particular attribute if they rate that feature high in both self-descriptiveness and importance to the self-concept. Although one can debate the role that self-descriptiveness and self-importance should play in identifying the self-schema (e.g., Burke, Kraut, & Dworkin, 1986; Nystedt, Smari, & Boman, 1991), one can well imagine a self-concept defined by that unique set of features for which the individual is "schematic."

In any case, the classical proper-set view of the self as a set with only a single instance aptly recognizes our experience of ourselves as unique—that we are not the same as anyone else. Research by McGuire and his colleagues has found that people who are in the minority with respect to age, birthplace, gender, ethnicity, and other physical, social, and demographic features are more likely to mention them when asked to describe themselves (e.g., McGuire & McGuire, 1988). Apparently, people notice aspects of themselves, and incorporate these attributes into their self-concepts, to the extent that these features render them distinctive.

On the other hand, philosophers and cognitive scientists have identified a number of problems with the classical view of concepts as proper sets, problems that have led to the progressive elaboration of a number of revisionist views of conceptual structure (e.g., Smith & Medin, 1981). Chief among these alternatives is the *probabilistic* view of concepts as *fuzzy* sets represented by summary prototypes whose characteristic features are only imperfectly correlated with category membership. Instead of sharing some set of singly necessary and jointly sufficient defining features, instances of a concept are related to each other by a principle of family resemblance.

The view of the self as a cognitive prototype quickly won wide acceptance within social cognition (Cantor & Mischel, 1979; Hampson, 1982), but it has never been clear what the self was a prototype *of*. On the one hand, it might be that there is a monolithic, unitary self-concept whose characteristic features permit us to distinguish ourselves probabilistically from other people. On the other hand, the notion of family resemblance suggests that there might well be more than one self represented in the individual's cognitive system. That is to say, the self-as-prototype might be abstracted from multiple, context-specific mental representations of self—self at work, self at home, self with friends, and the like. Clinical cases of multiple personality disorder (also known as dissociative identity disorder) bring the multiplicity of self into bold relief (Kihlstrom, 2001). But we do not have to be mentally ill to harbor in our minds a multiplicity of selves. Despite our tendency to describe each other in terms of stable traits, human social behavior is widely variable across time and place, and our self-knowledge must represent this kind of variability.[1]

Just as various problems with the classical view of concepts led to the development of an alternative prototype view, so problems with the prototype view have led to further revisionist views (e.g., Medin, 1989). For example, an exemplar-based view represents concepts as collections of instances instead of as summaries of the features of category members. In addition, a *theory-based* view holds that concept exemplars are related to each other by some theory of the domain in question, rather than by any kind of similarity. In principle, both these views can be applied to the self-concept, but as yet there has been no sustained effort to do so (Kihlstrom & Klein, 1994).[2]

The Self as Image

A large literature on mental images in *nonsocial* perception provides us with a starting point for perception-based mental representations of the self (e.g., Kosslyn, 1980, 1983, 1988; Shepard & Cooper, 1983). For example, perception-based representations in the nonsocial domain take at least three forms. First, and most familiar, are mental images per se, seen in "the mind's eye" and heard in "the mind's ear," which preserve sensory detail—what our faces and bodies look like, what our voices sound like, the feel of our skin and body hair (e.g., Farah, 1988). Then there are *spatial images,* which preserve information about the spatial relations among features and objects—up–down, left–right, front–back—in the absence of sensory details (e.g., Farah, Hammond, Levine, & Calvanio, 1988). Finally, there are representations of serial order, which preserve information about the temporal relations of events, such as first–last, before–after, early–late, and remote–recent (Mandler & Dean, 1969), and other rank-ordered features such as richer–poorer and taller–shorter (Trabasso & Riley, 1975)—again, independent of sensory modality. Knowledge of sensory details, spatial relations, and serial order may be verbally expressed, but because they are independent of meaning, they are properly classified as perception-based rather than meaning-based in nature.

Compared with meaning-based representations, perception-based representations of the self have not been much studied in social cognition (Kihlstrom & Klein, 1994). The anlage of the self-image may be found in the body schema postulated by Sir Henry Head to account for the ability of animals, including humans, to maintain stability of posture and adjust to their physical surroundings (Head, 1926), and in the *body image* defined by Schilder as "the picture of our own body which we form in our mind, that is to say, the way in which the body appears to ourselves" (Schilder, 1938, p. 11; see also Fisher & Cleveland, 1958). A number of clinical syndromes appear to involve pathologies of the body image, including autotopagnosia, phantom limb, schizophrenia, eating disorders such as anorexia and bulimia, and, of course, body dysmorphic disorder (Kihlstrom & Klein, 1994).

Procedures for the assessment of the body image and other perception-based representations of the self have not been well developed. One of the most popular instruments, the Body-Image Aberration Scale, is a verbal self-report questionnaire, not a perceptual task (Chapman, Chapman, & Raulin, 1978). Nonverbal, analog representations are more closely tapped by the Body-Image Assessment (Williamson, Davis, Goreczny, & Blouin, 1989) and similar tasks (Fallon & Rozin, 1985; Rozin & Fallon, 1988), in which subjects rate themselves on a set of line drawings of swimsuit-clad males and females. Distorting mirrors (Orbach, Traub, & Olson, 1966; Traub, Olson, Orbach, & Cardone, 1967; Traub & Orbach, 1964) and photographs (Yarmey & Johnson, 1982) have also been employed in the assessment of aspects of the self-image, although none of these procedures has been particularly well developed.

Despite the general lack of standardized assessment protocols, the literature contains a scattering of studies on the self-image as a perception-based knowledge representation. For example, although the failure to recognize one's own voice has been taken as evidence of self-deception (Gur & Sackeim, 1979; Sackeim & Gur, 1985; but see also Douglas & Gibbins, 1983; Gibbins & Douglas, 1985), infants as young as 5 months old are known to recognize their own voices, as well as their own faces (Legerstee, Anderson, & Schaffer, 1998). Moreover, people prefer left–right reversals of photos of themselves (i.e., as they would see themselves in a mirror), and they prefer unreversed photos of others (i.e., as they would view them head-on). Evidence such as this

clearly indicates that the self-image preserves both spatial relations and visual detail (Mita, Dermer, & Knight, 1977). Thus the little work that has been done in this area does seem to indicate that, in addition to verbal knowledge about our characteristic features, we also possess analog representations of what we look and sound like. However, research on the self-image (or, for that matter, on perception-based representations of other people) has yet to draw on experimental paradigms developed in the study of imagery in the nonsocial domain.

The Self as Memory

Whether perception-based or meaning-based, self-knowledge is represented in the individual's memory. Accordingly, in addition to viewing the self as a concept or as an image, it is useful to think of the self as one's memory for oneself (Klein, 2001). This is not an entirely new idea. In his *Essay Concerning Human Understanding* (1690, Book II, Chapter 27), John Locke famously identified the self with memory. Whereas Descartes had found the self in the immediate conscious experience of thinking ("I think, therefore I am"), Locke found identity in the extension of consciousness backward in time. In Locke's view, a person's identity extends to whatever of his or her past he or she can remember. Consequently, past experiences, thoughts, or actions that the person does not remember are not part of his identity. For Locke, identity and selfhood have nothing to do with continuity of the body or even continuity of mind. Selfhood consists entirely in continuity of memory. A person who remembers nothing of his or her past literally has no identity.

Because Locke identified self with identity, such a person will not have any sense of self, either. This conclusion may at first strike the reader as unreasonable. After all, even with no memory, there would still be the Cartesian self of immediate experience. However, it must be remembered that Locke was an empiricist, opposed in principle to Descartes's nativism. Like all knowledge, self-knowledge must be derived a posteriori from experiences of sensation and reflection. Without the capacity to record such experiences in memory, there can be no self—just an organism responding reflexively to environmental stimuli. On the other hand, the notion of self as memory makes no sense unless there is a person, namely oneself, to be represented in the memory. Perhaps the notion of *I, me,* and *mine* is derived empirically, but perhaps this primitive sense of the self, as distinct from other objects and people in the environment, is given a priori.

Despite these sorts of difficulties, Locke's identification of the self with memory proved very popular over the years. David Hume, in the *Treatise of Human Nature* (1739–1740, Book I, Part 4, Section 6), generally affirmed the connection between identity and memory, adding that the role of memory is to permit us to comprehend the causal relations among events. This ability, however, enables us to extend our identity beyond those acts and experiences that we can personally remember, so that our self-narrative also includes events that we know *must* have happened, given what we *do* remember—whether they actually happened or not. Thus, whereas Locke's view of the self-as-memory is based on our ability to *reproduce* our experiences *from* memory, Hume's is based also on our ability to *reconstruct* our experiences *in* memory. Freud, for his part, also adopted the Lockean view, with the proviso that the important memories are *unconscious,* as opposed to consciously accessible (Freud, 1916–1917/1963).

Identity and Forms of Memory

The Lockean view of the self is almost entirely empirical, because in his view people's identities are built up a posteriori from memories of their own sensory experiences, as well as their reflections on these experiences. But experiences do not exhaust the knowledge that is represented in memory (J. R. Anderson, 1976, 1983). For example, Endel Tulving distinguished between *episodic* and *semantic* memory (Tulving, 1983). *Episodic memory* is autobiographical memory for the events and experiences of one's past. Every episodic memory, by definition, entails a mental representation of the self as the agent or patient of some action or as the stimulus or experiencer of some state (Kihlstrom, 1997). Examples of

episodic memories are *I gave a present to Lucy on her birthday* and *Lucy made me very happy yesterday.* Because our sense of self is very much tied up with the "story" of what we have experienced and what we have done, the relevance of episodic memory to Locke's and Hume's concepts of the self is obvious.

By contrast, *semantic memory* is more generic, context-free knowledge about the world. In contrast to episodic knowledge, every bit of which necessarily entails some reference to the self, much semantic memory makes no reference to the self at all. Such items of knowledge as *Apples are red, green, or yellow fruits* or *Columbus discovered America in 1492* do not involve the self in any way. However, some items of semantic knowledge do relate to the self. The date and place of one's birth, the names of one's parents and siblings, ethnic identity and religious affiliation, and one's own personality and sociodemographic attributes do not refer to any discrete episodes in one's life: I don't *remember* being born, but I do *know* when and where it happened. Examples of semantic self-knowledge are *I am a member of the middle class, I am more than 6 feet tall,* and *I am a neurotic extravert.* Self-relevant semantic knowledge is also part of one's identity: It is tantamount to the self-concept and self-image, translated into the vocabulary of memory theory.

Episodic and semantic memories, in turn, are forms of *declarative knowledge* (Winograd, 1972, 1975). They constitute our fund of factual knowledge about the world; factual knowledge of this sort can be represented as sentence-like propositions. But declarative knowledge is not the only knowledge stored in the mind. There is also *procedural knowledge*: our cognitive repertoire of rules and skills, by which we manipulate and transform declarative knowledge. Procedural knowledge can be represented as a collection of *productions* specifying the actions (motor or mental) that will achieve some goal under specified conditions (J. R. Anderson, 1976, 1983). Examples of procedural knowledge, somewhat simplified for purposes of exposition, are *If the goal is to shift gears, then press down on the clutch* and *If the goal is to convert Fahrenheit to Celsius, then subtract 32 and multiply the result by 5/9.*

Note that there is no reference to the self in these productions. Moreover, in contrast to declarative knowledge, which is available (if not always accessible) to conscious awareness, procedural knowledge is, by definition, unavailable to direct conscious introspection under any circumstances (Kihlstrom, 1987). For this reason, it seems unlikely that procedural knowledge per se is included in the mental representation of the self. However, we can learn about our procedural knowledge indirectly, through informal and formal analyses of our own performances on cognitive and motor tasks. As we acquire skills and teach them to others, we become aware of the skills we have—which is not the same thing as being aware of the production systems that underlie skilled activity. Put another way, we acquire a form of *meta-knowledge* about our repertoire of cognitive and mental skills (Flavell, 1979, 1999; see also Mazzoni & Nelson, 1998; Metcalfe & Shimamura, 1994; Nelson, 1992; Reder, 1996)—declarative knowledge that is available to consciousness (Nelson, 1996) and that can therefore become part of the self-concept. All meta-knowledge is potentially relevant to the self, because all meta-knowledge concerns people's knowledge of they themselves know, including what they themselves know what to do. Meta-cognitions such as *I know how to drive a standard-shift car* and *I know how to tie a necktie in a Windsor knot* underlie self-efficacy expectations (Bandura, 1977, 2000; see also Mischel, 1973; Mischel, Shoda, & Rodriguez, 1989), part of a broader repertoire of social intelligence that makes up personality from a cognitive point of view (Cantor & Kihlstrom, 1987). But meta-knowledge is declarative, not procedural, in nature. Accordingly, the following discussion focuses entirely on declarative knowledge about the self and, particularly, on the relations between episodic and semantic knowledge about the self.[3]

Associative Network Models of the Self as Memory

Precisely how are episodic and semantic self-knowledge organized in memory? In a generic associative network model of memory, such as the various versions of the ACT model (ACT is an acronym for Adaptive Control of Thought or, perhaps tongue-in-cheek, Another Cognitive Theory; J. R. Anderson, 1983, 1993; J. R. Anderson & Lebière, 1998), the self (or each of a multiplicity of context-specific selves) can be represented as a node (which we might call the *ego node*) representing the self, just as there are other nodes in memory representing other people, places, and things with which we are familiar. Fanning out from this ego node would be other nodes corresponding to one's episodic and semantic knowledge about oneself. In this way, individual nodes representing self-relevant knowledge such as *I gave a present to Lucy on her birthday, Lucy made me happy yesterday, I am a member of the middle class, I am more than 6 feet tall, I am a neurotic extravert, I know how to drive a standard-shift car,* and *I know how to tie a necktie in a Windsor knot* would fan out from a central node representing oneself as the agent, patient, stimulus, or experiencer of all the events recorded in episodic memory, the object of all the self-descriptive statements recorded in semantic self-memory, and the possessor of all the knowledge indexed in meta-memory. In such a structure, the retrieval of self-knowledge begins by activating the ego node through perception or thought and then tracing the activation as it spreads through associated links to nodes representing various bits of episodic and semantic self-knowledge (Figure 4.1, Panel A).

Such a structure, known as an *independent storage model* because each piece of self-knowledge is stored independently of every other piece of self-knowledge, has the virtue of simplicity. But it also has one very big liability: the *fan effect* and the paradox of interference (J. R. Anderson, 1974; J. R. Anderson & Reder, 1999; Lewis & Anderson, 1976). Put briefly, retrieval latency increases as a function of the number of facts associated with a node in an associative network. In other words, the more one knows about a topic, the harder it is to gain access to any particular item of topic-relevant information. If, as seems likely, the self is a very large knowledge structure stored in memory, the fan effect would seem to imply that it would be relatively difficult to gain access to any particular item of self-knowledge stored in memory—a somewhat counterintuitive implication. To some extent, the

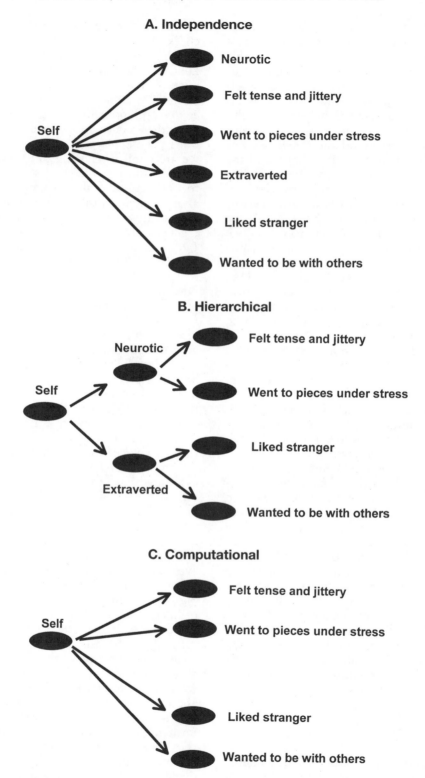

FIGURE 4.1. Possible relations among episodic and semantic self-knowledge in a generic associative-network model of memory, after Kihlstrom and Klein (1994). (A) Independence model. (B) Hierarchical model. (C) Computational model.

paradox of interference can be resolved by imposing hierarchical organization on memory, which creates considerable efficiencies in the process of information retrieval (E. E. Smith, Adams, & Schorr, 1978). For example, instead of each item of self-relevant information being separately and independently associated with the ego node, memories for individual actions and experiences could be organized by their trait implications. That is, all the neurotic behaviors would be grouped together, all the extraverted behaviors, and so forth (Figure 1, Panel B).

Such a hierarchically organized structure is consistent with what is known about the role of category clustering and organizational principles in memory and also congruent with some theoretical models of person memory in general (e.g., Hamilton, Katz, & Leirer, 1980; Ostrom, Lingle, Pryor, & Geva, 1980). In principle, the organization of episodic self-knowledge by semantic self-knowledge—and, for that matter, the hierarchical organization of semantic self-knowledge according to subordinate, basic-level, and superordinate trait categories—would make it easier to retrieve individual pieces of episodic (and semantic) self-knowledge. On the other hand, such an organizational structure also increases the risk of false recognition of conceptually similar behaviors (Reder & Anderson, 1980). Of course, this is precisely the kind of "false alarms effect" uncovered by Rogers, Rogers, and Kuiper (1979). So the hierarchical alternative gains credence both from abstract considerations of efficiency and empirical evidence such as the "false alarms" effect.

As it happens, the two models described here—independence and hierarchical—do not exhaust all the alternatives. It is possible that semantic self-knowledge is not stored in memory at all but rather is computed online as it is required (e.g., when completing personality self-ratings or describing oneself in a "personals" advertisement). Thus, when asked whether (or to what extent) they are neurotic or extraverted, people might first retrieve a sample of their behaviors from episodic memory. Then, employing "cognitive algebra," they might compute scores for neuroticism and extraversion by integrating across the values for

these traits associated with each of these behaviors (N. H. Anderson, 1974, 1981). For example, people might compute how likeable they are, a piece of semantic self-knowledge, based on episodic self-knowledge of whether, how often, and under what circumstances they have done likable things (N. H. Anderson, 1968). However, the results of these computations are not themselves stored in memory. Rather, they are computed anew each time they are needed. Memory stores only representations of behavior and experience (Figure 4.1, Panel C).

Such a computational scheme would be consistent with Bem's theory of self-perception of attitudes (Bem, 1967), which holds that people have no introspective access to their attitudes but rather infer them from observations of their own behaviors—just as they infer *other* people's attitudes from observations of their behaviors. A related view is that our social behaviors are generated automatically and unconsciously in response to eliciting stimuli in the environment, so that the reasons we give for our behaviors are little more than post hoc rationalizations (Bargh, 1984; see also Bargh, 1989, 1994, 1997; Bargh & Chartrand, 1999; Bargh & Ferguson, 2000; Nisbett & Wilson, 1977; Wilson, 1985; Wilson & Stone, 1985). In extending self-perception theory to traits and other psychosocial characteristics, we must consider whether people say that they are neurotic extraverts (for example) not because they have these traits encoded in semantic memory but because they retrieve episodic memories of themselves doing neurotic and extraverted things.

Empirical Studies of the Self as Memory

For most of its history, cognitive psychology has attempted to understand memory structures and processes by analyzing aspects of human performance such as savings in relearning (e.g., Ebbinghaus, 1885/1964), retroactive and proactive inhibition (e.g., Postman & Underwood, 1973), organization in free recall (e.g., Bower, 1970; Mandler, 1979), recall and recognition accuracy (e.g., Craik & Lockhart, 1972; Roediger & McDermott, 1994), response latencies (e.g., Reder & Anderson, 1980; Sternberg, 1969), and the like. This has also been true of research on the self as a memory structure, which has generally followed the paradigms established in the study of person memory within social cognition generally (e.g., Hastie & Carlston, 1980; Kihlstrom & Hastie, 1997; Srull, 1981; Wyer & Carlston, 1994).

The Self-Reference Effect

Perhaps the earliest empirical attempt to view the self as a memory structure was in work by Rogers and his colleagues on what has come to be known as the self-reference effect (for reviews, see Rogers, 1981; Kuiper & Derry, 1981). Extending the "levels of processing" paradigm introduced by Craik and Lockhart (1972), Rogers, Kuiper, and Kirker (1977) asked subjects to perform a self-referent encoding task: judging whether each of a set of trait adjectives was self-descriptive. On a later recall test, the subjects showed better memory for these items than for items studied under the structural and semantic orienting tasks of the standard levels-of-processing experiment . This *self-reference effect* has since been replicated many times (Figure 4.2, Panel A) and is so reliable that it can be used as a classroom demonstration (Symons & Johnson, 1997). Later studies showed that the recognition of

self-referenced material is likely to be accompanied by an experience of *remembering* as opposed to *knowing* (Conway & Dewhurst, 1995; Hirshman & Lanning, 1999)—further evidence that self-reference is a powerful encoding condition.

Based on the idea that the experimental conditions in the levels-of-processing experiment promote contact between studied items and increasingly rich and elaborate cognitive structures, Rogers and others (e.g., Keenan & Baillet, 1980) suggested that the self might be the richest, most elaborate knowledge structure in memory. However, this inference is undercut by the fact that reference to other people, particularly if they are well known, can produce equivalent effects (e.g., Bower & Gilligan, 1979). On the other hand, there is no reason why one's knowledge about, say, one's mother might not also constitute a rich and elaborate knowledge structure. More critical was a finding that the self-reference effect was an artifact of the organization of self-referent items into categories (Klein & Kihlstrom, 1986). In the semantic orienting task employed in the typical self-reference experiment, a different question is associated with each item. A word such as "neurotic" might be compared with "anxious," whereas a word such as "extraverted" might be compared with "outgoing." How-

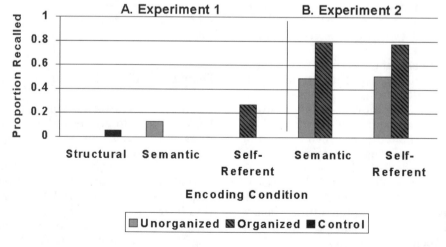

FIGURE 4.2. Influence of organizational processing on the self-reference effect, after Klein and Kihlstrom (1986, Experiments 1 and 2).

ever, in the self-reference condition the orienting question is always the same—whether the trait is self-descriptive. Accordingly, the self-reference orienting task tacitly encourages subjects to group the study items into two categories: those that are and those that are not self-descriptive. Based on the principle that organizational activity facilitates memory, the advantage of self-referenced items might be a function of organization rather than of self-reference.

To address this issue, Klein and Kihlstrom (1986) conducted a series of experiments that unconfounded self-reference and organization. Subjects were asked to study a list of words representing body parts in an experiment in which self-reference and organization were manipulated orthogonally. In a variant on the standard semantic/unorganized condition, the subject was asked if the target word fit in a sentence frame; different frames were used for each item. In the semantic/organized condition, however, the subjects were asked to make a dichotomous category judgment: whether the word referred to an internal or external body part. In a variant on the standard self/organized condition, the subjects were asked whether they had ever had an injury or illness to various body parts.

The results of these experiments were clear (Figure 4.2, Panel B). In the self/unorganized condition, each of the target words was referenced to a *different* self-descriptive question. Comparing the standard semantic and self-referent orienting tasks, the standard self-reference effect emerged. But reversing the organizational qualities of the two tasks also reversed the self-reference effect. In other words, the standard self-reference effect was due entirely to the organizational qualities of the standard self-reference task. Later research showed that elaborative, as well as organizational, activity was implicated in the self-reference effect but that the effects of elaboration were independent of self-reference (Klein & Loftus, 1988; Klein, Loftus, & Burton, 1989). The self may well be the richest, best organized, and most elaborate knowledge structure stored in memory; but because the self-reference effect is an artifact of organizational activity, experiments demonstrating the effect do not provide any evidence that this is the case.

Self-Relevance and Recognition

In their program of research, Rogers and his colleagues employed other aspects of memory performance to support their claim that the self is a schematically organized knowledge structure. For example, they showed that memory is enhanced for trait adjectives known to be self-descriptive, even when self-referent judgments are not made at the time of encoding (Kuiper & Rogers, 1979). Moreover, previous research in both nonsocial (Posner & Keele, 1970) and social (Cantor & Mischel, 1977) domains had shown that when subjects study a list of category-relevant words and then receive a memory test, they tend to falsely recognize new category exemplars as if they had been previously studied. This *false alarms effect* is generally interpreted as indicating that subjects routinely abstract categories from related instances that they encounter in experience. Something similar happens with self-relevant material. After subjects study a list of trait adjectives, they are more likely to falsely recognize new items that are self-descriptive than new items that are not self-descriptive (Rogers et al., 1979). In retrospect, this latter result can be viewed as a foreshadowing of the associative memory illusion (Roediger & McDermott, 1994), in which (for example) subjects who study a list of words associatively related to the word *needle* tend to falsely remember that word as having been studied as well. In any case, increases in both accurate and false memory for self-descriptive words, even when subjects do not make self-descriptive judgments at the time of encoding, suggests that self-relevant knowledge information is stored as such in memory.

Priming and Self-Referent Processing

Over the past decade, considerable research on the self has employed a *priming* paradigm (Meyer & Schvaneveldt, 1971) to address the question of how episodic knowledge of one's past behaviors and experiences and semantic memory for one's traits and other psychosocial characteristics can be represented in memory (Klein & Loftus, 1993a, 1993b). In associative network models of memory, information retrieval begins by activating nodes that represent cues (available in the environment or generated through thought); activation then spreads to associated nodes in the network. These nodes then remain activated for some period of time. So long as some level of activation persists, the information represented at that node is easier to retrieve and employ in ongoing cognitive tasks. This phenomenon is called "priming." So, for example, in a lexical identification task (in which the task is to determine whether a presented item is a legal word), prior presentation of the associatively related word "bread" makes it easier to judge that "butter" is a legal English word. In this way, the results of priming experiments can serve as a basis for inferring the underlying structure of memory. If "bread" primes "butter" but "nurse" does not, we can infer that "bread" and "butter" are associatively linked but that "nurse" and "butter" are not.

In a series of experiments, Klein and his colleagues have used a priming methodology to determine the underlying structure of the mental representation of self in memory (e.g., Klein & Loftus, 1993a). In a typical experiment of this sort, subjects are presented with trait words and asked to answer one of three questions: how the word is defined, whether the word describes themselves, and whether they can recall an incident in which they displayed trait-relevant behavior. For each trait term, two questions are asked in sequence: "describe" followed

by "recall," "define" followed by "recall," and "recall" followed by "describe." There are also control conditions in which each task is repeated. The initial trial of each task constitutes a further control condition in which there is no priming. If the hierarchical model is correct, asking people questions about their traits should facilitate their answers to questions about their behaviors (because activation has to pass through semantic nodes representing traits before it gets to episodic nodes representing behaviors). If the computational model is correct, asking people questions about their behaviors should facilitate their answers to questions about their traits (because nodes representing trait-relevant behaviors have already been activated). The absence of priming would constitute evidence for the independence model.

Figure 4.3 shows representative results of these experiments (Klein et al., 1989, Experiment 2). When the same task is repeated on two successive trials, there is a significant priming effect, compared with the task performed without any prime. However, there is no priming across tasks. Compared with the neutral definition task, describing oneself as extraverted does not prime the retrieval of extraverted behaviors from memory: This is inconsistent with the hierarchical model. Similarly, and in contrast to the predictions of the computational model, retrieving memories of extraverted behaviors

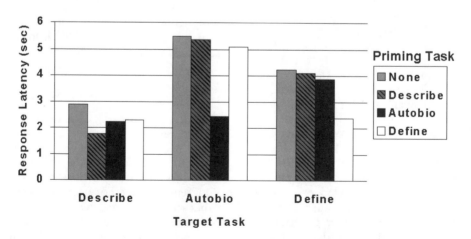

FIGURE 4.3. Priming effects in autobiographical and self-descriptive tasks, after Klein, Loftus, and Burton (1989, Experiment 2).

does not prime the description of oneself as extraverted. The absence of priming of either sort, a null result that has been consistently obtained across a large number of experiments, supports the independence model, in which episodic and semantic knowledge about the self are represented independently of each other. This model, however cumbersome it might seem, is consistent with evidence concerning the representation of other persons in memory (e.g., J. Anderson & Hastie, 1974; Hastie, 1988; Srull, 1981), as well as evidence about the organization of nonsocial knowledge in memory (e.g., J. R. Anderson, 1983).

One potential problem with this line of research is that it depends on the assumption that the "define" task used to establish baselines for priming is truly a control task. If the ostensibly impersonal act of defining a trait nevertheless activates trait-relevant episodic and semantic self-knowledge, then the absence of priming between the episodic and semantic tasks themselves becomes difficult to interpret. Accordingly, a further series of studies employed a control condition in which subjects simply read the words in question without performing any other cognitive operation (Klein, Babey, & Sherman, 1997). There was still no evidence of priming, strengthening the conclusion that items of episodic and semantic self-knowledge are represented independently. A final experiment found a reversed association between the episodic and semantic tasks, depending on the level of trait-descriptiveness—a dissociation that strengthens the inference that the two forms of self-knowledge are, indeed, represented independently.

Additional evidence on the structure of self-knowledge comes from memory experiments employing paradigms other than priming. For example, one study made use of the principle of encoding variability, which states that memory is best for items that are encoded in a number of different ways (Martin, 1968; Postman & Knecht, 1983). In an experiment, subjects encoded items during autobiographical and self-descriptive tasks, alone and in combination (Klein et al., 1989, Experiment 4). Items that were encoded with two different tasks were remembered better than items encoded twice with the same task, again suggesting that autobiographical memory and self-

description are two different ways of processing.

According to the encoding specificity principle (Tulving & Thomson, 1973), information is best remembered if the cues present at retrieval match those that were processed at the time of encoding. In one study, trait words encoded during an autobiographical task were better remembered when retrieved in an autobiographical context than in a self-descriptive context, whereas items encoded in a self-descriptive context showed the opposite pattern of results (Klein, Loftus, & Plog, 1992). This finding suggests that autobiographical retrieval and self-description are different cognitive tasks.

Interactions between Episodic and Semantic Self-Knowledge

The priming experiments, as well as studies employing paradigms other than priming, indicate that self-descriptions can be mediated by retrieval of semantic self-knowledge from semantic memory and need not be computed from information retrieved from episodic memory (e.g., Babey, Queller, & Klein, 1998; Klein et al., 1997; Klein, Loftus, & Sherman, 1993; Klein, Loftus, Trafton, & Fuhrman, 1992; Klein, Sherman, & Loftus, 1996; Schell, Klein, & Babey, 1996; Sherman & Klein, 1994). This is not to say, however, that episodic and semantic self-knowledge never interact. We know from the person memory literature that semantic memory for an individual's personality traits can affect the encoding and retrieval of episodic memory for that person's actions and experiences (Hastie, 1980, 1981; Hastie & Kumar, 1979; Srull, 1981). There is no reason to think that the situation is any different when the person represented in memory is oneself.

Moreover, episodic memory for behavioral exceptions can qualify self-descriptions retrieved from semantic memory. A person may generally think of him- or herself as extraverted, and this characteristic may be encoded in semantic memory as part of his or her self-concept, but a person who can remember engaging in some introverted behaviors may describe himself as less extraverted than one who cannot. In fact, research employing a variant on the priming paradigm indicates that self-descriptive processing will prime the retrieval of trait-*inconsistent* episodes, even if (as the earlier studies consistently showed) there is no priming of trait-*consistent* episodes (Babey et al., 1998; Klein, Cosmides, Tooby, & Chance, 2001). These results are consistent with a model of self-description in which subjects retrieve both summary information in semantic memory and episodic memories that are inconsistent with that summary (Klein, Cosmides, Tooby, & Chance, 2002). In this way, episodic memories constrain the scope of generalizations that people make about themselves.

The Self in Relation to Others

The research described thus far considers the mental representation of the self to be a single, monolithic entity, existing in isolation from mental representations of other people. However, this is probably not the case. Because we identify ourselves partly in terms of kinship and other interpersonal relations and group memberships, other people must form a substantial part of our self-concept (Markus & Cross, 1990; Ogilvie & Ashmore, 1991). It is known, for example, that we endorse traits in ourselves more quickly if they are also characteristic of our marital partners (Aron, Aron, Tudor, & Nelson, 1991; E. R. Smith, Coats, & Walling, 1999; E. R. Smith & Henry, 1996), or if they are also characteristic of groups of which we are members (E. R. Smith et al., 1999; E. R. Smith & Henry, 1996). Based on findings such as these, E. R. Smith and colleagues have developed a connectionist model of social memory in which activation spreads reciprocally between semantic-memory nodes representing oneself, one's partner, or other significant others, including groups. If self and partner possess the same trait, activation is increased at both self and partner nodes, facilitating both self- and other-judgments (E. R. Smith et al., 1999). As the closeness of the relationship decreases, indexed by diminishing the weight on the link between self and other nodes, the degree of self–other priming will also decrease.

Other people also play a role in defining the situations that distinguish one context-specific mental representation of self from another. In an extension of the priming paradigm employed by Klein and Loftus (e.g., Klein & Loftus, 1993a), a series of studies has examined episodic and semantic self-knowledge within various close relationships (Beer & Kihlstrom, 2001). In one study, for example, college students were presented with a set of interpersonal trait terms. For the priming task, they were asked to remember an incident in which they displayed each trait with their fathers, their mothers, or their romantic partners; a fourth condition, in which they simply defined the trait, served as a control. For the target task, they were asked whether the trait was characteristic of them when they were with their fathers, mothers, or romantic partners. Representative results are depicted in Figure 4.4. For self-with-mother and self-with-father, the first experiment revealed no priming from the episodic to the semantic task, in line with the results of Klein and Loftus (1993a; Panel A). For self-with-partner, however, there was a significant priming effect. The priming effect for self-with-partner was replicated in a second study (Figure 4.4, Panel B). However, no such priming occurred in tasks involving the self-with-best friend. The subjects in these studies being lower division college students, on average, their relationships with their best friends had been going on longer than their relationships with their romantic partners. The pattern of results suggests that the structure of the relational self may change over time. The mental representation of self in long-term relationships, whether with one's parents or with one's romantic partner, appear to be characterized by independent representations of episodic and semantic self-knowledge. For relationships with a shorter time course, however, relational self-knowledge may be organized in a more interdependent fashion.

Although the Beer and Kihlstrom (2001) studies focused on priming *within* each relational self, they also provided evidence about the relations *between* the context-specific mental representations of self. In addition to the episodic self-with-partner task, the semantic self-with-partner task was also preceded by the episodic self-with-mother and self-with-father tasks. When these two conditions were combined to create an aggregate "self-with-parents" condition, there

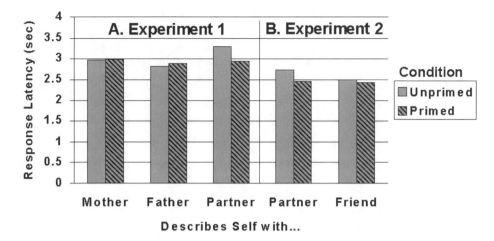

FIGURE 4.4. Priming effects in the relational self, after Beer and Kihlstrom (2001). (A) Self-with-mother, self-with-father, and self-with-romantic-partner (Experiment 1); (B) Self-with-romantic-partner and self-with-best friend (Experiment 2).

was no evidence of priming the mental representation of self-with-partner. Later studies in the series suggested that knowledge of self-with-partner is dependent on episodic information, whereas knowledge of self-with-parents and self-with-best friend is dependent on semantic information. On the surface, at least, the independence between mental relationships of self-with-parents and of self-with-partner would appear to be inconsistent with some forms of adult attachment theory, which suggest that mental representations of self-with-parents serve to filter and structure mental representations of self-with-romantic-partners. Given the ages of the subjects involved in these experiments, however, the critical factor determining the structure of the various mental representations of self may be time spent in the relationship, with the representation becoming more abstract, emphasizing semantic rather than episodic self-knowledge, as the relationship ages.

Neuropsychological Approaches to the Self as Memory

Taking traditional cognitive psychology as a model for the study of social cognition, a great deal has been learned about the mental representation of self from studies of the performance of normal human subjects in laboratory tasks derived from the study of nonsocial cognition. Over the past two decades, however, we have seen the emergence of another, complementary approach to the study of cognition: systematic studies of patients who experience specific cognitive deficits as a result of some insult, injury, or disease to the brain. Experimental studies of amnesia, aphasia, agnosia, and other neurological syndromes have offered a view of the cognitive system in dysfunction that, in turn, has shed light on its normal operations (Ellis & Young, 1988; Gazzaniga, 1999; Gazzaniga, Ivry, & Mangun, 1998; Rapp, 2001). Taking the success of cognitive neuropsychology as a model, Klein and Kihlstrom have argued that neuropsychological studies of brain-injured patients and brain-imaging studies of normal subjects, may provide new solutions to old problems and afford new theoretical insights for personality and social psychologists as well (Klein & Kihlstrom, 1998; Klein, Loftus, & Kihlstrom, 1996).[4]

Studies of Amnesia

Consider, for example, the relation between self and memory. If, as Locke argued, our sense of self and identity is intimately tied up with our recollection of our past, what happens in the case of an amnesic patient? This was, in fact, Bishop Butler's principal objection to Locke's proposal (Butler, 1791). Although the concept of amnesia was not yet prominent in the medical literature,[5] Locke himself anticipated Butler's objection when he imagined what would happen if a prince's mind, with all its memories, would enter a cobbler's body. H.M., the famous patient with the amnesic syndrome, cannot consciously remember anything that he did or experienced since the surgery that destroyed the hippocampus and other structures of his medial temporal lobes, but he still knows who he is. Of course, H.M.'s amnesia is primarily anterograde in nature, and his identity and sense of self would be maintained by whatever memories he retained from before his surgery. This is fine, so far as it goes, but H.M.'s surgery occurred when he was a young man, and he is aware that he is now much older (Hilts, 1995; Ogden & Corkin, 1991). When he looks in the mirror in the morning, he doesn't think, "Who the hell are you?"

Writing in the early 18th century, Locke did not fully appreciate the distinction between episodic and semantic memory. Although new knowledge is acquired through experience, the knowledge acquired through learning is not incorrigibly linked to a mental representation of the learning episode. We now know that amnesia reflects a specific failure of episodic memory that leaves the patient's semantic memory intact. Amnesic patients are unable to remember events from their lives, but they retain the ability to retrieve generic knowledge about themselves and the world around them (Schacter & Tulving, 1982). Moreover, amnesic patients retain some ability to learn new facts (Schacter, 1987), and this preserved function may permit their identities to be based on "updated" semantic self-knowledge, even if they are lacking a complete record of autobiographical memory. If episodic and semantic self-knowledge are represented independently, as seems to be the case from the research of Klein and Loftus (1993), then even a densely amnesic patient could preserve some sense of identity based on semantic self-knowledge.

The first attempt to address this hypothesis empirically employed patient K.C., who suffered a severe head injury as a result of a motorcycle accident (Tulving, 1993).[6] K.C. is especially interesting because he may be the most densely amnesic patient ever studied: whereas most other amnesics have at least some premorbid memory, K.C. has both a complete anterograde amnesia covering events since his accident and a complete retrograde amnesia covering his life before that time. Put another way, K.C. has no autobiographical memory at all. Moreover, the same accident that caused his amnesia also resulted in a profound personality change, from quite extraverted to rather introverted. Because of his amnesia, K.C. has no idea what he used to be like, as described by his mother; nor does he have any idea how he has changed. Nevertheless, he possesses a self-concept that accurately reflects his changed personality and comports fairly well with his mother's description of him. K.C. has acquired new semantic knowledge about himself, but he has not retained the experiences on which this self-knowledge is based; and his newly acquired self-knowledge has effectively replaced the knowledge he possessed before the accident.

Similar results were obtained by Klein and his colleagues in a study of W.J., a college freshman who suffered a temporary retrograde amnesia covering the period since her high school graduation as a result of a concussive blow to the head (Klein, Loftus, & Kihlstrom, 1996). Asked to describe herself while she was amnesic, W.J. showed a good appreciation of how she had changed since matriculating, as corroborated both by her boyfriend's ratings of her and her own self-ratings after her memory was restored. Findings such as these lend strength to the conclusion, based on experimental studies of priming, that semantic (trait) knowledge of the self is encoded independently of episodic (behavioral) knowledge.

Another patient studied by Klein and his colleagues yielded similar results: patient D.B., a 79-year-old man who was rendered profoundly amnesic as the result of a stroke (Klein, Cosmides, Costabile, & Mei, 2001; Klein, Loftus, & Kihlstrom, in press). Like Tulving's patient K.C., D.B. was apparently unable to recollect a single episode from any period in his life, either before or after the accident. Nevertheless, like K.C. and W.J., he was able to make reliable and valid ratings of his own personality characteristics. Interestingly, D.B. is also unable to imagine what his life might be like in the future, although he retained the capacity to predict future events in the public domain. Perhaps our ability to anticipate our futures is tied to our ability to consciously reflect on our pasts (Atance & O'Neill, 2001; Tulving, 1985, 1999). Patient M.L., who sustained a severe retrograde amnesia but little anterograde amnesia following a traumatic brain injury that affected the ventral portions of the right frontal cortex, has difficulty formulating goals and executing plans to achieve them, suggesting that impairments in self-regulation may be linked to impairments in episodic self-knowledge (Levine et al., 1998).

At the very least, these neuropsychological studies offer further evidence favoring the independence of episodic and semantic self-knowledge revealed by the priming experiments described earlier. In those studies, the independence model won by default after the failure of priming to occur in either direction eliminated the organizational and computational models from competition. In the neuropsychological studies, the performance of amnesic patients on self-description tasks consistently provides positive support for the independent-trace model.

Beyond Amnesia

Given Locke's ideas about the relationship between identity and memory, amnesia is an obvious place to begin a neuropsychological study of self-knowledge; but other clinical syndromes also promise to reveal important aspects of self-knowledge. In particular, in the syndrome known as anosognosia, patients appear to be unaware of their own cognitive deficits (McGlynn & Schacter, 1989; see also Prigatano & Schacter, 1991). Anosognosia is frequently observed in cases of hemiplegia resulting from frontal-lobe damage, although it can also occur in association with other syndromes resulting from damage to other locations. It is a genuine disruption in self-awareness, distinct from indifference and defensive denial. Because it can be attached to so many different neurological disorders but is not necessarily a characteristic of any of them, anosognosia may prove to be a specific deficit in self-awareness that offers a unique opportunity to confront issues pertaining to the mental representation of the self (Kihlstrom & Tobias, 1991).

Also potentially relevant to the self is a group of syndromes known collectively as the pervasive developmental disorders, including infantile autism, Asperger's disorder, and Williams syndrome. Although autism originally received its name because patients were generally withdrawn from the environment, it is now recognized that at least some forms of the disorder represent specific deficits in social as opposed to nonsocial cognition. Although the neurological basis of autism is unknown at present, it seems possible that autistic individuals have suffered damage to one or more brain modules or systems associated with understanding other people and relating self to others (e.g., Baron-Cohen, 1995; Frith & Frith, 1999; Happe, 1999).

Although experimental studies of autistic individuals have focused on their impaired understanding of other people, it may be that at least some forms of autism also involve impaired understanding of self. For example, a recent study of patient R.J., a 21-year-old autistic male, revealed that he, like the amnesic patients described previously, has a severe deficit in autobiographical memory (Klein, Chan, & Loftus, 1999). Nevertheless, he was able to make personality self-ratings that were both reliable (in terms of stability across testing sessions) and valid (compared with ratings of him made by his mother and by one of his teachers). This dissociation, like the one observed in amnesic patients, constitutes further evidence that episodic and semantic self-knowledge are stored independently. Moreover, R.J.'s spared semantic knowledge of self contrasts with his impaired semantic knowledge of other domains, including inanimate objects, animals, and food (Klein, Cosmides, Tooby, & Chance, 2001). If it should prove that R.J.'s semantic knowledge of other persons is also impaired, such evidence might suggest that there is a specific brain module for mediating self-knowledge whose operations are dissociable from whatever modules underlie knowledge of other people.

The idea is not far-fetched. For example, since the time of Phineas Gage, who, the phrenologists claimed, suffered damage to the lobes of veneration and benevolence, the frontal lobes have been implicated in social behavior (see also Damasio et al., 1994;

Macmillan, 1986, 2000), but they may be implicated in self-awareness, as well as self-regulation. Freeman and Watts (1942), the pioneering psychosurgeons, noted that "the greatest change induced in the individual by operation upon the frontal lobes is in the intimate relationship of the self with the self" (p. 5). More recent clinical and experimental studies indicate that patients with damage to the frontal lobes, and particularly the orbitofrontal cortex, appear to experience profound disruptions in self-reflection and other meta-cognitive functions (Stuss, 1991a, 1991b).

In addition, the central characteristic of frontotemporal dementia, resulting from degeneration of the prefrontal and anterior temporal regions, entails a severe impairment in the self-regulation of social behavior (Brun et al., 1994). Based on such observations, some neurologists are beginning to refer to the orbitofrontal lobes, amygdala, and anterior temporal lobes as a "social brain"—a module or system that regulates various aspects of social behavior (Miller, Hou, Goldberg, & Mena, 1999). Although formal neuropsychological research on these structures has focused primarily on aspects of social behavior, studies of self-knowledge and other aspects of social intelligence (Cantor & Kihlstrom, 1987; Kihlstrom & Cantor, 2000) may help define "social dementia" in cognitive terms (Perry et al., 2001).

Brain Imaging Studies

If indeed there are brain structures that constitute a module or system for maintaining a sense of self, these might be "visible," in a sense, using advanced brain-imaging techniques such as positron emission tomography (PET) or functional magnetic resonance imaging (fMRI). In fact, a recent study used PET to image the brain while subjects rated themselves on a list of trait adjectives (Craik et al., 1999). As comparison tasks, subjects rated the prime minister of Canada on the same traits; they also judged the social desirability of each trait and the number of syllables in each word. One analytic technique, known as statistical parametric mapping, indicated that the self-rating, other-rating, and desirability-rating tasks invoked the same areas of the brain—sites in the left

frontal cortex known to be associated with semantic processing. However, another analytic technique, known as a partial least-squares analysis, revealed activations of the right and left medial frontal lobe (Brodmann's Areas 9 and 10), the right middle frontal gyrus (BA 10), and the inferior frontal gyrus (BA 45). This provocative study, taken together with the evidence from the autistic patient R.J., suggests that different social-cognitive brain systems might well underlie self-knowledge and knowledge of others.

Another recent study used fMRI to image the brain while subjects viewed morphed pictures of their own faces (compared with an unfamiliar face) or when they read trait adjectives that were or were not self-descriptive (Kircher et al., 2000, 2001). Both tasks activated the left fusiform gyrus, whereas the face task also activated the right limbic and left prefrontal areas, and the trait task activated the left superior parietal area, anterior cingulate, and putamen. A subsequent study (Kircher et al., 2001) of facial self-perception also implicated the right limbic system and left prefrontal cortex, as well as the left superior temporal cortex.

The Self in Mind and Brain

Although these pioneering studies are provocative and interesting, it is probably too early to conclude that the self is located in the right cerebral hemisphere. Although cognitive neuroscience has generally embraced a doctrine of modularity, the neural representation of individual items of declarative knowledge is distributed widely across the cerebral cortex. Accordingly, whereas self-referent processing may be performed by a specialized brain module or system, declarative knowledge of the self—whether episodic or semantic—is likely to be widely distributed over the same neural structures that represent knowledge of other people, as well as objects in the nonsocial domain.

Brain imaging is not the royal road to the self, not least because interpretation of images of the functioning brain requires that we already have an adequate psychological theory of the task the subject is performing—a theory that can only be based on

studies of human performance. Nevertheless, neuropsychological and brain-imaging
research has offered cognitive psychologists
new perspectives on enduring problems.
This should be no less true for social and
personality psychologists seeking to understand the structure of self-knowledge in
memory and other problems of social cognition.

focus attention on the experiences, thoughts,
and actions of the individual person rather
than on the structures and functions of neural
systems.
5. The American physician (and signer of the Declaration of Independence) Benjamin Rush referred to amnesia in 1786, and Korsakoff first
described his eponymous syndrome in 1889.
6. K.C. is also sometimes referred to as patient
N.N. (Tulving, 1985).

Acknowledgments

The point of view represented in this chapter is based on research supported by Grant No. MH-35856 from the National Institute of Mental Health, a National Research Service
Predoctoral Fellowship from the National Science Foundation, and Academic Senate Research Grants from the University of California, Santa Barbara.

Notes

1. A software system, known as PERSPACE, has
been designed to elicit such information idiographically and (by means of cluster analysis)
produce a graphical portrayal of the relations
among an individual's context-specific selves
(Kihlstrom & Cunningham, 1991; Kihlstrom
& Olsen, 1992). For example, a subject
known as Adele (Kihlstrom, Marchese-Foster,
& Klein, 1997) evinced no less than seven different situationally specific self-concepts.
Adele's self-with-her husband was closely related to her "ideal self" (as defined by Higgins, 1987), and as far, psychometrically,
from her self-with-former-significant-other as
it was possible to be. Interestingly, however,
this latter self-concept was closely related to
both Adele's "actual self" and her "ought
self" (Higgins, 1987).
2. One exception is Epstein (1973).
3. For an early anticipation of this approach, see
Mancuso and Ceely (1980).
4. For the record, our proposal (Klein &
Kihlstrom, 1998; Klein et al., 1996) was inspired, in part, by Jackendoff's proposal that
certain aspects of social cognition might be
regulated by dedicated brain modules (Jackendoff, 1992; Jackendoff, 1994). Proper reference to Jackendoff's work was unaccount-
ably omitted from our paper, and we wish to
correct that error now. In the meantime, our
proposal has been echoed by a call for the development of a social-cognitive neuroscience
(e.g., Adolphs, 1999; Ochsner & Lieberman,
2001). Although the term "neuroscience" has
a certain appealing cachet, our use of the term
"neuropsychology" was intended to firmly

References

Adolphs, R. (1999). Social cognition and the human brain.
Trends in Cognitive Sciences, 3(12), 469–479.
Allport, G. W. (1937). *Personality: A psychological inter-
pretation.* New York: Holt, Rinehart & Winston.
Allport, G. W. (1961). *Pattern and growth in personality.*
New York: Holt, Rinehart & Winston.
Anderson, J., & Hastie, R. (1974). Individuation and refer-
ence in memory: Proper names and definite descriptions.
Cognitive Psychology, 6, 495–514.
Anderson, J. R. (1974). Retrieval of propositional informa-
tion from long-term memory. *Cognitive Psychology, 6,*
451–474.
Anderson, J. R. (1976). *Language, memory, and thought.*
Hillsdale, NJ: Erlbaum.
Anderson, J. R. (1983). *The architecture of cognition.*
Mahwah, NJ: Erlbaum.
Anderson, J. R. (1993). *Rules of the mind.* Hillsdale, NJ:
Erlbaum.
Anderson, J. R. (1995). *Cognitive psychology and its impli-
cations* (4th ed.). New York: Freeman.
Anderson, J. R., & Lebière, C. (1998). *The atomic compo-
nents of thought.* Mahwah, NJ: Erlbaum.
Anderson, J. R., & Reder, L. M. (1999). The fan effect:
New results and new theories. *Journal of Experimental
Psychology: General, 128*(2), 186–197.
Anderson, N. H. (1968). Likableness ratings of 555 person-
ality-trait words. *Journal of Personality and Social Psy-
chology, 9*(3), 272–279.
Anderson, N. H. (1974). Cognitive algebra: Integration the-
ory applied to social attribution. In L. Berkowitz (Ed.),
Advances in experimental social psychology (Vol. 7, pp.
1–101). New York: Academic Press.
Anderson, N. H. (1981). *Foundations of information integration theory.* New York: Academic Press.
Aron, A., Aron, E. N., Tudor, M., & Nelson, G. (1991).
Close relationships as including other in the self. *Journal of Personality and Social Psychology, 60,* 241–253.
Atance, C. M., & O'Neill, D. K. (2001). Episodic future
thinking. *Trends in Cognitive Sciences, 5*(12), 533–539.
Babey, S. H., Queller, S., & Klein, S. B. (1998). The role of
expectancy-violating behaviors in the representation of
trait knowledge: A summary-plus-exception model of
social memory. *Social Cognition, 16*(3), 287–339.
Bandura, A. (1977). Self-efficacy: Toward a unifying theory of behavioral change. *Psychological Review, 84*(2),
191–215.
Bandura, A. (2000). Self-efficacy: The foundation of
agency. In W. J. Perrig & A. Grob (Eds.), *Control of hu-*

man behavior, mental processes, and consciousness: Essays in honor of the 60th birthday of August Flammer (pp. 17–33). Mahwah, NJ: Erlbaum.

Bargh, J. A. (1984). Automatic and conscious processing of social information. In R. S. Wyer & T. K. Srull (Eds.), Handbook of social cognition (pp. 1–43). Hillsdale, NJ: Erlbaum.

Bargh, J. A. (1989). Conditional automaticity: Varieties of automatic influence in social perception and cognition. In J. S. Uleman & J. A. Bargh (Eds.), Unintended thought (pp. 3–51). New York: Guilford Press.

Bargh, J. A. (1994). The four horsemen of automaticity: Awareness, intention, efficiency, and control in social cognition. In R. S. Wyer & T. K. Srull (Eds.), Handbook of social cognition (pp. 1–40). Hillsdale, NJ: Erlbaum.

Bargh, J. A. (1997). The automaticity of everyday life. In R. S. Wyer (Ed.), Advances in social cognition (Vol. 10, pp. 1–61). Mahwah, NJ: Erlbaum.

Bargh, J. A., & Chartrand, T. L. (1999). The unbearable automaticity of being. American Psychologist, 54(7), 462–479.

Bargh, J. A., & Ferguson, M. J. (2000). Beyond behaviorism: On the automaticity of higher mental processes. Psychological Bulletin, 126(6), 925–945.

Baron-Cohen, S. (1995). Mindblindness: An essay on autism and theory of mind. Cambridge, MA: MIT Press.

Beer, J., & Kihlstrom, J. F. (2001). The relational self: Representations of self-with-others in close relationships. Unpublished manuscript, University of California, Berkeley.

Bem, D. J. (1967). Self-perception: An alternative interpretation of cognitive dissonance phenomena. Psychological Review, 74(3), 183–200.

Bower, G. H. (1970). Organizational factors in memory. Cognitive Psychology, 1, 18–46.

Bower, G. H., & Gilligan, S. G. (1979). Remembering information related to one's self. Journal of Research in Personality, 13, 420–432.

Brun, A., Englund, B., Gustafson, L., Passant, U., Mann, D. M. A., & Neary, D. (1994). Frontal lobe dementia of the Alzheimer's type revisited. Dementia, 4, 126–131.

Burke, P. A., Kraut, R. E., & Dworkin, R. H. (1984). Traits, consistency, and self-schemata: What do our measures measure? Journal of Personality and Social Psychology, 47, 568–579.

Butler, J. (1791). The analogy of religion. London: J. F. & C. Rivington.

Cantor, N., & Kihlstrom, J. F. (1987). Personality and social intelligence. Englewood Cliffs, NJ: Prentice-Hall.

Cantor, N., & Mischel, W. (1977). Traits as prototypes: Effects on recognition memory. Journal of Personality and Social Psychology, 35, 38–48.

Cantor, N., & Mischel, W. (1979). Prototypes in person perception. In L. Berkowitz (Ed.), Advances in experimental social psychology (Vol. 12, pp. 3–52). New York: Academic Press.

Chapman, L. J., Chapman, J. P., & Raulin, M. L. (1978). Body image aberration in schizophrenia. Journal of Abnormal Psychology, 87, 399–407.

Conway, M., & Dewhurst, S. (1995). The self and recollective experiences. Applied Cognitive Psychology, 9, 1–9.

Craik, F. I. M., & Lockhart, R. S. (1972). Levels of processing: A framework for memory research. Journal of Verbal Learning and Verbal Behavior, 11, 671–684.

Craik, F. I. M., Moroz, T. M., Moscovitch, M., Stuss, D. T., Winocur, G., Tulving, E., & Kapur, S. (1999). In search of the self: A positron emission tomography study. Psychological Science, 10(1), 26–34.

Damasio, H., Grabowski, T., Frank, R., Galaburda, A. M., Damasio, A. R., & Macmillan, M. B. (1994). The return of Phineas Gage: Clues about the brain from the skull of a famous patient. Science, 264, 1102–1105.

Douglas, W., & Gibbins, K. (1983). Inadequacy of voice recognition as a demonstration of self-deception. Journal of Personality and Social Psychology, 44(3), 589–592.

Ebbinghaus, H. (1964). Memory: A contribution to experimental psychology. New York: Dover. (Original work published 1885)

Ellis, A. W., & Young, A. W. (1988). Human cognitive neuropsychology Hove, UK: Erlbaum.

Epstein, S. (1973). The self-concept revisited: Or a theory of a theory. American Psychologist, 28, 404–416.

Fallon, A. E., & Rozin, P. (1985). Sex differences in perception of desirable body shape. Journal of Abnormal Psychology, 94, 102–105.

Farah, M. J. (1988). Is visual imagery really visual? Overlooked evidence from neuropsychology. Psychological Review, 95, 307–317.

Farah, M. J., Hammond, K. M., Levine, D. N., & Calvanio, R. (1988). Visual and spatial mental imagery: Dissociable systems of representation. Cognitive Psychology, 20, 439–462.

Fisher, S., & Cleveland, S. E. (1958). Body image and personality. Princeton, NJ: Van Nostrand.

Flavell, J. H. (1979). Metacognition and cognitive monitoring: A new area of cognitive-developmental inquiry. American Psychologist, 34(10), 906–911.

Flavell, J. H. (1999). Cognitive development: Children's knowledge about the mind. Annual Review of Psychology, 50, 21–45.

Freeman, W. J., & Watts, J. (1942). Psychosurgery: Intelligence, emotion, and social behaviour following prefrontal lobotomy for mental disorder. Baltimore: Thomas.

Freud, S. (1963). Introductory lectures on psycho-analysis. In J. Strachey (Ed. & Trans.), The standard edition of the complete psychological works of Sigmund Freud (Vols. 15–16). London: Hogarth Press. (Original work published 1916–1917)

Frith, C. D., & Frith, U. (1999). Interacting minds: A biological basis. Science, 286, 1692–1695.

Gallagher, S. (2000). Philosophical conceptions of the self: Implications for cognitive science. Trends in Cognitive Sciences, 4(1), 14–21.

Gallagher, S., & Shear, J. (Eds.). (1999). Models of the self. London: Imprint Academic.

Gazzaniga, M. S. (1999). The new cognitive neurosciences. Cambridge, MA: MIT Press.

Gazzaniga, M. S., Ivry, R. B., & Mangun, G. R. (1998). Cognitive neuroscience: The biology of the mind. New York: Norton.

Gibbins, K., & Douglas, W. (1985). Voice recognition and self-deception: A reply to Sackeim and Gur. Journal of Personality and Social Psychology, 48(5), 1369–1372.

Gur, R. C., & Sackeim, H. A. (1979). Self-deception: A concept in search of a phenomenon. Journal of Personality and Social Psychology, 37(2), 147–169.

Hamilton, D. L., Katz, L. B., & Leirer, V. O. (1980). Organizational processes in impression formation. In R. Hastie, T. M. Ostrom, E. B. Ebbesen, R. S. Wyer, D. L. Hamilton, & D. E. Carlston (Eds.), *Person memory: The cognitive basis of social perception* (pp. 121–153). Hillsdale, NJ: Erlbaum.

Hampson, S. E. (1982). Person memory: A semantic category model of personality traits. *British Journal of Psychology, 73*, 1–11.

Happe, F. (1999). Autism: Cognitive deficit or cognitive style. *Trends in Cognitive Sciences, 3*(6), 216–222.

Hastie, R. (1980). Memory for behavioral information that confirms or contradicts a personality impression. In R. Hastie, T. M. Ostrom, E. B. Ebbesen, R. S. Wyer, D. L. Hamilton, & D. E. Carlston (Eds.), *Person memory: The cognitive basis of social perception* (pp. 155–177). Hillsdale, NJ: Erlbaum.

Hastie, R. (1981). Schematic principles in human memory. In E. T. Higgins, C. P. Herman, & M. P. Zanna (Eds.), *Social cognition: The Ontario Symposium* (Vol. 1, pp. 39–88). Hillsdale, NJ: Erlbaum.

Hastie, R. (1988). A computer simulation model of person memory. *Journal of Experimental Social Psychology, 24*, 423–447.

Hastie, R., & Carlston, D. (1980). Theoretical issues in person memory. In R. Hastie, T. M. Ostrom, E. B. Ebbesen, R. S. Wyer, D. L. Hamilton, & D. E. Carlston (Eds.), *Person memory: The cognitive basis of social perception* (pp. 1–53). Hillsdale, NJ: Erlbaum.

Hastie, R., & Kumar, P. A. (1979). Person memory: Personality traits as organizing principles in memory for behaviors. *Journal of Personality and Social Psychology, 37*, 25–38.

Head, H. (1926). *Aphasia and kindred disorders of speech.* Cambridge, UK: University Press.

Higgins, E. T. (1987). Self-discrepancy: A theory relating self and affect. *Psychological Review, 94*, 319–340.

Hilts, P. J. (1995). *Memory's ghost: The strange tale of Mr. M and the nature of memory.* New York: Simon & Schuster.

Hirshman, E., & Lanning, K. (1999). Is there a special association between self judgments and conscious recollection? *Applied Cognitive Psychology, 13*, 29–42.

Jackendoff, R. (1992). Is there a faculty of social cognition? In R. Jackendoff (Ed.), *Languages of the mind: Essays on mental representation* (pp. 19–31). Cambridge, MA: MIT Press.

Jackendoff, R. S. (1994). Social organization. In R. S. Jackendoff (Ed.), *Patterns in the mind: Language and human nature* (pp. 204–222). New York: Basic Books.

James, W. (1980). *Principles of psychology.* Cambridge, MA: Harvard University Press. (Original work published 1890)

Keenan, J. M., & Baillet, S. D. (1980). Memory for personally and socially significant events. In R. S. Nickerson (Ed.), *Attention and performance* (Vol. 8, pp. 651–659). Hillsdale, NJ: Erlbaum.

Kihlstrom, J. F. (1987). The cognitive unconscious. *Science, 237*(4821), 1445–1452.

Kihlstrom, J. F. (1997). Consciousness and me-ness. In J. D. Cohen & J. W. Schooler (Eds.), *Scientific approaches to consciousness* (pp. 451–468). Mahwah, NJ: Erlbaum.

Kihlstrom, J. F. (2001). Dissociative disorders. In P. B. Sutker & H. E. Adams (Eds.), *Comprehensive handbook of psychopathology* (3rd ed., pp. 259–276). New York: Plenum.

Kihlstrom, J. F., & Cantor, N. (1984). Mental representations of the self. In L. Berkowitz (Ed.), *Advances in experimental social psychology* (Vol. 17, pp. 1–47). New York: Academic Press.

Kihlstrom, J. F., & Cantor, N. (2000). Social intelligence. In R. J. Sternberg (Ed.), *Handbook of intelligence* (pp. 359–379). New York: Cambridge University Press.

Kihlstrom, J. F., Cantor, N., Albright, J. S., Chew, B. R., Klein, S. B., & Niedenthal, P. M. (1988). Information processing and the study of the self. In L. Berkowitz (Ed.), *Advances in experimental social psychology: Vol. 21. Social psychological studies of the self: Perspectives and programs* (pp. 145–178). San Diego, CA: Academic Press.

Kihlstrom, J. F., & Cunningham, R. L. (1991). Mapping interpersonal space. In M. Horowitz (Ed.), *Person schemas and maladaptive interpersonal patterns* (pp. 311–336). Chicago: University of Chicago Press.

Kihlstrom, J. F., & Hastie, R. (1997). Mental representations of persons and personality. In R. Hogan, J. Johnson, & S. Briggs (Eds.), *Handbook of personality psychology* (pp. 711–735). San Diego, CA: Academic Press.

Kihlstrom, J. F., & Klein, S. B. (1994). The self as a knowledge structure. In R. S. Wyer, Jr., & T. K. Srull (Eds.), *Handbook of social cognition: Vol. 1. Basic processes* (2nd ed., pp. 153–208). Hillsdale, NJ: Erlbaum.

Kihlstrom, J. F., Marchese-Foster, L. A., & Klein, S. B. (1997). Situating the self in interpersonal space. In U. Neisser & D. A. Jopling (Eds.), *The conceptual self in context: Culture, experience, self-understanding* (pp. 154–175). New York: Cambridge University Press.

Kihlstrom, J. F., & Olsen, D. (1992). *User manual for the PERSPACE software system, Version 3.5* [Computer software and manual]. Available from http://socrates. berkeley.edu/~kihlstrm/Perspace.htm.

Kihlstrom, J. F., & Tobias, B. A. (1991). Anosognosia, consciousness, and the self. In G. P. Prigatano & D. L. Schacter (Eds.), *Awareness of deficit after brain injury: Clinical and theoretical issues* (pp. 198–222). New York: Oxford University Press.

Kircher, T. T. J., Senior, C., Phillips, M. L., Benson, P. J., Bullmore, E. T., Brammer, M., Simmons, A., Williams, S. C. R., Bartels, M., & David, A. S. (2000). Towards a functional neuroanatomy of self processing: Effects of faces and words. *Cognitive Brain Research, 10*(1–2), 133–144.

Kircher, T. T. J., Senior, C., Phillips, M. L., Rabe-Hesketh, S., Benson, P. J., Bullmore, E. T., Brammer, M., Simmons, A., Bartels, M., & David, A. S. (2001). Recognizing one's own face. *Cognition, 78*(1), B1–B15.

Klein, S. B. (2001). A self to remember: A cognitive neuropsychological perspective on how self creates memory and memory creates self. In C. Sedikides & M. B. Brewer (Eds.), *Individual self, relational self, collective self* (pp. 25–46). Philadelphia: Psychology Press/Taylor & Francis.

Klein, S. B., Babey, S. H., & Sherman, J. W. (1997). The functional independence of trait and behavioral self-knowledge: Methodological considerations and new empirical findings. *Social Cognition, 15*(3), 183–203.

Klein, S. B., Chan, R. L., & Loftus, J. (1999). Independence of episodic and semantic self-knowledge: The case from autism. *Social Cognition, 17,* 413–436.

Klein, S. B., Cosmides, L., Costabile, K. A., & Mei, L. (2001). *Is there something special about the self? A neuropsychological case study.* Unpublished manuscript, University of California, Santa Barbara.

Klein, S. B., Cosmides, L., Tooby, J., & Chance, S. (2001). Priming exceptions: A test of the scope hypothesis in naturalistic trait judgments. *Social Cognition, 19*(4), 443–468.

Klein, S. B., Cosmides, L., Tooby, J., & Chance, S. (in press). Decisions and the evolution of memory: Multiple systems, multiple functions. *Psychological Review.*

Klein, S. B., & Kihlstrom, J. F. (1986). Elaboration, organization, and the self-reference effect in memory. *Journal of Experimental Psychology: General, 115*(1), 26–38.

Klein, S. B., & Kihlstrom, J. F. (1998). On bridging the gap between social–personality psychology and neuropsychology. *Personality and Social Psychology Review, 2*(4), 228–242.

Klein, S. B., & Loftus, J. (1988). The nature of self-referent encoding: The contributions of elaborative and organizational processes. *Journal of Personality and Social Psychology, 55*(1), 5–11.

Klein, S. B., & Loftus, J. (1993a). The mental representation of trait and autobiographical knowledge about the self. In T. K. Srull & R. S. Wyer, Jr. (Eds.), *Advances in social cognition* (Vol. 5, pp. 1–49). Hillsdale, NJ: Erlbaum.

Klein, S. B., & Loftus, J. (1993b). Some lingering self-doubts: Reply to commentaries. In T. K. Srull & R. S. Wyer, Jr. (Eds.), *Advances in social cognition* (Vol. 5, pp. 171–180). Hillsdale, NJ: Erlbaum.

Klein, S. B., Loftus, J., & Burton, H. A. (1989). Two self-reference effects: The importance of distinguishing between self-descriptiveness judgments and autobiographical retrieval in self-referent encoding. *Journal of Personality and Social Psychology, 56*(6), 853–865.

Klein, S. B., Loftus, J., & Kihlstrom, J. F. (1996). Self-knowledge of an amnesic patient: Toward a neuropsychology of personality and social psychology. *Journal of Experimental Psychology: General, 125*(3), 250–260.

Klein, S. B., Loftus, J., & Kihlstrom, J. F. (in press). Memory and temporal experience: The effects of episodic memory loss on an amnesic patient's ability to remember the past and imagine the future. *Social Cognition.*

Klein, S. B., Loftus, J., & Plog, A. E. (1992). Trait judgments about the self: Evidence from the encoding specificity paradigm. *Personality and Social Psychology Bulletin, 18*(6), 730–735.

Klein, S. B., Loftus, J., & Sherman, J. W. (1993). The role of summary and specific behavioral memories in trait judgments about the self. *Personality and Social Psychology Bulletin, 19*(3), 305–311.

Klein, S. B., Loftus, J., Trafton, J. G., & Fuhrman, R. W. (1992). Use of exemplars and abstractions in trait judgments: A model of trait knowledge about the self and others. *Journal of Personality and Social Psychology, 63*(5), 739–753.

Klein, S. B., Sherman, J. W., & Loftus, J. (1996). The role of episodic and semantic memory in the development of trait self-knowledge. *Social Cognition, 14*(4), 277–291.

Kosslyn, S. M. (1980). *Image and mind.* Cambridge, MA: Harvard University Press.

Kosslyn, S. M. (1983). *Ghosts in the mind's machine.* New York: Norton.

Kosslyn, S. M. (1988). Aspects of a cognitive neuroscience of mental imagery. *Science, 240,* 1621–1626.

Kuiper, N. A., & Derry, P. A. (1981). The self as a cognitive prototype: An application to person perception and depression. In N. Cantor & J. F. Kihlstrom (Eds.), *Personality, cognition, and social interaction* (pp. 215–232). Hillsdale, NJ: Erlbaum.

Kuiper, N. A., & Rogers, T. B. (1979). Encoding of personal information: Self-other differences. *Journal of Personality and Social Psychology, 37,* 499–514.

Legerstee, M., Anderson, D., & Schaffer, A. (1998). Five- and eight-month-old infants recognize their faces and voices as familiar and social stimuli. *Child Development, 69*(1), 37–50.

Levine, B., Black, S. E., Cabeza, R., Sinden, M., McIntosh, A. R., Toth, J. P., Tulving, E., & Stuss, D. T. (1998). Episodic memory and the self in a case of isolated retrograde amnesia. *Brain, 121*(10), 1951–1973.

Lewis, C. H., & Anderson, J. R. (1976). Interference with real world knowledge. *Cognitive Psychology, 7,* 311–335.

Macmillan, M. (2000). *An odd kind of fame: Stories of Phineas Gage.* Cambridge, MA: MIT Press.

Macmillan, M. B. (1986). A wonderful journey through skulls and brains: The travels of Mr. Gage's tamping iron. *Brain and Cognition, 5,* 67–107.

Mancuso, J. C., & Ceely, S. G. (1980). The self as memory processing. *Cognitive Therapy and Research, 4,* 1–25.

Mandler, G. (1979). Organization, memory, and memory structures. In C. R. Puff (Ed.), *Memory organization and structure* (pp. 304–319). New York: Academic Press.

Mandler, G., & Dean, P. J. (1969). Seriation: Development of serial order in free recall. *Journal of Experimental Psychology, 81,* 207–215.

Markus, H. (1977). Self-schemata and processing information about the self. *Journal of Personality and Social Psychology, 35,* 63–78.

Markus, H., & Cross, S. (1990). The interpersonal self. In L. A. Pervin (Ed.), *Handbook of personality* (pp. 576–608). New York: Guilford Press.

Martin, E. (1968). Stimulus meaningfulness and paired-associate transfer: An encoding variability hypothesis. *Psychological Review, 75*(5), 421–441.

Mazzoni, G., & Nelson, T. O. (1998). *Metacognition and cognitive neuropsychology: Monitoring and control processes.* Mahwah, NJ: Erlbaum.

McGlynn, S. M., & Schacter, D. L. (1989). Unawareness of deficits in neuropsychological syndromes. *Journal of Clinical and Experimental Neuropsychology, 11,* 143–205.

McGuire, W. J., & McGuire, C. V. (1988). Content and process in the experience of the self. In L. Berkowitz (Ed.), *Advances in experimental social psychology* (Vol. 21, pp. 97–144). San Diego, CA: Academic Press.

The me millennium. (1999, October 17). *New York Times Magazine,* p. 20.

Medin, D. L. (1989). Concepts and conceptual structure. *American Psychologist, 44,* 1469–1481.

Metcalfe, J., & Shimamura, A. P. (1994). *Metacognition: Knowing about knowing.* Cambridge, MA: MIT Press.

Meyer, D. E., & Schvaneveldt, R. W. (1971). Facilitation in recognizing pairs of words: Evidence of a dependence between retrieval operations. *Journal of Experimental Psychology, 90,* 227–234.

Miller, B. L., Hou, C., Goldberg, M., & Mena, I. (1999). Anterior temporal lobes: Social brain. In B. L. Miller & J. L. Cummings (Eds.), *The human frontal lobes: Functions and disorders* (pp. 557–567). New York: Guilford Press.

Mischel, W. (1973). Toward a cognitive social learning reconceptualization of personality. *Psychological Review, 80*(4), 252–253.

Mischel, W., Shoda, Y., & Rodriguez, M. I. (1989). Delay of gratification in children. *Science, 244,* 933–938.

Mita, T. H., Dermer, M., & Knight, J. (1977). Reversed facial images and the mere-exposure hypothesis. *Journal of Personality and Social Psychology, 13,* 89–111.

Nelson, T. O. (1992). *Metacognition: Core readings.* Boston: Allyn & Bacon.

Nelson, T. O. (1996). Consciousness and metacognition. *American Psychologist, 51*(2), 102–116.

Nisbett, R. E., & Wilson, D. S. (1977). Telling more than we can know: Verbal reports on mental processes. *Psychological Review, 84,* 231–253.

Nystedt, L., Smari, J., & Boman, M. (1991). Self-schemata: Ambiguous operationalizations of an important concept. *European Journal of Personality, 5,* 1–14.

Ochsner, K. N., & Lieberman, M. D. (2001). The emergence of social cognitive neuroscience. *American Psychologist, 56*(9), 717–734.

Ogden, J. A., & Corkin, S. (1991). Memories of H. M. In W. C. Abraham, M. Corballis, & K. G. White (Eds.), *Memory mechanisms: A tribute to G. V. Goddard* (pp. 195–215). Hillsdale, NJ: Erlbaum.

Ogilvie, D. M., & Ashmore, R. D. (1991). Self-with-other representation as a unit of analysis in self-concept research. In R. C. Curtis (Ed.), *The relational self: Theoretical convergences in psychoanalysis and social psychology* (pp. 282–314). New York: Guilford Press.

Orbach, J., Traub, A. C., & Olson, R. (1966). Psychophysical studies of body-image: II. Normative data on the adjustable body-distorting mirror. *Archives of General Psychiatry, 14,* 41–47.

Ostrom, T. M., Lingle, J. H., Pryor, J. B., & Geva, N. (1980). Cognitive organization of person impressions. In R. Hastie, T. M. Ostrom, E. B. Ebbesen, R. S. Wyer, D. L. Hamilton, & D. E. Carlston (Eds.), *Person memory: The cognitive basis of social perception* (pp. 55—88). Hillsdale, NJ: Erlbaum.

Paivio, A. (1971). *Imagery and verbal processes.* New York: Holt, Rinehart & Winston.

Paivio, A. (1986). *Mental representations: A dual coding approach.* New York: Oxford University Press.

Perry, R. J., Rosen, H. R., Kramer, J. H., Beer, J. S., Levenson, R. L., & Miller, B. L. (2001). Hemispheric dominance for emotions, empathy and social behaviour: Evidence from right and left handers with frontotemporal dementia. *Neurocase, 7,* 145–160.

Posner, M. I., & Keele, S. W. (1970). Retention of abstract ideas. *Journal of Experimental Psychology, 83,* 304–308.

Postman, L., & Knecht, K. (1983). Encoding variability and retention. *Journal of Verbal Learning and Verbal Behavior, 22*(2), 133–152.

Postman, L., & Underwood, B. J. (1973). Critical issues in interference theory. *Memory and Cognition, 1,* 19–40.

Prigatano, G. P., & Schacter, D. L. (1991). *Awareness of deficit after brain injury: Clinical and theoretical issues.* New York: Oxford University Press.

Rapp, B. (2001). *The handbook of cognitive neuropsychology: What deficits reveal about the human mind.* Philadelphia: Psychology Press.

Reder, L. M. (1996). *Implicit memory and metacognition.* Mahwah, NJ: Erlbaum.

Reder, L. M., & Anderson, J. R. (1980). A partial resolution of the paradox of interference: The role of integrating knowledge. *Cognitive Psychology, 12*(4), 447–472.

Roediger, H. L., & McDermott, K. B. (1994). Creating false memories: Remembering words not presented in lists. *Journal of Experimental Psychology: Learning, Memory, and Cognition, 21,* 803–914.

Rogers, T. B. (1981). A model of the self as an aspect of the human information processing system. In N. Cantor & J. F. Kihlstrom (Eds.), *Personality, cognition, and social interaction* (pp. 193–214). Hillsdale, NJ: Erlbaum.

Rogers, T. B., Kuiper, N. A., & Kirker, W. S. (1977). Self reference and the encoding of personal information. *Journal of Personality and Social Psychology, 35,* 677–688.

Rogers, T. B., Rogers, P. J., & Kuiper, N. A. (1979). Evidence for the self as a cognitive prototype: The "false alarms effect." *Personality and Social Psychology Bulletin, 5,* 53–56.

Rozin, P., & Fallon, A. (1988). Body image, attitudes to weight, and misperceptions of figure preferences of the opposite sex: A comparison of men and women in two generations. *Journal of Abnormal Psychology, 97,* 342–345.

Sackeim, H. A., & Gur, R. C. (1985). Voice recognition and the ontological status of self-deception. *Journal of Personality and Social Psychology, 48*(5), 1365–1368.

Schacter, D. L. (1987). Implicit memory: History and current status. *Journal of Experimental Psychology: Learning, Memory, and Cognition, 13,* 501–518.

Schacter, D. L., & Tulving, E. (1982). Memory, amnesia, and the episodic semantic distinction. In R. L. Isaacson & N. E. Spear (Eds.), *The expression of knowledge* (pp. 33–65). New York: Plenum Press.

Schell, T. L., Klein, S. B., & Babey, S. H. (1996). Testing a hierarchical model of self-knowledge. *Psychological Science, 7*(3), 170–173.

Schilder, P. (1938). *Image and appearance of the human body.* London: Kegan, Paul, Trench, & Tribner.

Shepard, R. N., & Cooper, L. A. (1983). *Mental images and their transformations.* Cambridge, MA: MIT Press.

Sherman, J. W., & Klein, S. B. (1994). Development and representation of personality impressions. *Journal of Personality and Social Psychology, 67*(6), 972–983.

Smith, E. E., Adams, N., & Schorr, D. (1978). Fact retrieval and the paradox of interference. *Cognitive Psychology, 10,* 438–464.

Smith, E. E., & Medin, D. L. (1981). *Categories and concepts.* Cambridge, MA: MIT Press.

Smith, E. R., Coats, S., & Walling, D. (1999). Overlapping mental representations of self, in-group, and partner: Further response time evidence and a connectionist model. *Personality and Social Psychology Bulletin, 25*(7), 873–882.

Smith, E. R., & Henry, S. (1996). An in-group becomes

part of the self: Response time evidence. *Personality and Social Psychology Bulletin, 22,* 635–642.

Srull, T. K. (1981). Person memory: Some tests of associative storage and retrieval models. *Journal of Experimental Psychology: Human Learning and Memory, 7,* 440–463.

Sternberg, S. (1969). The discovery of processing stages: Extensions of Donders' method. In W. G. Koster (Ed.), *Attention and performance II* (Vol. 30, pp. 276–315). Amsterdam: North-Holland.

Stuss, D. T. (1991a). Disturbance of self-awareness after frontal-system damage. In G. Prigatano & D. L. Schacter (Eds.), *Awareness of deficit after brain injury: Clinical and theoretical issues* (pp. 63–83). New York: Oxford University Press.

Stuss, D. T. (1991b). Self, awareness, and the frontal lobes: A neuropsychological perspective. In J. Strauss & G. R. Goethals (Eds.), *The self: Interdisciplinary approaches* (pp. 255–278). New York: Springer-Verlag.

Symons, C. S., & Johnson, B. T. (1997). The self-reference effect in memory: A meta-analysis. *Psychological Bulletin, 121,* 371–394.

Trabasso, T. R., & Riley, C. A. (1975). The construction and use of representations involving linear order. In R. L. Solso (Ed.), *Information processing and cognition* (pp. 381–410). Hillsdale, NJ: Erlbaum.

Traub, A., Olson, R., Orbach, J., & Cardone, S. (1967). Psychophysical studies of body-image. *Archives of General Psychiatry, 17,* 664–670.

Traub, A. C., & Orbach, J. (1964). Psychophysical studies of body-image: I. The adjustable body-distorting mirror. *Archives of General Psychiatry, 11,* 53–66.

Tulving, E. (1983). *Elements of episodic memory.* Oxford, UK: Oxford University Press.

Tulving, E. (1985). Memory and consciousness. *Canadian Psychology, 26*(1), 1–12.

Tulving, E. (1993). Self-knowledge of an amnesic individual is represented abstractly. In T. K. Srull & R. S.

Wyer, Jr. (Eds.), *Advances in socil cognition* (Vol. 5, pp. 147–156). Hillsdale, NJ: Erlbaum.

Tulving, E. (1999). On the uniqueness of episodic memory. In T. K. Srull & R. S. Wyer, Jr. (Eds.), *Cognitive neuroscience of memory* (pp. 11–42). Seattle, WA: Hogrefe & Huber.

Tulving, E., & Thomson, D. M. (1973). Encoding specificity and retrieval processes in episodic memory. *Psychological Review, 80*(5), 359–380.

Williamson, D. A., Davis, C. J., Goreczny, A. J., & Blouin, D. C. (1989). Body-image disturbances in bulimia nervosa: Influences of actual body size. *Journal of Abnormal Psychology, 98,* 97–99.

Wilson, T. D. (1985). Strangers to ourselves: The origins and accuracy of beliefs about one's own mental states. In J. H. Harvey & G. Weary (Eds.), *Attribution: Basic issues and applications* (pp. 9–36). Orlando, FL: Academic Press.

Wilson, T. D., & Stone, J. I. (1985). Limitations of self-knowledge: More on telling more than we can know. In P. Shaver (Ed.), *Review of personality and social psychology* (Vol. 6, pp. 167–183). Beverly Hills, CA: Sage.

Winograd, T. (1972). *Understanding natural language.* New York: Academic Press.

Winograd, T. (1975). Frame representations and the declarative/procedural controversy. In D. Bobrow & A. Collins (Eds.), *Representations and understanding: Essays in cognitive science* (pp. 185–212). New York: Academic Press.

Wyer, R. S., Jr., & Carlston, D. E. (1994). The cognitive representation of persons and events. In R. S. Wyer, Jr., & T. K. Srull (Eds.), *Handbook of social cognition, Vol. 1: Basic processes* (2nd ed., pp. 41–98). Hillsdale, NJ: Erlbaum.

Yarmey, A. D., & Johnson, J. (1982). Evidence for the self as an imaginal prototype. *Journal of Research in Personality, 16,* 238–246.

5

The Reflected Self: Creating Yourself as (You Think) Others See You

DIANNE M. TICE
HARRY M. WALLACE

Denise likes to paint but doesn't think of herself as a very good painter. Because her family often jokes about her paintings, she believes that they don't think she is very good, either. One day Denise's rabbi asks her to paint a mural for the synagogue wall. Denise is surprised when the rabbi tells her, "We all think you are a terrific painter. Your father and sisters brag about you all the time." When Denise realizes that her family and friends think she is a good painter, she changes her view of herself and starts to think of herself as artistically talented.

This example demonstrates the *reflected self*—the idea that people come to see themselves as they believe others see them. Early psychologists and sociologists felt that the self was built on just such reflected appraisals (e.g., Cooley, 1902; James, 1890; Mead, 1934). In keeping with this long tradition, most researchers of the self have acknowledged the importance of social processes in constructing and modifying the self-concept (e.g., Baumeister, 1982, 1986; Goffman, 1959; Gollwitzer, 1986; Rhode-

walt, 1986; Schlenker, 1986; Wicklund & Gollwitzer, 1982).

Symbolic Interactionism and the Looking-Glass Self

As one of the earliest psychologists, William James (1890) set the stage for the idea of a reflected self. He strongly emphasized the social component of the self and maintained that the self was a product and reflection of social life (James, 1890). The idea of a reflected or "looking-glass self" was introduced by C. H. Cooley (1902), who is usually credited as the first symbolic interactionist. Cooley expanded the idea that the self develops in reference to other people in the social environment. He argued that the concept or idea of the "self" cannot be separated from social influences and suggested that the self is built by reflecting the views that others hold of the person. In Cooley's view, the person observes how others view him- or herself, and then incorporates those views into the self-concept. From early childhood, people see themselves in the "looking glass" of others' appraisals and build or constructs a self that is congruent with the appraisals of others. Our self-concepts develop and change by seeing how others respond to us and then incorporating those responses into the self. Cooley recognized that some people's judgments hold more weight than others'; close, important members of our social networks are more likely to elicit an effect on the looking-glass self than are strangers. Cooley felt that three elements are involved in constructing a looking-glass self that reflected the appraisals of the social network. First, one has to imagine how one appears to others; second, one has to imagine how others judge or appraise that appearance; and third, one feels some emotional response to the appraisal, such as pride or shame.

The major theorist of what later became known as symbolic interactionism was George Herbert Mead, who built on Cooley's (1902) work and greatly expanded the idea of the looking-glass self. A major advance introduced by Mead was the idea of a "generalized other" in eliciting a looking-glass effect on the self-concept. People are affected not only by how they think significant others respond to them (as Cooley, 1902, had suggested) but also by how they think their entire social group, in an abstract sense, responds to them. Thus, even if our parents and friends think we are attractive, we may still not see ourselves as attractive if we believe that society at large does not value our physical attributes. The idea of a generalized other in creating a reflected self from a looking-glass process is an important element of Kenny and DePaulo's (1993) analysis of reflected appraisals, which is discussed later.

Goffman (1959) further developed the idea that people actively attempt to create desired impressions or appraisals of themselves in the minds of the social audience. In his view, people behave in a certain way in front of others in order to elicit certain appraisals from them (in his words, to make certain impressions on them). By behaving differently in front of an audience than they might behave in private, people attempt to elicit feedback from others that is consistent with the way they would like others to see them. The use of self-presentations to change

the self-concept is discussed more fully in a later section.

Evaluating the Looking-Glass Self

Social psychologists and other symbolic interactionists have tested many of the ideas of the looking-glass self. In most cases they proceeded by collecting self-views from a person, appraisals (usually ratings or rankings) of that person by others, and/or reflected appraisals, defined as what the person believed others thought of him or her. Often these appraisals were collected from classrooms or families, making it possible to obtain information about many people who knew each other and could rate each other at one time.

Evidence for a Looking-Glass Self

Consistent with the notion of the looking-glass self, Cole (1991) found that both peer appraisals and teacher appraisals affected the self-images of fourth-graders with regard to academic and athletic competence. Peer evaluations also predicted change in self-evaluations of social competence over time. In a follow-up study, Cole, Maxwell, and Martin (1997) found that reflected appraisals were especially likely to be observed if the researchers focused on multiple domains (most researchers focus on competencies in only one domain) and if the researchers took into account the appraisals of multiple important others, such as parents, teachers, and peers. When aggregating across multiple domains and appraisers, these researchers found substantial evidence for the looking-glass self. In other words, perceived and even actual reflected appraisals highly influenced people's self-views.

Bartusch and Matsueda (1996; see also Matsueda, 1992) reported data that supported a symbolic interactionist theory of delinquency. They found evidence for a looking-glass self in adolescents for both males and females, reporting that parental appraisals of young people exert nontrivial effects on the youths' reflected appraisals. Youths who believed that others saw them as rule violators were more likely to engage in delinquent behavior. Believing that others saw them as sociable was also significantly related to delinquency. Those who believed that others saw them as well liked and socially skilled were *more* likely to engage in delinquent behavior (which contradicts the view of delinquents as isolated sociopaths). In another domain, Harter (1993, 1999; see also Harter, Waters, & Whitesell, 1998) found a positive correlation between reflected appraisals and children's self-esteem, especially in context-specific situations.

The imposter phenomenon describes people who think poorly of themselves but believe that others think well of them. If the imposter phenomenon exists, it would suggest that people sometimes perceive positive appraisals by others but fail to incorporate those reflected appraisals into the self-concept. However, Leary, Patton, Orlando, and Funk (2000) found little to no evidence for a real (private) imposter phenomenon, suggesting that people's self-appraisals were consistent with their perceptions of how they believed others perceived them.

The body-image literature also contains suggestive support for the looking-glass self theory of reflected self-appraisal, at least with respect to the evaluative quality of the self's attributes. Pinhey, Rubinstein, and Colfax (1997) found that, in cultures in which thinness was valued, overweight people were significantly less happy than in cultures in which obesity is common and accepted (and even a sign of high status). They found this to be true even when holding constant the effects of ethnicity, age, gender, education, income, employment status, marital status, parenthood, and body mass (see also Ross, 1994). Cioffi (2000) has argued that reflected appraisals are especially salient for stigmatized people. Thus, when a society derogates obesity, the self-concept of obese individuals may be affected in a way that reduces the obese individual's happiness. Specifically, fat people seem to internalize their society's attitude about obesity and in many cases learn to think poorly about themselves and become unhappy because the "generalized other" regards them negatively.

Clients undergoing psychotherapy also may be affected by the reflected appraisals of their therapists. Kelly (2000) found that psychotherapy clients who withhold relevant personal information from their therapists are able to hold more positive self-images and therefore make better therapeutic progress (even after controlling for the clients' initial level of pathology) because they are not hampered by negative perceived appraisals of the therapists. She was not proposing that therapy clients should make a habit of lying to their therapists, but she did conclude that therapeutic progress does depend to some extent on how the client internalizes the view of him or her held by the therapist. Thus some selective manipulation of information so as to sustain the therapist's favorable impression of the client can have value. For present purposes, the important point is that the reflected appraisal (of the client by the therapist) is an important factor in therapy and can help or hinder the client's efforts to change.

Low Self-Esteem and the Looking Glass

Robinson and Harter (1991) studied the effects of the looking-glass self on feelings of self-worth by examining individual differences in how much people endorse the idea that self-worth is based on peer approval. They found that those endorsing the looking-glass-self orientation reported lower self-worth and less approval than those who held the opposite belief, namely that their level of self-worth determines their level of social approval. In other words, people whose self-concepts reflect their beliefs about how they think others view them may have lower self-esteem than people who believe others should judge them based on their beliefs about themselves. In a subsequent study, Harter, Stocker, and Robinson (1996) distinguished between three types of self-worth orientations. In the first, perceived self-worth determines approval from others. In the second, approval from others determines perceived self-worth (the looking-glass-self view of the self-concept). In the last, there is no connection between self-worth and peer approval. Harter and colleagues found that adolescents with looking-glass selves (those who felt that peer approval determines self-worth) were more likely to suffer fluctuations in feelings of self-worth and received lower actual ratings of peer approval (based on evaluations of teachers and peers) than adolescents with a less peer-focused sense of self. Thus the looking-glass self may be somewhat self-defeating, in that children who based their self-worth on the approval of peers were least likely to have the approval of peers and had the lowest feelings of self-worth.

How the Looking Glass Operates (and Fails)

Through the Glass Darkly

One of the first big challenges to the idea of the reflected self was developed by Shrauger and Schoeneman (1979). They reviewed a large body of research findings pertaining to how self-appraisals matched (and failed to match) perceived and actual appraisals by others. Contrary to the main thrust of symbolic interactionist theory, Shrauger and Schoeneman concluded that people's self-perceptions were only weakly and crudely related to how they were regarded by others. In both naturalistic and laboratory settings, little support existed for the view that self-perceptions derived in a clear, straightforward fashion from others' appraisals.

On the positive side, however, Shrauger and Schoeneman (1979) found reasonably strong and close correspondence between self-perceptions and how people *believed* they were regarded by others. This pattern thus partially rehabilitated the symbolic interactionist view, insofar as it fits the idea that self-perceptions can derive from perceived appraisals by others. To be sure, most findings were correlational, so one could not rule out the alternative interpretation that self-appraisals cause people to make false assumptions about how they are viewed by others. That is, people's inferences of how they are appraised by others may be based on their self-views rather than on an accurate understanding of how others actually see them.

Thus the symbolic interactionist theory emerged from Shrauger and Schoeneman's (1979) review battered but not entirely demolished. The original theory suggested that appraisals by others would be discerned by the individual and would then be internalized so as to produce self-appraisals. The second step was supported, even though the first was not. Put another way, people did not seem to perceive accurately how others appraised them, but their (inaccurate) perceptions of the appraisals by others did correspond to self-appraisals. At best, then, people's self-appraisals could well be derived from how they thought others appraised them.

Shrauger and Schoeneman's (1979) research posed the agenda and challenge for further work on reflected appraisals. Two sets of questions were raised. First, why was there such a gap between actual other-appraisals and perceived other-appraisals? Second, what caused the close link between self-appraisals and perceived other-appraisals? Did perceived other-appraisals cause self-appraisals (as symbolic interactionist theory had proposed) or the other way around?

The Role of Self-Views in the Reflected Self

An important year for challenging the idea that self-images are created by reflected appraisals was 1993. Ichiyama (1993) found mixed evidence in support of the reflected-appraisal model with small-group interactions. In this study, self-appraisal, reflected appraisals (what participants think others think of them), and others' actual appraisals of interpersonal behavior were collected at two different points in time. First, Ichiyama found that others' actual appraisals were only moderately linked to self-appraisals and reflected appraisals, consistent with what Shrauger and Schoeneman (1979) had found. Second, Ichiyama provided some support for the symbolic interactionist view by showing that reflected appraisals at time 1 did predict self-appraisals at time 2 (although these effects were generally weak, they were significant for some dimensions), which suggests that people do internalize how they believe others regard them. Third, however, there was strong evidence that self-appraisals influence how people perceive they are regarded by others (reflected appraisals), which is the direction opposite to the symbolic interactionist hypothesis. The broader implication is that reflected appraisals do play some role in shaping the self-concept, but rather than being the passive product of such a process, the individual self actively chooses, shapes, and constructs the reflected appraisal.

In his 1993 review, Felson summarized his extensive body of work casting doubt on the importance of reflected appraisals as a major source of self-image. Based on the work he published throughout the 1980s (e.g., Felson, 1980, 1981, 1989, 1992), Felson (1993) suggested that people's initial self-views are stronger predictors of their subsequent self-views than are reflected appraisals. In a large number of studies, he found that people do not have accurate views of how others see them but rather think that others see them as they see themselves. In short, he too concluded that the main causal influence flows from self-perceptions to perceived other appraisals, contrary to the symbolic interactionist hypothesis.

Also in 1993, Kenny and DePaulo published a very influential paper that reviewed eight studies that employed the social relations model of interaction analysis (Kenny & Albright, 1987) to assess meta-perceptions and meta-accuracy in interpersonal domains. Kenny and DePaulo (1993) defined meta-accuracy as the extent to which people know how others see them, and they defined meta-perceptions (following Laing, Phillipson, & Lee, 1966) as the perceptions that people have about how people view one another. They concluded that meta-perceptions are more influenced by one's own self-conceptions than by the feedback provided by others. In other words, people determine how others view them not from the feedback they receive from others but from their own self-perceptions. People have some image of themselves, and they think others see them as they see themselves.

Kenny and DePaulo's (1993) conclusion is clearly consistent with what Felson (1993) concluded based on his large body of data and with what Ichiyama (1993) was reporting, and in combination these conclusions dealt another blow to the symbolic interactionist position. The part of the theory that was best supported in Shrauger and Schoeneman's (1979) critique—namely, that self-appraisals and perceived other-appraisals are highly correlated—was found to be to due to self-appraisals influencing the perception of appraisals by others, contrary to the view that self-perceptions derive from feedback received from others.

Kenny and DePaulo's (1993) analysis suggested that any given "other-appraisal"—defined as the way a particular other actually views a person—is not very influential on the self-concept because people are not very accurate at ascertaining what particular others think of them. Because people are poor at knowing how specific others actually see them, these specific impressions held by others have little impact on self-concepts. People's accuracy about how others view them varies in a systematic fashion. People are reasonably good at knowing how others in general view them, but they are not very good at knowing how any particular other individual views them.

The social relations approach to studying interpersonal processes offered a valuable tool for sorting the effects of self, specific others, and others in general. The essence of the method (as proposed by Kenny & Albright, 1987) is that a group of individuals have a series of dyadic interactions with each other. Each person interacts with each other one, and the resultant impressions are measured. In that way, one can discriminate between effects of the person (which should be consistent across interactions with different partners), effects of the partner (seen in interactions with other persons), and interactions (effects unique to the combination of person and partner). For example, if Joe forms an impression of Bob as clever, one can ascertain whether this is due to Bob (do other partners find him clever?), to Joe (does Joe think everyone clever?), or their interactive combination (does only Joe think Bob is clever?).

From their review of multiple studies using these methods, Kenny and DePaulo (1993) concluded that people overestimate the degree of consistency between different individuals' perceptions of them. This suggests that people are not basing their estimations of how others view them on the feedback they are given by any particular individual, because they think they are making the same impression on everyone, even if they had very different interactions and feedback with the different observers.

Although people have poor "dyadic meta-accuracy" (the ability to know how one is differentially regarded by particular other people), they do tend to have reasonably good "generalized meta-accuracy" (accuracy in determining how one is generally viewed by others). In other words, people are better at knowing how others generally view them than at knowing how they are uniquely viewed by specific individuals. Kenny and DePaulo (1993) suggested that perhaps this is why people's attempts at self-presentations sometimes go awry: People don't realize what views any particular person actually holds of them. People may be making a bad impression on others without even knowing it, because people often do not know how they are being perceived by specific others.

According to Kenny and DePaulo (1993), people's self-perceptions do not come from their beliefs about how others view them (i.e., their meta-perceptions). Instead, their meta-perceptions follow directly from their self-perceptions. In other words, people directly observe their own behavior and infer from it what others probably think of them. However, people are not totally oblivious to the feedback from others. Kenny and DePaulo suggested that people can achieve some degree of dyadic accuracy in their perceptions of how specific others view them. Occasionally, people do look to others for feedback, and when they do they can catch a glimpse of how others actually do view them.

The Kenny and DePaulo (1993) findings were further supported by Sedikides and Skowronski (1995), who found that, among college students, self-reflection (the self-view generated by focusing on and evaluating the self) was the primary source of self-knowledge, compared with social comparison and reflected appraisals (see also Schoeneman, 1981). Thus, once again, the self actively constructs its view of self rather than learning or internalizing passively the feedback from others.

Another follow-up study conducted by Malloy, Albright, Kenny, Agatstein, and Winquist (1997) examined how people detected appraisals in friends, family, and coworkers. Targets had to nominate three "informants" from each social group (friends, family, and coworkers). Informants in different social groups were not allowed to have met or have been together when observing the target. Results showed that targets were most accurately aware of how they were generally viewed by family members, and they were somewhat accurate about how they were regarded by friends.

Self–other agreement was strongest in the family group and at weaker levels in the friend and coworker groups. Targets believed that members of different social groups perceived them much more similarly then those persons actually perceived them, further supporting the Kenny and DePaulo (1993) analysis.

Not Getting the Message

Why are people so seemingly unaffected by how others appraise them? There are two possibilities: Either they disregard the feedback from others, or they fail to get the message. The latter explanation can be further divided into two possibilities: Either the message is not sent (that is, if people fail to express their views accurately and bluntly), or the person is somehow unable or unwilling to receive it.

The first possibility was addressed in a study by Shechtman and Kenny (1994). They identified a culture, namely Israel, that is generally regarded as favoring a clear, direct, no-nonsense style of communication. The possibility that people politely decline to express their views would therefore be less plausible in an Israeli sample than in an American sample. Schechtman and Kenny reasoned that meta-accuracy (the ability of people to know how others view them) might be better in Israel than in the United States, because of this cultural proclivity for blunt communication. However, the results replicated the findings reviewed by Kenny and DePaulo (1993). Israelis, like Americans, seem to use their own self-perceptions as evidence of how others view them. People of both cultures seem relatively blind to the feedback cues given by others (even when these cues might be more direct, as they are hypothesized to be in Israel). These findings suggest that the chasm between self-appraisals and appraisals by others cannot be blamed on the reticence of others.

Further evidence was provided by Jussim, Soffin, Brown, Ley, and Kohlhepp (1992), who conducted several experiments to test whether feedback influences self-perceptions through a process of internalization of reflected appraisals. Although their results were somewhat conflicting, they found that, when people were fully aware of how others viewed them, their self-perceptions were indeed affected by reflected appraisals. However, if there was insufficient information to know how others view oneself, people may assume that others see them much as they see themselves. When little information about how others view them is available, people project their self-views onto the others rather than changing their self-views based on the appraisals of others, at least partly because they are less aware of those appraisals.

Thus feedback from others can shape the self-concept if it is accurately received, but apparently it is often not received accurately. And the failure to get the message seems to be due more to people's reluctance to receive the message than to other people's willingness to express the feedback. Thus evidence converges on suggesting that people typically manage to avoid or disregard evaluative feedback from others.

That conclusion was supported in an investigation by O'Conner and Dyce (1993), who conducted a study of bar bands in which the band members were asked to rate their own musical ability, the ability of others in the band, and how other members perceived their ability. These authors suggested that the weak link in the looking-glass-self chain is not between actual appraisals and feedback given (thus people do say how they feel about the others) but between feedback given and feedback received, so that people are likely to distort what feedback they were given. Thus it is cognitive distortion on the receiver's part, not communications barriers, that darkened the reflected self in this study.

Summary

Our understanding of reflected appraisals has changed since the early conceptions by the symbolic interactionists. We now know that people do not see clearly through others' minds and eyes how they are viewed by these others, but, as Shrauger and Schoeneman (1979) put it, people see "through the glass darkly." People may see themselves more as they think others see them rather than as others really do see them, because people may not be accurate at knowing how others actually see them. Although people may be aware of how others in general see them, they are not as accurate at knowing

how specific others view them. Thus it is unlikely that their self-images reflect the views specific others hold of them. However, because people do know how they are viewed by others in general, their self-images may reflect the views their generalized social world holds of them.

The looking glass may be even darker than Shrauger and Schoeneman (1979) thought, however. Shrauger and Schoeneman (1979) recognized that people did not see themselves exactly as others saw them, but rather as they thought others saw them and that the perception of how others saw one was open to a great deal of cognitive distortion. In addition, people's own self-images may play a large role in how they see themselves. Kenny and DePaulo (1993) and Felson (1993) demonstrated that much of the distortion comes from self-views already held by the individual. People hold certain conceptions of themselves, and they think that others must see them in much the same way as they see themselves. Thus the reflected self, as perceived by the individual, often reinforces the individual's original view of himself or herself (Swann, 1987, 1990, 1996; Swann, De La Ronde, & Hixon, 1994; Swann & Ely, 1984; Swann & Hill, 1982; Swann, Stein-Seroussi, & Giesler, 1992). If a person holds a particular view of himself or herself as athletic, for example, he or she is likely to believe that others see him or her as athletic as well. (In a later section, we discuss how holding such a self-view can influence self-presentation and therefore reflect back on the self-image.) The reflected self is likely to be reflected through a biased prism of the person's own self-image and through the way the person believes that others see him or her.

Internalization and Self-Presentation

It is apparent from the preceding sections that people do not just view themselves as others actually see them but rather view themselves as they think others see them. In addition, self-views can influence the way people think others see them (through biased processing). In this section, we discuss an additional component of the reflected appraisal process: the role of self-presentations. Self-views can solidify themselves in a circular process by changing the way one is viewed by others (or at least the way one thinks others see him or her) through self-presentations and public behaviors. People often hold views of themselves that they attempt to communicate to others through self-presentations and public behaviors (see Schlenker, Chapter 25, this volume). People may (accurately or inaccurately) perceive reflected appraisals by others because they have actively tried to present themselves in a given manner. They assume that others view them as they believe they have presented themselves.

Other factors (besides self-views) that affect self-presentations can likewise affect the self-concept through the reflected appraisal process. Presenting oneself in an aggressive manner in order to avoid being taken advantage of, for instance, may lead a person to believe that others see him or her as aggressive. This perceived appraisal following the self-presentation may lead to a more aggressive self-concept (see Rhodewalt, 1998; Tice, 1998). Presenting oneself as depressed to a psychotherapist may likewise lead a person to come to feel and act more depressed (Kelly, 2000).

Cognitive Models of Self-Concept Change

The term "internalization" refers to changes in the self-concept that follow from overt behavior (Tice, 1992). Internalization is a matter of bringing one's private concept of self into agreement with one's recent behavior (e.g., Festinger & Carlsmith, 1959), changing the self-view as a result of public behavior. The public behavior may lead the actor to perceive an appraisal by the audience, and the perceived appraisal may be reflected in the self-concept.

Self-perception theory (Bem, 1972) suggests that this internalization occurs because people look to their behavior (which would certainly include self-presentations) to infer their attitudes and traits, especially when the self-presentations are not incompatible with their prior self-views or when the individuals are uncertain about their self-views on that dimension. Jones, Rhodewalt, Berglas, and Skelton (1981) and Fazio, Effrein, and Falender (1981) updated this self-perception view to add the cognitive dimension of biased scanning to the

process. According to the biased scanning understanding of internalization, when people self-present, they search their memories for information that is consistent with their self-presentation. This memory search makes some information salient in conscious awareness, and this salience leads to a shift in the self-view. Fazio and colleagues found that responding to situational constraints, such as answering loaded questions that pulled for introverted or extraverted responses, affected their participants' self-concepts. That is, when their participants were subsequently asked to rate themselves on an introversion–extraversion dimension, they rated themselves along the lines of their recent (induced) self-presentations. In fact, participants even behaved in a manner consistent with their presentations when they did not know they were being observed. Participants who had presented themselves as extraverts in response to the loaded questions sat closer to a confederate and talked to her more than participants who had presented themselves as introverts. Fazio and colleagues proposed that the loaded questions had produced a biased search of memory, thereby producing information consistent with one or the other view of self, and that the information from this biased memory search had in turn influenced the subsequent self-ratings and actual behavior. In an important sense, the individuals had been induced to present themselves in a certain way and had then "internalized" their behavior; the inner cognitive processes mediated the internalization.

Jones and colleagues (1981) and Rhodewalt and Agustsdottir (1986) also reported that induced behavior led to self-concept shifts so as to reflect an internalization of the overt behavior, and they suggested two cognitive mechanisms for these self-concept shifts. If one had been induced to behave in a manner inconsistent with one's beliefs about oneself, cognitive dissonance resulted. The dissonance resulting from the atypical behavior was reduced by changing the beliefs about the self. However, if one was induced to behave in a manner that was not inconsistent with one's self-views, biased scanning occurred. The induced behavior directed attention toward certain aspects of the self-concept, and so self-evaluations shifted in the direction of the salient cognitions. For example, an individual who just presented himself or herself positively to an audience was described as having more positive than negative information about the self immediately accessible in memory (Jones et al., 1981).

Similarly, Markus and Kunda (1986) induced participants to label themselves as "very unique" or "very similar to others." Subsequently, participants' self-concepts were subtly affected by the label. Markus and Kunda suggested that these effects resulted from a change in the accessibility of the self-conceptions.

The Interpersonal Dimension

What does biased scanning have to do with the reflected self? Subsequent follow-up work (Schlenker, Dlugolecki, & Doherty, 1994; Tice, 1992) to the biased scanning studies demonstrated that having an audience was crucial to the internalization of the behavior. In other words, only when people perceived that their self-presentation affected another's appraisal of them did the self-view change.

A set of studies by Tice (1992) attested to the importance of public circumstances and interpersonal contexts for producing self-concept change. In two experiments, identical behaviors produced consistently stronger impact on the self-concept when they had been performed publicly rather than privately. Public circumstances were operationally defined as the potential presence and knowledge of someone else; that is, people answered the same loaded questions either anonymously (for a tape recording) or to a live other person. Public behaviors led to substantial shifts in self-descriptions and even to consistent behavioral change found on unobtrusive measures in subsequent situations. In contrast, the same behaviors had little or no apparent impact on the self-concept when they were performed in a private, anonymous context. Internalization of behavior in the public conditions was robust, unlike the effects in the private conditions. Thus self-concept change appeared to occur only when participants believed the self-presentation was reflected in another person's appraisal of the participant.

In the first study (Tice, 1992), participants were induced to portray themselves in either an emotionally responsive or emotionally stable manner (or in an irrelevant manner in control conditions). The self-portrayals were either made in public, under highly identifiable conditions, or in private, under relatively anonymous conditions. Identical behaviors had greater impact on the self-concept when performed publicly rather than privately. That is, the first experiment indicated that the self-concept is more likely to change by internalizing public behavior than by internalizing behavior that is identical but lacks the interpersonal context of reflected appraisals. Using different self-portrayals, a second study replicated the findings of the first study and demonstrated that the self-concept change extends even to behavioral changes and even when participants are unaware of being observed.

Schlenker and colleagues (1994) likewise found that public, interpersonal behavior led to self-concept change and behavioral changes through a reflected appraisal process. They found that people who presented themselves as sociable to an interviewer demonstrated self-concept changes reflecting increased ratings in sociability and behavioral changes reflecting an increase in sociable behavior (such as speaking sooner, more frequently, and longer than people who had not presented themselves as sociable). Schlenker and colleagues also found that public commitment to the identity portrayed in the self-presentation was the crucial antecedent of changes in the self-concept; biased self-perceptions were not sufficient to produce the changes. Directing participants' thoughts toward congruent or incongruent prior experiences (thereby affecting the biased scanning of relevant information) also had no impact on self-concept changes. Changes in self-concept were produced only when participants had a public commitment to the behavior, including the perceived reflected appraisals of an audience. In addition, Schlenker and his colleagues have demonstrated that a key part of the internalization process involves the actor's performing self-presentations that he or she perceives are believable, accurate, and defensible representations of the self (Schlenker, 1986; Schlenker & Trudeau,

1990; Schlenker & Weingold, 1992; see also Swann, 1987, 1996; Swann & Ely, 1984; Swann & Hill, 1982).

Summary

Thus public, interpersonal behavior or public commitment to an identity appears to be very influential in affecting self-concept change. If one can change the public image of self first, the private self will follow along (as will behavior). Only when self-presentations are believed to be reflected in an audience's appraisals will the self-presenter change his or her self-image. Self-presentations and public behavior are one way in which actors create reflected selves that they themselves perceive. When the actors perceive reflected appraisals from the audience as a result of their self-presentations, these perceptions can affect the self-image. People may actively try to create desired selves through a self-presentational–reflected-self process. In other words, people may try to present themselves in an ideal manner (a presentation that is consistent with the ideal self) and may thereby come to see themselves as more similar to their ideal selves because they perceive (accurately or inaccurately) a reflection of their ideal selves in the eyes of others.

The Reflected Self in Close Relationships

The role of the reflected self in creating a self-concept may be stronger in closer relationships than in casual, less intimate relationships (see Tice, Butler, Muraven, & Stillwell, 1995). People are most accurate at knowing how they are appraised by close, intimate others (Malloy et al., 1997). De-Paulo, Kashy, Kinkendol, Wyer, and Epstein (1996) found a positive correlation between degree of closeness and frequency of social interaction, suggesting that people spend more time with those they know better and are closer to than with strangers. To the extent that self-concepts are shaped by internalization processes from social interactions, a high frequency of social interactions would result in a high amount of opportunity to shape the self-concept. Thus there is some reason to suspect that close others

may influence the self-concept through reflected appraisals more than casual acquaintances do (cf. Hensley, 1996).

Intimate Couples

Murray, Holmes, and Griffin (1996) followed dating partners over the course of a year and found considerable evidence for the looking-glass self. They found that the more the participants' partners idealized the participants, the more the participants came to have positive changes in their self-concept. Thus, when participants saw an idealized version of themselves reflected in their partners' appraisals of them, the participants changed their self-views to be more consistent with the partners' appraisals. When the participants knew that their partners held them in high regard, participants felt even more secure in their own sense of self-worth as these romances developed. According to Murray and colleagues, this increase in feelings of self-worth might then have allowed individuals to see their partners in an even more positive or generous light (because of the role of positive self-regard in fostering illusions). The authors suggested that this reciprocal process of mutual affirmation and reaffirmation could be the keystone for lasting satisfaction and security in romantic relationships.

In subsequent followups to the Murray and colleagues (1996) study, Murray, Holmes, and Griffin (2000) found that the reflected-self process was moderated by trait self-esteem. Participants with high self-esteem were more accurate at knowing how their partners felt about them. Participants with high self-esteem correctly believed that their partners saw them positively, whereas participants with low self-esteem incorrectly believed that their partners saw them relatively negatively. (These patterns suggest once again that a person's initial self-views end up exerting an influence on how the person believes that others regard him or her, as we emphasized earlier.) Murray, Holmes, MacDonald, and Ellsworth (1998) replicated the Murray and colleagues (1996) findings demonstrating the looking-glass self in relationships, and these authors also found that the effect was moderated by self-esteem. Participants with low self-esteem reacted to self-doubts (even self-doubts created by esteem-boosting feedback) by doubting their partners' regard for them, which then led them to have a lowered view of their partners (the contamination effect). In contrast, participants with high self-esteem reacted to self-doubts by becoming more convinced of their partners' high regard and continued acceptance. Participants with high self-esteem thus were able to use their relationships as a resource of support. Participants with low self-esteem seemed to react to self-doubt and consequent fears of rejection by diminishing the value of the very resource—a close interpersonal relationship—that they might have relied on as a source of comfort. Thus the symbolic interactionist view of the reflected self in close relationships was better supported for people with high self-esteem than for people with low self-esteem, because people with low self-esteem were less accurate in judging how their partners saw them. For people with high self-esteem, there was no discrepancy between self-views and the views of the partner, so self-views did not interfere with the reflection process, and a looking-glass-self process described the findings quite well. For people with low self-esteem, self-views were inconsistent with the appraisals of their partners, and their relatively negative self-views seemed to interfere with an accurate reading of their partners' appraisals.

Murray and Holmes (2000) further developed these ideas of a reflected self construed in intimate relationships, and they provided additional longitudinal support for the looking-glass self and for the idea that it is perceptions of how one is viewed, not how one is actually viewed, that drive the self-concept change. Their findings suggested that self models are constructed and anchored in a top-down fashion, incorporating images in the looking glass that are themselves distorted by existing levels of self-esteem.

In an interesting and influential article, Drigotas, Rusbult, Wieselquist, and Whitton (1999) introduced the concept of the Michelangelo phenomenon. The Michelangelo phenomenon is the means by which the self is shaped by a close partner's behavior. Drigotas and colleagues described the process whereby a loving partner's positive views of the target are consistent with the target's ideal self. When the target perceives that the partner views the target person the way the target person ideally likes to be seen, the target comes to act more like the ideal self, consistent with the way the partner views the target. Specifically, a person's movement toward the ideal self was described as a product of partner affirmation, or the degree to which a partner's perceptions of the target person and behavior toward the target person are congruent with the target person's ideal self. When the reflected appraisals of partners reflect the ideal self of the target person, the target comes to see himself or herself as more similar to his or her ideal self. Close partners sculpt one another to bring each person closer to his or her ideal self.

There are three steps to the Michelangelo phenomenon. Drigotas and colleagues (1999) referred to the first step as "partner perceptual affirmation," in which one holds views of one's partner that are in line with the partner's ideal self. For example, Mark holds beliefs about Kathy that are close to the way she would ideally like to be. Drigotas and colleagues referred to the second step as "partner behavioral affirmation," in which one behaves in a way that brings out the best in one's partner. For example, Mark elicits behaviors from Kathy that are highly congruent with Kathy's ideal self. The third step was called "self movement toward the ideal self," in which the partner comes to view himself or herself more in line with the ideal self, due to self-perception of the ideal self-behaviors she or he has been exhibiting. For example, Kathy increasingly comes to see herself as the person she ideally wishes to be because she has been behaving more like her ideal self.

Drigotas and colleagues (1999) suggested two other possible relationships between a partner's perceptions and the ideal self. Disaffirmation can also occur; for example, Mark may hold beliefs and behave in a manner that leads Kathy to stray from her ideal self. Partner perceptions may also be irrelevant to the ideal self. However, in many cases the reflected self may be strongly affected through the Michelangelo phenomenon.

Other research also supported the revised view of the reflected self in relationships, in which people's self-views affect their perceptions of others' appraisals and people are affected more by their perceptions of others' appraisals than by the others' actual appraisals because they tend to be inaccurate at reading specific others' appraisals. Aron, Paris, and Aron (1995) suggested that falling in love might be particularly influential on the self because it would likely involve the three conditions that Tice (1992) found to create greatest self-concept change: high choice, self-reference, and the expectation of future interaction with the observer. Aron and colleagues reported that participants who fell in love showed greater self-concept change and greater diversity of self-concept than participants who did not fall in love, supporting a reflected self-change in the self-image. Cast, Stets, and Burke (1999) examined the reflected self in new marriages and found that people of equal and higher status influence the self views of their partners more than people of lower status. Thus the status of the appraiser may be relevant to the reflected self.

Self-verification findings also provided some support for the revised reflection process in close relationships (see Swann, Rentfrow, & Guinn, Chapter 18, this volume). Swann, Hixon, and De La Ronde (1992) found that people with negative self-views were more committed to their spouses when they felt their spouses appraised them unfavorably. In contrast, people with positive self-views were more committed to those they felt appraised them positively. Pelham and Swann (1994) found that the relations between participants' self-views and the appraisals they received from their partners was especially strong for self-views that participants held with greater certainty (and was weak for participants' least certain self-views).

Other Close Relationships

McNulty and Swann (1994) found that self-views were influenced by students' roommates' appraisals and perceptions of those appraisals (either positive or negative appraisals) as the semester progressed. In addition to the looking-glass self, self-verification also occurred. Typically, dyads showed evidence of either appraisal or self-verification effects, not both.

Cook and Douglas (1998) used Kenny's (e.g., Kenny & Albright, 1987; Kenny, Bond, Mohr, & Horn, 1996) social relations model to investigate the accuracy of adolescents' and college students' perceptions of how they are viewed by their parents. They found that how young people think of themselves tends to be related to how they think they are perceived by their parents but that young people do not have an accurate perception of how they are perceived by their parents.

Thus close relationships and intimate others seem to provide an importance source of input for the reflected self. Turner and Onorato (1999), however, disagreed that close others are really separate from the self. They asserted that reflected appraisals have an impact on the self only when the appraising others are members of an ingroup; outgroup reflected appraisals should be rejected. Because ingroup others are part of the "collective self," it is inappropriate, in their view, to think of ingroup members as "others." If the people providing the looking-glass self are really other (that is, excluded from the working self of the perceiver), they can tell people only what they are not, through comparison and contrast. Defining what the self is not is not the same as an acquisition of self through a process of reflection and influence. Thus, Turner and Onorato dismissed the idea that intimates can create a reflected self because of the way they defined the self (including others in the collective self). However, Hensley (1996) suggested a curvilinear relationship between closeness and the impact of appraisals. In this view, casual acquaintances and friends provide the least distorted reflection of oneself. Strangers have the most distortion (due to lack of information), and intimates have a moderately distorted reflection of oneself (due to subjectivity and desire to protect oneself from harsh truths).

Summary

Close relationships are especially likely to affect the reflected self. The opinions of close others matter most to us, so our perceptions of how those close others view us have a significant impact on our self-concepts. If romantic partners view you in an idealized fashion, you may be able to move closer to those ideals and become more like your ideal selves. People with high self-esteem may be more likely than people with low self-esteem to move in the direction of partner ideals and thus exhibit the looking-glass self because their self-views are not inconsistent with idealized partner views. Self-verification may be found in relationships in which partners' idealized views were inconsistent with self-views.

Conclusions

The symbolic interactionist view of the reflected self may have been a bit simplified. The idea that people look through the minds and eyes of others and come to view themselves as others view them has not been totally supported. Instead, a revised view of the looking-glass self seems to have the most empirical support. People tend to hold certain views of themselves, and these views can bias their perceptions of how others view them. It is people's perceptions of how they are viewed, not how they are actually viewed by others, that have the strongest impact on people's self-concepts. People's perceptions of how they are viewed are strongly influenced by their own, prior beliefs about themselves.

People's self-presentations can also influence their self-concepts. People attempt to influence others' perceptions of them by behaving in certain ways in public, but these impression management strategies have significant effects on people's own self-views. People come to view themselves in a manner consistent with their public self-presentations.

Close, intimate relationships with important others are especially likely to create a looking-glass self. The views people believe their significant others hold of them come to be reflected in the people's own views of themselves. To the extent that partners hold idealized beliefs about the person, the person may move toward an ideal self.

Acknowledgments

The preparation of this chapter was supported by Grant No. MH-57039 from the National Institutes of Health.

References

Aron, A., Paris, M., & Aron, E. N. (1995). Falling in love: Prospective studies of self-concept change. *Journal of Personality and Social Psychology, 69,* 1102–1112.

Bartusch, D. J., & Matsueda, R. L. (1996). Gender, reflected appraisals, and labeling: A cross-group test of an interactionist theory of delinquency. *Social Forces, 75,* 145–177.

Baumeister, R. F. (1982). A self-presentational view of social phenomena. *Psychological Bulletin, 91,* 3–26.

Baumeister, R. F. (1986). *Identity: Cultural change and the struggle for self.* New York: Oxford University Press.

Bem, D. J. (1972). Self-perception theory. In L. Berkowitz (Ed.), *Advances in experimental social psychology* (Vol. 6, pp. 1–62). New York: Academic Press.

Cast, A. D., Stets, J. E., & Burke, P. J. (1999). Does the self conform to the views of others? *Social Psychology Quarterly, 62,* 68–82.

Cioffi, D. (2000). The looking-glass self revisited: Behavior choice and self-perception in the social token. In T. F. Heatherton, R. E. Kleck, M. R. Hebl, & J. G. Hull (Eds.), *The social psychology of stigma* (pp. 184–219). New York: Guilford Press.

Cole, D. A. (1991). Change in self-perceived competence as a function of peer and teacher evaluation. *Developmental Psychology, 27,* 682–688.

Cole, D. A., Maxwell, S. E., & Martin, J. M. (1997). Reflected self-appraisals: Strength and structure of the relation of teacher, peer, and parent ratings to children's self-perceived competencies. *Journal of Educational Psychology, 89,* 55–70.

Cook, W. L., & Douglas, E. M. (1998). The looking-glass self in family context: A social relations analysis. *Journal of Family Psychology, 12,* 299–309.

Cooley, C. H. (1902). *Human nature and the social order.* New York: Scribner's.

DePaulo, B. M., Kashy, D. A., Kinkendol, S. E., Wyer, M. M., & Epstein, J. A. (1996). Lying in everyday life. *Journal of Personality and Social Psychology, 70,* 979–995.

Drigotas, S. M., Rusbult, C. E., Wieselquist, J., & Whitton, S. W. (1999). Close partner as sculptor of the ideal self: Behavioral affirmation and the Michelangelo phenomenon. *Journal of Personality and Social Psychology, 77,* 293–323.

Fazio, R. H., Effrein, E. A., & Falender, V. J. (1981). Self-perceptions following social interactions. *Journal of Personality and Social Psychology, 41,* 232–242.

Felson, R. B. (1980). Communication barriers and the reflected appraisal process. *Social Psychology Quarterly, 43,* 116–126.

Felson, R. B. (1981). Ambiguity and bias in the self-concept. *Social Psychology Quarterly, 44,* 64–69.

Felson, R. B. (1989). Parents and reflected appraisal process: A longitudinal analysis. *Journal of Personality and Social Psychology, 56,* 965–971.

Felson, R. B. (1992). Coming to see ourselves: Social sources of self-appraisals. *Advances in Group Processes, 9,* 185–205.

Felson, R. B. (1993). The (somewhat) social self: How others affect self-appraisals. In J. Suls (Ed.), *The self in so-

cial perspective (Vol. 4, pp. 1–26). Hillsdale, NJ: Erlbaum.

Festinger, L., & Carlsmith, J. M. (1959). Cognitive consequences of forced compliance. *Journal of Abnormal and Social Psychology, 58,* 203–210.

Goffman, E. (1959). *The presentation of self in everyday life.* New York: Anchor Books.

Gollwitzer, P. M. (1986). Striving for specific identities: The social reality of self-symbolizing. In R. F. Baumeister (Ed.), *Public self and private self* (pp. 143–159). New York: Springer-Verlag.

Harter, S. (1993). Causes and consequences of low self-esteem in children and adolescents. In R. F. Baumeister (Ed.), *Self-esteem: The puzzle of low self-regard* (pp. 87–116). New York: Plenum Press.

Harter, S. (1999). *The construction of the self: A developmental perspective.* New York: Guilford Press.

Harter, S., Stocker, C., & Robinson, N. S. (1996). The perceived directionality of the link between approval and self-worth: The liabilities of a looking-glass self-orientation among young adolescents. *Journal of Research on Adolescence, 6,* 285–308.

Harter, S., Waters, P., & Whitesell, N. R. (1998). Relational self-worth: Differences in perceived worth as a person across interpersonal contexts among adolescents. *Child Development, 69,* 756–766.

Hensley, W. E. (1996). A theory of the valenced other: The intersection of the looking-glass-self and social penetration. *Social Behavior and Personality, 24,* 293–308.

Ichiyama, M. A. (1993). The reflected appraisal process in small-group interaction. *Social Psychology Quarterly, 56,* 87–99.

James, W. (1890). *The principles of psychology.* New York: Holt.

Jones, E. E., Rhodewalt, F., Berglas, S., & Skelton, J. A. (1981). Effects of strategic self-presentation on subsequent self-esteem. *Journal of Personality and Social Psychology, 41,* 407–421.

Jussim, L., Soffin, S., Brown, R., Ley, J., & Kohlhepp, K. (1992). Understanding reactions to feedback by integrating ideas from symbolic interactionism and cognitive evaluation theory. *Journal of Personality and Social Psychology, 62,* 402–421.

Kelly, A. E. (2000). Helping construct desirable identities: A self-presentational view of psychotherapy. *Psychological Bulletin, 126,* 475–494.

Kenny, D. A., & Albright, L. (1987). Accuracy in interpersonal perception: A social relations analysis. *Psychological Bulletin, 102,* 390–402.

Kenny, D. A., Bond, C. F., Mohr, C. D., & Horn, E. M. (1996). Do we know how much people like one another? *Journal of Personality and Social Psychology, 71,* 928–936.

Kenny, D. A., & DePaulo, B. M. (1993). Do people know how others view them? An empirical and theoretical account. *Psychological Bulletin, 114,* 145–161.

Laing, R. D., Phillipson, H., & Lee, A. R. (1966). *Interpersonal perception: A theory and method of research.* New York: Springer.

Leary, M. R., Patton, K. M., Orlando, A. E., & Funk, W. W. (2000). The imposter phenomenon: Self-perceptions, reflected appraisals, and interpersonal strategies. *Journal of Personality, 68,* 725–756.

Malloy, T. E., Albright, L., Kenny, D. A., Agatstein, F., &

Winquist, L. (1997). Interpersonal perception and metaperception in nonoverlapping social groups. *Journal of Personality and Social Psychology, 72,* 390–398.

Markus, H., & Kunda, Z. (1986). Stability and malleability of the self-concept. *Journal of Personality and Social Psychology, 51,* 858–866.

Matsueda, R. L. (1992). Reflected appraisals, parental labeling, and delinquent behavior: Specifying a symbolic interactionist theory. *American Journal of Sociology, 97,* 1577–1611.

McNulty, S. E., & Swann, W. B., Jr. (1994). Identity negotiation in roommate relationships: The self as architect and consequence of social reality. *Journal of Personality and Social Psychology, 67,* 1012–1023.

Mead, G. H. (1934). *Mind, self, and society.* Chicago: University of Chicago Press.

Murray, S. L., & Holmes, J. G. (2000). Seeing the self through a partner's eyes: Why self-doubts turn into relationship insecurities. In A. Tesser, R. B. Felson, & J. M. Suls (Eds.), *Psychological perspectives on self and identity* (pp. 173–197). Washington, DC: American Psychological Association.

Murray, S. L., Holmes, J. G., & Griffin, D. W. (1996). The self-fulfilling nature of positive illusions in romantic relationships: Love is not blind, but prescient. *Journal of Personality and Social Psychology, 71,* 1155–1180.

Murray, S. L., Holmes, J. G., & Griffin, D. W. (2000). Self-esteem and the quest for felt security: How perceived regard regulates attachment processes. *Journal of Personality and Social Psychology, 78,* 478–498.

Murray, S. L., Holmes, J. G., MacDonald, G., & Ellsworth, P. C. (1998). Through the looking glass darkly? When self-doubts turn into relationship insecurities. *Journal of Personality and Social Psychology, 75,* 1459–1480.

O'Conner, B. P., & Dyce, J. (1993). Appraisals of musical ability in bar bands: Identifying the weak link in the looking-glass-self chain. *Basic and Applied Social Psychology, 14,* 69–86.

Pelham, B. W., & Swann, W. B., Jr. (1994). The juncture of intrapersonal and interpersonal knowledge: Self-certainty and interpersonal congruence. *Personality and Social Psychology Bulletin, 20,* 349–357.

Pinhey, T. K., Rubinstein, D. H., & Colfax, R. S. (1997). Overweight and happiness: The reflected self-appraisal hypothesis reconsidered. *Social Science Quarterly, 78,* 747–755.

Rhodewalt, F. (1986). Self-presentation and the phenomenal self: On the stability and malleability of the self-concept. In R. F. Baumeister (Ed.), *Public self and private self* (pp. 117–142). New York: Springer-Verlag.

Rhodewalt, F. (1998). Self-presentation and the phenomenal self: The "carry-over effect" revisited. In J. Cooper & J. M. Darley (Eds.), *The legacy of Edward E. Jones* (pp. 409–421). Washington, DC: American Psychological Association.

Rhodewalt, F., & Agustsdottir, S. (1986). Effects on self-presentation on the phenomenal self. *Journal of Personality and Social Psychology, 50,* 47–55.

Robinson, N. S., & Harter, S. (1991, April). *Which comes first from the adolescent's point of view: Approval from others or liking oneself?* Paper presented at the meetings of the Society for Research in Child Development, Seattle, WA.

Ross, C. E. (1994). Overweight and depression. *Journal of Health and Social Behavior, 35,* 63–78.

Schlenker, B. R (1986). Self-identification: Toward an integration of the public and private self. In R. F. Baumeister (Ed.), *Public self and private self* (pp. 21–62). New York: Springer-Verlag.

Schlenker, B. R., Dlugolecki, D. W., & Doherty, K. (1994). The impact of self-presentations on self-appraisals and behavior: The power of public commitment. *Personality and Social Psychology Bulletin, 20,* 20–33.

Schlenker, B. R., & Trudeau, J. V. (1990). Impacts of self-presentations on private self-beliefs: Effects of prior self-beliefs and misattribution. *Journal of Personality and Social Psychology, 58,* 22–32.

Schlenker, B. R., & Weingold, M. F. (1992). Interpersonal processes involving impression regulation and management. *Annual Review of Psychology, 43,* 133–168.

Schoeneman, T. J. (1981). Reports of the sources of self-knowledge. *Journal of Personality, 49,* 284–294.

Sedikides, C., & Skowronski, J. J. (1995). On the sources of self-knowledge: The perceived primacy of self-reflection. *Journal of Social and Clinical Psychology, 14,* 244–270.

Shechtman, Z., & Kenny, D. A. (1994). Metaperception accuracy: An Israeli study. *Basic and Applied Social Psychology, 15,* 451–465.

Shrauger, J. S., & Schoeneman, T. J. (1979). Symbolic interactionist view of self-concept: Through the looking glass darkly. *Psychological Bulletin, 86,* 549–573.

Swann, W. B., Jr. (1987). Identity negotiation: Where two roads meet. *Journal of Personality and Social Psychology, 53,* 1038–1051.

Swann, W. B., Jr. (1990). To be adored or to be known: The interplay of self-enhancement and self-verification. In R. M. Sorrentino & E. T. Higgins (Eds.), *Handbook of motivation and cognition: Foundations of social behavior* (Vol. 2, pp. 408–448). New York: Guilford Press.

Swann, W. B., Jr. (1996). *Self-traps: The elusive quest for higher self-esteem.* New York: Freeman.

Swann, W. B., Jr., De La Ronde, C., & Hixon, J. G. (1994). Authenticity and positivity strivings in marriage and courtship. *Journal of Personality and Social Psychology, 66,* 857–869.

Swann, W. B., Jr., & Ely, R. J. (1984). A battle of wills: Self-verification versus behavioral confirmation. *Journal of Personality and Social Psychology, 46,* 1287–1302.

Swann, W. B., Jr., & Hill, C. A. (1982). When our identities are mistaken: Reaffirming self-conceptions through social interaction. *Journal of Personality and Social Psychology, 43,* 59–66.

Swann, W. B., Jr., Hixon, J. G., & De La Ronde, C. (1992). Embracing the bitter "truth": Negative self-concepts and marital commitment. *Psychological Science, 3,* 118–121.

Swann, W. B., Jr., Stein-Seroussi, A., & Giesler, R. B. (1992). Why people self-verify. *Journal of Personality and Social Psychology, 62,* 392–401.

Tice, D. M. (1992). Self-presentation and self-concept change: The looking-glass self is also a magnifying glass. *Journal of Personality and Social Psychology, 63,* 435–451.

Tice, D. M. (1998). Effects of self-presentation depend on the audience. In J. Cooper & J. M. Darley (Eds.), *The legacy of Edward E. Jones* (pp. 409–421). Washington, DC: American Psychological Association.

Tice, D. M., Butler, J. L., Muraven, M. B., & Stillwell, A. M. (1995). When modesty prevails: Differential favorability of self-presentation to friends and strangers. *Journal of Personality and Social Psychology, 69,* 1120–1138.

Turner, J. C., & Onorato, R. S. (1999). Social identity, personality, and the self-concept: A self-categorization perspective. In T. R. Tyler, R. M. Kramer, & O. P. John (Eds.), *The psychology of the social self* (pp. 11–46). Mahwah, NJ: Erlbaum.

Wicklund, R. A., & Gollwitzer, P. M. (1982). *Symbolic self-completion.* Hillsdale, NJ: Erlbaum.

6

Stability and Variability in Self-Concept and Self-Esteem

MICHAEL H. KERNIS
BRIAN M. GOLDMAN

Our focus in this chapter is on stability and variability in self-concept and self-esteem. Self-concept and self-esteem are components of the self-system, which also includes psychological needs and motives, and they are influenced by contextual factors such as feedback, the presence of others, and role salience. We begin with a discussion of self-concept stability and variability. As will be seen, this literature emphasizes general processes that presumably affect most people, and it is less concerned with individual differences per se. In contrast, the self-esteem literature emphasizes individual differences in stability and variability, the psychological implications of these individual differences, and the factors that promote them.

Self-Concept

Markus and Wurf (1987) describe the self-concept as consisting of multiple representations that vary in (1) their centrality or importance; (2) whether they reflect actual or potential achievements; (3) their temporal orientation—that is, past, present, or future;

and (4) their positivity or negativity. Moreover, they assert that this multifaceted self-concept has both components that are relatively stable (i.e., core self-conceptions) and those that are more malleable and contextually based (i.e., working self-concept). Self-aspects can be added to, or subtracted from, people's core conceptions as people acquire self-knowledge through sources such as social comparisons, performance feedback, adoption of new roles, physical maturation, and so forth. The working self-concept consists of a subset of one's core self-conceptions that is accessible at any given point in time. Other terms that have been used to refer to how people are thinking about themselves at any moment include the "phenomenal self" (Jones & Gerard, 1967), the "spontaneous self" (McGuire & McGuire, 1981, 1988), and "current self-appraisals" (Kernis & Johnson, 1990). How people think about themselves at any given moment is affected by such things as the immediate context, mood states, goals, cognitive priming, and so forth (for discussions, see Brown, 1998; Hoyle, Kernis, Leary, & Baldwin, 1999). Unfortunately, the distinction between the working self-concept and one's core self-concept is too often blurred in research examining self-concept variability. Whenever possible, we state explicitly to which aspect of the self theory and research findings pertain.

Our understanding of the self-concept is that it reflects how people think about themselves, that is, the content of their self-representations. This content may be purely descriptive in nature or it may have evaluative aspects that we term self-appraisals (e.g., "stupid," "unfriendly," "creative"). Most self-representations will have an evaluative component to them, as people are especially prone to attach positive and negative values to their self-aspects. Nonetheless, we believe that such self-appraisals more properly belong in the domain of self-concept rather than self-esteem. In a later section, we focus on self-esteem, which we take to reflect global feelings of self-worth, liking, and acceptance (see also Brown, 1993). Considerable research supports maintaining a distinction between global self-esteem and specific self-appraisals (for a review, see Brown, 1993). Although specific self-appraisals are predictive of global self-esteem, particularly if they are central to a person's self-definition (Kernis, Cornell, Sun, Berry, & Harlow, 1993, Study 2; Pelham, 1995), it is clear that combining them into a summary score (with or without weighting for importance or centrality) cannot substitute for global self-esteem or even serve as its proxy. For one thing, using specific self-appraisals to predict global self-esteem leaves unaccounted substantial self-esteem variance (Pelham, 1995). For another, specific self-appraisals are more closely related to cognitive than to affective reactions to performance outcomes, whereas the reverse is true for global self-esteem (Dutton & Brown, 1997). Finally, there are individual differences in the extent to which specific self-appraisals predict global self-esteem that are important in their own right (Crocker & Wolfe, 2001; Kernis et al., 1993, Study 2). In sum, we think that it is important to maintain the distinction between self-appraisals and self-esteem and to conceptualize self-appraisals as part of the self-concept that may or may not relate to global self-esteem.

We turn now to a review of the major theories and research findings that pertain to short-term changes or malleability in the self-concept. First, we focus on several of the most important factors that can produce these short-term changes. Next, we discuss theory and research pertaining to factors that promote self-concept stability. Following this, we discuss the relative adaptiveness of self-concept variability and stability and the implications of new cultural technologies such as the Internet.

Self-Concept Variability

Social Comparison

A wide variety of contextual or situational factors are implicated in self-concept variability. Prominent among these factors is the availability of *social comparison targets*. One compelling example of the impact of social comparison on self-concept malleability comes from the McGuires' (e.g., McGuire & McGuire, 1981) work on the "distinctiveness postulate." When children are asked to describe themselves using an unstructured Who am I ? task, they are especially likely to mention self-aspects that distinguish themselves from others in their immediate social mileau. For example, the greater the proportion of other-sex people in the home or in the classroom, the more likely children are to spontaneously mention their own sex. Conceptually similar findings have emerged on a wide variety of dimensions, including height, weight, hair color, and race (for a review, see McGuire & McGuire, 1988).

Feedback

Explicit feedback also has an impact on the way people think about and appraise themselves at any given moment. Sometimes people accept the implications of positive and negative feedback and incorporate it into their self-representations. Kernis and Johnson (1990) found that current self-appraisals[1] ("How do you rate yourself on various specific dimensions right now?") declined after people received negative feedback but became more favorable after positive feedback. Typical ("How do you generally, or typically, rate yourself on various specific dimensions?") appraisals were much more resistant to change, although the overall pattern of change was similar to that of current appraisals. In follow-up work, Kernis, Jadrich, Gibert, and Sun (1996) found that this pattern characterized individuals with low self-esteem better than it did individuals with high self-esteem.

Other research has shown that individuals with high self-esteem respond to public instances of failure and negative feedback by engaging in what is called *compensatory self-inflation* (Baumeister, 1982; Greenberg & Pysczynski, 1985). Suppose, for example, that an individual is told that he or she is not very socially skilled. Individuals with high, but not low, self-esteem buffer the blow of this feedback by publicly exaggerating their positive standing on dimensions irrelevant to the feedback, such as intelligence or athletic prowess.

Thus the self-concepts of individuals with either high or low self-esteem are affected by explicit feedback. The extent to which these effects hold for private self-views, as well as public self-presentations, is unknown, however. Moreover, although it is generally assumed that the self-concept changes that emerge are temporary, this assumption has yet to be rigorously examined. In any event, the processes involved in the reactions of individuals with low as opposed to high self-esteem to feedback (especially negative feedback) are likely to be multiple and complex. Among individuals with low self-esteem, the tendency to overgeneralize the negative implications of failure is one likely candidate (Brown & Dutton, 1995; Carver & Ganellen, 1983; Epstein, 1992; Kernis, Brockner, & Frankel, 1989). Specifically, some people take one negative occurrence as reflective of their general incompetence, which then exacerbates their negative affect and undermines their motivation to do better in the future.

Another factor that is likely to help account for the differences between how people with low as opposed to high self-esteem react to feedback is self-concept clarity (Campbell, 1990). Self-concept clarity refers to the extent to which one's self-concept is confidently held, internally consistent, and temporally stable. Research has shown that across a variety of indices, individuals with low self-esteem individuals are lower in self-concept clarity than are individuals with high self-esteem. For example, compared with individuals with high self-esteem, individuals with low self-esteem are less confident of their self-descriptions; they are more likely to endorse as self-descriptive adjectives constituting bipolar opposites; and their self-descriptions are less temporally stable over time. Campbell (1990) argues that low self-clarity increases one's sensitivity and responsiveness to external information and feedback and that this is one reason why individuals with low self-esteem show greater "plasticity" (Brockner, 1984) than individuals with high self-esteem. This hypothesis is highly intriguing and deserving of greater attention than it has received to date. Importantly, the extent to which the individual components of low confidence, low internal inconsistency, and temporal variability predict responsiveness to specific instances of feedback has yet to be examined.

In our view, self-concept clarity is an important aspect of the self that is likely to have implications for psychological functioning that are only beginning to be understood. A major step in this direction was taken by Campbell and her colleagues (1996) with the development of an individual difference measure of self-concept clarity (Self-Concept Clarity Scale, or SCC). Their findings indicated that low SCC scores related to low self-esteem, high depression, high neuroticism, low agreeableness, low conscientiousness, and ruminative forms of self-focused attention. Moreover, SCC scores predicted the stability and consistency of participants' self-descriptions. Other research on SCC is reported later in the chapter.

Among individuals with high self-esteem, self-affirmation processes (Steele, 1988) are likely to hold a prominent place in the processes associated with reactions to negative feedback. According to self-affirmation theory, failure or negative feedback poses a threat to the overall integrity of the self (Steele, 1988). As reported in a series of studies (Spencer, Josephs, & Steele, 1993) individuals with high self-esteem are better able than individuals with low self-esteem to draw on feedback-irrelevant positive self-aspects to restore their overall sense of self-integrity. This is particularly true when individuals are led to focus on their levels of self-esteem prior to responding to the threat (Spencer, Fein, & Steele, 1992, as cited in Spencer et al., 1993). In essence, engaging in self-affirmation processes results in short-term positive changes in feedback-irrelevant self-aspects, while simultaneously maintaining the stability of self-aspects directly relevant to the feedback. As such, these processes bear more than a passing resemblance to the compensatory inflation processes described earlier.

Unfortunately, little is known about how the self-concepts of individuals with low as opposed to high self-esteem are affected by positive feedback. In part, this lack is due to the absence of self-esteem differences that sometimes have emerged in studies that examined reactions to positive feedback (Brown, 1998). We believe, however, that this is an understudied issue deserving of greater attention in the future.

Actions

One's own actions may also promote variability in one's self-beliefs, particularly if these actions are undertaken in social contexts (Tice, 1992). In an interesting series of studies, Tice (1992) asked participants to portray themselves either as extraverted and outgoing or as introverted and thoughtful. Some participants did this in a very public context while being watched by a graduate student who knew their names, hometowns, and so forth, whereas others did this in a more private context in which they spoke into a tape recorder to be reviewed later by someone who was not aware of their individual identities. After completing this task, participants then rated themselves on dimensions such as talkativeness, shyness, and friendliness. As anticipated, participants' self-ratings were influenced by the nature of their self-presentation only in the public, highly social condition. That is, participants who acted in an extraverted manner in the presence of the graduate student rated themselves as more extraverted than did those who acted in an introverted manner. No such differences emerged when the self-presentation was done anonymously. In addition, among people in the "public presentation" conditions, their future behavior directed toward a conversation partner mapped onto the content of their self-presentation. Specifically, those who acted in an extraverted manner sat closer to their conversation partner than did those who acted in an introverted manner.

Several processes have been proposed to account for the internalization of public performances into one's self-beliefs. The present discussion relies heavily on Hoyle and colleagues (1999; see also Tice, 1992). The *biased scanning hypothesis* (Jones, Rhodewalt, Berglas, & Skelton, 1981) suggests that when people draw on a subset of their personal memories to present themselves in a particular way, this information can subsequently affect how they think about themselves. For example, if people are asked to present themselves in an extraverted manner, they can draw on previous experiences in which they acted that way. Given that most people can find instances in which they acted in ways consistent with either pole of a pair of bipolar adjectives (i.e., extraverted, introverted), retrieving memories consistent with their current performance is highly likely. Once accessed, these past memories influence people's self-judgments so that they are more in line with their current behavior than would be the case if these memories were not accessed. For example, individuals asked to publicly display extraversion probe their memories for past instances in which they acted extravertedly, whereas those asked to publicly display introversion can readily resurrect past instances of similar introverted displays. These retrieved instances then exert considerable influence over how people see themselves in the present. In biased scanning, people are not necessarily learning something new about themselves through their portrayals; they are looking for, and finding, confirmations of past instances of behavior similar to their present behavior. Ironically, this process would seem to work best in people who do possess well-developed, multifaceted belief systems. These individuals not only possess diverse self-information from which to draw on but also they presumably can do so with relative ease (due in part to the strength of associative linkages).

The *self-perception process* (Bem, 1972) suggests that presenting a particular public self can generate behavioral evidence that leads people to see what they are doing as accurately representing part of their true self. In this way, new identities can be constructed from one's self-presentational be-havior. That is, people's immediate self-beliefs may be based largely on their most recent behaviors, except in cases in which obvious external pressures cause a person to act in a particular way. For example, a woman who tends to consider herself re-served may think that she is more outgoing after jumping up on stage at a karaoke bar to join her friends in singing Madonna's "Like a Virgin." In short, individuals' self-views may fluctuate depending on how they have just behaved. This is thought to be par-ticularly true when individuals' self-beliefs are ambiguous or unclear.

Self-Concept Stability

Swann's self-verification theory (e.g, Swann, 1990) is the dominant theoretical frame-work that focuses on stability of the self-con-cept. According to this theory, once individ-uals' self-concepts are firmly formed, people use a wide variety of cognitive and behav-ioral strategies to maintain them. People gen-erally work hard to maintain the stability of their self-conceptions by creating, seeking out, and endorsing information that is con-sistent with their self-conceptions and by avoiding and rejecting information that is inconsistent with their self-conceptions (Swann, 1983). For example, at the cognitive level, people preferentially attend to infor-mation that they suspect will be consistent rather than inconsistent with their self-con-ception, they are better able to retrieve self-confirmatory information, and they inter-pret self-confirming feedback as more accurate than self-disconfirming feedback (Swann, Griffin, Predmore, & Gaines, 1987; Swann & Hill, 1982). Regarding behavioral strategies, people may display signs and sym-bols depicting core self-aspects (e.g., a lawyer driving a Jaguar or a physician dis-playing multiple diplomas and certifica-tions), may selectively affiliate with people who see them as they see themselves (e.g., en-joying cocktails at the "Martini Club" fre-quented only by young professionals), and may behave in certain ways so as to elicit the desired self-confirming reactions from others (e.g., a 65-year-"young" grandmother danc-ing at her grandchild's wedding).

According to Swann, people seek out and prefer self-verifying information for both *epistemic* and *pragmatic* reasons (Swann, Stein-Seroussi, & Giesler, 1992). *Epistemic* reasons refer to the fact that we feel more comfortable when we believe that others see us as we see ourselves. Self-verifying feedback bolsters our confidence in our own self-knowledge, that is, that we do, in fact, know ourselves. The alternative of re-ceiving nonverifying feedback may lead people to doubt that they are who they think they are, raising their anxiety levels and promoting confusion. *Pragmatic* rea-sons reflect the notion that our social inter-actions are likely to proceed more smoothly when self–other conceptions are consistent with each other.

Perhaps the most controversial aspect of self-verification theory is its contention that people with negative self-views will seek out and desire to interact with others who also view them negatively. For example, people who see themselves as submissive (and view this negatively) prefer to interact with some-one who also sees them as submissive (as opposed to dominant; Swann & Read, 1981), and depressed people prefer to inter-act with people who also see them as de-pressive (as opposed to nondepressive; Swann, Wenzlaff, Krull, & Pelham, 1992). Thus the tendency to be attracted to people who see oneself in a manner consistent with one's self-conception appears to be a very broad one. Other research shows that peo-ple with low self-esteem rate negative feed-back as more accurate than positive feed-back and that they view the negative evaluator as more competent than the posi-tive evaluator, *even though the receipt of negative feedback makes them feel bad emotionally* (Swann et al., 1987). Thus self-verification processes operate at the level of specific traits, as well as broad affective and personality dispositions. Although this work is not without its critics (e.g., Epstein & Morling, 1995), it provides a needed counterpoint to the preponderance of work that has emphasized self-enhancement (the desire to maintain a positive self-view) as the primary motive driving the acquisition of self-relevant feedback and information. To his credit, Swann recently has developed a model that incorporates both self-enhancement and self-verification motives (Swann & Schroeder, 1995). According to this framework, self-enhancement processes operate in a relatively automatic and primitive manner. On encountering positive self-relevant information, for example, people's initial and automatic reaction is affectively favorable. If people are prevented from processing the information further (either because they are distracted or cognitively overloaded) or are unmotivated to do so, the process stops. However, given sufficient time, the availability of cognitive resources, and sufficient motivation, people access their self-concepts and compare the new information with existing self-representations. For people with positive self-representations, the new positive information is embraced as accurate. In contrast, for people with negative self-representations, this new information is judged to be inaccurate, and self-verification processes then are activated (for further discussion, see Swann & Schroeder, 1995).

The Relative Adaptiveness of Self-Concept Variability versus Stability

As the foregoing review indicates, research has shown that the contents of individuals' self-concepts can be variable or stable. However, an important conceptual controversy exists that has yet to be fully resolved. The crux of this controversy revolves around the relative adaptiveness of contextually based self-concept variability. According to some (e.g., Gergen, 1991; Markus & Wurf, 1987; Sande, Goethals, & Radloff, 1988; Snyder, 1987), the ability to call into play multiple and perhaps contradictory self-aspects reflects the complexities of social life and people's ability to adjust to them. According to others (e.g., Campbell, 1990; Campbell et al., 1996), self-concept variability and malleability is likely to reflect confusion and lack of internal self-coherence. This controversy is further complicated by the advent of new technologies (to be discussed shortly) that allow people to present themselves in multiple and conflicting ways without being held accountable.

Paulhus's (Paulhus & Martin, 1988) distinction between "functional flexibility" and "situationalism" surely is relevant, although it has not received much attention.

Functional flexibility involves having confidence in one's ability to call into play multiple, perhaps contradictory, self-aspects in dealing with life situations. One who is high in functional flexibility believes that he or she would experience little anxiety in calling forth these multiple selves because they are well defined and can be enacted with confidence. In contrast, situationality involves the belief that one is not very capable at calling forth well-defined multiple self-aspects, but this belief is tempered by the sense that one's behaviors are called forth by situational contexts, which may require multiple conflicting self-actions. In Paulhus and Martin's (1988) research, functional flexibility was tied to a high sense of agency and was positively related to other measures of adaptive psychological functioning. In contrast, situationality was marked by self-doubt and other indices of psychological problems. Thus possessing a multifaceted self may be based either on strong self-beliefs and self-confidence (i.e., one based on a high sense of agency) or on self-doubts that heighten the impact of situational factors on one's actions and self-beliefs (i.e., one that is primarily reactive). In our view, future research on the adaptiveness of self-concept malleability will benefit from incorporating Paulhus's constructs of functional flexibility and situationality.

The breadth (or multiplicity) of the self-concept may further be enhanced by the diversity of self-relevant information made available through the interaction of people with mass-media-based popular culture. Increasingly, notions of the self and the accompanying self-concept have the opportunity to broaden their scope in response to an ever-expanding array of cultural communication technologies (Internet chat rooms, e-mail, digital photography, computer-based conferencing) that help meet the demands of existing in a pluralistic "postmodern" society. These contemporary technologies challenge our view of the self-concept because they actively embrace the myriad of possibilities that come from interacting with mass-media-based cultural technology (Markus & Nurius, 1986). In addition, they challenge individuals to incorporate into their self-concepts a myriad of "possible selves" that are derived from the pool of "categories made salient by the individual's particular sociocultural context and from the models, images, and symbols provided by the media and by the individual's immediate social experiences" (Markus & Nurius, 1986, p. 964).

A critical component of present-day cultural technologies is that they provide unprecedented opportunities for people to self-select from an enormous range of self-relevant information that previously was unavailable or inaccessible. These technologies allow for self-relevant information to be instantaneously accessed, refined, indeed, even fabricated before being assimilated into the self-system. Furthermore, cultural technologies have actively dissolved the physical constraints of space and time, as mass amounts of self-relevant information may be stored by personal computers and accessed at will (as opposed to watching one's favorite TV show at a time imposed by a network). This unprecedented access allows individuals to control when and for how long they interact with self-selected information in constructing their self-concepts.

What implications do "postmodern" cultural technologies have for the self-concept? Some theorists assert that the self is increasingly becoming a problem to define because the enormity of self-relevant information gives rise to uncertainty about the self and thereby destabilizes one's self-concept (Baumeister, 1987; Gergen, 1996). Put differently, as the self-concept is responding to the multitude of faces, languages, and relations inherent in the complex of "postmodern" life, there is a "permanent tension between the process of continuous redefinition of oneself and the need to stabilize one's boundaries" (Weber, 2000, p. 51).

Moreover, as individuals reconcile the complexities of contemporary societal challenges, there may be a shift in how individuals conceptualize themselves. Individuals may achieve harmony among the multifaceted components of the self by shifting their self-concepts from stable quantifiable self-categorizations based on traditional social roles to more contextually based self-knowledge that reflects one's highly personalized self-aspects. One way of doing this is to transform self-knowledge gained within any given context into a personalized story that gives rise to an individual's sense of

"voice" (see Hermans, 1996). Achieving unity in self-organization may be accomplished by a dialogical interchange within a multivoiced self, whereby seemingly disparate self-knowledge is synthesized into an internally generated singular narrative of the self (Hermans, 1996; McAdams 1997). By representing the self as the unifying narrative theme across the multiple contexts displayed in contemporary life, individuals may use a sort of internal storytelling to strategically codify the self and bring coherence to the self-concept. Moreover, interacting with cultural technology that exposes the self to diverse self-relevant information may be a compelling source of opportunity for personal growth, expansion, or experimentation.

One important characteristic of contemporary cultural technology is that anonymity may be preserved while individuals explore their self-concepts (e.g. through Internet chat rooms, e-mail, or newsgroups). As an example, McKenna and Bargh (1998) reported that participants in "marginalized" (i.e., subversive political beliefs, deviant sexual interest groups) newsgroups sought out such groups because there were no such equivalent groups in "real" life. In short, the information accessed via cultural technologies can serve to broaden the self-concept by exposing people to diverse self-knowledge information and by providing validation for the self-concept when one discovers that his or her beliefs are shared or popularized by others. Moreover, these technologies enable people to experiment with or explore self-aspects that potentially are socially undesirable without having to be concerned with issues of accountability.

Significant questions arise from this "postmodern" perspective. For example, what is the role of popular culture in creating identities and narratives? It seems that in recent years, many youth and young adults are dissatisfied with, or are not accurately represented by, the more traditional ways of defining the self, particularly those aspects pertaining to social identity. As described by Deaux and her colleagues (Deaux, Reid, Mizrahi, & Ethier, 1995), these traditional categories of social identity include (1) personal relationships, (2) vocations and avocations, (3) political affiliations, (4) ethnic and religious groups, and (5) stigmatized groups. Although this analysis is highly insightful, Deaux and colleagues' (1995) descriptions of the categories people use in defining group membership are not exhaustive. Moreover, many of the social categories identified by Deaux and colleagues represent social roles that people are born into or socialized to assume (e.g., the same religious affiliation as one's parents). Today's youth, in contrast, are turning to various nontraditional sources of identity such as movies and musical genres of rock, rap, and hip-hop as forms of self-expression that are then internalized. What are we to make of this? Are people who turn to such forms doing so out of "pure" growth motives as they strive toward their possible selves (Markus & Nurius, 1986), or are they turning to them as temporary way stations because of insecurities and self-doubts? Is the self-relevant information accessed by cultural technologies qualitatively different from the information attained by more traditional (perhaps more face-to-face) sources? If so, what implications does this pose for the stability versus variability of the self-concept? Many other issues can also be raised that hopefully will be the focus of sustained empirical efforts in the near future.

Self-Esteem Variability

Self-esteem variability (instability)[2] has been conceptualized both in terms of short- and long-term fluctuations (Rosenberg, 1986). When viewed as long-term fluctuations, self-esteem instability reflects change that occurs gradually over an extended period of time. Rosenberg (1986) referred to this as change in one's baseline self-esteem. Among children and adolescents, for example, many show a decrease in global self-esteem as they make the transition from the relatively safe confines of elementary school to the more turbulent middle school environment, which then is followed by a slow but steady increase in self-esteem through the high school years (e.g., Bachman, O'Malley, & Johnston, 1978; Demo & Savin-Williams, 1983; McCarthy & Hoge, 1982; O'Malley & Bachman, 1983; Savin-Williams & Demo, 1983).

Most research and theory, however, has focused on self-esteem variability as reflected in short-term fluctuations in one's contextually based global self-esteem. Rosenberg (1986) referred to these short-term fluctuations as barometric instability. He further suggested that for self-esteem to be considered unstable, these fluctuations must involve dramatic shifts between feelings of worthiness and worthlessness. In fact, his Stability of Self Scale (Rosenberg, 1965) requires individuals with unstable self-esteem to endorse items such as, "Some days I have a very good opinion of myself; other days I have a very poor opinion of myself."

Another perspective is that self-esteem instability may take numerous forms. Some people may in fact experience dramatic shifts from feeling very positively to very negatively about themselves. Others, however, may primarily fluctuate in the *extent* to which they feel positively or negatively about themselves. The precise nature of these fluctuations is likely to depend on a number of factors, including what self-aspects are salient and the valence of recently experienced self-relevant events (cf. Markus & Kunda, 1986; Morse & Gergen, 1970). The implications of various patterns of fluctuations has yet to be examined, but we suspect that in general they all will reflect an underlying fragility in feelings of self-worth. Kernis and his colleagues (Kernis et al., 1993) have argued that the essence of unstable self-esteem is the propensity to experience short-term fluctuations in contextually based feelings of self-worth that interact with situationally based factors to produce specific patterns of fluctuations. Thus these fluctuations may at times (or for certain people) be primarily unidirectional (e.g., within a relatively positive or negative range) or bidirectional (between positive and negative ranges; for a relevant discussion of this issue, see Vallacher & Novak, 2000).

Although both short- and long-term self-esteem instability are likely to have important implications for psychological functioning, most researchers have focused on short-term instability. The distinction between these two types of stability is important because people may exhibit considerable short-term fluctuations while manifesting little or no long-term change.

The most common way to assess short-term fluctuations in self-esteem (and the way that it has been assessed in the bulk of the research reviewed in this chapter) is to have respondents complete a self-esteem measure once or twice daily over a 4–7 day period under instructions to base their responses on how they feel *at the moment they are completing each form.* The standard deviation of each individual's total scores across these multiple assessments then is computed; the greater the standard deviation, the more unstable one's self-esteem. To measure self-esteem *level,* respondents are asked to complete the same self-esteem scale, but are asked to base their responses on how they *typically or generally feel about them-selves.*[3]

Correlations between level and stability of self-esteem generally range from the low teens to the low 30s, suggesting that they are relatively independent dimensions of self-esteem (for a summary of representative values, see Kernis & Waschull, 1995). Invariably, the direction of the correlation indicates that more unstable self-esteem is associated with lower levels of self-esteem. However, it is incorrect to presume that only individuals with low self-esteem possess unstable self-esteem. In fact, we frequently find that self-esteem stability has effects among individuals with either high or low self-esteem, and sometimes these effects are stronger among individuals high, not low, in self-esteem (e.g., Kernis, Grannemann, & Barclay, 1989).

Unstable self-esteem is thought to reflect fragile, vulnerable feelings of immediate self-worth that are influenced by potentially self-relevant events that are externally provided (e.g., a complement or insult) or self-generated (reflecting on one's appearance; Kernis et al., 1998; Kernis & Paradise, 2002; Kernis & Waschull, 1995). One core characteristic of people with fragile self-esteem is that they are highly responsive to events that have potential relevance to their feelings of self-worth—in fact, they may interpret events as being self-esteem relevant even when they are not (cf. Greenier et al., 1999). For example, a nonreturned greeting may be viewed as reflective of one's own unlikeableness and not the recipient's busyness. Evidence to be reviewed shortly indicates that individuals with unstable self-

esteem may respond by completely accepting, even exaggerating, an event's evaluative implications (e.g., they may feel incompetent and demoralized following a specific failure; Kernis et al., 1998). At the other extreme, they may respond very angrily and defensively by attacking the validity of the threatening information or the credibility of its source (Kernis et al., 1989). In contrast, people with relatively stable self-esteem typically have less extreme reactions to potentially evaluative events, precisely because these events have little impact on their immediate feelings of self-worth. (We use the terms "stable" and "unstable" self-esteem throughout this chapter for ease of exposition only. Conceptually and empirically, we treat stability of self-esteem as a continuous dimension along which people vary).

Several factors have been implicated in the reasons that the current self-esteem of some individuals is highly unstable. For example, overreliance on the evaluations, love, and approval of others, an impoverished self-concept, and excessive dependency needs are thought to promote unstable self-esteem (Butler, Hokanson, & Flynn, 1994; Kernis, Paradise, et al., 2000; Rosenberg, 1986; Tennen & Affleck, 1993). Unfortunately, data exist only with respect to the role of impoverished self-concepts (which we discuss shortly). In addition, people with unstable self-esteem may be especially prone to interpret everyday events as having relevance to their feelings of self-worth and to experience their self-esteem as "continually on the line" (i.e., heightened ego-involvement). These events may be external, environmentally based (e.g., being turned down for a date) or more internally based, such as reflecting on one's progress toward an important goal. Greenier et al. (1999) portrayed this heightened ego-involvement as an "evaluative set" composed of several interlocking components. First, an *attentional* component involves "zeroing in" on information or events that have potentially self-evaluative implications. Second, a *bias* component involves interpreting ambiguous or non-self-esteem relevant events as self-esteem relevant. Finally, a *generalization* component involves linking one's immediate global feelings of self-worth to specific outcomes and events (e.g., a poor math performance is taken to reflect low overall intelligence and worth). Each of these components may operate outside of one's awareness or be consciously and deliberately invoked (for further discussion, see Kernis & Paradise, 2002).

Although different in their specifics, each of the aforementioned factors implies that people with unstable self-esteem do not have a well-anchored sense of their self-worth. Also, they suggest that unstable self-esteem reflects fragile and vulnerable feelings of self-worth that are subject to the vicissitudes of externally provided and internally generated positive and negative experiences. A number of implications follow from this characterization, which we now discuss.

First, negative stressful events should be more likely to precipitate or exacerbate depressive symptoms among individuals with unstable as compared with stable self-esteem. According to a number of clinical theorists (e.g., Chodoff, 1973; Jacobson, 1975; for a review, see Tennen & Affleck, 1993), people who are vulnerable to depression are susceptible to substantial downward fluctuations in their feelings of self-worth, particularly in response to negative events. Consistent with this contention, several studies have shown that aversive events exacerbate depressive symptoms, especially among people with unstable self-esteem. Roberts and Monroe (1992) reported that among initially nondepressed individuals, failure on a college examination predicted increases in depression only among individuals with unstable self-esteem. Butler and colleagues (1994) examined the relationships between self-esteem instability, major life stressors, and depression. Their findings indicated that, as major life stressors increased, unstable self-esteem predicted greater depression among individuals with low, but not high self-esteem. Kernis and colleagues (1998) found that increases in depressive symptoms across a 4-week period were most apparent among individuals who reported experiencing considerable daily hassles and whose self-esteem was unstable.

Roberts and Gotlib (1997) reported that day-to-day variability in either global self-esteem or specific self-evaluations, in combination with stressful life events, predicted increases in depressive symptoms over a 6-week period, particularly in individuals who had a past history of depressive episodes. These findings emerged after controlling for other variables such as neuroticism and self-concept certainty. Importantly, neither variability in day-to-day affect nor any of the other predictor variables interacted with life stressors to predict depression. Finally, none of the predictor variables (including self-esteem stability) interacted with life stressors to predict increases in anxiety.

Although there are some differences in findings across these studies, they support the general conclusion that unstable self-esteem, in combination with aversive events, may precipitate or promote depressive symptoms. However, the precise mechanisms by which this occurs have not yet been definitively established. Some studies (Roberts & Monroe, 1992) demonstrate that threats to self-esteem interact with unstable self-esteem to promote depressive symptoms. These studies suggest that the particular vulnerability exhibited by individuals with unstable self-esteem pertains to the way they react to self-esteem threats, perhaps involving internalization or over-generalization processes. Other studies (e.g., Kernis et al., 1998; Roberts & Gotlib, 1997), however, show that daily hassles, irrespective of their direct self-relevant implications, interact with unstable self-esteem in promoting depressive symptoms. Two explanations of these latter findings exist. First, it is possible that people with unstable self-esteem interpret non-self-relevant events as relevant to their self-esteem, as suggested by the "evaluative set" described earlier. Second, it is possible that unstable self-esteem relates more generally to suboptimal coping strategies that are associated with susceptibility to depression.

One mechanism deserving of attention is the tendency to overgeneralize the implications of failure and other negative events (Carver & Ganellen, 1983). Kernis and colleagues (1998) found that, compared with participants with stable self-esteem, participants with unstable self-esteem were more prone to overgeneralize the negative implications of failure. That is, whereas people with unstable self-esteem react to a specific failure by feeling incompetent and stupid (the generalization component of the evaluative set described earlier), people with stable self-esteem have more localized reactions (i.e., if they question anything, it may be their ability to succeed at the task at hand). Moreover, these feelings of incompetence appear to contribute to a vicious cycle characterized by a lack of motivation and subsequent additional failures (Kernis, Brockner, & Frankel, 1989).

Second, everyday positive and negative events should have a greater immediate impact on the self-feelings of people with unstable self-esteem, compared with those of people with stable self-esteem. Although this hypothesis seems rather intuitive, evidence supporting it has important implications for the construct validity of the technique used to assess self-esteem stability. Specifically, skeptics can argue that unstable self-esteem as typically assessed merely measures unreliability in responding and that, apart from this, it has little or no implications for psychological functioning. However, if it can be shown that unstable self-esteem is related to reactivity to actual events, this would severely undermine the credibility of this assertion. Also, it is important to demonstrate that the heightened reactivity associated with unstable self-esteem is not limited to negative events but extends to positive events as well. To examine this reactivity, Greenier and colleagues (1999) had college students describe the most positive and most negative event they experienced each day, Monday through Thursday, for a period of 2 weeks. For each event, participants indicated how the event made them feel about themselves (on a scale ranging from "made me feel considerably worse about myself" to "made me feel considerably better about myself"). In addition, participants' stability and level of self-esteem were assessed. Importantly, for both positive and negative events, the more unstable individuals' self-esteem, the more these events affected how they felt about themselves. These effects emerged after controlling for the effect of self-esteem level, which related to reactivity to negative, but not positive, events.

Greenier and colleagues (1999) also had a team of coders rate each event for its degree of self-esteem relevance and implications for social acceptance. For negative events, the events reported by individuals with unstable self-esteem were rated as having greater self-esteem relevance and implications for one's social acceptance. No such effects emerged for positive events. Moreover, for negative events, both self-esteem relevance and social acceptance implications were found to mediate (i.e., account for) the relationship between unstable self-esteem and greater reactivity. Further analyses indicated that self-esteem relevance was a more powerful mediator. Thus the greater reactivity to negative events exhibited by individuals with unstable as opposed to stable self-esteem was accounted for by the greater self-esteem relevance (and to a lesser extent, their implications for social acceptance) of the negative events that they reported.

Does this mean that individual differences in self-esteem stability can be accounted for by differences in the frequency with which self-esteem-relevant daily events are experienced? This is an intriguing question that, unfortunately, cannot be definitively answered given our current knowledge. On the one hand, it does seem likely that differential exposure to self-esteem-relevant events contributes to individual differences in self-esteem stability. On the other hand, it seems unlikely that this differential exposure completely accounts for these individual differences. At the very least, it seems premature to draw the latter conclusion. First, participants in the Greenier and colleagues (1999) study reported only on one negative and one positive event each day. Therefore, these data are moot with respect to the frequency with which individuals with stable and unstable self-esteem experience self-esteem-relevant events. Second, differential exposure to self-esteem-relevant events cannot account for differences in how individuals with stable and unstable self-esteem respond to the same events (e.g., Kernis, Greenier, Herlocker, Whisenhunt, & Abend, 1997; Kernis, Paradise, & Goldman, 2002; Kernis et al., 1993, Study 1; Paradise & Kernis, in press). Third, Greenier and colleagues (1999) found no difference in the self-esteem relevance of daily positive events experienced by individuals with stable as compared with unstable self-esteem. Presumably, then, the reactivity to positive events evinced by individuals with unstable self-esteem is due to their heightened tendencies to link feelings of self-worth to positive outcomes regardless of the outcomes' self-esteem relevance. Fourth, it is possible that the "evaluative set" described earlier predisposed people with unstable self-esteem to focus on events that had self-esteem relevance or to report events in such a way that highlighted their self-esteem implications, which subsequently were picked up by coders (for a more extensive discussion, see Greenier et al., 1999).

These considerations notwithstanding, an important issue for future research is to determine precisely the role of environmental factors in promoting unstable self-esteem. Novel, highly evaluative environments (e.g., sorority "rush" weeks, beginning a new job) are likely to increase the magnitude of unstable self-esteem experienced by many individuals (as examined at the aggregate level). As people continue negotiating these environments and implicit and explicit evaluations become less frequent and/or salient, the magnitude of unstable self-esteem at the aggregate level is likely to decline as well. This is speculation, however, and it would be useful for future research to examine the extent to which it is true.

The crux of the issue, and one that cannot be resolved with Greenier and colleagues' (1999) data, is the relative strength of the evaluative set described earlier and of more objective event qualities (i.e., self-esteem relevance, social acceptance implications) as factors that promote unstable self-esteem. It seems likely that personal (interpretational) and environmental (objective) factors each plays a role, but this is an issue that can be resolved only with additional research.

Third, people with unstable self-esteem should be especially sensitive to, and concerned about avoiding, potential self-esteem threats. Waschull and Kernis (1996) examined how self-esteem level and self-esteem stability relate to children's intrinsic motivation in the classroom. Prior research (Ryan, 1993) indicates that situational factors that emphasize the link between specific outcomes and self-esteem often undermine intrinsic motivation. This research suggests that heightened concerns about one's self-esteem may undermine the desire to take on challenges and instead promote a more cautious but safer route to positive outcomes. Therefore, to the extent that unstable self-esteem reflects a heightened sensitivity and concern about avoiding potential self-

esteem threats, it should relate to lower levels of intrinsic motivation in children.

A sample of fifth-grade children completed Harter's (1981) Intrinsic versus Extrinsic Orientation in the Classroom Scale, as well as measures of stability and level of self-esteem. As anticipated, compared with children with stable self-esteem, children with unstable self-esteem reported lower Preference for Challenge (Does the child prefer challenging tasks or those that are easy?) and Curiosity/Interest scores (Is the child motivated by curiosity or to get good grades and please the teacher?). These findings suggest that unstable self-esteem in children is linked to a relatively cautious or strategic self-esteem-focused orientation toward learning rather than to an intrinsic orientation involving undertaking challenges for learning's sake.

Another goal of this study was to examine how self-esteem stability related to children's reasons for becoming angry at their peers. The findings indicated that children with unstable self-esteem, compared with their counterparts with stable self-esteem, were more likely to indicate that they would become angry because of the self-esteem-threatening aspects of aversive events depicted in a series of vignettes. Thus children with unstable self-esteem are especially sensitive to the self-esteem-threatening aspects of aversive environmental events (perhaps via the evaluative set described earlier).

Fourth, the magnitude of fluctuations that people experience in their global self-esteem will be associated with the magnitude of fluctuations that they experience in their domain specific self-evaluations. To the extent that unstable self-esteem is associated with individuals placing substantial weight on specific evaluative information or to their generalizing the implications of specific evaluative information to their feelings of self-worth, the magnitude of day-to-day fluctuations that they experience in self-perceived competence and social acceptance should be related to the magnitude of fluctuations they experience in global feelings of self-worth. To address this issue, Waschull and Kernis (1996) had participants indicate their felt competence and social acceptance each time they rated their current self-esteem (to assess self-esteem stability). Findings indicated that the magnitude of daily fluctuations in perceived competence and social acceptance each correlated with the magnitude of daily fluctuations in global self-esteem ($r = .59, .62$, respectively).

In related research involving college students, Kernis and colleagues (1993, Study 2) tested the hypothesis that variability in day-to-day evaluations of competence, social acceptance, and physical attractiveness would relate more strongly to self-esteem instability if the self-evaluative dimension was high rather than low in self-importance. As was found by Waschull and Kernis (1996), the magnitude of day-to-day variability along each dimension was significantly correlated with the magnitude of self-esteem instability. Additional analyses indicated that the relation between greater variability in perceived competence and self-esteem instability was especially strong among people who viewed competence as an important determinant of their overall self-worth. This pattern also emerged for the dimensions of physical attractiveness and social acceptance, but only among people who generally rated themselves relatively favorably along these dimensions. For people who generally rated themselves unfavorably on these dimensions, high daily variability was related to highly unstable self-esteem regardless of the dimension's importance. Kernis and colleagues suggested that the impact of personal importance may have been overridden by the substantial interpersonal consequences associated with low social acceptance and physical attractiveness.

Fifth, people with unstable self-esteem should have a weaker sense of self (i.e., be less self-determining, have relatively impoverished self-concepts) than people with stable self-esteem. The research discussed so far provides convergent, albeit indirect, evidence that unstable self-esteem is linked to a heightened tendency to be ego-involved in everyday events and, by extension, to the possession of an "evaluative set." Additional evidence comes from a recent study (Kernis, Paradise, Whitaker, Wheatman, & Goldman, 2000) that focused on the ways in which people regulate their everyday, recurrent goals, referred to as personal strivings (Emmons, 1986).

In their discussion of self-regulatory styles, Ryan and Connell (1989) proposed that people engage in goal-directed activities for reasons that reflect varying degrees of choice, self-determination, and integration with one's core self. External regulation reflects the absence of self-determination inasmuch as the impetus for action is external to the actor (e.g., another person's request that is tied implicitly or explicitly to reward or punishment). Introjected regulation involves the direct application of affective and self-esteem contingencies to motivate oneself (Ryan, Rigby, & King, 1993). Gaining the approval of self and others promotes behaviors that "are performed because one 'should' do them, or because not doing so might engender anxiety, guilt, or loss of self-esteem" (Ryan et al., 1993, p. 587). Introjected regulation goes hand in hand with heightened ego-involvement and, as such, involves only minimal self-determination. Considerably more self-determination is present in identified regulation, which involves the individual personally and freely identifying with the activity's importance for his or her functioning and growth. Intrinsic regulation is the prototypical form of self-determined regulation in that activities are chosen purely for the pleasure and enjoyment they provide.

Self-determination theory (e.g., Deci & Ryan, 1991; see Ryan & Deci, Chapter 13, this volume) holds that the self-regulatory styles of optimally functioning individuals consist primarily of identified and intrinsic regulation (i.e., that is highly self-determining) rather than introjected and external regulation (i.e., that involves little or no self-determination). Furthermore, Deci and Ryan (1995) suggest that contingent self-esteem (i.e., self-esteem that is dependent on specific outcomes) is anchored in external and introjected self-regulatory processes, controlling forms of regulation that gain their power through the linking of behaviors and outcomes to self- and other-based (dis)approval. In contrast, true self-esteem is posited to emerge naturally out of more agentic processes associated with identified and intrinsic self-regulation.

To our knowledge, the relations of contingent and true self-esteem to self-regulatory styles has not been directly examined. However, contingent and unstable self-esteem share a number of features, as do true and stable self-esteem (although they are not identical; see Kernis & Paradise, 2002). First, conceptualizations of both contingent and unstable self-esteem emphasize the link between feelings of self-worth and specific outcomes. Second, both describe enhanced tendencies to be caught up in the processes of defending, maintaining, and (in the case of unstable or contingent *high* self-esteem) maximizing one's positive, though tenuous, feelings of self-worth. (Although we focus here on different kinds of high self-esteem, this discussion should not be taken to suggest that individuals with low self-esteem are devoid of self-enhancement motives or strategies; for relevant research, see Wood, Giordano-Beech, Taylor, Michela, & Gaus, 1994). Likewise, both stable and true high self-esteem are taken to reflect secure, well-anchored feelings of self-worth that do *not* need continual validation. These considerations suggest that the more unstable individuals' self-esteem, the more they would engage in external and introjected self-regulation, and the less they would engage in identified and intrinsic self-regulation.

Kernis, Paradise, and colleagues (2000) had participants complete measures of stability and level of self-esteem, along with a measure of self-concept clarity (Campbell et al., 1996). In addition, participants generated a list of eight personal strivings, and they indicated the extent to which they engaged in each striving for reasons reflecting external, introjected, identified, and intrinsic self-regulatory processes. The results offered strong support for our hypotheses. After controlling for the effects of self-esteem level, we found that the more unstable individuals' self-esteem, the more external and introjected and the less identified and intrinsic were their self-regulatory styles. Moreover, the more unstable individuals' self-esteem, the more they recalled feeling tense and pressured when engaged in their goal strivings, emotions associated with heightened ego-involvement.

As noted earlier, participants also completed the Self-Concept Clarity Scale (Campbell et al., 1996), which contains 12 items (e.g., "My beliefs about myself often conflict with one another"; "In general, I have a clear sense of who I am and what I am"). Kernis and Waschull (1995) suggest-ed that having a poorly developed self-concept may contribute to unstable self-esteem by leading individuals to rely on and be more affected by specific evaluative information. In other words, the less confident and internally consistent one's self-knowledge, the less well anchored one's feelings of self-worth are likely to be. Again the results offered strong support, as unstable self-esteem was associated with lower self-concept clarity (after controlling for self-esteem level).

Summary

In sum, research has shown that, compared with people with stable self-esteem, people with unstable self-esteem (1) experience greater increases in depressive symptoms when faced with daily hassles (Kernis et al., 1998) or stressful life events (Roberts & Gotlib, 1997), (2) have self-feelings that are more affected by everyday negative and positive events (Greenier et al.,1999), (3) take a more self-esteem-protective (hence, less mastery-oriented) stance toward learning (Waschull & Kernis, 1996), (4) focus relatively more on the self-esteem-threatening aspects of aversive interpersonal events (Waschull & Kernis, 1996), (5) regulate their goal strivings in a relatively non-self-determined fashion (Kernis, Paradise, et al., 2000), and (6) have more impoverished self-concepts (Kernis, Paradise, et al., 2000). Importantly, each of these effects for self-esteem stability emerged after controlling for the role of self-esteem level.

The Development of Unstable Self-Esteem

Waschull and Kernis (1996) reported that meaningful individual differences in self-esteem stability emerge in children as young as 10 to 11 years old. Kernis and Waschull (1995) speculated that early childhood environments that involve considerable amounts of noncontingent (Berglas, 1985) and/or controlling (Deci & Ryan, 1987) feedback are likely to promote the development of unstable self-esteem. The essence of noncontingent feedback is that it is not subject to personal control (Berglas, 1985). Moreover, as Berglas notes, it is not a direct function of one's abilities and performances but rather is based on criteria such as the target's ascribed characteristics (e.g., family membership), the evaluator's mood, or criteria established by the evaluator but unknown to the recipient (see Kernis & Waschull, 1995, for an extended discussion).

Controlling feedback is experienced as (pressure to think, feel, or behave in specified ways) (Deci & Ryan, 1985, p. 95). This felt pressure leads individuals to govern their actions and internal states primarily on the basis of specific rewards and punishments rather than by an awareness of one's basic organismic needs and the desire to fulfill them. Over time, an excessive focus on playing into these contingencies is likely to lead to feelings of self-worth that are dependent on matching them. In Deci and Ryan's (1995) terminology, one's thoughts, feelings, and actions will primarily be regulated through introjects, and one's self-esteem will be contingent (unstable) rather than true (stable).

With one exception, to be discussed shortly, research on early childhood environments and self-esteem has focused on self-esteem level, not self-esteem stability. In a classic study, Coopersmith (1967) found that parents of children with high self-esteem exhibited substantial warmth and acceptance toward them, while at the same time setting clearly defined limits (i.e., authoritative parenting style; Baumrind, 1971). Other studies also have documented the importance of parental involvement, acceptance, and support and the establishment of clearly defined limits to children's high self-esteem and well-being (e.g., Buri, Louiselle, Misukanis, Mueller, 1988; Gecas & Schwalbe, 1986; Grolnick & Ryan, 1989).

As reviewed in this chapter, a growing literature indicates that unstable self-esteem reflects fragile feelings of self-worth that are associated with heightened reactivity to potentially self-esteem-relevant events and to relatively poor psychological adjustment. Thus one key to obtaining a better understanding of psychological well-being and adjustment may rest in identifying the factors in childhood and early adolescence that promote unstable and fragile, as opposed to stable, self-esteem. As a first step toward identifying such factors, Kernis, Brown, and

Brody (2000) examined how children's stability of self-esteem related to their perceptions of how their parents communicate with them. Participants were 11- to 12-year-old children, all of whom resided with both of their biological parents. Seventy-nine percent of this sample identified themselves as Caucasian; 21% identified themselves as African American.

The major findings indicated that children's perceptions of many aspects of parent–child communication patterns (especially fathers) were linked to the extent to which they possessed unstable self-esteem. For example, children who perceived their fathers to be highly critical, to engage in insulting name calling, and to use guilt arousal and love withdrawal as control techniques had more unstable (as well as lower) self-esteem than did children who did not perceive their fathers in this manner. Moreover, compared with children with stable self-esteem, children with unstable self-esteem indicated that their fathers less frequently talked about the good things that they (the children) had done and were less likely to use value-affirming methods when they did show their approval. Interestingly, perceptions of mothers' communication styles were more consistently related to children's self-esteem level than to their self-esteem stability. The findings for self-esteem stability that did emerge, however, were largely consistent with those that emerged for fathers.

To our knowledge, these findings are the first to relate parental communication styles to the instability of their children's self-esteem. It is disconcerting, though not entirely surprising, that derogatory name calling and criticism by parents appears to undermine both the stability and level of their children's self-esteem. Children tend to be very sensitive to evaluative information conveyed about them by parents and other significant individuals in their lives (Dweck & Goetz, 1978; Rosenberg, 1986). Also, when parents attempt to control children's unwanted behaviors by arousing guilt or withdrawing their love, they may set up contingencies whereby children feel worthy and valuable when they act appropriately but useless and unworthy when they act inappropriately. Called *conditions of worth* a number of years ago by Rogers (1959), such controlling contingencies are likely to promote self-regulatory styles that are *external* and *introjected* rather than *identified* and *intrinsic* (Deci & Ryan, 1985).

On a more positive note, the more value-affirming ways of approval fathers reportedly showed toward their children, the more stable and higher was their children's self-esteem. Spending time together, displaying physical affection, and so forth, provide opportunities to deepen the affective bonds between parent and child, and they signal to children that they are valued and appreciated. Instead of promoting an external or introjected self-regulatory style in children, value-affirming methods promote identified and intrinsic self-regulation (Ryan, 1993). In short, value affirmation encourages children to trust, value, and utilize their own internal states as guides for action, as well as to feel likeable.

Although intriguing, these findings are limited in that they focus entirely on children's perceptions of how their parents communicate with them. Therefore, the extent to which children with unstable self-esteem misperceive or are especially sensitive to certain aspects of parental communications is unknown. Future research can build on these findings by examining objective indices of parental communication styles, as well as other aspects of familial functioning.

Can a Consideration of Self-Esteem Stability Inform Us about the Nature of High Self-Esteem?

Considerable attention currently is focused on the nature of high self-esteem and its relation to optimal psychological functioning. Traditionally, high self-esteem was thought of in unequivocally positive terms. However, a "dark side" to high self-esteem has been increasingly recognized and its implications examined (Baumeister, Smart, & Boden, 1996). In fact, there now are two "competing" perspectives on the nature of high self-esteem (for extended discussions, see Kernis, in press; Kernis & Paradise, 2002). One perspective is that individuals with high self-esteem are very caught up in defending and promoting their positive self-feelings through the use of a wide variety of self-enhancing and self-protective strategies.

This perspective suggests that high self-esteem is *fragile* and that it may not always relate to adaptive functioning. The contrasting perspective is that individuals with high self-esteem are accepting of their weaknesses and not easily threatened and that they have little need to engage in self-protective or self-promotional activities. This perspective suggests that high self-esteem is *secure* and that it will positively relate to other measures of adaptive functioning. Which view is correct? Importantly, research on self-esteem stability has shown that both views are correct, in that each characterizes a subset of individuals with high self-esteem. Specifically, this research has demonstrated that the view of high self-esteem as *fragile* characterizes individuals with *unstable* high self-esteem, whereas the view of high self-esteem as *secure* characterizes individuals with *stable* high self-esteem.

People with unstable high self-esteem are more defensive and self-aggrandizing than are their counterparts with stable high self-esteem, and they are lower in psychological health and well-being. Defensiveness often manifests itself in feelings of anger and hostility directed toward others whom one believes is responsible for wrongdoing. These efforts may be somewhat successful in the short run by alleviating the individuals' immediate distress or by providing a sense of control, but in the long run they may undermine one's relationships with others, as well as stifle efforts to improve one's self-insight and personal growth (Deci & Ryan, 2000; Kernis, 2000; Crocker & Parke, Chapter 15, this volume). Kernis, Grannemann, and Barclay (1989) reported that individuals with unstable high self-esteem scored the highest on several well-validated anger and hostility inventories (e.g., the Novaco Anger Inventory; Novaco, 1975), individuals with stable high self-esteem scored the lowest, and individuals with stable or unstable low self-esteem scored between these two extremes. As evidence of self-aggrandizing tendencies, compared with individuals with stable high self-esteem, people with unstable high self-esteem say that they would be more likely to boast about a success to their friends (Kernis et al., 1997); after an actual success, they were also more likely to claim that they were successful in spite of the operation of performance-inhibiting factors

(Kernis, Grannemann, & Barclay, 1992). Also, Kernis and Waschull (1995) found that individuals with unstable as compared with stable high self-esteem reported taking greater pride in themselves and in their behaviors, as measured by the Test of Self-Conscious Affect (Tangney, Wagner, & Gramzow, 1989).

However, these enhanced tendencies toward self-glorification and self-defense do not appear to translate into greater psychological health and well-being. Paradise and Kernis (in press) administered Ryff's (1989) measure of psychological well-being to a sample of college students who also completed measures of level and stability of self-esteem. Importantly, differences among individuals with high self-esteem emerged as a function of self-esteem stability. Relative to individuals with stable high self-esteem, individuals with unstable high self-esteem reported lower autonomy, environmental mastery, purpose in life, self-acceptance, and positive relations with others. Stated differently, whereas individuals with stable high self-esteem reported that they functioned in a highly autonomous manner, possessed a clear sense of meaning in their lives, related effectively within both their physical and social environments, and were highly self-accepting, these reports were less likely to be true of individuals with unstable high self-esteem.

Unstable high self-esteem also appears to have adverse implications for how individuals function in their intimate relationships. Kernis, Paradise, and Goldman (2000) reasoned that individuals with stable high self-esteem would interpret and react to ambiguously negative actions by their partner by treating these events as innocuous, either by minimizing their negative aspects or by offering a benign interpretation of them. In contrast, individuals with unstable high self-esteem were expected to imbue these events with adverse self-relevant implications. Participants in this study read a series of scenarios that depicted ambiguously negative events that their partner might engage in. The findings that emerged provided strong support for our hypotheses. Specifically, individuals with *unstable* high self-esteem reported the most "personalizing" (i.e., magnifying the event's negative implications for the self) and "reciprocating" (i.e., resolving to get even with their partner as a way to deal with the self-esteem threat) reactions, whereas individuals with *stable* high self-esteem reported the least (individuals with low self-esteem fell between these two extremes). Conversely, individuals with *stable* high self-esteem reported the most "benign" (i.e., transient, external, usually partner-related) explanations and "minimizing" (i.e., taking the event at face value and not making a big deal of it) reactions, whereas individuals with *unstable* high self-esteem reported the least (individuals with low self-esteem again fell in between). These findings suggest that individuals with unstable high self-esteem are prone to interpret their partners' actions in ways that foster a vicious cycle of negativity within their intimate relationships. They are important because they point to the operation of dynamics associated with fragile high self-esteem that heretofore have been ascribed to individuals with low self-esteem (Murray, Holmes, MacDonald, & Ellsworth, 1998) or to those highly sensitive to rejection (Downey, Freitas, Michaelis, & Khouri, 1998).

In sum, the studies reviewed in this section indicate that not all people who report high levels of self-esteem are secure in their positive self-feelings and that, when they are not, defensiveness and self-aggrandizement are heightened, and psychological well-being and relationship functioning are diminished.

A Few Caveats

Before concluding this chapter, we note several caveats. First, not all research suggests that unstable self-esteem is invariably associated with relatively poor psychological functioning. In some studies, we have found that among individuals with low self-esteem, self-esteem instability is related to more, not less, adaptive outcomes (Kernis et al., 1992; Paradise & Kernis, in press). In Paradise and Kernis's (in press) study on fragile self-esteem and psychological well-being, self-esteem stability among individuals with low self-esteem exhibited a pattern of relations with some components of positive psychological functioning that was different from the pattern that emerged among individuals with high self-esteem. In some cases (i.e., relations with others and personal growth), individuals with unstable as compared with stable low self-esteem revealed more positive psychological functioning, whereas in the self-acceptance domain, there were no differences. Why does unstable self-esteem among individuals with low self-esteem (compared with individuals with stable low self-esteem) relate to better psychological functioning in some domains but not in others? One possibility is that fragile negative feelings of self-worth confer relatively more benefits than do secure negative self-feelings within the contexts of social relationships and personal improvements. Consistently maintaining negative self-feelings probably would be reflected in an interaction style that other people find undesirable; also, stable negative self-feelings may serve to undermine attempts at personal change and improvement. At times, individuals with unstable low self-esteem might present a positive self to others that is more endearing than a gloomy disposition, as well as positive self-feelings that may fuel efforts directed toward personal growth. In any event, unstable self-esteem appears to be associated with relatively better functioning among individuals with low self-esteem in some, but not all, aspects of well-being.

Also, inconsistent findings among individuals with low self-esteem as a function of self-esteem stability have emerged in the past (although the inconsistencies involved different samples of individuals). Apparently, unstable self-esteem sometimes operates differently among individuals with low as compared with high self-esteem. At times, possessing unstable low self-esteem might provide a temporary release from negative self-feelings that improves well-being in some domains. In contrast, fragile feelings of positive self-worth appear to consistently undermine psychological functioning (for further discussion of this issue, see Kernis, 1993; Kernis & Waschull, 1995).

Second, we should acknowledge that there are isolated instances in the literature of failure to replicate certain findings. Specifically, Kernis, Grannemann, and Mathis (1991) reported that self-esteem level predicted future depression only among individuals whose self-esteem is stable. Roberts, Kassel, and Gotlib (1995) conduct-ed several studies with different samples and failed to replicate this pattern once. A similar lack of convergence was reported by Gable and Nezlek (1998). There are numerous methodological differences between these three sets of studies that may account for the discrepancies, but none are especially salient and compelling.

Third, we have generally characterized the tendency to fluctuate in contextually based self-esteem in unfavorable terms, linking it to vulnerability, fragility, and suboptimal functioning. A contrasting view has been put forth to suggest that some degree of self-esteem fluctuations are desirable and that moderate self-esteem instability may be related to optimal psychological functioning. Leary's sociometer theory (Leary & Downs, 1995) holds that self-esteem fluctuations inform people about the degree to which they are socially accepted. A decline in state self-esteem (i.e., contextually based feelings of self-worth) in response to rejection is thought to be adaptive, for it signals that the organism is responsive to reality. Furthermore, these fluctuations may stimulate behavioral changes that will increase one's social acceptance. Although we believe that this theory is very important and that it has many positive features, we question whether linking negative outcomes to global self-feelings is either desirable or adaptive. From our vantage point, people can be responsive to feelings of rejection without feeling that they are less worthy individuals (see also Deci & Ryan, 1995). When rejected, there are instances in which people would benefit from questioning their social skills, presentational styles, and so forth. This would be adaptive in many instances. What we question is whether it is adaptive for people to link these relatively specific self-appraisals to their overall feelings of self-worth (so that their global self-esteem suffers). This apparent difference in perspectives is likely to generate considerable controversy in the near future, and we hope that it will stimulate an equal amount of careful empirical attention.

Conclusions

Self-concepts and self-esteem are imbedded within a complex self-system that includes multiple psychological needs (e.g., self-determination, self-enhancement, self-verification) and that is affected by a wide variety of contextual factors. These needs and contextual factors form the backdrop against which self-concept and self-esteem stability and variability can be understood. Research and theory on stability and variability in self-concept and self-esteem have important implications for the nature of the self and its role in various aspects of human functioning. With respect to self-concept variability (versus stability), these implications are complicated by the advent of new cultural technologies that allow people to construct temporary identities with little or no consequences. Self-concept variability is more likely to reflect flexibility and adaptiveness when it is accompanied by a strong sense of efficacy rather than an external focus on situational requirements per se. Even when based in feelings of high self-efficacy, however, it is unlikely that an infinite amount of self-concept variability will relate to optimal psychological functioning. As suggested by self-verification theory, people seem to desire stability in at least some of their core self-aspects. Research on self-esteem variability (instability) tells a somewhat different story. With few exceptions, the more unstable individuals' self-esteem, the less optimal their psychological functioning. Recent theoretical perspectives, however, raise the possibility that some degree of self-esteem instability is optimal. Additional research is needed to directly assess the viability of this possibility, as well as to increase our understanding of the role of unstable self-esteem among individuals with low self-esteem.

Acknowledgments

Preparation of this chapter was facilitated by National Science Foundation Grant No. SBR-9618882.

Notes

1. As noted earlier, we chose to discuss self-appraisals in the section on self-concept stability rather than in the section on self-esteem stability for two reasons. First, we wanted to emphasize that self-appraisals reflect judgments or ratings of one's standing along spe-cific dimensions, similar to descriptions of the content of one's self-concept. Second, we wanted to clearly distinguish self-appraisals from self-esteem, which refers to global feelings of self-worth, liking, acceptance, and so forth, irrespective of specific self-appraisals.
2. The terms "variability" and "instability" have each been used to refer to short-term fluctuations in self-esteem. Although we prefer the term "instability," we use the terms interchangeably throughout this chapter.
3. We also included Rosenberg's Stability of Self Scale in some of our early work (e.g., Kernis, Grannemann, & Barclay, 1992) but we had little success with it. Kernis and colleagues (1992) reported a nonsignificant correlation between scores on this scale and self-esteem stability as assessed through multiple assessments but a high correlation between these scores and self-esteem level ($r = -.58$). Other data from that study indicated that asking people to rate the extent to which their self-esteem fluctuates from day to day was more strongly related to scores on Rosenberg's scale than it was to observed self-esteem instability. We believe that people are not fully aware of how unstable their self-esteem may be and that, consequently, asking them how much their self-esteem fluctuates cannot substitute for a measure of self-esteem stability that is based on repeated assessments obtained in naturalistic contexts. Therefore, we limit our review to studies that used multiple assessments (for periods ranging from 4 to 30 days) to assess self-esteem stability.

References

Bachman, J. G., O'Malley, P. M., & Johnson, J. J. (1978). *Youth in transition: Volume 6. Adolescence to adulthood: A study of change and stability in the lives of young men.* Ann Arbor: Institute for Social Research, University of Michigan.

Baumeister, R. F. (1982). Self-esteem, self-presentation, and future interaction: A dilemma of reputation. *Journal of Personality, 50,* 29–45.

Baumeister, R. F. (1987). How the self became a problem: a psychological review of historical research. *Journal of Personality and Social Psychology, 52,* 163–176.

Baumeister, R. F., Smart, L., & Boden, J. M. (1996). Relation of threatened egotism to violence and aggression: The dark side of high self-esteem. *Psychological Review, 103,* 5-33.

Baumrind, D. (1971). Current patterns of parental authority. *Developmental Psychology Monographs, 4*(1, Pt. 2), 1–103.

Bem, D. (1972). Self-perception theory. In L. Berkowitz (Ed.), *Advances in experimental social psychology* (Vol. 6, pp. 1–62). New York: Academic Press.

Berglas, S. (1985). Self-handicapping and self-handicappers: A cognitive/attributional model of interpersonal self-protective behavior. In R. Hogan & W. H. Jones (Eds.), *Perspectives in personality* (Vol. 1, pp. 235–270). Greenwich, CT: JAI Press

Brockner, J. (1984). Low self-esteem and behavioral plasticity: Some implications for personality and social psychology. In L. Wheeler (Ed.), *Review of personality and social psychology* (Vol. 4, pp. 237–271). Beverly Hills, CA: Sage.

Brown, J. D. (1993). Self-esteem and self-evaluation: Feeling is believing. In J. Suls (Ed.), *Psychological perspectives on the self* (Vol. 4, pp. 27–58). Hillsdale, NJ: Erlbaum.

Brown, J. D. (1998). *The self.* Boston: McGraw-Hill.

Brown, J. D., & Dutton, K. A. (1995). The thrill of victory, the complexity of defeat: Self-esteem and people's emotional reactions to success and failure. *Journal of Personality and Social Psychology, 68,* 712–722.

Buri, J. R., Louiselle, P. A., Misukanis, T. M., & Mueller, R. A. (1988). Effects of parental authoritarianism and authoritativeness on self-esteem. *Personality and Social Psychology Bulletin, 14,* 271–282.

Butler, A. C., Hokanson, J. E., & Flynn, H. A. (1994). A comparison of self-esteem ability and low self-esteem as vulnerability factors for depression. *Journal of Personality and Social Psychology, 66,* 166–177.

Campbell, J. D. (1990). Self-esteem and clarity of the self-concept. *Journal of Personality and Social Psychology, 59,* 538–549.

Campbell, J. D., Trapnell, P. D., Heine, S. J., Katz, I. M., Lavallee, L. F., & Lehman, D. R. (1996). Self-concept clarity: Measurement, personality correlates, and cultural boundaries. *Journal of Personality and Social Psychology, 70,* 141–156.

Carver, C. S., & Ganellen, R. J. (1983). Depression and components of self-punitiveness: High standards, self-criticism, and overgeneralization. *Journal of Abnormal Psychology, 92,* 330–337.

Chodoff, P. (1973). The depressive personality: A critical review. *International Journal of Psychiatry, 11,* 196–217.

Coopersmith, S. (1967). *The antecedents of self-esteem.* San Francisco: Freeman.

Crocker, J., & Wolf, C. T. (2001). Contingencies of self-worth. *Psychological Review, 108,* 593–623.

Dact, G. L., & Ryan, R. M. (2000). The "what" and "why" of goal pursuits: Human needs and the self-determination of behavior. *Psychological Inquiry, 11,* 227–268.

Deaux, K., Reid, A., Mizrahi, K., & Ethier, K.A. (1995). Parameters of social identity. *Journal of Personality and Social Psychology, 68,* 280–291.

Deci, E. L., & Ryan, R. M. (1985). *Intrinsic motivation and self-determination in human behavior.* New York: Plenum Press.

Deci, E. L., & Ryan, R. M. (1987). The support of autonomy and the control of behavior. *Journal of Personality and Social Psychology, 53,* 1024–1037.

Deci, E. L., & Ryan, R. M. (1991). A motivational approach to self: Integration in personality. In R. Dienstbier (Ed.), *Nebraska Symposium on Motivation: Vol. 38. Perspectives on motivation* (pp. 237–288). Lincoln: University of Nebraska Press.

Deci, E. L., & Ryan, R. M. (1995). Human agency: The basis for true self-esteem. In M. Kernis (Ed.), *Efficacy,*

agency, and self-esteem (pp. 31–50). New York: Plenum Press.

Deci, E. L., & Ryan, R. M. (2000). The "what" and "why" of goal pursuits: Human needs and the self-determination of behavior. *Psychological Inquiry, 11,* 227–268.

Demo, D. H., & Savin-Williams, R. C. (1983). Early adolescent self-esteem as a function of social class: Rosenberg and Pearlin revisited. *American Journal of Sociology, 88,* 763–774.

Downey, G., Freitas, A. L., Michaelis, B., & Khouri, H. (1998). The self-fulfilling prophecy in close relationships: Rejection sensitivity and rejection by close partners. *Journal of Personality and Social Psychology, 75,* 545–560.

Dutton, K. A., & Brown, J. D. (1997). Global self-esteem and specific self-views as determinants of people's reactions to success and failure. *Journal of Personality and Social Psychology, 73,* 139–148.

Dweck, C., & Goetz, T. E. (1978). Attributions and learned helplessness. In J. Harvey, W. Ickes, & R. F. Kidd (Eds.), *New directions in attribution theory* (Vol. 2). Hillsdale, NJ: Erlbaum.

Emmons, R. A. (1986). Personal strivings: An approach to personal strivings and well-being. *Journal of Personality and Social Psychology, 51,* 1058–1068.

Epstein, S. (1992). Coping ability, negative self-evaluation, and overgeneralization: Experiment and theory. *Journal of Personality and Social Psychology, 62,* 826–836.

Epstein, S., & Morling, B. (1995). Is the self motivated to do more than enhance and/or verify itself? In M. H. Kernis (Ed.), *Efficacy, agency, and self-esteem* (pp. 9–30). New York: Plenum Press.

Gable, S. L., & Nezlek, J. B. (1998). Level and instability of day-to-day psychological well-being and risk for depression. *Journal of Personality and Social Psychology, 74,* 129–138.

Gecas, V., & Schwalbe, M. L. (1986). Parental behavior and adolescent self-esteem. *Journal of Marriage and the Family, 48,* 37–46.

Gergen, K. J. (1991). *The saturated self.* New York: Basic Books.

Gergen, K. J. (1996). Technology and the self: from the essential to the sublime. In D. Grodin & T. R. Lindloff (Eds.), *Constructing the self in a mediated world* (pp. 156–178). Thousand Oaks, CA: Sage.

Greenberg, J., & Pyszczynski, T. (1985). Compensatory self-inflation: A response to the self-regard of public failure. *Journal of Personality and Social Psychology, 49,* 274–280.

Greenier, K. G., Kernis, M. H., Whisenhunt, C. R., Waschull, S. B., Berry, A. J., Herlocker, C. E., & Abend, T. (1999). Individual differences in reactivity to daily events: Examining the roles of stability and level of self-esteem. *Journal of Personality, 67,* 185–208.

Grolnick, W. S., & Ryan, R. M. (1989). Parent styles associated with children's self-regulation and competence in school. *Journal of Educational Psychology, 81,* 143–154.

Harter, S. (1981). *A scale of intrinsic versus extrinsic orientation in the classroom.* Denver, CO: University of Denver Press.

Hermans, H. (1996) Voicing the self: from information processing to dialogical interchange. *Psychological Bulletin, 119,* 31–50.

Hoyle, R. H., Kernis, M. H., Leary, M. R., & Baldwin, M.

(1999). *Selfhood: Identity, esteem, regulation.* Boulder, CO: Westview Press.

Jacobson, E. (1975). The regulation of self-esteem. In E. J. Anthony & T. Benedek (Eds.), *Depression and human existence* (pp. 169–182). Boston: Little, Brown.

Jones, E. E., & Gerard, H. B. (1967). *Foundations of social psychology.* New York: Wiley.

Jones, E. E., Rhodewalt, F., Berglas, S., & Skelton, J. A. (1981). Effects of strategic self-presentation on subsequent self-esteem. *Journal of Personality and Social Psychology, 41,* 407–421.

Kernis, M. H. (1993). The roles of stability and level of self-esteem in psychological functioning. In R. F. Baumeister (Ed.), *Self-esteem: The puzzle of low self-regard* (pp. 167–182). New York: Plenum Press.

Kernis, M. H. (2000). Substitute needs and the distinction between fragile and secure high self-esteem. *Psychological Inquiry, 11,* 298–300.

Kernis, M. H. (in press). Toward a conceptualization of optimal self-esteem. *Psychological Inquiry.*

Kernis, M. H., Brockner, J., & Frankel, B. S. (1989). Self-esteem and reactions to failure: The mediating role of overgeneralization. *Journal of Personality and Social Psychology, 57,* 707–714.

Kernis, M. H., Brown, A. C., & Brody, G. H. (2000). Fragile self-esteem in children and its associations with perceived patterns of parent–child communication. *Journal of Personality, 68,* 225–252.

Kernis, M. H., Cornell, D. P., Sun, C., Berry, A., & Harlow, T. (1993). There's more to self-esteem than whether it's high or low: The importance of stability of self-esteem. *Journal of Personality and Social Psychology, 65,* 1190–1204.

Kernis, M. H., Grannemann, B. D., & Barclay, L. C. (1989). Stability and level of self-esteem as predictors of anger arousal and hostility. *Journal of Personality and Social Psychology, 56,* 1013–1023.

Kernis, M. H., Grannemann, B. D., & Barclay, L. C. (1992). Stability of self-esteem: Assessment, correlates, and excuse-making. *Journal of Personality, 60,* 621–644.

Kernis, M. H., Grannemann, B. D., & Mathis, L. C. (1991). Stability of self-esteem as a moderator of the relation between level of self-esteem and depression. *Journal of Personality and Social Psychology, 61,* 80–84.

Kernis, M. H., Greenier, K. D., Herlocker, C. E., Whisenhunt, C. R., & Abend, T. (1997). Self-perceptions of reactions to positive and negative outcomes: The roles of stability and level of self-esteem. *Personality and Individual Differences, 22,* 845–854.

Kernis, M. H., Jadrich, J., Gibert, P., & Sun, C. R. (1996). Stable and unstable components of self-evaluations: Individual differences in self-appraisal responsiveness to feedback. *Journal of Social and Clinical Psychology, 15,* 430–448.

Kernis, M. H., & Johnson, E. K. (1990). Current and typical self-appraisals: Differential responsiveness to evaluative feedback and implications for emotions. *Journal of Research in Personality, 24,* 241–257.

Kernis, M. H., & Paradise, A.W. (2002). Differentiating between fragile and secure forms of high self-esteem. In E. L. Deci & R. M. Ryan (Eds.), *Handbook of self-determination research* (pp. 339–360). Rochester, NY: University of Rochester Press.

Kernis, M. H., Paradise, A. W., & Goldman, B. N. (2002). *Overinvestment of self in relationships: Implications of fragile self-esteem.* Manuscript in preparation.

Kernis, M. H., Paradise, A.W., Whitaker, D., Wheatman, S., & Goldman, B. (2000). Master of one's psychological domain? Not likely if one's self-esteem is unstable. *Personality and Social Psychology Bulletin, 26,* 1297–1305.

Kernis, M. H., & Waschull, S. B. (1995). The interactive roles of stability and level of self-esteem: Research and theory. In M. P. Zanna (Ed.), *Advances in experimental social psychology* (Vol. 27, pp. 93–141). San Diego, CA: Academic Press.

Kernis, M. H., Whisenhunt, C. R., Waschull, S. B., Greenier, K. D., Berry, A. J., Herlocker, C. E., & Anderson, C. A. (1998). Multiple facets of self-esteem and their relations to depressive symptoms. *Personality and Social Psychology Bulletin, 24,* 657–668.

Leary, M. R., & Downs, D. L. (1995). Interpersonal functions of the self-esteem motive: The self-esteem system as a sociometer. In M. H. Kernis (Ed.), *Efficacy, agency, and self-esteem* (pp. 123–144). New York: Plenum Press.

Markus, H., & Kunda, Z. (1986). Stability and malleability of the self-concept. *Journal of Personality and Social Psychology, 51,* 858–866.

Markus, H., & Nurius, P. (1986). Possible selves. *American Psychologist, 41,* 954–969.

Markus, H., & Wurf, , E. (1987). The dynamic self-concept: A social psychological perspective. *Annual Review of Psychology, 38,* 299–337.

McAdams, D. P. (1997). The case for unity in the (post) modern self. In R.D. Ashmore & L. Jussim (Eds.), *Self and identity* (Vol. 1, pp. 46–80). New York: Oxford University Press.

McCarthy, J. D. , & Hoge, D. R. (1982). Analysis of age effects in longitudinal studies in longitudinal studies of adolescent self-esteem. *Developmental Psychology, 18,* 372-379.

McGuire, W. J., & McGuire, C. V. (1981). The spontaneous self-concept as affected by personal distinctiveness. In M. D. Lynch, A. A. Norem-Hebeisen, & K. Gergen (Eds.), *Self-concept: Advances in theory and research* (pp. 147–171). New York: Ballinger.

McGuire, W. J., & McGuire, C. V. (1988). Content and process in the experience of self. In L. Berkowitz (Ed.), *Advances in experimental social psychology* (Vol. 21, pp. 97–144). New York: Academic Press.

McKenna, K.Y.A., & Bargh, J.A. (1998). Coming out in the age of the Internet: Identity "demarginalization" through virtual group participation. *Journal of Personality and Social Psychology, 75,* 681–694.

Morse, S., & Gergen, K. J. (1970). Social comparison, self-consistency, and the concept of self. *Journal of Personality and Social Psychology, 16,* 148–156.

Murray, S. L., Holmes, J. G., MacDonald, G., & Ellsworth, P. C. (1998). Through the looking glass darkly? When self-doubts turn into relationship insecurities. *Journal of Personality and Social Psychology, 75,* 1459–1480.

Novaco, R. W. (1975). *Anger control: The development and evaluation of an experimental treatment.* Lexington, MA: Lexington Books.

O'Malley, P. M., & Bachman, J. G. (1983). Self-esteem: Change and stability between ages 13 and 23. *Developmental Psychology, 18,* 372–379.

Paradise, A. W., & Kernis, M. H. (in press). Self-esteem and psychological well-being: Implications of fragile self-esteem. *Journal of Social and Clinical Psychology.*

Paulhus, D. L., & Martin, C. L. (1988). Functional flexibility: A new conceptualization of interpersonal flexibility. *Journal of Personality and Social Psychology*, 55, 88–101.

Pelham, B. (1995). Self-investment and self-esteem: Evidence for a Jamesian model of self-worth. *Journal of Personality and Social Psychology, 69,* 1141–1150.

Roberts, J. E., & Gotlib, I. H. (1997). Temporal variability in global self-esteem and specific self-evaluation as prospective predictors of emotional distress: Specificity in predictors and outcomes. *Journal of Abnormal Psychology, 106*, 521–529.

Roberts, J. E., Kassel, J. D., & Gotlib, I. H. (1995). Level and stability of self-esteem as predictors of depressive symptoms. *Personality and Individual Differences, 19,* 217–224.

Roberts, J. E., & Monroe, S. M. (1992). Vulnerable self-esteem and depressive symptoms: Prospective findings comparing three alternative conceptualizations. *Journal of Personality and Social Psychology, 62*, 804–812.

Rogers, C. (1959). A theory of therapy, personality, and interpersonal relationships, as developed in the client-centered framework. In S. Koch (Ed.), *Psychology: A study of science* (Vol. 3, pp. 184–256). New York: McGraw-Hill.

Rosenberg, M. (1965). *Society and the adolescent self-image.* Princeton, NJ: Princeton University Press.

Rosenberg, M. (1986). Self-concept from middle childhood through adolescence. In J. Suls & A. G. Greenwald (Eds.), *Psychological perspectives on the self* (Vol. 2, pp. 107–136), Hillsdale, NJ: Erlbaum.

Ryan, R. M. (1993). Agency and organization: Intrinsic motivation, autonomy, and the self in psychological development. In J. Jacobs (Ed.), *Nebraska Symposium on Motivation: Vol. 40. Developmental perspectives on motivation* (pp. 1–56). Lincoln: University of Nebraska Press.

Ryan, R. M., & Connell, J. P. (1989). Perceived locus of causality and internalization: Examining reasons for acting in two domains. *Journal of Personality and Social Psychology, 57*, 749–761.

Ryan, R. M., Rigby, S., & King, K. (1993). Two types of religious internalization and their relations to religious orientations and mental health. *Journal of Personality and Social Psychology*, 65, 586–596.

Ryff, C. (1989). Happiness is everything, or is it? Explorations on the meaning of psychological well-being. *Journal of Personality and Social Psychology, 57*, 1069–1081.

Sande, G. N., Goethals, G. R., & Radloff, C. E. (1988). Perceiving one's own traits and others': The multifaceted self. *Journal of Personality and Social Psychology, 54,* 13–20.

Savin-Williams, R. C., & Demo, D. H. (1983). Situational and transsituational determinants of adolescent self-feelings. *Journal of Personality and Social Psychology, 44*, 924–833.

Snyder, M. (1987). *Public appearances/private realities: The psychology of self-affirmation.* New York: Freeman.

Spencer, S. J., Josephs, R. A., & Steele, C. M. (1993). Low self-esteem: The struggle for self-integrity. In R. F. Baumeister (Ed.), *Low self-esteem: The puzzle of low self-regard* (pp. 21–36). New York: Plenum Press.

Steele, C. M. (1988). The psychology of self-affirmation: Sustaining the integrity of the self. In L. Berkowitz (Ed.), *Advances in experimental social psychology* (Vol. 21, pp. 261–302). New York: Academic Press.

Swann, W. B., Jr. (1983). Self-verification: Bringing social reality into harmony with the self. In J. Suls & A. G. Greenwald (Eds.), *Psychological perspectives on the self* (Vol. 2, pp. 33–66). Hillsdale, NJ: Erlbaum.

Swann, W. B. Jr. (1990). To be adored or to be known? The interplay of self-enhancement and self-verification. In E. T. Higgins & R. M. Sorrentino (Eds.), *Handbook of motivation and cognition* (Vol. 2, pp. 408–448). New York: Guilford Press.

Swann, W. G., Jr., Griffin, J. J., Predmore, S., & Gaines, B. (1987). The cognitive–affective crossfire: When self-consistency confronts self-enhancement. *Journal of Personality and Social Psychology, 52*, 881–889.

Swann, W. B., Jr., & Hill, C. A. (1982). When our identities are mistaken: Reaffirming self-conceptions through social interaction. *Journal of Personality and Social Psychology, 43*, 59–66.

Swann, W. B., Jr., & Read, S. J. (1981). Acquiring self-knowledge: The search for feedback that fits. Journal of Personality and Social Psychology, 41, 1119-1128.

Swann, W. B., Jr., & Schroeder, D. G. (1995). The search for beauty and truth: A framework for understanding reactions to evaluations. *Personality and Social Psychology Bulletin, 21*, 1307–1318.

Swann, W. B., Jr., Stein-Seroussi, A., & Giesler, R. B. (1992). Why people self-verify. *Journal of Personality and Social Psychology, 62*, 392–401.

Swann, W. B., Jr., Wenzlaff, R. M., Krull, D. S., & Pelham, B. W. (1992). Allure of negative feedback: Self-verification strivings among depressed persons. *Journal of Abnormal Psychology, 101*, 293–306.

Tangney, J. P., Wagner, P., & Gramzow, R. (1989). *The Self-Conscious Affect (TOSCA).* Fairfax, VA: George Mason University.

Tennen, H., & Affleck, G. (1993). The puzzles of self-esteem: A clinical perspective. In R. F. Baumeister (Ed.), *Self-esteem: The puzzle of low self-regard* (pp. 37–54). New York: Plenum Press.

Tice, D. (1992). Self-presentation and self-concept change: The looking-glass self is also a magnifying glass. *Journal of Personality and Social Psychology, 63*, 435–451.

Vallachar, R. & Novak, A. (2000). Landscapes of self-reflection: Mapping the peaks and valleys of personal assessment. In A. Tesser, R. B. Felson, & J. M. Suls (Eds.), *Psychological perspectives on self and identity* (pp. 35–66). Washington, DC: American Psychological Association.

Waschull, S. B., & Kernis, M. H. (1996). Level and stability of self-esteem as predictors of children's intrinsic motivation and reasons for anger. *Personality and Social Psychology Bulletin, 22*, 4–13.

Weber, R. J. (2000). *The created self.* New York: Norton.

Wood, J. V., Giordano-Beech, M., Taylor, K. L., Michela, J. L., & Gaus, V. (1994). Strategies of social comparison among people with low self-esteem: Self-protection and self-enhancement. *Journal of Personality and Social Psychology, 67*, 713–731.

7

A Sociological Approach to Self and Identity

JAN E. STETS
PETER J. BURKE

Thoughts on Social Structure

A sociological approach to self and identity begins with the assumption that there is a reciprocal relationship between the self and society (Stryker, 1980). The self influences society through the actions of individuals, thereby creating groups, organizations, networks, and institutions. Reciprocally, society influences the self through its shared language and meanings that enable a person to take the role of the other, engage in social interaction, and reflect on oneself as an object. The latter process of reflection constitutes the core of selfhood (McCall & Simmons, 1978; Mead, 1934). Because the self emerges in and is reflective of society, the sociological approach to understanding the self and its parts (identities) means that we must also understand the society in which the self is acting, keeping in mind that the self is always acting in a social context in which other selves exist (Stryker, 1980). This chapter focuses primarily on the nature of self and identity from a sociological perspective. However, because the nature of the self and what individuals do depends to a large extent on the society within which they live, some discussion of society is warranted.

Sociologists are interested in understanding the nature of society and social structure, the latter being the more abstract forms and patterns that constitute groups, networks, organizations, and larger political units. They are interested in the ways in which society develops and is transformed. The traditional symbolic interactionist perspective, known as the *situational approach* to self and society, sees society as always in the process of being created through the interpretations and definitions of actors in situations (Blumer, 1969). Actors identify the things that need to be taken into account for themselves, act on the basis of those identifications, and attempt to fit their lines of action with others in the situation to accomplish their goals. From this perspective, the inference is made that individuals are free to define the situation in any way they care to, with the consequence that society is always thought to be in a state of flux, with no real organization or structure. As Stryker (2000, p. 27) recently remarked on this perspective:

"[It] tends to dissolve structure in a solvent of subjective definitions, to view definitions as unanchored, open to any possibility, failing to recognize that some possibilities are more probable than others. On the premise that self reflects society, this view leads to seeing self as undifferentiated, unorganized, unstable, and ephemeral."

Our view of self and society is rooted in the *structural approach* to the symbolic interactionist perspective (Stryker, 1980). Within this perspective, we do not see society as tentatively shaped. Instead, we assume that society is stable and durable as reflected in the "patterned regularities that characterize most human action" (Stryker, 1980, p. 65). Patterns of behavior within and between individuals have different levels of analysis, and this difference is key to understanding the link between self and society. At one level, we can look at the patterns of behavior of one individual over time and come to know that individual. By pooling several such patterns across similar individuals, we can come to know individuals of a certain type. At still another level, we can look at the patterns of behavior across individuals to see how these patterns fit with the patterns of others to create larger patterns of behavior. It is these larger, interindividual patterns that constitute social structure. We provide an illustration.

In this chapter, we discuss how people act to verify their conceptions of who they are. A scientist, for example, may act in ways that make it clear to herself, as well as to others, that she is careful, analytical, logical, and experimentally inclined. She may engage in a variety of actions and interactions to convey these images. These are individual patterns of behavior that help us to understand the individual scientist. These same patterns of behavior may be part of a larger social structure. We may find, for example, that scientists who are careful, analytical, logical, and experimentally inclined and who do these things well are elected to high positions in their scientific organizations. If we take a broader view, we may see that there is a flow of such persons into positions of prominence within their scientific societies and into positions of eminence in policy and governmental circles. The result is that their pronouncements about being scientists and their activities as scientists

help to maintain boundaries between themselves and nonscientists, as well as to keep resources flowing to the groups and organizations to which they belong. The flow of persons into positions of importance through the mechanism of elections and appointments is part of the social structure, as are the flows of resources they control and the mechanisms that support and sustain these flows.

Individuals act, but those actions exist within the context of the full set of patterns of action, interaction, and resource transfers among all persons, all of which constitute the structure of society. Social structures do emerge from individual actions, as those actions are patterned across individuals and over time, but individual actions also occur in the context of the social structure within which the individuals exist. In this way, social structure is a very abstract idea. It is not something we experience directly. We are not directly tuned to these patterns as they occur across persons and over time. Nevertheless, we can become aware of them and study them. Many of the patterns are well recognized, named, and attended to. They enter our everyday language as things such as General Motors, the New York Yankees, the Brown family, Milwaukee. Some are recognized but harder to point to, such as "the working class" or "the country club set" that do not have a legal status and do not maintain offices or locations. We can only point to individuals who may contribute to the patterns of behavior that constitute the structure. Some structures we tend not to see at all (without special effort or thought), such as the patterns of action that block access of African Americans to the education system or the patterns of actions that create the "glass ceiling" in organizations preventing qualified women from rising to positions of power and authority. Nevertheless, these too are parts of social structure, and it is the job of sociologists to discover, attend to, and understand these patterns.

The preceding implies that the basis for understanding social structure arises from the actions of individuals, keeping in mind that these agents (individuals) receive feedback from the structures they and others create to change themselves and the way they operate. In this chapter, we direct our attention to understanding selves that are producing actions, the patterns of which constitute social structure. However, as sociological social psychologists, we want the reader to keep in mind that persons are always embedded in the very social structure that is, at the same time, being created by those persons. It is this social context that is central in distinguishing sociological approaches to the study of the self.

Self and Identity in Sociology

Self

The symbolic interactionist perspective in sociological social psychology sees the self as emerging out of the mind, the mind as arising and developing out of social interaction, and patterned social interaction as forming the basis of social structure (Mead, 1934). The mind is the thinking part of the self. It is covert action in which the organism points out meanings to itself and to others. The ability to point out meanings and to indicate them to others and to itself is made possible by language, which encapsulates meanings in the form of symbols. When one's self is encapsulated as a set of symbols to which one may respond as an object, as one responds to any other symbol, the self has emerged. The hallmark of this process—of selfhood—is reflexivity. Humans have the ability to reflect back on themselves, taking themselves as objects. They are able to regard and evaluate themselves, to take account of themselves and plan accordingly to bring about future states, to be self-aware or achieve consciousness with respect to their own existence. In this way, humans are *processual* entities. They formulate and reflect, and this process is ongoing.

To be clear, the responses of the self as an object to itself come from the point of view of others with whom one interacts. By taking the role of the other and seeing ourselves from others' perspectives, our responses come to be like others' responses, and the meaning of the self becomes a shared meaning. Thus, paradoxically, as the self emerges as a distinct object, there is at the same time a merger of perspectives of the self and others and a becoming as one

with the others with whom one interacts. This becoming as one is possible through the shared meanings of the objects and symbols to which individuals respond in interaction. In using language, individuals communicate the same meanings to themselves as to others. The self is, thus, both individual and social in character. It works to control meanings to sustain itself, but many of those meanings, including the meanings of the self, are shared and form the basis of interaction with others and, ultimately, social structure.

Self-Concept

Over time, as humans point out who they are to themselves and to others, they come to develop a concept or view of who they are. Humans are entities that embody *content* and a *structure*. Sociologists have spent considerable time in understanding the content and structure of the self: one's self-concept. Early views of the self-concept were concerned only with self-evaluation. Self-concept often meant self-esteem (one's evaluation of oneself in affective—negative or positive—terms; cf., Rosenberg, 1979). To broaden this view, Rosenberg (1979) suggested that there was more to the self-concept than self-esteem. He defined the self-concept as the sum total of our thoughts, feelings, and imaginations as to who we are. Later conceptions elaborated and refined this view, suggesting that the self-concept was made up of cognitive components (given the collection of identities), as well as affective components or self-feelings, including self-esteem (both worth-based and efficacy-based self-esteem; Franks & Marolla, 1976; Stryker, 1980).

In general, the self-concept is the set of meanings we hold for ourselves when we look at ourselves. It is based on our observations of ourselves, our inferences about who we are gained from others' behavior toward us, our wishes and desires, and our evaluations of ourselves. The self-concept includes not only our idealized views of who we are that are relatively unchanging but also our *self-image* or *working copy* of our self-views that we import into situations and that is subject to constant change and revision based on situational influences (Burke, 1980). It is this *self-image* that guides moment-to-moment interaction, that is changed in situated negotiation, and that may act back on our idealized self-views.

For sociological social psychologists, the self-concept emerges out of the reflected-appraisal process (Gecas & Burke, 1995). Although some of our self-views are gained by direct experience with our environment, most of what we know about ourselves is derived from others. According to the reflected-appraisal process, which is based on the "looking-glass self" (Cooley, 1902),[1] significant others communicate their appraisals of us, and these appraisals influence the way we see ourselves. In a now-classic review of studies on the reflected-appraisal process, Shrauger and Schoeneman (1979) found that, rather than our self-concepts resembling the way others actually see us, our self-concepts are filtered through our perceptions and resemble how we *think* others see us.

Felson (1993) summarized a program of research in which he attempted to explain why individuals are not very accurate in judging what others think of them. Among the causes of the discrepancy is the apprehension of others about revealing their views. At best, they may reveal primarily favorable views rather than both favorable and unfavorable views. Consistent with other research (DePaulo, Kenny, Hoover, Webb, & Oliver, 1987; Kenny & Albright, 1987), Felson found that individuals have a better idea of how groups see them than of how specific individuals see them. Presumably, individuals learn the group standards and then apply those standards. In turn, when group members judge individuals, they use the same standards that individuals originally applied to themselves. Thus we find a correspondence in self-appraisals and others' appraisals of the self.

In our investigation of the reflected-appraisal process with newly married couples, we found that social status derived from one's position in the social structure also influences the appraisal process. The spouse with the higher status (education, occupation, and income) in the marriage is more likely to not only influence his or her partner's self-views but also the partner's views of him or her (Cast, Stets, & Burke, 1999). Spouses with a lower status in the marriage have less influence on the self-views of their higher status counterparts or on how their higher status counterparts view them.

Self-Evaluation

The aspect of the self-concept that has received a significant amount of attention in sociological social psychology is the evaluative part of the self-concept, better known as self-esteem (Rosenberg, 1979). Two dimensions of self-esteem have been identified: *efficacy-based* self-esteem (seeing oneself as competent and capable) and *worth-based* self-esteem (feeling that one is accepted and valued; Gecas & Schwalbe, 1983). Others have labeled the distinction *inner self-esteem* (being effective) and *outer self-esteem* (acceptance by others; Franks & Marolla, 1976). As Gecas and Burke (1995) pointed out, the significant interest in self-esteem is largely due to the assumption that high self-esteem is associated with good outcomes, such as personal success whereas low self-esteem is associated with bad outcomes, such as deviance. Although these associations are a bit misleading because research does not always show such consistency in these outcomes, part of the inconsistency may come from, among other things, measuring self-esteem in global terms rather than in more specific terms (Hoelter, 1986; Rosenberg, Schooler, Schoenbach, & Rosenberg, 1995).[2] Nevertheless, self-esteem remains a high-profile topic of investigation and has been examined from a variety of different viewpoints: as an outcome (Rosenberg, 1979), as a buffer against stress (Longmore & DeMaris, 1997), and as a motive that directs behavior (Kaplan, 1975; Tesser, 1988).

Cast and Burke (2002) used identity theory as a theoretical framework for the integration of these different conceptualizations of self-esteem. They argued that self-esteem is intimately tied to the identity verification process.[3] They point out that (1) high self-esteem has been founded to be an outcome of the identity verification process—people feel good about themselves when their identities are confirmed (Burke & Stets, 1999), (2) high self-esteem that is generated from the identity verification process can act as a buffer or resource when the verification process fails, and (3) the desire for self-esteem may be what motivates people to create and maintain situations or relationships that verify their identities. They also argue that the two components of self-esteem (worth based and efficacy based) are each rooted primarily in the different bases of identities. They argued that verification of group-based identities (acceptance of who one is) has a stronger impact on worth-based self-esteem, whereas verification of role-based identities (acceptance of one's performance) has a stronger impact on efficacy-based self-esteem. Analyzing data from a sample of newly married couples, their results support the integration of the different viewpoints on self-esteem into identity theory (Cast & Burke, 2002).

If (worth-based) self-esteem is a source of motivation, so too is self-efficacy (Bandura, 1982). Self-efficacy is seeing oneself as a causal agent in one's life. As Bandura (1995) pointed out, efficacy is a *belief* about one's causative capabilities. Whether one actually has control, objectively, is less relevant than what one perceives to be the case. Like self-esteem, positive outcomes have been associated with high self-efficacy, such as effectively coping with life's stresses and adopting good health habits (Bandura, 1995). Our own research has found that identity verification of the spousal role enhances not only feelings of self-worth, as noted previously (based on the group or "we" character of the spouse identity), but also feelings of control over one's environment (based on the performance character of the spouse identity; Burke & Stets, 1999). Some have also recently linked self-esteem with efficacy by arguing that people with high self-esteem should also tend to perceive themselves as competent and, in turn, exhibit more involvement in social movements to try to effect social change (Owens & Aronson, 2000).

Identity

Because the self emerges in social interaction within the context of a complex, organized, differentiated society, it has been argued that the self must be complex, organized, and differentiated as well, reflecting the dictum that the "self reflects society" (Stryker, 1980). This idea is rooted in James's (1890) notion that there are as many different selves as there are different positions that one holds in society and, thus, different groups who respond to the self. At this point identity enters into the overall self. The overall self is organized into multiple parts (identities), each of which is tied to aspects of the social structure. A person has an identity, an "internalized positional designation" (Stryker, 1980, p. 60), for each of the different positions or role relationships the person holds in society. Thus, self as father is an identity, as is self as colleague, self as friend, and self as any of the other myriad of possibilities corresponding to the various roles one may play. The identities are the meanings one has as a group member, as a role holder, or as a person. What it means to be a father, a colleague, or a friend forms the content of the identities.

Most interaction is not between whole persons but between aspects of persons having to do with their roles and memberships in particular groups or organizations: their identities. As a parent, we talk with our children. As a spouse, we talk to our partner. As a member of an organization, we talk to our employer. An assumption and implication of the foregoing is that any identity is always related to a corresponding counteridentity (Burke, 1980). When one claims an identity in an interaction with others, there is an alternative identity claimed by another to which it is related. The husband identity is enacted as it relates to the wife identity, the teacher identity is played out in relation to the student identity, and so forth. In each of these cases, there are things that are not talked about because they are not relevant to that identity, and there are things that are more likely to be talked about given the identity that is currently being claimed. There are various styles of interaction that are appropriate in each situation for each identity. We move into and out of these modalities very easily, and generally with very little thought. Often we operate in two or more identities at a time, as in being both a friend and a colleague.

In examining the nature of interaction between identities of different persons, we can take two different perspectives: *agency* and *social structure*. In terms of social structure, we can focus on the external and talk about actors taking a role or playing a role. Here, the social structure in which the identities are embedded is relatively fixed, and people play out the roles that are given to them. Teachers do the things that teachers are supposed to do. Variations across persons taking on the same identities are viewed as relatively minor, except insofar as they affect the success (or failure) of a group or organization. Essentially, the social structure persists and develops according to its own principles; individuals are recruited into positions and individuals leave positions, but for the most part the positions remain.

But there is also agency. As agents, individuals can make or create a role by making behavioral choices and decisions. For example, research finds that making roles and accumulating role identities fosters greater psychological well-being (Thoits, 2001). However, Thoits (2001) found that the reverse is also true: Greater psychological well-being allows individuals to actively acquire multiple role identities over time, particularly voluntary role identities such as neighbor and churchgoer. When individuals feel good about themselves, they take on more identities. In general, therefore, examining the nature of interaction between identities means addressing both social structure and agency. We must go back and forth and understand how social structure is the accomplishment of actors and also how actors always act within the social structure they create.

Identity Theory

Sociology contains multiple views of identity (Stryker, 2000). Some researchers take a cultural or collective view of identity in which the concept represents the ideas, beliefs, and practices of a group or collective. This view of identity is often seen in work on ethnic identity, although identity is often not defined, thus obscuring what is gained by using the concept (e.g., Nagel, 1995; Scheff, 1994). This view does not allow examination of individual variability in behavior, motivation, and interaction. Another view, growing out of the work of Tajfel (1981) and others (e.g., J. C. Turner, Hogg, Oakes, Reicher, & Wetherell, 1987) on social identity theory, sees identity as embedded in a social group or category. This view often collapses the group/category distinction and misses the

importance of within-group behavior such as role relationships among group members. A third view of identities grows out of the symbolic interactionist tradition, especially its structural variant (Stryker, 1980). This view takes into account individual role relationships and identity variability, motivation, and differentiation. It is this work that we present and elaborate in this chapter. In addition, as we have argued elsewhere, social identity theory may be seen as a special case of this variant of identity theory (Stets & Burke, 2000).

What the following views of identity theory have in common is a general set of principles that Stryker (1980) has enumerated as underlying the structural symbolic interaction perspective. These principles hold that (1) behavior is dependent on a named or classified world and that these names carry meaning in the form of shared responses and behavioral expectations that grow out of social interaction; (2) among the named classes are symbols that are used to designate positions in the social structure; (3) persons who act in the context of social structure name one another in the sense of recognizing one another as occupants of positions and come to have expectations for those others; (4) persons acting in the context of social structure also name themselves and create internalized meanings and expectations with regard to their own behavior; and (5) these expectations and meanings form the guiding basis for social behavior and, along with the probing interchanges among actors, shape and reshape the content of interaction, as well as the categories, names, and meanings that are used. The shared component of these views of identity theory is that negotiated meaning emerges from social interaction.

Identity theory that grows out of structural symbolic interaction has two slightly different emphases (Stryker & Burke, 2000). The work of Stryker and his colleagues (Serpe & Stryker, 1987; Stryker & Serpe, 1982, 1994) focuses on how social structure influences one's identity and, in turn, behavior. The work of Burke and his associates (Burke & Cast, 1997; Burke & Reitzes, 1981, 1991; Burke & Stets, 1999; Cast & Burke, 2002; Stets & Burke, 1996, 2000; Tsushima & Burke, 1999) emphasizes the internal dynamics within the self that influence behavior. Very similar to this version of identity theory is affect control theory, developed by Heise and his colleagues (Heise, 1979; MacKinnon, 1994; Smith-Lovin, 1988) that also focuses on the internal dynamics but draws more heavily on the shared cultural meanings of identities as opposed to individual, subcultural, or group meanings. A third form of identity theory is found in the work of McCall and Simmons (1978). Though a clear program of research has not come out of this version of identity theory, it does make some important theoretical contributions to understanding identities that are important to review. We discuss all of these perspectives.

To begin, we emphasize that the core of an identity is the categorization of the self as an occupant of a role and incorporating into the self the meanings and expectations associated with the role and its performance (Stets & Burke, 2000). Sociological social psychologists see persons as always acting within the context of social structure, in which they and others are labeled such that each recognizes the other as an occupant of positions or roles in society (Stryker, 1980). Thus one assumes a role identity, thereby merging the role with the person (R. H. Turner, 1978).

McCall and Simmons

McCall and Simmons (1978, p. 65) defined a role identity as "the *character* and the *role* [italics added] that an individual devises for himself as an occupant of a particular social position." This follows the conception of R. H. Turner (1962) that criticized the Lintonian (Linton, 1936) role-theoretic character of social roles as too rigid and not allowing for the individual variability and negotiation that exists. McCall and Simmons (1978, p. 68) indicated that a role identity has a "conventional" dimension and an "idiosyncratic" dimension. The former is the *role* of role identity that relates to the expectations tied to social positions, whereas the *identity* of role identity relates to the unique interpretations individuals bring to their roles. McCall and Simmons (1978) pointed out that the proportion of conventional versus idiosyncratic behavior tied to role identities varies across people and across identities for any one person.

Because the self typically has multiple role identities, McCall and Simmons (1978) saw the many different role identities as organized in a *hierarchy of prominence*. This organization reflects a person's "ideal self" (McCall & Simmons, 1978, p. 74). The prominence of an identity depends on the degree to which one (1) gets support from others for an identity, (2) is committed to the identity, and (3) receives extrinsic and intrinsic rewards from the role identity. The more prominent the role identity, the more likely it is that it will be activated and performed in a situation.

For successful enactment of a role in a situation, McCall and Simmons (1978) highlighted the importance of negotiation with others in the situation. Enacting a role identity is always done in relation to a corresponding counteridentity in the interaction, for example, husband to wife. One's expectations associated with a role identity, whether they are conventional or personal, may differ from the expectations others associate with that role identity in the situation. Each party is trying to enact a role that meshes with the other; each has self-conceptions (one's own identity), as well as conceptions of the other (the other's identity). This implies some degree of coordination and compromise between individuals so that smooth role performances can be achieved.

Research on the leadership role identity evidences this negotiation. When individuals cannot negotiate leadership performances in a group that match their leadership identities, they become less satisfied with their roles and are less inclined to remain in the group (Riley & Burke, 1995). Alternatively, when they can negotiate leadership performances consistent with their identities, they become more satisfied and more inclined to remain in the group. Other work shows that when different but interrelated and complementary role behaviors are negotiated by role partners, a strong attachment to the group develops (Burke & Stets, 1999).

Stryker

Although developed independently, Stryker's (1980) view of identities is somewhat similar to that of McCall and Simmons

(1978). He sees the many role identities that a person may have as organized in a hierarchy, but it is a *salience hierarchy* rather than a *prominence hierarchy*. A salient identity is an identity that is likely to be played out (activated) frequently across different situations.[4] Whereas the prominence hierarchy of McCall and Simmons (1978) addresses what an individual *values*, the salience hierarchy focuses on how an individual will likely *behave* in a situation. What one values may or may not be related to how one behaves in a situation, although there is a significant relationship between the two (Stryker & Serpe, 1994). However, there may be times at which one may not be able to express what one values in a situation given situational constraints, so Stryker and Serpe (1994) argued that identity prominence and identity salience should be kept as distinct concepts.

What importantly influences the salience of an identity is the degree of commitment one has to the identity. Commitment has two dimensions: a quantitative and a qualitative aspect (Stryker & Serpe, 1982, 1994). In the former, reflecting the individual's ties to the social structure, commitment reflects the number of persons that one is tied to through an identity. The greater the number of persons to whom one is connected through having a particular identity, the greater is the commitment to that identity. With respect to the qualitative dimension of commitment, the stronger or the deeper the ties to others based on a particular identity, the higher the commitment to that identity.[5] Stryker (1968, 1980) suggested that the greater the commitment to an identity, the higher the identity will be in the salience hierarchy. Once again, the relevance of social structure in understanding the self is made clear. Because people live their lives in social relationships, commitment takes these ties into account when explaining which identities persons are likely to invoke in a situation. For example, if a man's social network in terms of the number of others and the importance of those others is largely based on his occupying a particular role, such as father, then the father identity is likely to be invoked across various different situations.

Research strongly supports the link between commitment, identity salience, and behavior consistent with salient identities.

For example, Stryker and Serpe (1982) examined the religious role identity. Their 6-item commitment scale measures the extensiveness and intensiveness of relations with others in life based on being in the religious role. For example, "In thinking of the people who are important to you, how many would you lose contact with if you did not do the religious activities you do?" (extensiveness), or "Of the people you know through your religious activities, how many are close friends?" (intensiveness). The salience of the religious identity is measured by asking respondents to rank the religious role in relation to other roles they may assume, such as parent, spouse, and worker. Their measure of behavior is time in the religious role. Respondents are asked how many hours in an average week they spend doing things related to religious activities. Stryker and Serpe found that those committed to relationships based on religion have more salient religious identities that are associated with more time spent in religious activities.

In another study, Callero (1985) examined the blood-donor role identity. In separate measures of the salience of the blood-donor role identity (in relation to other identities one might claim), commitment to the blood-donor identity (borrowing Stryker and Serpe's [1982] commitment scale), and behavioral measure of the identity (number of blood donations given in a 6-month period), Callero reached similar conclusions to that of Stryker and Serpe (1982). The more relationships one has that are premised on the blood-donor identity, the higher the blood-donor role identity is in one's identity salience hierarchy, and the more this salient role identity is related to donating blood.

Multiple Identities

The image of a hierarchy of identities, used by both McCall and Simmons (1978) and Stryker (1980), highlights the fact that individuals have multiple role identities (which are ranked). This idea of multiple identities highlights the fact that individuals are always acting in the context of a complex social structure out of which these multiple identities emerge. Having multiple role identities may be good for the self. Indeed, self-complexity theory shows that selves that are more complex are better buffered from situational stresses (Linville 1985, 1987). Consistent with this idea, Thoits (1983, 1986) has shown that having multiple role identities is more beneficial than harmful to individuals because it gives their lives meaning and provides guides to behavior. Other studies have shown that the more one accumulates different role identities, the more positive these accumulated role identities on mental health (see Thoits, 2001, for a review).

The positive effect of multiple identities on mental health may be contingent on the kind of role identities being invoked. Thoits (1992) found that *obligatory* role identities, such as the parent identity, spouse identity, or worker identity, are beneficial to mental health only when chronic strains in each role are low. Alternatively, *voluntary* role identities, such as friend or neighbor, significantly reduce psychological distress because they are less demanding physically and psychologically and because they are easier to exit when their costs exceed their rewards.

More attention is being given to understanding the development of multiple role identities and their outcomes for individual behavior. Smith-Lovin (2001) generated a series of predictions, derived mostly from social ecology and network theory, to explain why some individuals develop multiple identities and, thus, more complex selves than others do. For example, she argued that the larger one's network of others and the less homophilous (similar) they are, the more complex the self will be. Higher status actors will also have more complex selves than lower status actors because they are likely to have more diverse networks that range further through the social system. In general, Smith-Lovin draws our attention to the social structures in which individuals are embedded, because they influence the complexity of the self that is formed.

Burke (2001) also examined how multiple identities are related to the social structure, but in a slightly different fashion. He examined how the same two identities play themselves out differently for persons who are in two structurally different locations in a group. Specifically, he compared individuals who occupy the coordinator role in a group with those who do not occupy this position. He found that those persons who hold the coordinator role in a group have task and social–emotional identity performances that are highly and positively correlated, whereas those who do not hold the position of coordinator have task and social–emotional identity performances that are relatively independent. This finding suggests that the multiple identities that one holds may come to share meanings in response to the structural conditions in which the identities are played out—again emphasizing the effect of structural location on identity processes.

Burke

If the work of Stryker focuses on the arrangement of identities and how they relate to social structure, Burke's work has focused more on the internal dynamics that operate for any one identity. In early work (Burke, 1980; Burke & Tully, 1977), it was argued that identity and behavior are linked through a common system of meaning. In order to predict how one behaves, we have to identify the meanings of the role identity for the individual. Drawing on the conceptualization of meaning developed by Osgood, Suci, and Tannenbaum (1957), Burke and Tully (1977) presented a method for the measurement of the self-meanings of a role identity. Burke (1980) suggested that a person learns the meanings of a role identity in interaction with others in which others act toward the self *as if* the person had an identity appropriate to their role behavior. Thus one's role identity acquires meaning through the reactions of others (Burke, 1980). This is not to say that persons do not import some of their own understandings into their role identities that may be different from others' understandings. These differences are worked out through the negotiation process in interaction.

Role identities generally contain a set of multiple meanings (Burke & Tully, 1977). For example, the male role identity for John may mean being independent, competitive, and self-confident. Additionally, different individuals may have different meanings for the same role identity. For example, a student may see him- or herself as, and be seen by others as, academic, if he or she regularly attends class, takes notes, passes exams, and finishes courses (Burke & Reitzes, 1981). Another student, however, may see him- or herself as sociable rather than academic if he or she finds opportunities to have fun with peers while at school, having friends over and going to parties. More generally, the meanings of identities have implications for how one behaves (with respect to the meanings of the behavior), and one's behavior confirms one's identity when they share meanings.

More recent conceptions of identity expand on the notion of a correspondence of meaning between identity and behavior and incorporate the idea of a perceptual *control system,* a cybernetic model, based on the work of Powers (1973). The internal dynamics of identities are most clearly seen in these conceptions (Burke, 1991, 1996; Burke & Reitzes, 1991; Riley & Burke, 1995). Because an identity is a set of meanings attached to the self in a social role, this set of meanings serves as a standard or reference for a person. When an identity is activated in a situation, a feedback loop is established. This loop has four components: (1) the standard (the self-meanings); (2) a perceptual input of self-relevant meanings from the situation, including how one sees oneself (meaningful feedback in the form of reflected appraisals); (3) a process that compares the perceptual input with the standard (the comparator); and (4) output to the environment (meaningful behavior) that is a result of the comparison (difference) of perceptions of self-meanings with actual self-meanings held in the standard. The system works by modifying outputs (behavior) to the social situation in attempts to change the input to match the internal standard. In this sense, the identity control system can be thought of as having a goal, that is, matching the situational inputs (perceptions) to the internal standards. This system attempts to control the perceptual input (to match the standard).

What is important about the cybernetic model of the identity process is that, instead of seeing behavior as strictly guided by the situation or strictly guided by internal self-meanings, behavior is seen to be the result of the relation between the two. It is goal-directed in that there is an attempt to change the situation in order to match perceived situational meanings with meanings held in the identity standard, that is, to bring about in the situation the meanings that are held in the standard. Thus the model has the interesting implication of making different predictions about behavior from the same identity meanings, depending on the (perceived) situation. When self-meanings in the situation match self-meanings in the identity, the meanings of the behaviors correspond to these meanings. However, if the self-meanings perceived in the situation fail to match, behavior is altered to counteract the situational meanings and restore perceptions. Thus, for example, if one views herself as strong and sees that others agree, she will continue to act as she has (strongly). But if she sees that others appear to view her as weak, she will increase the "strength" of her performance in an effort to restore perceptions of herself as strong, as seen in the reflected appraisals.[6]

Identities are tied to social structure in the sense that role performances are the meaningful behaviors produced by an identity. Role behaviors are a means by which one strives to keep perceptions of self-relevant meanings in the situation in line with the meanings held in the identity standard (in other words, one strives for self-verification).[7] Role behaviors are accomplished through interaction with others whose behavior is an output of their own identity processes that also strive for self-verification (Riley & Burke, 1995). All participants in the interactive setting mutually accomplish their respective self-verifications (if all goes well). Because each is motivated to match self-relevant meanings in the situation with self-meanings in their respective identity standards, and because the actions of each change or disturb the meanings in the situation, self-verification is accomplished only by the cooperative and mutually agreed-on arrangement of role performances. However, this does not happen automatically. Performances are stretched, identity standards are altered, and negotiations are conducted as the participants seek ways to accomplish self-verification—at worst, without disturbing the verification of others, and at best, helping them to verify themselves. When congruity between reflected appraisals and the identity standard occurs, ties to role partners are strengthened. More recently, we have argued that commitment results from the self-verifying aspect of the identity process (Burke & Stets, 1999). In studying married couples, we showed that the more the spousal roles of both partners are verified, the more it leads to the development of committed relationships, high levels of trust, and a perceived collective (group).

The cybernetic character of identity theory has led to a view of the nature of commitment that is slightly different from the view outlined earlier by Stryker (1980). In this slightly different view, commitment to an identity is the sum total of the pressure to keep perceptions of self-relevant meanings in the situation in line with the self-meanings held in the identity standard (Burke & Reitzes, 1991). One is more committed to an identity when one strives harder to maintain a match between self-in-situation (perceptual input) meaning and the meaning held in the identity standard. Commitment thus moderates the link between identity and behavior, making it stronger (high commitment) or weaker (low commitment). This process does not negate the importance of the structural side, shown in ties to role partners (Stryker & Serpe, 1982, 1994), but shows how those ties, as well as other factors such as rewards and praise one might receive for being in the role, bring about commitment as defined by Burke and Reitzes (1991) in terms of the strength of the self-verification response. The structural connection is maintained. For example, Burke and Reitzes showed that those who are highly committed to a student identity (by having more ties to others, as well as receiving rewards for having the identity) have a stronger link between identity meanings (for example, academic responsibility) and behavior meanings (for example, time in the student role or grade point average) than those with lower levels of commitment.

An extension that has been made to the identity model in identity theory concerns the nature of the meanings that are encapsulated in the identity standard. The notion of meaning was originally thought of in terms of symbols in the tradition of symbolic interaction (cf. Stryker, 1980). Freese and Burke (1994) extended the notion of meaning to include not only symbols (shared meanings) but also signs, drawing from earlier work in symbolic interaction that had not been fully developed (Lindesmith & Strauss, 1956). Signs are signals (stimuli) that convey meanings through which individuals relate directly to their environment and all of the "things" in the situation insofar as they are used, transferred, or transformed: clothing, food, objects, air, and so forth. There may be, in addition, symbolic meanings attached to the objects; for example, a very expensive fountain pen may convey wealth and prestige, but as a writing implement that is manipulated to put ink on paper, it is also simply an object in the environment. In this way, Freese and Burke (1994) introduced the idea of the control of resources (through sign meanings), an idea that is essential to sociology in understanding social structure. Thus role performances are not just symbolic interactions but also sign interactions. Persons manipulate signs (resources) and symbols in the situation to bring sign and symbolic meanings to match the sign and symbolic meanings held in their role identities. By using this expanded model of identities, Burke (1997) simulated the role of exchanging resources in verifying the identities of experimental participants as studied in network exchange theory (e.g., Skvoretz & Willer, 1993). These simulations produced predictions for the final distribution of resources and power that were observed in laboratory experiments.

The perceptual control system as it is applied to identities is a self-regulating system and is very similar to Carver and Sheier's (1981, 1998) theory of self-regulated behavior. In this way, sociologists and psychologists are thinking along similar lines with respect to understanding the self. We see that when the meanings of the self in the situation (based in part on feedback from others and in part on direct perception of the environment) are congruent with the meanings held in the identity standard, self-verification has occurred (Burke & Stets, 1999). This idea is also very similar to Swann's (1983, 1990) formulation of self-verification. We agree with Swann that people seek to verify their self-views in interaction, even if those self-views happen to be negative. Once again, sociologists and psychologists are thinking along similar lines in explaining the self.

A Variant of Identity Theory: Affect Control Theory

Affect control theory, independently developed by Heise and his colleagues (Heise, 1979; MacKinnon, 1994; Smith-Lovin, 1988) is very similar to the cybernetic model of the identity process. Affect control theory also views identities as containing self-meanings, with a focus on the fundamental dimensions of meanings identified by Osgood, Suci, and Tannenbaum (1957) of evaluation, potency, and activity (EPA). These self-views are the fundamental sentiments persons hold about themselves in a social role (like the identity standard of Burke). When events in the situation disturb the perceived self-meanings (called transients) so that they no longer match the fundamental sentiments, individuals act to create new events that restore the transients toward the fundamental sentiments.

Although these broad outlines show a high level of similarity between affect control theory and identity theory, there are some differences, and the two theories have each pursued slightly different questions. One difference is that affect control theory uses culturally defined (shared) views of what an identity means, whereas identity theory has not confined itself to necessarily shared meanings but has focused on the self-definition of self-meanings assessed along culturally shared dimensions (Burke & Tully, 1977). Identity theorists recognize that persons' meanings tied to a role may, in part, be idiosyncratic to those persons. Another difference is that affect control theory has considered only the EPA dimensions of meaning for defining all identities (as well as behaviors), thus allowing direct comparisons among different identities. Identity theory, on the other hand, has tried to find the dimensions of meaning most relevant to the occupants of the positions, though these may vary from one role identity to another, making direct comparisons more difficult.

Emotion in Identity Theory

In the identity cybernetic model, any discrepancy between perceived self-in-situation meanings and identity standard meanings is signaled in the comparator. This discrepancy reflects a problem in verifying the self, and as a result of this the individual experiences negative emotional arousal such as depression and distress (Burke, 1991; Burke & Stets, 1999), anger (Bartels, 1997), and hostility (Cast & Burke, 2002). The absence of an error or discrepancy is self-verification and results in positive emotional arousal such as high self-esteem and mastery (Burke & Stets, 1999; Cast & Burke, 2002).

The role of emotion in the identity control model is consistent with earlier arguments made by identity theorists on the relationship between identity and emotion. For example, McCall and Simmons (1978) argued that if a prominent identity has been threatened (by others not supporting one's role performance), an individual would experience a negative emotional response. Consistent with this idea, Ellestad and Stets (1998) reported that when nurturing behavior is linked to fathering rather than mothering, women whose mother identity is prominent report the negative emotion of jealousy.

Stryker (1987) discussed how emotion and identities are related given the salience hierarchy. He argued that identities that generate positive feelings should be played out more often and move up in the salience hierarchy, whereas identities that repeatedly cause negative feelings should be less likely to be played out and move down in the salience hierarchy. He also argued that identities that are inadequately played out should generate negative feelings, because poor role performance results in others not supporting one's identity claims. Therefore, identity theorists such as McCall and Simmons, Stryker, and Burke agree that negative emotion results from not meeting one's identity expectations and that positive emotion results from meeting one's identity expectations.

In a similar fashion, affect control theory (Heise, 1979; Smith-Lovin, 1995; Smith-Lovin & Heise, 1988) has posited emotional responses to the discrepancy between the self-meanings in the identity standard (fundamentals) and perceptions of self-relevant meanings in the situation (transients). Not only are particular emotions signaled in response to discrepancies of particular meanings, but also the display of emotion is itself an event that changes the meanings in the situation that can move transients back toward the fundamental sentiments. For example, Heise (1989) suggested that the negative implications of a deviant act can be forestalled by the appropriate display of shame by the perpetrator. One difference between affect control theory and identity theory with respect to emotions is that affect control theorists argue that a discrepancy can generate positive emotion when one exceeds the expectations tied to identities in a situation (MacKinnon, 1994).

Feelings vary in terms of their strength or intensity. Stryker (1987) argued that the strength of the emotional response to identity-related behaviors in situations should signal to individuals how important an identity is in their salience hierarchy, with more important identities producing a stronger emotion. This parallels McCall and Simmons's (1978) point as to the role of emotions in the prominence hierarchy. Burke (1991, 1996) hypothesized that repeated interruptions in the self-regulating identity process cause more negative emotion than occasional or infrequent interruptions.

Stets (2001) examined more closely the identity assumptions that (1) a discrepancy leads to negative emotion and (2) frequent interruptions in the identity process cause more intense or stronger negative emotion. These two assumptions are actually similar to Higgins's (1989) self-discrepancy theory. For Higgins, negative emotion results from a discrepancy between one's actual state and one's ideal state. The negative emotion becomes more intense and frequent as the magnitude of the discrepancy increases. Stets examined the identity theory assumptions by studying the distributive justice process and individuals' emotional responses to injustice in a laboratory setting that simulates a work situation. If we translate the idea of disruption of the self-verification process into being overrewarded or underrewarded in a justice situation (in either case, one's standard is not being met), negative emotion should result, and more intense negative emotions should occur as the inequitable distributive process persists.

Stets's (2001) findings show that an identity discrepancy does not always lead to negative emotion. When one is overrewarded, positive emotion results. Stets argued that when individuals receive rewards

(goods) rather than punishments (bads), their standard quickly adjusts in a positive direction to the new level if the overreward is relatively small. Making this adjustment has two consequences: The self is enhanced, and any discrepancy between one's standard and one's perceptions (reward) is removed. The degree of exceeding the standard is important because an outcome that significantly exceeds one's standard in a positive direction may lead to negative emotion, as the size of the discrepancy makes it too difficult to self-verify.

This resolves the self-enhancement–self-verification debate in the literature in a different fashion from that offered by Swann and his colleagues (Swann 1990; Swann, Griffin, Predmore, & Gaines, 1987). Swann and his associates claimed that self-enhancement was dependent on immediate affective reactions to social feedback, whereas self-verification was dependent on less immediate cognitive reactions to social feedback. Stets (2001) argued that what may be more important is the degree of disparity in meanings held in the input and identity standard. Self-enhancement may be more highly activated when a small discrepancy occurs in a positive direction. Self-verification may be more highly activated when a large discrepancy exists in a positive direction. Thus, rather than assuming that any discrepancy produces negative emotion because the information is not self-verifying, as is assumed in identity theory, it may depend on the size of the error registered in the comparator.

Stets (2001) also found that, as the inequitable distributive process is repeatedly experienced by participants, their emotions become less, not more, intense. This pattern again suggests that individuals are changing their standards, adjusting their standards to the level of rewards they received. Because a strong emotional response would signal a discrepancy between input meanings and standard meanings, a weaker emotional response over time would suggest a closer correspondence between input and identity standard meanings. In general, these unexpected findings have implications for modifying assumptions in identity theory about the relationship between identity expectations, emotion, and the repetitiveness of disrupting the identity process.

Another way in which the strength or intensity of an emotional response to identity disconfirmation has been examined is in the recent work of Stets and Tsushima (2001). Using a national probability sample, Stets and Tsushima found that more intense anger is associated with the lack of verification of *group-based* identities that are intimate, such as the family identity, and that meet our need to feel valuable, worthy, and accepted. Less intense anger is associated with *role-based* identities that are less intimate, such as the worker identity, and that fulfill our need to feel competent and effective. Burke (1991) has argued that greater distress will be felt by the individual when the self-verification process is interrupted by a significant other than by a casual acquaintance. The fact that Stets and Tsushima found intense angry feelings in the family identity compared with the worker identity is consistent with this thesis. Group-based identities that are socioemotional have strong ties that make others' views about the self important. If the self is not verified, the emotional response can be powerful.

According to identity theory, when negative emotion is felt, actors may either change what they are doing (the output end of the model) or they may think about the situation in a different way (the input side) in order to achieve greater congruence (Burke, 1991). In later work, Burke (1996) referred to these responses as different coping responses. One can modify the situation through some behavioral strategy or modify the meaning of the problem through some cognitive strategy.[8] Ellestad and Stets (1998) revealed that the more salient the identity, the more likely it is that persons devise behavioral strategies to reassert their role identity, thereby maintaining who they are to themselves and significant others. More recent work has found that disruption of self-verification for group-based identities that are more intimate, such as the family identity, leads to coping strategies that are cognitive (activity on the input side of the identity model), whereas disruption of self-verification for role-based identities that are less intimate, such as the worker identity, leads to behavioral strategies of coping (activity on the output side of the identity model; Stets & Tsushima, 2001).

The Hierarchy of Identity Control Systems and Identity Change

The identity control model has been further extended so that a particular identity standard is viewed as the output of a higher level perceptual control process, thus embedding the identity control process within a hierarchical control structure (Burke, 1997; Burke & Cast, 1997; Powers, 1973; Tsushima & Burke, 1999). For example, recent research has discussed the relationship between *principle-level* identity standards at a higher level of control and *program-level* identity standards at a lower level of control (Tsushima & Burke, 1999). Principle-level standards are abstract goal states such as values, beliefs, and ideals. Program-level standards are more concrete goals that are accomplished in situations. When the distinction of these two levels is applied to the parent identity, evidence reveals that some parents are more principle-oriented (e.g., they desire their child to be a critical thinker, loving, and autonomous) and some parents are more program-oriented (e.g., they are concerned that their child makes her bed and gets to school). Those parents with more fully developed principle-level components of the parent identity are able to relate the principle level to the program level to alter programs so that the programs not only accomplish the mundane goals (getting the child to complete her homework) but also the higher level goals (being independent). As a consequence, these parents experience higher efficacy and lower stress (Tsushima & Burke, 1999).

If we extend our analysis beyond one identity and consider multiple identities, the hierarchical model is a useful way of understanding the relationship among multiple identities (Burke, 2001). If we think of an identity as the set of all meanings held for oneself in terms of, for example, a particular role, then an identity standard might be thought of as a set or vector of meanings. Strictly, each meaning is part of a separate control system, but conceptually it is easier to think of the set or vector of meanings of an identity as part of a single control system. Thus, when multiple identities are enacted in a situation, separate control systems have been activated, each of which is acting to control self-in-situation meanings to match an identity standard. Because control systems can be arranged hierarchically, higher, more abstract identities, as well as lower, less abstract identities, may be activated in a situation.

This hierarchical model also helps us understand how identities change. Identity standards of lower level control systems are the outputs of higher level control systems. In other words, when a higher level control system behaves, it provides the reference standard to the control systems just below it. When a higher level system brings the higher level perceptions into alignment with the higher level standard, it does so by changing its outputs—thereby changing lower level standards. In this way the meanings contained in lower level standards are altered (Burke & Cast, 1997). Furthermore, because the overall perceptual control system is continuously operating to verify identity perceptions at all levels for identities that are activated, identity change is always going on, though at a much slower pace than behavior that alters the situation. Nevertheless, when actions cannot change the meanings in the situation to verify an identity, the identity standard itself will change toward the meanings in the situation.[9] For example, Burke and Cast (1997) showed that the birth of a child to a newly married couple provides a new set of meanings in the situation that is difficult to change. The consequence is that the gender identities of the husband and wife both change. Husbands become more masculine in their self-views, and their wives become more feminine.

Identity change has also been examined by Kiecolt (1994). She argued that a change occurs when a stressor such as chronic role strain or a life event disrupts valued role identities and when, among other things, people believe they can change, they see that the benefits of self-change outweigh the costs, and others provide support for their self-change. More recently, Kiecolt (2000) argued that involvement in social movements can result in change by changing one's salience hierarchy of identities. This can be done in three ways: (1) either adding or discarding an identity, (2) changing the importance of an identity without changing the ranking of the identity (for example, the "activist" identity can become more impor-

tant as one becomes more involved in a social movement, but its importance relative to other identities does not change), or (3) changing the importance and ranking of an identity. One could also change the meanings of an identity. Consistent with the idea that higher levels of the perceptual control system change more slowly, Kiecolt (2000) indicated that if social movement participation results in self-concept change, the change is gradual, not sudden.

Most recently, Burke (2002) has provided additional thoughts on identity change. Examining the spousal identities and behaviors of newly married couples over a 3-year period, he showed how both the spouse identity and the performance of the spouse role change in response to marital interaction. The spousal identities were measured in terms of the extent to which persons thought they should do various activities associated with the spousal role, such as cleaning the house, yardwork, and maintaining contact with parents and in-laws. Role performance was measured by daily diary indication of the extent to which participants reported doing these things over a 4-week period, collected at a later point. Burke found that when the spouse identity was not verified (because the actual role performance was either greater than or less than would be expected given one's self-views), the actual role performance shifted over time toward a closer correspondence with the standard contained in the spousal identity. At the same time, however, the spousal identity standard changed (though more slowly) toward the levels reflected in the actual performance in accordance with the theoretical expectations. Thus we see that behavior adjusts to conform to the meanings contained in the identity standard, and the identity standard also slowly shifts over time to conform to the meanings of the behavior.

Identity Theory as a Theory

The predictive power of identity theory can be tested against alternative theories. In doing this, we are in a better position to identify the scope of identity theory, that is, where it does and does not apply and the ways in which the theory can be extended. For example, in a series of studies (Stets, 1997;

Stets & Burke, 1996), we examined positive and negative emotion-based behavior among newly married couples. We compared predictions derived from expectation-states theory (Ridgeway & Walker, 1995; Webster & Foschi, 1988) with those of identity theory.

According to expectation-states theory, those with more power should use more negative behavior in interaction as a way of maintaining the system of stratification (Ridgeway & Johnson, 1990). Higher-status people such as men should use more negative behavior when they encounter challenges to their position, particularly illegitimate opposition from lower status people such as women. Alternatively, according to identity theory, those with a more masculine gender identity should be more likely to use negative behavior in interaction because the meaning of masculinity is related to dominance and competition, and this meaning is more consistent with a negative style than a positive style of interaction. In studying newly married couples, we found that although the data are consistent with identity theory, they are inconsistent with expectation-states theory (Stets & Burke, 1996). Wives rather than husbands use more negative behavior in conversation. Although the expectation-states predictions could be correct though inapplicable to intimate interactions, it might also be true that the predictions are wrong.

The finding that women are more likely to use negative behavior in interaction could be a gender specific finding, or it could be part of a more general pattern of how powerless persons act, perhaps in response to being discounted by others. To test this possibility, Stets (1997) conducted a follow-up study to examine whether the effects of negative behavior in marriage was confined to gender. Stets investigated individuals in other powerless groups in our society, such as the young, the less educated, and those having a low-status occupation, to investigate whether their status produced the same negative behavior. Consistent with the results on gender, Stets found that those with a low status on these other dimensions were also more likely to use negative behavior in marriage. Furthermore, the identity effects (that is, that those with a more masculine identity are more negative) remained. These results

identified ways in which one's structural position and self-meanings combine to produce action that maintains both the status hierarchy and the self. In general, the preceding results, together with the earlier results by Stets and Burke (1996), indicate that self-meaning tied to the identity may, in fact, be a better predictor of behavior than predictions laid out from expectation-states theory.

The previous statement must be qualified. Although expectation-states theory may not predict emotion-based behavior, it may provide insight into cognitive-based behavior, particularly how individuals see themselves. In yet another follow-up on the preceding research, we examined who is influential in how we see ourselves by investigating spouses' self-perceptions from their own viewpoints (self-views), as well as from the viewpoints of their spouses (Cast, Stets, & Burke, 1999). We found support for the expectation-states theory prediction that the views of the spouse with higher status in the marriage about their lower status partner influences how the lower status partner views himself or herself. Further, the higher status spouse influences the lower status spouse's views of the higher status person. Thus one's social structural position serves as a signal as to who is likely to have power in the interaction. In this way, one's position in the macro social order generalizes to the micro social order. This important process again reflects the social structurally contingent nature of identity processes that needs to be incorporated more fully into identity theory.

Another way in which the predictive power of identity theory has been tested against alternative theories is through an analysis of trust and commitment in marriage. Research has examined trust and commitment through the lens of exchange theory (Kollock, 1994; Lawler & Yoon, 1996). We argued that when a person's identity is repeatedly verified in interaction, several consequences will emerge, including positive feelings, increased trust for the other, commitment to the other, and a perception that one is part of a group (Burke & Stets, 1999). Exchange theory posits many of these same outcomes, but for different reasons. In exchange theory, commitment is influenced not by repeated self-verification but by repeated exchange agreements (Lawler & Yoon, 1996). Such agreements generate an emotional "buzz" between actors in the form of satisfaction or excitement. These mild positive emotions lead to relational cohesion or the perception that one is part of a group, and cohesion influences commitment.

On the one hand, there may be little difference between exchange theory and identity theory, as repeated exchange agreements may be viewed as self-verification. What is gained through the exchange is a confirmation of the self as needing the thing gained. On the other hand, in exchange terms, value preferences guide one's behavior, whereas in identity terms the identity standard sets the value. In exchange terms, we seek out rewards and avoid punishment. In identity terms, we are motivated to seek self-verification. We see identity theory as applying to a wider range of situations and relationships than those examined by exchange theorists. For example, identity theory can apply to individuals who have a history of interaction. Indeed, most of our daily interactions are characterized by such interactions. In general, we see that one of the ways of extending a theory is testing it with alternative theories. In doing this, we may arrive at a better sense of the strengths, as well as limitations, of our own theory.

Integrating the Identity Theory Versions

The program of research of Stryker and his colleagues, that of Heise, Smith-Lovin, and their colleagues, as well as Burke's program of research, offer important theoretical assumptions as to the nature of identities and how they operate. Stryker's work highlights the fact that identities exist within and reflect social structure. Identities are constrained by social structure, but they also maintain and facilitate the further development of social structure. Burke's work, along with that of Heise and Smith-Lovin, highlights the dynamic process that emerges when an individual claims an identity in a situation and what occurs when that claim is not verified. The ideas of the aforementioned researchers can be easily integrated (Stryker & Burke, 2000). For example, in thinking about the identity standard in the identity control model, we can conceptual-

ize it as reflecting the role meanings of particular groups to which one is committed in society. The more strongly a person is committed to one or more of these groups, the greater the salience of that identity. The greater the commitment and salience to a particular identity, the more likely those meanings will be perceived to be personally relevant in a situation, and the greater the motivational force inherent in a discrepancy to bring the identity standard and self-perception in line. The greater the difficulty in aligning the identity standard with self-in-situation meanings, the more likely it is that the identity will decrease in salience and result in decreased commitment to the relationships on which the identity is premised.

The integration of the aforementioned programs of research can be seen not only in the incorporation of committed and salient identities (from the social structure) into the identity control model but also in how functioning identities influence the social structure. For example, in some of our recent research, we found that when individuals verify each other's identities, commitment to each other increases, and a shift in cognition takes place such that the individuals come to see themselves as a collectivity or group, that is, a new social structure (Burke & Stets, 1999). On the other hand, when the individuals have problems verifying their identities, ties may be broken so that the structure comes apart. Indeed, Cast and Burke (2002) showed that husbands and wives whose spousal identities are not mutually verified in their marriages are more likely to be divorced.

Integrating Sociological and Psychological Identity Theory

Social and Role Identities

Identity theory in sociological social psychology has chiefly focused on *role* identities. However, individuals not only occupy roles in society, but they are also members of some groups (and not others) and therefore may take on particular *social* identities. Social identity theory in psychological social psychology has been instrumental in informing us as to the processes involved in social identity formation, activation, and motivation (Abrams & Hogg, 1990; J. C. Turner et al., 1987). Role identity theory and social identity theory have developed as disparate lines of research. Unlike Hogg and his colleagues (Hogg, Terry, & White, 1995), we see significant similarities between social identity theory and role identity theory. We recently called for a merger of the two theories that would yield a stronger social psychology, that is, a general theory of identity, as it would integrate the various bases by which individuals are tied to society (Stets & Burke, 2000).

We have argued that the overlap between identity theory and social identity theory is striking. For example, the process of self-categorization into groups in social identity theory (J. C. Turner et al., 1987) is analogous to the process of identification into roles in identity theory (McCall & Simmons, 1978). In self-categorization, people compare themselves with others, and those who are similar to the self are categorized with the self and are labeled the "ingroup," whereas those who are different from the self are categorized as the "outgroup." In identification, persons identify themselves as occupants of particular roles. Rather than seeing others as similar to oneself in interaction, individuals see themselves as set apart from others in the counterroles others assume in the interaction. For example, sons and daughters are different from the corresponding counterroles of mothers and fathers. Students are different from the corresponding counterrole of teachers. What theorists in both traditions share is the idea that when persons categorize themselves as members of a group or a role, they do so by seeing themselves as an embodiment of a (group or role) prototype or standard. This prototype or standard contains the societal meanings and norms about the social category or role, serving to guide behavior. Broadly speaking, then, theorists in both traditions recognize that individuals view themselves in ways defined by the social structure. Therefore, persons are born into a particular society with social categories preexistent to the individual (Hogg & Abrams, 1988; Stryker, 1980).

Although identity theorists and social identity theorists see somewhat different consequences when individuals take on an identity, these varying consequences are equally important in understanding the self. According to social identity theory, when individuals take on group-based identities, there is uniformity of perception and action among group members (Haslam, Oakes, McGarty, & Turner, 1996; Oakes, Haslam, & Turner, 1994). According to role identity theorists, taking on a role-based identity results in different perceptions and action between individuals, as roles interact with counterroles (Burke, 1980; Burke & Reitzes, 1981). As we pointed out, social identities and role identities can simultaneously exist in a situation, with the result that there are both similarities (social identities) and differences (role identities) with others (Stets & Burke, 2000). Within groups, individuals assume different roles (*intra*group relations), but persons also categorize themselves as members of one group (the ingroup) and not another (the outgroup; *inter*group relations). Whereas intergroup relations activate a sense of belongingness and *self-worth* for individuals (focusing on who one is), intragroup relations activate a sense of *self-efficacy* (what one *does*). Both self-worth and self-efficacy are important dimensions of self-esteem, and both appear to be fostered through their ties to social and role identities, respectively (Cast & Burke, 2002).

Personal Identities

Social identity and identity theorists have discussed personal identities, but they have remained peripheral in both theories. As another basis of the self, we think more attention should be given to personal identities, particularly as they relate to social and role identities. In social identity theory, the personal identity is the lowest level of self-categorization (Brewer, 1991; Hogg & Abrams, 1988). Categorizing oneself in terms of the personal identity means seeing the self as distinct and different from others. The person is guided by his or her own goals rather than the group's goals. The activation of a social identity rather than a personal identity in a situation is a product of accessibility and fit (Oakes, 1987). This is the process of depersonalization, shifting the perception of the self from being unique toward the perception of the self as a member of a social category (Hogg et al., 1995). The "Me" becomes a "We" (Thoits & Virshup, 1997). The person sees him- or herself as the embodiment of the ingroup prototype rather than as a unique individual. Depersonalization does not mean a loss of one's personal identity but rather a change in focus from the personal to the group basis of an identity. To social identity theorists, because the personal and social identities are mutually exclusive bases of self-definition, both cannot operate at the same time.

Deaux (1992) attempted to link the personal identity to the social identity. She indicated that, although social identities are expressed along normative lines, there is an aspect of social identities that may be expressed along personal, idiosyncratic lines. Thus personal identities may be linked to social identities by creating new ways of expressing one's membership in groups. Deaux also suggested that some personal identities may represent a general view of the self and therefore may pervade all the membership groups to which one belongs.

Our own work has addressed personal identities (Stets, 1995; Stets & Burke, 1994). We see personal identities as tied to an individual rather than being attached to a role in society. They operate across various roles and situations. In this sense, our conceptualization is very close to that of Deaux (1992). In the same way in which we regulate the meanings of our role identities and our social (group) identities, we also regulate the meanings of our personal identities. Thus personal identities are not dispositions to act in a certain way; rather, like role and group identities, they are maintained by a feedback control process. Like role and group identities, perceptions of one's personal identity in a situation are compared with one's meaning of the personal identity held in the standard. Any discrepancy between the two will register an error, and either behavior, perception, or the identity standard will be modified to resolve the discrepancy.

Another way of looking at these three bases of identity—group, role, and person—is in terms of the resources that are controlled by each (cf. Freese & Burke, 1994). Again, the distinction is analytic, being difficult to sort out in any empirical situation,

but one may think of group-based identities as controlling resources that support the group qua group sustaining it, its patterns of interaction, its boundaries, and so forth. Role identities, on the other hand, control resources that sustain the role. Because most roles exist within groups, such resources may also work ultimately to sustain the group. Finally, person identities control the resources needed to sustain the individual as a biological being, maintaining food, clothing, shelter, love, and so forth.

In the same way that Deaux (1992) attempted to link personal identities to social identities, Stets (1995) attempted to link personal identities to role identities. Stets argued that personal and role identities may be related to each other through a common system of meanings. In other words, the meanings of role identities may overlap with the meanings of personal identities. For example, Stets found that the masculine gender *role* identity is linked to the mastery *personal* identity through the shared meaning of "control." Stets observed that, when the meanings of role identities conflict with the meanings of personal identities, people may act without regard to their role identities in order to maintain their personal identities.

In general, attempts are continuing to be made to integrate these different identity bases. Most recently, Deaux and Martin (2001) offered a model that links social and role identities. They proposed that each large-scale group identity is linked to an interpersonal network of others. These interpersonal networks consist of people who share, to varying degrees, the category membership of which a person is a member and who provide, also in varying degrees, support for the group identity. Support comes in assuming reciprocal roles for the identity one claims, thereby producing role and counterrole identities.

Future Research

As we think about future research, a number of issues emerge: integrating the various bases of identities (group, role, and person), understanding how the multiple identities a person has are interrelated, and developing better measures of various aspects of identities, as well as the identity verification process. We briefly discuss each of these.

Integrating Social, Role, and Personal Identities

We suggest that future research examine all three bases of identities: person, role, and social (group) identities. This would lead to a more integrated and a stronger theory of identity. Within groups, there are roles and persons playing out those roles. All are operating in a situation, and we need to identify how they are related in the setting. For example, it would be important to investigate how much group and role identities are constrained by normative expectations. The less constrained the normative expectations, the more it may be that personal identities can influence not only behaviors but also the meanings of the role or social (group) identities, creating unique patterns of interaction. Looked at another way, we need to examine the conditions under and extent to which personal identities influence role identities and group identities without disrupting smooth social relations and social order. Part of the answer may be in how much one's role in the group carries with it power (a social structural characteristic) and thus increased freedom to express oneself according to one's personal identities. Alternatively, some groups may allow personal identities to influence group interaction more than others. Further, we might examine whether some identities are more malleable than others. For example, under some conditions, personal identities may shift in meaning to fit into situations rather than motivating behavior to modify structurally constrained role or group identities.

Another concern is the conditions under which group, role, and person identities compete in a situation or, alternatively, support one another. Are some personal identities an easier fit with some role and social identities than others? How much are individuals aware of this fit or lack of fit among identities? Just as individuals have multiple role identities (Thoits, 1983), they also have multiple personal identities (Deaux, 1992). Finally, there is the issue of the effect of

these identities among themselves over time. For example, it may be that personal identities influence role and group identities when they are first taken on but have little impact once a role or group identity becomes established (Stets, 1995).

Finally, the relationships between the different bases of identity (group, role, and person) and the varieties of self-esteem (self-worth self-efficacy, and self-authenticity) need to be explored. Cast and Burke (2002) have suggested that verification of identities based on group membership leads to self-worth, and that verification of identities based on role incumbency leads to self-efficacy. The third form of esteem, suggested by Turner and Billings (1991), may be the result of verification of person-based identities.

Integrating the various bases of the self is challenging given that there are multiple personal identities, multiple role identities, and multiple social identities. How can we conceptualize this interrelationship? We might demarcate the self-concept as having distinct salience hierarchies or distinct identity control systems that refer to these three different kinds of identities. The movement within the hierarchies across situations is influenced by situational factors, commitment to those identities, or both. At issue is how these hierarchies operate to produce particular combinations of identities in any one situation.

Multiple Identities

Future research needs to address more fully issues related to the occurrence of multiple identities in a situation. We expect that having two oppositional identities activated at the same time in a situation will result in much distress, because the verification of one identity necessarily increases the discrepancy for the other. For example, a person may have the identity "friend" to a peer and "daughter" to her parents. The two groups may intersect when the peer visits in the person's home while her parents are present. Should the overlap of the two sets of relationships regularly occur, we would hypothesize that there will occur some sort of change in the identity standards involved, with the more important, salient, or more committed identity shifting the least. This means that identities higher in the hierarchy of importance or salience should take preference in the verification process in a situation over identities lower in the hierarchy.

When two identities share common meanings, the situation is simpler. Controlling self-in-situation meanings to match the identity standard helps both identities. Verifying one of the identities will help verify the other.[10] For example, consider a married person with children. If the spousal identity includes standards for providing material support for one's spouse, and if the parent identity includes standards for providing material support for one's children, then getting a well-paying job will help verify both identities. We hypothesize that identities with common meanings will tend to be activated together. Identities that are often activated together should develop similar levels of salience and commitment.

Trying to understand how individuals manage their different identities in a situation becomes more complex when multiple personal, role, and social identities become activated, not just for any one person in a situation but for two or more persons in a situation. Furthermore, because this self is not a static entity but an entity that is dynamic and can change, it is important to examine how these different identities change over time and come to shape a new self-concept. Because of the complexity of this process, simulation of various theoretical formulations, such as those employed by Burke (1997) in studying the complex interactions of multiple identities in social networks, may be a viable start.

Measurement

The measurement of identity aspects beyond self-meanings needs further development. As Stryker and Burke (2000) pointed out, if we consider an identity as a person schema (how you see yourself as you move from one situation to the next), we might be able to measure identity salience by way of response latency measures (cf. Markus, 1977; Fazio, Sanbonmatsu, Powell, & Kardes, 1986). The idea is that greater responsiveness to identity cues increases the likelihood that identity-relevant behavior will be performed. The cues might be pictures that individuals can identify with. The quicker they identify the pictures, the higher the identity may be in their salience hierarchy, and the more likely it may be to be played out across situations. Additionally, following the idea of Burke and Reitzes (1991), commitment may be indicated by the (computer-measured) strength of response in bringing disrupted identity descriptions back in line with self-conceptions. In this case, not the latency of response but the strength and persistence in restoring the self-description would be measured.

Also needed are more direct measures of identity verification. In the past, self-verification has been assessed by the degree of agreement between how individuals thought they should behave and how others thought they should behave (Burke & Stets, 1999) or by how individuals thought they should behave and how they did behave (Burke, 2001). Drawing on the idea of reflected appraisals, we need to ask individuals what they think others' perceptions are of them. To the extent that the reflected appraisals are consistent with one's identity standard, then verification is more directly captured. Further, if emotion is an outcome of the verification process, we need to be able to measure both verification (or the lack of it) and emotional responses on a moment-by-moment basis, perhaps with procedures similar to those employed by Levenson and Gottman (1985).

Conclusion

The ideas contained in the various research programs on self and identity included under the rubric of identity theory have been gaining visibility in the discipline of sociology and are increasingly being incorporated into other ongoing research. Facilitating this process has been the ability of identity theory to build coherent and cumulative theory that has been able to bridge the gap between the individual and society, addressing issues of more macro concern, such as the origins of the patterns of activity that constitute social structure, as well as issues of more micro concern, such as understanding interaction in groups, individual choice behavior, and how resources are managed in exchanges.

Three characteristics of identity theory within sociology have been central to these endeavors: its focus on symbolic and sign meanings rather than behavior itself, its incorporation of the perceptual control system that uses behavior to control perceived meanings, and its recognition that perceptions, meaning, and behavior all occur within, are influenced by, and contribute to the patterns of meaning and behavior that constitute the social structure of society. As we have reviewed the ideas and work that have figured prominently in the sociological study of self and identity, we have tried to highlight these central characteristics and spell out some of their implications for future research and theory building.

Notes

1. Cooley's (1902) classic "reflected" or "looking-glass self" has three principal elements: "the imagination of our appearance to the other person, the imagination of his judgment of that appearance; and some sort of self-feeling, such as pride or mortification" (p. 184).
2. Rosenberg and colleagues (1995) argue that *specific* self-esteem is most relevant to *behavior*, whereas *global* self-esteem is most relevant to *psychological well-being*. Thus specific behavioral outcomes are best predicted by specific self-esteem that is somehow connected to that behavior, whereas psychological well-being is best predicted by global self-esteem.
3. Identity verification involves the cognitive process of matching self-relevant meanings in the situation to the meanings defined in the identity standard. A match signals self-verification or self-confirmation.
4. This idea of salience as the probability of enacting an identity in a situation separates this notion from that of activation and allows the separate consideration of factors such as context (for example, the existence of an appropriate role partner) that activate an identity in the situation separately from factors such as commitment that influence the probability of an identity being played out across situations. Social identity theory has tended to blend the ideas of activation and salience as conceptualized here (Stets & Burke, 2000).
5. Stryker (1980) speaks of commitment in terms of the costs of losing or giving up the identity, reminiscent of the idea of commitment as side bets introduced by Becker (1960).
6. Cast (2001) has recently argued that we need to examine situations in which behavior influences the self-meanings associated with an identity rather than those in which self-meanings influence behavior. She argues that when we adopt new role identities, it is likely that our understanding of the role identity meanings is vague and loosely organized. Trying out different behaviors may help us crystallize the standard meanings of role identity. Once we have settled in on those standard meanings of identity, then those meanings will chiefly direct future role behavior.
7. Another means by which self-verification is achieved is in the input side of the identity model, in which actors may modify what they perceive in the situation so that the resulting perceptions better match their identity standards.
8. Behavioral strategies and cognitive strategies are analogous to engaging in primary and secondary control, respectively (Rothbaum, Weisz, & Snyder, 1982). In primary control, one attempts to influence the situation. In identity theory, this attempt occurs on the output side. Individuals act in order to match self-in-situation meanings with the identity standard. If this action is ineffective, one may resort to cognitive strategies, making adjustment to the current perceptions—otherwise known as secondary control. For example, one may bias his or her perceptions in a direction that reduces any discrepancy between self-in-situation meanings and identity standard meanings. If this strategy is ineffective, one may change his or her identity standard as a last resort—another secondary control strategy.
9. Of course, another alternative is to leave the situation in order to deactivate the identity or to give up the identity entirely, as in the case of divorce.
10. There are situations in which two identities are unrelated to each other. An action of one identity leaves the other identity unaffected.

References

Abrams, D., & Hogg, M. A. (1990). *Social identity theory: Constructive and critical advances*. London: Harvester-Wheatsheaf.

Bandura, A. (1982). Self-efficacy mechanism in human agency. *American Psychologist, 37*, 122-147

Bandura, A. (1995). Exercise of personal and collective efficacy in changing societies. In A. Bandura (Ed.), *Self-efficacy in changing societies* (pp. 1–45). New York: Cambridge University Press.

Bartels, D. J. (1997). *An examination of the primary emo-*

tions of anger and sadness in marriage within the context of identity theory. Unpublished manuscript, Washington State University, Pullman, WA.

Becker, H. S. (1960). Notes on the concept of commitment. *American Journal of Sociology, 66*, 32–40.

Blumer, H. (1969). *Symbolic interactionism.* Englewood Cliffs, NJ: Prentice-Hall.

Brewer, M. B. (1991). The social self: On being the same and different at the same time. *Personality and Social Psychology Bulletin, 17*, 475–482.

Burke, P. J. (1980). The self: Measurement implications from a symbolic interactionist perspective. *Social Psychology Quarterly, 43*, 18–29.

Burke, P. J. (1991). Identity processes and social stress. *American Sociological Review, 56*, 836–849.

Burke, P. J. (1996). Social identities and psychosocial stress. In H. B. Kaplan (Ed.), *Psychosocial stress: Perspectives on structure, theory, life course, and methods* (pp. 141–174). Orlando, FL: Academic Press.

Burke, P. J. (1997). An identity model for network exchange. *American Sociological Review, 62*, 134–150.

Burke, P. J. (2001, April). *Relationships among multiple identities.* Paper presented at "The Future of Identity Theory and Research: A Guide for a New Century" conference, Bloomington, IN.

Burke, P. J. (2002). *Marital socialization and identity change.* Vancouver, BC, Canada: Pacific Sociological Association.

Burke, P. J., & Cast, A. D. (1997). Stability and change in the gender identities of newly married couples. *Social Psychology Quarterly, 60*, 277–290.

Burke, P. J., & Reitzes, D. C. (1981). The link between identity and role performance. *Social Psychology Quarterly, 44*, 83–92.

Burke, P. J., & Reitzes, D. C. (1991). An identity theory approach to commitment. *Social Psychology Quarterly, 54*, 239–251.

Burke, P. J., & Stets, J. E. (1999). Trust and commitment through self-verification. *Social Psychology Quarterly, 62*, 347-366.

Burke, P. J., & Tully, J. (1977). The measurement of role/identity. *Social Forces, 55*, 881–897.

Callero, P. L. (1985). Role-identity salience. *Social Psychology Quarterly, 48*, 203–214.

Carver, C. S., & Scheier, M. F. (1981). *Attention and self-regulation: A control-theory approach to human behavior.* New York: Springer-Verlag.

Carver, C. S., & Scheier, M. F. (1998). *On the self-regulation of behavior.* Cambridge, UK: Cambridge University Press.

Cast, A. D. (2001, April). *Identities and behavior.* Paper presented at "The Future of Identity Theory and Research: A Guide for a New Century" conference, Bloomington, IN.

Cast, A. D., & Burke, P. J. (2002). A theory of self-esteem, *Social Forces, 80*, 1041–1068.

Cast, A. D., Stets, J. E., & Burke, P. J. (1999). Does the self conform to the views of others? *Social Psychology Quarterly, 62*, 68–82.

Cooley, C. H. (1902). *Human nature and social order.* New York: Scribner's.

Deaux, K. (1992). Personalizing identity and socializing self. In G. M. Blackwell (Ed.), *Social psychology of* identity and the self-concept (pp. 9–33). London: Surry University Press.

Deaux, K., & Martin, D. (2001, April). *Which context?: Specifying levels of context in identity processes.* Paper presented at "The Future of Identity Theory and Research: A Guide for a New Century" conference, Bloomington, IN.

DePaulo, B. M., Kenny, D. A., Hoover, C. W., Webb, W., & Oliver, P. (1987). Accuracy of person perception: Do people know what kinds of impressions they convey? *Journal of Personality and Social Psychology, 52*, 303–315.

Ellestad, J., & Stets, J. E. (1998). Jealousy and parenting: Predicting emotions from identity theory. *Sociological Perspectives, 41*, 639–668.

Fazio, R. H., Sanbonmatsu, D. M., Powell, M. C., & Kardes, F. R. (1986). On the automatic activation of attitudes. *Journal of Personality and Social Psychology, 50*, 229–238.

Felson, R. B. (1993). The (somewhat) social self: How others affect self-appraisals. In J. M. Suls (Ed.), *The self in social perspective* (pp. 1–26). Hillsdale, NJ: Erlbaum.

Franks, D. D., & Marolla, J. (1976). Efficacious action and social approval as interacting dimensions of self-esteem: A tentative formulation through construct validation. *Sociometry, 39*, 324–341.

Freese, L., & Burke, P. J. (1994). Persons, identities, and social interaction. In B. Markovsky, K. Heimer, & J. O'Brien (Eds.), *Advances in group processes* (pp. 1–24). Greenwich, CT: JAI Press.

Gecas, V., & Burke, P. J. (1995). Self and identity. In K. Cook, G. A. Fine, & J. S. House (Eds.), *Sociological perspectives on social psychology* (pp. 41–67). Boston: Allyn & Bacon.

Gecas, V., & Schwalbe, M. L. (1983). Beyond the looking-glass self: Social structure and efficacy-based self-esteem. *Social Psychology Quarterly,.46*, 77-88.

Haslam, S. A., Oakes, P. J., McGarty, C., & Turner, J. C. (1996). Stereotyping and social influence: The mediation of stereotype applicability and sharedness by the views of in-group and out-group members. *British Journal of Social Psychology, 35*, 369–397.

Heise, D. R. (1979). *Understanding events: Affect and the construction of social action.* Cambridge, UK: Cambridge University Press.

Heise, D. R. (1989). Effects of emotion displays on social identification. *Social Psychology Quarterly, 52*, 10–21.

Higgins, E. T. (1989). Self-discrepancy theory: What patterns to self-beliefs cause people to suffer? In L. Berkowitz (Ed.), *Advances in experimental social psychology* (Vol. 22, pp. 93–136). New York: Academic Press.

Hoelter, J. W. (1986). The relationship between specific and global evaluations of the self: A comparison of several models. *Social Psychology Quarterly, 49*, 129–141.

Hogg, M. A., & Abrams, D. (1988). *Social identifications: A social psychology of intergroup relations and group processes.* London: Routledge.

Hogg, M. A., Terry, D. J., & White, K. M. (1995). A tale of two theories: A critical comparison of identity theory with social identity theory. *Social Psychology Quarterly, 58*, 255–269.

James, W. (1890). *Principles of psychology*. New York: Holt.

Kaplan, H. (1975). The self-esteem motive. In H. B. Kaplan (Ed.), *Self-attitudes and deviant behavior* (pp. 10–31). Pacific Palisades, CA: Goodyear.

Kenny, D. D., & Albright, L. (1987). Accuracy in interpersonal perception: A social relations analysis. *Psychological Bulletin, 102*, 390–402.

Kiecolt, K. J. (1994). Stress and the decision to change oneself: A theoretical model. *Social Psychology Quarterly, 57*, 49–63.

Kiecolt, K. J. (2000). Self change in social movements. In S. Stryker, T. Owens, & R. White (Eds.), *Identity, self, and social movements (pp. 110-131)*. Minneapolis: University of Minnesota Press.

Kollock, P. (1994). The emergence of exchange structures: An experimental study of uncertainty, commitment, and trust. *American Journal of Sociology, 100*, 313–345.

Lawler, E. J., & Yoon, J. (1996). Commitment in exchange relations: Test of a theory of relational cohesion. *American Sociological Review, 61*, 89–108.

Levenson, R. W., & Gottman, J. M. (1985). Physiological and affective predictors of change in relationship satisfaction. *Journal of Personality and Social Psychology, 49*, 85–94.

Lindesmith, A. R., & Strauss, A. L. (1956). *Social psychology*. New York: Holt, Rinehart & Winston.

Linton, R. (1936). *The study of man*. New York: Appleton-Century-Crofts.

Linville, P. (1985). Self-complexity and affective extremity: Don't put all of your eggs in one cognitive basket. *Social Cognition, 3*, 94–120.

Linville, P. (1987). Self-complexity as a cognitive buffer against stress-related illness and depression. *Journal of Personality and Social Psychology, 52*, 663-676.

Longmore, M. A., & DeMaris, A. (1997). Perceived inequity and depression in intimate relationships: The moderating effect of self-esteem. *Social Psychology Quarterly, 60*, 172–184.

MacKinnon, N. J. (1994). *Symbolic interaction as affect control*. Albany: State University of New York Press.

Markus, H. (1977). Self-schemata and processing information about the self. *Journal of Personality and Social Psychology, 35*, 63–78.

McCall, G. J., & Simmons, J. L. (1978). *Identities and interactions*. New York: Free Press.

Mead, G. H. (1934). *Mind, self, and society*. Chicago: University of Chicago Press.

Nagel, J. (1995). American Indian ethnic renewal: Politics and the resurgence of identity. *American Sociological Review, 60*, 947–965.

Oakes, P. (1987). The salience of social categories. In J. C. Turner, M. A. Hogg, P. J. Oakes, S. D. Reicher, & M. S. Wetherell, (Eds.), *Rediscovering the social group: A self-categorization theory* (pp. 117–141). New York: Basil Blackwell.

Oakes, P. J., Haslam, S. A., & Turner, J. C. (1994). *Stereotyping and social reality*. Oxford, UK: Blackwell.

Osgood, C. E., Suci, G. J., & Tannenbaum, P. H. (1957). *The measurement of meaning*. Urbana: University of Illinois Press.

Owens, T. J., & Aronson, P. J. (2000). Self-concept as a force in social movement involvement. In S. Stryker, T. J. Owens, & R. White (Eds.), *Self, identity, and social movements* (pp. 191–214). Minneapolis: University of Minnesota Press.

Powers, W. T. (1973). *Behavior: The control of perception*. Chicago: Aldine.

Ridgeway, C. L., & Johnson, C. (1990). What is the relationship between socioemotional behavior and status in task groups. *American Journal of Sociology, 95*, 1189–1212.

Ridgeway, C. L., & Walker, H. A. (1995). Status structures. In K. S. Cook, G. A. Fine, & J. S. House (Eds.), *Sociological perspectives on social psychology* (pp. 281–310). Boston: Allyn & Bacon.

Riley, A., & Burke, P. J. (1995). Identities and self-verification in the small group. *Social Psychology Quarterly, 58*, 61–73.

Rosenberg, M. (1979). *Conceiving the self*. New York: Basic Books.

Rosenberg, M., Schooler, C., Schoenbach, C., & Rosenberg, F. (1995). Global self-esteem and specific self-esteem: Different concepts, different outcomes. *American Sociological Review, 60*, 141–156.

Rothbaum, F., Weisz, J. R., & Snyder, S. S. (1982). Changing the world and changing the self: A two-process model of perceived control. *Journal of Personality and Social Psychology, 42*, 5–37.

Scheff, T. (1994). Emotions and identity: A theory of ethnic nationalism. In C. Calhoun (Ed.), *Social theory and the politics of identity* (pp. 277–303). Philadelphia: Temple University Press.

Serpe, R. T., & Stryker, S. (1987). The construction of self and reconstruction of social relationships. In E. Lawler & B. Markovsky (Eds.), *Advances in group processes* (pp. 41–66). Greenwich, CT: JAI Press.

Shrauger, J. S., & Schoeneman, T. J. (1979). Symbolic interactionist view of self-concept: Through the looking glass darkly. *Psychological Bulletin, 86*, 549–573.

Skvoretz, J., & Willer, D. (1993). Exclusion and power: A test of four theories of power in exchange networks. *American Sociological Review, 58*, 801–818.

Smith-Lovin, L. (1988). The affective control of events within settings. In L. Smith-Lovin & D. R. Heise (Eds.), *Analyzing social interaction: Research advances in affect control theory* (pp. 71–101). New York: Gordon & Breach.

Smith-Lovin, L. (1995). The sociology of affect and emotion. In K. S. Cook, G. A. Fine, & J. S. House (Eds.), *Sociological perspectives on social psychology* (pp. 118–148). Boston: Allyn & Bacon.

Smith-Lovin, L. (2001, April). *Self, identity and interaction in an ecology of identities*. Paper presented at "The Future of Identity Theory and Research: A Guide for a New Century" conference, Bloomington, IN.

Smith-Lovin, L., & Heise, D. R. (1988). *Analyzing social interaction: Advances in affect control theory*. New York: Gordon & Breach.

Stets, J. E. (1995). Role identities and person identities: Gender identity, mastery identity, and controlling one's partner. *Sociological Perspectives, 38*, 129–150.

Stets, J. E. (1997). Status and identity in marital interaction. *Social Psychology Quarterly, 60*, 185-217.

Stets, J. E. (2001, April). *Justice, emotion, and identity theory*. Paper presented at "The Future of Identity Theory and Research: A Guide for a New Century" conference, Bloomington, IN.

Stets, J. E., & Burke, P. J. (1994). Inconsistent self-views in the control identity model. *Social Science Research, 23,* 236–262.

Stets, J. E., & Burke, P. J. (1996). Gender, control, and interaction. *Social Psychology Quarterly, 59,* 193–220.

Stets, J. E., & Burke, P. J. (2000). Identity theory and social identity theory. *Social Psychology Quarterly, 63,* 224–237.

Stets, J. E, & Tsushima, T. M. (2001). Negative emotion and coping responses within identity control theory. *Social Psychology Quarterly, 64,* 283–295.

Stryker, S. (1968). Identity salience and role performance. *Journal of Marriage and the Family, 4,* 558–564.

Stryker, S. (1980). *Symbolic interactionism: A social structural version.* Menlo Park, CA: Benjamin/Cummings.

Stryker, S. (1987). *The interplay of affect and identity: Exploring the relationships of social structure, social interaction, self, and emotion.* Chicago: American Sociological Association.

Stryker, S. (2000). Identity competition: Key to differential social movement involvement. In S. Stryker, T. Owens, & R. White (Eds.), *Identity, self, and social movements* (pp. 21–40). Minneapolis: University of Minnesota Press.

Stryker, S., & Burke, P. J. (2000). The past, present, and future of an identity theory. *Social Psychology Quarterly, 63,* 284–297.

Stryker, S., & Serpe, R. T. (1982). Commitment, identity salience, and role behavior: A theory and research example. In W. Ickes & E. S. Knowles (Eds.), *Personality, roles, and social behavior* (pp. 199–218). New York: Springer-Verlag.

Stryker, S., & Serpe, R. T. (1994). Identity salience and psychological centrality: Equivalent, overlapping, or complementary concepts? *Social Psychology Quarterly, 57,* 16–35.

Swann, W. B., Jr. (1983). Self-verification: Bringing social reality into harmony with the self. In J. Suls & A. Greenwald (Eds.), *Psychological perspectives on the self* (pp. 33–66). Hillsdale, NJ: Erlbaum.

Swann, W. B., Jr. (1990). To be adored or to be known?: The interplay of self-enhancement and self-verification. In E. T. Higgins & R. M. Sorrentino (Eds.), *Handbook of motivation and cognition* (Vol. 2, pp. 408–448). New York: Guilford Press.

Swann, W. B., Jr., Griffin, J. J., Jr., Predmore, S. C., & Gaines, B. (1987). The cognitive–affective crossfire: When self-consistency confronts self-enhancement.

Journal of Personality and Social Psychology, 52, 881–889.

Tajfel, H. (1981). *Human groups and social categories: Studies in social psychology.* Cambridge, UK: Cambridge University Press.

Tesser, A. (1988). Toward a self-evaluation maintenance model of social behavior. In L. Berkowitz (Ed.), *Advances in experimental social psychology* (Vol. 21, pp. 181–228). New York: Academic Press.

Thoits, P. A. (1983). Multiple identities and psychological well-being: A reformulation and test of the social isolation hypothesis. *American Sociological Review, 49,* 174–187.

Thoits, P. A. (1986). Multiple identities: Examining gender and marital status differences in distress. *American Sociological Review, 51,* 259–272.

Thoits, P. A. (1992). Identity structures and psychological well-being: Gender and marital status comparisons. *Social Psychology Quarterly, 55,* 236–256.

Thoits, P. A. (2001, April). *Personal agency in the accumulation of role-identities.* Paper presented at "The Future of Identity Theory and Research: A Guide for a New Century" conference, Bloomington, IN.

Thoits, P. A., & Virshup, L. K. (1997). Me's and we's: Forms and functions of social identities. In R. D. Ashmore & L. J. Jussim (Eds.), *Self and identity: Fundamental issues* (pp. 106–133). New York: Oxford University Press.

Tsushima, T., & Burke, P. J. (1999). Levels, agency, and control in the parent identity. *Social Psychology Quarterly, 62,* 173–189.

Turner, J. C., Hogg, M. A., Oakes, P. J., Reicher, S. D., & Wetherell, M. S. (Eds.). (1987). *Rediscovering the social group: A self-categorization theory.* New York: Blackwell.

Turner, R. H. (1962). Role-taking: Process versus conformity. In A. M. Rose (Ed.), *Human behavior and social processes* (pp. 20-40). Boston: Houghton Mifflin.

Turner, R. H. (1978). The role and the person. *American Journal of Sociology, 84,* 1–23.

Turner, R. H., & Billings, V. (1991). The social contexts of self-feeling. In J. A. Howard & P. L. Callero (Eds.), *The self-society dynamic: Cognition, emotion, and action* (pp. 103–122). New York: Cambridge University Press.

Webster, M., Jr., & Foschi, M. (1988). Overview of status generalization. In M. Webster, Jr. & M. Foschi (Eds.), *Status generalization: New theory and research* (pp. 1–20). Stanford, CA: Stanford University Press.

8

Implicit Self and Identity

THIERRY DEVOS
MAHZARIN R. BANAJI

When William James (1890) wrote about the unique problem of studying self and identity, he immediately noted the peculiar blurring of the otherwise clear demarcation between the *knower* and the *known*. The object of scrutiny, the self, was also the agent doing the scrutinizing. This illicit merger of the knower and the known has created an epistemological unease that philosophers have worried about and psychologists have either ignored or turned into an assumption of their theorizing. The human ability for self-awareness and self-reflection is so unique that tapping it as a vital source of information about mind and social behavior has come at the expense of confronting the severe problems of the knower also being the known and of using introspection as the primary path to discovery. In this chapter, we argue that at least one circumstance can disentangle the knower from the known in the study of self: when self-as-knower does not have full introspective access to self-as-known. When knowledge about oneself resides in a form that is inaccessible to consciousness but can indeed be tapped indirectly, the self-as-knower and the self-as-known can be dissociated in a manner that is epistemologically more pleasing. In this chapter, we focus on states of un-

conscious thought and feeling—those marked by a lack of conscious awareness, control, intention, and self-reflection.

Over the past two decades, the study of implicit social cognition has created new paradigms for studying several traditional fields (for reviews, see Banaji, Lemm, & Carpenter, 2001; Greenwald & Banaji, 1995; Wegner & Bargh, 1998). At first sight, this trend, it would seem, has little to say about the topic of self and identity. Indeed, it is a common assumption that the studies of self centrally involve experiences of reflexive consciousness (Baumeister, 1998): Individuals reflect on their experiences, self-consciously evaluate the contents of consciousness, and introspect about the causes and meaning of things. In addition, the self is often viewed as playing a consciously active role in making meaning, implementing choices, pursuing goals, and initiating action. Studies that focus on unconscious modes of thinking and feeling, when applied to self and identity processes, question these assumptions, and they do so based on the discovery of mental acts that are fully meaningful and lawful but that appear to arise without introspective access or deliberative thought.

In this chapter, we provide an overview of

research on the implicit social cognition of self and identity. No attempt is made to exhaustively review the literature at hand. Rather, we focus on reflections of self and identity in a particular social context—the context in which thoughts and feelings about oneself are shaped by membership in a larger collective and in which such thoughts and feelings go beyond the self as target to represent and shape a view of the collective (Banaji & Prentice, 1994; Walsh & Banaji, 1997). Such a focus places us in the respectable company of others who also assume or demonstrate that the individual self is meaningfully considered in reference to social entities that transcend the individual self (Cooley, 1902; Mead, 1934; Turner, Oakes, Haslam, & McGarty, 1994). Our unique position limits the coverage to aspects of the self that emerge when (1) viewed in the context of social group memberships and (2) measured via unconscious expressions of thought and feeling. We begin with research paradigms that link the study of self with social group and proceed to specific analyses of basic preference for the ingroup and other attributes associated with the self. We then include analyses of implicit self and identity processes as viewed in research on self-evaluation, performance and behavior, and goal pursuit. In the next major section we attend to the top-down influence of societal and cultural influences on the construction of implicit self and identity. Together, the research we review reveals the plasticity of the self as it develops and exists in close response to the demands of social group and culture.

The term "implicit" is used to refer to processes that occur outside conscious awareness. Evaluations of one's self, for example, may be influenced by group membership, even though the individual is not aware of such an influence. An Asian woman may come to view herself as excelling in math when her ethnic identity is implicitly brought to the foreground but as weak in math skills when her gender is highlighted (see Shih, Pittinsky, & Ambady, 1999, for a demonstration of such group membership effects on math performance). There are multiple ways in which one may be unaware of the source of influence on thoughts, feelings, and behavior. For example, one may be unaware of the existence of the source of influence, whereas in other circumstances one may consciously and accurately perceive the source of influence while being unaware of its causative role in self-evaluation. The term "implicit" is also applied to those processes that occur without conscious control. Here, the circumstances are such that one may be perfectly aware of the contingencies that connect a particular stimulus to a response but be unable to change or reverse the direction of the thought, feeling, or action. A person may have a view of herself as egalitarian but find herself unable to control prejudicial thoughts about members of a group, perhaps including groups of which she is herself a member. Although empirical investigations focus on one or another of these aspects of unconscious social cognition, as well as on those that select intention and self-reflection, we use the term "implicit" here to encompass both processes that occur without conscious awareness and those that occur without conscious control.

Self and Social Group

Since at least the 1970s, self-concept has been profitably studied by representing it as an information structure with empirically tractable cognitive and affective features (for reviews, see Greenwald & Pratkanis, 1984; Kihlstrom & Cantor, 1984; Kihlstrom et al., 1988). From such a theoretical vantage point came the idea that the self-concept, like other representations, could be viewed as possibly operating in automatic mode and that aspects of self may be hidden from introspective awareness (e.g., Bargh, 1982; Bargh & Tota, 1988; Higgins, Van Hook, & Dorfman, 1988; Markus, 1977; Rogers, Kuiper, & Kirker, 1977; Strauman & Higgins, 1987).

Although strongly social in focus, research in the American social cognition tradition, focused on the interpersonal aspects of self and identity, whereas another tradition with European roots, emphasized the association between self and social group, resulting in an intergroup emphasis. The latter's most articulate and encompassing formulation, labeled self-categorization theory (Turner, 1985; Turner, Hogg, Oakes, Reicher, & Wetherell, 1987), holds that, under particular conditions, group members perceive themselves as exemplars of the group rather than as unique individuals. In this mode, they highlight the similarities between themselves and other ingroup members, and they apply characteristics typical of the ingroup to the self (self-stereotyping). In other words, the representations of self and ingroup become inextricably linked. Until recently, tests of this hypothesis mainly involved self-report measures (Biernat, Vescio, & Green, 1996; Hogg & Turner, 1987; Simon & Hamilton, 1994; Simon, Pantaleo, & Mummendey, 1995). However, several empirical investigations have revealed that the process by which the ingroup may be said to become part and parcel of the self can operate at an implicit level.

Adapting a paradigm developed by Aron, Aron, Tudor, and Nelson (1991), Smith and Henry (1996) examined people's psychological ties to significant ingroups. Participants were asked to rate themselves, their ingroup, and an outgroup on a list of traits. Next, they indicated, as quickly and accurately as possible, whether each trait was self-descriptive or not. Self-descriptiveness judgments were faster for traits on which participants matched their ingroup than for traits on which they mismatched. On the contrary, no such facilitation was observed for traits rated as matching or mismatching the outgroup. This finding has been taken to illustrate that the ingroup becomes part of the representation of self, and a follow-up study (Smith, Coats, & Walling, 1999) demonstrated that the reverse was also true: Characteristics of the self influenced evaluations of the ingroup. Using a similar procedure, Smith and colleagues (1999) found that participants were faster to make ingroup descriptiveness judgments for traits that matched their self-perceptions. As another example, fraternity or sorority members are faster to make liking judgments for attitude objects (e.g., parties, tattoos, science, beer) on which they match the ingroup rather than on those on which there is a mismatch with the ingroup (Coats, Smith, Claypool, & Banner, 2000). Together, these results support the idea of a mental fusion of the self and social group.

The Implicit Association Test (IAT; Greenwald, McGhee, & Schwartz, 1998) is a technique developed to assess the strength of implicit associations between concepts (e.g., self, group) and attributes (e.g., evaluation of good–bad, specific traits). The assumption underlying the technique is that the more closely related a concept and an attribute are (e.g., ingroup and good, outgroup and bad), the more quickly information representing the concept and the attribute should be paired. For purposes of obtaining a baseline with which such pairings can be compared, the task includes a measure of response time to contrasting pairs that are made simultaneously (ingroup and bad, outgroup and good).[1]

Recent experiments have used this technique and variations of it to investigate the strength of self + group association, referring to this pairing as a measure of automatic identity with the social group. For example, Devos and Banaji (2001) used this procedure to capture the strength of implicit national identity among citizens of the United States. Participants were asked to categorize, as quickly as possible, stimuli presented on a computer screen. Some stimuli were pictures of American or foreign symbols (e.g., flags, coins, maps, monuments), whereas other stimuli were pronouns frequently used to designate ingroups (e.g., "we," "ourselves") or outgroups (e.g., "they," "other"). Participants completed this task twice. In one case, American symbols were paired with words representing the ingroup (e.g., "we," "ourselves"), and foreign symbols were combined with words representing the outgroup (e.g., "they," "other"). In another case, American symbols were combined with outgroup words, and foreign symbols were paired with ingroup words. Results indicated that participants performed the categorization task more quickly when American symbols and ingroup words shared the same response key. In other words, it was easier to associate American symbols with items such as "we" or "ourselves" rather than with "they" or "other." American symbols may be seen here as automatically evoking belonging and implying that, at least when unable to control their responses, this sample of Americans strongly identified with their national group.

Using the same technique, other empirical investigations have demonstrated strong implicit associations between self and attributes, roles, or domains stereotypical of gender categories. For instance, female participants could more easily associate idiographic information (e.g., their names, their hometowns) or pronouns such as "me" or "mine" with feminine traits (e.g., gentle, warm, tender) rather than with masculine attributes (e.g., competitive, independent, strong), whereas the opposite was true for male participants (Greenwald & Farnham, 2000; Lemm & Banaji, 1998). Similarly, strong automatic associations between self and the concept "math" for men, and the concept "arts" for women have been obtained repeatedly (Nosek, Banaji, & Greenwald, 2002b). In addition, Lane, Mitchell, and Banaji (2001) have shown that implicit identification with a new ingroup could occur early on and without extensive contact with the group. As predicted, Yale students showed stronger implicit identity with Yale as an institution (rather than with Harvard), but strength of identity was equally strong among those who had been on campus for a few days and those who were starting their fourth and final year. Theories of implicit social cognition that assume slow learning (through long-term experience) need to explain the presence of such fast-to-form and fast-to-stabilize implicit identities.

The previous examples indicate that group membership comes to be automatically associated with self and that people automatically endorse attributes stereotypic of their group as also being self-descriptive. Recently, von Hippel, Hawkins, and Schooler (2001) identified circumstances under which the opposite is true: Counterstereotypic attributes become strongly associated to the self. For example, African Americans were more likely to endorse the trait "intelligent" rapidly (i.e., to be schematic for this attribute) than white Americans if they performed well academically, and white Americans were more likely than African Americans to be schematic for "athletic" if they performed well in that domain. These findings are consistent with the idea that characteristics or features that make one distinctive from others are particularly likely to be represented in the self-concept (McGuire & McGuire, 1988). Both sets of seemingly opposing results may be explained by theories that emphasize the strong association between self and social group. In both cases, one's knowledge or understanding of the association between group + attribute comes to influence implicit self-perception.

A Preference for Ingroups

The links between self and ingroup are not only visible in implicit knowledge and thought but also present in measures of attitude or evaluation. Tajfel (1974) emphasized this point when he defined "social identity as that part of an individual's self-concept which derives from his knowledge of his membership of a social group (or groups) together with the emotional significance attached to that membership" (p. 69). A growing body of research shows that people evaluate ingroup members more favorably than outgroup members (Brewer, 1979; Mullen, Brown, & Smith, 1992), and we examine those studies that used measure of implicit attitude or evaluation. The literature on implicit attitudes clearly suggests that groups unconsciously or automatically trigger more positive affective reactions when they are associated to self. Assessments of ethnic attitudes without perceivers' awareness or control consistently reveal that white Americans have more positive feelings toward white Americans than toward African Americans (Dasgupta, McGhee, Greenwald, & Banaji, 2000; Fazio, Jackson, Dunton, & Williams, 1995; Greenwald et al., 1998; Wittenbrink, Judd, & Park, 1997). Likewise, members of other groups also show implicit preference for the ingroup (Japanese Americans vs. Korean Americans; Greenwald et al., 1998), and findings such as these are expected to be obtained with a wide variety of groups (affiliations with nation, state, and city, with school and sports team, with family and friends). Some studies indicate that implicit intergroup biases in the realm of ethnic relations include both ingroup favoritism (positivity toward white Americans) and outgroup derogation (negativity toward black Americans) (Dovidio, Evans, & Tyler, 1986; Nosek & Banaji, 2001), whereas others suggest that individuals no longer differentially ascribe negative characteristics to ethnic groups but continue to associate positive attributes to a greater extent to whites than to blacks (Gaertner & McLaughlin, 1983). Research also shows that undergraduate students hold a more favorable attitude toward the category "young" than toward the category "old" (Nosek, Banaji, & Greenwald, 2002; Perdue & Gurtman, 1990; Rudman, Greenwald, Mellott, & Schwartz, 1999). Strong implicit preferences for American symbols have been revealed in several studies (Ashburn-Nardo, Voils, & Monteith, 2001; Devos & Banaji, 2001; Rudman et al., 1999). To this list of implicit ingroup preference we add findings that show implicit positive attitudes toward groups based on sexual orientation (Lemm & Banaji, 2000) or social class (Cunningham, Nezlek, & Banaji, 2001). In fact, Cunningham and colleagues (2001) have shown implicit positive associations to the category white (rather than black), rich (rather than poor), American (rather than foreign), straight (rather than gay) and Christian (rather than Jewish) among students known to be white, American, and Christian, a majority of whom were also assumed to be high on the social class dimension and to be heterosexual. Cunningham and colleagues have taken the extra step of claiming that these implicit preferences do not develop in isolation and that an individual difference marks the pattern: Those who show higher preference for one ingroup also show higher preference for all other ingroups, which is evidence for an implicit ethnocentrism dimension.

In most of the research described, researchers have assessed the implicit attitudes of only people belonging to one particular group. That is, white participants have been shown to have greater implicit liking for whites over blacks, but equivalent data from black participants have not always been available. Of the few studies that do measure both sides, symmetry has been found under some circumstances. Greenwald and colleagues (1998) reported data from both Japanese Americans and Korean Americans, each of whom showed a more positive implicit attitude toward their own ethnic group. The level of immersion in Asian culture moderated this pattern of implicit preferences. More precisely, partici-

pants who were immersed in their particular Asian culture (i.e., had a high proportion of family members and acquaintances who were from that culture and were familiar with the language) showed greater ingroup preference. Depending on their religious affiliation, individuals exhibit an implicit preference for Christian or Jewish people (Rudman et al., 1999). The relations between Bavarians and North Germans have also shown strong implicit ingroup bias (Neumann et al., 1998).

Using linguistic patterns to indicate intergroup bias, Maass, Salvi, Arcuri, and Semin (1989) revealed another interesting form of implicit ingroup favoritism. They show that individuals usually described positive behaviors in more abstract language terms ("X is helpful") when performed by an ingroup member than when performed by an outgroup member ("X gave them directions to go to the station"). The opposite held for negative behaviors (see also Karpinski & von Hippel, 1996; von Hippel, Sekaquaptewa, & Vargas, 1997). This linguistic bias does not appear to be under volitional control (Franco & Maass, 1996). Recent research indicates that participants from Belgium and Spain automatically attributed secondary emotions, such as affection, pride, and remorse, more to ingroups than to outgroups (Leyens et al., 2000). Given that such secondary emotions are also seen to be uniquely human characteristics, this finding is consistent with the idea that ingroups are viewed as being more human than outgroups.

The tendency to favor the ingroup attitudinally (e.g., along a good–bad dimension) sometimes underlies implicit stereotyping (e.g., the assignment of specific qualities that may also vary in evaluation). For example, both men and women hold similar implicit gender stereotypes, but they are exhibited to a stronger extent when they reflect favorably on their own group (Rudman, Greenwald, & McGhee, 2001). Male participants are more likely to differentiate men and women with respect to an attribute such as "power," whereas female participants are more likely to do so on a trait such as "warmth." In other words, each group emphasizes stereotypes in an ingroup-favorable direction. These findings parallel observations based on self-report measures as well (Lindeman & Sundvik, 1995; Peabody, 1968).

Using measures of consciously accessible cognition, the ingroup bias has been shown to emerge under minimal conditions: The mere categorization of individuals into two distinct groups elicits a preference for the ingroup (Diehl, 1990; Tajfel, Billig, Bundy, & Flament, 1971). There is now evidence that a minimal social categorization is sufficient to automatically or unconsciously activate positive attitudes toward self-related groups and negative or neutral attitudes toward non-self-related groups. For example, Perdue, Dovidio, Gurtman, and Tyler (1990) found that participants responded faster to pleasant words when primed with ingroup pronouns (such as "we" or "us") rather than with outgroup pronouns (such as "they" or "them"), even though they were unaware of the group-designating primes. Thus the use of words referring to ingroups or outgroups might unconsciously perpetuate intergroup biases. More recently, Otten and Wentura (1999) showed that neutral words automatically acquired an affective connotation, simply by introducing them as group labels and by relating one of them to participants' self-concepts. The self-related group label functioned equivalently to a priori positive primes, whereas the other label functioned similarly to a priori negative primes. In other words, as soon as a word designated an ingroup, it acquired a positive connotation, whereas words referring to an outgroup immediately conveyed a negative valence. Using a different procedure, Otten and Moskowitz (2000) also found evidence for implicit activation of positive affect toward novel ingroups. A minimal intergroup setting was combined with a well-established procedure measuring spontaneous trait inferences (Uleman, Hon, Roman, & Moskowitz, 1996). Results showed that when behaviors implied a positive trait about the ingroup, they were more likely to be categorized in a manner consistent with the implied trait than when the behaviors were performed by an outgroup member or when the traits implied were negative. These experiments suggest that the ingroup bias occurs automatically or unconsciously under minimal conditions (see also Ashburn-Nardo et al., 2001).

Preferences for Self Extend to Attributes Associated with Self

These findings are reminiscent of research showing that the mere ownership of an object or its association to the self is a condition sufficient enough to enhance its attractiveness. Nuttin (1985) found that when individuals were asked to choose a preferred letter from each of several pairs consisting of one alphabetical letter from their names and one not, they tended reliably to prefer alphabets that constitute their names. This finding, known as the "name letter effect" (NLE), has been replicated in many countries (Nuttin, 1987) and with samples from very different cultures (Hoorens, Nuttin, Herman, & Pavakanun, 1990; Kitayama & Karasawa, 1997). In addition, the preference for name letters has been shown to be stable over a 4-week period (Koole, Dijksterhuis, & van Knippenberg, 2001).

In order to test whether the preference for name letters depended on a conscious decision, Nuttin (1985) invited participants to search for a meaningful pattern in the pairs of letters presented. Despite the fact that no time limit was imposed and that a monetary award was promised to anyone who could correctly identify the prearranged pattern of letters, not a single participant could come up with the solution. This finding supports the idea that the NLE does not stem from a conscious recognition of the connection between the attribute and one's self. Several alternative interpretations of the effect have been ruled out. For instance, the NLE does not seem to be a remainder of the positive mastery affect most people experienced when they first succeeded in reading or writing their own names (Hoorens & Todorova, 1988; Hoorens et al., 1990). In addition, the NLE does not appear to be due to an enhanced subjective frequency of own name letters as compared with non-name letters (Hoorens & Nuttin, 1993). The most convincing interpretation of this effect at present is that preference for letters in one's name reflects an unconscious preference for self, and its generality is shown through research on preference for other similar self-related information, such as birthdates over other numbers (Kitayama & Karasawa, 1997; Koole et al., 2001). Finch and Cialdini (1989) showed that this effect extended to greater liking for otherwise undesirable characters (e.g., Rasputin), and Prentice and Miller (1992) showed that sharing a birthday with another person led participants to be more cooperative in a competitive situation. Recently, Pelham, Mirenberg, and Jones (2002) have shown that the extent of implicit positive evaluation of self influences where people choose to live and what people choose to do for a living. Across a dozen studies, they found that people are more likely to live in cities or states and to choose careers whose names share letters with their own first or last names. For example, a person named Louis is disproportionately likely to live in St. Louis and individuals named Dennis or Denise are overrepresented among dentists. If corroborated with continued evidence of such relationships, these findings suggest that personal choices may be constrained by linkage to self that is not noticed, not consciously sought, and even surprising.

Interesting as such research is in suggesting automatic attitude preference for self, the studies are quasi-experimental in that name letters and birth dates are not manipulated variables. Feys (1991) has provided experimental evidence for the idea that mere ownership of an object is a sufficient condition to enhance its attractiveness. Participants first learned to discriminate four computer-displayed graphic icons (which represented the participant in a computerized game) from four others that represented the participant's opponent (the computer). When participants subsequently judged all eight patterns for aesthetic attractiveness, the self-associated patterns received higher ratings. Thus individuals evaluated an object more favorably simply from the act of owning it (see also Beggan, 1992). Objects attached to the self are immediately endowed with increased value. These findings, along with the classic attitude-similarity effect, were interpretable as implicit self-esteem effects (Greenwald & Banaji, 1995); they reveal introspectively unidentified (or inaccurately identified) effects of the self-

attitude on evaluations of associated objects.

Balancing Self and Social Group

Work reviewed so far highlights the cognitive and affective ties between self and group memberships and stresses the fact that individuals are not necessarily fully aware of these bounds on their thinking or that they are aware but unable to control their operation. Now we turn to the relationships between the cognitive and affective components that make up the self system. Several theories predict some consistency between constructs that represent self and social group. For example, social identity theory (Tajfel, 1974; Tajfel & Turner, 1986) assumes some interrelations between self-esteem, group identification, and ingroup bias. According to the theory, social identification serves as a source of self-esteem. Generally speaking, individuals strive to maintain or increase their self-esteem. They can derive a sense of self-worth through favorable intergroup comparisons: Group membership contributes to positive self-esteem if the ingroup can be positively differentiated from outgroups. Thus self-esteem should be enhanced by membership in a valued group, and strong identification with the group should go hand in hand with positive evaluation of the ingroup. Evidence for the role of self-esteem in intergroup comparisons is mixed (Abrams & Hogg, 1988; Brown, 2000; Hogg & Abrams, 1990; Rubin & Hewstone, 1998). Moreover, support for the idea that there should be a positive correlation between group identification and ingroup favoritism is not overwhelming (Brown, 2000; Hinkle & Brown, 1990); this relationship is obtained only under specific circumstances (Brown et al., 1992). The absence of expected relationships has led to examinations of these constructs using implicit measures. For example, Knowles, Peng, and Levy (2001) found that the strength of the automatic association between self and whites (ingroup identification) was positively correlated with the intensity of the pro-white implicit attitude (ingroup favoritism) and also accounted for the extent to which individuals possessed a restrictive representation of their ethnic group (ingroup exclusiveness).

Recently, Greenwald and colleagues (2002; see also Greenwald et al., 2000) proposed a unified theory of social cognition that predicts patterns of interrelations between group identification, self-esteem, and ingroup attitude. Their approach draws its inspiration from theories of affective–cognitive consistency that dominated social psychology in the 1960s (Abelson et al., 1968) and allows them to integrate a range of otherwise isolated findings obtained with the IAT (Greenwald et al., 1998). This approach is based on the assumption that social knowledge (including knowledge about the self) can be represented as an associative structure. From this point of view, the structure of the self is a network of associations: The self is linked to traits, groups, concepts, or evaluations. A core principle of the theory is that attitudes toward self and concepts closely associated with self (i.e., components of self-concept or identity) should tend to be of similar valence. In other words, according to the *balance-congruity* principle, if someone holds a positive attitude toward the self and considers that a particular concept (e.g., a group, an attribute, or a domain) is part of his or her self-concept, this person should also hold a positive attitude toward that particular concept.

A study on women's gender identity illustrates this principle more concretely. For women, one would typically expect an association between self and the concept "female" (gender identity or self + female) and a positive association toward the self (positive self-esteem or self + good). Based on the balance-congruity principle, these two links should also be accompanied by a third link: a positive association toward the concept "female" (liking for female or female + good). More precisely, the strength of the positive attitude toward "female" should be a joint (or interactive) function of the strength of the associations between self and positive and between self and female. Data supported this prediction: As gender identity increased, so did the positive relation between self-esteem and liking for women (see also Farnham, Greenwald, & Banaji, 1999). Further support for similar hypotheses was found in studies on race and age identities. Interestingly, the balance-congruity principle always received stronger support when tested with implicit than with explicit measuring tools.

Another key principle of the theory, the *imbalance-dissonance* principle, is that the network resists forming new links that would result in a component being tied to pairs of bipolar-opposed constructs. A study on self-concept and gender stereotypes about mathematics demonstrates the heuristic value of this principle (Nosek et al., 2002b). Relative gender stereotypes link the concept "math" with "male," and the concept "arts" with "female." Both men and women displayed automatic associations fitting these stereotypes. Given that women also associate the self to the concept "female," the imbalance-dissonance principle leads to the prediction that women should therefore not associate themselves with "math." Using a variety of social groups and differing clusters of attributes that measure attitude, stereotype, and self-esteem, Greenwald and colleagues (2002) show evidence for balanced identities: The stronger the connection between self and social group, the more likely are the preferences and beliefs to follow in stereotypic fashion. Moreover, such effects were primarily obtained when implicit measures of self and group identity were used and appeared in weaker form on measures of conscious affect and cognition.

Self-Evaluation

Having shown the presence of self and social group connections on attitude and beliefs, we turn to research that demonstrates shifts in self-evaluation that also occur without conscious intention. For example, the unconscious activation of significant others has implications for self-evaluation. Baldwin (1992) proposed that the internalization of relationships involves the development of *relational schemas*; these cognitive structures represent regularities in patterns of interpersonal interactions. Often, the sense of self can be derived from such well-learned scripts of interpersonal evaluations. In other words, activated relational schemas shape self-evaluative reactions, even when these schemas are primed below the level of awareness. Indeed, subliminal exposure to the name of a critical versus an accepting significant other led participants to report more negative versus positive self-evaluations (Baldwin, 1994). Similarly, undergraduate students evaluated their own research ideas less favorably after being subliminally exposed to the disapproving face of their department chair rather than the approving face of another person (Baldwin, Carrell, & Lopez, 1990). These effects occurred only when the prime was a significant other. For instance, Catholic participants rated themselves more negatively after exposure to the disapproving face of the Pope, but not after exposure to the disapproving face of an unfamiliar person. In addition, if the Pope did not serve as a figure of authority, self-evaluation remained unaffected by the priming manipulation.

Mitchell, Nosek, and Banaji (2000) have shown that subtly varying the race and gender composition of the context in which a particular social group is evaluated strongly affected implicit attitudes. For example, they found that white women expressed a more negative attitude toward black females when race (rather than gender) was the distinctive categorization criterion. On the other hand, highlighting gender elicited a relatively negative attitude toward white males, whereas making race salient triggered a more positive attitude. Although these studies do not speak directly to the issue of self and identity, they lend support to the idea that intergroup biases vary as a function of the frame through which a given situation is filtered.

Unobtrusively making a social identity salient can also influence self-evaluation. S. Sinclair, Hardin, and Lowery (2001) asked participants to indicate how others and they themselves evaluated their verbal and math ability. Before they made these judgments, participants reported either their gender or ethnic identity. This subtle manipulation affected impressions attributed to others. For example, when their gender identity was salient, Asian American women reported that others evaluated them higher in verbal ability than math ability, but when their ethnic identity was salient, they stated that others evaluated them higher in math ability than verbal ability. This

social identity manipulation not only affected perceived evaluations of others but also translated into self-stereotyping effects: Changes in self-evaluations paralleled changes in evaluations of the self by others. In other words, individuals were more likely to endorse the stereotype associated with their group when their membership in that particular group was subtly implied. It is quite unlikely that participants were aware of the impact of the manipulation on their self-evaluations, and the results may be taken as evidence of implicit self-stereotyping. Internalized expectations about one's social group can shape self-evaluations, though perhaps only or especially when they are unobtrusively activated.

Research on implicit self-esteem also indicates that contextual variations can produce an effect on unconscious or automatic preferences. For example, Bylsma, Tomaka, Luhtanen, Crocker, and Major (1992) demonstrated that self-descriptive judgments were faster for positive adjectives after positive than after negative feedback. Using the name-letter test described earlier, a recent study shows that such an effect did not occur after participants had received failure feedback on an alleged IQ test but that it reemerged once participants were given the opportunity to affirm a personally important value (Koole, Smeets, van Knippenberg, & Dijksterhuis, 1999). Thus it appears that a failure on an alleged intelligence test increases the accessibility of failure-related cognitions and reduces, at least temporarily, participants' implicit self-esteem. Affirming an important aspect of one's self-concept permits counteracting the negative consequences of the feedback. Such work illustrates the dynamic nature of self-related processes (Markus & Wurf, 1987). It is a fact of modern life that people belong to a range of social groups, both chosen and given. As societies become more heterogeneous, the opportunity for comparing and contrasting oneself to others will only increase. Across time and situations, varying identities may come forward or recede from consciousness. Effects that appear to be unsystematic and unpredictable may be quite lawful when unconscious social influences on self-evaluations are considered. Routine use of measures of implicit social cognition will need to be considered in a wide range of research topics, rather than relegating them to a subset of research on particular topics, as appears to be the case at present.

Performance and Behavior

If thoughts and feelings are transformed by the activation of social group membership, it is expected that behavior should be influenced as well. Yet, because cognition and affect are much better understood systems than behavior, studies of the latter have been less frequently reported. Perhaps for this reason, and because behavior is the gold standard in this science, studies that show the influence of social group on self-relevant behavior are attention getting. This is certainly true of work on *stereotype threat*, or situations in which the presence of a negative stereotype about one's group can handicap the test performance of members of the group (Steele, 1997; Steele & Aronson, 1995). According to the proponents of this theoretical framework, when African American students perform a scholastic or intellectual task, they face the threat of confirming a negative stereotype about their group's intellectual ability. This threat, it is speculated, interferes with intellectual functioning and can lead to detrimental impact on performance. Support for this argument has now been obtained in many experiments showing the influence of subtle activation of race/ethnicity, gender, class, and age distinctions on performance on standardized tests. For example, Steele and Aronson (1995) found that stereotype threat can affect the performance of African American college students, who performed significantly worse than white Americans on a standardized test when the test was presented as diagnostic of their intellectual abilities. This effect did not occur when the test was presented as nondiagnostic of their ability. Other studies have demonstrated that women underperform on tests of mathematical ability when the stereotype associated with their group was made salient (Spencer, Steele, & Quinn, 1999). Shih and colleagues (1999) showed that activating gender identity or ethnic identity among Asian women shifted performances to be respectively inferior or superior on a math test. Students of low socioeconomic status

(SES) performed worse than students of high SES only when a test was presented as diagnostic of their intellectual abilities (Croizet & Claire, 1998). The manipulations producing these effects are often rather subtle. In some cases, it is sufficient to ask participants to indicate their group membership just prior to assessing their performance (Steele & Aronson, 1995). Using age as the social category, Levy (1996) showed that subliminally activated negative stereotypes about the elderly produced decrements in the memory performance of elderly participants. In contrast, the activation of positive stereotypes of the elderly improved their memory performance. Interestingly, the same manipulations did not affect the performance of young individuals, who should not be susceptible to the threat posed by the negative stereotype about elderly individuals.

There is now considerable evidence that the activation of trait constructs or stereotypes can automatically or unconsciously influence social behavior. When trait constructs or stereotypes are primed in the course of an unrelated task, individuals subsequently are more likely to act in line with the content of the primed trait construct or stereotype (Bargh, Chen, & Burrows, 1996). For instance, if participants were exposed to words related to rudeness, they were more likely to interrupt an ongoing conversation. If, instead, they were primed with words related to politeness, chances were higher that they would respond in a polite fashion, waiting for the conversation to end without interruption. Priming the stereotype of the elderly caused participants to walk more slowly down the hallway after leaving the experiment. Not only did the subliminal presentation of African American faces lead participants to behave with greater hostility, it also increased the hostility of the person they were interacting with (Chen & Bargh, 1997). Thus the effect is not restricted to commonly accepted social groups, such as gender, class, or race/ethnicity, but works through the meaningful activation of information (as in the polite–rude study). Yet social groups tend to be among the dimensions of social life that provide clear and consensual stereotypes and may be particularly effective at producing a connection to oneself.

For instance, studies showed that priming a stereotype of professors or the trait "intelligent" enhanced performance on a general knowledge task (similar to Trivial Pursuit) and that priming the stereotype of soccer hooligans or the trait "stupid" decreased performance on the test (Dijksterhuis & van Knippenberg, 1998). More important, recent findings suggest that these effects are mediated by passive perceptual activity and are direct consequences of environmental events (priming manipulations). Indeed, manipulations or factors known to produce changes in perception also affected behaviors. For example, priming stereotypes of social categories produced assimilation effects like the ones we just described, whereas activating specific exemplars of the same categories led to contrast effects (Dijksterhuis et al., 1998). More precisely, if participants were primed with the category "professors" (rather than "supermodels"), their own intellectual performance was enhanced (assimilation effect), but if they were primed with the exemplar "Albert Einstein" (rather than "Claudia Schiffer"), a decrement in their performance resulted (contrast effect). The strength of stereotypic associations also mediates the impact of experience on behavior (Dijksterhuis, Aarts, Bargh, & van Knippenberg, 2000). Those who report having high contact with the elderly showed a stronger association between the category "elderly" and the attribute "forgetful" than people who had less contact with the elderly. We speculate that such an effect of greater stereotyping that relies on direct experience can exist in the presence of a positive attitude toward the group. Those with a positive attitude toward the elderly but with experience that strengthens a stereotype (perceiving them to be forgetful) may have no recourse but to show the negative stereotype even in the face of a consciously positive attitude.

Other studies have demonstrated that individuals can fail to detect changes in their actions when those actions were induced implicitly. For example, people can be unaware that their behaviors shift in accordance with the behaviors of others. Chartrand and Bargh (1999) coined the term "chameleon effect" to describe the tendency to mimic unconsciously the postures, mannerisms, or facial expressions of one's interaction partners. They showed that the mere perception of another's behavior automatically increased the likelihood of engaging in that behavior oneself. Individuals were more likely to rub their faces or shake their feet if they interacted with someone who was performing that behavior. Such an effect is assumed to serve an adaptive function by facilitating smooth social interaction through increases in liking between individuals involved in the interactions.

Vorauer and Miller (1997) also observed that people engaged in behavior matching and that they were unaware of doing so. Individuals who read another's positive self-description conveyed more positive impressions of their own satisfaction with academic achievements and university experiences compared with those who first read another's negative self-description. Participants' own sense of the impression they had conveyed was not affected by this manipulation. Thus people failed to detect the extent to which they were induced to present a particular impression of their feelings and experiences. The extensive information that individuals possess about their general personal qualities, as well as about their feelings in the moment, may make it difficult to perceive social influence on their actions. In each of these cases, the irony is that, of all the special domains of knowledge, self-knowledge is assumed to be well known and well defended against intrusion. Such discoveries both highlight the pervasiveness of social influences on the self and point to the inadequacy of introspection as the only tool for obtaining self-knowledge. Indirect measures reveal the subtle but important ways in which the social construction of self unfolds and the lack of conscious access to the process.

Self-Motives and Goal Pursuits

In recent years, research on self and identity has put a greater emphasis on the motivational mechanisms that propel social behavior. In particular, the role of *self-enhancement* has been the focus (Baumeister, 1998; Kunda, 1990; Sedikides, 1993; Swann, 1990), with investigations of a desire for positive feedback about the self and self-protective reactions unleashed by threatening experiences. Several lines of research suggest that unconscious or automatic processes are triggered when the self or the ingroup is threatened. Spencer, Fein, Wolfe, Fong, and Dunn (1998) showed that threat to self-image can automatically activate stereotypes of social groups even under conditions that otherwise do not produce such activation (i.e., under cognitive load; see Gilbert & Hixon, 1991). Following negative feedback, participants were more likely to view others in stereotypic ways, and this reaction has been taken to suggest a dynamic process of restoring a positive self-image (Fein & Spencer, 1997). Recently, L. Sinclair and Kunda (1999) demonstrated that a self-enhancement motive not only prompted stereotype activation but also led to an inhibition of applicable stereotypes. Participants motivated to disparage a black doctor (because of his criticism of them) inhibited the stereotype of doctors and used a race stereotype, whereas participants motivated to esteem the same target (because of his praise of them) inhibited the race stereotype and relied on the doctor stereotype. In these examples, the threat was directed toward the self, but similar reactions might also be at stake when the ingroup is threatened. Maass, Ceccarelli, and Rudin (1996) showed that the linguistic intergroup bias (the propensity to describe in more abstract ways behaviors depicting the ingroup favorably) was intensified when an outgroup was seen to threaten the ingroup, supporting the idea that this bias is a result of a motivation to protect the ingroup. Pratto and Shih (2000) investigated the links between implicit intergroup biases and the personality variable captured by social dominance orientation (SDO), the degree to which people endorse ideologies that justify hierarchical relationships among groups in society (Pratto, Sidanius, Stallworth, & Malle, 1994). Using a priming technique, they found that individuals high in SDO exhibited stronger implicit intergroup biases than people who generally support group equality, but this difference occurred only following a threat to participants' social identity.

Individuals do not merely seek to preserve or establish a positive self-image; they also feel the need to be similar to others (need for *assimilation*) and to maintain their uniqueness (need for *differentiation*). According to the optimal distinctiveness model (Brewer, 1991), identity stems from a tension between these two needs. Individual security and well-being are threatened when one of these needs is not met: Excessive depersonalization no longer offers a basis for self-definition, and excessive individualization renders one vulnerable to isolation and stigmatization. These motives affect people's identification even at the implicit level. Using a measure of speed of response adapted by Smith and Henry (1996), Brewer and Pickett (1999) found that the need for assimilation increased students' implicit identification with their university, whereas the need for differentiation decreased their group identification.

Work based on Bargh's (1990) automotive model is centrally relevant to this discussion, beginning with the idea that pursuit of goals can occur automatically and nonconsciously. Goals activated outside of awareness, control, or intention are pursued similarly to goals chosen through deliberate or conscious means. For example, Chartrand and Bargh (1996) demonstrated that information processing goals, such as impression formation or memorization, can be automatically activated and pursued. Gardner, Bargh, Shellman, and Bessenhoff (2000) observed that the same brain region reacts whether an evaluation goal is consciously or unconsciously activated. Individuals primed nonconsciously with an achievement goal performed better on an achievement task and were more likely to persist at the task than individuals who were not primed with such a goal (Bargh, Gollwitzer, Lee-Chai, Barndollar, & Trötschel, 2001). In addition, Chartrand (2000) found that success or failure at a nonconsciously activated goal led to the same consequences that resulted from success or failure at conscious goal pursuit. Specifically, succeeding at a nonconscious goal improved people's mood, and failure depressed it, paralleling shifts in mood usually occurring in the presence of consciously activated goals.

This research highlights the similarities between conscious and nonconscious self-motives or goals. Other researchers have examined the extent to which implicit and explicit motives differ. McClelland, Koestner, and Weinberger (1989) investigated the differences between self-reported motives (explicit) and motives identified in associative thoughts (implicit). Among other things, they make the case that implicit motives predict spontaneous behavioral trends over time, whereas self-attributed motives predict immediate responses to specific situations. They also report evidence suggesting that implicit motives represent a more primitive motivational system derived from affective experiences, whereas self-attributed motives are based largely on more cognitively elaborated constructs. This finding is consistent with research by Woike (1995) on the relationship between implicit or explicit motives and most-memorable experiences. Implicit motives were associated with affective experiences about the implicit motive, whereas explicit motives were related to routine experiences corresponding to self-descriptions.

Levesque and Pelletier (2000) argued that automatic processes could regulate *intrinsic* and *extrinsic* motivations and that these processes were functionally distinct from their explicit counterparts. *Intrinsic* motivation involves doing activities for the pleasure and satisfaction inherent in doing them, whereas *extrinsic* motivation refers to behaviors that are performed for instrumental reasons, that is, in order to attain a goal or an outcome. They found that cognitive structures relevant to intrinsic and extrinsic motivations could temporarily be made accessible through priming of associated constructs and that they influenced self-reported motivation. In addition, explicit and implicit motivations predicted different outcomes: Self-reported intrinsic motivation predicted immediate intentions about long-term behavior, whereas chronically accessible intrinsic motivation predicted the actual long-term behavior.

Research on self and identity has documented the pervasiveness of self-presentational concerns (Baumeister, 1982; Leary, 1995), and a common claim is that techniques assessing implicit attitudes or beliefs are usually free of self-presentational concerns. However, such an argument assumes that when people try to make a good impression, they are fully aware of doing so. Research on implicit self-motives and goals raises the possibility that such motives or goals may operate unconsciously and that self-presentation itself is a complex process that could include components that are strategic but inaccessible to conscious awareness and control.

Societal and Cultural Foundations

We now turn our attention to the influence of societal and cultural realities on implicit identities. We have indicated already that stereotypes about social groups have a profound impact on the implicit self. Automatic associations involving the self often reflect an internalization of cultural stereotypes. Other lines of research bring to the fore the societal roots of implicit processes. We begin with the premise that more often than not, relations between groups are hierarchically organized (Sidanius & Pratto, 1999). In other words, social groups rarely occupy interchangeable positions, and groups that enjoy greater social favors usually remain in that position for extended periods, whatever may be the criteria that characterize the hierarchy (e.g., numerical status, social status, or power; Sachdev & Bourhis, 1991). What is the impact of these factors on social identities? To what extent do members of dominant and subordinate groups exhibit a preference for their own group? On this issue, contrasting predictions can be formulated. On one hand, one would expect that members of subordinate groups engage in more ingroup bias than members of dominant groups. This would be consistent with the idea that the former have a stronger need to achieve a positive social identity, which should be satisfied by increasing favorable intergroup distinctions. On the other hand, we might hypothesize that members of subordinate groups are less likely than members of dominant groups to display a preference for their group because social conditions consistently impose a less favorable evaluation of the subordinate group. At least in the case of natural groups, the evidence at hand seemed to support the first alternative. A meta-analysis conducted by Mullen and colleagues (1992) indicated that members of low-status groups had a tendency to exhibit a stronger ingroup bias than members of high-status groups. In the case of ethnic comparisons in the United

States, African Americans often display more ethnocentric intergroup perceptions than white Americans (Judd, Park, Ryan, Brauer, & Kraus, 1995).

However, a different pattern of findings has emerged with some regularity when implicit social identity has been examined. Data from a demonstration Web site, *www.yale.edu/implicit*, provide some insights on this issue (Nosek et al., 2002) that support those from more traditional laboratories (Greenwald et al., 2002). Web data show that on a measure of conscious feeling, white respondents report a preference for the group "white" over the group "black," and black respondents report an opposite and even stronger preference for their own group. This strong explicit liking reported by black respondents stands in sharp contrast to performances on the implicit measure. Unlike white respondents, who continue to show a strong preference for white over black on the implicit measure of liking, black respondents show no such preference. This pattern of results mimics laboratory data obtained with college students (Banaji, Greenwald, & Rosier 1997): Black students exhibited strong explicit liking and identification with their own ethnic group (compared with white students), whereas a reversed pattern was observed on implicit measures (with white students showing stronger implicit ingroup preference). In addition, Jost, Pelham, and Carvallo (2001) found that students from high- and low-status universities both implicitly associated academic characteristics with the higher status group and extracurricular activities with the lower status group. Moreover, students from the high-status university exhibited significant ingroup favoritism on an implicit measure, whereas students from the low-status university did not.

These findings illustrate that the expected ingroup preference effect is moderated by sociocultural evaluations of social groups. On explicit measures, disadvantaged group members exert effort to report positive attitudes, but the lower social standing of their group is internalized sufficiently so as to be detected in their failure to show an implicit preference for their own group. On the other hand, advantaged group members' preferences show the combined benefit of both ingroup liking and the sociocultural advantage assigned to their group. Such results are consistent with the notion of *system justification* (Jost & Banaji, 1994), or the idea that beyond ego justification and group justification lies the more insidious tendency to justify the system or status quo, even when it reflects poorly on one's self or group. Members of dominant groups share thoughts, feelings, and behaviors that reinforce and legitimize existing social systems, which is in their interest, but, surprisingly, so do members of less dominant groups. Examples reviewed in this section indicate that ideological bolstering can occur outside conscious awareness, and this prevents perceivers and even targets of prejudice from questioning the legitimacy of social arrangements.

It would be erroneous to claim that members of subordinate groups cannot display strong implicit preference for their group. It depends on the comparison group. Devos and Banaji (2001) found that Asian American and African American students showed only a slight implicit preference for their ethnic group when it was compared with white Americans. However, when their group was compared with another minority group, ingroup favoritism was more pronounced: Asians displayed strong preference for Asian Americans relative to African Americans, whereas African Americans showed the opposite effect. This finding is consistent with the idea that members of minorities seek to maintain a positive social identity through downward social comparisons (Tajfel & Turner, 1986; Wills, 1981). In addition, we should stress that members of ethnic minorities often display strong implicit preferences for the self relative to others (Banaji et al., 1997; Nosek, Banaji, & Greenwald, 2002a), suggesting that members of disadvantaged groups (who show low group esteem) do not show lower self-esteem; they are able to avail themselves of opportunities to protect self-esteem (Crocker & Major, 1989). Thus, to the degree that members of subordinate groups are influenced by cultural evaluations of their group, they may develop a negative social identity, but it may not necessarily translate into a negative view of self (Pelham & Hetts, 1999).

Very little research has analyzed the relationship between self and identities that may be in conflict. We have chosen to study these by viewing connections between national and ethnic identity (Devos & Banaji, 2001). The United States is a perfect testing ground, being, as it is, a pluralist society composed of identifiable ethnic groups that vary in length of association, immersion into mainstream culture, and conditions of immigration. We investigated the extent to which ethnic groups are implicitly conceived as being part of America in a culture, that explicitly holds that all groups be treated equally. We assumed that the hierarchy present in American society would structure implicit beliefs about the links between ethnicity and American identity. More precisely, we hypothesized that white Americans are unconsciously viewed as being more essentially American and as exemplifying the nation, whereas ethnic minorities are placed psychologically at the margins (Sidanius, Feshbach, Levin, & Pratto, 1997; Sidanius & Petrocik, 2001).

Using techniques developed to assess implicit attitudes or beliefs (Greenwald et al., 1998; Nosek & Banaji, 2001), we examined the extent to which various ethnic groups (white, Asian, and African Americans) were associated with the category "American" (relative to "foreign"). For example, we asked participants to pair, as quickly as possible, American or foreign symbols (e.g., flags, maps, coins, monuments) with faces that varied in ethnicity (white, Asian, and African Americans) but were clearly understood to be American.[2] Although participants were aware that all individuals were American, irrespective of ethnicity, consistently the data indicated that African and Asian Americans were less strongly associated with the category "American" than were white Americans. Participants categorized items faster when American symbols were paired with white American faces than with Asian or African American faces. These findings did not merely reflect the fact that members of ethnic minorities were viewed as more foreign; using the appropriate technique (Nosek & Banaji, 2001), we showed that they are excluded from the category "American." Such implicit associations are sometimes consistent with people's explicit beliefs. For example, Asian Americans are viewed as less American than white Americans at both explicit and implicit levels of responding. Indeed, people stated explicitly that they did not consider Asian and white Americans to be equally American even when both held citizenship; they also considered Asian Americans to have weaker ties to American culture than whites.

In other cases, we found strong discrepancies between explicit and implicit beliefs (Devos & Banaji, 2001). For instance, at the explicit level, African and white Americans were not differentiated. In particular, both groups were perceived to be strongly and equally tied to American culture. However, in sharp contrast to the parity expressed at the explicit level, African Americans were viewed unconsciously as less American than were white Americans. These implicit associations were revealed even when explicit beliefs or knowledge showed the contrary. For example, on explicit measures, in a domain such as track and field sports, in which black Americans dominate, we found that black athletes were more strongly associated with the category "American" than were white athletes. Participants explicitly endorsed the statement that black athletes represent to a greater extent than white athletes "what America is all about" or that they contribute to a greater extent "to the glory of the American nation." However, at the implicit level, black athletes were less strongly associated with the category "American" than were white athletes. In an attempt to find a condition that would surely remove this bias, we tested the association between ethnic and national category by blatantly selecting exemplars who are known Asian Americans and known white foreigners. We still could not shake off the strong implicit association between white and American: Participants were able to associate "American" with known white foreigners (e.g., Gérard Depardieu, Katarina Witt, Hugh Grant) more swiftly than with known Asian Americans (e.g., Connie Chung, Kristi Yamaguchi, Michael Chang). In other words, even though people were fully aware that someone like Gérard Depardieu is not American and that Connie Chung is American, it remained easier to make the white + American connection. We conclude from these studies that the national identity of being American is associated with the ethnic identity of being white—and sufficiently intimately so as to be irremovable even when it is consciously rejected.

In the previous studies, participants were all white Americans. In separate data collections (Devos & Banaji, 2001) we examined the role of group membership and found that Asian American participants displayed very similar implicit associations. Among other things, they viewed their own group as being less American than the group "white," showing an internalization that is detrimental to their personal and group interests. Indeed, such implicit association potentially hurts their national identity. African Americans, on the other hand, did not display the same pattern of associations. Although viewed by white participants to be less American, they themselves perceived their own group to be as American as the group "white" and more American than the group "Asian American." Implicit associations are rooted in experiences, they bear the mark of cultural socialization, and they reflect differences between ethnic groups at these levels. African Americans, perhaps because of the presence of other minorities who may be seen as less American, do not internalize the belief that resides in the minds of the advantaged majority, whereas Asian Americans do.

In sum, despite declarations of equality before the law, under a variety of circumstances, white Americans are unconsciously conceived of as being more American than Asian Americans or African Americans. Such implicit beliefs both reflect the hierarchy between ethnic groups within American society and contribute to the preservation of existing social arrangements (Jost & Banaji, 1994).

Research on culture and self-concept shows that members of different cultures often define and evaluate the self in different ways. A major distinction in cross-cultural psychology is the opposition between *collectivist* and *individualist* societies (Triandis, Bontempo, Villareal, Asai, & Lucca, 1988; Triandis, McCusker, & Hui, 1990). In *collectivist* cultures, people define themselves as members of groups, subordinate their personal goals to group goals, and show strong emotional attachment to the group. In *individualist* cultures, people place a strong emphasis on self-reliance, individual achievement, and personal goals. In their work on the self-concept, Markus and Kitayama (1991, 1994) argued that the self is

defined in terms of interdependence in Asian cultures. In other words, the self is inherently collective in these cultures. In contrast, the typically Western conception of self is one in which individuals see themselves as distinct and independent from others. Hetts, Sakuma, and Pelham (1999; see also Pelham & Hetts, 1999) used this distinction to compare the implicit and explicit self-concepts of people who varied in their exposure to individualistic cultures but who were currently living in the *same* culture. More precisely, they examined to what extent explicit and implicit self-evaluations of recent Asian immigrants differed from those of European Americans and Asian Americans reared in the United States. At the explicit level, they found little difference between these groups. In particular, Easterners emigrating to a Western culture seemed to endorse the kind of self-concept promoted in individualistic societies. However, a different picture emerged at the implicit level. Using response latency and word-completion techniques, Hetts and colleagues found strong differences between groups in terms of personal versus group regard. For people reared in an individualistic culture, ideas that were automatically associated with the individual and collective identities were relatively positive. For people socialized in a collectivist culture, the group or collective identity automatically elicited positive thoughts, but ideas tied to individual identity were neutral, ambivalent, or even negative. Such discoveries are consistent with the idea that the need for positive regard is expressed through social or collective identities in some cultures and in individualistic ways in others.

In sum, the cultural context can overshadow differences in cultural experiences when measured through explicit self-evaluations, but implicit self-evaluations continue to reveal the mark of cultural socialization. These results could be taken as evidence that implicit self-evaluations are less influenced by normative demands than their explicit counterparts. More fundamentally, they also suggest that implicit self-evaluations are slower to change. Because they are overlearned associations rooted in experiences, it may take substantial or highly salient contradictory experiences to shift them. Consistent with this argument, Hetts and colleagues (1999) report that implicit self-evaluations of recent immigrants to the United States become increasingly individualistic over time.

Implicit and Explicit Self-Concept

So far, we have placed the emphasis on research demonstrating that self-related processes do occur unconsciously or automatically. On several occasions, we pointed out that findings at the implicit level were convergent with observations based on self-report measures. In other cases, we stressed the fact that investigations of unconscious or automatic processes revealed a different picture from what we knew based on assessments of explicit self-concepts or identities. In this section, we examine more carefully how implicit and explicit self-related processes might be intertwined.

This issue has been addressed mostly in the domain of self-esteem or self-evaluation. For example, Bosson, Swann, and Pennebaker (2000) examined systematically the correlations between various measures of implicit and explicit self-esteem. Although some implicit measures correlated significantly with explicit measures, the magnitude of the observed correlations was relatively small (all $rs < .27$). Using confirmatory factor analysis, Greenwald and Farnham (2000) demonstrated that implicit self-esteem and explicit self-esteem were distinct constructs (positively, but weakly, correlated). Research by Hetts and colleagues (1999) on the influence of culture on the self-concept also indicated that measures of implicit self-regard or group-regard were generally uncorrelated with explicit measures of self-concept. Spalding and Hardin (1999) found a correlation of −.05 between the Rosenberg Self-Esteem Scale (Rosenberg, 1965) and a priming technique designed to assess implicit self-esteem. In addition, they showed that implicit self-esteem predicted some behavioral consequences, whereas explicit self-esteem did not. In their study, participants took part in either a self-relevant or a self-irrelevant interview and were then rated by the interviewer on their anxiety. When the interview was self-relevant, participants low in implicit self-esteem appeared more anxious than participants

high in implicit self-esteem. Explicit self-esteem did not predict participant's apparent anxiety. Interestingly, individuals' own ratings of anxiety were linked to explicit self-esteem but not to implicit self-esteem.

Several studies support the idea that, under some circumstances, self-descriptions may switch from a controlled mode to an automatic mode. One would expect automatic self-evaluations to be much more positive than controlled self-evaluations because people have a lifetime of practice describing themselves mostly in positive terms. Paulhus and Levitt (1987) demonstrated that a shift in self-description occurred when people were emotionally aroused. Participants were asked to indicate the self-descriptiveness of a set of traits. These traits were presented on a computer screen, along with emotional or nonemotional distractors. The presence of emotional distractors induced participants to claim more of the positive and fewer of the negative traits than they did in the presence of nonemotional distractors. A similar positivity effect was found when participants' attentional capacity was reduced (Paulhus, Graf, & Van Selst, 1989).

Koole and colleagues (2001) demonstrated that encouraging participants to rely on their feelings clearly led to implicit self-esteem effects (positivity biases for name letters and birthdate numbers). In contrast, these forms of implicit self-esteem were no longer apparent when participants were encouraged to find reasons why they felt the way they did. Thus deliberative forms of processing can overrule automatic self-evaluations. In addition, Koole and colleagues found that the ability to engage in conscious self-reflection affected the degree of congruence between implicit self-esteem and self-reported evaluations of the self. For example, slow self-evaluations were less congruent with implicit self-evaluation than fast self-evaluations. Similarly, when participants' cognitive resources were deprived (high cognitive load), implicit self-evaluations predicted self-reported evaluations, but that was not the case when cognitive resources were available (low cognitive load). These findings support the idea that when the capacity or the motivation to engage in conscious self-reflection is lacking, implicit self-evaluations will be the prevailing influence on phenomenological experience. In sum, the evidence at hand suggests that implicit and explicit self-concepts are distinct constructs, although, at least under some circumstances, connection may also be detected.

Conclusions

The question of how we know ourselves and what we know about ourselves is of fundamental interest to understanding how personal knowledge is represented, the degree to which such knowledge is constructed in social context, and its implications for health and well-being. Yet the epistemological quagmire inherent in the empirical assessment of knowledge about oneself has always posed a problem, as noted at the start of this chapter. We recommended that analyses of unconscious self-processes may assist in this regard, and we focused on the social aspect of self and identity, restricting our attention to a particular aspect of the self—one that emerges in the context of social group membership. From the initial research using implicit or indirect measures of self and identity, we already have evidence about the visible role of social group membership in creating a sense of self and self-worth.

The work reviewed in this chapter raises several possible issues that need to be incorporated into an understanding of self. Processes that capture group identity can operate without introspective access or deliberative thought. Such group identity and even knowledge about social groups (that is automatically learned even if consciously denied) can have indirect influence on assessments of the self. An unspoken assumption has been that implicit attitudes, beliefs, and motives about oneself are hard to change given that they are overlearned associations about a well-known object. Several findings reported in this chapter would suggest, to the contrary, that implicit associations are not rigid and that shifts in self-definitions or self-evaluations can occur without conscious awareness or intention. Situational or contextual manipulations reveal the plasticity of self-related implicit social cognition. Finally, several lines of research reported in this chapter show the

subtle but crucial ways in which sociocultural realities shape self-related mental processes. In many instances, the impact of sociostructural influences on psychological processes become more obvious when research is focused on the nitty-gritty of mental processes that are not consciously accessible but may nevertheless be found using indirect measures. In that regard, work on implicit processes offers the promise to renew thinking about the obvious interplay between the psychological and the social, the individual and the collective.

Notes

1. For a sample of such tasks, readers may vist www.yale.edu/implicit or www.tolerance.org.
2. A sample task is available at www.tolerance.org or may be obtained by writing to the authors.

Acknowledgments

Preparation of this chapter was supported by grants from the National Institute of Mental Health (No. MH-57672) and from the National Science Foundation (No. SBR-9709924) to Mahzarin R. Banaji and by a Swiss National Science Foundation Fellowship (No. 8210-056562) to Thierry Devos.

References

Abelson, R. P., Aronson, E., McGuire, W. J., Newcomb, T. M., Rosenberg, M. J., & Tannenbaum, P. (Eds.). (1968). *Theories of cognitive consistency: A sourcebook*. Chicago: Rand-McNally.

Abrams, D., & Hogg, M. A. (1988). Comments on the motivational status of self-esteem in social identity and intergroup discrimination. *European Journal of Social Psychology, 18*, 317–334.

Aron, A., Aron, E. N., Tudor, M., & Nelson, G. (1991). Close relationships as including other in the self. *Journal of Personality and Social Psychology, 60*, 241–253.

Ashburn-Nardo, L., Voils, C. I., & Monteith, M. J. (2001). Implicit associations as the seeds of intergroup bias: How easily do they take root? *Journal of Personality and Social Psychology, 81*, 789–799.

Baldwin, M. W. (1992). Relational schemas and the processing of social information. *Psychological Bulletin, 112*, 461–484.

Baldwin, M. W. (1994). Primed relational schemas as a source of self-evaluative reactions. *Journal of Social and Clinical Psychology, 13*, 380–403.

Baldwin, M. W., Carrell, S. E., & Lopez, D. F. (1990). Priming relationship schemas: My advisor and the Pope are watching me from the back of my mind. *Journal of Experimental Social Psychology, 26*, 435–454.

Banaji, M. R., Greenwald, A. G., & Rosier, M. R. (1997, October). *Implicit esteem: When collectives shape individuals.* Paper presented at the Second Annual SESP Preconference on the Self, Toronto, Ontario, Canada.

Banaji, M. R., Lemm, K. M., & Carpenter, S. J. (2001). The social unconscious. In A. Tesser & N. Schwartz (Eds.), *Blackwell handbook of social psychology: Intraindividual processes* (pp. 138–158). Oxford, UK: Blackwell.

Banaji, M. R., & Prentice, D. A. (1994). The self in social contexts. *Annual Review of Psychology, 45*, 297–232.

Bargh, J. A. (1982). Attention and automaticity in the processing of self-relevant information. *Journal of Personality and Social Psychology, 43*, 425–436.

Bargh, J. A. (1990). Auto-motives: Preconscious determinants of social interaction. In E. T. Higgins & R. M. Sorrentino (Eds.), *Handbook of motivation and cognition* (Vol. 2, pp. 93–130). New York: Guilford Press.

Bargh, J. A., Chen, M., & Burrows, L. (1996). Automaticity of social behavior: Direct effects of trait construct and stereotype activation on action. *Journal of Personality and Social Psychology, 71*, 230–244.

Bargh, J. A., Gollwitzer, P. M., Lee-Chai, A., Barndollar, K., & Trötschel, R. (2001). The automated will: Nonconscious activation and pursuit of behavioral goals. *Journal of Personality and Social Psychology, 81*, 1014–1027.

Bargh, J. A., & Tota, M. E. (1988). Context-dependent automatic processing in depression: Accessibility of negative constructs with regard to self but not others. *Journal of Personality and Social Psychology, 54*, 925–939.

Baumeister, R. F. (1982). A self-presentational view of social phenomena. *Psychological Bulletin, 91*, 3–26.

Baumeister, R. F. (1998). The self. In D. T. Gilbert, S. T. Fiske, & G. Lindzey (Eds.), *The handbook of social psychology* (Vol. 1, pp. 680–740). Boston: McGraw-Hill.

Beggan, J. K. (1992). On the social nature of nonsocial perception: The mere ownership effect. *Journal of Personality and Social Psychology, 62*, 229–237.

Biernat, M., Vescio, T. K., & Green, M. L. (1996). Selective self-stereotyping. *Journal of Personality and Social Psychology, 71*, 1194–1209.

Bosson, J. K., Swann, W. B., Jr., & Pennebaker, J. W. (2000). Stalking the perfect measure of implicit self-esteem: The blind men and the elephant revisited. *Journal of Personality and Social Psychology, 79*, 631–643.

Brewer, M. B. (1979). Ingroup bias in the minimal intergroup situation: A cognitive-motivational analysis. *Psychological Bulletin, 86*, 307–324.

Brewer, M. B. (1991). The social self: On being the same and different at the same time. *Personality and Social Psychology Bulletin, 17*, 475–482.

Brewer, M. B., & Pickett, C. L. (1999). Distinctiveness motives as a source of the social self. In T. R. Tyler & R. M. Kramer (Eds.), *The psychology of the social self* (pp. 71–87). Mahwah, NJ: Erlbaum.

Brown, R. (2000). Social identity theory: Past achievements, current problems and future challenges. *European Journal of Social Psychology, 30*, 745–778.

Brown, R., Hinkle, S., Ely, P. G., Fox-Cardamone, L., Maras, P., & Taylor, L. A. (1992). Recognizing group diversity: Individualist–collectivist and autonomous–relational social orientations and their implications for intergroup processes. *British Journal of Social Psychology, 31*, 327–342.

Bylsma, W. H., Tomaka, J., Luhtanen, R., Crocker, J., & Major, B. (1992). Response latency as an index of temporary self-evaluation. *Personality and Social Psychology Bulletin, 18*, 60–67.

Chartrand, T. L. (2000). *Mystery moods and perplexing performance: Consequences of succeeding or failing at a nonconscious goal.* Manuscript submitted for publication.

Chartrand, T. L., & Bargh, J. A. (1996). Automatic activation of impression formation and memorization goals: Nonconscious goal priming reproduces effects of explicit task instructions. *Journal of Personality and Social Psychology, 71*, 464–478.

Chartrand, T. L., & Bargh, J. A. (1999). The chameleon effect: The perception–behavior link and social interaction. *Journal of Personality and Social Psychology, 76*, 893–910.

Chen, M., & Bargh, J. A. (1997). Nonconscious behavioral confirmation processes: The self-fulfilling consequences of automatic stereotype activation. *Journal of Experimental Social Psychology, 33*, 541–560.

Coats, S., Smith, E. R., Claypool, H. M., & Banner, M. J. (2000). Overlapping mental representations of self and ingroup: Reaction time evidence and its relationship with explicit measures of group identification. *Journal of Experimental Social Psychology, 36*, 304–315.

Cooley, C. H. (1902). *Human nature and social order.* New York: Scribner's.

Crocker, J., & Major, B. (1989). Social stigma and self-esteem: The self-protective properties of stigma. *Psychological Review, 96*, 608–630.

Croizet, J.-C., & Claire, T. (1998). Extending the concept of stereotype and threat to social class: The intellectual underperformance of students from low socioeconimic backgrounds. *Personality and Social Psychology Bulletin, 24*, 588–594.

Cunningham, W. A., Nezlek, J. B., & Banaji, M. R. (2001). *Conscious and unconscious ethnocentrism: Revisiting the ideologies of prejudice.* Manuscript submitted for publication.

Dasgupta, N., McGhee, D. E., Greenwald, A. G., & Banaji, M. R. (2000). Automatic preference for White Americans: Eliminating the familiarity explanation. *Journal of Experimental Social Psychology, 36*, 316–328.

Devos, T., & Banaji, M. R. (2001). *Who is American? Implicit and explicit beliefs about ethnicity and American identity.* Manuscript in preparation.

Diehl, M. (1990). The minimal group paradigm: Theoretical explanations and empirical findings. In W. Stroebe & M. Hewstone (Eds.), *European review of social psychology* (Vol. 1, pp. 263–292). Chichester, UK: Wiley.

Dijksterhuis, A., Aarts, H., Bargh, J. A., & van Knippenberg, A. (2000). On the relation between associative strength and automatic behavior. *Journal of Experimental Social Psychology, 36*, 531–544.

Dijksterhuis, A., Spears, R., Postmes, T., Stapel, D., Koomen, W., van Knippenberg, A., & Scheepers, D. (1998). Seeing one thing and doing another: Contrast effects in automatic behavior. *Journal of Personality and Social Psychology, 75*, 862–871.

Dijksterhuis, A., & van Knippenberg, A. (1998). The relation between perception and behavior, or how to win a game of Trivial Pursuit. *Journal of Personality and Social Psychology, 74*, 865–877.

Dovidio, J. F., Evans, N., & Tyler, R. B. (1986). Racial stereotypes: The contents of their cognitive representations. *Journal of Experimental Social Psychology, 22*, 22–37.

Farnham, S. D., Greenwald, A. G., & Banaji, M. R. (1999). Implicit self-esteem. In D. Abrams & M. A. Hogg (Eds.), *Social identity and social cognition* (pp. 230–248). Malden, MA: Blackwell.

Fazio, R. H., Jackson, J. R., Dunton, B. C., & Williams, C. J. (1995). Variability in automatic activation as an unobstrusive measure of racial attitudes: A bona fide pipeline? *Journal of Personality and Social Psychology, 69*, 1013–1027.

Fein, S., & Spencer, S. J. (1997). Prejudice as self-image maintenance: Affirming the self through derogating others. *Journal of Personality and Social Psychology, 73*, 31–44.

Feys, J. (1991). Briefly induced belongingness to self and preference. *European Journal of Social Psychology, 21*, 547–552.

Finch, J. F., & Cialdini, R. B. (1989). Another indirect tactic of (self-) image management: Boosting. *Personality and Social Psychology Bulletin, 15*, 222–232.

Franco, F. M., & Maass, A. (1996). Implicit versus explicit strategies of outgroup discrimination: The role of intentional control in biased language use and reward allocation. *Journal of Language and Social Psychology, 15*, 335–359.

Gaertner, S. L., & McLaughlin, J. P. (1983). Racial stereotypes: Associations and ascriptions of positive and negative characteristics. *Social Psychology Quarterly, 46*, 23–30.

Gardner, W., Bargh, J. A., Shellman, A., & Bessenhoff, G. (2000). *This is your brain on primes: Lateralized brain activity is the same for nonconscious and conscious evaluative processing.* Manuscript submitted for publication.

Gilbert, D. T., & Hixon, J. G. (1991). The trouble of thinking: Activation and application of stereotypic beliefs. *Journal of Personality and Social Psychology, 60*, 509–517.

Greenwald, A. G., & Banaji, M. R. (1995). Implicit social cognition: Attitudes, self-esteem, and stereotypes. *Psychological Review, 102*, 4–27.

Greenwald, A. G., Banaji, M. R., Rudman, L. A., Farnham, S. D., Nosek, B. A., & Mellot, D. S. (2002). Unified theory of implicit social cognition. *Psychological Review, 109*, 3–25.

Greenwald, A. G., Banaji, M. R., Rudman, L. A., Farnham, S. D., Nosek, B. A., & Rosier, M. (2000). Prologue to a unified theory of attitudes, stereotypes, and self-concept. In J. P. Forgas (Ed.), *Feeling and thinking: The role of affect in social cognition* (pp. 308–330). New York: Cambridge University Press.

Greenwald, A. G., & Farnham, S. D. (2000). Using the implicit association test to measure self-esteem and self-concept. *Journal of Personality and Social Psychology, 79*, 1022–1038.

Greenwald, A. G., McGhee, D. E., & Schwartz, J. L. K. (1998). Measuring individual differences in implicit

cognition: The implicit association test. *Journal of Personality and Social Psychology, 74*, 1464–1480.

Greenwald, A. G., & Pratkanis, A. R. (1984). The self. In R. S. Wyer & T. K. Srull (Eds.), *Handbook of social cognition* (pp. 129–178). Hillsdale, NJ: Erlbaum.

Hetts, J. J., Sakuma, M., & Pelham, B. W. (1999). Two roads to positive regard: Implicit and explicit self-evaluation and culture. *Journal of Experimental Social Psychology, 35*, 512–559.

Higgins, E. T., Van Hook, E., & Dorfman, D. (1988). Do self-attributes form a cognitive structure? *Social Cognition, 6*, 177–206.

Hinkle, S., & Brown, R. (1990). Intergroup comparisons and social identity: Some links and lacunae. In D. Abrams & M. A. Hogg (Eds.), *Social identity theory: Constructive and critical advances* (pp. 48–70). New York: Harvester Wheatsheaf.

Hogg, M. A., & Abrams, D. (1990). Social motivation, self-esteem and social identity. In D. Abrams & M. A. Hogg (Eds.), *Social identity theory: Constructive and critical advances* (pp. 28–47). New York: Harvester Wheatsheaf.

Hogg, M. A., & Turner, J. C. (1987). Intergroup behaviour, self-stereotyping and the salience of social categories. *British Journal of Social Psychology, 26*, 325–340.

Hoorens, V., & Nuttin, J. M. (1993). Overvaluation of own attributes: Mere ownership or subjective frequency? *Social Cognition, 11*, 177–200.

Hoorens, V., Nuttin, J. M., Herman, I. E., & Pavakanun, U. (1990). Mastery pleasure versus mere ownership: A quasi-experimental cross-cultural and cross-alphabetical test of the name letter effect. *European Journal of Social Psychology, 20*, 181–205.

Hoorens, V., & Todorova, E. (1988). The name letter effect: Attachment to self or primacy of own name writing? *European Journal of Social Psychology, 18*, 365–368.

James, W. (1890). *The principles of psychology.* New York: Holt.

Jost, J. T., & Banaji, M. R. (1994). The role of stereotyping in system-justification and the production of false consciousness. *British Journal of Social Psychology, 33*, 1–27.

Jost, J. T., Pelham, B. W., & Carvallo, M. R. (2001). *Nonconscious forms of system justification: Cognitive, affective, and behavioral preferences for higher status groups.* Manuscript submitted for publication.

Judd, C. M., Park, B., Ryan, C. S., Brauer, M., & Kraus, S. (1995). Stereotypes and ethnocentrism: Diverging interethnic perceptions of African American and white American youth. *Journal of Personality and Social Psychology, 69*, 460–481.

Karpinski, A., & von Hippel, W. (1996). The role of the linguistic intergroup bias in expectancy maintenance. *Social Cognition, 14*, 141–163.

Kihlstrom, J. F., & Cantor, N. (1984). Mental representation of the self. In L. Berkowitz (Ed.), *Advances in experimental social psychology* (Vol. 17, pp. 1–47). Orlando, FL: Academic Press.

Kihlstrom, J. F., Cantor, N., Albright, J. S., Chew, B. R., Klein, S. B., & Niedenthal, P. M. (1988). Information processing and the study of the self. In L. Berkowitz (Ed.), *Advances in experimental social psychology*

(Vol. 21, pp. 145–178). San Diego, CA: Academic Press.

Kitayama, S., & Karasawa, M. (1997). Implicit self-esteem in Japan: Name letters and birthday numbers. *Personality and Social Psychology Bulletin, 23*, 736–742.

Knowles, E. D., Peng, K., & Levy, T. H. (2001). *Ingroup overexclusion and identity protection in the categorization of sex and race.* Unpublished manuscript.

Koole, S. L., Dijksterhuis, A., & van Knippenberg, A. (2001). What's in a name: Implicit self-esteem and the automatic self. *Journal of Personality and Social Psychology, 80*, 669–685.

Koole, S. L., Smeets, K., van Knippenberg, A., & Dijksterhuis, A. (1999). The cessation of rumination through self-affirmation. *Journal of Personality and Social Psychology, 77*, 111–125.

Kunda, Z. (1990). The case for motivated reasoning. *Psychological Bulletin, 108*, 480–498.

Lane, K., Mitchell, J. P., & Banaji, M. R. (2001, February). *Formation of implicit attitudes: Direct experience not required.* Poster presented at the annual meeting of the Society for Personality and Social Psychology, San Antonio, TX.

Leary, M. R. (1995). *Self-presentation: Impression management and interpersonal behavior.* Madison, WI: Brown & Benchmark.

Lemm, K. M., & Banaji, M. R. (1998, April). *Implicit and explicit gender identity and attitudes toward gender.* Paper presented at the annual meeting of the Midwestern Psychological Association, Chicago.

Lemm, K. M., & Banaji, M. R. (2000, February). *Motivation to control moderates the relationship between implicit and explicit prejudice.* Poster presented at the annual meeting of the Society for Personality and Social Psychology, Nashville, TN.

Levesque, C., & Pelletier, L. G. (2000). *On the investigation of conscious and nonconscious regulatory processes underlying intrinsic and extrinsic motivation.* Manuscript submitted for publication.

Levy, B. (1996). Improving memory in old age through implicit self-stereotyping. *Journal of Personality and Social Psychology, 71*, 1092–1107.

Leyens, J.-P., Paladino, P. M., Rodriguez-Torres, R., Vaes, J., Demoulin, S., Rodriguez-Perez, A., & Gaunt, R. (2000). The emotional side of prejudice: The attribution of secondary emotions to ingroups and outgroups. *Personality and Social Psychology Review, 4*, 186–197.

Lindeman, M., & Sundvik, L. (1995). Evaluative bias and self-enhancement among gender groups. *European Journal of Social Psychology, 25*, 269–280.

Maass, A., Ceccarelli, R., & Rudin, S. (1996). Linguistic intergroup bias: Evidence for ingroup-protective motivation. *Journal of Personality and Social Psychology, 71*, 512–526.

Maass, A., Salvi, D., Arcuri, L., & Semin, G. R. (1989). Language use in intergroup contexts: The linguistic intergroup bias. *Journal of Personality and Social Psychology, 57*, 981–993.

Markus, H. (1977). Self-schemata and processing information about the self. *Journal of Personality and Social Psychology, 35*, 63–78.

Markus, H., & Wurf, E. (1987). The dynamic self-concept: A social psychological perspective. *Annual Review of Psychology, 38*, 299–337.

Markus, H. R., & Kitayama, S. (1991). Culture and the self: Implications for cognition, emotion, and motivation. *Psychological Review, 98*, 224–253.

Markus, H. R., & Kitayama, S. (1994). The cultural construction of self and emotion: Implications for social behavior. In S. Kitayama & H. R. Markus (Eds.), *Emotion and culture: Empirical studies of mutual influence* (pp. 89–130). Washington, DC: American Psychological Association.

McClelland, D. C., Koestner, R., & Weinberger, J. (1989). How do self-attributed and implicit motives differ? *Psychological Review, 96*, 690–702.

McGuire, W. J., & McGuire, C. V. (1988). Content and process in the experience of self. In L. Berkowitz (Ed.), *Advances in experimental social psychology* (Vol. 21, pp. 97–144). San Diego: Academic Press.

Mead, G. H. (1934). *Mind, self and society.* Chicago: University of Chicago Press.

Mitchell, J. P., Nosek, B. A., & Banaji, M. R. (2000). *Contextual variations in implicit evaluation.* Manuscript submitted for publication.

Mullen, B., Brown, R., & Smith, C. (1992). Ingroup bias as a function of salience, relevance, and status: An integration. *European Journal of Social Psychology, 22*, 103–122.

Neumann, R., Ebert, M., Gabel, B., Guelsdorff, J., Krannich, H., Lauterbach, C., & Wiedl, K. (1998). Vorurteile zwischen Bayern und Norddeutschen: Die Anwendung einer neuen Methode zur Erfassung evaluativer Assoziationen in Vorurteilen [Prejudice between Bavarians and North Germans: Applying a new method for assessing evaluative association within prejudice]. *Zeitschrift Für Experimentelle Psychologie, 45*, 99–108.

Nosek, B., & Banaji, M. R. (2001). Measuring implicit social cognition: The go/no-go association task. *Social Cognition, 19*, 625–666.

Nosek, B., Banaji, M. R., & Greenwald, A. G. (2002a). Harvesting implicit group attitudes and beliefs from a demonstration website. *Group Dynamics, 6*, 101–115.

Nosek, B. A., Banaji, M. R., & Greenwald, A. G. (2002b). Math = male, me = female, therefore math ≠ me. *Journal of Personality and Social Psychology, 83*, 44–59.

Nuttin, J. M. (1985). Narcissism beyond Gestalt and awareness: The name letter effect. *European Journal of Social Psychology, 15*, 353–361.

Nuttin, J. M. (1987). Affective consequences of mere ownership: The name letter effect in twelve European languages. *European Journal of Social Psychology, 17*, 381–402.

Otten, S., & Moskowitz, G. B. (2000). Evidence for implicit evaluative ingroup bias: Affect-biased spontaneous trait inference in a minimal group paradigm. *Journal of Experimental Social Psychology, 36*, 77–89.

Otten, S., & Wentura, D. (1999). About the impact of automaticity in the Minimal Group Paradigm: Evidence from affective priming tasks. *European Journal of Social Psychology, 29*, 1049–1071.

Paulhus, D. L., Graf, P., & Van Selst, M. (1989). Attentional load increases the positivity of self-presentation. *Social Cognition, 7*, 389–400.

Paulhus, D. L., & Levitt, K. (1987). Desirable responding

triggered by affect: Automatic egotism? *Journal of Personality and Social Psychology, 52*, 245–259.

Peabody, D. (1968). Group judgments in the Philippines: Evaluative and descriptive aspects. *Journal of Personality and Social Psychology, 10*, 290–300.

Pelham, B. W., & Hetts, J. J. (1999). Implicit and explicit personal and social identity: Toward a more complete understanding of the social self. In T. R. Tyler & R. M. Kramer (Eds.), *The psychology of the social self* (pp. 115–143). Mahwah, NJ: Erlbaum.

Pelham, B. W., Mirenberg, M. C., & Jones, J. K. (2002). Why Susie sells seashells by the seashore: Implicit egotism and major life decisions. *Journal of Personality and Social Psychology, 82,* 469–487.

Perdue, C. W., Dovidio, J. F., Gurtman, M. B., & Tyler, R. B. (1990). Us and them: Social categorization and the process of intergroup bias. *Journal of Personality and Social Psychology, 59*, 475–486.

Perdue, C. W., & Gurtman, M. B. (1990). Evidence for the automaticity of ageism. *Journal of Experimental Social Psychology, 26*, 199–216.

Pratto, F., & Shih, M. (2000). Social dominance orientation and group context in implicit group prejudice. *Psychological Science, 11*, 515–518.

Pratto, F., Sidanius, J., Stallworth, L. M., & Malle, B. F. (1994). Social dominance orientation: A personality variable predicting social and political attitudes. *Journal of Personality and Social Psychology, 67*, 741–763.

Prentice, D., & Miller, D. T. (1992). *The psychology of ingroup attachment.* Paper presented at the Conference on the Self and the Collective, Princeton, NJ.

Rogers, T. B., Kuiper, N. A., & Kirker, W. S. (1977). Self-reference and the encoding of personal information. *Journal of Personality and Social Psychology, 35*, 677–688.

Rosenberg, M. (1965). *Society and the adolescent self-image.* Princeton, NJ: Princeton University Press.

Rubin, M., & Hewstone, M. (1998). Social identity theory's self-esteem hypothesis: A review and some suggestions for clarification. *Personality and Social Psychology Review, 2*, 40–62.

Rudman, L. A., Greenwald, A. G., & McGhee, D. E. (2001). Implicit self-concept and evaluative implicit gender stereotypes: Self and ingroup share desirable traits. *Personality and Social Psychology Bulletin, 27*, 1164–1178.

Rudman, L. A., Greenwald, A. G., Mellott, D. S., & Schwartz, J. L. K. (1999). Measuring the automatic components of prejudice: Flexibility and generality of the Implicit Association Test. *Social Cognition, 17*, 437–465.

Sachdev, I., & Bourhis, R. Y. (1991). Power and status differentials in minority and majority group relations. *European Journal of Social Psychology, 21*, 1–24.

Sedikides, C. (1993). Assessment, enhancement, and verification determinants of the self-evaluation process. *Journal of Personality and Social Psychology, 65*, 317–338.

Shih, M., Pittinsky, T. L., & Ambady, N. (1999). Stereotype susceptibility: Identity salience and shifts in quantitative performance. *Psychological Science, 10*, 80–83.

Sidanius, J., Feshbach, S., Levin, S., & Pratto, F. (1997). The interface between ethnic and national attachment: Ethnic pluralism or ethnic dominance? *Public Opinion Quarterly, 61*, 102–133.

Sidanius, J., & Petrocik, J. R. (2001). Communal and national identity in a multiethnic state: A comparison of three perspectives. In R. D. Ashmore, L. Jussim, & D. Wilder (Eds.), *Social identity, intergroup conflict, and conflict resolution.* New York: Oxford University Press.

Sidanius, J., & Pratto, F. (1999). *Social dominance: An intergroup theory of social hierarchy and oppression.* New York: Cambridge University Press.

Simon, B., & Hamilton, D. L. (1994). Self-stereotyping and social context: The effects of relative ingroup size and ingroup status. *Journal of Personality and Social Psychology, 66*, 699–711.

Simon, B., Pantaleo, G., & Mummendey, A. (1995). Unique individual or interchangeable group member? The accentuation of intragroup differences versus similarities as an indicator of the individual self versus the collective self. *Journal of Personality and Social Psychology, 69*, 106–119.

Sinclair, L., & Kunda, Z. (1999). Reactions to a Black professional: Motivated inhibition and activation of conflicting stereotypes. *Journal of Personality and Social Psychology, 77*, 885–904.

Sinclair, S., Hardin, C. D., & Lowery, B. (2001). *Self-stereotyping in the context of multiple social identities.* Manuscript submitted for publication.

Smith, E. R., Coats, S., & Walling, D. (1999). Overlapping mental representations of self, ingroup, and partner: Further response time evidence and a connectionist model. *Personality and Social Psychology Bulletin, 25*, 873–882.

Smith, E. R., & Henry, S. (1996). An ingroup becomes part of the self: Response time evidence. *Personality and Social Psychology Bulletin, 22*, 635–642.

Spalding, L. R., & Hardin, C. D. (1999). Unconscious unease and self-handicapping: Behavioral consequences of individual differences in implicit and explicit self-esteem. *Psychological Science, 10*, 535–539.

Spencer, S. J., Fein, S., Wolfe, C. T., Fong, C., & Dunn, M. A. (1998). Automatic activation of stereotypes: The role of self-image threat. *Personality and Social Psychology Bulletin, 24*, 1139–1152.

Spencer, S. J., Steele, C. M., & Quinn, D. M. (1999). Stereotype threat and women's math performance. *Journal of Experimental Social Psychology, 35*, 4–28.

Steele, C. M. (1997). A threat in the air: How stereotypes shape intellectual identity and performance. *American Psychologist, 52*, 613–629.

Steele, C. M., & Aronson, J. (1995). Stereotype threat and the intellectual test performance of African Americans. *Journal of Personality and Social Psychology, 69*, 797–811.

Strauman, T. J., & Higgins, E. T. (1987). Automatic activation of self-discrepancies and emotional syndromes: When cognitive structures influence affect. *Journal of Personality and Social Psychology, 53*, 1004–1014.

Swann, W. B., Jr. (1990). To be adored or to be known?: The interplay of self-enhancement and self-verification. In E. T. Higgins & R. M. Sorrentino (Eds.), *Handbook of motivation and cognition* (Vol. 2, pp. 408–448). New York: Guilford Press.

Tajfel, H. (1974). Social identity and intergroup behaviour. *Social Science Information, 13*, 65–93.

Tajfel, H., Billig, M. G., Bundy, R. P., & Flament, C. (1971). Social categorization and intergroup behaviour. *European Journal of Social Psychology, 1*, 149–178.

Tajfel, H., & Turner, J. C. (1986). The social identity theory of intergroup behavior. In S. Worchel & W. G. Austin (Eds.), *Psychology of intergroup relations* (pp. 7–24). Chicago: Nelson-Hall.

Triandis, H. C., Bontempo, R., Villareal, M. J., Asai, M., & Lucca, N. (1988). Individualism and collectivism: Cross-cultural perspectives on self-ingroup relationships. *Journal of Personality and Social Psychology, 54*, 323–338.

Triandis, H. C., McCusker, C., & Hui, C. H. (1990). Multimethod probes of individualism and collectivism. *Journal of Personality and Social Psychology, 59*, 1006–1020.

Turner, J. C. (1985). Social categorization and the self-concept: A social cognitive theory of group behaviour. In E. J. Lawler (Ed.), *Advances in group processes: Theory and research* (Vol. 2, pp. 77–122). Greenwich, CT: JAI Press.

Turner, J. C., Hogg, M. A., Oakes, P. J., Reicher, S. D., & Wetherell, M. (1987). *Rediscovering the social group: A self-categorization theory*. Oxford, UK: Blackwell.

Turner, J. C., Oakes, P. J., Haslam, S. A., & McGarty, C. (1994). Self and collective: Cognition and social context. *Personality and Social Psychology Bulletin, 20*(5), 454–463.

Uleman, J. S., Hon, A., Roman, R. J., & Moskowitz, G. B. (1996). On-line evidence for spontaneous trait inferences at encoding. *Personality and Social Psychology Bulletin, 22*, 377–394.

von Hippel, W., Hawkins, C., & Schooler, J. W. (2001). Stereotype distinctiveness: How counter-stereotypic behavior shapes the self-concept. *Journal of Personality and Social Psychology, 81*, 193–205.

von Hippel, W., Sekaquaptewa, D., & Vargas, P. (1997). The linguistic intergroup bias as an implicit indicator of prejudice. *Journal of Experimental Social Psychology, 33*, 490–509.

Vorauer, J. D., & Miller, D. T. (1997). Failure to recognize the effect of implicit social influence on the presentation of self. *Journal of Personality and Social Psychology, 73*, 281–295.

Walsh, W. A., & Banaji, M. (1997). The collective self. In J. G. Snodgrass & R. L. Thompson (Eds.), *The self across psychology: Self-recognition, self-awareness, and the self concept* (pp. 193–214). New York: New York Academy of Sciences.

Wegner, D. M., & Bargh, J. A. (1998). Control and automaticity in social life. In D. T. Gilbert, S. T. Fiske, & G. Lindzey (Eds.), *The handbook of social psychology* (Vol. 2, pp. 446–496). Boston: McGraw-Hill.

Wills, T. A. (1981). Downward comparison principles in social psychology. *Psychological Bulletin, 90*, 245–271.

Wittenbrink, B., Judd, C. M., & Park, B. (1997). Evidence for racial prejudice at the implicit level and its relationship with questionnaire measures. *Journal of Personality and Social Psychology, 72*, 262–274.

Woike, B. A. (1995). Most-memorable experiences: Evidence for a link between implicit and explicit motives and social cognitive processes in everyday life. *Journal of Personality and Social Psychology, 68*, 1081–1091.

PART III

AGENCY, REGULATION, AND CONTROL

9

Self-Awareness

CHARLES S. CARVER

When you think about yourself, what comes to mind? When your attention drifts to yourself while you're working on something, does it change anything about what you're doing, or how you do it? When you see yourself in the gaze of a group of others, what are your reactions? When you set out to make a particular impression on a stranger, what are the processes that underlie your self-portrayal? These are some of the questions that underlie the study of self-awareness processes.

Today's interest in the concept of self-awareness has deep roots in the literature of psychology and sociology, tracing back at least as far as the writings of William James (1890) and the sociological school of symbolic interactionism (Cooley, 1902; Mead, 1934). James pointed out that the self has what appears to be a unique capacity that he termed "reflexivity": the ability to somehow turn around and take itself as the object of its own view. Thus the self has both a "process" aspect—the self as the knower of things—and a "content" aspect—the self as that which is known. In the language of the first person singular, the self is both the "I"—the active subject engaged in human experience—and also potentially the "me"—the object of its own experience (Mead, 1934).

This property of reflexivity does not always dominate the flow of subjective experience. Rather, it enters the flow to a greater degree at some times and to a lesser degree at other times. People's awareness can gravitate to a wide range of possible stimuli. Sometimes people are especially aware of things that lie outside themselves. Sometimes, however, their attention is drawn to experiences occurring inside themselves or to themselves as entities in the social matrix. These differences in the content that is being processed or thought about appear to have several influences on what happens next. When attention is directed to the self instead of to the outside world, experience changes. Just exactly how experience changes when attention is self-directed has been the matter of some debate over the past 30 years. In this chapter I describe some of the ideas that have been proposed in that regard.

From Philosophy to Experimental Social Psychology

What happens when attention is self-focused? Responses to that question have come from several directions, with several

179

different underlying rationales. Given the diversity of the starting points, the various responses that people have suggested have some overtones that differ fairly substantially from one to another.

James

James (1890) wrote about a wide range of topics concerning the self. In so doing, he provided suggestions about at least one of the things that can happen when people become aware of themselves. Elsewhere in his writings he noted that self-esteem (feeling good or bad about the self) is dependent on both pretensions (aspirations) and successes (perceived accomplishments). For example, if a young man has no aspiration to play football well, the fact that he is not good at football has no adverse implications for his self-esteem. However, if he does have aspirations for excellence at football, the extent to which those aspirations are presently being fulfilled in his behavior is quite relevant for his self-esteem.

Self-esteem thus can be defined by the extent of discrepancy between pretensions and present behavior. It would seem to follow that such discrepancies become noticeable only to the extent that the person's attention is directed toward this aspect of the self. This principle raises the possibility that self-directed attention can create negative feelings, if the person's present behavior does not correspond to his or her pretensions or aspirations. If behavior *does* correspond to those aspirations, in contrast, the result should be pride and satisfaction.

Cooley and Mead

The symbolic interactionist view also dealt with the property of reflexivity (Cooley, 1902; Mead, 1934). This view dealt primarily with how the self comes to exist, as opposed to how self-focus influences subsequent experience, though it does have some implications for the latter as well. This view holds that there is no sense of self at birth but rather that the self develops as a function of interaction with others. As we observe that other people react to us in an evaluative way (praising and rewarding, or criticizing and punishing), we gradually become aware of the fact that there is a perspective other than our own subjective impression of the world. Gradually, we become able to take this outside perspective; more particularly, we become able to take this perspective on ourselves.

Because we interact with many different people as this viewpoint develops, Mead (1934) called it the "perspective of the generalized other." When we reflect on ourselves, from then on, we do so from that perspective, and we evaluate ourselves in the same way as those other people had done earlier. Thus we come to evaluate ourselves from the point of view of the social standards that are held by people we are exposed to in growing up.

This view resembles that of James in assuming that when attention is self-directed (when a person takes the perspective of the generalized other), there will be an evaluation of the self with respect to some comparison point. From the view that James articulated, that comparison value will be a personal aspiration. From the view of the symbolic interactionists, it is more likely to be a social value that has been internalized from exposure to others.

It is a little more explicit from the symbolic interactionist view than from the view of James that the resultant evaluation can be positive, as well as negative. That is, if the self that one sees when taking the perspective of the generalized other is failing to live up to a social value, the evaluation will be self-critical. If the self is nicely embodying that value, however, the evaluation will be positive and self-congratulatory.

Duval and Wicklund

These early writings about the self and its reflexive property were theoretical in nature. Indeed, they represented philosophical statements as much as psychological ones. Although a lot of research was conducted on a related psychological phenomenon—self-esteem—during the mid-20th century, it was not until later that systematic studies of the effects of self-awareness per se were undertaken.

In 1972 Shelley Duval and Robert Wicklund, a pair of experimental social psychologists, published a book that detailed their initial explorations in the effects of experimentally manipulated self-awareness. Their conceptual view drew in some respects on the history of ideas just outlined, and in other respects diverged from that history. Consistent with the earlier writings, Duval and Wicklund (1972) assumed that when attention gravitated to the self (or was induced to the self), the person would become aware of salient standards or values, and would be drawn to notice any discrepancy between his or her present state and whatever standard was salient. However, their view of the consequences of becoming aware of such discrepancies was also informed by another set of influences from within social psychology during that period.

Specifically, Duval and Wicklund (1972) made use of a motivational principle that had become common in social psychology in the 1950s and 1960s, deriving from the earlier work of Hull (1943) and Spence (1956). This principle was that behavior and even cognitive processes are responsive to aversive drive states of motivation. Following dissonance theory (Festinger, 1957) and reactance theory (Brehm, 1966), both of which made use of the drive principle, Duval and Wicklund's self-awareness theory postulated that the awareness of a discrepancy between one's present state or behavior and a salient standard would create an aversive drive state. People in such a situation would be motivated to avoid self-awareness; if they could not avoid self-awareness, they would be motivated to try to reduce the discrepancy and thus reduce the drive state.

This motive principle was consistent with the idea from James and Mead that failing to conform to a salient aspiration or social value would lead to negative self-evaluation. Wicklund (1975) later added a statement to the effect that if the person was at or above the salient standard, the result could instead be positive self-evaluation, again consistent with the ideas of James and Mead.

A large number of studies make the case that self-focus causes closer conformity to salient standards. Induction of self-focus has caused effects as diverse as these: Students conformed more closely to the instruction to work fast on a clerical task (Wicklund & Duval, 1971); students conformed more to their personal attitudes about punishment when those attitudes had

been made salient (Carver, 1975) and rated erotica more consistently with their own standards (Gibbons, 1978); people opposed to stereotyping restrained themselves from doing so, whereas those who condoned it stereotyped even more (Macrae, Bodenhausen, & Milne, 1998); men conformed more to an implicit social standard of "chivalry" when giving punishment to a woman (Scheier, Fenigstein, & Buss, 1974); students allocating group earnings responded more to equity and equality norms when each was salient (Greenberg, 1980; Kernis & Reis, 1984); children in the midst of trick-or-treating conformed more to the instruction to take one (implicitly *only* one) piece of candy from a bowl (Beaman, Klentz, Diener, & Svanum, 1979).

Two points should be emphasized about these studies: First, in all cases, self-focused attention caused participants to conform more closely to the standard that was salient as being appropriate in that situation. Second, this effect of self-focus is an influence on a *process*, not a direct effect on the *content* of behavior. That is, being self-aware can make you *less* punitive if the salient standard is to be so (Scheier et al., 1974), but it can also make you *more* punitive if the standard calls for it (Carver, 1974, 1975). The content of behavior when self-focus is high depends on the reference value. People often can easily plug in one standard or another, and the effect of self-focus on overt action changes correspondingly.

Attribution

Duval and Wicklund's (1972) adoption of the concept of standards of comparison had great conceptual resonance with the ideas of James and Mead. However, Duval and Wicklund also added at least one other principle, based in part on the foundation of ideas from Heider (1944), whose work in social psychology had also stimulated Duval and Wicklund's thinking. An idea that would prove to be important later on in the self-awareness literature was that self-focused attention would make the self more prominent as a causal agent. To the extent that the self was prominent as a causal agent, the self would receive proportionally greater causal attribution regarding events in which it was involved. That is, the self would be blamed or credited with the outcomes of those events to a greater degree when attention was self-directed than when it was not.

In one early study (Duval & Wicklund, 1973) research participants made causal attributions for hypothetical outcomes in states of high or lower self-awareness. Greater attributions to the self were made when attention was self-directed. Using a variety of paradigms, this general finding has been replicated repeatedly, showing that self-aware persons ascribe greater responsibility to themselves for various kinds of events, including the plights of other people (e.g., Arkin & Duval, 1975; S. Duval, Duval, & Neely, 1979; see also Carver & Scheier, 1981, pp. 102–103).

Additional Contributors and Further Principles

The early work by Duval and Wicklund drew a good deal of interest from others in personality and social psychology. As is often the case, this interest eventually resulted in the addition of new hypotheses and the development of several differences of opinion. These differences of opinion helped to direct subsequent research efforts in several directions. They also led to conceptualizations of the nature of self-awareness and its consequences that had very different metatheoretic underpinnings.

Salience of Various Self Elements

One idea that was soon added was drawn fairly directly from intuition, although it also seems to be implied by the attributional principle just discussed. Specifically, it was suggested that whatever aspect of the self was salient at the moment that attention was directed to the self would have a disproportionate influence on the person's subsequent subjective experience and behavioral response (e.g., Buss, 1980). Sometimes a behavioral standard is what is salient; sometimes the self as a causal agent is what is salient; and sometimes yet other aspects of the self are salient.

For example, the physical self constantly generates internal stimuli—emotions, aches and pains, sensations of hunger, daydreams.

If one of those internal stimuli is salient, perhaps self-focused attention would selectively pick that stimulus out, and it would seem subjectively more intense or subjectively more prominent than it otherwise would. If so, perhaps it would influence behavior more than it otherwise would. This "salience of self" hypothesis led to several studies.

Scheier and Carver (1977) used this idea to predict that affective experience would feel more intense when attention was self-focused than when it was not. They induced an affective state, then increased self-awareness. When participants were then asked to report on their feelings, they reported feelings of greater intensity than did participants who were less self-aware.

Scheier (1976) also used this line of thought to predict that greater awareness of an affect would make the person more responsive behaviorally to that affect. He generated a state of anger in some research participants through a staged provocation, then gave them an opportunity to retaliate against the person who had provoked them. Participants who were higher in self-focus reported more anger and were also more aggressive than those who were lower in self-focus.

Another derivation from this line of thought turned it on its head: What would happen if a person was led to expect an internal event, but the event failed to occur? What would self-focus do in such a case? The hypothesis was posed that the self-aware state in this case would make the person more aware of the *absence* of the anticipated sensation.

This hypothesis was confirmed in several studies. In one of them (Gibbons, Carver, Scheier, & Hormuth, 1979), participants were led to expect that a powder they ingested (actually a placebo, which had no effect) would produce symptoms of physical arousal—sweaty palms, racing heart, and so forth. After an intervening task, the participants were asked to make ratings of their symptom levels. Those lower in self-focus reported the anticipated symptoms. Those who were made higher in self-focus reported (correctly) that they were *not* experiencing symptoms. Ancillary data indicated that the self-aware participants had engaged in a search for the specific symptoms that they had been led to expect, revealing to them the absence of the sensations.

These findings were conceptually replicated in further studies, focusing on other kinds of suggestibility phenomena. In one such study (Scheier, Carver, & Gibbons, 1979, Study 1), male undergraduates were shown slides of nude women, chosen as being moderately attractive. An off-handed remark prior to the viewing of the slides suggested to the participant that previous viewers had found them to be either extremely attractive or extremely unattractive. Not surprisingly, this remark had a strong influence on the ratings that participants later made of the women in the slides. However, the impact of the remark was actually less among self-aware participants, whose ratings were in the intermediate range of attractiveness.

Self-Knowledge from Recurrent Self-Focus

Nasby (1985, 1989a, 1989b) suggested what amounts to a longer term function of having spent a given amount of time in a state of self-awareness. Rather than examine the momentary effects of directing attention to the self, Nasby considered the consequences of such focusing of attention over many repeated instances, or perhaps a tendency to probe more deeply over time.

This might be a good place to point out that the term "self-awareness" has different connotations in different contexts. The research literature under discussion uses it in a way that differs from its meaning in other contexts (and perhaps differs from the meaning that comes most readily to your own mind). The term "self-awareness" as used here does not typically imply a prolonged or penetrating self-examination or self-absorption. Nor does it usually connote self-knowledge beyond the ordinary. *Attention* is selective processing of particular aspects of the available informational field, such that some information is more salient or more fully processed than others. Self-awareness is usually regarded as self-focused *attention,* selective processing of information about the self.

Nasby (1985, 1989a, 1989b) has pointed out, however, that such selective processing of self-knowledge also lies behind the development of the self-concept. He has further

argued that people who spend a good deal of their time engaged in that kind of selective processing naturally develop a view of themselves that is more elaborated and more firmly anchored than do other people. He has also produced research findings that are consistent with this view (see also Hjelle & Bernard, 1994). In a similar vein, Turner (1978) found that people who tend to think about themselves process self-relevant information more quickly than people who tend not to think about themselves. Specifically, they are quicker to decide whether trait terms apply to them or not.

In a way, the idea discussed here follows fairly directly from the logic behind the salience of self findings just described. That is, if one pores over the information one has about oneself, whether from repeated subjective experience or from more consolidated stores of information, one gains a clearer and more internally consistent view of the subject one is viewing.

Indeed, self-awareness may also enhance people's ability to access such information about themselves from memory. Gibbons and colleagues (1985) asked persons with clinical disorders to report on aspects of their health problems. Self-focus led to more accurate self-reports of their hospitalization history, as compared with hospital records and staff judgments.

Self-Awareness and Selective Processing of Self-Related Information

The notion that self-awareness is involved in the processing of personally relevant information was also proposed by Hull and Levy (1979). Their view is very different, however, in at least one important respect, from the self-awareness model of Duval and Wicklund (1972) and from other models to follow. Specifically, Hull and Levy argued that self-awareness is not a matter of *attentional focus*; rather, it is a matter of selective processing and *encoding* of aspects of the information that has already been brought in by attentional processes. In this view, when people are self-focused, they are selectively encoding information that pertains to the self. This selective encoding renders the person especially sensitive to aspects of the environment that are potentially self-relevant.

Hull and Levy (1979) conducted a series of laboratory tasks to examine predictions from their model. One of these was an incidental encoding paradigm, in which people are presented with a series of words and asked to answer different questions about different words. Later, in a surprise recall task, people are asked to remember the words they had been presented with. A common finding is that being asked whether a descriptive word applies to oneself makes it more likely to be recalled. Hull and Levy found that people who tend to think about themselves a lot are especially prone to such incidental encoding of the self-relevance of personality traits.

In another study, Hull and Levy (1979) found that self-awareness results in more self-blame for hypothetical bad outcomes, but only if the judgment was made publicly. Presumably, self-focus in the private-judgment condition sensitized participants to the issue of self-esteem protection, whereas self-focus in the public-judgment condition sensitized participants to the public-display aspects of the situation.

Principles Arising from Matching to Standard

In many ways, the most interesting of the initial self-awareness effects was the self-awareness-induced behavioral conformity to salient standards of behavior. Duval and Wicklund (1972) viewed these effects in terms of a drive reduction process. A different interpretation of those effects was offered a few years later (Carver, 1979; Carver & Scheier, 1981). This alternate interpretation placed the self-awareness effect within the framework of a very different motivational dynamic than the one that was assumed by Duval and Wicklund.

Specifically, this view treated self-awareness-induced conformity to salient standards as an example of the operation of a discrepancy-reducing cybernetic feedback loop. Discrepancy-reducing feedback processes had already been used for some time as a depiction of a class of self-regulatory dynamics in both artificial and living systems (MacKay, 1956; Miller, Galanter, & Pribram, 1960; Wiener, 1948). Carver and Scheier (1981) adopted that construct and

applied it to the discrepancy-reducing consequence of self-awareness.

Cybernetics and Discrepancy-Reducing Feedback Processes

The feedback loop as a construct is a mainstay of today's understanding of how physiological systems function. The elements of such a feedback loop (whether in a living or artificial system) are a reference value (or set point, or goal), a perceptual input channel, a comparator that checks the fit between reference and input, and an output channel that serves to change present conditions in a way that induces closer conformity between reference and input. In a homeostatic physiological system, the loop serves to counter disruptive influences from outside the system, keeping some quality stable (e.g., body temperature, heart rate). In a more dynamic system, the reference value is a moving target, and the feedback process tracks that moving target. For example, when a person engages in strenuous physical activity, the reference value for heart rate goes up, and the physiological system activating the heart keeps the actual rate higher than it otherwise would. When the activity ceases, the reference rate diminishes.

What makes the motivational dynamic of this model different from that of the drive theory model is that this one does not assume an aversive drive state behind the regulatory processes. Rather, feedback loops are considered to be naturally occurring self-regulatory organizations within living systems. They keep sensed values within relatively constrained ranges in the natural course of events, operating fairly automatically. Adopting this view with respect to even consciously mediated human behavior raises a number of questions, of course, including (but not limited to) whether this view dispenses with the concept of "will" (Ryan & Deci, 1999).

Carver and Scheier (1981; Carver, 1979) found this view on self-awareness processes compelling in part because many of the elements of self-awareness theory line up neatly against those of the feedback loop. Duval and Wicklund (1972) had said that self-awareness induces a tendency to compare one's present behavior or state against whatever standard of comparison is salient in the situation (a tendency that was later verified by Scheier and Carver, 1983). This is exactly what happens in the comparator function of a feedback loop. Duval and Wicklund also had allowed for the possibility that the awareness of a discrepancy between present condition and standard would lead to a behavioral effort to reduce the discrepancy. That discrepancy reduction process is the function of a feedback loop taken as a whole.

Indeed, the idea that this construct could be applied to the experience of self-awareness turns out not to have been so new after all. MacKay had foreshadowed this interpretation of self-awareness effects as feedback processes in 1963. He wrote then (1963, p. 227) that "an artifact capable of receiving and acting on information about the state of its own body can begin to parallel many of the modes of activity we associate with self-consciousness."

Carver and Scheier (1981) took this view on self-awareness and joined it with ideas from other literatures (e.g., Powers, 1973) to argue for the existence of a hierarchical assembly of feedback loops (see also Vallacher & Wegner, 1987). Together, the elements of the hierarchical organization account for how concrete physical motions take place in response to the relatively abstract intention to act. This view is addressed in more detail later in the chapter.

Discrepancy-Enlarging Feedback Processes

The idea that self-awareness engages a feedback process also suggested another hypothesis, which does not seem directly implied by other theoretical derivations. Specifically, although the discrepancy-reducing feedback loop is the most common sort of feedback process, it is not the only one. There also exist discrepancy-enlarging feedback processes (cf. Shibutani, 1961). These loops act to create and increase a discrepancy between a sensed condition and a reference value.

Several studies were conducted to determine whether there were conditions under which self-focus would produce this discrepancy-enlarging effect rather than the discrepancy-reducing effect. One of them made use of a phenomenon known as a negative reference group (Newcomb, 1950). A negative reference group is a group to which people compare themselves for the purpose of maintaining and even emphasizing differences. A negative reference group is a group you want *not* to resemble. The easiest example is the tendency of many adolescents to treat their parents as a group to diverge from in every possible way. Behavior that manifests a contrary quality thus helps the adolescent differ from the standard of the parents.

Carver and Humphries (1981) used this idea to test the possibility that self-focus would enhance the discrepancy-enlarging tendency. They chose a group of participants who had a readily identifiable negative reference group: Cuban American college students. These persons had been raised in an exile community and had been taught all their lives to treat the Castro government in Cuba as a negative reference group. Carver and Humphries presented these students with a set of policy statements ostensibly made by representatives of the Castro government. Participants then were asked to report their own opinions on the issue of each policy statement. Participants who were higher in self-focus made reports that deviated more from those of the negative reference group than did those who were lower in self-focus.

This is not the only case of discrepancy enlargement through self-focus. Several further studies used reactance paradigms to examine this phenomenon. Reactance occurs when a person feels pressured to believe something or do something—when the perceived freedom of choice is being infringed on (Brehm, 1966). Of most importance at present is the fact that the typical response to reactance is to behave contrarily—to do the opposite of what one is being pressured to do. This looks very much like a discrepancy-enlarging process, and it turns out that this process is also enhanced by higher levels of self-focus (see Carver & Scheier, 1981, pp. 157–162).

Carver and Scheier (1998) have more recently argued that the discrepancy-reducing and discrepancy-enlarging processes are also manifest in two kinds of social comparison phenomena (Buunk & Gibbons, 1997; Helgeson & Taylor, 1993; Wood, 1989, 1996). Social comparison sometimes involves comparing oneself to someone else who is better off than oneself (called upward comparison); it sometimes involves comparing oneself to someone else who is worse off than oneself (called downward comparison). Carver and Scheier suggested that when people engage in upward comparison, their primary motivation for doing so involves using the point of comparison as a positive reference value. It provides something to shoot for, something positive to become. When people engage in downward comparison, in contrast, their primary motivation is to push themselves away from those negative values. They actively try not to become like the persons to whom they are comparing themselves.

Role of Expectancies

Another theoretical derivation in the developing literature of self-awareness stemmed from the fact that the Carver and Scheier (1981) model did not assume a negative emotional response to self-awareness when there was a discrepancy between self and standard. This view raised a number of questions.

One very obvious question concerned the fact that Duval and Wicklund (1972) had posited two potential responses to the presumed aversiveness of self-focus. Indeed, they had argued that the behavioral discrepancy reduction was not even first in line. First would be the attempt to avoid self-awareness, if this could be done. Because Carver and Scheier (1981) did not assume an aversive drive state, they did not expect an attempt to avoid self-focus to dominate. Indeed, they argued that such a response would occur only under certain fairly specific conditions.

Several studies bearing on this issue were conducted during that period. For example, Steenbarger and Aderman (1979) pointed out that in previous work the experimentally created discrepancies that led to avoidance were always inflexible. That is, the discrepancies were fixed because of some aspect of the situation faced by the research participants. With no opportunity to do anything about reducing them, participants chose to avoid facing them. Steenbarger and Aderman argued that this avoidance might not occur if participants thought they could do something to reduce the discrepancy.

They set up a situation in which that possibility was made salient for some of the participants. The result was that self-focus was aversive—and led to avoidance—only among participants in whom the discrepancy was set up to be irreducible. If the discrepancy was potentially reducible, these effects did not obtain.

At about the same time, Carver and Scheier (1981) had conceived the idea that which of the two responses would be made to self-awareness was dependent on people's *expectancies* of being able to reduce the discrepancy. If people expect to be successful, they strive to reach their goals, even if that involves a struggle. If people expect to fail, they experience a tendency to disengage effort and sometimes even disengage from the goal itself. This depiction fit the pattern that had emerged from the work just described.

It also had a considerable resonance with other ideas appearing elsewhere during that period. For example, Wortman and Brehm (1975) had devised an integration between reactance and helplessness theories. This proposed integration rested on the idea that reactance (which is sometimes expressed as renewed efforts to attain a goal) occurs when the person feels able to carry out an intention, whereas helplessness (which is expressed as abandonment of effort) occurs when the person feels unable to succeed in the effort. In the same vein, Carver and Scheier (1981) came to refer to the avoidance response not as an avoidance of self-awareness, but rather as a disengagement of effort from action directed at attaining that particular goal (cf. also Klinger, 1975).

Several further studies (reviewed in Carver & Scheier, 1981, 1998) provided support for this line of reasoning. In one such study (Carver & Scheier, 1981), participants who reported being moderately afraid of snakes were asked to approach and pick up a live snake. These persons had all reported the same level of fear but slightly differing levels of confidence about being able to execute the behavior in question. Self-focus interacted with confidence, such that persons higher in confidence reacted to self-focus by intensifying their efforts, whereas persons lower in confidence quit the attempt sooner in the approach sequence.

Another study (Carver & Scheier, 1981) created a behavioral discrepancy by a manipulation in which all persons performed poorly at an initial task said to reflect intelligence. Expectancies of being able to do better on a second task (also related to intelligence) were then manipulated, and the participants attempted the second task. This second task, however, was actually a measure of persistence. The item that participants attempted first was impossible to solve correctly, and the question was which participants would try hardest (longest). Again self-focus interacted with expectancies, causing greater persistence among those led to be confident and lower persistence among those led to be doubtful.

More recent work appears to show that responses to self-focus depend partly on the size of the discrepancy being confronted. One project (T. S. Duval, Duval, & Mulilis, 1992) conceptually replicated the pattern just described for persistence but added such a qualifier. In their studies, self-focus led to enhanced persistence among participants who had been led to perceive themselves as able to close a relatively small discrepancy between present condition and standard of comparison. But among those with very large discrepancies, even the perception of constant movement toward the goal did not lead to persistence under self-focus. Only when the rate of progress was adequate—relative to the discrepancy—did the facilitation occur.

Optimism and Emotion

This set of ideas about expectancies and effort versus disengagement has subsequently been expanded in two other directions that deserve some brief mention, although it takes us away from the self-awareness literature per se. First, Scheier and Carver (1985, 1992) proposed that individual differences in generalized expectancies for good versus bad outcomes in important life domains represent the essence of the well-known personality quality of optimism versus pessimism. A very substantial literature now demonstrates that optimists (with their favorable expectancies for the future) tend to respond to adversity with continued efforts to reach their goals, whereas pessimists (with their unfavorable expectancies for the future) tend to display signs of disengagement and greater distress (for reviews of

various aspects of this literature, see Carver & Scheier, 2001; Scheier, Carver, & Bridges, 2001). These findings are consistent with the points made just earlier about more specific expectancies.

The optimism extrapolation derives from the assumption that expectancies are an important determinant of subsequent behavior. The other extrapolation derives from further thought regarding the feedback construct, taken together with the pattern of findings concerning the conditions under which self-awareness leads to negative feelings. This other extrapolation is a theory about the source of affect (Carver & Scheier, 1990, 1998).

The essence of this theory is the argument that a different feedback loop from the one already discussed monitors the effectiveness, over time, of movement toward incentives and (separately) movement away from threats. An analogy may help this make sense. The feedback loop that was discussed earlier in the chapter (which controls behavior) manages a psychological quality that is analogous to the physical quality of distance. In effect, the feedback loop that relates to affect controls a psychological quality that is analogous to velocity—distance over time.

This second feedback system is assumed to compare a signal corresponding to rate of progress against a reference rate. Discrepancies noticed by this system are manifest subjectively as affect. If the rate of progress is too low, negative affect arises. If the rate is just acceptable but no more, there is no affect. If the rate exceeds the criterion, positive affect arises. In essence, the argument is that positive feelings mean you are doing better than you need to, and negative feelings mean you are doing worse than you need to (for broader discussion and a review of evidence, see Carver & Scheier, 1998, Chapters 8 and 9).

This line of thought is consistent with previously discussed findings that self-focus is aversive when the behavioral discrepancy cannot be reduced, but is not aversive when it looks as though the behavioral discrepancy can be reduced. That is, given the desire to reduce a discrepancy that is presently not being reduced, velocity is zero, which is guaranteed to be below the criterion rate. This line of thought goes farther than the previously discussed findings, however. It suggests that even moving forward in the act of discrepancy reduction will be associated with negative feelings if the rate of progress is too slow. Carver and Scheier (1998) expanded this notion into a more general view of how feelings come to exist and what their functions are. Although that development goes well beyond the self-awareness concept, it is interesting to note how a principle from the self-awareness literature connects to ideas in a much broader domain.

Aspects of Self

Another theoretical contribution to the self-awareness domain took the literature in a very different direction, although this direction also had several precedents in the history of ideas bearing on this topic. This contribution came about as a side consequence of the effort to create an analog in individual differences to the experimental variation of self-awareness (Fenigstein, Scheier, & Buss, 1975). This effort resulted in a self-report measure called the Self-Consciousness Scale, which had subscales measuring people's tendencies to be aware of two different aspects of the self.

Public and Private Aspects of the Self

Private self-consciousness is the tendency to ruminate about covert, personal aspects of the self. Public self-consciousness is the tendency to be cognizant of the self as a social object. The subscales are distinct, though usually positively correlated. Thus a person can be high in one tendency or high in both—there is no assumption of an opposition between these two contents of awareness. This distinction echoed a distinction made by James (1890) between social and spiritual aspects of the self and a distinction made by Wylie (1968) between social and private aspects of the self.

A variety of studies soon examined these differences among people (for a review, see Carver & Scheier, 1985). Some studies also extended the logic to experimental manipulations. The latter studies make the case that some manipulations make people selectively aware of private self-aspects, whereas other manipulations make people selectively aware of public self-aspects (see Carver & Scheier, 1998).

An example of the latter is a project by Froming, Walker, and Lopyan (1982). They selected people who reported having personal attitudes about the use of punishment that either tended to oppose it or tended to favor it. These people also reported having subjective norms (beliefs about what most people believe) that differed from their own attitudes. These people were later placed into a situation in which they had to teach another person using punishments for incorrect responses but could freely choose the level of punishment. Compared with a control condition, a manipulation believed to direct attention preferentially to private self-aspects (a small mirror) caused behavior to shift in the direction of the participant's personal attitude. A manipulation believed to direct attention preferentially to public self-aspects (an evaluative audience) caused behavior to shift toward the subjective norm.

The public–private distinction, taken together with ideas discussed previously concerning confidence and doubt, is also embedded in models proposed by other theorists for more specific domains of behavior. For example, Schlenker and Leary (1982) suggested that the deficits of socially anxious persons reflect doubts about their ability to attain desired self-presentational goals. The effects of such doubts are presumably amplified by focusing attention on public aspects of the self—the self as it is being displayed to others in the social group.

Despite a wide adoption of the public–private distinction, there has been disagreement about its value. Wicklund and Gollwitzer (1987) argued (in part) that public self-awareness was not a valuable construct. To them, taking public pressure into account while behaving could not be a self-awareness phenomenon because the resultant behavior does not involve the self. This raises the question of what the self consists of, a question that is very interesting in its own right. Carver and Scheier (1987) replied that the self is very much involved in such behaviors, because it is the self that chooses to take into account the social context and the preferences of others. Thus, for example, self-presentational acts are attempts by the self to create certain displays to other people, for the self's own reasons.

The idea that people can take into account their own needs and desires and the needs and desires of a social group at different times (or in different cultures) is one that has been used by many theorists in the past two decades. Carver and Scheier (1998) have reviewed a variety of applications of those ideas, including further distinctions that have been made within both public and private domains.

Although the Self-Consciousness Scale has been useful as an individual-differences measure of self-focus, recent work suggests that it blurs some important distinctions. Trapnell and Campbell (1999) distinguished between what they called *reflective* and *ruminative* facets of private self-consciousness. They did so from the assumption that two different motives underlie focus on the private self as operationalized in the Self-Consciousness Scale. One motive is curiosity, the other is the mental probing of negative feeling states.

Trapnell and Campbell (1999) found (as have others) that items measuring private self-consciousness split into two subsets. Both subsets relate to the trait of openness to experience, but one also relates to neuroticism. The two item sets behaved differently enough to cause Trapnell and Campbell to develop their own measure of reflection and rumination. The items of their scales are explicitly aimed at those two tendencies: Rumination items all incorporate language about thinking back, rethinking, being unable to put something behind oneself. Reflection items all incorporate language about being fascinated, meditative, philosophical, and inquisitive.

The main point here is that these new scales both reflect individual differences in the awareness of some aspect of the self. Thus both are self-consciousness measures, though they differ from each other in a way quite different from that reflected in the measure of Fenigstein and colleagues (1975). But this work makes an even broader point: The experience of the self has a very great deal of diversity. It is possible to assess individual differences in the tendency to focus on any particular one of those experiences of the self. The number of potential scales is endless. Perhaps, in the future, more such differences will be revealed to be important.

Hierarchicality

In talking about the various aspects of the self, I am also starting to get back to the notion that the self is partly about the pursuit of goals, the matching of actions to salient standards. I turn now to another issue that pertains to that notion.

Some goals are broader in scope than others. How to think about the difference in breadth can be hard to put your finger on. Sometimes it is a difference in the time span involved in the action. That is, some goals (to get a college degree) take a long time; other goals (to mow the lawn) take a short time. Often the difference in breadth is more than a matter of time. It is a difference in the goal's level of abstraction. For example, the goal of following an experimenter's instructions for engaging in a task is fairly concrete; the goal of living up to your potential as a human being is more abstract.

In a 1973 book, William Powers argued that a hierarchical organization of feedback loops underlies the self-regulation of behavior. Because feedback loops imply goals, this argument also constituted a model of hierarchical structuring among the goals used in creating actions. His general line of thinking ran as follows: In a hierarchical organization of feedback systems, the output of a high-level system consists of the resetting of reference values at the next lower level of abstraction. To put it somewhat differently, higher order or superordinate systems "behave" by providing goals to the systems just below them (see also the action identification theory of Vallacher & Wegner, 1987).

The values specified as behavioral outputs become more concrete and restricted as one moves from higher to lower levels of the hierarchy. Control at each level reflects regulation of a quality that contributes to the quality controlled at the next higher level. Each level monitors input at a level of abstraction that is appropriate to its own functioning, and each level adjusts output so as to minimize discrepancies at that level.

Powers (1973) focused particularly on low levels of abstraction, saying less about the levels of abstraction that are of most interest to personality and social psychologists, other than to suggest labels for several levels whose existence makes intuitive sense. *Sequences* are strings of acts that run off directly once cued. *Programs* are activities that require conscious decisions at various points. The level above that is *principles*, qualities that are abstracted from (or, alternatively, implemented by) programs. These are qualities at the level of abstraction of trait labels. Powers gave the not-very-euphonious name *system concepts* to the highest level he considered, but goal representations at this level reduce essentially to the idealized overall sense of self, relationship, or group identity.

A simple way of portraying this hierarchy is illustrated in Figure 9.1. This diagram omits the loops of feedback processes, using lines to indicate only links among goal values. The lines imply that moving toward a particular lower level goal contributes to the attainment of some higher level goal (or even several at once). Multiple lines leading to a given goal indicates that several lower

level action qualities can contribute to its attainment. As indicated previously, there are goals to "be" a particular way and goals to "do" certain things (and at lower levels, goals to create physical movement).

Another point arising from the notion of hierarchical organization concerns the fact that goals are not equivalent in importance. The higher you go into the organization, the more fundamental to the overriding sense of self are the qualities encountered. Thus, in general, goal qualities at higher levels are intrinsically more important than those at lower levels.

An issue that was raised in the preceding section is what the self consists of. It was raised there with regard to the question of whether the self is involved in self-presentational phenomena or conformity to social pressures. My own opinion (described there) is that some goals of the self are explicitly goals for self-presentation and impression management. These kinds of goals fall under principles that involve taking oth-

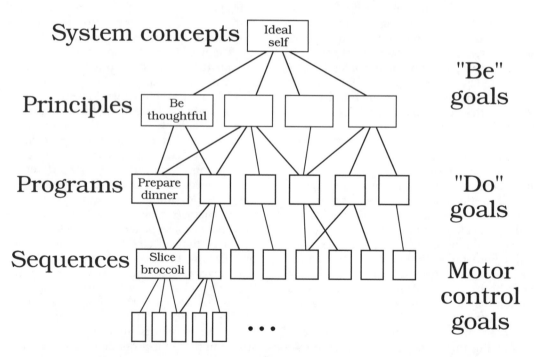

FIGURE 9.1. A hierarchy of goals (or of feedback loops) within the self. Lines indicate the contribution of lower level goals to specific higher level goals. They can also be read in the opposite direction, indicating that a given higher order goal specifies more-concrete goals at the next lower level. The hierarchy described in text involves goals of "being" particular ways, which are attained by "doing" particular actions. From C. S. Carver and M. F. Scheier (1998). *On the self-regulation of behavior.* Copyright 1998 by Cambridge University Press. Reprinted by permission.

ers' opinions into account. Other goals of the self are more personal and take others into account less. These fall under different sorts of orienting principles.

A question that is interesting to pose but hard to answer is, How many layers of a person's goals should be considered to fall under the label *self*? Most would certainly agree that the ideal self belongs under that label. The broad idealized sense of self readily translates into principles of conduct, and it seems likely that most people would agree that one's guiding principles are also elements of the self.

But where are the limits? How far down the hierarchy of goals can you go and have it still be sensible to think about the goals as part of the self? Are the goals that define programs of action part of the self? Certainly each person individualizes the pattern of goals that make up even such a common activity as doing the laundry or taking a holiday trip. Furthermore, people differ from one another in terms of the programs in which they engage. But does that make these goal structures part of the self? I have no clear answer to this question.

There is some precedent, though, for equating a reduction in self-focus (for example, via alcohol use; Hull, 1981) with suspension of self-regulation at the principle level and higher, and sometimes even the program level. Does this mean there is no self at lower levels? The answer may be a matter of definition. The sequences programmed into people's repertoires differ from one person to another, implying a distinctiveness that may connote selfhood. On the other hand, these bits of information are so concrete and minimal that it may not be useful to think of them as elements of the self.

The discussion of how many of these layers constitute the self also raises another question, related but different: Are all these layers of the hierarchy involved in behavior all the time? No, almost certainly not. There appear to be many times in life when people mindlessly engage in sequences of action or programs of behavior with little or no regard to whether these actions conform to particular principles or the ideal self. Indeed, it is arguable that the sense of the ideal self comes into play relatively infrequently in most people's lives. To put it a different way, it appears that the upper levels of control come into play only when the person focuses on them. In contrast, all levels lower than the one being focused on are presumably engaged at all times.

Recent Directions

The self-awareness area has recently enjoyed something of a resurgence of research interest. T. S. Duval and Silvia and their colleagues (T. S. Duval & Silvia, 2001; Silvia & Duval, 2001; Silvia & Gendolla, 2001) have raised a number of questions regarding the prior literature on self-awareness effects. They have also gone on to argue that some of the principles introduced early in the developing literature have greater importance than is commonly realized.

Salience of the Self

One of the questions raised by Silvia and Gendolla (2001) concerns a set of findings described earlier in the chapter in the context of "salience of self" effects. That is, several studies seemed to indicate that self-focused attention causes an increase in the subjective intensity of internal sensations. Further, self-focused attention appeared to enhance awareness of the absence of sensations that the person expected to occur but which actually were not present. Silvia and Gendolla argue that these effects actually represent a different phenomenon: that they are attempts to behave in line with salient standards, to increase consistency among aspects of the self. In their view, in situations in which self-focus led people to report judgments of more intense affect, the participants in the research were conforming to a standard favoring emotional expression.

In an intriguing set of studies (reviewed in Silvia & Gendolla, 2001), Silvia induced affect along with a variety of different sorts of situational and personal cues (in different studies), thereby making different kinds of standards salient. In general (though there are variations from study to study), he found that when standards emphasizing the appropriateness of feeling and expressing emotions were salient, self-focus led to reports of stronger emotions. When standards emphasizing the inhibition of emotions were salient, self-focus led to reports of less emotion (or had no influence on reports of emotion).

What of the findings that self-focus reduces suggestibility effects? Silvia and Gendolla (2001) interpret these effects as also reflecting the principle of conformity. Rather than conformity to a behavioral standard, though, these effects are said to reflect conformity—consistency—within the self. Silvia and Gendolla argue that participants in these studies all knew that the information they had been given was incorrect, but that only the self-aware participants were motivated to point it out. These people were motivated by the desire for consistency between internal experience and the judgments they made. Again, then, the findings can be interpreted in terms of matching an aspect of behavior to a standard, in this case an internal reference value (the perception).

Although the Silvia and Gendolla article is interesting, it is also somewhat misleading in one respect. Specifically, throughout the article, the authors refer to a perceptual "accuracy" hypothesis: that is, that self-focus makes people more *accurate* in their perceptions. However, my reading of the earlier articles is that the studies more typically focused on the *subjective intensity* of the experience, rather than accuracy per se (an exception being Gibbons, 1983). My interpretation of the earlier work has been that self-focus in that context expands the mental image of the focal region of a dimension of experience, much as a thumbnail image on a Web site expands to a larger size when clicked. This does not necessarily argue for greater accuracy, though. Instead, there may be a sharper view of a more limited region of experience (looking very closely at one inch instead of an entire foot). The person looking at the larger subjective image (e.g., presence of affect) may exaggerate what is there rather than being more accurate about it. The person looking at a small subjective image (e.g., absence of arousal) may exaggerate how little of the experience there is. This issue renders some of the points made by Silvia and Gendolla less compelling, though other points remain well taken.

Throughout these recent accounts of self-awareness phenomena threads the idea that self-awareness effects are more about cognitive consistency than about anything else (T. S. Duval & Duval, 1983; T. S. Duval & Silvia, 2001; Silvia & Duval, 2001; Silvia & Gendolla, 2001). Thus these authors interpret a good many other findings in terms of the consistency principle. For example, Duval and Silvia (2001) told people they had passed or failed on a cognitive task, under conditions of higher or lower self-focus. Manipulation checks showed that the groups were equivalently aware of having met or failed to meet the standard. However, only the more self-focused group made defensive attributions for the failure and showed a loss of self-esteem. The researchers concluded that it requires self-focus to engage the desire for consistency, thus yielding such effects.

Attributions and Behavior

Another aspect of this more recent work on self-awareness is a renewed interest in the attributional consequences of self-awareness. This interest has, in part, taken the form of closer scrutiny of the effects of situational constraints on the attributions that are made under high self-focus (see Silvia & Gendolla, 2001). For example, participants in some of this research worked on mental rotation tasks, which had been described as reflecting people's ability at three-dimensional problem solving. In some studies, participants were told their performance was substandard. Half of these were led to believe that they could rapidly improve; the other half were told their chances of improving were slim. Persons high in self-focus made attributions for their failure that differed from those of control participants in the following pattern. When they expected to improve, they attributed failure internally; when they expected to be unable to improve, they attributed the failure externally. It appears from findings such as these that self-defensiveness in response to a failure emerges when the chances of making up for the failure are low but not when the chances are higher.

To account for findings of this sort, T. S. Duval and Duval (1983) argued for a confluence of the principles of attribution and consistency. They suggested that making an internal attribution for the failure to meet a standard prompts the matching-to-standard process, but that this kind of attribution also creates a problem for self-esteem management. This problem would be minimal if the failure were easy to correct. However, it would be far more troublesome if the failure were a permanent one. In the latter case, the cost of the permanent self-discrepancy outweighs any cost that might arise from making an inaccurate attribution. Thus, in the case of the permanent failure, the person is likely to make a more external attribution under self-focus. Several studies have produced findings that are consistent with this reasoning (see Silvia & Duval, 2001).

Another extension of this reasoning came from Dana, Lalwani, and Duval (1997). They argued that sometimes people shift their behavior so it conforms to the standard and sometimes they shift the standard to be more like their behavior. They told research participants that they had failed to meet a performance standard and then led them to focus either on the standard itself or on their performance. Among those who were attending to the standard, self-focus led them to derogate the standard and not try to improve their performance in a subsequent task period. Among those who were attending to their performances, however, self-focus caused greater efforts during the second task period, with no derogation of the standard.

T. S. Duval and Lalwani (1999) proposed that attributional processes underlie this difference between groups. The argument is that focusing on the standard leads people to attribute the cause of the discrepancy to the standard. Focusing on their own performance leads people to attribute the cause of the discrepancy to themselves. Self-focus, then, causes people to act on what they see as the cause of the discrepancy. In the one case, this means changing the standard; in the other case, it means changing their behavior.

Brain Functioning, Self-Awareness, and Self-Regulation

A final topic I want to mention briefly, although I will not go into it deeply, is a body of brain research that bears on some of the processes described in this chapter. It has been argued for some time that the prefrontal cortex controls phenomena captured by the term *self-awareness* (e.g., Stuss, 1991; Stuss & Alexander, 2000; Stuss, Alexander, & Benson, 1997; Stuss & Levine, 2002). Stuss (1991) argued that the frontal cortex has three levels of function. The first involves the ability to organize and maintain information in meaningful sequences. The second is an executive function involved in moving toward goals in novel or nonroutine situations. This function is divisible into processes such as goal selection, means–end analysis, reflective evaluation of behavioral outcomes, and performance maintenance in light of those evaluations. The third level of frontal function is consciousness itself, the ability to be aware of oneself and one's relationship to the environment.

Much of this argument rests on studies of persons with frontal lobe damage. Stuss and colleagues (Stuss, 1991; Stuss & Alexander, 2000; Stuss et al., 1997; Stuss & Levine, 2002) have reviewed portions of this literature and concluded that several themes can be extracted from it. First, many patients display a dissociation between knowledge and its use. For example, although they can detect errors, they do not use this knowledge appropriately. Second, patients with frontal lobe damage often show a loss of the sense of temporal order, a sense that is obviously necessary to implement plans or to experience the continuity of the self (see also Tulving, 1989). A third theme, more diffuse, is that there are differing levels of awareness of self, with higher levels being more likely to be disturbed by frontal lobe damage.

A very different kind of evidence bearing on a related idea has been reported by Gehring, Goss, Coles, Meyer, and Donchin (1993). Participants in this study performed a long series of simple choices while electroencephalogram (EEG) data were recorded to assess aspects of their brain activity. Of particular interest was what occurred on trials in which participants made errors. The errors were associated with a particular pattern in the EEG, which indicated that a brain mechanism was noting the error even as it was being made. Further, this pattern was also associated with several measures indicating attempts at error correction. Taken together, the data suggest the existence of a brain system that detects errors and attempts to compensate for them.

Although these links between neuropsychology and social–personality psychology are fairly tenuous, they are also exciting. They suggest that in work such as this there may emerge a better understanding of the physiological mechanisms within which the phenomena described in this chapter take place.

Conclusion

This chapter has reviewed a variety of ideas and research about the effects of self-awareness on people's subjective experience and on ongoing behavior. The sources of this work have ranged from the 19th to the 21st centuries. The ideas themselves have ranged in their nature from drive theories to cybernetic theories.

One theme that has run fairly strongly through the literature of ideas on this topic is the principle of attaining consistency between elements of the self and between the self and the actions that it engages in. The human mind appears to have a mechanism that operates to compare mental elements with each other (self and experience, goal and behavior) and to bring them into greater consistency, if that can be done without too much difficulty. If it cannot be done fairly easily, other things may happen: perhaps an avoidance of further consideration of the elements, or perhaps even an effort to move the elements farther from each other, as though to place them in different parts of the mental organization of the self. Whether this reflects an internal drive state or whether it is a natural consequence of the way living systems are organized remains a matter of debate.

Although *this* chapter is finished, it is very unlikely that the *final* chapter on this topic has been written. Research on the consequences of self-awareness is alive and well, and theoretical models of how the effects emerge continue to evolve and grow. As is true of all literatures that concern the self, the topic is one that is complex and deep. With much more to be known, there will also be much more for future authors to chronicle.

Acknowledgment

Preparation of this chapter was facilitated by NCI Grant Nos. CA64710, CA78995, and CA84944.

References

Arkin, R., & Duval, S. (1975). Focus of attention and causal attributions of actors and observers. *Journal of Experimental Social Psychology, 11*, 427–438.

Beaman, A. L., Klentz, B., Diener, E., & Svanum, S. (1979). Self-awareness and transgression in children: Two field studies. *Journal of Personality and Social Psychology, 37*, 1835–1846.

Brehm, J. W. (1966). *A theory of psychological reactance.* New York: Academic Press.

Buss, A. H. (1980). *Self-consciousness and society anxiety.* San Francisco: Freeman.

Buunk, B. P., & Gibbons, F. X. (Eds.). (1997). *Health, coping, and well-being: Perspectives from social comparison theory.* Mahwah, NJ: Erlbaum.

Carver, C. S. (1974). Facilitation of physical aggression through objective self-awareness. *Journal of Experimental Social Psychology, 10*, 365–370.

Carver, C. S. (1975). Physical aggression as a function of objective self-awareness and attitudes toward punishment. *Journal of Experimental Social Psychology, 11*, 510–519.

Carver, C. S. (1979). A cybernetic model of self-attention processes. *Journal of Personality and Social Psychology, 37*, 1251–1281.

Carver, C. S., & Humphries, C. (1981). Havana daydreaming: A study of self-consciousness and the negative reference group among Cuban Americans. *Journal of Personality and Social Psychology, 40*, 545–552.

Carver, C. S., & Scheier, M. F. (1981). *Attention and self-regulation: A control-theory approach to human behavior.* New York: Springer-Verlag.

Carver, C. S., & Scheier, M. F. (1985). Aspects of self, and the control of behavior. In B. R. Schlenker (Ed.), *The self and social life* (pp. 146–174). New York: McGraw-Hill.

Carver, C. S., & Scheier, M. F. (1987). The blind men and the elephant: Selective examination of the public–private literature gives rise to a faulty perception. *Journal of Personality, 55*, 525–541.

Carver, C. S., & Scheier, M. F. (1990). Origins and functions of positive and negative affect: A control-process view. *Psychological Review, 97*, 19–35.

Carver, C. S., & Scheier, M. F. (1998). *On the self-regulation of behavior.* New York: Cambridge University Press.

Carver, C. S., & Scheier, M. F. (2001). Optimism, pessimism, and self-regulation. In E. C. Chang (Ed.), *Optimism and pessimism: Implications for theory, research, and practice* (pp. 31–51). Washington, DC: American Psychological Association.

Cooley, C. H. (1902). *Human nature and the social order.* New York: Scribner's.

Dana, E. R., Lalwani, N., & Duval, T. S. (1997). Objective self-awareness and focus of attention following awareness of self-standard discrepancies: Changing self or changing standards of correctness. *Journal of Social and Clinical Psychology, 16*, 359–380.

Duval, S., & Wicklund, R. A. (1972). *A theory of objective self-awareness*. New York: Academic Press.

Duval, S., & Wicklund, R. A. (1973). Effects of objective self-awareness on attribution of causality. *Journal of Experimental Social Psychology, 9,* 17–31.

Duval, S., Duval, V. H., & Neely, R. (1979). Self-focus, felt responsibility, and helping behavior. *Journal of Personality and Social Psychology, 37,* 1769–1778.

Duval, T. S., & Duval, V. H. (1983). *Consistency and cognition*. Hillsdale, NJ: Erlbaum.

Duval, T. S., Duval, V. H., & Mulilis, J.-P. (1992). Effects of self-focus, discrepancy between self and standard, and outcome expectancy favorability on the tendency to match self to standard or to withdraw. *Journal of Personality and Social Psychology, 62,* 340–348.

Duval, T. S., & Lalwani, N. (1999). Objective self-awareness and causal attributions for self-standard discrepancies: Changing self or changing standards of correctness. *Personality and Social Psychology Bulletin, 25,* 1220–1229.

Duval, T. S., & Silvia, P. J. (2001). *Self-awareness and causal attribution: A dual-systems theory*. Boston: Kluwer Academic.

Fenigstein, A., Scheier, M. F., & Buss, A. H. (1975). Public and private self-consciousness: Assessment and theory. *Journal of Consulting and Clinical Psychology, 43,* 522–527.

Festinger, L. (1957). *A theory of cognitive dissonance*. Stanford, CA: Stanford University Press.

Froming, W. J., Walker, G. R., & Lopyan, K. J. (1982). Public and private self-awareness: When personal attitudes conflict with societal expectations. *Journal of Experimental Social Psychology, 18,* 476–487.

Gehring, W. J., Goss, B., Coles, M. G. H., Meyer, D. E., & Donchin, E. (1993). A neural system for error detection and compensation. *Psychological Science, 4,* 385–390.

Gibbons, F. X. (1978). Sexual standards and reactions to pornography: Enhancing behavioral consistency through self-focused attention. *Journal of Personality and Social Psychology, 36,* 976–987.

Gibbons, F. X. (1983). Self-attention and self-report: The "veridicality" hypothesis. *Journal of Personality, 51,* 517–542.

Gibbons, F. X., Carver, C. S., Scheier, M. F., & Hormuth, S. E. (1979). Self-focused attention and the placebo effect: Fooling some of the people some of the time. *Journal of Experimental Social Psychology, 15,* 263–274.

Gibbons, F. X., Smith, T. W., Ingram, R. E., Pearce, K., Brehm, S. S., & Schroeder, D. J. (1985). Self-awareness and self-confrontation: Effects of self-focused attention on members of a clinical population. *Journal of Personality and Social Psychology, 48,* 662–675.

Greenberg, J. (1980). Attentional focus and locus of performance causality as determinants of equity behavior. *Journal of Personality and Social Psychology, 38,* 579–585.

Heider, F. (1944). Social perception and phenomenal causality. *Psychological Review, 51,* 358–374.

Helgeson, V. S., & Taylor, S. E. (1993). Social comparisons and adjustment among cardiac patients. *Journal of Applied Social Psychology, 23,* 1171–1195.

Hjelle, L. A., & Bernard, M. (1994). Private self-consciousness and the retest reliability of self-reports. *Journal of Research in Personality, 28,* 52–67.

Hull, C. L. (1943). *Principles of behavior*. New York: Appleton-Century-Crofts.

Hull, J. G. (1981). A self-awareness model of the causes and effects of alcohol consumption. *Journal of Abnormal Psychology, 90,* 586–600.

Hull, J. G., & Levy, A. S. (1979). The organizational function of the self: An alternative to the Duval and Wicklund model of self-awareness. *Journal of Personality and Social Psychology, 37,* 756–768.

James, W. (1890). *The principles of psychology*. New York: Holt.

Kernis, M. H., & Reis, H. T. (1984). Self-consciousness, self-awareness, and justice in reward allocation. *Journal of Personality, 52,* 58–70.

Klinger, E. (1975). Consequences of commitment to and disengagement from incentives. *Psychological Review, 82,* 1–25.

MacKay, D. M. (1956). The epistemological problem for automata. In C. E. Shannon & J. McCarthy (Eds.), *Automata studies* (pp. 235–251). Princeton, NJ: Princeton University Press.

MacKay, D. M. (1963). Mindlike behavior in artefacts. In K. M. Sayre & F. J. Crosson (Eds.), *The modeling of mind: Computers and intelligence* (pp. 225–241). Notre Dame, IN: University of Notre Dame Press.

Macrae, C. N., Bodenhausen, G. V., & Milne, A. B. (1998). Saying no to unwanted thoughts: Self-focus and the regulation of mental life. *Journal of Personality and Social Psychology, 74,* 578–589.

Mead, G. H. (1934). *Mind, self, and society*. Chicago: University of Chicago Press.

Miller, G. A., Galanter, E., & Pribram, K. H. (1960). *Plans and the structure of behavior*. New York: Holt, Rinehart & Winston.

Nasby, W. (1985). Private self-consciousness, articulation of the self-schema, and recognition memory of trait adjectives. *Journal of Personality and Social Psychology, 49,* 704–709.

Nasby, W. (1989a). Private and public self-consciousness and articulation of the self-schema. *Journal of Personality and Social Psychology, 56,* 117–123.

Nasby, W. (1989b). Private self-consciousness, self-awareness, and the reliability of self-reports. *Journal of Personality and Social Psychology, 56,* 950–957.

Newcomb, T. M. (1950). *Social psychology*. New York: Dryden Press.

Powers, W. T. (1973). *Behavior: The control of perception*. Chicago: Aldine.

Ryan, R. M., & Deci, E. L. (1999). Approaching and avoiding self-determination: Comparing cybernetic and organismic paradigms of motivation. In R. S. Wyer, Jr. (Ed.), *Advances in social cognition* (Vol. 12, pp. 193–215). Mahwah, NJ: Erlbaum.

Scheier, M. F. (1976). Self-awareness, self-consciousness, and angry aggression. *Journal of Personality, 44,* 627–644.

Scheier, M. F., & Carver, C. S. (1977). Self-focused attention and the experience of emotion: Attraction, repulsion, elation, and depression. *Journal of Personality and Social Psychology, 35,* 625–636.

Scheier, M. F., & Carver, C. S. (1983). Self-directed attention and the comparison of self with standards. *Journal of Experimental Social Psychology, 19,* 205–222.

Scheier, M. F., & Carver, C. S. (1985). Optimism, coping,

and health: Assessment and implications of generalized outcome expectancies. *Health Psychology, 4,* 219–247.

Scheier, M. F., & Carver, C. S. (1992). Effects of optimism on psychological and physical well-being: Theoretical overview and empirical update. *Cognitive Therapy and Research, 16,* 201–228.

Scheier, M. F., Carver, C. S., & Bridges, M. W. (2001). Optimism, pessimism, and psychological well-being. In E. C. Chang (Ed.), *Optimism and pessimism: Implications for theory, research, and practice* (pp. 189–216). Washington, DC: American Psychological Association.

Scheier, M. F., Carver, C. S., & Gibbons, F. X. (1979). Self-directed attention, awareness of bodily states, and suggestibility. *Journal of Personality and Social Psychology, 37,* 1576–1588.

Scheier, M. F., Fenigstein, A., & Buss, A. H. (1974). Self-awareness and physical aggression. *Journal of Experimental Social Psychology, 10,* 264–273.

Schlenker, B. R., & Leary, M. R. (1982). Social anxiety and self-presentation: A conceptualization and model. *Psychological Bulletin, 92,* 641–669.

Shibutani, T. (1961). *Society and personality: An interactionist approach to social psychology.* Englewood Cliffs, NJ: Prentice-Hall.

Silvia, P. J., & Duval, T. S. (2001). Objective self-awareness theory: Recent progress and enduring problems. *Personality and Social Psychology Review, 5,* 230–241.

Silvia, P. J., & Gendolla, G. H. E. (2001). On introspection and self-perception: Does self-focused attention enable accurate self-knowledge? *Review of General Psychology, 5,* 241–269.

Spence, K. W. (1956). *Behavior theory and conditioning.* New Haven, CT: Yale University Press.

Steenbarger, B. N., & Aderman, D. (1979). Objective self-awareness as a nonaversive state: Effect of anticipating discrepancy reduction. *Journal of Personality, 47,* 330–339.

Stuss, D. T. (1991). Self, awareness, and the frontal lobes: A neuropsychological perspective. In J. Strauss & G. R. Goethals (Eds.), *The self: Interdisciplinary approaches* (pp. 255–278). New York: Springer-Verlag.

Stuss, D. T., & Alexander, M. P. (2000). Executive functions and the frontal lobes: A conceptual view. *Psychological Research/Psychologische-Forschung, 63,* 289–298.

Stuss, D. T., Alexander, M. P., & Benson, D. F. (1997). Frontal lobe functions. In M. R. Trimble & J. L. Cummings (Eds.), *Contemporary behavioral neurology: Blue books of practical neurology* (Vol. 16, pp. 169–187). Woburn, MA: Butterworth-Heinemann.

Stuss, D. T., & Levine, B. (2002). Adult clinical neuropsychology: Lessons from studies of the frontal lobes. *Annual Review of Psychology, 53,* 401–433.

Trapnell, P. D., & Campbell, J. D. (1999). Private self-consciousness and the five-factor model of personality: Distinguishing rumination from reflection. *Journal of Personality and Social Psychology, 76,* 284–304.

Tulving, E. (1989). Memory: Performance, knowledge, and experience. *European Journal of Cognitive Psychology, 1,* 3–26.

Turner, R. G. (1978) Self-consciousness and speed of processing self-relevant information. *Personality and Social Psychology Bulletin, 4,* 456–460.

Vallacher, R. R., & Wegner, D. M. (1987). What do people think they're doing? Action identification and human behavior. *Psychological Review, 94,* 3–15.

Wicklund, R. A. (1975). Objective self-awareness. In L. Berkowitz (Ed.), *Advances in experimental social psychology* (Vol. 8, pp. 233–275). New York: Academic Press.

Wicklund, R. A., & Duval, S. (1971). Opinion change and performance facilitation as a result of objective self-awareness. *Journal of Experimental Social Psychology, 7,* 319–342.

Wicklund, R. A., & Gollwitzer, P. M. (1987). The fallacy of the private-public self-focus distinction. *Journal of Personality, 55,* 491–523.

Wiener, N. (1948). *Cybernetics: Control and communcation in the animal and the machine.* Cambridge, MA: MIT Press.

Wood, J. V. (1989). Theory and research concerning social comparisons of personal attributes. *Psychological Bulletin, 106,* 231–248.

Wood, J. V. (1996). What is social comparison and how should we study it? *Personality and Social Psychology Bulletin, 22,* 520–537.

Wortman, C. B., & Brehm, J. W. (1975). Responses to uncontrollable outcomes: An integration of reactance theory and the learned helplessness model. In L. Berkowitz (Ed.), *Advances in experimental social psychology* (Vol. 8, pp. 277–336). New York: Academic Press.

Wylie, R. C. (1968). The present state of self theory. In E. F. Borgatta & W. W. Lambert (Eds.), *Handbook of personality theory and research* (pp. 728–787). Chicago: Rand McNally.

10

Self-Regulation and the Executive Function of the Self

ROY F. BAUMEISTER
KATHLEEN D. VOHS

The self is not a passive, indifferent, or unresponsive entity. Rather, the self is active, involved, and responsive, intentionally engaging in volitional processes to change, alter, or modify itself. Processes such as altering one's own behavior, resisting temptation, and changing one's moods are characterized by the terms "self-control" and "self-regulation." More broadly, the self takes action, selects a response from numerous options, filters irrelevant information, and is responsible for response selection and enactment. The aspect of the self that initiates behaviors and makes selections is called the executive function.

Defined as such, executive functioning and self-regulation are ubiquitous. Activities as varied as inhibiting a triumphant smile or snide remark, choosing what sweater to wear, suppressing undesired thoughts, running a marathon, practicing safe sex, and being attentive during boring meetings involve self-control and self-regulation.

Psychologists invoked the term "self-regulation" to apply learning theories to human behavior, which is often self-directed and volitional (although self-regulation does not have to be consciously initiated; see Chartrand & Bargh, 1996). Some researchers, such as Deci and Ryan (1991), Higgins (1989), and Banaji and Prentice (1994), have focused on the willful, intentional acts in which people engage to align themselves with the person they ideally want to be or should be. Although most of the empirical research covered in this review involves carefully crafted experimental situations that assess self-regulation within a short time period, in actuality, people's self-regulatory efforts are often aimed at both short- and long-term goals. Thus human behavior goes beyond the stimulus–response models that are well-suited to animal learning theories. Rather, contemporary self-regulation theories aim to understand how, over periods of days, weeks, and years, people resist temptations, effortfully persist, and carefully weigh options to choose the optimal course of action to reach their goals.

Theories of self-regulation and self-control flourished in the 1980s and 1990s, followed by a wealth of empirical research to test the validity of these ideas. During the past two decades, the field has made great strides in understanding self-regulation by refining theories of self-regulatory processes and amassing vast amounts of data to test our theories. Consequently, the importance of self-regulation now appears immediate and obvious. Some recent works have begun to treat executive functioning as one of the most important functions of the self (Baumeister, 1998; Carver & Scheier, 1998; Higgins, 1997). In addition to scientific advances (e.g., theories, empirical evidence) that have illuminated the significance of self-regulation in maximizing the capabilities of the self, historical changes also illustrate the considerable role that self-regulation plays in people's everyday lives.

The role of self-regulation is especially acute in modern cultures, insofar as people may now be faced with more choices and decisions every day than people of times past were faced with in a year (see Schwartz, 2000, p. 81, on the so-called "tyranny of choice"). Moreover, identity in contemporary society is very much a product of self-regulation, especially in relation to people of premodern cultures (see Baumeister, 1997). Looking back to premodern cultures, we see that people's identities were formed in relation to a group with which they were intimately associated. Moreover, identity was created through a sequence of established rites, rituals, ceremonies, and other cultural experiences. It was once common and normative for people to live among the same group of others from birth until death, and in such a context a person's identity was defined by the group and sustained by it, with little opportunity for choice or change. In contrast, the increasing individualization and mobility of Western societies have shifted the burden of responsibility for creating and sustaining identity to the individual. It is now unusual for a person in a modern Western society to spend an entire life in the same town, whereas once it may have been commonplace. Moreover, even if a person does happen to remain in one place for a lifetime, friends and neighbors are likely to move away, and, hence, the person's social network would likely undergo significant change regardless of their stationary state. One scholar described the increasing indi-

vidualization of the United States over the 20th century as a "gradual release . . . in which the individual's linkages to traditional social collectivities (e.g., extended family, local community, status group) have tended to weaken" (Buchmann, 1989; p. 21). The inevitable changing of one's social network frees the person from many external constraints that once required stability of identity. In its place are both an opportunity to change and often even a necessity of reinventing and redefining oneself.

Indeed, one of the most celebrated cultural stories of the United States is the tale of the person who overcame trials and tribulations to become a great individual—a mighty athlete, an international scholar, a successful entrepreneur, or president of the United States. Now that a person's identity is almost wholly self-determined (or so Americans prefer to believe) and people are given more choice in determining their life course, each aspect of the self has the appearance of being intentionally developed. Furthermore, a lack of ties to extended family and local community and the high degree of mobility of modern lives suggest that people not only have to establish their identities but may do so over and over again with each new setting. The process demands much from the self, in terms of developing and maintaining a coherent sense of identity—especially if people are forced to repeatedly re-create a sense of who they are with each change in environment. Thus the link between self-regulation and identity in modern Western cultures certainly adds to the burden of selfhood.

Definitional Matters and Conceptual Distinctions

Our review focuses on the executive function of the self, with emphasis on self-regulation and self-control, which are considered subcomponent processes of the executive function. In this section, we first distinguish among these concepts by providing definitions and examples, and then we detail some theories on the purpose of having these functions as part of the self.

The active, intentional aspect of the self is referred to as the *executive function* of the self or in terms of the *agentic* nature of the self (see Baumeister, 1998; Gazzaniga, Ivry, & Mangun, 1998). The executive function of the self can be thought of as the aspect of the self that is ultimately responsible for the actions of the individual. We prefer to use "executive function" because the term "agent" is somewhat misleading, at least with respect to its common usage of someone acting on behalf of another party. When speaking of the agentic nature of the self, there is an implied reflexiveness in terms of who is acting on behalf of whom: The self is acting on itself, on behalf of its own selfhood. It could be said, however, that the use of the word "agent" in English parallels the "agentic" aspects of the self if one recalls the distinction between self as subject ("I") and self as object ("me") as described by William James (1890/1950).

To define the executive function of the self as the self-aspect that initiates behavior suggests that it is all-encompassing or omnipresent. On the contrary, there is a host of human responses and behaviors that do not invoke the executive function. Examples of nonexecutive functioning behaviors are coordination of motor movements, reflexively turning away from a flame, or jiggling one's leg back and forth. In contrast, many actions do require executive functioning. Signing up for a dance class, getting divorced, and asking for a raise are tasks that come from the executive function. Behavior can occur without much in the way of a self, after all, as is shown by the behaviors of many psychologically simpler creatures. Human organisms would also behave if they did not have selves. The self is, however, a structure that can exert considerable "steering" control over behavior, such as by altering the course of behavior, refraining from some responses, and initiating behavior that would not otherwise be activated by the immediate stimulus environment. The self's executive function thus dramatically increases the range, complexity, and diversity of human behavior. It is involved, for instance, in making the deliberate (but often inconsequential) decisions that are required to move through everyday life, such as what color socks to wear, what to cook for dinner, and what movie to see.

Less broad than the concept of executive functioning, self-regulation involves the self acting on itself to alter its own responses with the (conscious or nonconscious) goal of producing a desired outcome. Hence, the process of self-regulation involves overriding a natural, habitual, or learned response by altering behavior, thoughts, or emotions. This process includes interrupting a response by changing or modifying it, substituting another response in its place, or blocking an additional response from occurring (Baumeister, 1998; Baumeister, Heatherton, & Tice, 1994). The process of self-regulation has been broken down into three components: establishing a goal or desired state, engaging in appropriate behaviors to obtain one's goals (Baumeister et al., 1994; Carver & Scheier, 1981), and monitoring progress toward the goal (which requires tracking the distance between one's current state and the desired state). In the realm of nonconscious self-regulation, for example, one could repeatedly—but unconsciously—be exposed to situational cues that prime a certain goal (e.g., Chartrand & Bargh, 1996), could experience affective consequences as a result of perceived progress toward the nonconscious goal (e.g., Chartrand, Tesser, & Cheng, 2001), and could use regulatory resources to achieve the unstated goal (Vohs & Baumeister, 2001).

The terms "self-regulation," "self-control," and "self-discipline" are often used interchangeably, although some authors draw distinctions among them. The term "self-regulation" is generally given the broadest usage, as it encapsulates both the conscious and nonconscious forms of altering the self. The term "self-control" is close to the term "self-regulation," but typically it implies a more deliberate, conscious process of altering the self. Some authors use "self-control" to refer specifically to the processes by which the self inhibits unwanted responses (e.g., resisting temptation or holding one's tongue when angry). "Self-discipline" is a yet more narrow and specific term that refers to people's intentional plans to improve or better themselves, most likely in accordance with cultural norms or mores. Thus the focus of this chapter is on research and theory relating to self-regulation generally, under which the other two terms are subsumed.

Evolutionarily, the ultimate purpose of the executive function is probably to improve the fit between the self and the environment (Gazzaniga et al., 1998). Because it is extremely difficult—in fact, probably impossible until modern times—to significantly modify aspects of the environment to fit the self, the goal of achieving the tightest fit between the self and the surroundings was best achieved by having a self that is capable of change. Thus creatures with a flexible self would be most likely to pass on their genes because they would be able to adapt to changes in setting (e.g., nomadic life), changes in environmental contingencies, and changes in interpersonal relationships. Conversely, creatures without a flexible self would be left to the mercy of the environment, with any and all changes lowering their chances of survival, or such creatures would spend excessive amount of time and energy trying futilely to create the perfect environment for themselves. Probably one of the most crucial and adaptive aspects of the executive function is the ability to guide current behavior according to long-term goals that lie well beyond the immediate situation. Delaying gratification, making long-term plans (and pursuing them), and preparing for possible events all involve self-regulation, and all of them probably contributed greatly to the survival and reproductive success of the first human beings to develop the requisite capacity.

Similarly, Sedikides and Skowronski (1997) posit that the modern self emerged during the Pleistocene epoch as the result of social and ecological demands that created a need for a symbolic self. (Leary, 2001, has suggested a more recent origin, based on a more sophisticated definition of self.) Part of the core aspects of a symbolic self are the abilities to (1) set goals; (2) engage in goal-directed behaviors; and (3) assess whether progress toward the goal has been made—that is, to engage in self-regulatory processes so as to alter the self in response to environmental pressures (Sedikides & Skowronski, 1997).

From an evolutionary perspective, there may also have been certain types of stimuli or information that promoted self-regulation. Specifically, recent postulates suggest that the presence of negative feedback or stimuli may have served as a catalyst for change (see Baumeister, Bratslavsky, Finkenauer, & Vohs, 2001). If an organism perceives something negative in the environment—whether through direct perceptual contact (e.g., seeing the snarling face of a tiger) or indirectly, perhaps via a negative emotional state (see Schwarz & Clore, 1983)—this information may trigger self-regulatory processes aimed at changing the self in some way so as to decrease (or eradicate) the negativity. From this perspective, creatures that could and would change themselves in response to negative or threatening stimuli would likely live to pass along their genes. Conversely, creatures that did not change themselves in response to environmental threats were less likely to live and to reproduce. The self is required in this process insofar as the changes in behavior as a result of negative or aversive stimuli are not merely reflexive but rather involve actively changing the self to avoid the presence of future negative stimuli. Thus different evolutionary factors—social and ecological pressures (Sedikides & Skowronski, 1997) and negative or threatening stimuli (Baumeister et al., 2001)—may have played a role in the development of self-regulatory capacities in modern-day humans.

Review of Theories and Empirical Evidence

Social psychologists have studied the concept of self-regulation using a variety of approaches, such as developmental models, (e.g., Mischel & Ebbesen, 1970), cybernetic models (Carver & Scheier, 1982), personality trait models (e.g., Funder, Block, & Block, 1983), cognitive factors (e.g., Metcalfe & Mischel, 1999), and the role of the self in the environment (e.g., Baumeister, 1998). For instance, classic experiments by Walter Mischel and colleagues (e.g., Mischel & Ebbesen, 1970; Mischel, Shoda, & Peake, 1988) illustrate the difficulty inherent in delaying gratification. Likewise, test–operate–test–exit (TOTE) models of self-regulation (e.g., Carver & Scheier, 1982) have emphasized the role of feedback loops in self-regulatory processes. Social psychologists have used empirical methods to address aspects of self-regulation such as appropriate goal setting (see Baumeister et al., 1994), the effects of pursuing competing—and sometimes conflicting—goals (e.g., Emmons & King, 1988), and the importance of affect and motivation (e.g., Pervin, 1989).

Recent advances in the study of self-regulation include theoretical reconceptualizations (e.g., Baumeister et al., 1994; Gollwitzer, 1999; Richards & Gross, 2000), refinements of current theories of self-regulatory processes (e.g., Carver & White, 1994; Metcalfe & Mischel, 1999), extensions of self-regulation theories into areas of study outside of the intrapsychic self (e.g., interpersonal functioning; Ciarocco, Sommer, & Baumeister, 2001; Finkel & Campbell, in press; Vohs, Ciarocco, & Baumeister, 2001), and a plethora of empirical studies on the processes of self-regulation. Hence, we think that a summary of the current status of self-regulation and self-control literature is particularly timely.

Control and Efficacy

We begin our review of the executive function of the self by summarizing the literature on control. Psychologists have long contended that people have a need for control (or need to believe they have control; see Langer, 1975; Taylor, 1983). Researchers brought to light the psychological effects of perceived control in studies on the deleterious effects of lack of control over one's environment (e.g., Glass, Singer, & Friedman, 1969). The results of these studies showed that humans possess a powerful drive to feel in control of a variety of outcomes, from controlling aversive noise bursts (Alloy & Abramson, 1982) and picking a winning lottery ticket (Langer, 1975; Langer & Roth, 1975) to believing in unproven practices to stop disease (Taylor, 1983).

Studies assessing the desire for control found that when people perceived that they lacked control, they fought back to regain it (Brehm, 1966). Brehm's (1966) theory of reactance states that people will resist having control taken away because they have a deeply rooted motivation to maintain the freedom to exercise a broad range of options. Resistance comes in the form of attempts to reassert control or to aggress against the source of their loss of control, a response that is usually performed in cases in which people are unable to regain control. For example, reactance may be seen in

the responses of teenagers who have been told by their parents that they are not allowed to date a certain person. Instead of seeing that their parents are being lovingly protective of them or instead of seeing the would-be date as the undesirable partner that he or she may be, teenagers are notorious for acting out by not only dating this person but also professing their undying love for him or her.

When people are repeatedly deprived of control, they may give up and show a pattern of learned helplessness (Seligman, 1975). Seligman's research shows that when organisms are not given the opportunity to see that their actions have desired consequences—that is, when there is a perception of lack of personal control—they fail to acquire new response patterns. One of the most serious consequences of learned helplessness is that eventually people are unable and unwilling to attempt to escape from a maladaptive situation that has become avoidable.

In reality, however, people do not have direct control over most contingencies in their lives. It is, to say the least, dismaying to recognize and appreciate this fact. Perhaps not surprisingly, then, research has found that people with chronic—or even temporary—depression hold very accurate perceptions of their personal control (see Alloy & Abramson, 1979). In contrast, nondepressed people are overly optimistic about their ability to control life outcomes, well beyond the degree of control they truly possess.

These overestimations have been deemed "illusions of control" (Langer, 1975), and humans seem to be unique in their preference for such self-delusions. In fact, humans would make better choices and be more rational if they did not believe that they personally could control what are, in actuality, chance outcomes. For instance, in paradigms that ask participants to predict which of two lights will flash next, humans reliably perform worse than animals—even when participants are told that the sequence of the lights is randomly determined (Wolford, Miller, & Gazzaniga, 2000). Humans use a strategy of frequency matching, in which the probabilities of each light flashing are detected independently and then used to predict which light will appear next. Animals, conversely, use a maximization strategy, which involves detecting which light flashes more often and consistently choosing that light as the one to appear next.

Humans, then, do appear to be less rational creatures than rats (at least as measured by the ability to predict a series of flashing lights), which suggests that our illusions of control are probably rooted in our perception of complex patterns. Neuroscientists believe that the human brain (specifically, the left hemisphere) is innately prepared to interpret and transform incoming information into meaningful patterns (Gazzaniga, 1997). Thus, even in cases in which predictability (and, hence, control) is not possible, humans seek to establish illusions to the contrary.

Nevertheless, there are benefits to having illusions of control. As mentioned, there is a relation between seeing oneself as not having much control and depression. Moreover, believing one has control can improve one's outcomes through self-efficacy processes. Research by Bandura (e.g., 1977, 1989) demonstrates that when people feel they can produce the behaviors necessary to bring about life changes, they are more successful in achieving their goals.

The distinction between the processes of primary and secondary control (e.g., Rothbaum, Weisz, & Snyder, 1982) relates not only to executive functioning but also to current theories of self-regulation. Rothbaum and colleagues' (1982) analysis of control differentiated between primary control, which is aimed at altering the environment for the self, versus secondary control, which is aimed at altering the self to fit the environment. Although people do engage in both types of control, there are circumstances in which one form is more appropriate than the other. Situations that allow for change, such as tasks within one's home, may respond well to primary control processes. In contrast, situations that do not allow for much change respond best to secondary control (Band & Weisz, 1988; Shaw, 1992; Weisz, McCabe, & Dennig, 1994). Consistent with the definitions of self-control and self-regulation stated previously, we believe that situations that call for secondary control processes are more prevalent than those requiring primary control and, moreover, that changing the self is a more

adaptive approach to solving most environment–self discrepancies.

A related issue to perceptions of control is having to make a series of decisions. Researchers have noted that the incidence of self-regulation failure (e.g., criminal acts, overeating, losing patience with others) increases late in the day (Baumeister & Heatherton, 1996), after people have spent the entire day making decisions. To investigate this link further, researchers asked some people to make a series of binary choices, such as deciding whether they would rather have a lemon or a vanilla candle, whereas others were asked to merely rate how often they would use such a product. Subsequent tests of self-regulatory ability showed that people who were asked to make multiple choices showed decrements in self-regulation (Twenge, Tice, Schmeichel, & Baumeister, 2001). Thus the act of making decisions robs the self of the ability to self-regulate. This may explain some of the negative effects of control that other authors have noted. For example, Burger (1989) showed that many people seemed to shirk or avoid control when they could exert it, and Iyengar and Lepper (2000) found that people exhibit negative reactions to having too many options to decide among.

Another approach to studying issues of personal control has arisen from self-determination theory (Deci & Ryan, 1991, 1995). Self-determination theory emphasizes three different motives of the self—competence, autonomy, and relatedness—as being central to achieving personally satisfying and rewarding goals. The motive for competence involves feeling efficacious and able to obtain intrinsically driven goals; the motive for autonomy involves feeling as if one's actions come from within the self and are not driven by exterior pressures; and the motive for relatedness involves establishing and sustaining interpersonal connections that satisfy a person's need to belong.

Self-determination theory has been used to predict the consequences of pursuing life goals related to intrinsic rewards versus the consequences of pursuing goals that are promoted by outside forces. Kasser and Ryan (1993, 1996) found that when people pursued goals that were extrinsically motivated (i.e., that were not self-determined, such as money and physical attractiveness), they showed higher levels of anxiety and depression and were less well off on other mental health indices. Conversely, people who were self-determined (i.e., who pursued intrinsically motivated goals, such as personal growth and satisfying interpersonal relations), exhibited better mental health.

Thus the literature on efficacy and control points to the importance of several factors in determining the likelihood of obtaining valued outcomes. Perceptions of control are of supreme importance, such that there is an almost instinctive desire for control which, consequently, leads people to overestimate their ability to exert control (e.g., Langer, 1975). People do not, however, use the most rational strategies when choosing and making decisions (Wolford et al., 2000), and, moreover, the act of making repeated decisions leaves people fatigued and less able to perform subsequent regulatory acts (Twenge et al., 2001). The types of goals that people attempt to achieve (e.g., Deci & Ryan, 1991) and perceptions of their ability to perform goal-directed behaviors (e.g., Bandura, Caprara, Barbaranelli, Pastorelli, & Regalia, 2001) also play a role in the cognitive and affective processes that accompany self-regulatory functions. Findings that there are limitations (e.g., fatigue) and biases (e.g., overestimations of control) are especially informative because they give indications as to the nature of the executive function. Next we review the extensive body of research on delay of gratification, as it provides a particularly illustrative example of the significance of self-control for immediate and long-term outcomes.

Delay of Gratification

The importance of self-regulation and self-control—both in daily life and over time—has been highlighted by research on delay of gratification by Walter Mischel and colleagues (e.g., Mischel & Ebbesen, 1970; Mischel, Shoda, & Peake, 1988). Delay of gratification is an important form of self-regulation because it requires overriding one's most pressing and salient impulses, namely to do whatever will bring immediate gratification, in order to pursue other goals and outcomes that may objectively be more desirable but that will not materialize for some time.

Mischel and others have illustrated the difficulty inherent in delaying gratification under tempting conditions. In these studies, children are presented with the choice between an immediately available treat or a more attractive treat at a later time. Successful delay of gratification involves several factors, most notably the use of effective cognitive strategies. In their hot–cold model of self-regulation, Metcalfe and Mischel (1999) posit that "hot" cognitions focus on the rewarding, pleasurable, appetizing aspects of objects, whereas "cold" cognitions focus on conceptual or symbolic meanings. Thus engaging in cognitive transformations—changing consummatory "hot" cognitions (e.g., thinking of how yummy marshmallows taste) into informational "cool" cognitions (e.g., imagining marshmallows as little clouds)—predicts delay of gratification in children (see Metcalfe & Mischel, 1999). Other successful strategies involve distraction (e.g., singing a song to oneself; although note that the song must not be about the yumminess of the marshmallows or it does not serve as a successful distracter) and removing the marshmallows from one's line of sight (e.g., by covering one's eyes or turning away; see Mischel et al., 1988). Thus delay of gratification experiments not only provided a paradigm within which to study self-regulation but also demonstrated that the seemingly simple act of self-stopping is extremely difficult.

Furthermore, ability to delay gratification affects personal well-being. Mischel and colleagues investigated the long-term importance of ability to delay gratification by using delay of gratification scores obtained at age 4 to predict social and cognitive outcomes assessed at ages 14–15 (Mischel et al., 1988). Being able to resist the temptations of available cookies or other enticing treats in childhood predicted successful adjustment in adolescence. That is, children who were good at delaying gratification at an early age were more likely to do well academically, be socially skilled, and deal with setbacks and frustrations more easily. Even more impressive is the finding that delay of gratification ability at age 4 predicts higher SAT scores, a finding that was stronger than using intelligence scores at age 4 to predict later SAT scores (Shoda, Mischel, & Peake, 1990).

More recently, Metcalfe and Mischel (1999) have proposed a refinement of executive function theories by proposing a hot–cold theory of self-regulation. As stated, Metcalfe and Mischel draw distinctions between construing an object or goal in terms of its rewarding, pleasurable, appetizing aspects (i.e., construe the object in "hot" terms) and construing an object or goal conceptually or symbolically (i.e., construe the object in "cool" terms). Moreover, Metcalfe and Jacobs (1998) have proposed that threatening stimuli activate hot memory systems and deactivate cold memory systems. Hence, when the appetitive "hot" system is activated (e.g., by food cues for chronic dieters), it is more difficult to delay gratification. Metcalfe and Mischel propose that the hot–cold distinction is based on how information is processed in the brain, with the hot system being amygdala-based and the cold system being hippocampus-based. According to this theory, the amygdala processes the appetitive and reward features of biologically significant stimuli. Conversely, the hippocampus is related to making plans, strategies, and goals, and is therefore responsible for self-control. Relating this theory back to the delay-of-gratification paradigm, it may be that temptation arises when an object's mental representation is transformed from cold to hot (or from hot to hotter), thereby activating neurological substrates related to appetitive behaviors and deactivating those related to goal attainment.

Feedback Loops

One prominent conceptualization of self-regulatory processes is feedback loops, most notably the test–operate–test–exit (TOTE) models proposed by Carver and Scheier (e.g., Carver & Scheier, 1981, 1982, 1998; based on Powers, 1973) as a supervisory process (cf. Norman & Shallice, 1986). In the initial "test" phase, a person evaluates his or her current status on some dimension (e.g., current body weight) in comparison with a desired end state (e.g., ideal body weight). The "operate" phase involves efforts to bring the self into line with the standard, and progress toward that goal is monitored by further "test" phases. When a test finally reveals that the standard has been met, the process is terminated, which constitutes the "exit" phase of the loop.

The act of setting standards itself can be a regulatory problem because, on the one hand, setting standards that are too high means increased likelihood that one will not achieve the goal. On the other hand, setting standards that are too low only ensures that one obtains the goal, even at the expense of rendering the goal less desirable. Research on the self-regulatory effects of self-esteem is relevant here: Under conditions of threat, people with high self-esteem set lofty goals that are less obtainable, whereas people with low self-esteem are more cautious, setting moderate goals that are less daring but also more readily achieved (Baumeister, Heatherton, & Tice, 1993; see also a conceptual replication of these results that measured participants' grenade-throwing estimates and actual distance after failure on a military test of leadership; Smith, Norrell, & Saint, 1996).

Research on perceived discrepancies also relates to personality traits. Perfectionism is a personality trait that strongly relates to—and, in fact, is defined by—habitually establishing lofty or unrealistic standards. As an example, research on women and their perceptions of their bodies has shown that women who are high in perfectionism are more likely to see themselves as overweight (Vohs, Bardone, Joiner, Abramson, & Heatherton, 1999) and to be dissatisfied with their bodies (Vohs et al., 2001). That women high and low in perfectionism do not differ in actual body weight indicates that women high in perfectionism set standards for thinness that are higher than their current body weight. These unachievable standards increase the likelihood of failure, the result of which can be the development of bulimic symptoms.

Recent research demonstrates that the self-regulatory goals people attempt to obtain are sometimes outside of their awareness. Work by Chartrand and Bargh (1996) shows that goals can be activated and acted on automatically. This line of research follows from Bargh's (1990) auto-motive theory, which states that conscious awareness of goals is not necessary for their stimulation and operation. Thus, with repeated pairings between an environment and certain goals, the mental representation of the goal may become automatically linked to the cognitive representation of the situation. Then, when aspects of the situation arise again, they can activate the relevant goal. According to this approach, the plans people have to reach the goal, as well as the subsequent actions they engage in, may also be initiated nonconsciously, thereby placing the whole cycle of goal activation and operation outside of the person's awareness. This model, then, suggests that a person may possess a self-regulatory goal, enact plans to achieve this goal, and exhibit behavior relevant to the goal, all without one's intention or perception.

Empirical research using this model has shown that goals can be activated nonconsciously through the use of primes (e.g., Chartrand & Bargh, 1996) and, moreover, that success or failure at a nonconscious goal may affect mood. According to work on so-called mystery moods (e.g., Tesser, Martin, & Cornell, 1996), nonspecific negative mood states are often present when people engage in self-enhancement. To further investigate the underlying mechanisms, Chartrand and colleagues (Chartrand, Tesser, & Cheng, 2001) investigated whether success versus failure at a nonconscious goal predicted self-enhancement. Chartrand and colleagues (2001) found that participants who failed at an anagram task after being nonconsciously primed with an achievement goal self-enhanced more than participants who failed but who were not primed and more than those who were given an explicit achievement goal.

Additional research on nonconscious processes has confirmed their effects on subsequent behavior. Vohs and Baumeister (2001) asked participants to perform either a flexing motion that involved bringing the arm up toward the body (as if performing a bicep curl) or an extending motion that involved pushing the arm down and away from the body. These motions were selected because they are considered nonconscious activators of approach and avoidance motivations, respectively (e.g., Neumann & Strack, 2000). Participants were given prompts every 2 minutes to perform their assigned motion while they worked on an unsolvable task of finding strings of numbers within a large grid of numbers and were told that they could stop working on the task whenever they desired. The type of motion participants were randomly assigned to perform significantly predicted length of time spent on the task, such that the flexing motion predicted more persistence than the extending motion, indicating increased motivation among participants in the flex condition. Thus research indicates that nonconsciously activated goals can have considerable influence on subsequent emotions, thoughts, and motivations.

With regard to TOTE models, a more specific definition of the "test" aspect of the model involves the process of assessing whether one has reached the established standard. If not, and if a discrepancy between one's current and desired state is perceived, then people move into the next step of the model, the "operate" mode. This component of the TOTE model has received less attention than the other components, although theories and empirical findings are beginning to accumulate (see also the subsequent section, "Self-Regulatory Resource Model").

One promising theory of effective ways in which to change the self to reach a goal is Gollwitzer's (e.g., 1993, 1999) implementation intentions theory. Gollwitzer conceptualizes the obtainment of goals in terms of action intentions that enable people to cope with obstacles or initiate behaviors. These implementation intentions are separate from goal intentions, which specify the end state the person desires to reach. Implementation intentions instead focus on the means by which people will achieve the goal; thus they underlie goal intentions. Implementation intentions take more of a conditional form, stating that when certain situations or conditions arise, certain behaviors will be performed. For instance, when trying to maintain a diet, a person might think, "When pieces of cake are passed around, I will say that I am too full to eat." Gollwitzer's (1999) empirical research shows that implementation intentions—either self-directed or situationally induced—help people to start on their goals. For instance, participants who were asked to write a report on how they spent Christmas Eve were either induced to think about when and where they would write the report or were simply asked to write the report. Within 48 hours of Christmas Eve (the time frame within which the reports were to be written), 75% of participants induced to make implementation intentions wrote a report, whereas only 33% of control participants completed the assignment (Gollwitzer & Brandstätter, 1997).

Gollwitzer (e.g., 1993) proposed that the mechanisms responsible for the beneficial effects of implementation intentions are (1) forming a mental representation of the hypothesized situation and (2) making the actions to be implemented more automatic. With respect to the former, Gollwitzer (1996) has found heightened perceptual and attentional responses among people who form implementation intentions relative to those who do not, suggesting that after implementation intentions are enacted, situations that contain the anticipated criteria garner more attention and, hence, promote the intended actions. With respect to the second mechanism, automatization, Gollwitzer's research (Gollwitzer & Brandstätter, 1997) has found that people who have been induced to form implementation intentions against racist remarks were quicker to initiate their counterarguments than were participants who only had the goal (not the implementation) intention to provide counterarguments.

Another theoretical approach to the study of the mechanisms of self-regulation has been proposed by Gross (1999), who conceptualizes emotion regulation in terms of antecedent-focused versus response-focused strategies. Antecedent-focused regulation comes before (or early in) the emotion-provoking process and involves four different methods of preemptively managing one's emotional state. Gross labels these four methods situation selection, situation modification, attentional deployment, and cognitive change. Situation selection involves choosing specific types of people, places, and objects that optimize one's emotional state. Situation modification involves intentionally changing a situation in order to modify its effects on one's emotions. Attentional deployment refers to an effortful emphasis on certain aspects of the situation that will best suit one's emotional goals. The fourth method, cognitive change (also called reappraisal), is used when the other three options are not available, because it involves reconstruing the situation to make

it less emotion provoking. As an example, if a couple wants to have a nice evening out, they might select a restaurant known to have a romantic setting (situation selection), ask to be moved if the mood is less than romantic because they are seated next to the kitchen (situation modification), look into each others' eyes when talking (attentional deployment), and relabel the situation as humorous when the waiter spills wine all over the man's shirt (reappraisal). In contrast, response-focused methods occur after a full emotional reaction. Gross lists response modulation, the act of directly controlling emotional responses (e.g., suppressing disappointment and amplifying relief when one is not chosen for a high-level executive position), as the primary response-focused regulation strategies.

Research by Gross (1999) and others shows that there exists specificity in terms of the effects of different emotion-regulation strategies. For instance, pretending that gruesome pictures of dead people come from the set of a movie rather than from police files dampens self-reported emotional experience and facial expressiveness (Kramer, Buckhout, Fox, Widman, & Tusche, 1991). Additionally, appraising environmental demands as challenging rather than threatening produces reliable cognitive, affective, and physiological consequences (Tomaka, Blascovich, Kibler, & Ernst, 1997) relevant to self-regulation. Appraisals of challenge, in which people believe they have the ability to cope with the stressor, lead to positive affect, low negative affect, and increased cardiovascular activity, combined with decreased vascular resistance ("efficient" and "organized" physiological reactions). Conversely, appraisals of threat, in which people believe that the stressor is too great for their perceived abilities, lead to negative affect and to "disorganized" physiological reactions such as moderate cardiac activity combined with an increase in vascular resistance. Furthermore, research by Richards and Gross (2000) shows that relative to controlling emotions through cognitive reappraisal, suppressing emotions results in decrements in memory. These results suggest that regulating emotions after an emotional response has been triggered requires regulatory resources that would otherwise be devoted to cognitive tasks, such as focusing attention.

To determine whether the behaviors one has enacted to close the discrepancy between current and desired goals have been successful, one must monitor his or her progress. Reduced monitoring is a prime cause of self-regulatory failure because it is easy to stop regulating if one fails to evaluate oneself relative to the goal (e.g., Kirschenbaum, 1987). For instance, dieters are often taught to keep a journal of their daily food intake and exercise to help them recognize their current caloric intake and expenditures. In support of the effectiveness of monitoring, research has shown that chronic dieters who are aware of their caloric intake eat significantly less than dieters who are inattentive (Polivy, Herman, Hackett, & Kuleshnyk, 1986). Deindividuation has also been cited as an example of reduced monitoring, wherein people lose awareness of the self as an individual and instead become another component of a larger movement (e.g., Diener, 1979). When people are deindividuated, they are more likely to engage in behaviors that violate their personal morals, such as committing violent acts as part of a lynch mob (Mullen, 1986).

In addition to setting appropriate and valued standards, engaging in goal-directed behaviors, and monitoring oneself with regard to a single objective, in actuality, people attempt to achieve multiple, distinct goals; as a result, some of these goals may be in conflict with each other. For instance, a woman may have the goal of eating healthy foods but also have the goal of being nice to her husband. Hence, when her husband brings home greasy hamburgers and french fries for dinner, her goals may be in conflict. Research by Emmons and King (1988) shows that when people possess multiple, conflicting goals, the resulting state is rumination and a lack of progress toward any of them.

Recent work has extended the notion of feedback loop models to incorporate a theory of motivational processes as related to the type of goal states being attained. One class of goals involves attempts to reach desired states by concentrating on the distance between one's current self and one's ideal self. A second class of goals involves attempting to avoid undesired states by concentrating on the distance between one's current self and one's undesired self. These approach and avoidance motivations have been named the behavioral activation system (BAS) and the behavioral inhibition system (BIS), respectively (e.g., Gray, 1982). The BIS is engaged when perceiving punishment and nonreward signals, whereas the BAS is engaged when perceiving reward and nonpunishment signals. This model has been used, for example, to define the personality characteristics of anxiety (BIS) and impulsivity (BAS; Gray, 1982), to understand disinhibition processes (i.e., failing to correct behavior after negative feedback; Patterson & Newman, 1993), and to predict affective states in the presence of contingent feedback (Carver & White, 1994). In addition, several self-report scales have been created to assess BIS/BAS sensitivity (e.g., Carver & White, 1994). Conceptualizing differential motivations in terms of the interaction of the affectability of rewards and punishments and features of the situation that activate these motivations looks to be a promising area for future self-regulation research.

In sum, TOTE models (e.g., Carver & Scheier, 1981, 1982) have provided an influential framework within which to study self-regulatory processes. New theories and related empirical research have advanced our understanding of the establishment and maintenance of appropriate standards (e.g., Baumeister et al., 1993; Vohs et al., 2001), the assessment of one's current state relative to one's desired end state (e.g., Polivy et al., 1986), the formation of plans and intentions (e.g., Gollwitzer, 1993), and the engagement of operations, such as situational reappraisal to control emotions (see Gross, 1999) or nonconscious strategies (see Chartrand & Bargh, 1996), to reach a goal.

Trait Self-Control

Chronic, habitual, or preferred level of self-control has been shown to have direct effects on functioning in a broad range of domains. Previous research suggests that people vary in their predetermined self-regulatory faculties, with some people being naturally more efficacious than others (e.g., Funder et al., 1983). More recently, Tangney and Baumeister (2000) showed that trait self-control (as measured by a 36-item self-report questionnaire) is significantly associated with a variety of physical and mental health indices. For instance, people higher in trait self-control report fewer disordered eating and alcohol abuse symptoms, reduced anger proneness, higher self-esteem, more secure attachment style, and even higher grade point averages. In a study of Dutch adolescents (Engels, Finkenauer, Den Exter Blokland, & Baumeister, 2001), high trait self-control was linked to fewer transgressions, such as fighting, theft, and vandalism, and also to more positive relationships with parents.

These findings, in combination with the recognition of the importance and influence of self-regulation on a personal and societal level (e.g., Higgins, 1996), have prompted psychologists to call for a national movement toward raising self-control abilities instead of raising self-esteem (e.g., Baumeister, 2001).

Self-Regulatory Resource Model

We view the study of self-regulatory resources as one of the most important contributions to the understanding of self-regulation. As noted in the section on feedback loops and TOTE models, only recently have psychologists begun to investigate what enables people to perform the behaviors that bring them toward their goals. Empirical studies (e.g., Gilbert, Krull, & Pelham, 1988) and theoretical postulates (e.g., Mischel, 1996) suggest that resource models in which self-regulation draws on an expendable psychological energy or resource are appropriate representations of self-regulatory mechanisms.

A recent conceptualization views self-regulation as a limited resource that controls impulses and desires (Baumeister & Heatherton, 1996; Heatherton & Baumeister, 1996). Consider a person who sets an obtainable goal, accurately assesses current and goal states, and tracks his or her progress. This person may still fail to achieve the goal because of an inability to alter cognitive, emotional, or behavioral responses due to depleted regulatory resources. According to this model, self-regulatory resources can be temporarily depleted or fatigued by self-regulatory demands, such as when people try to resist temptation (Vohs & Heatherton, 2000). The self-regu-

latory resource model (Baumeister & Heatherton, 1996; Heatherton & Baumeister, 1996) views the capacity to self-regulate as governed by a finite pool of resources. Thus the resource model posits that the ability to self-regulate is a limited resource that acts much like a muscle, such that the availability of its strength is lower with each individual act of self-control; but, with judicious use over time, its strength grows.

Support for the resource model comes from research linking self-stopping to temporary energy expenditure (e.g., Gilbert et al., 1988; Gross & Levenson, 1997; Wegner, Shortt, Blake, & Page, 1990). For instance, Gilbert and colleagues (1988) demonstrated that cognitive load can hinder self-regulation by showing that self-stopping reduces the availability of cognitive resources. In this research, participants watched an actor on videotape who they knew to be discussing topics that would likely affect her behavior. Participants who watched the video while simultaneously trying to ignore meaningless words on the screen made more dispositional inferences about the actor than those who viewed the same display without attempting to ignore the meaningless words. Gilbert and colleagues proposed that purposeful regulation of attention consumes cognitive operations, thereby impairing participants' ability to correct for situational inducements in the actor's behavior. Research by Wegner and colleagues (1990) relates physiological arousal to mental control abilities. Wegner and colleagues compared levels of physiological arousal between participants who were asked to suppress ideas about sex and participants who were asked to engage in sexual thoughts. They found that suppression of thrilling sexual thoughts consumed more physical energy (as indicated by heightened skin conductance) than directed thinking about them.

Direct evidence for a resource model of self-regulation has been tested using a two-task paradigm in which participants are asked to engage in an act of self-regulation (e.g., mental control or regulation of emotional expression). Subsequently, participants' self-regulatory capacity on a separate task (e.g., physical stamina) is assessed. The results of these studies, which have been conducted by Baumeister, Bratslavsky, Muraven, and Tice (1998), Muraven, Tice, and

Baumeister (1998), and Vohs and Heatherton (2000), indicate that the second act of self-regulation is often impaired as a result of the initial act, suggesting that both acts require some common resource that was depleted by the initial act.

Most experimental studies of self-regulatory resources have involved manipulating situational demands to induce self-regulatory behaviors. This method of inducing self-regulatory endeavors—which, it could be argued, are far less demanding and meaningful than the self-initiated self-regulatory tasks in which people engage in their daily lives—has shown robustly that one route to self-regulatory failure involves prior self-regulatory endeavors. For example, Muraven, Tice, and Baumeister (1998) asked participants first to engage in a form of self-regulation (e.g., mental control, emotional expression regulation); later, participants' self-regulatory strength was assessed by performance on a separate volitional task (e.g., physical stamina). This design illustrates that even externally created self-regulatory demands can temporarily affect global self-regulatory strength (see also Baumeister et al., 1998).

Related research has emphasized the importance of habitual inhibitions in activating depleting situational factors. Vohs and Heatherton (2000) studied chronic dieters to demonstrate that the presence of inhibitions (e.g., dietary restraint) was necessary for situational manipulations (e.g., proximity of tempting foods) to deplete self-regulatory resources and subsequently affect self-regulation. Chronic dieters were used as participants because these women engage in classic self-regulatory behaviors when attempting to override the desire to eat by focusing on long-term weight-loss goals. In these experiments, demand on self-regulatory resources was manipulated by exposing dieters to a situation that was either strongly depleting (i.e., sitting next to a bowl of candies) or weakly depleting (i.e., sitting far from a bowl of candies). Subsequent ability to self-regulate on a second self-regulatory task was poorer among those who had been strongly depleted, such that these dieters ate more ice cream (Study 1) and persisted less on a cognitive task (Study 2). Nondieters, conversely, were not affected—and, by implication, not depleted—by the situational manipulations involving the candies, again

confirming the importance of chronic inhibitions. These studies take an individual-difference approach to studying self-regulatory depletion, emphasizing the role of chronic differences among people that may render them vulnerable to self-regulatory depletion in certain regulation-relevant situations.

Assessing passivity is a particularly germane method of studying self-regulation. In the course of daily life, there is often the option to either engage in self-directed, willful action or to permit things to proceed without interruption. Investigating the circumstances that lead people to put forth the effort to exert volitional control over themselves and their environment and those circumstances that render people unable or unwilling to do so has been one of the goals of self-regulation research.

According to the self-regulatory resource model, when the self's resources are depleted, people become more passive. Passivity may also contribute to the patterns in which people give up more rapidly at a difficult or strenuous task when they have expended resources in previous self-regulation. For example, people who were required by experimental manipulations to override the desire to eat delicious chocolates and cookies (and had to make themselves eat radishes instead) gave up more rapidly than control participants on a subsequent puzzle (Baumeister et al., 1998). Similarly, participants who actively and willfully chose to make a counterattitudinal speech, the method used to induce dissonance (e.g., Linder, Cooper, & Jones, 1967), also exhibited reduced persistence on a task involving unsolvable geometric puzzles relative to participants who had been led to passively (i.e., had been told to) make a counterattitudinal speech (Baumeister et al., 1998). As noted, dieters persist less on an unsolvable embedded figures task after having to override the temptation to eat nearby candies (Vohs & Heatherton, 2000). Likewise, efforts to regulate emotional states while watching an upsetting video made people give up faster on a subsequent test of physical stamina (handgrip) task (Muraven et al., 1998). Collectively, these findings suggest that active, self-directed behaviors require self-regulatory resources such that people become passive when their self-regulatory resources are depleted.

These results run contrary to other, alternate models of self-regulation. For example, an information-processing, skill, or schematic model might predict that the initial act of self-regulation would prime the regulatory schema and hence improve (instead of impair) performance on the second act. Conceptualizing self-regulation as a skill implies no change between the two tasks, as skills are relatively resistant to situational demands. Thus the implication of these findings is that all acts of self-regulation depend on a shared resource that operates like an energy or strength. In practical terms, the ability of the self to regulate itself is severely limited (see also Muraven et al., 1998; Vohs & Baumeister, 2000).

Emotion regulation may hold a special place in self-management strategies. Findings from two different sets of experiments point to the conclusion that people first direct their efforts to regulating emotion, with other types of self-regulation relegated to secondary status. For instance, Tice, Bratslavsky, and Baumeister (2001) found that when people are put into a negative mood, they prioritize their subsequent regulatory tasks so as to focus on elevating their emotional state before attending to other tasks, such as practicing for an upcoming performance task. More serious consequences of emotion regulation strategies were investigated by Bushman, Baumeister, and Phillips (2001), who found that people who were induced to believe in catharsis, as well as people who had high tendencies toward venting anger, reacted to an insult with higher aggression (i.e., by choosing longer duration and greater intensity of an aversive noise given to an opponent). Despite people's beliefs about the utility of engaging in emotion regulation, existing evidence indicates that emotion regulation attempts often are unsuccessful. Whether in the form of suppressing depressive thoughts (e.g., Wenzlaff, Wegner, & Roper, 1988) or trying not to dwell on setbacks (Nolen-Hoeksema, 1998), attempts to control one's affective state are not easy or wholly successful. Moreover, as noted, research has demonstrated that controlling emotional responses depletes self-regulatory resources (Muraven et al., 1998; Vohs & Heatherton, 2000). Therefore, attempts to regulate emotional distress, which decrease self-regulatory resources, may hinder the capacity for subsequent acts of self-control and, unfortunately, may be ultimately ineffective. Notably, however, success-versus-failure feedback—which is often used a form of manipulating affect—does not "restore" self-regulatory depletion (Wallace & Baumeister, in press). This research found that self-regulatory ability on a second task was a function of prior self-regulatory exertion, thereby supporting the resource model, but was unaffected by intervening success-versus-failure feedback.

From a resource-model perspective, self-regulatory resource depletion may occur either suddenly or gradually. If a catastrophic event occurs and elicits devastating negative affect, self-regulatory resources may be so overwhelmed that the person immediately becomes passive or disinhibited or exhibits other forms of escaping the self. The process of escaping the self, particularly as it applies to suicide attempts, has been linked to depletion of self-regulatory resources (see Vohs & Baumeister, 2000). In contrast to an immediately depleted state, regulatory resources may erode gradually with multiple attempts at self-regulatory control, thereby becoming more depleted with each endeavor. In this case, the consequences may appear more gradually, perhaps escalating with time. Career burnout, for example, may be the result of an erosion of self-regulatory depletion over time—especially when one considers, for example, the medical or social service professions in which attempts to aid people often are met with disappointment and frustration.

Self-Regulation and Interpersonal Functioning

Just as it is well established that self-regulation is crucial to personal functioning, self-regulation is similarly important for interpersonal relations. Accordingly, researchers do not yet understand how self-regulation affects—and is affected by—interpersonal processes. Given that a variety of societal ills related to interpersonal problems are linked to failures of self-regulation (e.g., interpersonal violence, overcoming shyness, extradyadic sexual relations) and given the known detrimental effects of failed relationships, it is crucial that psychologists begin to investigate the association between these central aspects of the self.

An overview of the research on interpersonal processes reveals the significance of self-regulation. For instance, Gilbert's model of social inference (e.g., Gilbert et al., 1988) proposes that when viewing others' behavior, people initially "characterize" others by inferring stable personality traits and then must cognitively "correct" this dispositional judgment to account for situational influences. Thus the act of correction requires self-regulation to override initial characterization. Also, Nolen-Hoeksema and Davis (1999) showed that after a traumatic event, ruminators—who are unsuccessful in their mental control attempts—desired more social support than nonruminators but were less likely to receive it. Baumeister, Smart, and Boden (1996) concluded that interpersonal violence, an urge normally suppressed with emotional, cognitive, or behavioral control, is more likely to occur when a person's high (especially if inflated) opinion of himself or herself receives a blow from an external source. Several self-regulatory explanations can be given regarding the emanation of aggressive behaviors among people with high self-esteem after threat: It may be that the response to the threat is an urge too great to resist; it may be that attempting to cope with the threat in a nonaggressive manner quickly depletes regulatory resources, thereby allowing aggressive tendencies to emerge; or it may be that the emotional component of the threat is so aversive that feeling better—by any means—becomes the top priority. Whatever the root cause, people with high self-esteem do not show appropriate self-regulation in response to ego threats, as evidenced by their higher rate of interpersonal violence. Thus indirect evidence indicates that a variety of interpersonal processes involve the regulation of emotions, thoughts, or behaviors.

Direct tests of the relation between self-regulation and interpersonal functioning are beginning to accrue. Research by Ciarocco and colleagues (in press) investigated the role of self-regulation in ostracism by testing whether being the source (as opposed to the target) of ostracism affected ability to self-regulate on a later task. In one study, they found that people who were induced to refuse to speak to a confederate subsequently showed significant decreases in length of persistence on unsolvable cognitive prob-

lems. A second study confirmed these findings by showing that after having to ostracize someone, people are less able to exert physical effort on a handgrip task (Ciarocco et al., in press). These results are all the more remarkable when considering that participants in these studies were asked to ignore someone with whom they were not previously acquainted (as opposed to almost all real-life cases of ostracism, which involve ignoring an acquaintance or close other) and that they were asked to do so for only 3 minutes. Thus giving someone the silent treatment depletes the self's resources and makes it less able to carry out its other functions.

To maintain a close, romantic relationship, partners must override or suppress some feelings or exert effort for the betterment of the dyad. One such act is accommodation, which is the ability to react constructively—not destructively—to potentially destructive behaviors from a partner. In a set of studies assessing the association between self-regulation and acts of accommodation, Finkel and Campbell (2001) found that on both a trait and state level, high self-regulation was related to more accommodation. That is, people who reported higher levels of trait self-control also reported more accommodative tendencies. Moreover, the results of a laboratory study in which people were randomly assigned to be depleted of self-regulatory resources showed that depletion led to weaker tendencies toward accommodation.

A series of studies assessing the role of self-regulation across a broad spectrum of interpersonal processes was conducted by Vohs, Ciarocco, and Baumeister (2001). They investigated how self-regulatory depletion affects desire to self-disclose to an unacquainted partner. Participants were either given instructions to regulate their emotions by exaggerating their responses to a comedic video or were given no instructions regarding their responses. Subsequently, participants were asked to rate a list of topics in terms of their desirability for an upcoming conversation with a same-sex participant. The results showed that being depleted of self-regulatory resources led to differences in desire to self-disclose, but only as a function of trait attachment style. Specifically, participants who rated themselves as avoidantly attached showed the least desire to disclose, whereas participants with an anxious/ambivalent attachment style showed substantial increases in desire to disclose. Securely attached participants reported wanting to disclose somewhat more after depletion, relative to controls. In a second study, Vohs and colleagues found that self-presentational demands can deplete self-regulatory resources. Manipulating self-presentational goals of being modest or very positive about the self with either a stranger or a friend affected subsequent self-regulatory abilities, such that having to be modest with a stranger or very positive with a friend led to reduced persistence on an arduous arithmetic task. The reason these tasks were depleting is because they violate habitual or preferred self-presentational strategies in which people are self-enhancing among strangers and modest among friends (Tice, Butler, Muraven, & Stillwell, 1995).

The ability to engage in accommodative behaviors in the context of a romantic relationship has also been investigated within a self-regulation framework. Finkel and Campbell (in press) reported that both dispositional and situational self-regulatory abilities predicted people's willingness to engage in constructive responses in the face of a partner's destructive behaviors. Vohs and colleagues (2001) have also confirmed this finding and have even found that self-regulatory depletion leads to decreased accommodative tendencies among people who are not currently involved in a romantic relationship. This suggests, then, that the ability to put aside the self for the well-being of the dyad is severely compromised when self-regulatory resources are scarce.

Even in its early stages, this emergent area of research between self-regulation and interpersonal processes has yielded intriguing findings. These studies indicate that many of the interpersonal behaviors in which people engage every day are governed by some of the same processes that affect intrapersonal functioning. We look forward to following this growing area of investigation in the coming years.

Neuropsychological Research on Self-Regulation

Neuroscientists also study self-regulation and executive functioning. In neuroscience,

the term "executive function" is mainly used to denote cognitive mechanisms performed by the frontal lobes. Such operations including planning, volition, effortful and purposeful action, and maximizing performance (Lezak, 1983). From a neuroscientific perspective, executive function tasks require effortful acts, such as shifting between cognitive sets, problem solving, and strategic planning. In addition, executive function tasks often include a goal, which then necessitates self-regulation.

One popular method of testing executive functioning is the Wisconsin Card Sorting Task, in which participants sort cards that have multidimensional characters (e.g., red stars, blue stars, and red squares). Participants are asked to place the cards into piles according to an unstated experiment-defined rule (e.g., all stars; all red cards). This aspect of the task is not difficult, as most people learn the sorting dimension after negative feedback from the experimenter. After participants have learned the rule, however, the experimenter suddenly changes the sorting dimension, and the participant is then required to detect the new rule. It is the shifting of attention from one dimension to another, as well as the filtering of irrelevant information, that involves the frontal lobes. Indeed, patients with frontal lobe damage cannot learn a new rule after the initial rule has been learned. Instead they perseverate and continue to apply the old rule again and again (see Gazzaniga, Ivry, & Mangum, 1998).

Although the frontal lobes govern multiple aspects of self-regulation, specific areas appear to be involved in enabling a person to reach a goal. Within the prefrontal cortex, the dorsolateral prefrontal area has been linked to the representation of goal states, as well as to the active process of filtering irrelevant information (Davidson & Irwin, 1999; Koziol, 1993). Research has also suggested that the anterior cingulate is related to response modification demands, especially with regard to tasks that require divided attention (e.g., Corbetta, Miezin, Dobmeyer, Shulman, & Petersen, 1991). Norman and Shallice (1986) developed a model of goal-oriented behaviors. In their model, the anterior cingulate is hypothesized to monitor information on a variety of levels, possibly providing the basis for the so-called supervisory attentional system (SAS; Norman & Shallice, 1986) that oversees the executive functions of the brain. The SAS governs controlled, effortful behaviors and is activated during situations that involve planning, novel contingencies, difficult choices, or overriding habitual responses. The SAS is likely activated during social psychological research on self-regulation, as suggested by the types of paradigms found to be sensitive to assessing the effects of depleted self-regulatory resources (e.g., Baumeister et al., 1998; Vohs & Heatherton, 2000). These paradigms present participants with difficult choices (e.g., temptation) that require overriding a lower level response (e.g., eating the tempting foods) while in a novel situation. Thus neuropsychological research strongly suggests that the anterior cingulate is involved in tasks that deplete self-regulatory resources via the coordination of divided attention. Additionally, the dorsolateral prefrontal cortex appears to be necessary for the activation, maintenance, and modification of goal-directed responses.

A bridge between cognitive neuroscience and social psychology is being formed, in part by research on self-regulation and executive functioning. Each perspective can only serve to strengthen our understanding of executive functioning, and we encourage research to move toward an integration of these two approaches.

Conclusions

Many of life's greatest challenges involve attempting to achieve goals. Be it to run a marathon before turning 40, maintaining our current weight, raising happy children, or not ending up like a despised cousin, humans are constantly trying to improve their lives through self-regulation. The executive function, under which self-control and self-regulation are subsumed, is an indispensable facet of selfhood in its ability to make a better fit between the person and the environment. As seen in our review, the ability to self-regulate is an integral component of mental and physical well-being.

Some have questioned whether a person can have too much self-control. From our perspective, little empirical evidence has been found to support a curvilinear view of self-control. Rather, it is more likely that when people exert self-control and still fail to achieve their goals, they miscalculated at some step in the process or used an erroneous strategy to reach the desired state (Baumeister et al., 1994). Systematic efforts by Tangney and Baumeister (2000) to find maladaptive correlates of high levels of self-control repeatedly failed: The benefits of self-control were linear, not curvilinear.

Our review points to several advances in the study of self-regulation and self-control. We especially encourage the use of a self-regulation framework to study interpersonal processes, further investigations of the role of nonconscious goal activation and operations, and the neural correlates of self-regulatory functions. Furthermore, we cannot understate the importance of self-regulatory resources in understanding mechanisms of self-control. Without the ability to engage in successful responses to change the self, one cannot get from the current state to the desired end state, despite setting appropriate goals, understanding where one currently stands, or having the best intentions.

As the findings described in this chapter attest, the problems that result from a lack of or breakdown in self-control are consequential. Self-regulation failure taxes the self, the health of one's relationships, and the state of our society. Conversely, strong self-regulatory abilities could yield great achievements, at both the personal and societal level. Remarkable accomplishments will be achieved, however, only by developing, using, and strengthening self-regulatory processes to the utmost of our capacities.

Acknowledgments

We would like to thank the National Institutes of Health for Grant No. MH-57039, which supported this work.

References

Alloy, L. B., & Abramson, L. Y. (1979). Judgment of contingency in depressed and nondepressed students: Sadder but wiser? *Journal of Experimental Psychology: General, 108*, 441–485.

Alloy, L. B., & Abramson, L. Y. (1982). Learned helplessness, depression, and the illusion of control. *Journal of Personality and Social Psychology, 42*, 1114–1126.

Banaji, M. R., & Prentice, D. A. (1994). The self in social contexts. *Annual Review of Psychology, 45,* 297–332.

Band, E. B., & Weisz, J. R. (1988). How to feel better when it feels bad: Children's perspectives on coping with everyday stress. *Developmental Psychology, 24,* 247–253.

Bandura, A. (1977). Self-efficacy: Toward a unifying theory of behavior change. *Psychological Review, 84,* 191–215.

Bandura, A. (1989). Human agency in social cognitive theory. *American Psychologist, 44,* 1175–1184.

Bandura, A., Caprara, G. V., Barbaranelli, C., Pastorelli, C., & Regalia, C. (2001). Sociocognitive self-regulatory mechanisms governing transgressive behavior. *Journal of Personality and Social Psychology, 80,* 125–135.

Bargh, J. A. (1990). Goal not = intent: Goal directed thought and behavior are often unintentional. *Psychological Inquiry, 1,* 248–251.

Baumeister, R. F. (1997). Identity, self-concept, and self-esteem: The self lost and found. In R. Hogan & J. A. Johnson (Eds.), *Handbook of personality psychology* (pp. 681–710). San Diego, CA: Academic Press.

Baumeister, R. F. (1998). The self. In D. T. Gilbert, S. T. Fiske, & G. Lindzey (Eds.), *Handbook of social psychology* (4th ed., pp. 680–740). New York: McGraw-Hill.

Baumeister, R. F. (2001). Ego depletion and self-control failure: An energy model of the self's executive function. *Self and Identity, 1,* 129–136.

Baumeister, R. F., Bratslavsky, E., Finkenauer, C., & Vohs, K. D. (2001). Bad is stronger than good. *Review of General Psychology, 5,* 323–370.

Baumeister, R. F., Bratslavsky, E., Muraven, M., & Tice, D. M. (1998). Ego depletion: Is the active self a limited resource? *Journal of Personality and Social Psychology, 74,* 1252–1265.

Baumeister, R. F., & Heatherton, T. F. (1996). Self-regulation failure: An overview. *Psychological Inquiry, 7,* 1–15.

Baumeister, R. F., Heatherton, T. F., & Tice, D. M. (1993). When ego threats lead to self-regulation failure: Negative consequences of high self-esteem. *Journal of Personality and Social Psychology, 64,* 141–156.

Baumeister, R. F., Heatherton, T. F., & Tice, D. M. (1994). *Losing control: How and why people fail at self-regulation.* San Diego, CA: Academic Press.

Baumeister, R. F., Smart, L., & Boden, J. M. (1996). Relation of threatened egotism to violence and aggression: The dark side of high self-esteem. *Psychological Review, 103,* 5–33.

Brehm, J. (1966). *A theory of psychological reactance.* New York: Academic Press.

Buchmann, M. (1989). *The script of life in modern society: entry into adulthood in a changing world.* Chicago: University of Chicago Press.

Burger, J. M. (1989). Negative reactions to increases in perceived personal control. *Journal of Personality and Social Psychology, 56,* 246–256.

Bushman, B. J., Baumeister, R. F., & Phillips, C. M. (2001). Do people aggress to improve their mood? Catharsis beliefs, affect regulation opportunity, and aggressive responding. *Journal of Personality and Social Psychology, 81,* 17–32.

Carver, C. S., & Scheier, M. F. (1981). *Attention and self-regulation: A control theory approach to human behavior.* New York: Springer-Verlag.

Carver, C. S., & Scheier, M. F. (1982). Control theory: A useful conceptual framework for personality-social, clinical and health psychology. *Psychological Bulletin, 92,* 111–135.

Carver, C. S., & Scheier, M. F. (1998). *On the self-regulation of behavior.* New York: Cambridge University Press.

Carver, C. S., & White T. L. (1994). Behavioral inhibition, behavioral activation, and affective responses to impending reward and punishment: The BIS/BAS scales. *Journal of Personality and Social Psychology, 67,* 319–333.

Chartrand, T. L., & Bargh, J. A. (1996). Automatic activation of impression formation and memorization goals: Nonconscious goal priming reproduces effects of explicit task instructions. *Journal of Personality and Social Psychology, 71,* 464–478.

Chartrand, T. L., Tesser, A., & Cheng, C. M. (2001). *Consequences of failure at nonconscious goals for self-enhancement and stereotyping.* Unpublished manuscript, Ohio State University.

Ciarocco, N. J., Sommer, K. L., & Baumeister, R. F. (2001). Ostracism and ego depletion: The strains of silence. *Personality and Social Psychology Bulletin, 27,* 1156–1163.

Corbetta, M., Miezin, F. M., Dobmeyer, S., Shulman, G. L., & Petersen, S. E. (1991). Selective and divided attention during visual discriminations of shape, color, and speed: Functional anatomy by positron emission tomography. *Journal of Neuroscience, 11,* 2382–2402.

Davidson, R. J., & Irwin, W. (1999). The functional neuroanatomy of emotion and affective style. *Trends in Cognitive Neuroscience, 3,* 11–21.

Deci, E. L., & Ryan, R. M. (1991). A motivational approach to self: Integration in personality. In R. Dienstbier (Ed.), *Nebraska Symposium on Motivation: Vol. 38. Perspectives on motivation* (pp. 237–288). Lincoln: University of Nebraska Press.

Deci, E. L., & Ryan, R. M. (1995). Human autonomy: The basis for true self-esteem. In M. Kernis (Ed.), *Efficacy, agency, and self-esteem* (pp. 31–49). New York: Plenum Press.

Diener, E. (1979). Deindividuation, self-awareness, and disinhibition. *Journal of Personality and Social Psychology, 37,* 1160–1171.

Emmons, R. A., & King, L. A. (1988). Personal striving conflict: Immediate and long-term implications for psychological and physical well-being. *Journal of Personality and Social Psychology, 54,* 1040–1048.

Engels, R., Finkenauer, C., Den Exter Blokland, E., & Baumeister, R. F. (2001). *Parental influences on self-control and juvenile delinquency.* Unpublished manuscript, Utrecht University, Netherlands.

Finkel, E. J., & Campbell, W. K. (2001). Self-control and accommodation in close relationships: An interdependence analysis. *Journal of Personality and Social Psychology, 81,* 263–271.

Funder, D. C., Block, J. H., & Block, J. (1983). Delay of gratification: Some longitudinal personality correlates.

Journal of Personality and Social Psychology, 44, 1198–1213.

Gazzaniga, M. S. (1997). Why can't I control my brain? Aspects of conscious experience. In M. Ito & Y. Miyashita (Eds.) *Cognition, computation, and consciousness* (pp 69–79). New York: Oxford University Press.

Gazzaniga, M. S., Ivry, R. B., & Mangun, G. R. (1998). *Cognitive neuroscience: The biology of mind.* New York: Norton.

Gilbert, D. T., Krull, D. S., & Pelham, B. W. (1988). Of thoughts unspoken: Social inference and the self-regulation of behavior. *Journal of Personality and Social Psychology, 55,* 685–694.

Glass, D. C., Singer, J. E., & Friedman, L. N. (1969). Psychic cost of adaptation to an environmental stressor. *Journal of Personality and Social Psychology, 12,* 200–210.

Gollwitzer, P. M. (1993). Goal achievement: The role of intentions. In W. Stroebe & M. Hewstone (Eds.), *European review of social psychology* (Vol. 4, pp. 141–185). Chichester, UK: Wiley.

Gollwitzer, P. M. (1996). The violational benefits of planning. In P. M. Gollwitzer & J. A. Bargh (Eds.), *The Psychology of action: Linking cognition and motivation to behavior* (pp. 287–312). New York: Guilford Press.

Gollwitzer, P. M. (1999). Implementation intentions: Strong effects of simple plans. *American Psychologist, 54,* 493–503.

Gollwitzer, P. M., & Brandstätter, V. (1997). Implementation intentions and effective goal pursuit. *Journal of Personality and Social Psychology, 73,* 186–199.

Gray, J. A. (1982). *The neuropsychology of anxiety: An enquiry into the functions of the septo-hippocampal system.* New York: Oxford University Press.

Gross, J. J. (1999). Emotion and emotion regulation. In L. A. Pervin & O. P. John (Eds.), *Handbook of personality: Theory and research* (2nd ed., pp. 525–552). New York: Guilford Press.

Gross, J. J., & Levenson, R. W. (1997). Hiding feelings: The acute effects of inhibiting negative and positive emotion. *Journal of Abnormal Psychology, 106,* 95–103.

Heatherton, T. F., & Baumeister, R. F. (1996). Self-regulation failure: Past, present, and future. *Psychological Inquiry, 7,* 90–98.

Higgins, E. T. (1989). Self-discrepancy theory: What patterns of self-beliefs cause people to suffer? In L. Berkowitz (Ed.) *Advances in experimental social psychology* (Vol. 22, pp. 93–136). New York: Academic Press.

Higgins, E. T. (1996). Knowledge activation: Accessibility, applicability, and salience. In E. T. Higgins & A. W. Kruglanski (Eds.), *Social psychology: Handbook of basic principles* (pp. 133–168). New York: Guilford Press.

Higgins, E. T. (1997). Biases in social cognition: "Aboutness" as a general principle. In C. McGarty & S. A. Haslam (Eds.), *The message of social psychology: Perspectives on mind in society* (pp. 182–199). Malden, MA: Blackwell.

Iyengar, S. S., & Lepper, M. R. (2000). When choice is demotivating: Can one desire be too much of a good thing? *Journal of Personality and Social Psychology, 79,* 995–1006.

James, W. (1950). *The principles of psychology* (Vol. 2). New York: Dover. (Original work published 1890)

Kasser, T., & Ryan, R. M. (1993). A dark side of the American dream: Correlates of financial success as a central life aspiration. *Journal of Personality and Social Psychology, 65,* 410–422.

Kasser, T., & Ryan, R. M. (1996). Further examining the American dream: Differential correlates of intrinsic and extrinsic goals. *Personality and Social Psychology Bulletin, 22,* 280–287.

Kramer, T. H., Buckhout, R., Fox, P., Widman, E., & Tusche, B. (1991). Effects of stress on recall. *Applied Cognitive Psychology, 5,* 483–488.

Kirschenbaum, D. S. (1987). Self-regulatory failure: A review with clinical implications. *Clinical Psychology Review, 7,* 77–104.

Koziol, L. F. (1993). The neuropsychology of attention deficit and obsessive compulsive disorder: Towards an understanding of the cognitive mechanisms of impulse control. In L. F. Koziol, C. E. Stout, & D. H. Ruben (Eds.), *Handbook of childhood impulse disorders and ADHD: Theory and practice* (pp. 5–24). Springfield, IL: C. Thomas.

Langer, E. J. (1975). The illusion of control. *Journal of Personality and Social Psychology, 32,* 311–328.

Langer, E. J., & Roth, J. (1975). Heads I win, tails it's chance: The illusion of control as a function of the sequence of outcomes in a purely chance task. *Journal of Personality and Social Psychology, 32,* 951–955.

Leary, M. R. (2001, January). *The curse of the self.* Paper presented at the Preconference on Self of the Society for Personality and Social Psychology, San Antonio, TX.

Lezak, M. (1983). *Neuropsychological assessment* (2nd ed.). New York: Oxford University Press.

Linder, D. E., Cooper, J., & Jones, E. E. (1967). Decision freedom as a determinant of the role of incentive magnitude in attitude change. *Journal of Personality and Social Psychology, 6,* 245–254.

Metcalfe, J., & Jacobs, W. J. (1998). Emotional memory: The effects of stress on "cool" and "hot" memory systems. *Psychology of Learning and Motivation, 38,* 187–222.

Metcalfe, J., & Mischel, W. (1999). A two-system analysis of delay of gratification. *Psychological Review, 106,* 3–19.

Mischel, W. (1996). From good intentions to willpower. In P. M. Gollwitzer & J. A. Bargh (Eds.), *The psychology of action: Linking cognition and motivation to behavior* (pp. 197–218). New York: Guilford Press.

Mischel, W., & Ebbesen, E. B. (1970). Attention in delay of gratification. *Journal of Personality and Social Psychology, 16,* 329–337.

Mischel, W., Shoda, Y., & Peake, P. K. (1988). The nature of adolescent competencies predicted by preschool delay of gratification. *Journal of Personality and Social Psychology, 54,* 687–696.

Mullen, B. (1986). Atrocity as a function of lynch mob composition: A self-attention perspective. *Applied and Social Psychology Bulletin, 12,* 187–197.

Muraven, M., Tice, D. M., & Baumeister, R. F. (1998). Self-control as limited resource: Regulatory depletion patterns. *Journal of Personality and Social Psychology, 74,* 774–789.

Neumann, R., & Strack, F. (2000). Approach and avoidance: The influence of proprioceptive and exteroceptive cues on encoding of affective information. *Journal of Personality and Social Psychology, 79,* 39–48.

Nolen-Hoeksema, S. (1998). The other end of the continuum: The costs of rumination. *Psychological Inquiry, 9,* 216–219.

Nolen-Hoeksema, S., & Davis, C. G. (1999). "Thanks for sharing that": Ruminators and their social support networks. *Journal of Personality and Social Psychology, 77,* 801–814.

Norman, D., & Shallice, T. (1986). Attention to action: Willed and automatic control of behavior. In R. J. Davidson, G. E. Schwartz, & D. Shapiro (Eds.), *Consciousness and self-regulation* (pp. 1–18). New York: Plenum Press.

Patterson, C. M., & Newman, J. P. (1993). Reflectivity and learning from adverse events: Toward a psychological mechanism for the syndromes of disinhibition. *Psychological Review, 100,* 716–736.

Pervin, L. A. (1989). Psychodynamic-systems reflections on a social-intelligence model of personality. In R. S. Wyer & T. K. Srull (Eds.), *Advances in social cognition: Vol. 2. Social intelligence and cognitive assessments of personality* (pp. 153–161). Hillsdale, NJ: Erlbaum.

Polivy, J., Herman, C. P., Hackett, R., & Kuleshnyk, I. (1986). The effects of self-attention and public attention on eating in restrained and unrestrained subjects. *Journal of Personality and Social Psychology, 50,* 1253–1260.

Powers, W. T. (1973). *Behavior: The control of perception.* Chicago: Aldine.

Richards, J. M., & Gross, J. J. (2000). Emotional regulation and memory: The cognitive costs of keeping one's cool. *Journal of Personality and Social Psychology, 79,* 410–424.

Rothbaum, F., Weisz, J. R., & Snyder, S. S. (1982). Changing the world and changing the self: A two-process model of perceived control. *Journal of Personality and Social Psychology, 42,* 5–37.

Schwartz, B. (2000). Self-determination: The tyranny of freedom. *American Psychologist, 55,* 79–88.

Schwarz, N., & Clore, G. L. (1983). Mood, misattribution, and judgments of well-being: Informative and directive functions of affective states. *Journal of Personality and Social Psychology, 45,* 513–523.

Sedikides, C., & Skowronski, J. A. (1997). The symbolic self in evolutionary context. *Personality and Social Psychology Review, 1,* 80–102.

Seligman, M. E. P. (1975). *Helplessness: On depression, development, and death.* San Francisco: Freeman.

Shaw, R. J. (1992). Coping effectiveness in nursing home residents: The role of control. *Journal of Aging and Health, 4,* 551–563.

Shoda, Y., Mischel, W., & Peake, P. K. (1990). Predicting adolescent cognitive and self-regulatory competencies from preschool delay of gratification: Identifying diagnostic conditions. *Developmental Psychology, 26,* 978–986.

Smith, S. M., Norrell, J. H., & Saint, J. L. (1996). Self esteem and reactions to ego threat: A (battle)field of investigation. *Basic and Applied Social Psychology, 18,* 395–404.

Tangney, J. P., & Baumeister, R. F. (2000). *High self-control predicts good adjustment, less pathology, better grades, and interpersonal success.* Unpublished manuscript, George Mason University.

Taylor, S. E. (1983). Adjustment to threatening events: A theory of cognitive adaptation. *American Psychologist, 38,* 1161–1173.

Tesser, A., Martin, L. L., & Cornell, D. P. (1996). On the substitutability of self-protective mechanisms. In P. M. Gollwitzer & J. A. Bargh (Eds.), *The psychology of action: Linking cognition and motivation to behavior* (pp. 48–68). New York: Guilford Press.

Tice, D. M., Bratslavsky, E., & Baumeister, R. F. (2001). Emotional distress regulation takes precedence over impulse control: If you feel bad, do it! *Journal of Personality and Social Psychology, 80,* 53–67.

Tice, D. M., Butler, J. L., Muraven, M. B., & Stillwell, A. M. (1995). When modesty prevails: Differential favorability of self-presentation to friends and strangers. *Journal of Personality and Social Psychology, 69,* 1120–1138.

Tomaka, J., Blascovich, J., Kibler, J., & Ernst, J. M. (1997). Cognitive and physiological antecedents of threat and challenge appraisal. *Journal of Personality and Social Psychology, 73,* 63–72.

Twenge, J. M., Tice, D. M., Schmeichel, B. J., & Baumeister, R. F. (2001). *Decision fatigue: Making multiple personal decisions depletes the self's resources.* Unpublished manuscript, Case Western Reserve University.

Vohs, K. D., Bardone, A. M., Joiner, T. E., Jr., Abramson, L. Y., & Heatherton, T. F. (1999). Perfectionism, perceived weight status, and self-esteem interact to predict bulimic symptoms: A model of bulimic symptom development. *Journal of Abnormal Psychology, 108,* 695–700.

Vohs, K. D., & Baumeister, R. F. (2000). Escaping the self consumes regulatory resources: A self-regulatory model of suicide. In T. E. Joiner, Jr. & M. D. Rudd (Eds.), *Suicide science: Expanding boundaries* (pp. 33–42). Boston: Kluwer Academic.

Vohs, K. D., & Baumeister, R. F. (2001). *Nonconscious goal priming and self-regulatory capacities.* Unpublished manuscript, Case Western Reserve University.

Vohs, K. D., Ciarocco, N., & Baumeister, R. F. (2001). *Interpersonal functioning requires self-regulatory resources.* Unpublished manuscript, Case Western Reserve University.

Vohs, K. D., & Heatherton, T. F. (2000). Self-regulatory failure: A resource-depletion approach. *Psychological Science, 11,* 249–254.

Vohs, K. D., Voelz, Z. R., Pettit, J. W., Bardone, A. M., Katz, J., Abramson, L. Y., Heatherton, T. F., & Joiner, T. E., Jr. (2001). Perfectionism, body dissatisfaction, and self-esteem: An interactive model of bulimic symptom development. *Journal of Social and Clinical Psychology, 20,* 476–497.

Wallace, H. M., & Baumeister, R. F. (in press). Effects of success versus failure feedback on further self-control. *Self and Identity.*

Wegner, D. M., Shortt, J. W., Blake, A. W., & Page, M. S. (1990). The suppression of exciting thoughts. *Journal of Personality and Social Psychology, 58,* 409–418.

Weisz, J. R., McCabe, M. A., & Dennig, M. D. (1994). Primary and secondary control among children undergoing medical procedures: Adjustment as a function of coping style. *Journal of Consulting and Clinical Psychology, 62,* 324–332.

Wenzlaff, R. M., Wegner, D. M., & Roper, D. W. (1988). Depression and mental control: The resurgence of un-

wanted negative thoughts. *Journal of Personality and Social Psychology, 55,* 882–892.

Wolford, G., Miller, M. B., & Gazzaniga, M. (2000). The left hemisphere's role in hypothesis formation. *Journal of Neuroscience, 20,* RC64.

11

Self-Efficacy

JAMES E. MADDUX
JENNIFER T. GOSSELIN

"Self" and "identity" are concerned largely with the question, "Who am I?" So often people answer the question, "Who am I?" by asking, "What am I good at?" The study of self-efficacy is concerned with understanding this important aspect of self and identity—people's beliefs about their personal capabilities and how these beliefs influence what they try to accomplish, how they try to accomplish it, and how they react to successes and setbacks along the way.

Since the publication of Albert Bandura's "Self-Efficacy: Toward A Unifying Theory of Behavior Change" (1977), the term "self-efficacy" has become ubiquitous in psychology and related fields. Hundreds of articles on every imaginable aspect of self-efficacy have appeared in journals devoted to psychology, sociology, kinesiology, public health, medicine, nursing, and other fields. This research can be only summarized here and cannot be discussed in detail. Thus the goal of this chapter is breadth of coverage, not depth. The first section of this chapter discusses the definition and measurement of self-efficacy. The second section discusses how self-efficacy beliefs develop. The third section discusses the importance of self-efficacy and the application of self-efficacy the-

ory to a number of areas of human adaptation and adjustment.

We begin with some "big picture" information that may provide a context for a better understanding of self-efficacy. Understanding what self-efficacy beliefs are and how they develop requires understanding its theoretical foundation. Self-efficacy is best understood in the context of *social cognitive theory*—an approach to understanding human cognition, action, motivation, and emotion that assumes that people actively shape their environments, rather than simply react to them (Bandura, 1986, 1997, 2001; Barone, Maddux, & Snyder, 1997). Social cognitive theory has at least four basic premises.

First, people have powerful cognitive or symbolizing capabilities that allow them to create internal models of experience. Because of this capacity, people can observe and evaluate their own thoughts, behavior, and emotions. They also can develop new plans of action, make predictions about outcomes, test and evaluate their predictions, and communicate complex ideas and experiences to others.

Second, environmental events, inner personal factors (cognition, emotion, and biological events), and behaviors are reciprocal influences. People respond cognitively, emotionally, and behaviorally to environmental events. Also, through cognition, people can exercise control over their own behavior, which then influences not only the environment but also their cognitive, emotional, and biological states.

Third, self and identity are socially embedded. They are perceptions (accurate or not) of one's own and others' patterns of social cognition, emotion, and action as they occur in patterns of situations. Because they are socially embedded, self and identity are not simply what people *bring* to their interactions with others; they are created in these interactions, and they change through these interactions.

Fourth, the self-reflective capacities noted here set the stage for self-regulation. People choose goals and regulate their behavior in the pursuit of these goals. At the heart of self-regulation is the ability to anticipate or develop expectancies—to use past knowledge and experience to form beliefs about future events or states, one's abilities, and one's behavior. (The role of self-efficacy beliefs in self-regulation is addressed in greater detail in a later section.)

What Is Self-Efficacy?

Self-efficacy beliefs are beliefs about the ability to "organize and execute the courses of action required to produce given attainments" (Bandura, 1997, p. 3). Thus self-efficacy theory and research are concerned with people's beliefs about personal control and agency. Of course, notions about personal control and agency were not unknown before 1977 but had been discussed by philosophers and psychologists for many years. Spinoza, Hume, Locke, William James, and (more recently) Gilbert Ryle have all struggled with understanding the role of "volition" and "the will" in human behavior (Russell, 1954; Vessey, 1967). In psychology, effectance motivation (White, 1959), achievement motivation (McClelland, Atkinson, Clark, & Lowell, 1953), locus of control (Rotter, 1966), learned helplessness (Abramson, Seligman, & Teasdale, 1978), and other constructs are concerned with perceptions of personal competence

and the relationship between these perceptions and personal effectiveness, achievement, and psychological well-being (see also Skinner, 1995). Most of these models did not distinguish clearly between beliefs that specific behaviors will lead to specific outcomes and the belief that one will be able to perform successfully the behaviors in question, although this distinction had been alluded to before Bandura's 1977 article (Kirsch, 1985). One of the Bandura's major contributions in his 1977 article was that he offered relatively specific definitions of these familiar and commonsense notions and embedded them in a comprehensive theory of behavior. The essential idea of self-efficacy was not new; what were new were the concept's theoretical grounding and the empirical rigor with which it could now be examined.

Defining Self-Efficacy

One way to get a clearer sense of how self-efficacy is defined and measured is to understand how it differs from other concepts that deal with the self, identity, and perceptions of competence and control.

Self-efficacy beliefs are not *competencies*. Competencies are what people know about the world and what they know how to do in the world. They include "the quality and range of the cognitive constructions and behavioral enactments of which the individual is capable" (Mischel, 1973, p. 266) and the ability to "construct (generate) diverse behaviors under appropriate conditions" (Mischel, 1973, p. 265). Self-efficacy beliefs are beliefs (accurate or not) about one's competencies and one's ability to exercise these competencies in certain domains and situations.

Self-efficacy beliefs are not concerned with perceptions of skills and abilities *divorced from situations*; they are concerned, instead, with what people believe they can do with their skills and abilities under certain conditions. In addition, they are concerned not simply with the ability to perform trivial motor acts but with the ability to coordinate and orchestrate skills and abilities in changing and challenging situations.

Self-efficacy beliefs are not simply *predictions* about behavior. They are concerned not with what people believe they *will* do but with what they believe they *can* do under certain circumstances, especially challenging and changing circumstances.

Self-efficacy beliefs are not *intentions* to behave or intentions to attain particular goals. Intentions are what people say they are committed to doing or accomplishing, not just expectations or predictions of future actions (Bandura, 2001). Intentions are influenced by a number of factors, including but not limited to self-efficacy beliefs (Maddux, 1999a; Maddux & DuCharme, 1997). In addition, self-efficacy beliefs can influence behavior both directly and through their influence on intentions (Bandura, 1997; Maddux & DuCharme, 1997).

Self-efficacy beliefs are not *outcome expectancies* (Bandura, 1997) or *behavior-outcome expectancies* (Maddux, 1999b). Self-efficacy is an evaluation of how well one can mobilize one's resources to accomplish goals. An outcome expectation is a "judgment of the likely consequence such performances will produce" (Bandura, 1997, p. 21). Thus, as people contemplate a goal and approach a task, they consider what behaviors and strategies are necessary to produce the outcome they want, and they evaluate to what extent they can perform those behaviors and implement those strategies.

Self-efficacy is not *perceived control*. The perception of control depends on the belief that (1) certain behaviors will allow one to control what one wants to control (behavior-outcome expectancies) and (2) that one can enact those behaviors (self-efficacy expectancies; Kirsch, 1999; Maddux, 1999b; see also Baumeister & Vohs, Chapter 10, this volume, and Ryan & Deci, Chapter 13, this volume).

Self-efficacy beliefs are not *causal attributions*. Causal attributions are explanations for events, including one's own behavior and its consequences. Self-efficacy beliefs can influence causal attributions and vice versa because beliefs about competencies can influence explanations of success and failure and because explanations for success and failure will, in turn, influence perceptions of competence. For example, people with low self-efficacy for an activity are more likely than people with high self-efficacy to attribute success in that activity to external factors rather than to personal capabilities (Bandura, 1986, 1989; Schunk, 1995).

Self-efficacy is not *self-concept* or *self-esteem*. Self-concept is what people believe about themselves, and self-esteem is how people feel about what they believe about themselves. Self-efficacy beliefs are an important aspect of self-concept (e.g., Deci & Ryan, 1995), but self-concept includes many other beliefs about the self that are unrelated to self-efficacy, such as beliefs about physical attributes and personality traits. Self-efficacy beliefs in a given domain will contribute to self-esteem only in direct proportion to the importance one places on that domain. My (J. E. M.) self-efficacy beliefs for playing basketball are very low (and accurately so), but my self-efficacy for playing basketball rarely affects my self-esteem, because I usually care very little about whether or not I am good at playing basketball. My self-efficacy for teaching and writing chapters and articles, however, is an entirely different matter. The impact of self-efficacy beliefs on self-esteem also will depend on their accessibility under given circumstances (Showers, 1995). Take me out of the classroom and put me on a basketball court, and my self-esteem probably will be temporarily somewhat deflated (see also the chapters in Part II of this volume, on content, structure, and organization of the self).

Self-efficacy is not a *trait*. Most conceptions of competence and control—locus of control (Rotter, 1966), optimism (Carver & Scheier, 2002), hope (Snyder, Rand, & Sigmon, 2002), hardiness (Kobasa, 1979), learned resourcefulness (Rosenbaum, 1990) —are conceived of as traits or trait-like. Self-efficacy beliefs are important in all of these constructs, but self-efficacy is defined and measured not as a trait but as beliefs about the ability to coordinate skills and abilities to attain desired goals in particular domains and circumstances. Self-efficacy beliefs can generalize from one situation or task to another, depending on the similarities between the task demands and the skills and resources required to meet those demands (e.g., Samuels & Gibbs, in press), but self-efficacy in a specific domain does not emanate from a general sense of efficacy. Measures of traits, such as optimism and perceived control, seem to predict behavior only to the extent to which they overlap with the measurement of self-efficacy (Cozzarelli, 1993; Dzewaltowski, Noble, & Shaw, 1990). In addition, measures of global efficacy beliefs have been developed (e.g., Schwarzer, Baessler, Kwiatek, Schroder, & Zhang, 1997; Sherer at al., 1982; Tipton & Worthington, 1984) and are used frequently in research, but they have not demonstrated predictive value above that of domain-specific self-efficacy measures (Martin & Gill, 1991; Pajares & Johnson, 1996).

Are There Different Types of Self-Efficacy?

The variety of ways in which self-efficacy beliefs have been measured by various researchers and the various domains and levels of specificity or generality with which self-efficacy has been measured might lead one to conclude that there are different "types" of self-efficacy (e.g., Cervone, 2000; Mone, 1994; Schwarzer & Renner, 2000). The confusion arises partly because the term "self-efficacy" has been used in at least two different ways in research: (1) as the perceived ability to perform a particular behavior, which Kirsch (1995) has called *task self-efficacy*; and (2) the perceived ability to prevent, control, or cope with potential difficulties that might be encountered when engaged in a performance, which Kirsch called *coping self-efficacy* (see also Schwarzer & Renner, 2000; Williams, 1995). Kirsch's task self-efficacy is similar to Bandura's original (1977) definition of self-efficacy as "the conviction that one can successfully execute the behavior required to produce the outcomes" (p. 193). Kirsch's coping self-efficacy is more similar to Bandura's more recent (1997) definition of self-efficacy as the ability to "organize and execute the courses of action required to produce given attainments" (p. 3).

Of course, the names researchers give measures can be misleading. Just because two researchers use the term "self-efficacy" for two different measures does not mean that those measures are measuring two different "types" of self-efficacy or even that they are measuring self-efficacy at all. Self-efficacy should not be viewed as a construct with different "types"; rather, measures of self-efficacy are tailored for different types

of behaviors and performances in different domains and situations, ranging from relatively simple motor acts (Kirsch's task self-efficacy) to complex and challenging behavioral sequences and orchestrations (Kirsch's coping self-efficacy). For example, "hammering nails" and "sawing wood" may be simple (but not always easy) motor acts, but "building a house" is a complex undertaking that requires abilities beyond the effective manipulation of tools. One can have a self-efficacy belief for each of these motor acts, and one can have self-efficacy beliefs for building a house. Each requires some generative capability, although the generative capability required for hammering a nail is relatively small, whereas the generative capability required for building a house is relatively large. Likewise, "self-efficacy for condom use" could have two very different meanings—one trivial, one important. A person could have strong self-efficacy for slipping a condom over a penis but weak self-efficacy for "using a condom." Convincing a resistant partner to wear a condom requires complex social skills and self-management skills that go far beyond the ability to slip a vinyl casing over a shaft of flesh (e.g., Siegel, Mesagno, Chen, & Christ, 1989). Beliefs concerning the ability to execute these different behaviors and sequences are not different types of self-efficacy; rather, they are self-efficacy beliefs for different types of performances.

Is the belief that one can attain one's goal, as opposed to the belief that one can execute certain strategies for attaining goals, a type of self-efficacy, as some suggest (e.g., Cervone, 2000)? Should researchers use the term "self-efficacy" to refer to expectancies for attaining outcomes and goals and to expectancies for engaging in behaviors and performances to attain outcomes and goals (e.g, Bandura, 1995; Mone, 1994)? The answer depends on how the terms "performance," "goal," and "outcome" are defined. For example, getting an A in a course is neither a behavior nor a performance; it is an outcome that results from engaging in many behaviors and performances. Because a goal is a desired outcome, getting an A can certainly be a goal. Furthermore, getting an A is a marker of performance attainment (Bandura, 1995) because the A is the marker that indicates that one's performances were ultimately successful. The A, however, is a measure of the success of the performance, not the performance itself. Therefore, talking about "self-efficacy for getting an A" expands the meaning of self-efficacy from beliefs about performing behaviors and mobilizing resources to beliefs about attaining goals and outcomes. We should not use the term "self-efficacy" to refer to the expectancy for attaining an outcome (goal, performance marker) if we also use the term "self-efficacy" to refer to the expectancy engaging in the performances that lead to the goal. What we call this expectancy for attaining a goal is less important than acknowledging that it is not the same as the expectancy for performing behavior or mobilizing the resources that might lead to the goal. Kirsch's (1995) "personal outcome expectancy" and McClelland's (1984) "probability of success" are reasonable names for the former construct.

Measuring Self-Efficacy Beliefs

To be useful in research and practice, concepts need to be translated into operational definitions or measurement strategies. In addition, concepts will be most useful when their operational definitions are consistent across studies. Unfortunately, self-efficacy has been measured in such a variety of ways that comparing findings from one study with those of another often is difficult, as Forsyth and Carey (1998) point out regarding research on self-efficacy and safe sex behavior. For this reason, a few guidelines for measuring self-efficacy beliefs might be useful.

As noted previously, self-efficacy is not a trait and should not be measured as such. Instead, self-efficacy measures should be specific to the domain of interest (e.g., social skills, exercise, dieting, safe sex, arithmetic skills). Within a given domain, self-efficacy beliefs can be measured at varying degrees of behavioral and situational specificity, depending on what one is trying to predict. Thus the measurement of self-efficacy should be designed to capture the multifaceted nature of behavior and the context in which it occurs. Specifying behaviors and contexts improves the predictive power of self-efficacy measures, but such specificity can reach a point of diminishing returns if

carried too far. Therefore, the researcher must "know the territory" and have a thorough understanding of the behavioral domain in question, including the types of abilities called on and the range of situations in which they might be used (Bandura, 1997).

Self-efficacy measures can err in the direction of being not specific enough. For example, a poor measure of self-efficacy for dieting would be, "How confident are you that you will be able to stick to your diet when tempted to break it?" (Typically a scale of 1 to 7, 1 to 10, or 1 to 100 is used.) A good measure would be, "How confident are you that you will be able to stick to your diet when watching television?" (also "when depressed," "when someone offers you high fat food," "when eating breakfast at a restaurant"). These items should include a range of situations that offer a range of challenge from very easy to very difficult. Self-efficacy measures also can err in the direction of excessive specificity. For example, an assessment of self-efficacy for engaging in safe sex might include the item, "How confident are you that you could resist your partner's insistence that using a condom isn't necessary?" But an item that asks, "How confident are you that you could open the wrapper?" probably is neither necessary nor useful. Likewise, a good measure of self-efficacy for exercise might include an item concerning confidence in "your ability to fit a short walk or run into a busy day," but asking about confidence in "your ability to tie your running shoes" probably is going a little too far.

The information about behaviors and situations that is essential for constructing good self-efficacy measures can be acquired through interviews and surveys with people for whom the problem domain at hand is relevant, such as people who are trying to lose weight or engage in regular exercise (Bandura, 1997). (For additional guidelines, see Bandura, 1997, pp. 42–50, and Bandura, 1995.)

How Self-Efficacy Beliefs Develop

Major Sources of Self-Efficacy Beliefs

Self-efficacy beliefs are the result of information integrated from five sources: performance experience, vicarious experience, imaginal experience, verbal persuasion, and affective and physiological states.

One's own *performance experiences* are the most powerful source of self-efficacy information (Bandura, 1977, 1997). Successful attempts at control that one attributes to one's own efforts will strengthen self-efficacy for that behavior or domain. Perceptions of failure at control attempts usually diminish self-efficacy.

Self-efficacy beliefs also are influenced by *vicarious experiences*—observations of the behavior of others and the consequences of that behavior. People use these observations to form expectancies about their own behavior and its consequences, depending primarily on the extent to which a person believes that he or she is similar to the person he or she is observing. Vicarious experiences generally have weaker effects on self-efficacy expectancy than do performance experiences (Bandura, 1997).

People can influence their self-efficacy beliefs by *imagining* themselves or others behaving effectively or ineffectively in hypothetical situations. Such images can be inadvertent ruminations, or they can be an intentional self-efficacy enhancement strategy. These images may be derived from actual or vicarious experiences with situations similar to the one anticipated, or they may be induced by verbal persuasion, as when a psychotherapist guides a client through imagination-based interventions such as systematic desensitization and covert modeling (Williams, 1995). Simply imagining oneself doing something well, however, is not likely to have as strong an influence on self-efficacy as will an actual success experience (Williams, 1995).

Self-efficacy beliefs are influenced by *verbal persuasion*—what others say to one about one's abilities and probability of success. The potency of verbal persuasion as a source of self-efficacy beliefs is influenced by such factors as the expertness, trustworthiness, and attractiveness of the source, as suggested by decades of research on verbal persuasion and attitude change (e.g., Eagly & Chaiken, 1993). Verbal persuasion is a less potent source of enduring change in self-efficacy than are performance experiences and vicarious experiences.

Physiological and emotional states influence self-efficacy when people learn to associate poor performance or perceived failure with aversive physiological arousal and success with pleasant emotions. Thus, when people become aware of unpleasant physiological arousal, they are more likely to doubt their competence than if their physiological states are pleasant or neutral. Likewise, comfortable physiological sensations are likely to lead people to feel confident in their ability to deal with the situation at hand. Physiological indicants of self-efficacy expectancy, however, extend beyond autonomic arousal. For example, in activities involving strength and stamina, such as exercise and athletic performances, perceived efficacy is influenced by such experiences as fatigue and pain (Bandura, 1997).

Self-efficacy beliefs for a given performance in a given situation will be the result of the confluence of proximal (current) and distal (past) information from these five sources. For example, social self-efficacy during an ongoing interaction, such as a job interview or conversation with someone to whom one is attracted, will be determined by a variety of proximal and distal sources of information about one's social self-efficacy. Distal sources include past perceived successes and failures in similar interactions, evaluations about one's social skills made by important others, and recollection of one's physiological and emotional states during these similar interactions. Thus the person enters the new situation with well-formed beliefs about his or her ability to negotiate the situation successfully—beliefs that can lead to emotional comfort or to distress. Proximal sources of social self-efficacy might include one's physiological and emotional states (e.g., relaxed vs. anxious, happy vs. sad); one's own evaluation of one's ongoing performance; comments from others in the interaction; and interpretations of the reactions of others, which together may suggest, on a moment-to-moment basis, whether or not one is moving toward achieving one's goals in the situation, including self-presentational goals (Leary & Kowalski, 1995; Maddux, Norton, & Leary, 1988). Just as proximal consequences usually exert greater control over behavior than distal (future) consequences, proximal information about self-efficacy is likely to have a more powerful immediate effect on current self-efficacy and performance than distal past sources (see Kihlstrom, Beer, & Klein, Chapter 4, this volume).

Developmental Aspects of Self-Efficacy Beliefs

Self-efficacy beliefs develop over time through experience and through the interactions among the factors and forces noted previously. The process begins in infancy and continues throughout life. The early development of self-efficacy beliefs is influenced primarily by the development of the capacity for symbolic thought; the development of a sense of a "self" that is separate from others; and the reciprocal interaction of one's own behavior, the environment's responsiveness to one's behavior, and self-appraisal of one's performance (Bandura, 1997).

Infants who are only a few months old show some understanding of cause-and-effect relationships (Leslie, 1982; Mandler, 1992). As the infant's capacity for symbolic thought and memory increase, she comes to realize that she is distinct from others and from objects. He learns that biting his teddy bear's hand does not hurt but that biting his own hand does. She develops a sense of personal agency by performing the few actions of which she is capable, such as flailing her arms and legs, cooing, and grabbing and shaking objects. With repeated observations of actions and their consequences, he learns that he can affect his environment. As it becomes increasingly clear that outcomes are contingent on her behavior, the infant will attempt novel actions and examine their outcomes. These observations give her an understanding of the control she has over her surroundings.

On the other hand, if the infant repeatedly experiences delays in or absence of behavior-outcome contingency, such as observing a mechanical mobile that moves regardless of his behavior, he is less likely to come to understand and employ cause-and-effect relationships (Watson, 1977). Parents' responses to a child's attempts at exercising agency can influence greatly the development of efficacy beliefs (Bandura, 1997; Maxwell, 1998).

Thus the development of a sense of personal agency begins in infancy and moves from the perception of the causal relationship between events to an understanding that actions produce results to the recognition that one can produce actions that cause results (Bandura, 1997). As children's understanding of language increases, so does their capacity for symbolic thought and, therefore, their capacity for self-awareness and a sense of personal agency (Bandura, 1997; see also Harter, Chapter 30, this volume).

With each subsequent developmental period, the individual faces new demands and challenges that can build or diminish self-efficacy in the major domains of life. For example, in childhood, social self-efficacy beliefs are related to greater prosocial coping and less antisocial coping with interpersonal difficulties, and they predict how children manage or regulate their emotions (Denham, 1998). With adolescence comes the need to manage the demands of academics and peer relationships, physiological changes that result in sexual urges, and demands for increasing autonomy and responsibility—such as making decisions about sex and substance use. Making responsible decisions requires self-regulatory skills, whereby individuals guide their own actions by comparing what they are about to do with self-standards and develop plans and strategies to meet these standards (Bandura, 1997). For adolescents, an important aspect of self-regulation is the ability to think and act independently of others and to balance this ability with strong needs to affiliate. Thus adolescents who have a strong enough sense of self-efficacy to overcome peer pressure are less likely to abuse substances or to engage in unsafe sexual or in delinquent behavior (Caprara et al., 1998; Ludwig & Pittman, 1999).

Adulthood brings additional concerns and demands, primarily in the domains of work and relationships. Beliefs about personal abilities influence occupational choices, career paths, job-seeking behavior, and job performance (Bandura, 1997). Following job loss, job-seeking behavior can be enhanced by improving self-regulatory behavior and developing effective coping and problem-solving techniques (Vinokur, van Ryn, Gramlich, & Price, 1991). Individuals who have low self-efficacy in the area of vocational skills discourage themselves from applying for more appealing jobs (Wheeler, 1983).

Emerging adults also develop beliefs about their ability to fulfill certain roles, such as parenthood, and these beliefs influence how these roles are carried out (Bandura, 1997). For example, parents with higher goals for their children and who feel highly efficacious about their ability to advance their children's intellectual growth produce children with greater academic achievement (Bandura, Barbaranelli, Caprara, & Pastorelli, 1996). Efficacy beliefs can influence emotions experienced while performing adult roles. For example, mothers with higher parenting self-efficacy report less distress about parenting (Halpern & McLean, 1997). Parenting efficacy is influenced by a number of factors, such as the child's temperament and physical health and the social support available to the parent. Hence, the reciprocal interplay of a variety of factors influences the development of parental self-efficacy, which in turn influences parenting behaviors and the child's responses (Bandura, 1997).

In later life, self-efficacy often diminishes in a wide array of major life domains, including health, relationships, and cognitive tasks such as memory (McAvay, Seeman, & Rodin, 1996; McDougal, 1995). Self-efficacy for memory in older adults is malleable through experimental induction, and these induced positive changes in memory self-efficacy can facilitate recall of information (Gardiner, Luszcz, & Bryan, 1997). Although age-related declines in efficacy beliefs may reflect actual declines in ability, providing incentives to exercise one's memory might enhance subsequent memory performance. Among the infirm aged, the structure and organization of institutions (e.g., nursing homes) may actually diminish self-efficacy in important domains by limiting mastery experiences (Welch & West, 1995).

How and Why Self-Efficacy Beliefs Are Important

Self-efficacy plays a crucial role in our everyday lives in countless ways. Seven important areas that have received considerable attention from researchers are (1) self-regulation, (2) psychological well-being and adjustment, (3) physical health, (4) psychotherapy, (5) education, (6) occupational choice and performance, and (7) collective efficacy among groups and organizations. We begin by describing the role of self-efficacy beliefs in self-regulation because it is from self-efficacy's effect of self-regulatory ability that all of its other effects flow.

Self-Efficacy and Self-Regulation

One of the most important consequences of the development of self-efficacy beliefs (either strong ones or weak ones) is the development of capacity for self-regulation. Like self-efficacy, the capacity for self-regulation is not a fixed and generalized personality trait; instead, it is a set of skills that, like self-efficacy beliefs, develop in particular domains. As we have all seen in our own behavior and that of others, people can be relatively good self-regulators in some aspects of their lives and relatively poor self-regulators in others. Witness the highly disciplined athlete or the driven and committed public servant who makes a mess of his or her personal life or finances through careless, impulsive behavior. Yet studies of otherwise unexceptional people who have overcome difficult behavioral problems without professional help provide compelling evidence for people's capacity for self-regulation under even highly challenging circumstances (e.g., Prochaska, Norcross, DiClemente, 1994). Research on self-efficacy has added greatly to our understanding of how people guide their own behavior in the pursuit of their goals and how they sometimes fail to do so effectively.

Self-regulation (simplified) depends on four interacting components (Bandura, 1986, 1997; Barone, Maddux, & Snyder, 1997): goals or standards of performance; feedback; self-evaluative reactions to performance; and self-efficacy beliefs (see also Baumeister & Vohs, Chapter 10, this volume).

Goals are essential to self-regulation because people attempt to regulate their actions, thoughts, and emotions to achieve desired outcomes. The ability to envision desired future events and states allows people to create incentives that motivate and guide their actions. Goals also provide people with personal standards against which to monitor their progress and evaluate both their progress and their abilities.

Feedback is information about progress toward or away from a goal. This information can be provided by the physical environment, by other people, or by oneself. Feedback is essential to the effectiveness of goals (Locke & Latham, 1990).

People do not simply perceive information; they *interpret* it. Likewise, feedback about progress toward or away from a goal is interpreted, and different people will interpret the same feedback in different ways and react to it in different ways. Thus *self-evaluative reactions* are important in self-regulation because people's beliefs about the progress they are making (or not making) toward their goals are major determinants of their emotional reactions during goal-directed activity. These emotional reactions, in turn, can enhance or disrupt self-regulation. The belief that one is inefficacious and making poor progress toward a goal produces distressing emotional states (e.g., anxiety, depression) that can lead to cognitive and behavioral ineffectiveness and self-regulatory failure. Strong self-efficacy beliefs and strong expectations for goal attainment, however, usually produce adaptive emotional states that, in turn, enhance self-regulation.

Self-efficacy beliefs influence self-regulation in several ways. First, they influence the tasks people decide to tackle. The higher one's self-efficacy in a specific achievement domain, the loftier will be the goals that one sets for oneself in that domain.

Second, self-efficacy beliefs influence people's choices of goal-directed activities, expenditure of effort, persistence in the face of challenge and obstacles (Bandura, 1986, Locke & Latham, 1990), and reactions to perceived discrepancies between goals and current performance (Bandura, 1986). In the face of difficulties, people with weak self-efficacy beliefs easily develop doubts about their ability to accomplish the task at hand, whereas those with strong efficacy beliefs continue their efforts to master a task when difficulties arise. Perseverance usually produces desired results, and this success then strengthens the individual's self-efficacy beliefs. Motivation to accomplish difficult tasks and accomplish lofty goals is en-

hanced by overestimates of personal capabilities (i.e., positive illusions; Taylor & Brown, 1988), which then become self-fulfilling prophecies when people set their sights high, persevere, and surpass their previous levels of accomplishments. People with strong efficacy beliefs in a given domain will be relatively resistant to the disruptions in self-regulation that can result from difficulties and setbacks. As a result, they will persevere. Perseverance usually produces desired results, and this success then increases one's sense of efficacy.

Through the monitoring of their behavior and the situation, people develop beliefs not only about their current level of competence but also about the *rate* of improvement in competence and the rate of progress toward their goals. Motivation is not static, and at any given time, self-efficacy, affect, and behavior will be influenced not only by beliefs about one's current level of competence but also by the expected rate of change in competence or movement toward a goal. For example, a person learning a new skill will be concerned not just with whether or not he or she will attain a certain level of proficiency but also with how quickly he or she will attain that level of proficiency. People are more likely to persist in developing a skill or persist in efforts toward a goal if they believe that proficiency in the skill or attainment of the goal will come sooner rather than later.

Third, self-efficacy for solving problems and making decisions influences the efficiency and effectiveness of problem solving and decision making. When faced with complex decisions, people who have confidence in their ability to solve problems use their cognitive resources more effectively than do those people who doubt their cognitive skills (e.g., Bandura, 1997). Such efficacy usually leads to better solutions and greater achievement. In the face of difficulty, a person with high self-efficacy is more likely to remain *task-diagnostic* and continue to search for solutions to problems. Those with low self-efficacy, however, are more likely to become *self-diagnostic* and reflect on their inadequacies, which distracts them from their efforts to assess and solve the problem (Bandura, 1997).

Most of the research on the effect of self-efficacy on self-regulation suggests that "more is better"—that is, the higher one's self-efficacy, the more effective one's self-regulation in pursuit of a goal. But can self-efficacy be too high? Perhaps so, in at least two ways. First, as Bandura (1986) has suggested, "a reasonably accurate appraisal of one's capabilities is . . . of considerable value in effective functioning" and people who overestimate their abilities may "undertake activities that are clearly beyond their reach" (p. 393). Certainly, an important feature of effective self-regulation is to know when to disengage from a goal because one's efforts are not paying off. Although strong self-efficacy beliefs usually contribute to adaptive tenacity, if these beliefs are unrealistically high, they may result in the relentless pursuit of an obviously (to observers) unattainable goal. Thus high self-efficacy beliefs that are not supported by past experience or rewarded by positive goal-related feedback can result in wasted effort and resources that might be better directed elsewhere. As of yet, however, we have no way of determining when self-efficacy is "too high" and at what point people should give up trying to achieve their goals.

Second, the way in which strong self-efficacy beliefs develop can be important. Strong self-efficacy beliefs that are attained too quickly and easily may lead to complacency and diminished effort and performance. People who develop strong efficacy beliefs without effort and struggle may set lower goals than do those who attain strong efficacy beliefs through hard work. In addition, those who too easily attain strong efficacy beliefs may alter their performance standards and be too easily satisfied by performance feedback, including declining performance (Bandura & Jourdan, 1991). As a result, progress toward a goal may be hindered.

Psychological Well-Being and Adjustment

The belief that one has good self-regulatory skills is an important contributor to good psychological health and adjustment. Most philosophers and psychological theorists agree that a sense of control over one's behavior, one's environment, and one's own thoughts and feelings is essential for happiness and a sense of well-being. When the world seems predictable and controllable, and when behaviors, thoughts, and emotions seem within their control, people are better able to meet life's challenges, build healthy relationships, and achieve personal satisfaction and peace of mind. Feelings of loss of control are common among people who seek the help of psychotherapists and counselors.

Self-efficacy beliefs play a major role in a number of common psychological problems. Low self-efficacy expectancies are an important feature of depression (Bandura, 1997; Bandura, Pastorelli, Barbaranelli, & Caprara, 1999; Kavanaugh, 1992; Maddux & Meier, 1995). Depressed people usually believe they are less capable than other people of behaving effectively in many important areas of life. They usually doubt their ability to form and maintain supportive relationships and therefore may avoid potentially supportive people during periods of depression. Dysfunctional anxiety and avoidant behavior are often the direct result of low self-efficacy expectancies for managing threatening situations (Bandura, 1997; Williams, 1995; Williams, Kinney, Harap, & Liebmann, 1997). People who have strong confidence in their abilities to perform and manage potentially difficult situations will approach those situations calmly and will not be unduly disrupted by difficulties. On the other hand, people who lack confidence in their abilities will either avoid potentially difficult situations or approach them with apprehension, thereby reducing the probability that they will perform effectively. Thus they will have fewer success experiences and fewer opportunities to increase their self-efficacy. People with low self-efficacy also will respond to difficulties with increased anxiety, which usually disrupts performance, thereby further lowering self-efficacy, and so on. Stressful events often result in physical symptoms (e.g., headache), as well as psychological symptoms, and self-efficacy beliefs influence the relationship between stressful events and physical symptoms (Arnstein, Caudill, Mandle, Norris, & Beasley, 1999; Marlowe, 1998). Self-efficacy beliefs also predict effective coping with traumatic life events such as homelessness (Epel, Bandura, & Zimbardo, 1999) and natural disasters (Benight, Swift, Sanger, Smith, & Zeppelin, 2000).

Among people recovering from substance abuse, self-efficacy for avoiding relapse in high-risk situations and for recovery from relapse play a powerful role in successful abstinence (Bandura, 1999; DiClemente, Fairhurst, & Piotrowski, 1995; Mudde, Kok, & Strecher, 1996; Oei, Fergusson, & Lee, 1998). The same is true in the successful treatment of people with eating disorders (Goodrick et al., 1999) and of male sex offenders (Pollock, 1996).

Self-Efficacy and Physical Health

Health and medical care in our society gradually has been shifting from an exclusive emphasis on the treatment of disease to an emphasis on the prevention of disease and the promotion of good health. Most strategies for preventing health problems, enhancing health, and hastening recovery from illness and injury involve changing behavior. In addition, psychology and physiology are tightly intertwined such that affective and cognitive phenomena are influenced by physiological phenomena and vice versa (e.g., Bandura, 1986). Thus beliefs about self-efficacy influence health in two ways—through their influence on the behaviors that affect health and through their direct influence on physiological processes.

First, self-efficacy influences the adoption of healthy behaviors, the cessation of unhealthy behaviors, and the maintenance of behavioral changes in the face of challenge and difficulty. Research on self-efficacy has greatly enhanced our understanding of how and why people adopt healthy and unhealthy behaviors and of how to change behaviors that affect health (Bandura, 1997; Maddux, Brawley, & Boykin, 1995; O'Leary & Brown, 1995). All of the major theories of health behavior, such as protection motivation theory (Maddux & Rogers, 1983; Rogers & Prentice-Dunn, 1997), the health belief model (Strecher, Champion, & Rosenstock, 1997), and the theory of reasoned action–planned behavior (Ajzen, 1988; Fishbein & Ajzen, 1975; Maddux & DuCharme, 1997) include self-efficacy as a key component (see also Maddux, 1993; Weinstein, 1993). In addition, self-efficacy beliefs are crucial to successful change and maintenance of virtually every behavior crucial to health: exercise, diet, stress management, safe sex, smoking cessation, overcoming alcohol abuse, compliance with treatment and prevention regimens, and detection behaviors such as breast self-lexaminations (AbuSabha & Achterberg, 1997; Bandura, 1997; Bryan, Aiken, & West, 1997; Dawson & Brawley, 2000; Ewart, 1995; Holman & Lorig, 1992; Maddux et al., 1995; Schwarzer, 1992).

Second, self-efficacy beliefs influence a number of biological processes that, in turn, influence health and disease (Bandura, 1997). Self-efficacy beliefs affect the body's physiological responses to stress, including the immune system (Bandura, 1997; O'Leary & Brown, 1995) and the physiological pathways activated by physical activity (Rudolph & McAuley, 1995). Lack of perceived control over environmental demands can increase susceptibility to infections and hasten the progression of disease (Bandura, 1997). Self-efficacy beliefs also influence the activation of catecholamines, a family of neurotransmitters important to the management of stress and perceived threat, along with the endogenous painkillers referred to as endorphins (Bandura, 1997; O'Leary & Brown, 1995).

Self-Efficacy and Psychotherapy

The term "psychotherapy" refers to professionally guided interventions designed to enhance psychological well-being, although it must be acknowledged that the client's *self*-regulation plays an important role in all such interventions. In fact, most professionally guided interventions are designed to enhance self-regulation because they are concerned with helping people gain or regain a sense of efficacy over important aspects of their lives (Frank & Frank, 1991). Different interventions, or different components of an intervention, may be equally effective because they equally enhance self-efficacy for crucial behavioral and cognitive skills (Bandura, 1997; Maddux & Lewis, 1995).

Self-efficacy theory emphasizes the importance of arranging experiences designed to increase the person's sense of efficacy for specific behaviors in specific problematic and challenging situations. Self-efficacy theory suggests that formal interventions should not simply resolve specific problems but should provide people with the skills and sense of efficacy for solving problems themselves. Some basic strategies for enhancing self-efficacy are based on the five sources of self-efficacy previously noted.

Performance Experience

In facilitating self-efficacy, few things are more important than having people provide themselves with tangible evidence of their success. When people actually can see themselves coping effectively with difficult situations, their sense of mastery is likely to be heightened. These experiences are likely to be most successful when both goals and strategies are specific. Goals that are concrete, specific, and proximal (short range) provide greater incentive, motivation, and evidence of efficacy than goals that are abstract, vague, and set in the distant future (Locke & Latham, 1990). Specific goals allow people to identify the specific behaviors needed for successful achievement and to know when they have succeeded (Locke & Latham, 1990). For example, the most effective interventions for phobias and fears involve *guided mastery—in vivo* experience with the feared object or situation during therapy sessions, or between sessions as "homework" assignments (Williams, 1995). In cognitive treatments of depression, clients are provided structured guidance in arranging success experiences that will counteract low self-efficacy expectancies (Hollon & Beck, 1994).

Verbal Persuasion

Most formal psychological interventions rely strongly on verbal persuasion to enhance a client's self-efficacy by encouraging small risks that may lead to small successes. In cognitive and cognitive-behavioral therapies, the therapist engages the client in a discussion of the client's dysfunctional beliefs, attitudes, and expectancies and helps the client see the irrationality and self-defeating nature of such beliefs. The therapist encourages the client to adopt new, more adaptive beliefs and to act on these new beliefs and expectancies. As a result, the client experiences the successes that can lead to more enduring changes in self-efficacy beliefs and adaptive behavior (see Hollon & Beck, 1994; and In-

gram, Kendall, & Chen, 1991, for reviews). People also rely daily on verbal persuasion as a self-efficacy facilitator by seeking the support of other people when attempting to lose weight, quit smoking, maintain an exercise program, or summon up the courage to confront a difficult boss or loved one.

Vicarious Experience

Vicarious learning strategies can be used to teach new skills and enhance self-efficacy for those skills. For example, modeling films and videotapes have been used successfully to encourage socially withdrawn children to interact with other children. The child viewing the film sees the model child, someone much like himself, experience success and comes to believe that he too can do the same thing (Conger & Keane, 1981). Modeling can be particularly effective if models demonstrate or describe their struggle and success with managing difficult task demands rather than model a seemingly effortless, flawless performance (Bandura, 1997). *In vivo* modeling has been used successfully in the treatment of phobic individuals. This research has shown that changes in self-efficacy beliefs for approach behaviors mediate adaptive behavioral changes (Bandura, 1986; Williams, 1995). Common everyday (nonprofessional) examples of the use of vicarious experiences to enhance self-efficacy include advertisements for weight-loss and smoking cessation programs that feature testimonials from successful people. The clear message from these testimonials is that the listener or reader also can accomplish this difficult task. Formal and informal "support groups"—people sharing their personal experiences in overcoming a common adversity such as addiction, obesity, or illness—also provide forums for the enhancement of self-efficacy.

Imaginal Experience

Live or filmed models may be difficult to obtain, but the imagination is an easily harnessed resource. Imagining oneself engaging in feared behaviors or overcoming difficulties can be used to enhance self-efficacy. For example, cognitive therapy for anxiety and fear problems often involves modifying visual images of danger and anxiety, including images of coping effectively with the feared situation. Imaginal (covert) modeling has been used successfully in interventions to increase assertive behavior and self-efficacy for assertiveness (Kazdin, 1979). Systematic desensitization and implosion are traditional behavioral therapy techniques that rely on the ability to image coping effectively with a difficult situation (Emmelkamp, 1994). Because maladaptive distorted imagery is an important component of anxiety and depression, various techniques have been developed to help clients modify distortions and maladaptive assumptions contained in their visual images of danger and anxiety. A client can gain a sense of control over a situation by imagining a future self that can deal effectively with the situation.

Physiological and Emotional States

People usually feel more self-efficacious when calm than they do when aroused and distressed. Thus strategies for controlling and reducing emotional arousal (specifically anxiety) while attempting new behaviors should increase self-efficacy and increase the likelihood of successful implementation. Hypnosis, biofeedback, relaxation training, meditation, and medication are the most common strategies for reducing the physiological arousal typically associated with low self-efficacy and poor performance.

Enhancing the Impact of Success

Success is subjective, and accomplishments that are judged "successful" by observers are not always judged so by the performer. People often discount self-referential information that is inconsistent with current self-views (Barone et al., 1997; Fiske & Taylor, 1991). Thus, when people feel distressed and believe they are incompetent and helpless, they are likely to ignore or discount information from therapists, family, friends, and their own behavioral successes that is inconsistent with their negative self-beliefs (Barone et al., 1997; Fiske & Taylor, 1991). Therefore, therapists need to make concerted efforts to increase success experiences, but they also must encourage clients to interpret that success *as success* and as the result of their own efforts. Success experiences can be made more effective in two ways.

First, people who view competence as a set of skills to be performed in specific situations rather than as a trait and as *incremental* (acquirable through effort and experience) rather than *fixed* are more likely to persist in the face of obstacles (Dweck, 2000). The development of an incremental view of competence can be encouraged by the comparison of recent successful behaviors with past ineffective behaviors. Therefore, therapists need to teach clients to be eternally vigilant for success experiences and to actively retrieve past successes in times of challenge and doubt.

Second, changes in *causal attributions* can result in changes in self-efficacy. Self-efficacy can be enhanced by attributing successes to one's own effort and ability rather than to environmental circumstances or to the expertise and insights of others (Forsterling, 1986; Goldfried & Robins, 1982; Thompson, 1991). In addition, an individual who holds strong self-efficacy beliefs will be more resilient when setbacks occur and will be more likely to attribute failure to inadequate effort rather than to personal inability. Therefore, therapists should encourage clients to attribute successful change to their own efforts and abilities, not to the therapist's power or expertise.

Education

Children's educational efficacy beliefs are powerful predictors of their educational achievements (e.g., Schunk, 1995; Schunk & Zimmerman, 1997), although the pathways through which efficacy operates are diverse and complex (Bandura et al., 1996). Measures of academic self-efficacy are more powerful predictors of educational achievement than are global measures of academic self-concept (Bong & Clark, 1999).

A stronger sense of academic self-efficacy is associated with a greater likelihood of seeking help from teachers (Ryan, Gheen, & Midgley, 1998). The unfortunate paradox here is that the students with the least confidence in their abilities—the ones who may be most in need of help—are the least likely to seek help, an avoidance strategy that can only serve as a barrier to both skill acquisition and efficacy enhancement.

A child's academic success depends not only on his or her sense of efficacy but also on the efforts (or lack thereof) of his or her parents. Successful parental involvement in a child's education appears to be influenced strongly by the parents' sense of efficacy for helping their children succeed academically (Bandura et al., 1996; Hoover-Dempsey & Sandler, 1997).

Occupational Choice and Performance

Few choices have greater impact on life satisfaction than one's choice of occupation or career. These choices are often limited not by deficiencies in skills and abilities but by deficiencies in one's beliefs about one's skills and abilities. Such self-efficacy beliefs are important predictors of what occupations people choose to enter (the content of career choices) and how people go about making their choices (the process of career choices; Hackett & Betz, 1995), above and beyond what can be predicted from people's vocational interests (Donnay & Borgen, 1999). Most of the research on self-efficacy and occupational or career choice has focused on understanding the choices of women and members of minority groups, partly because these groups have traditionally been more restrained in their career and occupational roles and choices by societal norms (e.g., Byars & Hackett, 1998). Men and women usually express equivalent efficacy beliefs for most (but not all) traditionally female-dominated occupations, but women usually express lower self-efficacy for traditionally male-dominated occupations than for traditionally female-dominated occupations (Hackett & Betz, 1995). Perceptions of self-efficacy, outcome expectancies, and social forces (i.e., stereotyping) are associated with the underrepresentation of women and ethnic minorities in careers dominated by white males (Hackett & Betz, 1995). For example, women and African Americans tend to avoid classes and careers involving math and science, depriving themselves of the exposure to these areas (Betz, 1997). In addition, based on stereotypes that women and certain ethnic minorities are not as successful in these areas, they may not perform to the best of their ability, creating a "self-fulfilling prophecy," as they undermine their own performances in accordance with their expectancies. Without success experiences, these individuals' self-efficacy for perfor-

mance in these areas may remain low, leading to further avoidance of these kinds of tasks.

In addition, women and minorities have less access to self-efficacy-enhancing experiences for traditionally nonfemale and nonminority careers (Hackett & Byars, 1996). They generally have fewer positive models—particularly in science and technology careers—through which they can gain vicarious efficacy-enhancing experiences, and they may receive less encouragement from others to pursue nontraditional careers. When they encounter potentially efficacy-building experiences, if they believe in negative gender or ethnic stereotypes, their performances are likely to suffer due to avoidance of tasks, lack of focus on the task, or negative emotional arousal such as anxiety (Hackett & Byars, 1996). Even when members of a minority group develop strong self-efficacy beliefs, they may maintain low expectancies that their performances will lead to desired outcomes due to discrimination (Bandura, 1997). For example, African American children hold lower outcome expectancies for themselves than for Caucasian children, despite their beliefs that they can engage in the same behaviors as middle-class Caucasian children (Mickelson, 1990; Ogbu, 1991).

Self-efficacy beliefs predict not only what occupations people choose but also how well they perform those occupations. A recent meta-analysis of 144 studies on self-efficacy and work-related performance (Stajkovic & Luthans, 1998) found a weighted average correlation of .38 between self-efficacy measures and measure of work performance. This relationship is stronger than what has been shown for the effect on performance of goal-setting, feedback interventions, organizational behavior modifications, and personality trait-like constructs (Stajkovic & Luthans, 1998). The effects of self-efficacy beliefs on work-related performance seem to operate through their influence on task-related strategies, task focus, and early skill acquisition (Stajkovic & Luthans, 1998).

Collective Efficacy

Accomplishing important goals among groups, organizations, and societies always has depended on the ability of individuals to identify the abilities of other individuals and to harness these abilities to accomplish common goals. Thus a concept of perceived mastery that considers only individuals has limited utility. Social cognitive theory recognizes that the individual is embedded in a social network and a cultural milieu. Thus self-efficacy theory recognizes that there are limits to what individuals can accomplish alone. This idea is captured in the notion of *collective efficacy*, "a group's shared belief in its conjoint capabilities to organize and execute the courses of action required to produce given levels of attainments (Bandura, 1997, p. 477; also Zaccaro, Blair, Peterson, & Zazanis, 1995). Simply stated, collective efficacy is the extent to which people believe that they can work together effectively to accomplish their shared goals. Just as personal agency involves beliefs about personal abilities, collective agency involves a collective sense of efficacy. As does self-efficacy, collective efficacy influences collective motivation, planning and decision making, effective use of group resources, and persistence in goal pursuit (Bandura, 1997; Zaccaro et al., 1995).

Because collective efficacy is a relatively new term, researchers have not reached a consensus on its measurement. Some posit that collective efficacy consists of the individuals' perceptions of the group's abilities (e.g, Weldon & Weingart, 1993) or the individual's beliefs about the group's beliefs about its abilities (Paskevich, Brawley, Dorsch, & Widmeyer, 1999). Others have added together group members' individual responses to determine collective efficacy (Zacarro et al., 1995). Still others contend that collective efficacy includes beliefs that are shared among group members about how well the individual members can perform the actions necessary for success, as well as beliefs about how well they can orchestrate their combined efforts (Zaccaro et al, 1995). As with all social constructions, a consensus on the definition and measurement of collective efficacy will develop gradually as theorists and researchers debate the merits of the various alternatives (Maddux, 1999a).

Despite a lack of consensus on its measurement (Bandura, 1997; Maddux, 1999a), collective efficacy has been found to be important to a number of "collectives." The more efficacious spouses feel about their shared ability to accomplish important shared goals, the more satisfied they are with their marriages (Kaplan & Maddux, 2001). The individual and collective efficacy of teachers for effective instruction seems to affect the academic achievement of schoolchildren (Bandura, 1993, 1997). The effectiveness of self-managing work teams (Little & Madigan, 1997) and group "brainstorming" (Prussia & Kinicki, 1996) also seems to be related to a collective sense of efficacy. In neighborhoods, lower collective efficacy is associated with violent crime rates above and beyond the factors of lower family income; higher proportions of minorities, immigrants, and single-parent families; and previous homicide rates (Sampson, Raudenbush, & Earls, 1997). Finally, collective efficacy has become an important construct in the study of team sports and has facilitated a shift in research from a focus on individual motivation to group motivation (George & Feltz, 1995; Marks, 1999). For example, research has found that the collective efficacy of an athletic team can be raised or lowered by false feedback about ability and can subsequently influence its success in competitions (Hodges & Carron, 1992).

As cultural variations become more widely studied, research indicates, collective efficacy may be a more useful predictor of emotion and behavior in some cultures than in others. For example, collective efficacy is negatively correlated with depression, anxiety, and the desire to leave employment for workers in Hong Kong, but not among American workers (Schaubroeck, Lam, & Xie, 2000). An explanation for this difference is that collective efficacy may be a more important contributor to group achievements in groups that are higher in collectivism (Gibson, 1995). Nonetheless, individuals will differ in their collectivist and individualist leanings regardless of the group or cultural norms, and these individual differences may be more important than the group or cultural norm.

Researchers also are beginning to understand how people develop a sense of collective efficacy for promoting social and political change (Fernandez-Ballesteros, Diez-Nicolas, Caprara, Barbaranelli, & Bandura, 2000). Of course, personal efficacy and collective efficacy go hand in hand because a "collection of inveterate self-doubters is not easily forged into a collectively efficacious force" (Bandura, 1997, p. 480). In addition to self-efficacy and collective efficacy, other factors play a role in social change, such as preexisting sociocultural standards, outcome expectations (i.e., perceived benefit or cost of changes to particular groups), and perceived obstacles to change (Bandura, 1997).

The distinction between self-efficacy and collective efficacy should not be confused with the dimension of cultural orientation usually referred to as individualism–collectivism, the extent to which a culture values the individual relative to the group, competition versus cooperation, and individual goals and achievements versus collective goals and achievements. In even the most individualistic cultures, collective goals are important, and a sense of collective efficacy is essential for the attainment of those goals. Likewise, in even the most collectivist cultures, individuals set personal goals that may not require collective effort and group cooperation, and self-efficacy will be crucial in the attainment of those goals.

The ability of businesses, organizations, communities, and governments (local, state, and national) to achieve their goals will increasingly depend on their ability to coordinate their efforts, particularly because their goals often may conflict. In a world in which communication across the globe often is faster than communication across the street and in which cooperation and collaboration in commerce and government is becoming increasingly common and increasingly crucial, understanding collective efficacy will become increasingly important.

Summary

> The very little engine looked up and saw the tears in the dolls' eyes. And she thought of the good little boys and girls on the other side of the mountain who would not have any toys or good food unless she helped. Then she said, "I think I can. I think I can. I think I can."
> —*The Little Engine that Could* (Piper, 1930/1989)

Some of the most powerful truths also are the simplest—so simple that a child can un-

derstand them. The concept of *self-efficacy* deals with one of these truths—one so simple it can be captured in a children's book of 37 pages (with illustrations), yet so powerful that fully describing its implications has filled thousands of pages in scientific journals and books over the past 25 years. This truth is that an unshakable belief in one's ideas, goals, and capacity for achievement is essential for success. Strong self-efficacy beliefs are important because they lead to effective self-regulation and persistence, which in turn lead to success. Most people see only the extraordinary accomplishments of athletes, artists, and others but do not see "the unwavering commitment and countless hours of perseverant effort that produced them" (Bandura, 1997, p. 119). They then overestimate the role of "talent" in these accomplishments, while underestimating the role of determination and self-regulation. Because research on self-efficacy is concerned with understanding those factors that people can control rather than those that they cannot control, it is the study of human potential and possibilities, not human limitations.

References

Abramson, L. Y., Seligman, M. E. P., & Teasdale, J. D. (1978). Learned helplessness in humans: Critique and reformulation. *Journal of Abnormal Psychology, 87,* 49–74.

AbuSabha, R., & Achterberg, C. (1997). Review of self-efficacy and locus of control for nutrition- and health-related behavior. *Journal of the American Dietetic Association, 97,* 1122–1133.

Ajzen, I. (1988). *Attitudes, personality, and behavior.* Chicago: Dorsey Press.

Arnstein, P., Caudill, M., Mandle, C. L., Norris, A., & Beasley, R. (1999). Self efficacy as a mediator of the relationship between pain intensity, disability and depression in chronic pain patients. *Pain, 80,* 483–491.

Baker, L., & Wigfield, A. (1999). Dimensions of children's motivation for reading and their relations to reading activity and reading achievement. *Reading Research Quarterly, 34,* 452–477.

Barone, D., Maddux, J. E., & Snyder, C. R. (1997). *Social cognitive psychology: History and current domains.* New York: Plenum Press.

Bandura, A. (1977). Self-efficacy: Toward a unifying theory of behavioral change. *Psychological Review, 84,* 191–215.

Bandura, A. (1986). *Social foundations of thought and action.* New York: Prentice-Hall.

Bandura, A. (1989). Regulation of cognitive processes through perceived self-efficacy. *Developmental Psychology, 25,* 729–735.

Bandura, A. (1993). Perceived self-efficacy in cognitive development and functioning. *Educational Psychologist, 28*, 117–148.

Bandura, A. (1995). *Self-efficacy in changing societies.* New York: Cambridge University Press.

Bandura, A. (1997). *Self-efficacy: The exercise of control.* New York: Freeman.

Bandura, A. (1999). A sociocognitive analysis of substance abuse: An agentic perspective. *Psychological Science, 10*, 214–217.

Bandura, A. (2001). Social cognitive theory: An agentic perspective. *Annual Review of Psychology, 52*, 1–26.

Bandura, A., Barbaranelli, C., Caprara, G. V., & Pastorelli, C. (1996). Multifaceted impact of self-efficacy beliefs on academic functioning. *Child Development, 67*, 1206–1222.

Bandura, A., & Jourdan, J. F. (1991). Self-regulatory mechanisms governing the impact of social comparison on complex decision-making. *Journal of Social and Clinical Psychology, 60*, 941–951.

Bandura, A., Pastorelli, C., Barbaranelli, C., & Caprara, G. V. (1999). Self-efficacy pathways to childhood depression. *Journal of Personality and Social Psychology, 76*, 258–269.

Barone, D., Maddux, J. E., & Snyder, C. R. (1997). *Social cognitive psychology: History and current domains.* New York: Plenum Press.

Benight, C. C., Swift, E., Sanger, J., Smith, A., & Zeppelin, D. (2000). Coping self-efficacy as a mediator of distress following a natural disaster. *Journal of Applied Social Psychology, 29*, 2443–2464.

Betz, N. (1997). What stops women and minorities from choosing majors in science and engineering? In D. Johnson (Ed.), *Minorities and girls in school: Effects on achievement and performance.* Thousand Oaks, CA: Sage.

Bong, M. (1998). Tests of the internal/external frames of reference model with subject-specific academic self-efficacy and frame-specific academic self-concepts. *Journal of Educational Psychology, 90*, 102–110.

Bong, M., & Clark, R. E. (1999). Comparison between self-concept and self-efficacy in academic motivation research. *Educational Psychologist, 34*, 139–153.

Brouwers, A., & Tomic, W. (2000). A longitudinal study of teacher burnout and perceived self-efficacy in classroom management. *Teaching and Teacher Education, 16*, 239–253.

Bryan, A. D., Aiken, L. S., & West, S. G. (1997). Young women's condom use: The influence of acceptance of sexuality, control over the sexual encounter, and perceived susceptibility to common STDs. *Health Psychology, 16*, 468–479.

Burger, J. M. (1999). Personality and control. In V. J. Derlega, B. A. Winstead, & W. H. Jones (Eds.), *Personality: Contemporary theory and research* (2nd ed., pp. 282–306). Chicago: Nelson-Hall.

Byars, A. M., & Hackett, G. (1998). Applications of social cognitive theory to the career development of women of color. *Applied and Preventive Psychology, 7*, 255–267.

Caprara, G. V., Scabini, E., Barbaranelli, C., Pastorelli, C., Regalia, C., & Bandura, A. (1998). Impact of adolescents' perceived self-regulatory efficacy on familial communication and antisocial conduct. *European Psychologist, 3*, 125–132.

Carver, C. S., & Scheier, M. F. (2002). Optimism. In C. R. Snyder & S. J. Lopez (Eds.), *Handbook of positive psychology* (pp. 231–243). New York: Oxford University Press.

Cervone, D. (1989). Effects of envisioning future activities on self-efficacy judgments and motivation: An availability heuristic interpretation. *Cognitive Therapy and Research, 13*, 247–261.

Cervone, D. (2000). Thinking about self-efficacy. *Behavior Modification, 24*, 30–56.

Chwalisz, K., Altmaier, E. M., & Russell, D. W. (1992). Causal attributions, self-efficacy cognitions, and coping with stress. *Journal of Social and Clinical Psychology, 11*, 377–400.

Coldarci, T. (1992). Teachers' sense of efficacy and commitment to teaching. *Journal of Experimental Education, 60*, 323–337.

Conger, J. C., & Keane, S. P. (1981). Social skills intervention in the treatment of isolated or withdrawn children. *Psychological Bulletin, 90*, 478–495.

Conn, V. S. (1998). Older women: Social cognitive theory correlates of health behavior. *Women and Health, 26*, 71–85.

Cowan, R., Logue, E., Milo, L., Britton, P. J., & Smucker, W. (1997). Exercise stage of change and self-efficacy in primary care: Implications for intervention. *Journal of Clinical Psychology in Medical Settings, 4*, 295–311.

Cozzarelli, C. (1993). Personality and self-efficacy as predictors of coping with abortion. *Journal of Personality and Social Psychology, 65*, 1224–1236.

Dawson, K. A., & Brawley, L. R. (2000). Examining the relationship between exercise goals, self-efficacy, and overt behavior with beginning exercisers. *Journal of Applied Social Psychology, 30*, 315.

Deci, E. L., & Ryan, R. M. (1995). Human autonomy: The basis for true self-esteem. In M. H. Kernis (Ed.), *Efficacy, agency, and self-esteem* (pp. 31–49). New York: Plenum Press.

Denham, S. A. (1998). *Emotional development in young children.* New York: Guilford Press.

DiClemente, C. C., Fairhurst, S. K., & Piotrowski, N. A. (1995). Self-efficacy and addictive behaviors. In J. E. Maddux (Ed.), *Self-efficacy, adaptation, and adjustment: Theory, research, and application* (pp. 109–142). New York: Plenum Press.

Diener, E., Suh, E. M., Lucas, R. E., & Smith, H. L. (1999). Subjective well-being: Three decades of progress. *Psychological Bulletin, 125*, 276–302.

Donnay, D. A. C., & Borgen, F. H., (1999). The incremental validity of vocational self-efficacy: An examination of interest, self-efficacy, and occupation. *Journal of Counseling Psychology, 46*, 432–447.

Ducharme, J., & Bachelor, A. (1993). Perception of social functioning in dysphoria. *Cognitive Therapy and Research, 17*, 53–70.

Dweck, C. S. (2000). *Self-theories: Their role in motivation, personality, and development.* Philadelphia: Taylor & Francis.

Dzewaltowski, D. A., Noble, J. M., & Shaw, J. M. (1990). Physical activity participation: Social cognitive theory versus the theories of reasoned action and planned behavior. *Journal of Sport and Exercise Psychology, 12*, 388–405.

Eagly, A. H., & Chaiken, S. (1993). *The psychology of attitudes.* Dallas, TX: Harcourt Brace Jovanovich.

Emmelkamp, P. M. G. (1994). Behavior therapy with adults. In A. E. Bergin & S. L. Garfield (Eds.), *Handbook of psychotherapy and behavior change* (4th ed.; pp. 379–427). New York: Wiley.

Epel, E. S., Bandura, A., & Zimbardo, P. (1999). Escaping homelessness: The influences of self-efficacy and time perspective on coping with homelessness. *Journal of Applied Social Psychology, 29,* 575–596.

Ewart, C. K. (1995). Self-efficacy and recovery from heart attack: Implications for a social–cognitive analysis of exercise and emotion. In J. E. Maddux (Ed.), *Self-efficacy, adaptation, and adjustment: Theory, research, and application* (pp. 203–226). New York: Plenum Press.

Feltz, D. L., & Lirgg, C. D. (1998). Perceived team and player efficacy in hockey. *Journal of Applied Psychology, 83,* 557–564.

Fernandez-Ballesteros, R., Diez-Nicolas, J., Caprara, G. V., Barbaranelli, C., & Bandura, A. (2000). *Determinants and structural relation of personal efficacy to collective efficacy.* Unpublished manuscript, Stanford University.

Fishbein, M., & Ajzen, I. (1975). *Belief, attitude, intention, and behavior: An introduction to theory and research.* Reading, MA: Addison-Wesley.

Fiske, S. T., & Taylor, S. E. (1991) *Social cognition* (2nd ed.). New York: McGraw-Hill.

Forsterling, F. (1986). Attributional conceptions in clinical psychology. *American Psychologist, 41,* 275–285.

Forsyth, A. D., & Carey, M. P. (1998). Measuring self-efficacy in the context of HIV risk reduction: Research challenges and recommendations. *Health Psychology, 17,* 559–568.

Frank, J. D., & Frank, J. B. (1991). *Persuasion and healing: A comparative study of psychotherapy* (3rd ed.). Baltimore: Johns Hopkins University Press.

Gardiner, M., Luszcz, M. A., & Bryan, J. (1997). The manipulation and measurement of task-specific memory self-efficacy in younger and older adults. *International Journal of Behavioral Development, 21,* 209–227.

George, T. R., & Feltz, D. L. (1995). Motivation in sport from a collective efficacy perspective. *International Journal of Sport Psychology, 26,* 98–116.

Gibson, C. B. (1995). Determinants and consequences of group efficacy beliefs in work organizations in the United States, Hong Kong, and Indonesia. *Dissertation Abstracts International, 56*(6), 2318A.

Giles, M., & Rea, A. (1999). Career self-efficacy: An application of the theory of planned behaviour. *Journal of Occupational and Organizational Psychology, 72,* 393–399.

Goldfried, M. R., & Robins, C. (1982). On the facilitation of self-efficacy. *Cognitive Therapy and Research, 6,* 361–380.

Goodrick, G. K., Pendleton, V. R., Kimball, K. T., Poston, W. S. C., Reeves, R. S., & Foreyt, J. P. (1999). Binge eating severity, self-concept, dieting self-efficacy and social support during treatment of binge eating disorder. *International Journal of Eating Disorders, 26,* 295–300.

Guzzo, R. A., Yost, P. R., Campbell, R. J., & Shea, G. P. (1993). Potency in groups: Articulating a construct. *British Journal of Social Psychology, 32,* 87–106.

Hackett, G., & Betz, N., (1995). Self-efficacy and career choice and development. In J. E. Maddux (Ed.), *Self-efficacy, adaptation, and adjustment: Theory, research, and application* (pp. 249–280). New York: Plenum Press.

Hackett, G., & Byars, A. M. (1996). Social cognitive theory and the career development of African American women. *Career Development Quarterly, 44,* 322–340.

Halpern, L. F., & McLean, W. E., Jr. (1997). "Hey mom, look at me!" *Infant Behavior and Development, 20,* 515–529.

Hodges, L., & Carron, A. V. (1992). Collective efficacy and group performance. *International Journal of Sport Psychology, 23,* 48–59.

Hollon, S. D., & Beck, A. T. (1994). Cognitive and cognitive–behavioral therapies. In A. E. Bergin & S. L. Garfield (Eds.), *Handbook of psychotherapy and behavior change* (4th ed., pp. 428–466). New York: Wiley.

Holman, H. R., & Lorig, K. (1992). Perceived self-efficacy in self-management of chronic disease. In R. Schwarzer (Ed.), *Self-efficacy: Thought control of action* (pp. 305–324). Washington: Hemisphere.

Hoover-Dempsey, K. V., & Sandler, H. M. (1997). Why do parents become involved in their children's education? *Review of Educational Research, 67,* 3–42.

Ingram, R. E., Kendall, P. C., & Chen, A. H. (1991). Cognitive–behavioral interventions. In C. R. Snyder & D. R. Forsyth (Eds.), *Handbook of social and clinical psychology* (pp. 509–522). New York: Pergamon.

Kaplan, M., & Maddux, J. E. (2001). Goals and marital satisfaction: Perceived support for personal goals and collective efficacy for collective goals. *Journal of Social and Clinical Psychology, 21,* 157–164.

Kasimatis, M., Miller, M., & Marcussen, L. (1996). The effects of implicit theories on exercise motivation. *Journal of Research in Personality, 30,* 510–516.

Kavanaugh, D. (1992). Self-efficacy and depression. In R. Schwartzer (Ed.), *Self-efficacy: Thought control of action* (pp.177–194). Washington, DC: Hemisphere.

Kazdin, A. E. (1979). Imagery elaboration and self-efficacy in the covert modeling treatment of unassertive behavior. *Journal of Consulting and Clinical Psychology, 47,* 725–733.

Kirsch, I. (1985). Self-efficacy and expectancy: Old wine with new labels. *Journal of Personality and Social Psychology, 49,* 824–830.

Kirsch, I. (1995). Self-efficacy and outcome expectancies: A concluding commentary. In J. E. Maddux (Ed.), *Self-efficacy, adaptation, and adjustment: Theory, research, and application* (pp. 173–202). New York: Plenum Press.

Kirsch, I. (Ed.). (1999). *How expectancies shape behavior.* Washington, DC: American Psychological Association.

Kobasa, S. C. (1979). Stressful life events, personality and health: An inquiry into hardiness. *Journal of Personality and Social Psychology, 37,* 1–11.

Kozub, S. A., & McDonnell, J. F. (2000). Exploring the relationship between cohesion and collective efficacy in rugby teams. *Journal of Sport Behavior, 23,* 120–129.

Langer, E. J., & Rodin, J. (1976). The effects of choice and enhanced personal responsibility for the aged: A field experiment in an institutional setting. *Journal of Personality and Social Psychology, 34,* 191–198.

Leary, M. R., & Kowalski, R. M. (1995). The self-presentation model of social phobia. In R. G. Heimberg, M. R. Liebowitz, D. A. Hope, & F. R. Schneier (Eds.), *Social phobia: Diagnosis, assessment, and treatment* (pp. 94–112). New York: Guilford Press.

Leslie, A. M. (1982). The perception of causality in infants. *Perception, 11,* 173–186.

Little, B. L., & Madigan, R. M. (1997). The relationship between collective efficacy and performance in manufacturing work teams. *Small Group Research, 28,* 517–534.

Locke, E. A., & Latham, G. P. (1990). *A theory of goal setting and task performance.* Englewood Cliffs, NJ: Prentice-Hall.

Ludwig, K. B., & Pittman, J. F. (1999). Adolescent prosocial values and self-efficacy in relation to delinquency, risky sexual behavior, and drug use. *Youth and Society, 30,* 461–482.

Maddux, J. E. (1993). Social cognitive models of health and exercise behavior: An introduction and review of conceptual issues. *Journal of Applied Sport Psychology, 5,* 116–140.

Maddux, J. E. (1999a). The collective construction of collective efficacy: Comment on Paskevich, Brawley, Dorsch, and Widmeyer. *Group Dynamics: Theory, Research, and Practice, 3,* 223–226.

Maddux, J. E. (1999b). Expectancies and the social–cognitive perspective: Basic principles, processes, and variables. In I. Kirsch (Ed.), *How expectancies shape behavior* (pp. 17–40). Washington, DC: American Psychological Association.

Maddux, J. E., Brawley, L., & Boykin, A. (1995). Self-efficacy and healthy decision-making: Protection, promotion, and detection. In J. E. Maddux (Ed.), *Self-efficacy, adaptation, and adjustment: Theory, research, and application* (pp. 173–202). New York: Plenum Press.

Maddux, J. E., & DuCharme, K. A. (1997). Behavioral intentions in theories of health behavior. In D. Gochman (Ed.), *Handbook of health behavior research: I. Personal and social determinants* (pp. 133–152). New York: Plenum Press.

Maddux, J. E., & Lewis, J. (1995). Self-efficacy and adjustment: Basic principles and issues. In J. E. Maddux (Ed.), *Self-efficacy, adaptation, and adjustment: Theory, research, and application* (pp. 37–68). New York: Plenum Press.

Maddux, J. E., & Meier, L. J. (1995). Self-efficacy and depression. In J. E. Maddux (Ed.), *Self-efficacy, adaptation, and adjustment: Theory, research and application* (pp. 143–169). New York: Plenum Press.

Maddux, J. E., Norton, L. W., & Leary, M. R. (1988). Cognitive components of social anxiety: An investigation of the integration of self-presentation theory and self-efficacy theory. *Journal of Social and Clinical Psychology, 6,* 180–190

Maddux, J. E., & Rogers, R. W. (1983). Protection motivation and self-efficacy: A revised theory of fear appeals and attitude change. *Journal of Experimental Social Psychology, 19,* 469–479.

Mandler, J. M. (1992). How to build a baby: II. Conceptual primitives. *Psychological Review, 99,* 587–604.

Marks, M. (1999). A test of the impact of collective efficacy in routine and novel performance enviornments. *Human Performance, 12,* 295–309.

Marlowe, N. (1998). Self-efficacy moderates the impact of stressful events on headache. *Headache, 38,* 662–667.

Martin, J. J., & Gill, D. L. (1991). The relationships among

competitive consultation, sport-confidence, self-efficacy, anxiety, and performance. *Journal of Sport and Exercise Psychology, 13,* 149–159.

Maxwell, E. (1998). "I can do it myself!" Reflections on early self-efficacy. *Roeper Review, 20,* 183–187.

McAvay, G., Seeman, T. E., & Rodin, J. (1996). A longitudinal study of change in domain-specific self-efficacy among older adults. *Journals of Gerontology: Series B. Psychological Sciences and Social Sciences, 51B,* 243–253.

McClelland, D. C. (1984). *Motives, personality, and society: Selected papers.* New York: Praeger.

McClelland, D. C. (1985). How motives, skills, and values determine what people do. *American Psychologist, 40,* 812–825.

McClelland, D. C., Atkinson, J. W., Clark, R. W., & Lowell, E. L. (1953). *The achievement motive.* New York: Appleton-Century-Croft.

McDougall, G. J. (1995). Memory self-efficacy and strategy use in successful elders. *Educational Gerontology, 21,* 357–373.

Mischel, W. (1973). Toward a cognitive social learning reconceptualization of personality. *Psychological Review, 80,* 252–284.

Mone, M. A. (1994). Comparative validity of two measures of self-efficacy in predicting academic goals and performance. *Educational and Psychological Measurement, 54,* 516–529.

Mudde, A. N., Kok, G., & Strecher, V. J. (1995). Self-efficacy as a predictor for the cessation of smoking: Methodological issues and implications for smoking cessation programs. *Psychology and Health, 10,* 353–367.

Oei, T. P., Fergusson, S., & Lee, N. K. (1998). The differential role of alcohol expectancies and drinking refusal self-efficacy in problem and nonproblem drinkers. *Journal of Studies on Alcohol, 59,* 704–711.

Ogbu, J. U. (1991). Minority coping responses and school experience. *Journal of Psychohistory, 18,* 433–456.

O'Leary, A., & Brown, S. (1995). Self-efficacy and the physiological stress response. In J. E. Maddux (Ed.), *Self-efficacy, adaptation, and adjustment: Theory, research and application* (pp. 227–248). New York: Plenum Press.

Pajares, F. (1996). Self-efficacy beliefs in academic settings. *Review of Educational Research, 66,* 543–578.

Pajares, J., & Johnson, M. J. (1996). Self-efficacy beliefs and the writing performance of entering high school students. *Psychology in the Schools, 33,* 163–175.

Paskevich, D. M., Brawley, L. R., Dorsch, K. D., & Widmeyer, W. N. (1999). Relationship between collective efficacy and team cohesion: Conceptual and measurement issues. *Group Dynamics: Theory, Research, and Practice, 3,* 210–222.

Piper, W. (1989). *The little engine that could.* New York: Platt & Monk. (Original work published 1930)

Pollock, P. H. (1996). Self-efficacy and sexual offending against children: Construction of a measure and changes following relapse prevention treatment. *Legal and Criminology Psychology, 1,* 219–228.

Prochaska, J. O., Norcross, J. C., & DiClemente, C. C. (1994). *Changing for good.* New York: Morrow.

Prussia, G. E., & Kinicki, A. J. (1996). A motivational investigation of group effectiveness using social cognitive theory. *Journal of Applied Psychology, 81,* 187–198.

Rogers, R. W., & Prentice-Dunn, S. (1997). Protection motivation theory. In D. S. Gochman (Ed.), *Handbook of health behavior research: I. Personal and social determinants* (pp. 113–132). New York: Plenum Press.

Rosenbaum, M. (Ed.). (1990). *Learned resourcefulness: On coping skills, self-control, and adaptive behavior.* New York: Springer.

Rotter, J. B. (1966). Generalized expectancies for internal versus external control of reinforcement. *Psychological Monographs, 80* (1, Whole No. 609).

Rudolph, D. L., & Butki, B. D. (1998). Self-efficacy and affective responses to short bouts of exercise. *Journal of Applied Sport Psychology, 10,* 268–280.

Rudolph, D. L., & McAuley, E. (1995). Self-efficacy and salivary cortisol responses to acute exercise in physically active and less active adults. *Journal of Sport and Exercise Psychology, 17,* 206–213.

Russell, B. (1954). *A history of Western philosophy.* New York: Simon & Schuster.

Ryan, A. M., Gheen, M. H., & Midgley, C. (1998). Why do some students avoid asking for help? An examination of the interplay among students' academic efficacy, teachers' social–emotional role, and the classroom goal structure. *Journal of Educational Psychology, 90,* 528–535.

Sampson, R. J., Raudenbush, S. W., & Earls, F. (1997). Neighborhoods and violent crime: A multilevel study of collective efficacy. *Science, 277,* 918–924.

Samuels, S. M., & Gibbs, R. W. (in press). Self-efficacy assessment and generalization in physical education courses. *Journal of Applied Social Psychology.*

Schaubroeck, J., Lam, S. S. K., & Xie, J. L. (2000). Collective efficacy versus self-efficacy in coping responses to stressors and control: A cross-cultural study. *Journal of Applied Psychology, 85,* 512–525.

Schunk, D. H. (1995). Self-efficacy and education and instruction. In J. E. Maddux (Ed.), *Self-efficacy, adaptation, and adjustment: Theory, research, and application.* (pp. 281–304). New York: Plenum Press.

Schunk, D. H., & Zimmerman, B. J. (1997). Social origins of self-regulatory competence. *Educational Psychologist, 32,* 195–208.

Schwarzer, R. (1992). Self-efficacy in the adoption and maintenance of health behaviors: Theoretical approaches and a new model. In R. Schwarzer (Ed.), *Self-efficacy: thought control of action* (pp. 217–243). Washington, DC: Hemisphere.

Schwarzer, R., Bassler, J., Kwiatck, P., Schroder, K., & Zhang, J. X. (1997). The assessment of optimistic self-beliefs: Comparison of the German, Spanish, and Chinese versions of the General Self-Efficacy Scale. *Applied Psychology: An International Review, 46,* 69–88.

Schwarzer, R., & Renner, B. (2000). Social-cognitive predictors of health behavior: Active self-efficacy and coping self-efficacy. *Health Psychology, 19,* 487–495.

Sherer, M., Maddux, J. E., Mercandante, B., Prentice-Dunn, S., Jacobs, B., & Rogers, R. W. (1982). The self-efficacy scale: Construction and validation. *Psychological Reports, 51,* 633–671.

Showers, C. J. (1995). The evaluative organization of self-knowledge: Origins, processes, and implications for self-esteem. In M. H. Kernis (Ed.), *Efficacy, agency, and self-esteem* (pp. 101–120). New York: Plenum Press.

Siegel, K., Mesagno, F. P., Chen, J., & Christ, G. (1989).

Factors distinguishing homosexual males practicing risky and safer sex. *Social Science and Medicine, 28,* 561–569.

Skinner, E. A. (1995). *Perceived control, motivation, and coping.* Thousand Oaks, CA: Sage.

Snyder, C. R., Rano, K. L., & Sigmon, D. R. (2002). Hope theory: A member of the positive psychology family. In C. R. Snyder & S. J. Lopez (Eds.), *Handbook of positive psychology* (pp. 257–276). New York: Oxford University Press.

Sorensen, M. (1997). Maintenance of exercise behavior for individuals at risk for cardiovascular disease. *Perceptual and Motor Skills, 85,* 867–881.

Spink, K. S. (1990). Group cohesion and collective efficacy of volleyball teams. *Journal of Sport and Exercise Psychology, 12,* 301–311.

Smith, P. L., & Fouad, N. A. (1999). Subject-matter specificity of self-efficacy, outcome expectancies, interests, and goals: Implications for the social–cognitive model. *Journal of Counseling Psychology, 46,* 461–472.

Stanjovic, A. D., & Luthans, F. (1998). Self-efficacy and work-related performance: A meta-analysis. *Psychological Bulletin, 124,* 240–261.

Stanley, K. D., & Murphy, M. R. (1997). A comparison of general self-efficacy with self-esteem. *Genetic, Social, and General Psychology Monographs, 123,* 79–99.

Strecher, V. J., Champion, V. L., & Rosenstock, I. M. (1997). The health belief model and health behavior. In D. Gochman (Ed.), *Handbook of health behavior research: I. Personal and social determinants* (pp. 71–92). New York: Plenum Press.

Tabernero, C., & Wood, R. E. (1999). Implicit theories versus the social construal of ability in self-regulation and performance on a complex task. *Organizational Behavior and Human Decision Processes, 78,* 104–127.

Taylor, S. E., & Brown, J. D. (1988). Illusion and well-being: A social psychological perspective on mental health. *Psychological Bulletin, 2,* 193–210.

Thompson, S. C. (1991). Intervening to enhance perceptions of control. In C. R. Snyder & D. R. Forsyth (Eds.), *Handbook of social and clinical psychology* (pp. 607–623). New York: Pergamon.

Tipton, R. M., & Worthington, E. L. (1984). The measurement of generalized self-efficacy: A study of construct validity. *Journal of Personality Assessment, 48,* 545–548.

Vessey, G. N. A. (1967). Volition. In P. Edwards (Ed.), *Encyclopedia of philosophy* (Vol. 8). New York: Macmillan.

Vinokur, A. D., van Ryn, M., Gramlich, E. M., & Price, R. H. (1991). Long-term follow-up and benefit–cost analysis of the jobs program: A preventive intervention for the unemployed. *Journal of Applied Psychology, 76,* 213–219.

Wang, A. Y., & Richarde, R. S. (1988). Global versus task-specific measures of self-efficacy. *Psychological Record, 38,* 533–541.

Watson, J. S. (1977). Depression and the perception of control in early childhood. In J. G. Schulterbrandt & A. Raskin (Eds.), *Depression in childhood: Diagnosis, treatment, and conceptual models* (pp. 129–139). New York: Raven Press.

Watson, J. S., Hayes, L. A., & Vietze, P. (1982). Response-contingent stimulation as a treatment of developmental failure in infancy. *Journal of Applied Developmental Psychology, 3,* 191–203.

Weinstein, N. D. (1993). Testing four competing theories of health-protective behavior. *Health Psychology, 12,* 324–333.

Welch, D. C., & West, R. L. (1995). Self-efficacy and mastery: Its application to issues of environmental control, cognition, and aging. *Developmental Review, 15,* 150–171.

Weldon, E., & Weingart, L. R. (1993). Group goals and group performance. *British Journal of Social Psychology, 32,* 307–334.

Wheeler, K. G. (1983). Comparisons of self-efficacy and expectancy models of occupational preferences for college males and females. *Journal of Occupational Psychology, 56,* 73–78.

White, R. W. (1959). Motivation reconsidered: The concept of competence. *Psychological Review, 66,* 297–333.

Williams, S. L. (1995). Self-efficacy, anxiety, and phobic disorders. In J. E. Maddux (Ed.), *Self-efficacy, adaptation, and adjustment: Theory, research, and application* (pp. 69–107). New York: Plenum Press.

Williams, S. L., Kinney, P. J., Harap, S. T., & Liebmann, M. (1997). Thoughts of agoraphobic people during scary tasks. *Journal of Abnormal Psychology, 106,* 511–520.

Yeung, R. R., & Hemsley, D. R. (1997). Exercise behavior in an aerobics class: The impact of personality traits and efficacy cognitions. *Personality and Individual Differences, 23,* 425–431.

Zaccaro, S., Blair, V., Peterson, C., & Zananis, M. (1995). Collective efficacy. In J. E. Maddux (Ed.), *Self-efficacy, adaptation, and adjustment: Theory, research, and application* (pp. 305–330). New York: Plenum Press.

Zimmerman, B. J. (1989). A social cognitive view of self-regulated academic learning. *Journal of Educational Psychology, 81,* 329–339.

12

Self-Systems Give Unique Meaning to Self Variables

CAROL S. DWECK
E. TORY HIGGINS
HEIDI GRANT-PILLOW

Research in the field of self and identity has increasingly moved away from a focus on purely static qualities (such as chronic self-esteem) and toward an emphasis on more dynamic variables. This is clearly seen in work on motivated self-completion (Brunstein & Gollwitzer, 1996; Wicklund & Gollwitzer, 1982), contingencies of self-esteem (Crocker, 1999), stability of self-esteem (Kernis, Cornell, Sun, Berry, & Harlow, 1993), and self-evaluation maintenance theory (Tesser & Campbell, 1982). All of this work, implicitly or explicitly, brings motivation to the forefront of the self by showing the strong motivational power of self variables, as well as the dynamic properties of self variables as they respond to motivation-relevant events and situations. Thus this body of work highlights the critical importance of understanding the self in a motivational context, as individuals pursue their goals.

In this chapter we show how the contents of the self—self-defining beliefs and values—come to life through people's goals. We demonstrate that goals are what give the term "self-system" real and important meaning and that a goal approach can capture the dynamic (but also coherent) nature of the self, illuminating both individual differences and situational influences. In short, we propose that the contents of the self gain their importance and exert their influence through the motivational value they possess—through their ability to shape and energize people's goals.

However, we go on to make perhaps an even more dramatic claim: that self variables such as expectancies, self-efficacy, self-attributions, and self-esteem, cannot be properly studied or understood outside the context of self-systems. We show that all these variables can have entirely different meanings and modes of operation within different self-systems.

Thus we propose that goals form the core of self-systems and that these goal-driven self-systems give unique meaning to self variables. We use evidence from our own research programs to illustrate and support these proposals.

Self-Beliefs Come to Life through Goals

In their work, Dweck and her colleagues have identified beliefs about the self that orient people toward different self-relevant goals. Basically, when people believe that their personal traits, such as their intelligence, are fixed entities (an "entity" theory), they are highly concerned with documenting these traits and judging them positively (through "performance" goals—i.e., wanting to validate or demonstrate an attribute; Dweck & Leggett, 1988; Dweck & Sorich, 1999; Erdley, Cain, Loomis, Dumas-Hines, & Dweck, 1997; Hong, Chiu, Dweck, Lin, & Wan, 1999; Mueller & Dweck, 1998; see Dweck, 1999). That is, when a valued attribute is believed to be a fixed and limited commodity, people are eager to prove that the amount they have is an amount that they can be proud of and that will serve them well. In contrast, when people believe that their personal traits are potentialities that can be developed (an "incremental" theory), they are more oriented toward activities that will allow them to master new tasks and expand their skills (through "learning" goals—i.e., wanting to acquire or develop an attribute). That is, when a valued attribute is seen as something expandable, people are eager to do what it takes to cultivate it.

Although everyone values and engages in both performance goals and learning goals, the balance appears to shift depending on people's implicit theories—whether they view these attributes as fixed traits or malleable qualities. For example, when offered a choice between a task that will make them look smart and a task that will foster important learning (but entails confusion and mistakes), students holding an entity theory of their intelligence tend to opt for the former, whereas those holding an incremental theory tend to opt for the latter (Dweck & Leggett, 1988; Stone & Dweck, 1998).

In studies with both junior high school students (Dweck & Sorich, 1999) and college students (Mueller & Dweck, 1998; see Dweck, 1999; see also Robins & Pals, 1998), entity theorists of intelligence agreed significantly more than incremental theorists with statements that put the priority on performance over learning goals: "Although I hate to admit it, I would rather do well in a class than learn a lot" or "If I knew I wasn't going to do well at a task, I probably wouldn't do it even if I might learn a lot from it." In contrast, those holding an incremental theory agreed more with statements that put the priority on learning over performance goals, such as, "It's much more important for me to learn things in my classes than it is to get the best grades." In a study of college students at the University of Hong Kong, Hong and colleagues (1999) showed how these tendencies can play themselves out in real life. At the University of Hong Kong, one of the most prestigious universities in Hong Kong, all classes are conducted in English, and all assignments and exams are in English. Yet not all students arrive there already proficient in English. Would students pursue an English proficiency course to remedy any deficiencies? Students who held an incremental theory of their intelligence indicated that they would, whereas those holding an entity theory did not express this intention. In fact, entity theorists who had marked deficiencies were no more likely to want this course than those who were already proficient. In other words, entity theorists did not feel such a course would help them improve or perhaps were not willing to expose a deficiency in order to remedy it.

In experiments in which people were (temporarily) taught an entity or incremental theory (see Dweck & Leggett, 1988; Hong et al., 1999) , the same pattern of results was obtained. In these studies, students were given "scientific articles" that espoused either an entity or an incremental view of intelligence. Those who read that intelligence is fixed wanted to look smart and those who read that it is malleable wanted to learn. This same pattern has also been obtained in other domains: Those who have a fixed theory of their personalities are more concerned with validating their qualities than those who hold a malleable theory (Erdley et al., 1997; Kamins, Morris, & Dweck, 1997). For example, in a study with college students (Kamins et al., 1997), entity theorists primarily wanted partners who would validate them (make them look good, think they were perfect, enhance their self-esteem), whereas incremental theorists primarily wanted partners who would challenge them to grow.

It is important to note that people with different theories do not necessarily start out with different skill levels or different levels of self-esteem. They simply have different conceptions of self—different fundamental beliefs about the nature of their personal qualities—and these different conceptions spawn very different motivations. In one case, the motivation to validate the self through outcomes and judgments is heightened; in the other case, the motivation to grow is heightened. Thus these self-beliefs come to life and play themselves out through the different goal emphases they foster.

It is also important to note that both classes of goals can be powerful motivators. The desire to validate the self and the desire to develop the self can both energize activity in every domain of one's life. However, the character of that activity will differ. In the sections that follow, we show how these goals go on to foster different psychological worlds, with different affective experiences, cognitive construals, and attendant behavior.

Research by Higgins and his colleagues on self-discrepancy theory (Higgins, 1987) and regulatory focus theory (Higgins, 1997) illustrates another way in which self beliefs come to life through goals. Self-discrepancy theory distinguishes between two different styles of self-regulatory socialization children can receive, which in turn influence the self-conceptualizations that guide their behavior. When the caretaker's message to the child is, "This is what I would ideally *like* you to do," the child develops a strong *ideal* self-guide. Ideal self-guides are conceptualizations of the self that involve the individual's hopes, wishes, and aspirations. When the caretaker's message to the child is, "This is what I think you *ought* to do," the child develops a strong *ought* self-guide. Ought self-guides are conceptualizations of the self that involve the individual's duties, obligations, and responsibilities. An ideal or ought self-guide not only functions as a self-conceptualization but also determines the nature of the *goals* one pursues.

Although everyone has both types of self-conceptualizations and thus is both ideal-oriented and ought-oriented, reliable chronic differences across individuals have been shown to exist. These differences in strength of ideal or ought guide—through the different goals they foster—predict unique patterns of affect, cognition, and behavior, as well as differences in the strategic and motivational character of goal pursuit. Specifically, strong ideal self-guides result in an overall *promotion focus*, creating goals that concern aspirations, advancement, and accomplishments (or, more generally, the presence or absence of positive outcomes). Strong ought self-guides, in contrast, result in an overall *prevention focus*, creating goals that concern responsibilities, safety, and security (or, more generally, the presence or absence of negative outcomes). Momentary situations are also capable of temporarily inducing either a promotion focus or a prevention focus, such as task instructions or health messages that are represented in terms of the presence or absence of positive outcomes (i.e., gain or nongain) or the presence or absence of negative outcomes (i.e., loss or nonloss; Shah & Higgins, 1997; Shah, Higgins, & Friedman, 1998).

When a person has a promotion focus, his or her motivation is best characterized as *eagerness*, and, in pursuing a particular goal, eagerness is increased by actual or anticipated gain and decreased by actual or anticipated nongain (Idson, Liberman, & Higgins, 2000). In contrast, when a person has a prevention focus, his or her motivation is best characterized as *vigilance*, and, in pursuing a particular goal, he or she is sensitive to the presence or absence of negative outcomes (loss or nonloss). Vigilance is increased by actual or anticipated loss and decreased by actual or anticipated nonloss (Idson et al., 2000). Several studies have found that the promotion focus concern with advancement and accomplishment involves the strategic inclination to *approach matches* to desired end states, whereas the prevention focus concern with protection and safety involves the strategic inclination to *avoid mismatches* to desired end states (see Higgins, Roney, Crowe, & Hymes, 1994; Shah, Higgins, & Friedman, 1998).

Thus beliefs about the self in the form of self-guides come to life through promotion and prevention goals, which, as we show, significantly influence the ways in which people organize their experience and the nature of strategy, construal, affect, and motivation in goal pursuit.

Different Goals Are Associated with Different Affective Experiences

It can be argued that most important affective experiences are shaped by valued goals. People's ups and downs are typically associated with events that relate to their valued goals, but these goals, we propose, affect not only the valence of the affect but also its very nature.

Learning and performance goals, for example, have been identified with a host of different affective experiences as people contemplate, confront, and pursue a task. For example, within a learning goal, a challenge is more often greeted with excitement rather than apprehension or anxiety (see Dweck, 1999). The focus in this section, however, is on the ways in which learning goals can foster the maintenance of intrinsic motivation in the face of obstacles, because intrinsic motivation is widely seen as central to people's well-being and effectiveness (see Sansone & Harackiewicz, 2000).

Most often, intrinsic motivation is assessed following a manipulation that involves different kinds of rewards or different kinds of instructions. As Molden and Dweck (2000) point out, less often do researchers examine the factors that lead to hardy or lasting intrinsic motivation, that is, intrinsic motivation that will see people through repeated setbacks or prolonged difficulties. In the work of Dweck and her colleagues (Baer & Dweck, 2001; Dweck & Sorich, 1999; Grant, 2001; Mueller & Dweck, 1998), both learning and performance goals are compatible with high intrinsic motivation as people embark on a task. Whether people's naturally existing preferences for learning or performance goals are measured (Dweck & Sorich, 1999; Grant, 2001) or whether people's goal focus is manipulated experimentally (Baer & Dweck, 2001; Mueller & Dweck, 1998), those holding performance goals often start out having levels of intrinsic motivation that are just as high as those holding learning goals. This is true whether one assesses reported enjoyment or the desire to engage in the task as a free-choice activity.

However, after a meaningful setback, those holding performance goals often report substantial decreases in intrinsic motivation, whereas those holding learning goals do not. For example, after a manipulation that induced learning versus performance goals, Mueller and Dweck (1998) gave students a highly difficult series of problems. Following these problems, students in the condition that produced performance goals reported significantly and substantially lower levels of enjoyment and desire to take the problems home to practice than did students in the condition that produced learning goals. The latter maintained their high levels of intrinsic motivation, showing no decrement at all.

In a real-life analog, Grant (2001) followed students through a premed college chemistry course that was highly challenging and in which many students experienced their exam grades as disappointing. Although both learning and performance goals were associated with initial levels of intrinsic motivation, only learning goals were predictive of high intrinsic motivation by the end of the course. Thus an orientation toward learning allows students to enjoy a task even when they are not doing well at it. In contrast, when a task is used as a means of validating the self, that enjoyment appears to be sharply compromised when performance is not high. Indeed, in two studies involving scenarios that depict failure (Dweck & Sorich, 1999; Grant, 2001), students with performance goals told us directly that they would no longer be interested in a subject in which they did poorly on an exam, even if it was the first exam in a subject they had previously enjoyed.

Finally, Baer and Dweck (2001) induced performance versus learning goals and gave students a very difficult set of problems. Following these problems, those in the learning-goal condition rated themselves as being significantly more "motivated" and "determined" than those in the performance-goal condition. In essence, difficulty can be a natural part of learning and, as such, does not undermine interest and mastery motivation. On the other hand, difficulty within a performance goal—in which one is trying to validate one's ability—is often the equivalent of failure and, as we will see, often carries the implication of inadequacy.

It would be difficult to maintain enjoyment and enthusiasm under these circumstances.

Research on self-discrepancy theory (see Higgins, 1987, 1996) illustrates another way in which different self goals are associated with different emotional experiences. People's represented actual selves (or self-concepts) can be congruent with or discrepant from their ideal self-guides and can be congruent with or discrepant from their ought self-guides. The emotional impact of an "actual-self–goal" discrepancy (or congruency) has been found to vary depending on whether the goal is part of an ideal or an ought guide (see Higgins, 1987, 1996; see also Carver & Scheier, 1990, 1998).

A discrepancy between actual-self attributes and ideal goals is a meaningful pattern of self-beliefs that represents a particular psychological situation. When a person possesses this discrepancy, the current state of his or her actual attributes is discrepant from the ideal goals that someone (self of significant other) wishes or hopes that he or she would attain. Thus an *actual–ideal discrepancy* as a whole represents *the absence of positive outcomes*. In contrast, when a person possesses a discrepancy between his or her actual-self attributes and ought goals, there is a violation of prescribed duties or obligations that is associated with sanctions such as punishment or criticism. Thus an *actual–ought discrepancy* as a whole represents the *presence of negative outcomes*. Because an actual–ideal discrepancy pattern represents the absence of positive outcomes, individuals possessing this self-belief pattern are likely to experience emotions related to this psychological situation; specifically, dejection-related emotions such as feeling sad, disappointed, or discouraged. Because an actual–ought discrepancy represents the presence of negative outcomes, individuals possessing this self-belief pattern are likely to experience emotions related to this psychological situation; specifically, agitation-related emotions such as feeling tense, nervous, or worried (see Higgins, 1997, for a more detailed discussion).

The distinct relations between type of actual-self–goal discrepancy and emotional distress has been examined both dispositionally and situationally. Individuals' chronic actual-self beliefs and ideal and ought goals are obtained from the Selves Questionnaire (Higgins, 1987). This questionnaire asks respondents to list 8 or 10 attributes for each of a number of different self-states—their current actual selves, their ideal selves, and their ought selves. In addition to listing attributes for each state, they rate the extent to which they actually possess, ideally want to possess, or believe they should possess each attribute. Magnitude of actual–ideal discrepancy or actual–ought discrepancy is measured in terms of the extent to which actual-self attributes are discrepant from (or congruent with) each type of goal.

Several studies using this questionnaire have found that actual–ideal discrepancies (controlling for actual–ought discrepancies) predict individuals' dejection-related emotions as measured weeks later and that actual–ought discrepancies (controlling for actual–ideal discrepancies) predict individuals' agitation-related emotions (see Higgins, 1987, 1996; see also Higgins, 1999; Higgins, Grant, & Shah, 1999; Tangney, Niedenthal, Covert, & Barlow, 1998). Studies have also found that emotional reactions to real or imagined events varies depending on individuals' self-discrepancies. In an early study by Higgins, Bond, Klein, and Strauman (1986, Study 1), for example, undergraduates were asked to imagine a negative event in which performance failed to match a common standard (e.g., receiving a grade of D in a course that was necessary for obtaining an important job). Participants' mood was measured both before and after they imagined the negative event. The study found that the magnitude and type of actual-self–goal discrepancy possessed by the participants, as measured *weeks earlier*, predicted the amount and kind of emotional change they experienced when imagining the negative event—dejection-related emotions for actual–ideal discrepant participants and agitation-related emotions for actual–ought discrepant participants.

Strauman and Higgins (1987) used a covert, idiographic priming technique to activate self beliefs in a task supposedly investigating the "physiological effects of thinking about other people." The participants were given phrases of the form, "A(n) X person is _____" (where X is a trait adjective such as "friendly" or "intelligent") and were asked to complete each sentence as quickly as possible. For each sentence, each participant's total verbalization time and skin conductance amplitude were recorded. Their emotions were also measured at the beginning and end of the session. Participants were selected who were either high in actual–ideal discrepancy and low in actual–ought discrepancy or high in actual–ought discrepancy and low in actual–ideal discrepancy. Discrepant actual-self attributes were primed for each participant. The study found a dejection-related syndrome (i.e., mood, skin conductance amplitude, and total verbalization time all changing in the dejection-related direction) for the actual–ideal discrepant participants and an agitation-related syndrome for the actual–ought discrepant participants. These findings were later replicated by Strauman (1989) in a study using depressed and social phobic clinical samples.

Different Goals Are Associated with Different Cognitive Construals

Performance and learning goals are both related to the self, but in one case the goal is to validate a valued attribute of the self, and in the other the goal is to foster its growth. It is plausible to expect that given these different aims, similar events might be construed in very different ways and with very different consequences. In this section we look at how outcomes, particularly failure outcomes, are differently construed within the two goal frameworks and, in turn, differently affect people's expectancies or sense of self-efficacy.

In a number of studies, participants' naturally existing goal preferences were assessed (Dweck & Sorich, 1999; Grant, 2001) or participants' goal focus was induced, for example, by telling them that the task measured an inherent aptitude (performance goal condition) or involved an acquirable skill (learning goal condition; e.g., Kasimatis, Miller, & Marcussen, 1996; Martocchio, 1994; Tabernero & Wood, 1999; cf. Hong et al., 1999; Mueller & Dweck, 1998). The findings indicate that within a performance-goal framework—in which abilities are at issue—setbacks are often interpreted as signaling low ability. This low-ability attribution is then predictive of de-

clining expectancies of success or a decreased sense of self-efficacy (see also Dykman, 1998). It is particularly telling to note that this occurs even when people are in fact learning or mastering a task over time. However, the fact that the road is paved with obstacles signals to them that they lack ability (Tabernero & Wood, 1999; see also Robins & Pals, 1998).

In contrast, when people are aiming to acquire skills rather than to prove their inherent ability, effort attributions are more common (e.g., Hong et al., 1999). That is, setbacks or difficulties are seen as stemming from insufficient effort or as calling for stepped-up effort or new strategies. This, then, is accompanied by the maintenance of high expectancies and, when progress is evident, a growing sense of self-efficacy.

Attributions to ability or effort have been studied for many years and have been shown repeatedly to be important mediators of affect and persistence following outcomes. Although we are in agreement with attribution theorists on the central role of attributions in motivation, it is important to point out a major difference in perspective. In our view, these attributions grow organically out of the self-theories and the self-related goals people bring into the situation. When traits of the self are being measured (as in the entity theory–performance-goal system), it makes sense to view outcomes as reflecting on those attributes (see also Erdley et al., 1997, for self-theories, goals, and attributions in social situations). When, instead, one is striving to expand one's abilities (as in the incremental theory–learning-goal system), it makes sense to view outcomes as reflecting on the means one is using to do so. Thus our view places attributions and self-efficacy squarely within the systems of meaning and motivation that are created by people's self-conceptions and goals (see also Grant & Dweck, 2001).

Not only do self-related attributions (ability vs. effort) and expectancies (increasing vs. decreasing with effortful learning) differ within the two self-systems, but even the *same* attributions and expectancies can mean very different things and operate in different ways. In a study by Stone and Dweck (1998), grade school students were introduced to a task that was said to measure an important intellectual ability. Some time later, the students were probed for their understanding of what the task measured and what difficulty on the task would mean. Students who took an entity perspective on their intelligence thought that the task measured not only an important intellectual ability (as they had been told) but also how intelligent they were overall and how intelligent they would be when they grew up. Those who took an incremental perspective on their intelligence saw the task as reflecting only the task-relevant abilities, not their general or permanent intelligence. Thus even if the two groups made the "same" attribution on the task—a low-ability attribution—that attribution would carry importantly different implications.

In a related vein, self-efficacy expectations appear to operate differently within these two self-systems, such that even when people have the same efficacy expectations, the impact can differ. Elliott and Dweck (1988) showed that when students were given low-efficacy expectations (by means of low-ability feedback on a pretest), those in the learning-goal conditions still showed a hardy, mastery-oriented pattern of persistence in the face of failure. For those in the performance-goal conditions, the low-efficacy expectations led to a helpless reaction. In summary, these different self-systems can lead to different patterns of attributions and expectancies, but even when attributions and expectancies seem similar, they may have different meaning and impact (see also Grant & Dweck, 1999a).

Self-systems involving ideal-self and ought-self beliefs also influence people's construals of and attributions for events in the world. The distinction between ideal and ought self-regulation suggests that sensitivity to events involving the presence and absence of positive outcomes should be greater when ideal concerns predominate, whereas sensitivity to events involving the absence and presence of negative outcomes should be greater when ought concerns predominate. Like Kelly's (1955) personal-construct systems, which individuals use as a scanning pattern that sweeps back and forth across the perceptual field and "picks up blips of meaning" (p. 145), such chronic sensitivities should influence how stimulus information is processed and remembered. Higgins and Tykocinski (1992) tested this

prediction at the chronic level of ideal-self versus ought-self beliefs.

Undergraduate participants read the same essay about the life of a target person in which events reflecting the four different types of psychological situations occurred, that is (1) "I found a 20-dollar bill on the pavement of Canal Street near the paint store" (the presence of positive outcomes); (2) "I've been wanting to see this movie at the 8th Street theater for some time, so this evening I went there straight after school to find out that it's not showing anymore" (the absence of positive outcomes); (3) "I was stuck in the subway for 35 minutes with at least 15 sweating passengers breathing down my neck" (the presence of negative outcomes); and (4) "This is usually my worst school day. Awful schedule, class after class with no break. But today is election day—no school!" (the absence of negative outcomes). Ten minutes after reading the essay the participants were asked to reproduce the essay word for word. The study found that participants who had predominant actual–ideal discrepancies tended to remember target events representing the presence and absence of positive outcomes better than did participants who had predominant actual–ought discrepancies, whereas participants who had predominant actual–ought discrepancies tended to remember target events representing the absence and presence of negative outcomes better than did participants who had predominant actual–ideal discrepancies.

The results of the Higgins and Tykocinski (1992) study support the proposal that self-regulation in relation to ideal-self beliefs is motivationally distinct from self-regulation related to ought-self beliefs. The results of studies by Higgins and colleagues (1994) also support this general proposal and, in addition, indicate that ideal and ought self-regulation differ in sensitivity to events involving eagerness versus vigilance strategies. As we mentioned earlier, regulation in relation to ideal-self beliefs involves a promotion-focus concern with aspirations and accomplishments, whereas regulation in relation to ought-self beliefs involves a prevention-focus concern with responsibilities and security (Higgins, 1996, 1997). There is a natural fit between promotion-focus concerns and the use of eagerness strategies because eagerness strategies ensure the presence of positive outcomes (ensure hits; look for means of advancement) and ensure against the absence of positive outcomes (ensure against errors of omission; do not close off possibilities). There is also a natural fit between prevention-focus concerns and the use of vigilance strategies because vigilance strategies ensure the absence of negative outcomes (ensure correct rejections; be careful) and ensure against the presence of negative outcomes (ensure against errors of commission; avoid mistakes; Crowe & Higgins, 1997; Higgins, 1997).

In a study by Higgins and colleagues (1994), undergraduate participants were first asked to report either on how their hopes and aspirations have changed over time (activating ideal-self beliefs) or on how their sense of duty and obligation has changed over time (activating ought-self beliefs). Later, in a supposedly unrelated study, they read about several episodes that occurred over a few days in the life of another student. After a delay, they were asked to recall the story. In each of the episodes, the target used either an eagerness strategy of goal pursuit or a vigilance strategy, as in the following examples: (1) "Because I wanted to be at school for the beginning of my 8:30 psychology class, which is usually excellent, I woke up early this morning" (eagerness strategy); and (2) "I wanted to take a class in photography at the community center, so I didn't register for a class in Spanish that was scheduled at the same time" (vigilance strategy). The study found that the participants remembered episodes involving eagerness strategies better when ideal beliefs were activated than when ought beliefs were activated, whereas the reverse was true for remembering episodes involving vigilance strategies.

Attributional processes have also been found to vary depending on whether ideal-self or ought-self beliefs predominate. The eagerness strategy of a promotion focus inclines people to generate many hypotheses in order to maximize the number of "hits" or correctly identified causes, whereas the vigilance strategy of a prevention focus inclines people to generate only the few that are necessary in order to avoid "false alarms" or incorrectly identified causes. In

an object-naming task in which participants had to guess what the object was in each unusual picture they were given, Liberman, Molden, Idson, and Higgins (2001) found that participants with stronger ideal-self beliefs generated more hypotheses about what the object was in each picture, and, independently, participants with greater ought-self beliefs generated fewer hypotheses.

Liberman and colleagues (2001) predicted that this difference would also be associated with different attributional processes, because generation of hypotheses is a fundamental part of such processes. When observing an event that has multiple possible causes, individuals who have a vigilant prevention focus should attempt to find a necessary cause and reject the rest, as postulated by standard attribution models. On the other hand, individuals who have an eager promotion focus should keep all causal possibilities alive in order not to omit a "hit," thereby discounting fewer possibilities than would be predicted by standard attribution models. These hypotheses were supported in two studies in which regulatory focus varied as both a chronic personality variable (strong ideal-self beliefs versus strong ought-self beliefs) and as a situationally manipulated variable (by priming ideal-self beliefs versus ought-self beliefs; Liberman et al., 2001).

Different Goals are Associated with Different Behavioral Strategies

It makes sense that people will develop strategies that best serve their goals. If the goal is to validate one's attributes (and avoid invalidating them), this suggests very different strategies than does the goal of developing one's attributes. And indeed this is what is found.

We have already seen that when people bring performance goals to a situation or when performance goals are induced in the situation, people avoid tasks that might risk failure or reveal inadequacies (e.g., Elliott & Dweck, 1988). It is also true that they engage in other strategies, such as self-handicapping, that are aimed at preventing negative judgments of their ability. Rhodewalt (1994), for example, has shown that when people are concerned about fixed ability judgments, they are more likely to self-handicap, that is, to pursue strategies that prevent true judgments of their abilities (e.g., not starting a paper until the last minute, partying the night before an exam). Unfortunately, these strategies may also decrease the probability of success. In other words, in order to avoid negative judgments about their ability, some people put their achievement at risk. This can happen in relationships as well, when people may court the rejection that they fear but in a way that preserves their judgment of their underlying personalities and worth (Erdley et al, 1997; cf. Downey & Feldman, 1996).

Other findings as well speak to how important an outcome can be as a reflection of an underlying trait to people with performance goals and to the strategies they may employ as a result. Mueller and Dweck (1998) found that 45% of their participants in a performance-goal condition lied about their scores on a failure trial when they were reporting those scores to someone else. In contrast, very few participants in the learning-goal condition falsified this evidence. In a study by Dweck and Sorich (1999), students with performance goals reported far more often than those with learning goals that, were they to do poorly on a test in a new subject, they would seriously consider cheating the next time around. This latter finding may reflect not only the importance of looking smart (and the strategies to which they would resort in order to do so) but also the paucity of strategies that may appear available to them if their past performance was seen as indicating low ability.

Pronounced differences are also apparent in the strategies people with learning versus performance goals bring to bear on a task in which they are engaged. The goal of developing one's abilities appears to lead to deeper processing of material than does the goal of validating one's ability, whereas the latter appears to lead to more brute-force strategies, such as rote memorization, that are presumably aimed at test performance rather than understanding (Ames & Archer, 1988; Elliot, McGregor, & Gable, 1999; Farrell & Dweck, 1985; Graham & Golon, 1991; Grant, 2001; Pintrich & Garcia, 1991). Not surprisingly, deeper strategies often yield better performance than surface ones (e.g., Farrell & Dweck, 1985; Grant,

2001). In summary, it is not surprising that different goals would spawn different strategies. What might be more surprising is that performance goals spawn strategies that, although often self-protective, are also often self-defeating.

Learning and performance goals are also associated with different patterns of performance. As we have noted, both goals can be highly motivating. In fact, it looks as though, under conditions in which a task is not overly difficult, such as a fun game or an introductory psychology course (Elliot & Harackiewicz, 1996; Harackiewicz, Baron, Carter, Lehto, & Elliot, 1997), performance goals may give people an advantage. That is, because their intelligence is on the line, people with performance goals may work really hard when good outcomes are likely (see Grant, 2001). However, when the task is very difficult, such as a difficult problem-solving task or a premed chemistry course (Elliott & Dweck, 1988; Grant, 2001), then a learning goal is predictive of superior performance, whereas performance goals are predictive of vulnerability in the face of setbacks. Thus, just as with intrinsic motivation, knowing the self-system in which people are operating allows us to understand the different circumstances in which performance may be facilitated or impaired.

We discussed earlier how the ideal-self system functions with eagerness strategies and the ought-self system functions with vigilance strategies, and we described how this affects hypothesis generation and attributional processes. This strategic difference between the two self-systems has also been shown to have a major impact on people's problem solving and decision making. As just one example, the interactive effect of expectancy and value on decisions has been found to vary as a function of the strength of individuals' ideal-self versus ought-self beliefs.

A basic assumption of expectancy-value models is that, in addition to main effects of expectancy and value on goal commitment, there is also an effect from their multiplicative combination (Lewin, Dembo, Festinger, and Sears, 1944; Vroom, 1964; for a review, see Feather, 1982). The multiplicative assumption is that, as either expectancy or value increases, the impact of the other variable on commitment increases. This assumption reflects the notion that goal commitment involves a motivation to *maximize* the product of value and expectancy. Goal pursuit, with the strategic eagerness associated with ideal-self beliefs involves ensuring hits and advancement. This implies trying to maximize outcomes. In contrast, goal pursuit with the strategic vigilance associated with ought-self beliefs involves being careful not to make mistakes. This implies doing only what is necessary. How would this difference in strategies influence the multiplicative relation between expectancy and value?

Shah and Higgins (1997) suggested that making a decision with a promotion focus is more likely to involve the motivation to maximize the product of value and expectancy. Goal pursuit with eagerness strategies would involve pursuing highly valued goals with the highest expected utility, which maximizes value × expectancy. In contrast, goal pursuit with vigilance strategies would involve avoiding all unnecessary risks by striving to meet only responsibilities that are either clearly necessary (i.e., high value prevention goals) or safely attainable (i.e., high expectancy of attainment). When goal pursuit becomes a necessity, such as in ensuring the safety of one's child, one *must* do whatever one can to succeed regardless of the ease or likelihood of goal attainment. That is, although expectancy information would always be relevant, it would become relatively *less* relevant as goal pursuit becomes more a necessity. Thus, Shah and Higgins predicted that, as strength of prevention focus increased, the interactive effect of value and expectancy would become *negative*.

To summarize, Shah and Higgins (1997) hypothesized that, as strength of ideal beliefs increased (strong promotion focus), the positive interactive effect of value and expectancy would increase; but as strength of ought beliefs increased (strong prevention focus), the interactive effect of value and expectancy would decrease. These predictions were tested in a set of studies in which participants were asked to make decisions about taking a class in their major or taking an entrance exam for graduate school. In one study, for example, participants were asked to evaluate the likelihood that they would take a course in their major for which the value of doing well and the expectancy of doing well in the course were experimentally manipulated, and participants' promotion strength and prevention strength were measured. High versus low value was established as a 95% versus 51% acceptance rate of previous majors into their honor societies with a grade of B or higher in the course. High versus low expectancy was established as a rate of 75% versus 25% of previous majors receiving a grade of B or higher in the course. The study found that the contrast representing the expectancy × value effect on the decision to take the course was *positive* for individuals with a strong ideal-self beliefs but was *negative* for individuals with strong ought-self beliefs.

Different Self-Systems Give Different Meaning to Self-Esteem

In a fundamental way, we have been talking about different self-systems built around different self-beliefs and their allied goals. Each self-system involves a coordinated set of variables that give each a qualitatively different dynamic. As we have seen, the entity-theory–performance-goal system (that is built around judgments of the enduring self) gives rise to a different pattern of intrinsic motivation, attributions, expectancies, and behavior than does the incremental-theory–learning-goal system (that is built around development of a dynamic self). As we have also seen, the self-regulatory system associated with ought-self beliefs produces different emotions, memories, attributional processes, and decision-making processes than the self-regulatory system associated with ideal-self beliefs.

Insofar as these different self-systems imply different definitions of the self and different self-relevant motivation, they also imply different ways of feeling good about the self. In fact, the different classes of goals can be seen as different ways of pursuing and maintaining self-esteem or self-security within the different self-systems.

Specifically, when people conceive of the self as a set of fixed traits, the way they can feel good about this self is to validate the quality of these traits. In contrast, when people conceive of the self as a dynamic system of qualities that can be cultivated, then the way to feel good about this self is to strive to develop those qualities. Indeed, when students of all ages were asked when they felt good about their intelligence ("Sometimes students feel smart in school, and sometimes they don't. When do you feel smart?"), students with the fixed and malleable theories gave very different answers (see Dweck, 1999). Those with the fixed theory, more often than those with the malleable theory, named performance-goal successes as the times they felt smart. For example, they said they felt smart when they outperformed other students, made no mistakes, or found a task or a subject to be easy.

In contrast, those with a malleable theory of their intelligence, more often than those with the fixed theory, said they felt smart when they pursued learning goals. For example, they felt smart when things were hard but they were making progress or when they struggled but then mastered a task. Interestingly, they also said they felt smart when they put their knowledge to work helping others to learn. Thus those with fixed and those with malleable self-theories experienced high self-esteem under essentially opposite circumstances—tasks that were easy for them versus hard for them; peers whom they outperformed versus helped. That is, they experienced high self-esteem when they attained the goal that appears to be associated with their self-theory.

The difference between the ideal-self system and the ought-self system is also associated with different ways of feeling effective and different achievement motivations. Individuals with a subjective history of success in attaining ideal goals would have promotion pride, and individuals with a subjective history of success in attaining ought goals would have prevention pride. The Regulatory Focus Questionnaire (RFQ; Higgins et al., 2000) independently measures individuals' amount of promotion pride and amount of prevention pride. The promotion pride subscale measures individuals' subjective histories of promotion success with items such as, "How often have you accomplished things that got you 'psyched' to work even harder?" and the prevention pride subscale measures individuals' subjective histories of prevention success with items such as "Not being careful has gotten me into trouble at times" (reverse scored).

Higgins and colleagues (2000) found that individuals with high promotion pride were more inclined to use strategic eagerness in goal pursuit than individuals with low promotion pride and that, independently, individuals with high prevention pride were more inclined to use strategic vigilance than individuals with low prevention pride. For example, higher promotion pride was associated with using more means to pursue each goal (eagerly pursuing all means of advancement) and, independently, higher prevention pride was associated with using fewer mean to pursue each goal (only necessary means). This pattern was replicated when memories of promotion success or failure or prevention success or failure were primed in an experimental study. In addition, there is also evidence that promotion pride is associated with a sense of joy in one's life, whereas prevention pride is associated with a sense of peace in one's life (Higgins et al., 2000).

Self-Systems and Personal Stability versus Individual Variation

One great advantage of a goal approach to the self is that the same constructs can be used to understand the stabilities in people's self-systems and the ways people might vary over situations or change over time (see Mischel & Shoda, 1995; see also Cervone & Shoda, 1999; Grant & Dweck, 1999b). We have dealt extensively with how individuals might differ substantially in the goals that are chronically most accessible to them, but we have also shown how clear situational cues can induce particular goals along with their allied affects, cognitions, and strategies. Thus we can see how our goal-based self-systems can capture both stable individual differences (and how they can play out in people's lives) and the dynamic nature of self-construction in response to powerful situational forces. In summary, both the individual-difference approach to the self and the dynamic, constructivist approach to the self have had powerful insights to offer the field. We believe that our goal-based self-systems perspective can integrate the merits of these approaches.

Conclusion

In this chapter, based on evidence from our research programs, we proposed (1) that self-defining beliefs and values come to life through people's goals, (2) that goals give the term "self-system" real and important meaning, and (3) that key self-variables, such as self-efficacy, self-attributions, and self-esteem, cannot be properly understood outside of the goal-based self-systems in which they occur. Indeed, we showed how the very same self-variables (for example, the same self-efficacy expectancy or the same attribution) can take on entirely different meanings, operate in entirely different ways, and have entirely different impact in different self-systems. Throughout, we showed how these self-systems can be assessed as individual differences but can also be produced experimentally by manipulating the beliefs and goals that are at their core. Thus we ended by proposing that our self-system approach can capture both the enduring aspects of the self and the more dynamic, constructivist nature of the self.

References

Ames, C., & Archer, J. (1988). Achievement goals in the classroom: Students' learning strategies and motivation processes. *Journal of Educational Psychology, 80(3),* 260–267.

Baer, A., & Dweck, C. S. (2001). [Rumination, depressed affect, and coping: A meaning system approach.] Unpublished raw data.

Brunstein, J. C., & Gollwitzer, P. M. (1996). Effects of failure on subsequent performance: The importance of self-defining goals. *Journal of Personality and Social Psychology, 70,* 395–407.

Carver, C. S., & Scheier, M. F. (1990). Origins and functions of positive and negative affect: A control-process view. *Psychological Review, 97,* 19–35.

Carver, C. S., & Scheier, M. F. (1998). *On the self-regulation of behavior.* New York: Cambridge University Press.

Cervone, D., & Shoda, Y. (Eds.). (1999). *The coherence of personality: Social-cognitive bases of consistency, variability, and organization.* New York: Guilford Press.

Crocker, J. (1999). Social stigma and self-esteem: Situational construction of self-worth. *Journal of Experimental Social Psychology, 35(1),* 89–107.

Crowe, E., & Higgins, E. T. (1997). Regulatory focus and strategic inclinations: Promotion and prevention in decision-making. *Organizational Behavior and Human Decision Processes, 69,* 117–132.

Downey, G., & Feldman, S. I. (1996). Implications of rejection sensitivity for intimate relationships. *Journal of Personality and Social Psychology, 70,* 1327–1343.

Dweck, C. S. (1999). *Self-theories: Their role in motivation, personality, and development.* Philadelphia: Psychology Press.

Dweck, C. S., & Leggett, E. L. (1988). A social-cognitive approach to motivation and personality. *Psychological Review, 95,* 256–273.

Dweck, C. S., & Sorich, L. (1999). Mastery-oriented thinking. In C. R. Snyder (Ed.). *Coping* (pp. 232–25). New York: Oxford University Press.

Dykman, B. M. (1998). Integrating cognitive and motivational factors in depression: Initial tests of a goal-orientation approach. *Journal of Personality and Social Psychology, 74,* 139–158.

Elliot, A. J., & Harackiewicz, J. M. (1996). Approach and avoidance achievement goals and intrinsic motivation: A mediational analysis. *Journal of Personality and Social Psychology, 70,* 461–475.

Elliot, A. J., McGregor, H., & Gable, S. (1999). Achievement goals, study strategies, and exam performance: A mediational analysis. *Journal of Experimental Psychology, 91(3),* 549–563.

Elliott, E. S., & Dweck, C. S. (1988). Goals: An approach to motivation and achievement. *Journal of Personality and Social Psychology, 54,* 5–12.

Erdley, C. A., Cain, K. M., Loomis, C. C., Dumas-Hines, F., & Dweck, C. S. (1997). The relations among children's social goals, implicit personality theories, and responses to social failure. *Developmental Psychology, 33,* 263–272.

Farrell, E., & Dweck, C. S. (1985). *The role of motivational processes in transfer of learning.* Unpublished manuscript, Harvard University.

Feather, N. T. (1982). Actions in relation to expected consequences: An overview of a research program. In N. T. Feather (Ed.), *Expectations and actions: Expectancy-value models in psychology* (pp. 53–95). Hillsdale, NJ: Erlbaum.

Graham, S., & Golen, S. (1991). Motivational influences on cognition: Task involvement, ego involvement, and depth of information processing. *Journal of Educational Psychology, 83,* 187–194.

Grant, H. (2001). *Clarifying achievement goals and their impact: A new, multidimensional scale and a unified framework.* Unpublished doctoral dissertation, Columbia University

Grant, H., & Dweck, C. S. (2001). Cross-cultural response to failure: Considering outcome attributions with different goals. In F. Salili, C. Chiu, & Y. Y. Hong (Eds.), *Student motivation: The culture and context of learning* (pp. 203–220). Hong Kong: University of Hong Kong Press.

Grant, H., & Dweck, C. S. (1999a). Content vs. structure in motivation and self-regulation. In R. Wyer (Ed.), *Advances in social cognition* (Vol. 12, pp. 161–174). Mahwah, NJ: Erlbaum.

Grant, H., & Dweck, C. S. (1999b). A goal analysis of personality and personality coherence. In D. Cervone & Y. Shoda (Eds.), *The coherence of personality* (pp. 345–371). New York: Guilford Press.

Harackiewicz, J. M., Baron, K. E., Carter, S. M., Lehto, A. T., & Elliot, A. J. (1997). Predictors and consequences of achievement goals in the college classroom: Maintaining interest and making the grade. *Journal of Personality and Social Psychology, 73,* 1284–1295.

Higgins, E. T. (1987). Self-discrepancy: A theory relating self and affect. *Psychological Review, 94,* 319–340.

Higgins, E. T. (1996). The "self digest": Self-knowledge serving self-regulatory functions. *Journal of Personality and Social Psychology, 71,* 1062–1083.

Higgins, E. T. (1997). Beyond pleasure and pain. *American Psychologist, 52,* 1280–1300.

Higgins, E. T. (1999). When do self-discrepancies have specific relations to emotions?: The second-generation question of Tangney, Niedenthal, Covert, and Barlow (1998). *Journal of Personality and Social Psychology, 77,* 1313–1317.

Higgins, E. T., Bond, R. N., Klein, R., & Strauman, T. (1986). Self-discrepancies and emotional vulnerability: How magnitude, accessibility, and type of discrepancy influence affect. *Journal of Personality and Social Psychology, 51,* 5–15.

Higgins, E. T., Friedman, R. S., Harlow, R. E., Idson, L. C., Ayduk, O. N., & Taylor, A. (2000). Achievement orientations from subjective histories of success: Promotion pride versus prevention pride. *European Journal of Social Psychology, 30,* 1–23.

Higgins, E. T., Grant, H., & Shah, J. (1999). Self-regulation and quality of life: Emotional and non-emotional life experiences. In D. Kahneman, E. Diener, & N. Schwarz (Eds.), *Well-being: The foundations of hedonic psychology* (pp. 244–266). New York: Russell Sage.

Higgins, E. T., Roney, C., Crowe, E., & Hymes, C. (1994). Ideal versus ought predilections for approach and avoidance: Distinct self-regulatory systems. *Journal of Personality and Social Psychology, 66,* 276–286.

Higgins, E. T., & Tykocinski, O. (1992). Self-discrepancies and biographical memory: Personality and cognition at the level of psychological situation. *Personality and Social Psychology Bulletin, 18,* 527–535.

Hong, Y., Chiu, C., Dweck, C. S., Lin, D. M., & Wan, W. (1999). Implicit theories, attributions, and coping: A meaning system approach. *Journal of Personality and Social Psychology, 77*(3), 588–599.

Idson, L. C., Liberman, N., & Higgins, E. T. (2000). Distinguishing gains from non-losses and losses from non-gains: A regulatory focus perspective on hedonic intensity. *Journal of Experimental Social Psychology, 36*(3), 252–274.

Kamins, M. L., Morris, S. M., & Dweck, C. S. (1997). Implicit theories as predictors of goals in dating relationships. Paper presented at the annual meeting of the Eastern Psychological Association, Washington, DC.

Kasimatis, M., Miller, M., & Marcussen, L. (1996). The effects of implicit theories on exercise motivation. *Journal of Research in Personality, 30*(4), 510–516.

Kelly, G. A. (1955). *The psychology of personal constructs.* New York: Norton.

Kernis, M. H., Cornell, D. P., Sun, C., Berry, A., & Har-

low, T. (1993). There's more to self esteem than whether it is high or low: The importance of stability of self-esteem. *Journal of Personality and Social Psychology, 65*(6), 1190–1204.

Lewin, K., Dembo, T., Festinger, L., & Sears, P. S. (1944). Level of aspiration. In J. McHunt (Ed.), *Personality and the behavior disorders* (Vol. 1, pp. 333–378). New York: Ronald Press.

Liberman, N., Molden, D. C., Idson, L. C., & Higgins, E. T. (2001). Promotion and prevention focus on alternative hypotheses: Implications for attributional functions. *Journal of Personality and Social Psychology, 80,* 5–18.

Martocchio, J. (1994). Effects of conceptions of ability on anxiety, self-efficacy, and learning in training. *Journal of Applied Psychology, 79*(6), 819–825.

Mischel, W., & Shoda, Y. (1995). A cognitive-affective system theory of personality: Reconceptualizing situations, dispositions, dynamics, and invariance in personality structure. *Psychology Review, 102*(2), 246–268.

Molden, D., & Dweck, C. S. (2000). Meaning and motivation. In C. Sansone & J. Harackiewicz (Eds.), *Intrinsic and extrinsic motivation: The search for optimal motivation and performance* (pp. 131–161). San Diego, CA: Academic Press.

Mueller, C. M., & Dweck, C. S. (1998). Praise for intelligence can undermine children's motivation and performance. *Journal of Personality and Social Psychology, 75*(1), 33–52.

Pintrich, P. R., & Garcia, T. (1991). Student goal orientation and self-regulation in the college classroom. In M. L. Maehr & P. R. Pintrich (Eds.), *Advances in motivation and achievement* (Vol. 7, pp. 371–402). Greenwich, CT: JAI Press.

Rhodewalt, F. (1994). Conceptions of ability, achievement goals, and individual differences in self-handicapping behavior: On the application of implicit theories. *Journal of Personality, 62*(1), 67–85.

Robins, R. W., & Pals, J. (1998). *Implicit self-theories of ability in the academic domain: A test of Dweck's model.* Unpublished manuscript.

Sansone, C., & Harackiewicz, J. M. (Eds.). (2000). *Intrinsic and extrinsic motivation: The search for optimal motivation and performance.* San Diego, CA: Academic Press.

Shah, J., & Higgins, E. T. (1997). Expectancy × value effects: Regulatory focus as a determinant of magnitude and direction. *Journal of Personality and Social Psychology, 73,* 447–458.

Shah, J., Higgins, E. T., & Friedman, R. (1998). Performance incentives and means: How regulatory focus influences goal attainment. *Journal of Personality and Social Psychology, 74*(2), 285–293.

Stone, J., & Dweck, C. S. (1998). *Theories of intelligence and the meaning of achievement goals.* Unpublished manuscript, Columbia University.

Strauman, T. J. (1989). Self-discrepancies in clinical depression and social phobia: Cognitive structures that underlie emotional disorders? *Journal of Abnormal Psychology, 98,* 14–22.

Strauman, T. J., & Higgins, E. T. (1987). Automatic activation of self-discrepancies and emotional syndromes: When cognitive structures influence affect. *Journal of Personality and Social Psychology, 53,* 1004–1014.

Tabernero, C., & Wood, R. (1999). Implicit theories versus the social construal of ability in self regulation and performance on a complex task. *Organizational Behavior and Human Decision Processes, 78,* 104–127.

Tangney, J. P., Niedenthal, P. M., Covert, M. V., & Barlow, D. H. (1998). Are shame and guilt related to distinct self-discrepancies? A test of Higgins' (1987) hypothesis. *Journal of Personality and Social Psychology, 75,* 256–268.

Tesser, A., & Campbell, J. (1982). Self-evaluation maintenance and the perception of friends and strangers. *Journal of Personality, 50,* 261–279.

Vroom, V. H. (1964). *Work and motivation.* New York: Wiley.

Wicklund, R. A., & Gollwitzer, P. M. (1982). *Symbolic self-completion.* Hillsdale, NJ: Erlbaum.

13

On Assimilating Identities to the Self: A Self-Determination Theory Perspective on Internalization and Integrity within Cultures

RICHARD M. RYAN
EDWARD L. DECI

When human beings emerge into the world, they have no identity. That is, infants are not yet defined in terms of institutional affiliations, self-representations, and social roles by which others recognize them. The identity that a child will later have, perhaps as an athlete, a religious adherent, a physician, a collectivist, or all of these, results from a developmental process that takes place within a cultural context. Plainly put, individuals *acquire* identities over time, identities whose origins and meanings derive from people's interactions with the social groups and organizations that surround them. In turn, these identities, once adopted, play a significant role in the organization and regulation of people's everyday lives.

Identity Formation in the Modern World

The problem of identity is more salient today than at any time in history. The reasons for this are clear. In modern market-based societies (1) the range of possible identities available to any individual is larger than ever before, and (2) the latitude given to individuals to pursue different identities is considerable. No longer is it as common as it once was for identities to be conferred on people by relatively fixed factors such as birthrights, social and religious orders, or parental status. Furthermore, in market economies, because individual identities are not preordained or even self-apparent, individuals can at least superficially define themselves to others through their selection of clothes, commodities, media idols, and other markers of interests, status, and affiliations. That is, people are encouraged to consume their way into identities. Finally, the exposure of individuals to varied identities and role models, whether fabricated or real, has been exponentially expanded by media and Web-based communications, further complicating the process of adopting identities. In sum, in the absence of strong identity constraints and with the widening of apparent models and choices and the pressure for self-commodification, the developmental task of finding oneself within a social world has become among the most salient and difficult of life's challenges.

That identity formation has become, for historical, cultural, and economic reasons, a central developmental task in our age does not mean it is an entirely new issue. No doubt people have, throughout history, struggled with identity issues, such as dealing with having been forced into roles or lifestyles somehow unsuited to them. However, many of today's youth are facing the even greater risk of failing to negotiate the not-so-clear pathways to the adult roles, responsibilities, and relationships that secure identities afford. Often, in the face of this struggle, many end up adopting darker identities, such as drug abusers, sexual risk takers, or compulsive shoppers, as a compensatory method of experiencing aliveness or staving off depression and meaninglessness. Thus, although identity has been a perennial feature of persons within all human groups, the concept is more salient and the struggle more obvious today than ever before, precisely because identity is so frequently an open question.

Identity formation is a lifelong process, one that comes especially to the foreground when the individual shifts between social contexts. However, the major struggles of identity fall primarily on adolescents, for whom the establishment of secure identities is critical for passage into the adult world (Adams & Marshall, 1996; Erikson, 1968). Through the peer groups toward which they gravitate, the celebrities they admire, the logos they wear, the lifestyles they emulate, and the career interests they espouse, adolescents attempt to define a place for themselves within society. Both their motivation and their capacity for grappling with different identities are exacerbated by the advent of adolescent egocentrism (Elkind, 1985; Piaget, 1967). Specifically, with adolescence comes the propensity to view oneself from the perspective of others and thus to be conscious of the "place" one has within social contexts. This leads to greater self-awareness, but it also engenders considerable anxiety and conformity in order to avoid feelings of rejection (Ryan & Kuczkowski, 1994). Thus it is often amidst an atmosphere of social pressures, both real and imagined, that teens attempt to lay the foundation of adult identity.

In Search of Need Satisfaction

To discover why some available identities are accepted whereas others are ignored or wither, we must ask why identities are adopted at all and what functions the adoption of identities serves for individuals. The most general answer is that identities are adopted in the service of basic psychological needs. People develop identities first and foremost to help them secure, maintain, and solidify their connectedness to social groups. In acquiring identities people find a way to fit into social contexts, adopting roles, beliefs, and practices that are recognized and appreciated by others. In short, the principal function of identity formation is fostering the experience of secure belongingness or *relatedness* (Baumeister & Leary, 1995; Deci & Ryan, 2000; Ryan, 1993). Identities can fill other psychological needs as well, and, optimally, they do. In some cases identities are selected because they support feelings of *competence*. That is, people gravitate toward identities within which they can engage optimal challenges, gain skills and knowledge, and feel generally effective. Identities can also fulfill the need for *autonomy*, for they can provide a forum through which people develop and express personal interests, values, and capacities.

In some cases, identities are taken on more defensively, as when people adopt identities or group affiliations to avoid feelings of vulnerability or to gain power over others. Similarly, identities may be taken on reactively, as when people adopt identities in order to oppose the values of controlling authorities (Deci & Ryan, 2000). Because identities are typically selected and formed in the service of people's psychological needs (or in reaction to need deprivation), their acquisition and maintenance is considered dynamic and must be understood as a complex expression of the interaction between needs and affordances.

Self-Determination Theory

In this chapter our focus is on this process through which identities are acquired and organized within the individual. It begins, however, with the recognition that each individual has multiple identities and that each of these identities is more or less well assimilated to the self of the individual. Our perspective is that of self-determination theory (SDT; Deci & Ryan, 1985; Ryan & Deci, 2000b), a theory of motivation and personality within which the relative assimilation of goals, values, and identities has been a focal issue. SDT describes variations in the relative assimilation of identity to the self and argues that these variations have empirically testable and clinically relevant implications for human functioning. More specifically, SDT proposes that the identities we "wear" can vary: They may be forced on us by the contingencies of our social context; they may be partially assimilated as introjects; or they may be well integrated into the self so that they serve as personally meaningful and abiding guides to life. Further, the theory suggests that the more one's life roles and pursuits remain only partially assimilated to the self, the more they fail to fulfill psychological needs, a fact that in large part accounts for the relation between less internalization and poorer mental health and well-being. We believe that this conceptualization of internalization and the findings associated with it have relevance to the understanding of identity development and provide links both to theories of mental health and vitality and to practical approaches to socialization, education, and psychotherapy.

To introduce this perspective and the hypotheses that derive from it, we proceed as follows. First, we discuss the motivational basis of identity formation, focusing on the roles of intrinsic and extrinsic motivation. Second, elaborating the importance of extrinsic motivation, we outline a theoretical model of internalization and integration of identities. Third, we review empirical evidence concerning the functional outcomes associated with different types of internalization. Fourth, we examine the social–contextual factors that facilitate the assimilation of identities, values, and goals, as well as those that forestall it. Fifth, we consider the cross-cultural generalizability of our model of internalization and autonomy in the regulation of values and identities. A sixth issue we address is that of multiple identities and how the relative integration of personal identifications influences action and well-being. Finally, we examine some specific identities or life goals that influence well-being as a function of the degree to which they facilitate or thwart satisfaction of the basic psychological needs for relatedness and autonomy.

Acquiring Identities: The Contributions of Intrinsic Motivation and Extrinsic Motivation

The acquisition of identities, like the acquisition of any other psychological structure, occurs primarily through the process of assimilation. People are naturally inclined to imitate, explore, and take on ambient social roles and practices and to transform those into aspects of themselves. However, because people cannot assimilate every ambient identity and because families and societies discourage some roles for some individuals, the process of identity acquisition is clearly a complex one that is codetermined by individual proclivities and interests as they interact with social pressures, constraints, and reward systems. It is through the interaction of individuals with these social forces that identities are forged and anchored within the self, to whatever extent they are.

In some cases identities appear to grow directly from natural inclinations, interests, and curiosities. In other words, the enactment of some identities seems to be *intrinsically motivated*. Intrinsic motivation is the prototype for autonomous or self-determined activity. When people are intrinsically motivated, they experience their actions as inherently enjoyable or satisfying (Ryan & Deci, 2000a). Although intrinsic motivation is often a spontaneous experience associated with novel and interesting activities, it is nonetheless relevant to the selection and maintenance of identities. Thus a child who enjoys building and manipulating objects may become a craftsperson; one who loves to climb, run, and jump could become an athlete; and a musically inclined child might become a musician. In these examples, early experiences of intrinsic motivation supply the impetus for a person's choice of an avocation, career, or lifestyle that ultimately becomes part of his or her identity (Krapp, 2002). Thus opportunities to experience intrinsic motivation can play an important role in how people find and maintain some of the identities they adopt.

The transformation of inclinations, interests, and curiosities into identities is no simple process, however. Even activities that are intrinsically motivated require definite environmental affordances or supports if they are to be sustained over time and over life's natural obstacles. Thus children's general curiosity and fascination with the world around them will gradually become channeled into interests in particular subject areas or activities with which they come to identify, be those activities reading psychology, studying art history, or watching birds. This will be most likely to happen, however, only for activities that the individuals have found optimally challenging, for which they have received effectance-related supports and positive feedback, and that have not been overly controlled by others. That is, interpersonal supports facilitate the elaboration of inclinations and curiosities, allowing them to develop into identities. Within SDT we refer to this process in which general interest and curiosity become focused in particular areas or activities and thus contribute to identity formation as the differentiation of *intrinsic motivation* (Deci, 1975; Deci & Ryan, 1985).

However, although early inclinations and intrinsic interests can sometimes be the source of, or impetus toward, subsequent identities, many if not most of the identities adults adopt are not direct outgrowths of the things they loved to do as children. In fact nearly every adult identity carries with it certain roles, responsibilities, or tasks that are not, in themselves, intrinsically motivated (Ryan, 1995). Instead, over the course of socialization, people are exposed to identities, or aspects of them, that may or may not be intrinsically appealing but that may have instrumental value or importance. As these roles, tasks, and duties are modeled and taught, children take them in or accept them to differing degrees. Within SDT we use the concept of *internalization* to refer to this process of taking in and transforming external regulations and transmitted values into self-regulations and personally endorsed values (Deci & Ryan, 1985; Ryan & Connell, 1989; Vallerand, 1997). SDT further posits that variation in the extent and quality of people's internalization of extrinsic motivation for various identities explains the difference between authentic, vital, and committed living that some individuals exhibit and the alienated, halfhearted, or conflicted enactment of identities that afflicts others.

To illustrate, consider that a vast majority of Americans identify themselves as Christians. Among them, however, there is considerable variability in the extent to which that identity is experienced as authentic and is fully and congruently expressed in everyday life (Batson, 1976; Ryan, Rigby, & King, 1993). It is, in fact, easy to find Christians for whom the label is merely skin deep and thus describes nothing of what they really value and do, just as one can find persons for whom the label captures their essential core values and thus deeply describes their abiding concerns and lifestyles. Take any identity—student, Republican, spouse, businessperson, sports fan—and the following rule will apply: Identities vary in the extent to which they are assimilated to the self of the individual and therefore receive the person's full endorsement and engagement.

A Model of Internalization and Integration of Goals and Identities

When one observes various individuals engaged in a similar domain of activity, one cannot help but be impressed by variations in the spirit that animates these individuals and moves them into action. For instance, when two adolescent girls take on the identity of gymnast, they could engage this role or identity in different ways. One might, for example, merely be doing it to please her athletically oriented parents, in which case she would compliantly go through the motions of practice and performance with minimal enthusiasm or inspiration and perhaps with the experience of pressure and conflict. The other might fully embrace the identity of being a gymnast, viewing it as a personally valued avocation and engaging in it energetically on an everyday basis. Both examples are of young people who, from the outside, have an identity as gymnasts but who have clearly adopted the identity differently, resulting in different manners of engagement and different degrees to which the identity has permeated their lives. From the perspective of SDT, the different reasons for enacting a behavior or possessing an identity can be understood in terms of different degrees to which the behavioral regulations that underlie them have been internalized and integrated into one's sense of self.

Taking on the identity of gymnast is, of course, typically a voluntary matter, and many people either do not have the facility for it or might not find gymnastics relevant or interesting. For them, gymnastics plays no role in their identity, and they internalize nothing with respect to it. Within SDT, they would be described as "amotivated" with respect to gymnastics, and, provided they found other venues for constructive activity, it would have little consequence for their well-being. With some identities, however, significant others—one's parents, teachers, maybe even society as a whole—care very much about whether young people internalize them. Thus a given culture might heavily weigh in on the side of developing specific identities such as being a good student, a heterosexual, or a loyal soldier. In such cases, successfully adopting the favored identities (or failing to take them on) may have a variety of immediate and long-term consequences for people's place in the culture and feelings about themselves. Thus people assume identities under a varied landscape of interpersonal and tangible pressures, threats, and rewards

Internalization and Regulation of Identities

According to SDT, any characteristic behavior, role, or identity, if it is adopted at all, can be understood as being adopted by individuals for different reasons, and these reasons in turn can be understood as reflecting differing degrees to which the behavior or identity has been internalized to the self.

Insofar as an individual finds identity-relevant behaviors that are valued by a salient reference group to yield no desired outcomes or to be too difficult to enact, there will be an absence of internalization and intentionality, and the person will be amotivated with respect to that identity. For instance, a young person who does not find

school relevant or who feels unable to meet the demands of school may be amotivated in that domain. That is, if the person either does not care or just gives up, amotivation or nonregulation will be in evidence.

If, however, the person is able to enact the behaviors and finds them instrumental for desired outcomes, some degree of internalization will occur. The least internalized form of motivation is labeled "external regulation." This type of regulation involves intentionality and behavioral enactment, but the initiation and causation of the action is largely external to the person. Thus, when a person is externally regulated, he or she acts in accord with, and because of, rewards and punishments administered by others. When a person's actions are controlled by external contingencies, the only internalization required for such engagement is the internalization of information relevant to negotiating the contingencies successfully. From an attributional standpoint, the *perceived locus of causality* (deCharms, 1968) of the activity is fully external and is therefore dependent on the continued presence of the external causes for its persistence.

External regulation is a powerful form of motivation, a fact that has been amply demonstrated in more than five decades of operant research. However, as work both in that tradition and in the SDT tradition has shown, the problem with external regulation is maintenance and transfer (Deci & Ryan, 1985), because internalization is impaired under conditions of strong demands and salient contingencies. To the extent that contingencies are emphasized and that one's behavior is dependent on the external rewards and punishments, there is a lesser tendency for internalization to occur and for the behavior to be enacted in new situations and future times. When the controls are no longer present, adherence will be poor. Thus there is an inverse relation between the strength of someone's experience of being externally controlled and the likelihood that the person will, over time, internalize and identify with the relevant behavior or value. For example, a teenage boy who goes to religious services only because his parents pressure him to has *de facto* not internalized his faith nor assumed an identity as a religious person. The true test of this failure of internalization will be the degree of adherence he shows after he has left home and is not under close parental surveillance. Self-determination theory predicts that the stronger the pressures that were brought to bear on the teenager while he was externally regulated, the less likely he will be to adhere once the external contingencies are removed. As such, external controls undermine the development of a personal value for the endeavor, which would be the basis of sustained activity without external pressure or reward.

A greater degree of internalization is represented by external values and motivators that have been introjected. *Introjection* is a form of internalization—a kind of partial internalization—in which a regulation has been taken in but not accepted as one's own. Initially external contingencies are now represented internally, such that the person applies intrapsychically what had initially been applied interpersonally by socializing agents. In so doing, the person experiences rewards and punishments, typically in the form of self-esteem-related feelings and appraisals, and it is these contingent self-evaluations and their affective consequences that regulate behavior. For example, with introjected regulation, a person engages in an activity or adopts a role in order to enhance, maintain, or avoid losing self-esteem. In other words, introjected regulation involves pressuring oneself with contingencies of self-regard resulting from having been externally controlled by contingent love and regard (Assor, Roth, & Deci, 2001). A teen who attends religious services because not doing so would incur feelings of guilt and anxiety is regulated through introjection. Similarly, a young gymnast whose participation is based on feeling generalized approval and the self-aggrandizement that accompanies it is similarly operating from introjected regulation (Frederick & Ryan, 1993).

Even greater internalization is represented when a person's activities are regulated by *identifications*. A person who identifies with a role or activity has consciously endorsed or assented to its personal value and importance. A teenager who identifies with her religion thus attends services with volition and initiative because she consciously evaluates that activity as important and meaning-ful to herself. Activities regulated through identification are therefore to a large degree autonomous, that is, they are accompanied by an experience of volition and freedom in acting. According to SDT, being regulated in this more volitional way, relative to external and introjected motives, will result not only in a higher quality of engagement (e.g., greater persistence, effort, etc.) but also in more positive experiences such as enjoyment, sense of purpose, and well-being (Ryan & Deci, 2001).

SDT further proposes, however, that identifications can be either relatively isolated or compartmentalized within the psyche or relatively integrated and unified with other identifications, values, and needs of the self. For instance, suppose in the workplace a man identifies with the role of "ruthless entrepreneur," and in his religious life he aspires to follow the "Golden Rule." Both might be values or roles that he adopted as meaningful and which he experienced as personally valued identities. However, because of their inherent inconsistency, he must keep them compartmentalized from one another—following the Golden Rule at work would certainly constrain his entrepreneurial possibilities, while awareness of his cutthroat activities in business might engender guilt and anxiety when he is in his religious/moral mode of identity. Thus SDT suggests that identifications can be more or less compartmentalized and that only those that are well integrated within the psyche represent the full endorsement of the self. Accordingly, *integrated regulation* represents the most autonomous form of intentional, extrinsically motivated behavior.

It is worth noting that a fully integrated form of extrinsic motivation, although it regulates autonomous activity, is still different from intrinsic motivation. Specifically, intrinsic motivation involves doing an activity because the activity itself is interesting and enjoyable for its own sake, whereas extrinsic motivation involves doing a behavior because it is important for an instrumental outcome. As extrinsic motivation becomes more fully internalized, the instrumentality becomes more a part of one's sense of self so that the person is behaving because the activity is personally important for his or her value system and self-selected goals. But the motivation is still considered extrinsic because the behavior is instrumental for some separate, nonspontaneous outcome. In short, intrinsic motivation and well-integrated extrinsic motivation are similar in that they both represent fully autonomous or self-determined behavior, but they are different in that intrinsic motivation stems from an activity's interest value, whereas integrated regulation stems from its instrumental values or utility. Of course, it is possible that one could become intrinsically interested in an activity that had initially been extrinsically motivated, a phenomenon that Allport (1937) referred to as functional autonomy. However, it is important to keep the concepts of intrinsic motivation and integrated extrinsic motivation separate because it is possible for an activity to be autonomously regulated even when people do not find it interesting and enjoyable.

The Relative Autonomy Continuum

It should be obvious from these descriptions that one way in which these various forms of regulation differ is the relative autonomy experienced by the person within each. A person who is amotivated has a complete lack of volition, whereas a person who is externally regulated for a behavior is motivated but experiences very little autonomy with respect to the behavior. The person who has introjected a regulation experiences some autonomy, but not a lot; the person who has identified with its importance experiences still more; and the person who has integrated an initially external regulation is highly autonomous. Finally, a person who is intrinsically motivated experiences a similarly high or even higher degree of autonomy. As such, underlying this taxonomy of motives or regulatory processes is a *continuum of relative autonomy*. This continuum is displayed in the first column of Table 13.1, arranged vertically such that the regulatory process described in the first row is the least autonomous, that in the second row is slightly more autonomous, and so on. There is one caveat, however. Specifically, although both integrated regulation and intrinsic motivation are considered highly autonomous, intrinsic motivation does not require the internalization of motivation because interest is inherent (e.g., curiosity among children); integrated regulation re-

sults from the most complete internalization of extrinsic motivation. The rule in the table between integrated regulation and intrinsic motivation is intended to convey this, whereas the rule between amotivation and external regulation is intended to separate the lack of motivation from the various types of motivation.

Empirical Evidence for the Internalization Model and Its Outcomes

Support for the model of internalization and types of regulation has been manifold. First, we established that the subscales representing different types of motivation fell along a continuum as theorized. We looked for a simplex-like structure in which those subscales theorized to be closer together on the continuum were more strongly correlated than those theorized to be farther apart. In an initial demonstration, Ryan and Connell (1989) assessed children's regulatory styles for both prosocial and school-related activities and showed that the types of regulation within each domain did conform to the expected pattern of ordered correlations, thus providing evidence for an underlying continuum. The conceptual continuum and simplex-like pattern has been replicated numerous times, in domains as diverse as sport, religion, school, health care, and politics, among others (see, e.g., Deci & Ryan, 2000; Ryan & Deci, 2000b; Vallerand, 1997, for reviews).

Consequences of the Types of Internalization

We then explored relations between each subscale and other constructs that are theoretically related. Further, because the model was established in part to assess the overall degree to which an individual is autonomous in domain-specific behavioral regulation, Ryan and Connell (1989) proposed the use of an index of relative autonomy, created by algebraically combining the subscales. Several studies have used this index to predict various behavioral and psychological outcomes. Rather than reiterate comprehensive reviews of this research (e.g., Deci & Ryan, 2000; Ryan, 1995), we draw on a few examples of internalization studies so as to show the import of this model for identity formation and its enactment. In

TABLE 13.1. The Relative Autonomy Continuum With Types of Identity-Related Regulation, the Processes through Which They Develop, and the Contexts That Promote Their Development and Operation

	Types of regulation	Developmental processes	Social contextual facilitators
Complete lack of autonomy	*Amotivation* Lacking intentionality; behaving as a function of an unregulated drive, emotion, or external force.	Complete absence of internalization, interest, or belief in relevance of behavior.	Inconsistent responses from others; noncontingencies between behavior and outcomes; indicators of incompetence; irrelevance of behavior or outcomes.
	External regulation Intentional responding controlled primarily by external contingencies.	Internalization only of information relevant to operating within the controlling contingencies.	Coercive or strongly pressuring practices that emphasize reward and punishment contingencies.
	Introjected regulation Behavior controlled by internal contingencies related to self-worth and generalized approval, accompanied by the experience of pressure and anxiety.	Internalization of contingencies of worth and information about the activities and attributes that are instrumental for approval from significant others.	Relatively controlling contexts characterized by conditional affection and regard.
	Identified regulation Relatively volitional action regulated by one's sense of the importance of the activity or role for one's values and self-selected goals.	Internalization of the personal importance of the activity through consciously identifying with its meaning and value.	Autonomy-supportive context relating to target individual from his or her perspective and supporting choice and initiation.
	Integrated regulation Acting autonomously from an integrated sense of self, in accord with a coherent identity.	The reciprocal assimilation of the target identification with other identities, needs, and aspects of an integrated self.	Autonomy-supportive context that not only supports initiating but also encourages a mindful consideration and exploration of values, needs, and regulatory processes.
Highly autonomous	*Intrinsic motivation* Volitional engagement in activities out of interest and spontaneous satisfaction.	Differentiation of one's general interests and skills within specific activities or domains and then integration of those with other aspects of the self.	Affordances provided that allow one's interests to be pursued and sharpened in the context of optimal challenge, informational feedback, and supports for exploration and autonomy in action.

particular, we focus on the contrast between introjected regulation, in which people perform a behavior because they think they have to in order to feel like a good person, and identified or integrated regulation, in which people perform the behavior because it is personally important for their own goals. This distinction represents the most theoretically interesting, yet subtle, differences in internalization styles.

First, consider a study of people's religious identities. Ryan and colleagues (1993) assessed several diverse samples of individuals who described themselves as Christian. The focus of these assessments was the extent to which the motivation underlying their Christian activities, such as going to church, praying, or evangelizing, was introjected (e.g., because one is supposed to) versus identified (e.g., because I find it personally satisfying). Findings revealed that Christians did indeed vary in their reasons for religious participation, with both introjected and identified regulation appearing to foster church attendance, as expected. However, whereas introjected religiosity was associated with more negative psychological adjustment, identified religiosity was associated with greater mental health. This fits with the notion that, particularly for important life identities, the more they are assimilated to the self, the more positively they will be related to psychological well-being. Similar results were obtained by Strahan and Craig (1995) in a large-scale study of Seventh Day Adventists. Here, too, introjected regulation was associated with more inner conflict and poorer well-being, relative to identified regulation. Strahan and Craig also found that autonomy-supportive rather than controlling parenting styles were associated positively with identification and negatively with introjection, an issue to which we return in the next section.

Koestner, Losier, Vallerand, and Carducci (1996) compared people whose involvement in political concerns was based on either introjected or identified forms of internalization. They found that identification was associated with more actively seeking out information relevant to decisions, having a more complex or differentiated viewpoint, and actually being more likely to vote. Introjected regulation was associated with vulnerability to persuasion, reliance on oth-

ers' opinions, and conflicting emotions about outcomes. Thus identified versus introjected ways of embracing political concerns yielded not only different experiences but also different qualities of involvement.

The relation between style of internalization and the quality of involvement has been shown most clearly in the domain of schooling. Studies have repeatedly shown self-esteem, perceived competence, self-motivation, and well-being advantages to being autonomously regulated (see, e.g., Ryan & La Guardia, 1999, for a review). In one study, Grolnick and Ryan (1989) found that introjection and identification were equally strong predictors of working hard in school but that introjection was associated with anxiety and poor coping with failure, whereas identification was associated with enjoyment of school and positive coping. Increasingly, these same types of relations between autonomous regulation and school engagement, learning, and well-being have been shown to exist in non-Western nations (Chirkov & Ryan, 2001; Hayamizu, 1997; Tanaka & Yamauchi, 2000; Yamauchi & Tanaka, 1998).

An illustrative study (Black & Deci, 2000) with relevance for identity issues was conducted in university organic chemistry classes, a traditional gateway to professions such as medicine that have salient corresponding identities. It was found that autonomous, versus controlling, forms of regulation were associated with greater perceived competence, more interest in the course material, less anxiety, and better course performance, even when controlling for ability.

Internalization and Well-Being

Well-being is a complex construct, differentially construed by different theorists. A mainstream position in this area has been labeled the "hedonic" viewpoint (Kahneman, Diener, & Schwarz, 1999), in which well-being is equated with happiness or pleasure. A second, and somewhat divergent position is the "eudaimonic" viewpoint (Waterman, 1993), in which well-being is understood in terms of self-realization and meaning. There does, however, appear to be a convergence of results concerning the relation of identity and its regulation to well-being. Specifically, we have repeatedly found that the greater the internalization of one's values, practices, and goals—that is, those things that compose identity—the greater one's well-being, as reflected both in hedonic indicators, such as positive affect and life satisfaction, and in the more eudaimonic outcomes, such as vitality, self-actualization, freedom from inner conflict, and various qualities of relationships and experience (Ryan & Deci, 2001).

Regulation and Identities

To summarize, the SDT perspective suggests that the more fully a value or role has been internalized and thus accepted as one's own, the more it will represent a deeply held and flexibly enacted aspect of one's identity and self. It is useful to recognize, however, that the term "identity" is used to refer to roles or values that differ in their degree of generality. For example, a man might hold the identity of a psychologist, which is a relatively general identity; any identity this general will typically have several components. The identity of psychologist may include the component roles of teaching psychology, doing research, applying for grants, and writing books, among others. Of course, one could argue that each of these is a separate identity, but the point is that an identity, however broadly defined, can have different components, and it is possible that the behaviors associated with these different components or aspects of an identity can be regulated differently. The psychologist might, for example, do research because he thinks he should to attain generalized approval and respect (introjected); teach out of an intrinsic interest; apply for grants only because he thinks it will help him get tenure (external); and write books because he has identified with the importance and value of the activity. Thus, within a general identity, which will have been more or less fully assimilated to one's self, there can be different components that vary in the degree to which they are integrated and thus will be regulated by different processes.

Socializing Environments and the Regulation of Identity

As noted, internalization refers to the processes through which individuals take in and transform, to varying degrees, what is transmitted by their culture (Deci & Ryan, 1985; Ryan, Connell, & Deci, 1985). When that same process is considered from the standpoint of the social environment, the applicable term is "socialization." That is, socialization is the process of fostering internalization, and accordingly we expect a correspondence between the ways in which a social group regulates its members and the intrapsychic forms of regulation that develop within those members. In other words, the types of socializing practices used by a group are predicted to influence the degree to which values and norms are internalized by group members.

SDT views internalization as a motivated process, based in human psychological needs. That is to say, identities, which represent organized systems of goals and affiliations, are formed and adopted in the service of basic human needs (Deci & Ryan, 2000). Through forging their identities, individuals find their places within social organizations, and by internalizing and identifying with group values—that is, by making the values part of their identities—group members achieve a greater sense of belonging (Baumeister & Leary, 1995) or relatedness (Ryan, 1993). Accordingly, people will typically internalize the beliefs, practices, and values that are endorsed by people or groups whom they want to emulate or to whom they wish to be more closely connected. SDT suggests, therefore, that in order for any internalization to occur, there must be some form of individual attraction or attachment to socializing agents or institutions. Beyond that, it is largely the dynamic interplay of relatedness and autonomy that determines the form of internalization likely to occur.

SDT recognizes that some identities are not internalized at all; in other words, that some people remain amotivated with respect to various societally valued identities. To the extent, for example, that parents place no value on particular activities, are inconsistent or punishing when their children attempt the activities, or convey incompetence with respect to the children's attempts, the children are likely to become amotivated for the activities and to fail to internalize the activities' value as part of their identities.

SDT postulates that coercive forms of social regulation, such as the use of rewards and punishments to control behavior, will engender some motivation for the relevant behaviors but will result in the most impoverished forms of internalization, both of specific behaviors and of the more general organization of behaviors associated with identity. If socialization practices are highly controlling, people are likely to enact identity-relevant behaviors only when they are directly controlled to do so. That is, controlling socialization practices tend to occasion external regulation, represented by compliance when the demands or contingencies are operative. However, such practices also tend to forestall further identification with and assimilation of the activities' regulation.

SDT further proposes that moderately controlling socialization practices such as those involving what Rogers (1951) would have labeled "conditions of worth" are likely to promote introjection but not the fuller forms of internalization. In other words, if socializers contingently bestow and withdraw love or emotional security as a way of motivating particular behaviors and attributes, introjected regulation of the relevant behaviors and attributes is likely to follow, such that enactment of these identity-relevant behaviors will be pressured by self-esteem contingencies. In fostering introjection, affection and regard are made contingent on one's success, however defined, and thus provide intermittent satisfaction of the relatedness need. In the process, however, autonomy suffers a serious blow.

Finally, SDT hypothesizes that both identified and integrated regulation are fostered by autonomy-supportive socialization practices. Autonomy support involves minimal use of external controls, concern with the socializee's frame of reference, empathic limit setting, provisions of rationales, and affordance of relevant choice with respect to the behaviors, roles, or domains being cultivated (Grolnick, Deci, & Ryan, 1997; Koestner, Ryan, Bernieri, & Holt, 1984; Reeve, Bolt, & Cai, 1999). Indeed, facilitation of commitment and interest in an activity is predicted to occur the more socialization agents are autonomy supportive and noncontingently related or connected with their children, students, or subordinates.

Dynamically, identification is a particularly interesting form of internalization. Characterized by a conscious endorsement of a value or action, identified regulation is accompanied by the phenomenological experience of autonomy. Thus we expect identification to be fostered under autonomy-supportive conditions. However, it is important to recognize that some identifications are little more than "introjects in disguise," for they are adopted as positive representations of a "way to be" but are not necessarily holistically representative of the self. In other words, SDT suggests that identifications can be more or less integrated into personality. For example, consider a man who identifies with the importance of defending human rights and acts freely in support of political prisoners. If he became aware of the fact that much of the production of chocolate is done with enslaved labor but ignored that fact when purchasing chocolate, this suggests that his identity as a human rights advocate is not well integrated. The process of integration—of assimilating one's identifications into a more coherent sense of self—requires awareness of a person's multiple identities and a mindful consideration of their relations to other aspects of one's self. Still, although identifications may be more or less well integrated, when operating from an identification, the person experiences a high level of personal involvement.

Finally, the explication of how environments support or undermine intrinsic motivation is perhaps the most thoroughly accomplished (Deci, Koestner, & Ryan, 1999; Ryan & Deci, 2000a). Considerable research has suggested that autonomy support, optimal challenge, and informational (noncontrolling) feedback help foster and maintain intrinsic motivation and interest for any given pursuit. Regarding identities, we predict that when an intrinsic interest flowers into an identity, considerable support for autonomy and competence will have been afforded.

This overall model depicting relations among environmental supports, internalization, and outcomes is presented in Table 13.1. As the table indicates, there is considerable isomorphism between socializing forms on the one hand and self-regulatory forms on the other.

Empirical Support for the Socializing Model

A growing body of evidence supports the SDT model (see Deci & Ryan, 2000). For example, Grolnick and Ryan (1989) interviewed parents in a rural community concerning their socialization practices with respect to school and achievement, and the researchers also obtained teacher and child ratings of the children's motivation and performance. They found that children whose parents were rated by interviewers as more autonomy supportive than controlling expressed greater autonomy with respect to school. Specifically, these children were higher in both identified and intrinsic regulation than were the children of controlling parents. Subsequently, Grolnick, Ryan, and Deci (1991) used children's reports about their parents, rather than interviewer ratings, and replicated the findings in both urban and suburban samples.

In a different domain, Gagné, Ryan, and Barghman (2001) conducted a longitudinal diary-based study of young female gymnasts. These girls were participants in an elite club, and many aspired to bright futures in the sport. Interestingly, those who perceived their coaches or parents as more autonomy supportive than controlling reported more identification and intrinsic motivation with respect to gymnastics and greater well-being. In contrast, the young athletes whose socializing adults were more controlling reported greater external regulation and lower well-being. Parental and coach involvement—that is, their dedication of time, resources, and support to the girls' endeavor—were also positively associated with identification and intrinsic motivation. In turn, the athletes' internalization levels predicted their attitudes with respect to practice, performance, and teammates.

A laboratory experiment by Deci, Eghrari, Patrick, and Leone (1994) yielded comparable results. Specifically, they found, first, that a relatively autonomy-supportive induction, which provided a rationale, reflected feelings, and offered choice, led to greater internalization and subsequent behavioral enactment than a relatively controlling one, which used pressuring language and provided neither a rationale nor acknowledgment of feelings. Furthermore, internalization that occurred in the relatively autonomy-supportive context was more integrated, as reflected in positive correlations between the subsequent behavior and self-reports of feeling free and enjoying the activity, whereas internalization that occurred in the controlling context was merely introjected, as reflected in negative correlations between the behavior and the same self-reported feelings.

Assor and colleagues (2001) assessed college students' reports of how their parents had typically responded to their achievements (or lack thereof) in various domains. The researchers found that, when children experienced their parents' attention and affection as being conditional on certain behavioral accomplishments, the children enacted the relevant domain-specific behaviors in a pressured, self-esteem-based way. In other words, this relatively controlling socialization approach tended to foster introjection rather than a fuller integration of the value and regulations. Accompanying the introjection were student reports of feeling compelled to act, having contingent self-esteem (Deci & Ryan, 1995; Kernis & Paradise, 2002), and experiencing only fleeting satisfaction following successful enactment of the behaviors. As well, the more the parents were experienced as contingent in their approval and regard, the more the children felt a general sense of rejection, and the more negative the children's feelings toward their parents were. In short, this study confirmed that contingent regard can lead to internalization, as Sears, Maccoby, and Levin (1957) had suggested, but that the form of internalization will be introjection, which carries with it relative rigidity of action (Hoffmann, 1970) and a variety of emotional costs.

A second study by Assor and colleagues (2001) provided evidence for the intergenerational transmission of introjection. A sample of mothers reported the degree to which their parents were contingently loving. More perceived contingent love was associated with various emotional costs, as it had been for participants in the first study. Further, despite these negative consequences experienced by the mothers, they themselves, in turn, used contingent love as a socializing technique. Specifically, the mothers' reports of the degree to which their parents had used contingent affection in raising them was positively associated with the reports of the mothers' daughters about the degree to which the mothers had used this same parenting technique. It seems, therefore, that introjection is a communicable style of regulation.

A paradox of controlling socialization is that, the more controlling or authoritarian its form, the poorer the internalization that results. Thus controlling parents, rather than anchoring identities solidly in their offspring, at best seem to produce introjected or external forms of regulation for the values they transmit. They also appear in many instances to catalyze rejected identities—that is, their children move away from those things the parents had tried to promote. We have found that cold, controlling parents, relative to autonomy-supportive ones, have children who are susceptible to peer pressure (Ryan & Lynch, 1989), act out in school (Grolnick & Ryan, 1989), engage in risky sex and drug use (Williams, Cox, Hedberg, & Deci, 2000), and place high value on materialism and low value on prosocial behavior (Kasser, Ryan, Zax, & Sameroff, 1995). In other words, control seems to rupture relationships with socializers, leading children to seek out peers for guidance and approval and/or to engage in compensatory activities that fulfill the deprived needs that the children experienced in nonnurturing home environments. Similarly, we have repeatedly found that excessive control by teachers, bosses, and other socializers leads people, at best, to be externally regulated or introjected in their roles and, at worst, to reject the roles and responsibilities expected of them. In large part, this is a simple reflection of people's needs. The more that control processes are the basis for role performance, the less the role will satisfy the person's basic psychological need for autonomy. The result will typically be either passive compliance or active resistance to the socially transmitted identities.

In short, SDT has hypothesized and found support for a somewhat unconventional idea. The more pressure and control that is used in the socialization of identity, the less well anchored that identity will be in the self of the individual. For any internalization to occur, people must experience relatedness, and for more integrated internalization to occur they must also experience support for autonomy. Heavy external control, by contrast, produces poor internalization, alienation, and sometimes outright resistance to what socializers intend to foster.

Cross-Cultural Issues Regarding Autonomy and Internalization

The SDT view of internalization is built around the continuum of autonomy. We have argued that people are more engaged, committed, and healthy if the roles they adopt are more fully assimilated into the self so as to provide the basis for more autonomous enactment of those identities. Our emphasis on autonomy with respect to internalization has not been without controversy. For example, SDT has been portrayed by some theorists as being a Western theory, applicable only to individualistic cultures, which, the critics say, are the only ones that value autonomy. Markus, Kitayama, and Heiman (1996), for example, argued that SDT is not applicable to collectivistic cultures in which autonomy is considered a less salient social concern, and Oishi (2000) has gone further to argue that autonomy is not related to well-being outside of a very few highly individualistic nations. Miller (1997) similarly argued that in more authoritarian, vertically oriented, and/or tradition-bound countries, autonomy is not a valued attribute, so predictions based on SDT's internalization model should not hold

The emerging data have, however, provided strong support for SDT. As already mentioned, a spate of research generated by Japanese scholars suggests that in that collectivistic culture, measures of internalization based on SDT predict significant differences in both role-related performance and well-being (Hayamizu, 1997; Tanaka & Yamauchi, 2000; Yamauchi & Tanaka, 1998). Similar results have been obtained for comparisons of Asian Americans with Caucasian Americans (Asakawa & Csikszentmihalyi, 2000). Regarding Miller's argument concerning totalitarian cultures, Chirkov and Ryan (2001) recently examined the parenting and teaching styles experienced by both Russian and U.S. youths. As expected, they found controlling styles of socialization to be more pervasive among Russians, but, more importantly, in both Russian and U.S. samples, the effects of control versus autonomy support were the same. The more controlling parent and teacher styles fostered more external regulation and less au-tonomous regulation, and in both nations parental autonomy support (versus control) was positively related to overall mental health. Finally, Sheldon, Elliot, Kim, and Kasser (2001) investigated the attributes of events that were experienced as fulfilling and satisfying to individuals from both Ko-rea and the United States. They found, as would be predicted by SDT, that among the 10 candidate needs examined, autonomy was consistently in the top 4 for both coun-tries (as were competence and relatedness). Such results do not support the view that autonomy has no relevance outside of indi-vidualistic nations.

We understand the basis for this theoreti-cal conflict between SDT and some cultural relativistic perspectives in two ways. First, some cross-cultural theorists tend to equate autonomy with independence and claim that it is relevant only to individualistic cul-tures. Thus they view autonomy as resis-tance to influence or self-assertion over and against others (see, e.g., Oishi, 2000). How-ever, this definition fails to capture the meaning of autonomy as volition and self-endorsement, which is how it is defined within SDT. For us, people can just as readi-ly be autonomously collectivistic as they can be autonomously individualistic. That is, people can fully internalize and integrate collectivistic beliefs and goals and, there-fore, experience full volition or autonomy when acting in accord with those beliefs and goals. As such, we see no inherent conflict between collectivism and autonomy as we construe autonomy. We agree that there are huge differences in the values and patterns of living expressed within different cultures, but SDT maintains that fuller internaliza-tion of any cultural values, and thus more autonomous enactment of those values, is relevant to humans regardless of their cul-ture.

These points were illustrated in a study by Iyengar and Lepper (1999). They found, first, that both Asian American and Cau-casian American children were more intrin-sically motivated when they made personal choices about what to do than when the de-cisions were made by an experimenter, thus replicating a study by Zuckerman, Porac, Lathin, Smith, and Deci (1978) and sup-porting the importance of choice for East-

ern, as well as Western, children. However, the researchers also found that when in-group members (e.g., mothers) made the choices, the intrinsic motivation of Asian Americans was higher than when they made their own choices, whereas the intrinsic mo-tivation of Caucasian Americans was com-parable to that from experimenter-imposed decisions. This result suggests that Asian Americans, relative to Caucasian Ameri-cans, had more fully internalized and inte-grated the values for accepting ingroup in-puts, so they might have been acting autonomously when the ingroup members made the choices for them.

At another level of analysis, because SDT posits the basic and universal human needs for autonomy, competence, and relatedness, we stand at odds with the "standard social science model," as it is referred to by Tooby and Cosmides (1992), in which human na-ture is seen as culturally constructed, highly plastic, and contextually relative. In our view, despite manifold differences in the manifestation and opportunities to fulfill needs in different cultures, we view some psychological needs as invariantly influen-tial in all countries and contexts. Thus we know of no nation in which feelings of be-longing, feelings of effectance, or feelings of autonomy and self-congruence are not im-portant for well-being of cultural members. No matter how different the content of a culture that is being transmitted, a culture's capacity to meet the basic psychological needs of its members is critical if the content is to be effectively transmitted (Inghilleri, 1999).

In an illustrative project, Chirkov, Kim, Kaplan, and Ryan (in press) used four sam-ples, one each from Korea, Turkey, Russia, and the United States, to examine the rela-tive internalization of values and practices related to the cultural dimensions of hori-zontal collectivism, vertical collectivism, horizontal individualism, and vertical indi-vidualism. They found, as expected by cul-tural theorists such as Triandis (1995), that these nations differed in terms of their citi-zens' perceptions of which practices were dominant within their cultures. For exam-ple, Koreans and Russians perceived their cultures to be more collectivistic than Amer-icans perceived theirs to be, and Russians perceived their culture to be vertically oriented, whereas Americans emphasized more horizontal practices. However, despite such differences in the mean level of certain practices, the degree to which participants in each of the nations were autonomous in enacting the practices was a positive predictor of their mental health. For example, the degree to which the Turks enacted collectivist practices autonomously and the degree to which they enacted individualistic practices autonomously both predicted their well-being; findings were similar for the other three nations. Thus being merely introjected as a collectivist yields the same negative outcomes as being introjected as an individualist, regardless of which culture the participants were from. In sum, results suggested that in all four nations, and for men and women alike, autonomy with respect to enacting culturally prescribed behaviors mattered in terms of the participants' mental health. It thus appears that the need for autonomy may indeed be universally important.

Multiple Identities and Their Coherence within the Person

Although people often speak of the problem of identity, in truth the individual is faced throughout the life span with a problem of *identities*. In modern societies, the social fabric into which daily lives are woven is complex and multilayered. Often, people find themselves working, playing, loving, and learning in different social contexts within which it is possible for them to take on different identities. In fact, it seems that among the major psychological challenges of our era is the multiplicity of roles and identities that individuals must adopt.

Gergen (1991) and other postmodernists have claimed that multiple selves are an adaptive response to a world of multiple demands. Through this lens, as cultural evolution is carrying human nature toward a more autoplastic, docile structure of personality, the idea of an integrated identity or personality appears to be an ideological holdover from an earlier historical era. Similarly, Greenwald (1982) speculated that the idea of integrity or unity in personality, so central to classical theories of personality and psychotherapy (Ryan, 1995), may be a myth. For the postmodernist, the adoption

of identities is a more chameleon-like process. People enact different identities to fit in within different contexts (Gergen, 1991). These claims about the plasticity, changeability, and variability in identity run against the grain of many clinical and developmental perspectives in which the integration, harmony, and internal consistency of life roles and identities has been seen as a hallmark of maturity and mental health (Donahue, Robins, Roberts, & John, 1993; Ryan, 1995; Sheldon & Kasser, 1995). Accordingly, an interesting line of study concerns the effects of having different, discrepant identities or styles of living when one is in different roles.

Donahue and colleagues (1993) studied variability in personality characteristics across life roles by contrasting the view that variability across roles is adaptive with the view that such variability is indicative of fragmentation in personality. Using adjective checklists of attributes, completed with respect to what one is like in different life roles, they found that greater variability (lower correlations) across life roles of self-attributes was associated with lower well-being, suggesting support for the fragmentation view.

Using measures of the Big Five personality traits, Sheldon, Ryan, Rawsthorne, and Ilardi (1997) examined the cross-role consistency of personality. In two studies, they replicated the general findings of Donahue and colleagues (1993) that greater inconsistency was associated with lower well-being. Furthermore, they showed that discrepancies from one's general self-ratings were in large part a function of inauthenticity (assessed by low scores on items such as, "I experience this aspect of myself as an authentic part of who I am"). In other words, to the extent that people find themselves in life roles in which authenticity is not supported, they depart from their integrated selves and pay a cost in well-being for doing so. In addition to authenticity, conflict between roles also contributed to role-to-role discrepancies, in line with the fragmentation view of Donahue and colleagues and others.

In more recent research, Ryan, La Guardia, and Rawsthorne (2001) assessed multiple self-aspects, following procedures outlined by Linville (1987). With Linville's procedure, people spontaneously construct self-aspects, or features of the self, which they then sort into various categories. According to Linville, having more distinct categories of self-aspects indicates a more differentiated self, and she has shown that more differentiated selves can help to buffer stressful events. Presumably, a blow to any one self-aspect is less threatening if a person has more self-aspects in which to be invested. Ryan and colleagues, although replicating this buffering effect, argued and showed that there is also a main effect of self-complexity on well-being—albeit a negative main effect. They suggested that greater self-complexity, despite the buffing phenomenon, is characteristic of fragmentation and betrays a lack of coherence and integrity in personality. Supporting this reasoning, they showed that whatever the self-complexity of a person, it was the relative autonomy of self-aspects that was important for well-being. Thus even for complex identities, a critical issue is one's autonomy regarding those multiple self-aspects.

Sheldon and his colleagues (Sheldon & Elliot, 1998; Sheldon & Kasser, 1998) have proposed a *self-concordance model* of personality integration that applies well to these findings concerning multiple selves and differing role identities. According to the model, self-concordant identities would be those that fulfill basic needs for autonomy, competence, and relatedness and that are experienced as authentic, in the sense of being fully internalized and integrated within the self. Non-self-concordant identities are typically introjected and may even be externally regulated, and they are likely to be only indirect routes to basic need satisfactions. Sheldon and Elliot (1998) used longitudinal methods to show that goal attainment of self-concordant goals relative to non-self-concordant goals resulted in greater enhancement of well-being. Similarly, Sheldon and Kasser (1998) showed that the impact of goal progress on well-being was moderated by goal concordance, with goals that were less well integrated into the self, yielding fewer well-being benefits.

The idea of self-concordance relates to a fundamental proposition regarding identity, namely, that identities are adopted in the service of basic needs. SDT specifically proposes that there are three basic psychological needs—for relatedness, competence, and autonomy—and that each of them must be fulfilled for well-being and integrity to prevail, a view also reflected in the self-concordance model. These views suggest that what makes an identity satisfying is its relation to fulfillment of the three basic needs. A person who identifies herself as a political activist would therefore be expected to adhere to and find satisfaction in that identity to the extent that it (1) helps her feel connected to others and to society, (2) potentiates feelings of effectiveness and staves off helplessness, and (3) provides a vehicle for the expression of her true self and her authentic views. To the extent that any of these needs is compromised, SDT predicts that the identity in question will be less stable and less conducive to personal well-being.

Compensatory Identities: Not All Identities Are Created Equal

Research grounded in the SDT view of needs has, in line with the foregoing comments, confirmed that some life goals and identities may be less facilitative of well-being than others as a function of their relation to basic needs. The most systematic research on this topic is that by Kasser and his colleagues, who have examined what they call the "dark side of the American dream." In the initial studies on this topic, Kasser and Ryan (1993, 1996) hypothesized that some life goals are directly related to, and therefore likely to fulfill, basic psychological needs. Thus, people who hold central life goals of growing and learning in a personal sense, forming deep enduring relationships, and giving to their communities are pursing goals closely related to basic or intrinsic psychological needs. By contrast, people who pursue material goods, wealth, and other forms of acquisitiveness are argued to be pursuing a compensatory goal. The goal of wealth, and others such as fame and attractiveness, are referred to as extrinsic because they do not provide direct satisfaction of the basic psychological needs for relatedness and autonomy and can even interfere with such satisfaction if pursuing them interferes with satisfaction of the more intrinsic goals of relationships and generativity. Kasser and Ryan (1993, 1996) speculated, for example, that the pursuit of wealth and fame may be, dynamically speaking, an indirect attempt to capture admiration, approval, and positive regard from others. It is thus compensatory for more basic satisfaction of the relatedness need and thus, if too salient in a person's life, is expected to be associated with lower mental health and well-being. In their studies, Kasser and Ryan (1993, 1996) supported this formulation, showing that the more salient were materialism and other extrinsic goals in people's lives relative to the more intrinsic goals, the poorer was mental health and adjustment.

Further support for the dynamic interpretation of materialism was provided by developmental research. Kasser and colleagues (1995) investigated differences in the strength of materialism among a diverse set of 18-year-olds. As expected, more materialistic teenagers had lower well-being and community adjustment, as well as greater risk for psychopathology. However, Kasser and colleagues further hypothesized, and found, that those who had become materialists were significantly more likely to have experienced need-depriving home environments. Evidence from child and mother questionnaires and from maternal interviewers converged to suggest that children who adopted more materialistic values had mothers who had been more cold and controlling during their childhoods, thus creating deficits in felt autonomy and relatedness. Kasser and colleagues speculated that materialism often represents a compensatory attempt to gain feelings of worth through acquisition of material goods that many view as symbols of worth. Subsequent work by Williams and colleagues (2000) using other samples of teenagers similarly showed that less autonomy-supportive parenting was associated both with more extrinsic values in youths and with greater involvement in high-risk behaviors such as smoking and alcohol use.

This research supports a point we made earlier that the etiology of identities is a multifaceted process. Specifically, identities can be an outgrowth of interests and aptitudes that receive nurturing support from others with whom one is connected, and they can be taken on and integrated within a similarly supportive context. However, at times, the adoption of an identity may represent an attempt to garner satisfactions that have not been obtained, as with the case of materialism being a substitute for a solid experience of autonomy and lovability. Further empirical exploration of the relations of needs to goals will undoubtedly reveal manifold additional dynamic phenomena of this type.

Conclusion: The Need-Related Basis of Identity Formation

In this chapter we have argued that identity formation is a salient feature of our historical epoch. Although identity struggles may have always existed in human groups, the fluidity and commodification of identities in the modern age leaves individuals with a formidable task of selecting and engaging multiple identities and thereby defining for themselves a place in society.

If identity is especially salient today, what has not changed in human nature over the past few millennia are basic psychological needs. We have argued herein that the function of identities—the reasons we form them—is to fulfill our basic needs. First and foremost, identities facilitate relatedness by helping individuals connect with others and experience belonging in society. Beyond that critical need, identities, when they function most effectively, also facilitate the experience and expression of the other basic needs for competence and autonomy by providing vehicles for self-development and self-expression, as well as outlets for the vital engagement of self in social activities.

It is the case, however, that the roles and behaviors people appear to adopt as identities can vary greatly in terms of whether they are poorly or well internalized and integrated into the self. Self-determination theory provides a taxonomy of regulatory styles, ranging from external regulation to integrated regulation, which describe this variation in assimilation. SDT further proposes that the poorer the internalization of an identity, the less stably held and positively engaged that identity is likely to be, and the less it functions to foster well-being. Thus SDT provides an analysis of how identities are actually anchored in the selves of individuals, as well as an analysis of the social forces that produce the variations in the quality and level of internalization.

Finally, as a need-based theory, SDT suggests that identity formation is a dynamic process that includes a consideration of compartmentalization and compensatory formations that involve deprivation or conflict between different basic psychological needs. In particular, the struggle between attaining the contingent approval that identities often bestow and finding a fit between those identities and one's true self represents a central dialectical tension in development and in societies. Under conditions in which the identities offered individuals are both supported by significant others and allow fulfillment of the psychological needs for competence and autonomy, a healthy integration of the individual is possible. Still, no matter how strong the social pressures, if the identities available to individuals either fail to fulfill or conflict with basic psychological needs, then those who enact them will suffer alienation and ill-being, and their relation to the societal fabric will weaken.

References

Adams, G. R., & Marshall, S. K. (1996). A developmental social psychology of identity: Understanding the person in context. *Journal of Adolescence, 19,* 429–442.

Allport, G. (1937). *Personality: A psychological interpretation.* New York: Holt.

Asakawa, K., & Csikszentmihalyi, M. (2000). Feelings of connectedness and internalization of values in Asian American adolescents. *Journal of Youth and Adolescence, 29,* 121–145.

Assor, A., Roth, G., & Deci, E. L. (2001). *The emotional costs of perceived parental contingent regard: A self-determination theory analysis.* Unpublished manuscript, Ben Gurion University of the Negev.

Batson, C. D. (1976). Religion as prosocial: Agent or double agent? *Journal for the Scientific Study of Religion, 15,* 29–46.

Baumeister, R., & Leary, M. R. (1995). The need to belong: Desire for interpersonal attachments as a fundamental human motivation. *Psychological Bulletin, 117,* 497–529.

Black, A. E., & Deci, E. L. (2000). The effects of instructors' autonomy support and students' autonomous motivation on learning organic chemistry: A self-determination theory perspective. *Science Education, 84,* 740–756.

Chirkov, V. I., Kim, Y., Kaplan, U., & Ryan, R. M. (in press). Differentiating autonomy and individualism: A self-determination theory perspective on internalization of cultural orientations and well-being. *Journal of Personality and Social Psychology.*

Chirkov, V. I., & Ryan, R. M. (2001). Effects of parent and teacher control versus autonomy support in Russia and the U.S. *Journal of Cross Cultural Psychology, 32,* 618–635.

deCharms, R. (1968). *Personal causation: The internal affective determinants of behavior.* New York: Academic Press.

Deci, E. L. (1975). *Intrinsic motivation.* New York: Plenum Press.

Deci, E. L., Eghrari, H., Patrick, B. C., & Leone, D. R. (1994). Facilitating internalization: The self-determination theory perspective. *Journal of Personality, 62,* 119–142.

Deci, E. L., Koestner, R., & Ryan, R. M. (1999). A meta-analytic review of experiments examining the effects of extrinsic rewards on intrinsic motivation. *Psychological Bulletin, 125,* 627–668.

Deci, E. L., & Ryan, R.M. (1985). *Intrinsic motivation and self-determination in human behavior.* New York: Plenum Press.

Deci, E. L., & Ryan, R. M. (1995). Human autonomy: The basis for true self-esteem. In M. Kernis (Ed.), *Efficacy, agency, and self-esteem* (pp. 31–49). New York: Plenum Press.

Deci, E. L., & Ryan, R. M. (2000). The "what" and "why" of goal pursuits: Human needs and the self-determination of behavior. *Psychological Inquiry, 11,* 227–268.

Donahue, E. M., Robins, R. W., Roberts, B. W., & John, O. P. (1993). The divided self: Concurrent and longitudinal effects of psychological adjustment and social roles on self-concept differentiation. *Journal of Personality and Social Psychology, 64,* 834–846.

Elkind, D. (1985). Egocentrism redux. *Developmental Review, 5,* 218–226.

Erikson, E. H. (1968). *Identity: Youth and crisis.* New York: Norton.

Frederick, C. M., & Ryan, R. M. (1993). Differences in motivation for sport and exercise and their relations with participation and mental health. *Journal of Sport Behavior, 16,* 124–146.

Gagné, M., Ryan, R. M., & Barghman, K. (2001). *The effects of parent and coach autonomy support on need satisfaction and well-being of gymnasts.* Unpublished manuscript, University of Rochester.

Gergen, K. J. (1991). *The saturated self: Dilemmas of identity in contemporary life.* New York: Basic Books.

Greenwald, A. G. (1982). Is anyone in charge? Personalysis versus the principle of personal unity. In J. Suls (Ed.), *Psychological perspectives on the self* (Vol. 1, pp. 151–181). Hillsdale, NJ: Erlbaum.

Grolnick, W. S., Deci, E. L., & Ryan, R. M. (1997). Internalization within the family. In J. E. Grusec & L. Kuczynski (Eds.), *Parenting and children's internalization of values: A handbook of contemporary theory* (pp. 135–161). New York: Wiley.

Grolnick, W. S., & Ryan, R. M. (1989). Parent styles associated with children's self-regulation and competence in school. *Journal of Educational Psychology, 81,* 143–154.

Grolnick, W. S., Ryan, R. M., & Deci, E. L. (1991). The inner resources for school achievement: Motivational mediators of children's perceptions of their parents. *Journal of Educational Psychology, 83,* 508–517.

Hayamizu, T. (1997). Between intrinsic and extrinsic motivation: Examination of reasons for academic study based on the theory of internalization. *Japanese Psychological Research, 39,* 98–108.

Hoffmann, M. L. (1970). Moral development. In P. H. Mussen (Ed.), *Carmichael's manual of child psychology* (Vol. 2, pp. 261–359). New York: Wiley.

Inghilleri, P. (1999). *From subjective experience to cultural change* (E. Bartoli, Trans.). New York: Cambridge University Press.

Iyengar, S. S., & Lepper, M. R. (1999). Rethinking the value of choice: A cultural perspective on intrinsic motivation. *Journal of Personality and Social Psychology, 76,* 349–366.

Kahneman, D., Diener, E., & Schwarz, N. (Eds.). (1999). *Well-being: The foundations of hedonic psychology.* New York: Russell Sage Foundation.

Kasser, T., & Ryan, R. M. (1993). A dark side of the American dream: Correlates of financial success as a central life aspiration. *Journal of Personality and Social Psychology, 65,* 410–422.

Kasser, T., & Ryan, R. M. (1996). Further examining the American dream: Differential correlates of intrinsic and extrinsic goals. *Personality and Social Psychology Bulletin, 22,* 80–87.

Kasser, T., Ryan, R. M., Zax, M., & Sameroff, A. J. (1995). The relations of maternal and social environments to late adolescents' materialistic and prosocial values. *Developmental Psychology, 31,* 907–914.

Kernis, M. H., & Paradise, A. W. (2002). Distinguishing between secure and fragile forms of high self-esteem. In E. L. Deci & R. M. Ryan (Eds.). *Handbook of self-determination research* (pp. 339–360). Rochester, NY: University of Rochester Press.

Koestner, R., Losier, G. F., Vallerand, R. J., & Carducci, D. (1996). Identified and introjected forms of political internalization: Extending self-determination theory. *Journal of Personality and Social Psychology, 70,* 1025–1036.

Koestner, R., Ryan, R. M., Bernieri, F., & Holt, K. (1984). Setting limits on children's behavior: The differential effects of controlling versus informational styles on intrinsic motivation and creativity. *Journal of Personality, 52,* 233–248.

Krapp, A. (2002). An educational–psychological theory of interest and its relation to SDT. In E. L. Deci & R. M. Ryan (Eds.), *Handbook of self-determination research* (pp. 405–427). Rochester, NY: University of Rochester Press.

Linville, P. (1987). Self-complexity as a cognitive buffer against stress-related illness and depression. *Journal of Personality and Social Psychology, 52,* 663–676.

Markus, H. R., Kitayama, S., & Heiman, R. J. (1996). Culture and basic psychological principles. In E. T. Higgins & A. W. Kruglanski (Eds.), *Social psychology: Handbook of basic principles* (pp. 857–913). New York: Guilford Press.

Miller, J. G. (1997). Cultural conceptions of duty: Implication for motivation and morality. In D. Munro, J. F. Shumaker, & A. C. Carr (Eds.), *Motivation and culture* (pp. 178–192). New York: Routledge.

Oishi, S. (2000). Goals as cornerstones of subjective well-being: Linking individuals and cultures. In E. Diener & E. M. Sub (Eds.), *Culture and subjective well-being* (pp. 87–112). Cambridge, MA: Bradford Books.

Piaget, J. (1967). The mental development of the child. In D. Elkind (Ed.) & A. Tenzer (Trans.), *Six psychological studies* (pp. 3–73). New York: Vintage Books.

Reeve, J., Bolt, E., & Cai, Y. (1999). Autonomy-supportive teachers: How they teach and motivate students. *Journal of Educational Psychology, 91,* 537–548.

Rogers, C. (1951). *Client centered therapy.* Boston: Houghton-Mifflin.

Ryan, R. M. (1993). Agency and organization: Intrinsic motivation, autonomy and the self in psychological development. In J. Jacobs (Ed.), *Nebraska Symposium on Motivation: Vol. 40. Developmental perspectives on motivation* (pp. 1–56). Lincoln: University of Nebraska Press.

Ryan, R. M. (1995). Psychological needs and the facilitation of integrative processes. *Journal of Personality, 63,* 397–427.

Ryan, R. M., & Connell, J. P. (1989). Perceived locus of causality and internalization: Examining reasons for acting in two domains. *Journal of Personality and Social Psychology, 57,* 749–761.

Ryan, R. M., Connell, J. P., & Deci, E. L. (1985). A motivational analysis of self-determination and self-regulation in education. In C. Ames & R. E. Ames (Eds.), *Research on motivation in education: The classroom milieu* (pp. 13–51). New York: Academic Press.

Ryan, R. M., & Deci, E. L. (2000a). Intrinsic and extrinsic motivations: Classic definitions and new directions. *Contemporary Educational Psychology, 25,* 54–67.

Ryan, R. M., & Deci, E. L. (2000b). Self-determination theory and the facilitation of intrinsic motivation, social development, and well-being. *American Psychologist, 55,* 68–78.

Ryan, R. M., & Deci, E. L. (2001). To be happy or to be self-fulfilled: A review of research on hedonic and eudaimonic well-being. *Annual Review of Psychology, 52,* 141–166.

Ryan, R. M., & Kuczkowski, R. (1994). The imaginary audience, self-consciousness, and public individuation in adolescence. *Journal of Personality, 62,* 219–238.

Ryan, R. M., & La Guardia, J. G. (1999). Achievement motivation within a pressured society: Intrinsic and extrinsic motivations to learn and the politics of school reform. In T. Urdan (Ed.), *Advances in motivation and achievement* (Vol. 11, pp. 45–85). Greenwich, CT: JAI Press.

Ryan, R. M., La Guardia, J. G., & Rawsthorne, L. J. (2001). *Self-complexity and the relative autonomy of self-aspects: Effects on well-being and resilience to stressful events.* Unpublished manuscript.

Ryan, R. M., & Lynch, J. (1989). Emotional autonomy versus detachment: Revisiting the vicissitudes of adolescence and young adulthood. *Child Development, 60,* 340–356.

Ryan, R. M., Rigby, S., & King, K. (1993). Two types of religious internalization and their relations to religious orientations and mental health. *Journal of Personality and Social Psychology, 65,* 586–596.

Sears, R. R., Maccoby, E., & Levin, H. (1957). *Patterns of child rearing.* Evanston, IL: Row, Peterson.

Sheldon, K. M., & Elliot, A. J. (1998). Not all personal goals are "personal": Comparing autonomous and controlling goals on effort and attainment. *Personality and Social Psychology Bulletin, 24,* 546–557.

Sheldon, K. M., Elliot, A. J., Kim, Y., & Kasser, T. (2001). What's satisfying about satisfying events? Comparing ten candidate psychological needs. *Journal of Personality and Social Psychology, 80*, 325–339.

Sheldon, K. M., & Kasser, T. (1995). Coherence and congruence: Two aspects of personality integration. *Journal of Personality and Social Psychology, 68*, 531–543.

Sheldon, K. M., & Kasser, T. (1998). Pursuing personal goals: Skills enable progress but not all progress is beneficial. *Personality and Social Psychology Bulletin, 24*, 1319–1331.

Sheldon, K. M., Ryan, R. M., Rawsthorne, L., & Ilardi, B. (1997). Trait self and true self: Cross-role variation in the Big Five traits and its relations with authenticity and subjective well-being. *Journal of Personality and Social Psychology, 73*, 1380–1393.

Strahan, B. J., & Craig, B. (1995). *Marriage, family and religion*. Sydney, Australia: Adventist Institute of Family Relations.

Tanaka, K., & Yamauchi, H. (2000). Influence of autonomy on perceived control beliefs and self-regulated learning in Japanese undergraduate students. *North American Journal of Psychology, 2*, 255–272.

Tooby, J., & Cosmides, L. (1992). The psychological foundations of culture. In J. H. Barkow, L. Cosmides, & J. Tooby (Eds.), *The adapted mind: Evolutionary psychology and the generation of culture* (pp. 19–136). New York: Oxford University Press.

Triandis, H. C. (1995). *Individualism and collectivism*. Boulder, CO: Westview Press.

Vallerand, R. J. (1997). Toward a hierarchical model of intrinsic and extrinsic motivation. In M. P. Zanna (Ed.), *Advances in experimental social psychology* (Vol. 29, pp. 271–360). San Diego, CA: Academic Press.

Waterman, A. S. (1993). Two conceptions of happiness: Contrasts of personal expressiveness (eudaimonia) and hedonic enjoyment. *Journal of Personality and Social Psychology, 64*, 678–691.

Williams, G. C., Cox, E. M., Hedberg, V., & Deci, E. L. (2000). Extrinsic life goals and health risk behaviors in adolescents. *Journal of Applied Social Psychology, 30*, 1756–1771.

Yamauchi, H., & Tanaka, K. (1998). Relations of autonomy, self-referenced beliefs and self-regulated learning among Japanese children. *Psychological Reports, 82*, 803–816.

Zuckerman, M., Porac, J., Lathin, D., Smith, R., & Deci, E. L. (1978). On the importance of self-determination for intrinsically motivated behavior. *Personality and Social Psychology Bulletin, 4*, 443–446.

PART IV

EVALUATION, MOTIVATION, AND EMOTION

14

Self-Evaluation

ABRAHAM TESSER

This chapter presents a discussion of the nature of evaluation, including its antecedents, correlates and consequences, with particular emphasis on evaluation of the self. I suggest that evaluation is among the most primary and important reactions we have to "noun-like" things, such as persons (particularly ourselves), places, ideas, and objects. I also argue that evaluation is often associated with goal satisfaction or dissatisfaction and focus on some goals that have been identified as being particularly self-relevant. One such goal, the goal of maintaining a positive evaluation of the self, turns out to be particularly robust. Many qualitatively different mechanisms for maintaining a positive self-evaluation have been described in the psychological literature. In spite of the notable differences among these mechanisms, they seem to be substitutable for one another in meeting this goal. Self-evaluation turns out to be remarkably general in the processes by which it is served.

Evaluation

According to *Webster's* dictionary (1999), "evaluate" means "1. To determine or fix the value of; 2. To examine carefully: ap-

praise" (p. 388). So an evaluation refers to the value placed on something. The definition that emerges from the psychological literature on evaluation only partially overlaps the dictionary definition. It is like the dictionary definition in that evaluation refers to the value placed on something. However, the psychological definition does not refer to the monetary or exchange value but the psychological value, that is, the extent to which the object is good or bad, valuable or worthless, pleasant or unpleasant. Also like the dictionary definition, as in definition 2 preceding, evaluation can be a very deliberative, conscious activity (e.g., Ajzen & Fishbein, 1980). However, in contradiction to definition 2 preceding, evaluation is often the result of nonconscious, automatic processes that happen quickly. Indeed, evaluation is often so quick that we can be confident that all the relevant information has not even been apprehended (LeDoux, 1995; Zajonc, 1980)

Seminal work on the psychology of evaluation was done by Charles Osgood and his colleagues (e.g., Osgood, Suci, & Tannenbaum, 1957). Osgood was an experimental psychologist interested in psychology of meaning—not meaning in the precise, dictionary sense, but rather the connotative meaning of things, the feelings they evoke, the metaphors they recruit, and so forth. He believed that there might be a relatively small number of connotative dimensions of meaning. If that were the case, then meaning could be quantified and communicated as a set of scores on these dimensions. In such a system, apples could be compared to oranges by simply observing their similarities and differences on the primary meaning dimensions.

Osgood (Osgood et al., 1957) tested his ideas by developing a technique that is known as the "semantic differential." He presented a variety of concepts—for example, "mother," "beach," "Cuba"—to research participants. The participant's job was to indicate the connotative meaning of the concept by putting a check mark on a series of 7-point scales defined on each end by adjectives with opposite meanings. In order to thoroughly cover the potential connotative domain, he used a large number of such scales. Here are some examples of the opposite adjectives that Osgood used: "good–bad," "strong–weak," "active–passive," "nice–awful." The meaning of concepts could be compared by noting the similarity and differences of their average scores on each dimension. However, with so many dimensions, comparison would be difficult to understand. Moreover, the dimensions are not independent. For example, if we know how a concept is rated on the good–bad scale, we have a very good idea about how it will be rated on the nice–awful scale.

Osgood and colleagues (1957) used factor analysis to solve both of these problems, that is, reduce the number of dimensions and reduce the correlation among dimensions. Their solution is noteworthy in several ways. First, even when a large number of adjective pairs are used, only a few dimensions emerge—usually three, sometimes two. Second, these results are remarkably replicable over concepts, over participant samples, over cultures, and even over the specific adjective pairs used to capture connotative meaning. Finally, particularly important to this discussion, there is a consistent ordering of the importance of the factors. The factor that regularly emerges as the most important is what the researchers called the Evaluative factor. They called it

Evaluative because the scales that load highly on this factor are good–bad, nice–awful, pleasant–unpleasant, and valuable–worthless. The remaining factors were termed "Strength," that is, strong–weak, and "Activity," that is, active–passive. In some studies, the strength and activity dimensions fuse into a single factor that Osgood and colleagues termed "Potency." Note again that the Evaluative factor regularly emerges and regularly accounts for the largest portion of the connotative meaning domain. In short, the most important aspect of the meaning of "things" is our evaluation of them—evaluation colors our ratings on the largest number of scales, and it is the most important dimension for discriminating among concepts (Osgood et al., 1957).

Arguably, one of the most important things in our lives is our selves. When an evaluation is attached to the self, it is often termed self-esteem (Tesser, 2001). Self-esteem is among the most studied constructs in social psychology (Banaji & Prentice, 1994; Tesser, 2000; Wylie, 1974, 1979; see also the following chapters in this volume: Leary & MacDonald, Chapter 20; Dunning, Chapter 21; and Pyszczynski, Greenberg, & Goldenberg, Chapter 16). However, most research under the rubric of self-esteem is approached from an individual-difference point of view. It focuses on the correlates and consequences of chronic differences in self-evaluation. Although I occasionally touch on chronic individual differences in this chapter, the general concern is to understand evaluation of the self from a situational point of view. This point of view emphasizes the extent to which circumstances influence moment-to-moment self-evaluation, and it attempts to understand those dynamics.

Self-Evaluation and Affect

Osgood and colleagues' (1957) semantic differential analysis gives us some idea of what evaluation is, but it also raises some questions. For example, it is not difficult to interpret the judgment of valuable–worthless as a relatively cool, cognitive response; but the scale pleasant–unpleasant begins to shade into the warmer, affective domain. This observation raises the question of whether evaluation is a cognitive response, an affective response, or both. Clearly, we can logically distinguish a rational, cognitive judgment about something from an affective response to that same thing. Indeed, for nonpersonal objects, it is easy to demonstrate this distinction empirically. Martin, Abend, Sedikides, and Green (1997) used movies to put research participants into either pleasant (positive) or unpleasant (sad) moods. The participants then read stories that were intended to be either uplifting or sad. If affect or mood and evaluation are inseparable, then, regardless of the intent of the story, people in good moods should evaluate the story more favorably than people in bad moods. In fact, that was the case for uplifting stories. People in good moods evaluated them more favorably than people in unpleasant moods; and the more positive the mood, the more favorable the evaluation. However, the hypothesis that evaluation has an inseparable affective component and the hypothesis that affect and cognition are separate make the same prediction in this case. The critical case involves the stories intended to be depressing. Here the two hypotheses make different predictions. The data support the hypothesis that affect need not be a crucial part of evaluation. In this case, when the story was intended to be depressing, people in bad moods evaluated the story most favorably; and the worse their moods, the more favorable were their evaluations. Clearly, then, affective and cognitive responses to the same object can be quite different.

The distinction between affect and evaluation is obvious in the nonpersonal case. However, it is not nearly so clear when the object of judgment is the self. Indeed, some of the most prominent researchers in the area of the self have argued quite persuasively that affect clearly appears in self-evaluation and may even be the most psychologically interesting part of self-evaluation. For example, "Brown (1994) compared self-esteem to a parent's esteem for his or her child: the affective response seems to appear strongly and immediately, without waiting for detailed cognitive appraisals" (as cited in Baumeister, 1998, p. 695; see also Brown, 1993). Leary and his associates are even clearer in their statement of this point of view: "Precisely speaking, people

do not suffer negative emotions because their self-esteem is damaged. Rather, decreased self-esteem and negative affect are co-effects of the [same] system" (Leary & Downs, 1995, p. 134). Correlations between chronic measures of self-evaluation (self-esteem) and a variety of affective measures support the position that self-evaluation and affect are linked. For example, self-esteem correlates positively with life satisfaction (Myers & Diener, 1995) and positive affect (Brockner, 1984) but correlates negatively with anxiety (Brockner, 1984), hopelessness (Crocker, Luhtanen, Blaine, & Broadnax, 1994) and depression (Tennon & Hertzberger, 1987).

It is easy to see why scholars posit a close relationship between affect and self-evaluation. Just think about how you feel (affect) when you believe (cognition) that you are associated with something bad or have done something poorly or wrong. Now contrast that with how you feel when you are associated with something good or believe that you have done something well or upstanding. There is an obvious connection between what we believe and how we feel. But, as everyone who has taken a psychology "methods" course knows, a correlation between two things has an ambiguous interpretation (Crocker & Wolfe, 2001; Heatherton & Polivy, 1991). It could mean (1) that the beliefs cause the feeling, as in the thought experiment you just did; or (2) that our feelings about ourselves drive our self-beliefs; or (3) that feelings and beliefs are not causally related at all but, rather, are caused by a common third variable. Finally, it is important to bear in mind that these are not mutually exclusive alternatives. The correlations we observe between beliefs and feelings in connection with self-evaluation could result from all three possibilities, that is, beliefs influencing feelings, feelings influencing beliefs, and something else directly influencing both. There is research evidence for all three of these possibilities.

Beliefs have a causal impact on feelings. For example, if I learn that the plate from which I am eating is dirty, my feelings about the food change very quickly. There is a large literature documenting the causal role of beliefs on feelings (e.g., Tesser & Martin, 1996), but because this effect is so intuitively compelling I will spare you the detail. On the other hand, the idea that some vague feeling state can affect what we believe is not nearly so obvious, yet the evidence is no less compelling. One of my favorite demonstrations of this is a study by Milton Rosenberg (1960). He measured evaluative beliefs about the United States giving aid to foreign countries. A few days later, he hypnotized some of the participants in the experiment and told them, "After you awake, and continuing until our next meeting, you will feel very strongly opposed to the United States policy of giving economic aid to foreign nations. The mere idea of the United States giving economic aid to foreign nations will make you feel very displeased and disgusted" (Rosenberg, 1960, p. 38). Notice that this induction targets *feelings* about foreign aid and that there is no *cognitive* content regarding foreign aid. If this induction changes beliefs, it cannot be because the induction provided particular belief changes. All participants' beliefs about foreign aid were measured immediately, 2, and 4 days after the hypnotic induction. Although the hypnotic induction never mentioned any specific attributes of foreign aid, the beliefs of the experimental participants changed more than the beliefs of participants who had not had the hypnotic induction: The experimental participants saw foreign aid as less likely to promote their values. In short, changes in affect induced changes in cognition, even in the absence of any new information. Indeed, there is evidence that affect changes even the way in which we process information. Positive affect tends to make us more expansive and creative in our thinking (Isen, 1987; Frederickson, 1998; Frederickson & Levenson, 1998); negative affect often induces us to process information more deeply (Bless, Bohner, Schwarz, & Strack, 1990; Mackie & Worth, 1989).

So evaluative beliefs about the self can drive feelings, and feelings about the self can drive evaluative beliefs. Is there any evidence that both beliefs and feelings are correlated because they both derive from some third variable? From a theoretical perspective, this is certainly the case. Recall the previous quote from Leary and Downs (1995): "decreased self-esteem and negative affect are co-effects of the [same] system" (p. 134). According to Leary and his colleagues, human beings have evolved as so-cial creatures with strong needs to be with others (Baumeister & Leary, 1995). Maintenance of social bonds was important not only for mating but for defense and the acquisition of food, shelter, and so forth. Indeed, our survival depended on belonging with and being acceptable to others. Self-esteem evolved as a way of tracking our acceptability to others. Leary and Downs (1995) suggest that self-esteem is a "sociometer," that is, a kind of gauge of how acceptable we are to others. Any self-attribute or action that would cause one to be rejected by others should result in lowered self-evaluative beliefs and negative feelings. Just as a lowered reading on the gas gauge in the car signals us to refuel, these negative changes in self-evaluation function to signal the self to do reparative work to make ourselves more acceptable to others. Self-esteem functions "as a sociometer that (1) monitors the social environment for cues indicating disapproval, rejection, or exclusion and (2) alerts the individual via negative affective reactions when such cues are detected" (Leary & Downs, 1995, p. 129).

Evidence for any specific evolutionary path or for the innateness of any particular need, even the need to belong, is difficult to collect. But there is some evidence for the sociometer idea. For example, Leary, Tanbor, Terdal, and Downs (1995) had participants rate the extent to which others would reject them if they engaged in a number of different behaviors. Later, the participants rated the extent to which they would experience esteem-deflating emotions, for example, shame, dejection, and worthlessness, if they engaged in the behavior. There was a substantial positive correlation between these two sets of ratings, such that the more that participants thought that they would be rejected, the worse they felt. In another study (Leary et al., 1995), participants reported on personal events that had a positive or negative impact on their self-feelings. The correlation between self-feelings and the extent to which each of the situations involved social exclusion was significant. In additional research (Leary et al., 1995) participants were randomly assigned to be either accepted or rejected by a group or another person. Rejected participants showed greater negative self-feelings. We know little about the cognitive aspects of self-evaluation from these studies, but they clearly document the role of social acceptance on the affective component of self-evaluation. From the theoretical perspective of the sociometer model, it is the affective component that is particularly important because it is the affect that does the signaling.

In sum, self-evaluation has both cognitive and affective components or facets. These facets tend to be consistent with one another, that is, negative evaluative beliefs about the self tend to be accompanied by negative self-feelings or emotions. There is evidence that this consistency is overdetermined: negative cognitions about the self tend to produce negative feelings about the self; negative feelings about the self tend to produce negative cognitions about the self; and self-relevant experiences can, independently, produce both negative cognitions and negative feelings. It is the latter source of consistency, self-relevant experiences, which we focus on in the remainder of the chapter.

The Motive to Maintain a Positive Self-Evaluation

In examining the relationship between affect and cognition in evaluation, there appeared to be a qualitative difference between the evaluation of nonself objects and the evaluation of self. An inconsistency between feelings and beliefs was much easier to imagine for nonself objects than for the self. Why? At least part of the reason has to do with motivation. Our experiences generate both understanding (cognition) and feelings (affect). If we understand our experience as moving us toward our goals at a satisfactory rate, we experience positive affect; if we understand our experience as moving us away from our goals or toward our goal too slowly, then we experience negative affect (cf. Carver, Lawrence, & Scheier, 1996; Hsee & Abelson, 1991). It is not difficult to imagine experiencing positive feelings while believing negative things about a nonself object, because it is easy to imagine circumstances in which a nonself object with negative attributes serves our own goals. For example, to learn that a competitor's product is flawed and worthless is likely to make us feel good; to learn

that the competitor's product is outstanding is likely to make us feel bad. It is difficult to imagine this kind of inconsistency for the self because we tacitly ascribe to the assumption that an important goal for most of us is to maintain a positive evaluation of the self. So if the goal itself is a positive evaluation, then an understanding of any situation that reflects positively on the self will produce positive affect, and an understanding of any situation that reflects negatively on the self will produce negative affect. Regarding the self, cognition and affect will be tightly consistent.

I noted a tacit or implicit assumption that individuals are motivated to maintain a positive self-evaluation. From a scientific point of view, tacit assumptions, regardless of their plausibility, warrant theoretical analysis and empirical scrutiny. The assumption that people are motivated to maintain a positive self-evaluation has undergone such scrutiny. The empirical evidence supporting the idea that people are motivated to maintain a positive self-evaluation is overwhelming. Because the evidence for this proposition has been reviewed in numerous places (e.g., Dunning, 2001; Taylor, 1989; Tesser, 2001), I provide only a few examples. There is a strong bias in the way that we understand our own successes and failures. We tend to see successes as internally caused, that is, stemming from our ability or effort, and our failures as externally caused, that is, due to luck or task difficulty (for a review, see Zuckerman, 1979). We tend to remember our own participation in various situations as more central, more influential, and more capable than would an objective observer (Greenwald, 1980); we tend to be overly optimistic about our own futures (Tiger, 1979); we tend to overestimate our own contributions to joint tasks (Ross & Sicoly, 1979); and we tend to overestimate our level of control over events (Langer, 1975). In short, the motive for a positive self-evaluation has a strong empirical base.

Additional Self-Motives

From a theoretical point of view, two additional self-motives have been posited. These motives are not tied to assessments of one's value per se. One is the motive for self-knowledge, that is, a *self-assessment motive*, and the other is a consistency or *self-verification motive*. Proponents of the self-assessment motive suggest that feeling good about the self can take us only so far. From a functional point of view, we must have accurate knowledge about the self (Trope, 1986). Positive distortions and selective biases can be dysfunctional in a world with real outcomes. An accurate self-appraisal should allow us to avoid potential failures and seek out potential successes. In a seminal paper, Leon Festinger (1954) also suggested that we have a drive to evaluate our opinions and abilities. We seek out circumstances in which to learn more about ourselves. Indeed, that is one of the reasons we seek out others: We do so to compare our abilities and opinions in order to evaluate them. A motive to evaluate ourselves positively might predict that we seek out circumstances that will lead to positive feedback. The self-assessment point of view suggests that we should seek out situations that are objectively diagnostic of our skill, abilities, and other attributes regardless of how flattering or deflating. There is evidence for this perspective (e.g., Trope, 1980). However, exposure to negative diagnostic feedback about the self is preferred to flattering feedback only under some circumstances. For example, individuals are willing to expose themselves to negative information when they are uncertain about themselves and when the negative feedback is diagnostic (Trope, 1982). Prior success or being in a good mood is also a condition that makes individuals willing to expose themselves to diagnostic negative information (Trope & Neter, 1994). In sum, there is evidence that people are interested in accurate assessment, at least under certain circumstances.

According to the self-verification point of view, people are motivated to confirm the self-views that they already have (see Swann, Rentfrow, & Guinn, Chapter 18, this volume). They will seek out persons and situations that provide belief-consistent feedback. If a person has a positive view of self, he or she will seek out others who also evaluate them positively and situations in which they can succeed. Note that this is exactly the same expectation that could be derived from a self-enhancement point of view. However, self-verification and self-

enhancement predictions diverge when a person has a negative view of self. The interesting self-verification hypothesis predicts that persons with a negative self-view will seek out others who also perceive them negatively and situations that will lead to poor performance. Swann (e.g., 1983) and his students and associates (e.g., Swann, Stein-Seroussi, & Geisler, 1992) have provided ample evidence for the existence of a self-verification motive. However, this motive, like the self-assessment motive, is conditional; it only shows itself under certain circumstances. In this chapter, I have distinguished cognitive (belief) aspects and affective (feeling) aspects of self-evaluation. Self-verification seems limited to cognitive responses—people tend to believe feedback that confirms their current self-views, but they tend to feel good as a result of positive feedback about the self[1] (Shrauger, 1975). We can distinguish automatic behavior (quick, effortless) from controlled behavior (deliberate, effortful). Self-verification may be limited to circumstances that allow for controlled behavior (Swann, Hixon, Stein-Seroussi, & Gilbert, 1990). (See Dunning, 2001, and Swann, Rentfrow, & Guinn, Chapter 18, this volume, for more complete reviews of self-verification.)

It seems clear from this abbreviated review of the literature and from our intuition that persons are often motivated by concerns for accuracy (self-assessment) and by motives to maintain a belief system about the self (self-verification). Regrettably, many of the demonstrations of self-assessment and self-verification motives have been undertaken in a kind of contested atmosphere in which one motive is pitted against the other. Often evidence for one motive is construed, *ipso facto*, as evidence against another motive. Sometimes setting up research this way is necessary in order to develop distinctive evidence for a motive. As noted previously, if someone sought out confirming information about a positive self-aspect, we would not know whether the motive was self-enhancement or self-verification. If someone sought out diagnostic information that she believed would be flattering, then we would not know whether the motive was self-enhancement or self-assessment. Nevertheless, from an epistemological point of view, evidence for one motive does not have any implications for another motive unless there is a negative the-oretical link between the motives. An exam-ple of such a link might be that if a self-veri-fication motive exists, then there can be no motive to maintain a positive self-evalua-tion. I know of no such theoretical linkage. Further, setting up competing experimental circumstances does not solve the problem. To show that people prefer unflattering in-formation that agrees with their beliefs to flattering information that contradicts them provides evidence for self-verification but does not provide evidence against self-enhancement. It may simply mean that for this particular information, in this particular circumstance, the self-enhancement motive was stronger than the self-evaluation main-tenance motive.

In sum, at least three self-motives have garnered research attention. There is evi-dence that persons seek out accurate infor-mation about the self, and there is evidence that people seek out confirmatory informa-tion about the self. It is worth noting again that these self-motives are not directly relat-ed to the valuation of self-attributes. Main-taining a positive evaluation of the self is a motive for which there is a particularly strong research base. In the next section I examine some of the strategies by which people attempt to maintain a positive self-evaluation.

Self-Evaluation Maintenance Dynamics: Social Comparison, Inconsistency Reduction, and Value Expression

The number and variety of strategies that people use to maintain a positive self-evalu-ation is large. It is so large and varied that the collection of such strategies has been re-ferred to as the "self zoo" (Tesser, Martin, & Cornell, 1996). A detailed account of the research documenting all of these strategies is beyond the scope of this chapter. Howev-er, many of them can be grouped into one of three broad categories: social comparison, inconsistency reduction, and value expres-sion.

Social Comparison

With the publication of Leon Festinger's theory of social comparison processes in 1954, research on social comparison as a source of self-evaluation took a particularly important place in social psychological re-search. The heuristic value of this approach has continued unabated. (Detailed reviews of research on this topic can be found in Biernat & Billings, 2001; Dunning, 2001; Wood, 1989; Wood & Wilson, Chapter 17, this volume. Suls & Wheeler, 2000, have re-cently edited a complete volume on this top-ic.) This theory has been so popular among social psychologists over the years that one commentator calls it "everybody's second favorite theory" (Goethals, 1986).

Festinger's (1954) original theory put par-ticular emphasis on the self-assessment mo-tive. He suggested that people have a drive to evaluate their opinions and their abilities. Often, the only means of validating an opin-ion is to learn whether (similar) other peo-ple agree with it. To evaluate an ability, often, one must compare one's own perfor-mance in the ability domain with the perfor-mances of others. What makes this theory relevant to the motive to maintain a positive evaluation is Festinger's assertion that in the case of abilities there is a unidirectional dri-ve upward. That is, people do not want to suffer by comparison with others in the ability domain. This self-evaluation mainte-nance aspect of social comparison has at-tracted much of the research attention.

Festinger (1954) did a beautiful job of systematizing the idea that other people are a potent source of information. Indeed, by comparing ourselves with other people, we learn or validate what we are and what we are not. Earlier I introduced Leary's (e.g., Leary & Downs, 1995) suggestion that be-longing with other people is so fundamental that self-esteem evolved as a kind of inter-personal gauge or sociometer. Both Fes-tinger and Leary (e.g., Leary & Downs, 1995) suggest that other people are crucial to self-understanding and to self-evaluation. If we push these ideas to the limit, they im-ply that social comparison may be an inte-gral and inevitable accompaniment to thinking about the self. Indeed, just as it is not possible to view a figure without ground, it may not be possible to think about the self without some form of social comparison.

Recent research (Stapel & Tesser, 2001) is consistent with the idea that simply making the self salient increases interest in social comparison. In one study (Stapel & Tesser, 2001) the extent to which people tended to think about themselves was measured. Participants also responded to a scale intended to measure their interest in social comparison (Gibbons & Buunk, 1999). The results indicated that people who tended to think about themselves more scored higher on the social comparison scale than people who tended to think about themselves less. In other studies (Stapel & Tesser, 2001), the self was activated by randomly assigning some participants to describe themselves. The self was not activated in other participants. The participants who described themselves showed a greater interest in social comparison than did the control participants. It could be that activating the self leads to feelings of uncertainty. We already know that uncertainty about the self is often associated with social comparison. However, additional studies replicated the relationship between self-activation and interest in social comparison even when uncertainty about the self was controlled. In short, simply making the self salient seems to increase interest in social comparisons.

How do people use social comparison processes to maintain positive self-evaluations? The self-evaluation maintenance (SEM) model[2] (e.g., Tesser, 1988) provides one approach to answering this question. The SEM model assumes that people want to maintain a positive self-evaluation and that self-evaluation is influenced by the performances of other people. The theory recognizes that the effects of another's outstanding performance on self-evaluation are complex. It can lower self-evaluation because we suffer by comparison; or it can raise self-evaluation through a kind of basking in reflected glory (Cialdini et al., 1976). The SEM model also suggests that the performance of some people is more consequential for self-evaluation than the performance of others. People who are psychologically close to us in some way, for example, in the same class in school, from our own family, or from our hometown (cf. Heider's [1958] discussion of unit relatedness) are more likely to be targets of comparison or sources of reflected glory than are more distant people, people with whom we have no connection. So the closer the

other, the greater the threat to self-evaluation by comparison or the greater the potential boost to self-evaluation through reflection. Because the consequences of the comparison process and the reflection process are very different, it is important to specify when one or the other process will be more active.

The importance of the comparison process relative to the reflection process is determined by the personal relevance of the performance domain. Following William James (1907), the theory recognizes that not all performance dimensions are equally important. Each of us has an idiosyncratic set of performance domains in which we aspire to excellence. If a close other person's outstanding performance is in one of the personally relevant domains, then there will be a tendency to compare ourselves and be threatened. Suppose the performance domain is low in personal relevance. Here we are likely to take pride in the accomplishments of the person to whom we are close, that is, to bask in the reflected glory of the close other's outstanding performance.

This model makes a variety of predictions. Many of these have been confirmed. For example, the model predicts when we might help another. Being outperformed on a personally relevant dimension is threatening, and the closer the comparison person, the greater the threat. Therefore, when the performance domain is important, the closer the other person, the *less* helpful we should be. On the other hand, if the performance domain is low in relevance, we should bask in the reflected glory of the other person's better performance, particularly if the other is psychologically close. Therefore, when the performance domain is low in relevance, the closer the other person, the *more* helpful we should be. Tesser and Smith (1980) gave participants an opportunity to facilitate the performance of either a friend or a stranger on a task that was described as relating to either personally important attributes or as not relating to important attributes. As predicted, when the task was described as unrelated to important attributes, the participants were more helpful to their friends than to the stranger; when the task was described as being related to important attributes, participants were actually more helpful to strangers than they were to their friends. Much of this work is reviewed in Tesser (1988). Its implications for married and romantic couples are spelled out in Beach and Tesser (1995); some speculation on its heuristic value for understanding the biological evolution of interpersonal relationships is provided in Beach and Tesser (2000); and important extensions and caveats are described by Alicke, LoSchiavo, Zerbst, and Zhang (1997), by Lockwood and Kunda (1997) and by Pemberton and Sedikides (2001).

Cognitive Consistency

One can think of self-esteem as an evaluation of the self or one's attitude toward the self. A second approach to understanding self-evaluation maintenance processes grows out of the attitude literature. There are many progenitors of this approach in social psychology (e.g., Heider, 1958; Newcomb, 1961; Osgood, Suci, & Tannenbaum, 1957). A comprehensive summary of the early work in this tradition can be found in Abelson and colleagues (1968) a review of the more recent work can be found in Eagly and Chaiken (1993). The particular framework I use to explore this approach to self-evaluation maintenance is cognitive dissonance theory. The seminal voice for this theory, as for social comparison theory, was Leon Festinger. His 1957 monograph turned out to be one of the most stimulating documents in the history of contemporary social psychology. It spawned hundreds of studies, generated numerous controversies, and attracted some of the brightest, most creative people to the area.

The theory of cognitive dissonance made some surprising predictions that were confirmed in some ingenious experimental demonstrations. The general idea is that persons are motivated to be consistent in their beliefs and their behavior. Inconsistency generates a noxious feeling that persons strive to reduce by changing either their beliefs or their behavior. In the "forced choice" (or "induced compliance") paradigm, persons are led to behave in a way that contradicts their beliefs or feelings. For example, college students who are opposed to adding a required senior thesis to their curriculum may be induced to agree to write an essay in favor of such a requirement. In

order to vary the amount of inconsistency or dissonance the participants are experiencing, the inducement to engage in this counterattitudinal behavior—the amount of reward (e.g., Festinger & Carlsmith, 1959), the level of threat for not engaging in the behavior (e.g., Aronson & Carlsmith, 1963), or the level of perceived choice (e.g., Linder, Cooper, & Jones, 1967)—is manipulated. One way to reduce the inconsistency is attitude change. A person who agrees to write in favor of a senior thesis may come to believe that a senior thesis is really a good idea after all. Time and again, over many studies, what we find is consistent with the dissonance theory prediction. The amount of attitude change varies inversely with the inducement. Rather than more attitude change with greater reward or threat, the greater inducement (reward, threat of punishment, lack of choice) produces *less* dissonance and less attitude change. (See Harmon-Jones & Mills, 1999, for a recent review of current controversies and trends associated with this theory.)

One of the leading exponents of dissonance theory, Elliot Aronson, suggests that dissonance is not about inconsistency in general but rather about inconsistency between our actions and our self-concept (Aronson, 1969, 1992). Most people have positive self-concepts. Therefore, they will experience cognitive dissonance when they behave in ways that are incompetent, immoral, or irrational. Indeed, even consistent behavior can produce dissonance-like changes in behavior when it reflects negatively on the self. For example, most sexually active college students think that using condoms is a good idea, yet they do not always do so. Students given an opportunity to espouse their beliefs in the use of condoms and also given an opportunity to think of their own, perhaps hypocritical, behavior in this domain tend to become more likely to use condoms in the future than do control participants (Aronson, Fried, & Stone, 1991). In sum, cognitive dissonance plays an important role in self-evaluation maintenance.

Value Expression

A third approach to the maintenance of self-evaluation is simply expressing the values we hold. In a seminal paper on the functions that attitudes serve, Katz and Stotland (e.g., 1959; see also Smith, Bruner, & White, 1956) suggested that some of our attitudes are intended to help us understand the world; that others may be important in securing rewards and avoiding punishment; and that still others are important because they validate who we are. Simply expressing those values seems to boost self-evaluation. Examples of this kind of mechanism are easy to see. People wear clothing that indicates the teams they support, the hobbies they pursue, the social groups to which they belong. Nothing in particular seems to be necessary to trigger the expression of our values. We seem to give our opinions and identify ourselves in various ways with no apparent provocation whatsoever. Some of the nicest work demonstrating the relationship between simply expressing our values and self-esteem has been done by Claude Steele and his students and colleagues (e.g., Steele, 1988) under the rubric of self-affirmation. I describe some of that work a little later in this chapter.

One Self-Evaluation or Many?

I chose to describe the social comparison, dissonance, and value expression modes of self-evaluation maintenance for two reasons. First, these approaches do a good job of representing current research, and, second, they are very different from one another. The circumstances that initiate these mechanisms and the outcomes of the operation of these mechanisms differ substantially among the approaches. Social comparison is basically interpersonal. It is initiated when the self is outperformed by similar or psychologically close others. Dissonance is intrapersonal. It is initiated when there is an inconsistency, particularly an inconsistency with one's self-concept. There appear to be no special circumstances that set the stage for value expression or self-affirmation. The outcomes of these three processes are also quite different. For example, when outperformed by another, the individual can change his distance from the other: He or she can increase the distance to reduce the threat of comparison or can reduce the distance to the other to bask in reflected glory. A typical outcome in reducing cognitive dissonance is attitude change to reduce the discrepancy. The result of self-affirmation seems to be more diffuse. It seems to boost self-esteem without any other predetermined interpersonal or belief changes.

Because these mechanisms are so different from one another, the question of whether they are all serving the same self-evaluation maintenance goal is difficult to avoid. It is possible, for example, that changes in consistency have little to do with expressing one's values. That is, cognitive dissonance and value expression may both have something to do with the self but still be independent of one another. How might we know if these mechanisms are serving the same or different goals? Kurt Lewin (1935) and his student Ovsiankina (1928) have provided a strategy for finding out. They suggested that if one activity, for example, self-affirmation, substitutes for or turns off the tendency to complete another mechanism, for example, dissonance reduction, then the two mechanisms must be serving the same goal. (See Tesser, 2000, and Tesser, Martin, & Cornell, 1996, for an elaboration of this logic.) Here is a thought experiment. Suppose a group of students are induced to "choose" to agree to write a counterattitudinal essay (in favor of raising tuition) and are then given an opportunity to affirm themselves by completing a questionnaire about an important personal value. We then measure the groups' attitudes about raising tuition and compare that to the attitudes of a couple of control groups. If self-affirmation is serving a different goal from the goal served by dissonance reduction, we should find that having affirmed the self does not affect dissonance reduction. That is, the experimental group will show (1) as much favorable attitude change toward a tuition increase as do controls who did not affirm themselves and (2) more attitude change than a low-dissonance control group. Suppose, however, that self-affirmation is linked to the same goal as cognitive dissonance. Expressing one's values should help restore the positive self-evaluation that was threatened by behaving inconsistently. If self-evaluation is restored, there would be little need for attitude change and the experimental group (1) should show less attitude change than a high-dissonance no-self-affirmation group and (2) should be similar in attitude change to the low-dissonance group.

The conditions I just described were actually run in a groundbreaking experiment by Steele and Liu (1983). The results followed the substitution pattern of expectations. Self-affirmation substituted for or turned off the need to reduce cognitive dissonance. These very different mechanisms appear to be serving the same, general self-evaluation maintenance goal.

How robust or generalizable is the substitutability of one self-evaluation mechanism for another? Can self-affirmation also substitute for or turn off social comparison mechanisms? Participants in a relevant study (Tesser & Cornell, 1991) reported to the laboratory with a friend. When they arrived, another friendship pair was also present. All participants ranked a number of values for their personal importance and then were asked to write a short essay indicating why one of the values was important. To manipulate self-affirmation, half the participants wrote about a value that they had ranked as personally very important and half wrote about a value that was ranked as less important. Their joint task was then described: Each person would have an opportunity to identify a target word from clues. Participants in half of the sessions were told that the task was related to abilities that were personally important; the others were told that performance was unrelated to important abilities. Participants, one at a time, were given an opportunity to identify words while the other three participants submitted clues from a list of clues graded in difficulty. The choice of more or less difficult clues could affect the performance of the person trying to guess the target word: To prevent the other from doing better than oneself, one would give difficult clues; to facilitate the other's performance, one would give easy clues. The level of difficulty chosen for each of the other participants served as the dependent variable (Tesser & Cornell, 1991).

The SEM prediction is complex: When the task is related to personally important attributes, the better performance of another, particularly a close other, is threatening. Therefore, we expected that when the task was described as important, participants would give more difficult clues, and their friends would get more difficult clues than would the stranger. On the other hand, if task performance is not personally important, then another's good performance provides an opportunity to bask in reflected glory. The better the close other's performance, the easier it is to bask. We predicted that when the task was unimportant, one would give easier clues to the friend than to the stranger.

The left panel of Figure 14.1 shows the results for participants who did not affirm themselves, that is, they wrote about unimportant values. In this panel, the complicated set of predictions derived from the social comparison model was obtained. Persons were kinder to a stranger than to a friend when the task was personally relevant but kinder to their friends than to the stranger when the task was not personally relevant. For people who had not affirmed themselves, the social comparison mechanism of self-evaluation maintenance provides a well-understood route to self-evaluation. However, self-affirmation clearly seems to turn off the comparison mechanism. As can be seen in the right panel of the figure, for participants who had the opportunity to affirm themselves by writing about an important value, there is no evidence of the social comparison pattern displayed in the left panel. Indeed, there are no significant differences among the means in the left panel. Clearly, self-affirmation substitutes for or turns off self-evaluation maintenance via social comparison.

The case for a single self-evaluation is beginning to be made. So far it is clear that self-affirmation can substitute for or turn off cognitive dissonance reduction and that it can substitute for or turn off social comparison mechanisms. Perhaps substitutability is not general. Perhaps there is something special about self-affirmation. To address the question of general substitutability, Tesser, Crepaz, Collins, Cornell, and Beach (2000) attempted to affect social comparison processes by inducing cognitive dissonance. To manipulate cognitive dissonance, participants were induced to agree to write an essay in favor of requiring a senior thesis of all students. Participants in the high-dissonance condition were given much choice in the matter, and participants in the low-dissonance condition were given little

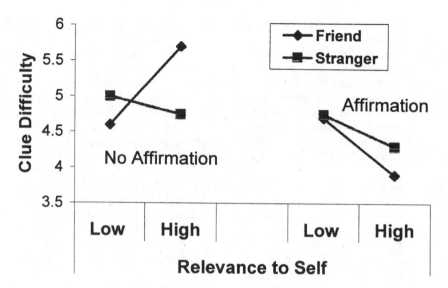

FIGURE 14.1. Difficulty of clues given to friends and strangers as a function of importance of task, that is, relevance and whether or not the participant had an opportunity to self-affirm. Adapted from Tesser and Cornell (1991). Copyright 1991 by Academic Press. Adapted by permission.

choice. All the participants were then asked to write an essay describing an instance in which another person outperformed them. Half the participants were asked to write about an instance in which they personally wanted to do well, and half were asked to write about an instance in which it was not particularly important for them personally to do well. Participants were then asked to fill out a questionnaire indicating how close or distant they felt from the person who had outperformed them.

One is potentially threatened by the better performance of a close other in a personally important domain; there is the potential of basking in the better performance of a close other in a personally less important domain. Therefore, we expected people in the personally important condition to distance themselves from the other; people in the less important condition were expected to draw themselves closer to the other. If cognitive dissonance and social comparison are serving the very same self-evaluation goal, then participants with high dissonance, more in need of restoring self-esteem, should engage in the social comparison strategy more vigorously than participants with low dissonance. Concretely, the difference in rated closeness should be greater for the participants with high than for the par-

ticipants with low dissonance. The results were consistent with this expectation. Participants experiencing high cognitive dissonance showed greater engagement in self-protective or self-enhancing social comparison than participants experiencing low cognitive dissonance.

The case for a single self-evaluation goal is building. We have seen that self-affirmation substitutes for cognitive dissonance and for social comparison; cognitive dissonance substitutes for (or turns on) social comparison. Indeed, the evidence for generality is much more extensive. There are now specific data to indicate that both cognitive dissonance and social comparison affect the extent to which people engage in self-affirmation; that both self-affirmation and social comparison affect the extent to which people engage in cognitive dissonance reduction; and that both cognitive dissonance and self-affirmation affect social comparison. (See Tesser et al., 2000, for some of the experiments and a discussion.) The case being made for a single, general self-evaluation is an inductive one. Therefore, we cannot know for certain how general it will turn out to be. However, as of this writing, the case is looking good.

The substitutability results suggest a confluence metaphor. Self-esteem seems to be fed by many self-evaluation mechanisms. It can rise or fall depending on the inflow from tributaries as different as social comparison, cognitive consistency, and value expression. Once a tributary affects self-evaluation, however, its specific identity is lost and the flow from any one mechanism can substitute for the flow from any other. This substitutability raises a number of questions that psychologists are only beginning to grapple with. There are a number of promising leads (e.g., Chartrand, Tesser & Chen, in preparation) and interesting controversies (Cooper, 1999; Stone, 1999; Tesser, 2000).

Summary

One of the first and most important responses we have to anything is evaluation. Judgments of how good, valuable, or attractive something is can frequently be distinguished from positive or negative feelings. On the other hand, the distinction between evaluative thoughts and feelings is more difficult to make when the object is the self. This difficulty arises at least in part because we are generally motivated to maintain a positive self-evaluation.

Current research has examined at least three self-motives. These include self-assessment, a motive for accurate information about the self; and self-verification, the motive to confirm one's beliefs about the self. However, the motive that has attracted the most attention in the literature is the motive to maintain a positive self-evaluation.

A large number of psychological mechanisms have been identified as having an impact on how we evaluate ourselves. Social comparison processes suggest that the better performance of similar or psychologically close others can affect self-evaluation; cognitive consistency mechanisms imply that inconsistent behavior can threaten self-evaluation; and value expressive mechanisms suggest that simply avowing or affirming one's important values can boost self-evaluation.

A close look at self-evaluation mechanisms suggests that they are qualitatively different from one another: The conditions that trigger these mechanisms and the responses associated with these mechanisms

are quite different. Nevertheless, evidence is accumulating to suggest that they are remarkably substitutable in their impact on self-evaluation. For example, a threat to self-esteem from social comparison can be addressed by self-affirmation. Although the specific mechanisms underlying this substitutability are not yet well understood, the results reviewed here imply that self-evaluation maintenance is a remarkably broad, catholic, and efficient set of interchangeable processes.

Notes

1. This seems consistent with the idea that the affective self-evaluative response is the result of a goal to maintain a positive self-evaluation. People appear to seek out information that verifies their point of view. If they have a negative view of some aspect of the self, then information that verifies that view is accepted; but because the goal is to maintain a positive self-evaluation, their feeling tone to that information is negative.

2. I focus on this approach because it the one with which I am most familiar and because I use it as a prototypical example of comparison approaches later in this chapter. The reader should note that there are other theoretical and empirical research programs that take a social comparison approach; see Biernat and Billings (2001) and Dunning (2001) for recent reviews.

References

Abelson, R. P., Aronson, E., McGuire, W. J., Newcomb, T. M., Rosenberg, M. J., & Tannenbaum. P. H. (Eds.). (1968). *Theories of cognitive consistency: A source book.* Chicago: Rand McNally.

Ajzen, I., & Fishbein, M. (1980). *Understanding attitudes and predicting social behavior.* Englewood Cliffs, NJ: Prentice-Hall.

Alicke, M. D., LoSchiavo, F. M., Zerbst, J., & Zhang, S. (1997). The person who outperforms me is a genius: Maintaining perceived competence in upward social comparison. *Journal of Personality and Social Psychology, 73,* 781–789.

Aronson, E. (1969). The theory of cognitive dissonance: A current perspective. In L. Berkowitz (Ed.), *Advances in experimental social psychology* (Vol. 4, pp. 2–32). New York: Academic Press.

Aronson, E. (1992). The return of the repressed: Dissonance theory makes a comeback. *Psychological Inquiry, 3,* 303–311.

Aronson, E., & Carlsmith, J. M. (1963). The effect of

severity of threat on the valuation of forbidden behavior. *Journal of Abnormal and Social Psychology, 66,* 584–588.

Aronson, E., Fried, C., & Stone, J. (1991). Overcoming denial and increasing the intention to use condoms through the induction of hypocrisy. *American Journal of Public Health, 81,* 1636–1638.

Banaji, M. R., & Prentice, D. A. (1994). The self in social contexts. *Annual Review of Psychology, 45,* 297–332.

Baumeister, R. F. (1998). The self. In D. T. Gilbert, S. T. Fiske, & G. Lindzey (Eds.), *Handbook of social psychology* (4th ed., pp. 680–740). New York: McGraw-Hill.

Baumeister, R. F., & Leary, M. R. (1995). The need to belong: Desire for interpersonal attachments as a fundamental human motivation. *Psychological Bulletin, 117,* 497–529.

Beach, S. R. H., & Tesser, A. (1995). Self-esteem and the extended self-evaluation maintenance model: The self in social context. In M. Kernis (Ed.), *Efficacy, agency, and self esteem* (pp. 145–170). New York: Plenum Press.

Beach, S. R. H., & Tesser, A. (2000) Self-evaluation maintenance and evolution: Some speculative notes. In J. Suls & L. Wheeler (Ed.), *Handbook of social comparison* (pp. 123–140). Mahwah, NJ: Erlbaum.

Biernat, M., & Billings, L. S. (2001). Standards, expectancies and social comparison. In A. Tesser & N. Schwarz (Eds.), *Blackwell handbook of social psychology: Intraindividual processes* (pp. 257–283). Oxford, UK: Blackwell.

Bless, H., Bohner, G., Schwarz, N., & Strack, F. (1990). Mood and persuasion: A cognitive response analysis. *Personality and Social Psychology Bulletin, 16,* 331–345.

Brockner, J. (1984). Low self-esteem and behavioral plasticity: Some implications for personality and social psychology. In L. Wheeler (Ed.), *Review of personality and social psychology* (Vol. 4, pp. 237–271). Beverly Hills, CA: Sage.

Brown, J. D. (1993). Self-esteem and self-evaluation: Feeling is believing. In J. Suls (Ed.), *Psychological perspectives on the self* (Vol. 4, pp. 27–58). Hillsdale, NJ: Erlbaum.

Brown, J. D. (1994, October). *Self-esteem: It's not what you think.* Paper presented at the meeting of the Society for Experimental Social Psychology, Lake Tahoe, NV.

Campbell, J. D., Trapnell, P. D., Heine, S. J., Katz, I. M., Lavallee, L. F., & Lehman, D. R. (1996). Self-concept clarity: Measurement, personality correlates, and cultural boundaries. *Journal of Personality and Social Psychology 70*(1), 141–156.

Carver, C. S., Lawrence, J. W., & Scheier, M. F. (1996). A control-process persective on the origins of affect. In L. L. Martin & A. Tesser (Eds.), *Striving and feeling: Interactions between goals and affect* (pp. 11–52). Hillsdale, NJ: Erlbaum.

Chartrand, T., Tesser, A., & Chen, C. (2001). *Mystery moods and self-evaluation maintenance.* Manuscript in preparation.

Cialdini, R. B., Borden, R. J., Thorne, A., Walker, M. R., Freeman, S., & Sloan, L. R. (1976). Basking in reflected glory: Three (football) field studies. *Journal of Personality and Social Psychology, 34,* 366–375.

Cooper, J. (1999). Unwanted consequences and the self: In search of the motivation for dissonance reduction. In E. Harmon-Jones & J. Mills (Eds.), *Cognitive dissonance: Progress on a pivotal theory in social psychology.* Washington, DC: American Psychological Association.

Crocker, J., Luhtanen, R. K., Blaine, B., & Broadnax, S. (1994). Collective self-esteem and psychological well-being among Black, White, and Asian college students. *Personality and Social Psychology Bulletin, 20,* 503–513.

Crocker, J., & Wolfe, C. (2001). Rescuing self-esteem: A contingencies of worth perspective. *Psychological Review, 108,* 593–623.

Dunning, D. (2001). On the motives underlying social cognition. In A. Tesser & N. Schwarz (Eds.), *Blackwell handbook of social psychology: Intraindividual processes* (pp. 348–374). Oxford, UK: Blackwell.

Eagly, A. H., & Chaiken, S. (1993). *The psychology of attitudes.* Fort Worth, TX: Harcourt Brace Jovanovich.

Festinger, L. (1954). A theory of social comparison processes. *Human Relations, 7,* 117–140.

Festinger, L. (1957). *A theory of cognitive dissonance.* Stanford, CA: Stanford University Press.

Festinger, L., & Carlsmith, J. M. (1959). Cognitive consequences of forced compliance. *Journal of Abnormal and Social Psychology, 58,* 203–210.

Frederickson, B. L. (1998). What good are positive emotions? *Review of General Psychology, 2,* 300–319.

Frederickson, B. L., & Levenson, R. W. (1998). Positive emotions speed recovery from the cardiovascular sequelae of negative emotions. *Cognition and Emotion, 12,* 191–220.

Gibbons, F. X., & Buunk, B. P. (1999). Individual differences in social comparison: Development of a scale of social comparison orientation. *Journal of Personality and Social Psychology, 76,* 129–141.

Goethals, G. R. (1986). Social comparison theory: Psychology from the lost and found. *Personality and Social Psychology Bulletin, 1*(2), 261–278.

Greenwald, A. G. (1980). The totalitarian ego: Fabrication and revision of personal history. *American Psychologist, 35,* 603–618.

Harmon-Jones, E., & Mills, J. (Eds.). (1999). *Cognitive dissonance: Progress on a pivotal theory in social psychology.* Washington, DC: American Psychological Association.

Heatherton, T. F., & Polivy, J (1991). Development and validation of a scale for measuring state self-esteem. *Journal of Personality and Social Psychology, 60,* 895–910.

Heider, F. (1958). *The psychology of interpersonal relations.* New York: Wiley.

Hsee, C. K., & Abelson, R. P. (1991). Velocity relation: Satisfaction as a function of the first derivative of outcome over time. *Journal of Personality and Social Psychology, 60,* 341–347.

James, W. (1907). *The principles of psychology.* New York: Holt.

Katz, D., & Stotland, E. (1959). A preliminary statement of a theory of attitude structure and change. In S. Koch (Ed.), *Psychology: A study of a science* (Vol. 3, pp. 423–475). New York: McGraw-Hill.

Langer, E. J. (1975). The illusion of control. *Journal of Personality and Social Psychology, 32,* 311–328.

Leary, M. R., & Downs, D. L. (1995). Interpersonal functions of the self-esteem motive: The self-esteem system as a sociometer. In M. Kernis (Ed.), *Efficacy, agency, and self-esteem* (pp. 123–144.) New York: Plenum Press.

Leary, M. R., Tandor, E. S., Terdal, S. K., & Downs, D. L. (1995). Self-esteem as an interpersonal monitor: The sociometer hypothesis. *Journal of Personality and Social Psychology, 68*, 518–530.

LeDoux, J. E. (1995). Emotions: Clues from the brain. *Annual Review of Psychology, 46*, 209–235.

Lewin, K. (1935). *A dynamic theory of personality: Selected papers* (D. E. Adams & K. E. Zener Trans.). New York: McGraw-Hill.

Linder, D. E., Cooper, J., & Jones, E. E. (1967). Decision freedom as a determinant of the role of incentive magnitude in attitude change. *Journal of Personality and Social Psychology, 6*, 245–254.

Lockwood, P., & Kunda, Z. (1997). Superstars and me: Predicting the impact of role models on the self. *Journal of Personality and Social Psychology, 73*(1), 91–103

Mackie, D. M., & Worth, L. T. (1989). Processing deficits and the mediation of positive affect in persuasion. *Journal of Personality and Social Psychology, 57*, 27–40.

Martin, L. L., Abend, T., Sedikides, C., & Green, J. D. (1997). How would it feel if . . .? Mood as input to a role fulfillment evaluation process. *Journal of Personality and Social Psychology, 73*(2), 242–253.

Myers, D. G., & Diener, E. (1995). Who is happy? *Psychological Science, 6*, 10–19.

Newcomb, T. M. (1961). *The acquaintance process.* New York: Holt, Rinehart & Winston.

Osgood, C. E., Suci, G. J., & Tannenbaum, P. H. (1957). *The measurement of meaning.* Urbana: University of Illinois Press.

Ovsiankina, M. (1928). Die Wiederaufnahme unterbrochener Handlugen [The resumption of interrupted acts]. *Pyschologische Forschung, 11*, 302–379.

Pemberton, M., & Sedikides, C. (2001). When do individuals help close others improve?: The role of information diagnosticity. *Journal of Personality and Social Psychology, 81*, 234–246.

Rosenberg, M. J. (1960). A structural theory of attitude dynamics. *Public Opinion Quarterly*, 24, 319–341.

Ross, M., & Sicoly, F. (1979). Egocentric biases in availability and attribution. *Journal of Personality and Social Psychology, 37*, 322–336.

Shrauger, J. S. (1975). Responses to evaluation as a function of initial self-perceptions. *Psychological Bulletin, 82*, 581–596.

Smith, M. B., Bruner, J. S., & White, R. W. (1956). *Opinions and personality.* New York: Wiley.

Stapel, D., & Tesser, A. (2001) Self-activation increases social comparison. *Journal of Personality and Social Psycholgy, 81*, 742–750.

Steele, C. M. (1988). The psychology of self-affirmation: Sustaining the integrity of self. In L. Berkowitz (Ed.), *Advances in experimental social psychology* (Vol. 21, pp. 261–302). New York: Academic Press.

Steele, C. M., & Liu, T. J. (1983). Dissonance processes as self-affirmation. *Journal of Personality and Social Psychology, 45*, 5–19.

Stone, J. (1999). What exactly have I done? The role of self-attribute accessibility in dissonance. In E. Harmon-Jones & J. Mills (Eds.), *Cognitive dissonance: Progress on a pivotal theory in social psychology* (pp. 175–200). Washington, DC: American Psychological Association.

Suls, J., & Wheeler, L. (Eds.). (2000). *Handbook of social comparison: Theory and research.* New York: Kluwer Academic/Plenum Press.

Swann, W. B., Jr. (1983). Self-verification: Bringing social reality into harmony with the self. In J. Suls & A. G. Greenwald (Eds.), *Psychological perspectives on the self* (Vol. 2, pp. 33–66). Hillsdale, NJ: Erlbaum.

Swann, W. B., Jr., Hixon, J. G., Stein-Seroussi, A., & Gilbert, D. T. (1990). The fleeting gleam of praise: Cognitive processes underlying behavioral reactions to self-relevant feedback. *Journal of Personality and Social Psychology, 59*, 17–26.

Swann, W. B., Jr., Stein-Seroussi, A., & Geisler, R. B. (1992). Why people self verify. *Journal of Personality and Social Psychology, 62*, 392–401.

Taylor, S. E. (1989). *Positive illusions: Creative self-deception and the healthy mind.* New York: Basic Books.

Tennon, H., & Hertzberger, S. (1987). Depression, self-esteem, and the absence of self-protective attributional biases. *Journal of Personality and Social Psychology, 52*, 72–80.

Tesser, A. (1988). Toward a self-evaluation maintenance model of social behavior. In L. Berkowitz (Ed.), *Advances in experimental social psychology* (Vol. 21, pp. 181–227). New York: Academic Press.

Tesser, A. (2000). On the confluence of self-esteem maintenance mechanisms. *Personality and Social Psychology Review, 4*, 290–299.

Tesser, A. (2001). Self-esteem. In A. Tesser & N. Schwarz (Eds.), *Blackwell handbook of social psychology: Intraindividual processes* (pp. 479–498). London: Blackwell.

Tesser, A. (in press). Psychology of self-evaluative processes. In N. J. Smelser & P. B. Baltes (Eds.), *International encyclopedia of the social and behavioral sciences.* Amsterdam: Pergamon.

Tesser, A., & Cornell, D. P. (1991). On the confluence of self-processes. *Journal of Experimental Social Psychology, 27*, 501–526.

Tesser, A., Crepaz, N., Collins, J. C., Cornell, D., & Beach, S. R. H. (2000). Confluence of self-defense mechanisms: On integrating the self zoo. *Personality and Social Psychology Bulletin, 26*, 1476–1489.

Tesser, A., & Martin, L. (1996). The psychology of evaluation. In E. T. Higgins & A.W. Kruglanski (Eds.), *Social psychology: Handbook of basic principles* (pp. 400–432). New York: Guilford Press.

Tesser, A., Martin, L. L., & Cornell, D. P. (1996). On the substitutability of self-protective mechanisms. In P. M. Gollwitzer & J. A. Bargh (Eds.), *The psychology of action: Linking cognition and motivation to behavior* (pp. 48–68). New York: Guilford Press.

Tesser, A., & Smith, J. (1980). Some effects of friendship and task relevance on helping: You don't always help the one you like. *Journal of Experimental Social Psychology, 16*, 582–590.

Tiger, L. (1979). *Optimism: The biology of hope.* New York: Simon & Shuster.

Trope, Y. (1980). Self-assessment, self-enhancement and task preference. *Journal of Experimental Social Psychology, 16*, 116–129.

Trope, Y. (1982). Self-assessment and task performance.

Journal of Experimental Social Psychology, 18, 201–215.

Trope, Y. (1986). Self-enhancement and self-assessment in achievement behavior. In R. M Sorrentino & E. T. Higgins (Eds.), *Handbook of motivation and cognition: Foundations of social behavior* (Vol. 1, pp. 350–378). New York: Guilford Press.

Trope, Y., & Neter, E. (1994). Reconciling competing motives in self-evaluation: The role of self-control in feedback seeking. *Journal of Personality and Social Psychology, 66,* 646–657.

Wood, J. V. (1989). Theory and research concerning social comparison of personal attributes. *Psychological Bulletin, 106*(2), 231–248.

Wylie, R. C. (1974). *The self-concept* (Rev. ed., Vol. 1). Lincoln: University of Nebraska Press.

Wylie, R. C. (1979). *The self-concept* (Rev. ed., Vol. 2). Lincoln: University of Nebraska Press.

Zajonc, R. B. (1980). Feeling and thinking: Preferences need no inferences. *American Psychologist, 35,* 151–175.

Zuckerman, M. (1979). Attribution of success and failure revisited, or: The motivational bias is alive and well in attribution theory. *Journal of Personality, 47,* 245–287.

15

Seeking Self-Esteem: Construction, Maintenance, and Protection of Self-Worth

JENNIFER CROCKER
LORA E. PARK

It is almost axiomatic in social psychology that people seek to maintain, enhance, and protect their self-esteem. Although there may be cultural variability in its expression (Heine, Lehman, Markus, & Kitayama, 1999), the tendency to seek self-esteem is well established in Western cultures in which individualism is a dominant ideology. In this chapter, we consider how people arrive at the judgment that they are worthwhile, that is, how they arrive at a sense of self-worth. We explore how the desire to be a person of worth influences the ways people organize their lives and spend their time. We examine what makes people vulnerable to feelings of worthlessness, and we consider the strategies people use to avoid feeling worthless. Our central proposition is that people seek to maintain, protect, and enhance self-esteem by attempting to obtain success and avoid failure in domains on which their self-worth has been staked. Contingencies of self-worth, then, serve a self-regulatory function, influencing the situations people select for themselves, their ef-

forts in those situations, and their reactions to successes and failures. Finally, we conclude with a consideration of the costs of living one's life in the pursuit of self-esteem.

Constructing Self-Esteem: Contingencies of Self-Worth

How do people decide that they are worthy or unworthy human beings? Do we need to excel at all things to be worthy, or are we selective in the domains on which we stake our self-worth? In his seminal discussion of self-esteem, William James (1890) made two points that have shaped our contemporary understanding of global self-esteem. First, James argued that global self-esteem has the qualities of both a state and a trait. Specifically, he argued that people tend to have average levels of self-esteem that are "direct and elementary endowments of our nature" (James, 1890, p. 43). This "average tone of self-feeling which each one of us carries about with him . . . is independent of the objective reasons we may have for satisfaction or discontent" (p. 43). On the other hand, James believed that the *state* of self-esteem rises and falls as a function of achievements and setbacks. As James put it, "the normal *provocative* of [state] self-feeling is one's actual success or failure, and the good or bad position one holds in the world" (James, 1890, p. 43, italics in original). Thus, according to James, although one's typical level of self-esteem is independent of one's objective circumstances or achievements, fluctuations around one's typical level will reflect changed circumstances, successes, and failures.

If any success or failure, acceptance or rejection, good deed or bad deed had the power to affect our self-esteem, we would spend each day with our state self-worth totally at the mercy of events. Yet not all successes and failures have the same effect on self-esteem, and this is a second major contribution of James's (1890) analysis. James argued that, instead, people are highly selective about the domains on which they stake their self-worth, concluding that "our self-feeling in this world depends entirely on what we *back* ourselves to be and do" (p. 45). In other words, people differ in the contingencies they must satisfy to attain high self-esteem. A contingency of self-worth is a domain or category of outcomes on which a person has staked his or her self-esteem, so that that person's view of his or her worth depends on perceived successes, failures, or adherence to self-standards in that domain. For some people, self-esteem may depend on being attractive, loved, or competent. For others, self-esteem may depend on being virtuous, powerful, or self-reliant.

We have developed a measure of common contingencies of self-worth in college students, called the Contingencies of Self-Worth Scale (CSW; Crocker, Luhtanen, & Bouvrette, 2001). The current version of the measure assesses seven contingencies of self-worth: appearance, others' approval, outdoing others in competition, academic competency, love and support from family, virtue, and God's love. Each subscale of the measure has high internal consistency (Cronbach's α's range from .82 to .97), high test–retest reliability (ranging from .63 to .89 over an 8.5-month interval), and is distinct from other constructs, such as level of self-esteem, social desirability, and the Big Five dimensions of personality. The highest loading item on each subscale of the measure is included in the Appendix 15.1.

We believe that James (1890) intended his two hypotheses to be taken together and not in isolation from one another. This assumption leads to an important but overlooked statement about the nature of self-esteem: *global state self-esteem rises and falls relative to its typical trait level in response to achievements, setbacks, and altered circumstances related to one's contingencies of self-worth.* We think that James overstated the extent to which a person's typical level of self-esteem (i.e., trait self-esteem) is independent of objective circumstances, achievements, and contingencies of self-worth. Nonetheless, fluctuations of state self-esteem relative to a person's typical level of trait self-esteem are crucially important to understanding the role of self-esteem in our daily lives (see also Kernis and Goldman, Chapter 6, this volume).

A Model of Contingencies of Self-Worth

Building on and extending James's (1890) insights, Crocker and Wolfe (Crocker & Wolfe, 2001; Wolfe & Crocker, 2002) developed a model of contingencies of self-worth and its relation to affect, motivation, and cognition. Central to our model is the contention that the impact of events and circumstances on self-esteem depends on the perceived relevance of those events to one's contingencies of self-worth. Self-esteem is both more vulnerable to and more defended in response to events that are relevant to one's contingencies of self-worth. It is the person's interpretation of the event or circumstance and of its relevance to his or her contingencies of self-worth, rather than the objective event or circumstance as categorized by an independent observer, that determines whether and how strongly the event will affect state self-esteem (McFarland & Ross, 1982).

Contingencies of Self-Worth and State Self-Esteem

State self-esteem rises and falls relative to its trait level in response to construals of external events such as achievements, setbacks, altered circumstances, and internal events (Greenier et al., 1999; Levine, Wyer, & Schwarz, 1994), but only when those events are relevant to one's contingencies of self-worth. For example, an imagined insult, a success at work, or a memory of a kind remark may all lead to temporary increases or decreases in state self-esteem if those events are perceived to be related to one's contingencies of self-worth. Furthermore, events in domains of contingencies of self-worth are particularly likely to affect state self-esteem when the events are clearly positive or negative and are important to people's lives.

A study of college seniors applying to graduate school provides support for this view (Crocker, Sommers, & Luhtanen, in press). Participants first completed a measure of contingencies of self-worth (this was an early version of our measure, assessing appearance, others' approval, academic competence, love of friends and family, power, self-reliance, virtue, and God's love as contingencies of self-worth). Then, for the next 2 months (from February 15 to April 15), they accessed a Web page twice a week (and any day on which they heard from a graduate school to which they had applied), completed a state version of the Rosenberg (1965) self-esteem scale, and reported on contacts from graduate programs. At the conclusion of the study, participants again completed the Contingencies of Self-Worth Scale. According to a contingencies of self-worth view, the impact of acceptances and rejections from graduate programs should be greater the more these college seniors based their self-esteem on being good at school. Consistent with this prediction, relative to baseline days on which students received no news from the graduate programs to which they had applied, self-esteem increased more on acceptance days and decreased more on rejection days the more students based their self-esteem on being good at school. Furthermore, only the school-competency contingency, none of the eight other contingencies assessed in this study, moderated both changes in response to acceptances and changes in response to rejections. The specificity of the effect supports the view that fluctuations in self-esteem are not due to a general characteristic of contingent self-esteem but rather to the specific match of life events with a particular contingency of self-worth. This study thus supports the central hypothesis that successes and failures lead to increases and decreases in state self-esteem relative to a person's typical level to the degree that self-esteem is contingent on that domain.

Contingencies and Trait Self-Esteem

James (1890) believed that a person's typical trait level of self-esteem is a direct and elementary endowment of his or her nature and is therefore unrelated to how successful that person is in domains of contingencies of self-worth. A person's trait level of self-esteem may be influenced by a variety of factors, such as biologically based dispositions to experience positive or negative affect. However, trait self-esteem is also influenced by people's enduring circumstances, their contingencies of self-worth, and their chronic tendency to construe the self as satisfying or not satisfying contingencies. High trait self-esteem may result from enduring environments, relationships, and activities that enable people to satisfy, or to believe they satisfy, their contingencies of self-worth. Low trait self-esteem may result from choosing or being trapped in enduring environments, relationships, or activities in which it is difficult to satisfy one's contingencies of self-worth, chronically engaging in behaviors that make it less likely that those contingencies will be satisfied, or consistently interpreting events in a negative light.

Evidence for this view is provided by a study of African American and European American freshmen on a predominantly white college campus (Crocker et al., 2001; Crocker & Wolfe, 2002). Predominantly white campuses may threaten African American students' self-esteem and depress academic performance because of negative stereotypes about their intellectual ability (Steele, 1997), prejudice and discrimination (Crocker & Major, 1989), and failure to live up to standards of attractiveness or worthiness that tend to be based on the values and norms of the majority culture (Steele, 1992). Unless they are able to define their own standards of success in these domains and ignore the standards of the dominant group, contingencies of self-worth may increase vulnerability of African American students to low self-esteem. The more African American students' self-esteem is based on others' approval, school competency, physical attractiveness, or other interpersonal contingencies of self-worth, the more vulnerable they should be to low levels of trait self-esteem. Indeed, this is what Crocker and colleagues (2001) found: For African American students, basing self-esteem on others' approval, physical appearance, being good at school, or outdoing others in competition were negatively correlated with level of trait self-esteem—more negatively than was the case for students from European American backgrounds. Although these data may suggest that *any* contingency of self-worth is more negatively related to trait self-esteem for black than for white students on a predominantly white campus, this was not the case. Basing self-esteem on love and support from one's family, on God's love, or on being a moral, virtuous person did not differ in its link to trait self-esteem for black and white students. These data indicate that trait self-esteem depends on both a person's contingencies of self-worth and on whether the person's circumstances enable him or her to satisfy those contingencies. Does it matter which contingencies of self-worth a person uses as the standards for evaluating self-worth? We believe the answer is a resounding yes. As the study of African American and European American students suggests, interpersonal contingencies of self-worth can be difficult to satisfy, particularly in certain contexts. Consequently, these contingencies may be more strongly associated with low trait self-esteem, as well as with unstable state self-esteem. For example, basing self-esteem on others' approval may result in either low trait self-esteem or unstable state self-esteem or both, because it is difficult to always avoid disapproval from a wide range of people and easy to interpret ambiguous or absent feedback as disapproval (Murray, Holmes, & Griffin, 1996; Murray, Holmes, MacDonald, & Ellsworth, 1998). On the other hand, basing self-esteem on being a virtuous person depends more on one's own standards, although they may be influenced by others. Consistent with this view, basing self-esteem on being virtuous is positively correlated with trait self-esteem, whereas basing self-esteem on the approval of others, on physical appearance, or on outdoing others in competition are all negatively correlated with level of trait self-esteem (Crocker & Wolfe, 2001). This does not mean that it is impossible for people whose self-esteem is dependent on approval from others to maintain a high level of self-esteem. However, in order to do so, they may need to constantly impress others or surround themselves with admirers.

Where Do Contingencies of Self-Worth Come From?

How do people arrive at their contingencies of self-worth? Do we choose to base our self-esteem only on domains that we expect to succeed at? Some research indicates that people are adept at basing their self-worth, or choosing as relevant to the self, only those things on which they tend to outperform others, particularly close others (Tesser, 1988; see also Tesser, Chapter 14, this volume). In our view, this is not so easy to do. We argue, along with others, that contingencies of self-worth develop over the course of time in response to many forms of socialization and social influence (Bandura, 1986, 1991), such as parent–child interactions (e.g., Bartholomew, 1990; Moretti & Higgins, 1990), cultural norms and values (e.g., Solomon, Greenberg, & Pyszczynski, 1991), and observational learning (Bandura, 1991). It is possible that contingencies of self-worth develop in those domains in which people have experienced acceptance or rejection from others (Leary & Baumeister, 2000). For example, a child who receives parental attention only when he or she has won some academic award or recognition may conclude that to be worthwhile, he or she must be smart. In addition, contingencies of self-worth such as self-reliance may develop based on experiences of being physically unsafe. For example, in a recent case, a 3-year-old child whose mother was a drug addict was responsible not only for his own physical well-being but for that of his two younger siblings as well (C. Bellamy, personal communication, October 30, 1995). As a result, this child might develop self-esteem that is contingent on his ability to be self-reliant.

More generally, we suspect that contingencies of self-worth develop based on personal or vicarious experiences that lead people to believe that they will be safe and secure (and accepted by others) if they succeed in those domains. Because contingencies of self-worth develop over the life span, they are relatively stable, but not immutable.

How can we reconcile this view with research indicating that people decide that areas in which they are outperformed by close others are irrelevant to the self? This apparent contradiction can be resolved if we consider that higher order, superordinate contingencies are relatively stable, whereas the more specific and subordinate contingencies are more amenable to change (Crocker & Wolfe, 2001). In our view, it is easier to shift from one subordinate contingency of self-worth to another (e.g., from being good at chemistry to being good at psychology) than to shift from one superordinate contingency to another (e.g., from being smart to being virtuous). Thus many academic couples may base their self-worth on intellectual abilities yet define their areas of specialization differently so as not to be outperformed by their spouses in an area of expertise. We return to the issue of when and under what circumstances people shift their contingencies of self-worth to protect self-esteem in a later section.

Implications for Cognition, Affect, Motivation, and Behavior

Contingencies of self-worth, once developed, have implications for much of people's experience. In particular, they shape interpretations of situations, emotional reactions to events, and personal goals.

Cognition

Consistent with recent cognitive interpretations of personality (Kihlstrom & Cantor, 1988; Kihlstrom & Hastie, 1997), we argue that contingencies of self-worth provide one of the mental schemas through which people filter their daily experience. Contingencies of self-worth are hypothesized to direct attention to contingency-relevant information and events, to guide interpretation of those events, and, consequently, to shape emotional reactions to those events (see Taylor &

Crocker, 1981, for a review). Preliminary support for this view was provided by a study in which participants read a description of an incident and were asked to imagine that it had happened to them (Sommers & Crocker, 2000). In the incident, a person found a wallet and returned it (with cash and credit cards) to the owner. The recipient of this good deed, however, was quite ungrateful and berated the unfortunate do-gooder. Sommers and Crocker (2000) hypothesized that this event would be interpreted positively by people who based their self-esteem on being virtuous but negatively by people who based their self-esteem on others' approval. As predicted, the more participants based their self-esteem on being virtuous, the more virtuous they said the event would make them feel; the more they based their self-esteem on others' approval, the less they would feel approved of. To examine effects on self-esteem, a difference score was calculated to assess how much more participants based their self-esteem on virtue than on others' approval. This difference in contingencies of self-worth predicted participants' reports of how their self-esteem and affect would be influenced by the event. The more participants' contingencies were weighted toward others' approval instead of toward virtue, the more they reported that their self-esteem would decrease and negative affect would increase as a result of this event.

Affect

Because contingencies of self-worth reflect the domains in which people have invested their self-worth and because people typically strive to be worthy rather than unworthy, contingencies of self-worth are linked to a person's goals and self-standards (see Wolfe & Crocker, 2002, for a discussion). Consequently, affective reactions to events are more intense the more relevant those events are to one's contingencies of self-worth. Previous research has demonstrated that goal-related events elicit stronger emotional responses than do goal-unrelated events (Cantor et al., 1991; Emmons, 1991; Lavallee & Campbell, 1995). If being a person of worth is a goal for most people, then affective reactions to events in a domain should be stronger the more self-esteem is based on doing well in that domain. The study of seniors applying to graduate school described previously (Crocker et al., in press) provided an opportunity to test this hypothesis. Specifically, in addition to completing daily self-reports of self-esteem, participants also completed a measure of positive and negative affect (Larsen & Diener, 1992). Hierarchical linear modeling analyses examined within-person effects of acceptances and rejections from graduate programs on affect (positive minus negative), relative to baseline days. As expected, the results indicated that positive affect rose in response to acceptances from graduate schools and fell in response to rejections. Furthermore, the more participants staked their self-worth on being good at school, the greater the affective increases and decreases were.

Thus both changes in self-esteem and changes in positive affect in response to successes and failures are more intense the more that self-esteem is contingent on the domain. This does not mean, however, that state self-esteem and positive affect are identical. Positive affect and self-esteem should be more strongly linked in domains in which self-esteem is highly contingent, because positive events will lead to both happiness and high self-esteem. In noncontingent domains, however, positive events may lead to happiness without self-esteem increases. Consistent with this view, self-esteem and positive affect were more strongly linked the more that students in the study of graduate school applicants based their self-esteem on being good at school (Crocker et al., 2000). In other words, for students high in this contingency, admissions to graduate school tended to raise self-esteem and affect together, whereas rejections tended to lower them. For students whose self-worth was not at stake, however, acceptances led to positive affect without raising self-esteem, and rejections led to negative affect without lowering self-esteem. Thus it seems that self-esteem and affect function independently in response to events that are irrelevant to one's contingencies of self-worth.

Motivation and Behavior

Contingencies of self-worth have motivational implications: People will generally try to avoid the drops in self-esteem and increases in negative affect that follow from failing in domains on which self-worth has been staked, and they will seek the increases in self-esteem and positive affect that follow from succeeding in domains of contingency. Although the level of a person's trait self-esteem is strongly related to affect and life satisfaction, it is relatively unimportant as a cause of behavior (see Baumeister, 1998, for a discussion). As the baseline of self-worth, trait self-esteem and the positive or negative affect that typically accompanies it has little motivational power. Trait self-esteem by definition is unlikely to change in response to temporarily falling short of or fulfilling one's standards. Because it tends to be stable, trait self-esteem lacks the power to provide internally generated rewards and punishments for behavior. State self-esteem, on the other hand, fluctuates in response to events that are relevant to one's contingencies and is also associated with heightened affective reactions to events. Consequently, fluctuations of state self-esteem and accompanying affect have the power to shape behavior. Indeed, the strongest influence on whether people in the United States find events satisfying or unsatisfying is the effect of those events on self-esteem (Sheldon, Elliot, Kim, & Kasser, 2001). Because fluctuations of state self-esteem depend on the contingencies of self-worth a person has, a focus on contingencies of self-worth may provide deeper insights into the link between self-esteem and behavior than a focus on trait self-esteem.

There are several routes through which contingencies of self-worth may influence behavior. First, people with different contingencies may choose to be in different situations, and the pressures or forces that operate on behavior in those situations may affect behavior. Second, contingencies of self-worth may serve as self-standards for behavior, motivating behaviors that help people to satisfy their contingencies or to avoid failing to live up to them. Third, people with different contingencies of self-worth may actually create different situations and circumstances in their lives.

Contingencies of Self-Worth, Situations, and Behavior

In our view, people organize their lives around their contingencies of self-worth.

Conclusion

They do this for two reasons: first, to have their beliefs about what makes them people of worth validated by others who share their contingencies, and, second, to increase their chances of avoiding the pain of drops in state self-esteem and obtaining the pleasure of increases in state self-esteem.

Selecting Situations

People select for themselves situations, settings, and circumstances in which their contingencies of self-worth are widely shared and valued. Thus people whose self-esteem is based on being smart are likely to apply to selective colleges or graduate programs in which other people share their view of what constitutes a worthy person. People whose self-esteem is based on their religious belief that God loves them are likely to join religious organizations in which others share this contingency. People who base their self-esteem on their physical appearance may seek out settings in which a high value is placed on attractiveness. For example, college students who base their self-esteem on God's love are more likely to join religious organizations, and college women who base their self-esteem on their appearance are more likely to join sororities (Crocker et al., 2001). Selecting situations in which others share their contingencies of self-worth may provide reassurance that the domains on which people have staked their own self-worth really do determine who is worthy and who is not. Furthermore, these situations may provide opportunities to satisfy one's contingencies. It is important to note, however, that selecting situations in which others share one's contingencies of self-worth does not guarantee that one will experience high self-esteem. Indeed, in addition to providing validation of one's contingencies and opportunities to succeed in those domains, these situations may also provide opportunities for failure in domains of contingency. For example, the person who bases self-esteem on being smart and who seeks out situations in which this contingency is widely shared may find himself or herself surrounded by people who all also want to be smart. The resulting struggle to be the smartest affords many opportunities for both increases and decreases in self-esteem.

Once people select situations based on their contingencies of self-worth, these situations, in turn, may influence behavior. For example, in our study of college freshmen, we found that women (particularly European American women) who base their self-esteem on their appearance are more likely to join sororities. Even after controlling for their contingencies of self-worth, women who join sororities spend more time partying, use drugs and alcohol more often, and show more symptoms of disordered eating than women who do not join sororities (Crocker et al., 2001). Thus, by shaping the situations people choose for themselves, contingencies of self-worth may indirectly shape behaviors.

Choosing How to Spend One's Time

Each of us has only 24 hours in a day, and we make choices each day about how to use that time. One influence on those choices is our contingencies of self-worth. Contingencies serve an important self-regulatory function by shaping people's goals and directing their behavior as they attempt to achieve those goals. Our study of college freshmen examined how contingencies of self-worth that students had before they entered college affected their use of time over the course of their freshman year (Crocker et al., 2001). After the end of both their first and second semesters of college, students were asked to report how much time they spent in a variety of activities, including studying, volunteering, going to church or synagogue, partying, socializing, exercising, shopping for clothes, and grooming. Controlling for differences associated with students' gender, race, and socioeconomic status, contingencies of self-worth prior to entering college significantly predicted how much time students spent in each of these activities. Furthermore, specific contingencies predicted specific activities. For example, students who based their self-esteem on school competency reported spending more time studying, students who based their self-esteem on virtue spent more time volunteering and less time partying, students who based their self-esteem on God's love spent more time in religious activities and less time partying, students who based their self-esteem on love and support from their families spent more time with or talking to their families, and students who based their self-esteem on their appearance spent more time grooming, exercising, shopping for clothes, socializing, and partying.

Thus it appears that contingencies of self-worth shape people's goals and how they spend their time—people spend more time on activities that enable them to satisfy their contingencies. But does it work? Does this self-regulatory function result in success at achieving one's goals? For example, is a student who spends more time volunteering really more virtuous than his or her peers? Is a student who exercises and spends more time grooming really more attractive than his or her peers? One area in which we can examine the success of this self-regulatory strategy is in the domain of school competency. The more students based their self-esteem on being good at school, the more hours per week they reported studying. Did this extra effort result in higher GPAs? To address this question, students reported their GPAs each semester of their freshman year. (A subset of students gave their permission to have their freshman year transcripts examined. Self-reported GPA was highly correlated with actual GPA, particularly for the first semester, when students reported their GPAs after they had received their fall term grades, $r = .88$; second semester grade reports were mailed after students completed the third session of our study.) Interestingly, although students who studied more had higher GPAs, the correlation between the school-competency contingency and GPA was non-significant ($r = .06$, n.s.) after controlling for SAT scores. Thus the extra time students spend studying because their self-esteem is at stake may not be particularly helpful in actually increasing their GPAs. Perhaps their studying is less efficient, impeded by anxiety because of what is at stake or by thoughts of how terrible they would feel if they do not succeed in school (Deci & Ryan, 1991). Or perhaps they are more concerned with *appearing* to be academically serious than with actually *being* competent. We cannot say for sure what accounts for this interesting but unexpected effect. But it suggests a larger point, to which we return later: The motivation that comes from having self-worth on the line does not necessarily result in greater success.

Contingencies Create Our Reality

At various points in this chapter, we have noted that contingencies of self-worth serve as the filters through which people interpret their experience; they shape people's selection of situations and serve a self-regulatory function, motivating behavior in an attempt to satisfy those contingencies. The result of these various processes is that contingencies of self-worth actually shape the situations—the reality—that we experience. The general idea that beliefs can create reality is a cornerstone of social psychology (Merton, 1948; Snyder, 1984). Of course, beliefs do not completely create reality, and contingencies of self-worth are not the only beliefs at play as we create our reality. Nonetheless, it is important to acknowledge the ways in which the creation of our reality is a function of our contingencies of self-worth.

Although we do not have data to support this point, a simple thought experiment about a type of person familiar to most academics should convey its plausibility. Consider, for example, a person we'll call John, whose self-worth is based on being smart. John tends to interpret situations through the filter of his contingency and therefore tends to see all situations as opportunities either to be smart or to be stupid. Because John wants to be a worthy person, he will try to be smart in those situations—perhaps by making insightful comments or asking tough questions, by appearing knowledgeable, by pointing out the flaws in others' comments, by being argumentative, and by always needing to be right or to win arguments. John's behavior, directed at the goal of feeling worthy by being smart, is likely to have an effect on those around him—especially if they also need to be smart to feel worthy. They may respect and admire his intelligence, as John probably desires. But it is more likely that they will feel that John's need to be smart, perhaps even the smartest person in the room, threatens their own need to be smart. Consequently, they may counterargue, put down John's ideas, and generally engage in intellectual one-upmanship. They may not like him and may even avoid him. It is probably hard for John to see the extent to which he has created the intellectually combative, unsupportive, even hostile environment in which he quite regularly finds himself. John may indeed feel worthy because he is smart in these situations. On the other hand, the repeated criticism he receives from those around him may wear on his self-esteem. In either case, it seems likely that John may not like the reality he has created for himself.

Maintaining, Protecting, and Enhancing Self-Esteem

Contingencies of self-worth represent the domains in which self-esteem is vulnerable—in which successes or failures can lead to increases or decreases in self-esteem. This, along with the increases and decreases in affect that accompany changes in self-esteem, is what gives contingencies of self-worth their motivational impetus and leads people whose self-esteem is based on school competency to study more; those whose self-esteem is based on attractiveness to spend more time exercising, grooming, and shopping for clothes; and so on. Thus people attempt to maintain the belief that they are worthy by achieving success in the domains on which their self-worth is staked. However, working to achieve success is not the only way people attempt to maintain and enhance their self-esteem or to protect it from failure in domains of contingency. Sometimes, people lack the time, energy, or ability to be successful in a domain on which their self-esteem has been staked, and it is inevitable that each of us will occasionally experience failure in domains of contingency. Consequently, people develop additional strategies for avoiding the drop in self-esteem that accompanies failure in domains of contingency. Some of these are a priori strategies that people use to avoid potential failure or to cushion the consequent blow to self-esteem. Others represent post hoc strategies that people use after experiencing failure in a domain of contingency. In the following sections, we consider both a priori and post hoc strategies for maintaining and protecting self-esteem.

In these sections, the research we review tends not to explicitly consider the role of contingencies of self-worth. Rather, most studies assume that these self-protective strategies will not be elicited unless self-esteem is threatened, and they expose participants to actual or anticipated success or failure in domains that are assumed to be important to nearly everyone. Thus studies of self-esteem maintenance and protection typically expose college students to the possibility of failure on an intellectual task or rejection in a social circumstance on the assumption that this failure or rejection threatens the self-esteem of participants. In each of the studies, there is likely to be unmeasured variance in the contingencies on which participants base their self-esteem, so the failure or rejection may be more threatening to some participants than to others. But in general, researchers implicitly select tasks or feedback relevant to the contingencies of self-worth of most of their participants. Thus we interpret these studies as demonstrating the effects of actual or anticipated threats in domains of contingency.

Avoiding Threats to Self-Esteem

The research we have reviewed thus far in this chapter suggests that people generally try to perform to the best of their ability on domains in which their self-esteem is contingent and that they spend their time in ways that they think will maximize their chances of success. Yet there are times at which people are more motivated to avoid the drops in self-esteem and negative affect associated with actual or anticipated failure than they are to enjoy the increases in self-esteem associated with success; that is, there are times at which people are focused more on prevention than on promotion (Higgins, 1998). When outcomes are highly desirable but uncertain, people tend to protect themselves from disappointment by engaging in a variety of cognitive and behavioral strategies (Pyszczynski, 1982).

Avoiding the Situation

The first line of defense when failure in a domain of contingency is anticipated is avoiding the situation altogether. Thus, in addition to selecting situations in which their contingencies are shared by others and that provide opportunities for succeeding in domains of contingency, people will generally avoid situations in which failure in domains of contingency seems likely. This strategy of avoiding situations is not studied much in social psychology because it is less amenable to laboratory methods. However, it is an important way in which people limit the risk of failure in domains of contingency, at the cost of limiting the range of their experience. Students who base their self-esteem on doing well in school tend to avoid challenges (Covington, 1984). For example, they may avoid taking courses reputed to have tough grading curves or in areas far removed from their specialization.

Lowering Expectations

When people cannot avoid the situation altogether, they may try to buffer the impact of anticipated failure on self-esteem by lowering their expectations to avoid being disappointed by failure (Pyszczynski, 1982). This strategy, called defensive pessimism, is focused on managing the anxiety generated by the possibility of failure and its consequent effects on self-esteem (Cantor & Norem, 1989; Norem & Cantor, 1986a, 1986b). Although low expectations are sometimes associated with poor performance, the strategy of setting low expectations in order to reduce anxiety is not usually associated with poor performance (Cantor & Norem, 1989; Norem & Cantor, 1986a, 1986b). Rather, it appears to reduce anxiety to a manageable level so that it is not debilitating. When their strategy of defensive pessimism is interfered with, people actually perform worse (Norem & Cantor, 1986b).

Self-Handicapping

Another strategy to cope with the possibility of failure is to engage in various forms of self-handicapping. Self-handicapping is an ironic phenomenon in that it increases people's chances of failure by creating obstacles to their performance, such as not trying or practicing, consuming alcohol or drugs, or procrastinating (Baumeister, 1998). Self-handicapping provides an excuse for failure so that, when a person self-handicaps, a poor performance is unlikely to be attributed to a lack of ability. It has the added ad-

vantage of making one appear particularly talented if one manages to perform well in spite of the self-handicap. Therefore, people may be motivated to self-handicap because it can provide an excuse for failure or make one's success seem particularly remarkable (Tice, 1991). Most self-handicapping occurs only when others know about the self-handicapping (Kolditz & Arkin, 1982). Thus it seems that self-handicapping is primarily a strategy for managing the attributions others will make about one's performance. This suggests that self-handicapping is particularly likely to be used by people whose self-esteem is highly contingent on others' approval.

Perfectionism

An alternative strategy to avoid losses of self-esteem associated with anticipated failure is perfectionism. Perfectionists are people who are imprisoned rather than served by their rigid demands for perfection (e.g., must get the top score, make no mistakes, win the first prize) instead of excellence. To avoid drops in self-esteem, they must strive to be perfect (Blankenstein, Flett, Hewitt, & Eng, 1993; Frost, Marten, Lahart, & Rosenblate, 1990). Perfectionism has high costs, in terms of both time and anxiety. Although perfectionism sometimes increases one's chances of success, it is also linked to procrastination, which may ultimately serve as a self-handicapping strategy and undermine performance (Frost et al., 1990).

Reacting to Threats to Self-Esteem

When people are optimistic about their chances of success in domains on which their self-worth is staked, they are less likely to engage in a priori strategies that buffer the self from possible failure (Norem & Cantor, 1986a). But how do people cope when failure, rejection, or other negative outcomes in domains of contingency cannot be avoided or have not been prepared for in advance? People have at their disposal several lines of defense against these threats to self-esteem, including cognitive strategies that minimize or discount the threat and its implications for self-esteem or that restore a general sense of self-worth (Greenberg, Pyszczynski, & Solomon, 1986). In addition, evidence is accumulating that people respond to such threats with anger and hostility and often lash out against others following threats to their self-worth (Baumeister, Smart, & Boden, 1996).

Dismissing the Threat

Perhaps the most effective response to threats in domains of contingency is to reduce the threat by attributing failure to something else—an invalid test, another's mistake, and so on. People are more likely to derogate a test as invalid or inaccurate when they fail than when they succeed (Frey, 1978; Greenberg, Pyszczynski, & Solomon, 1982; Shrauger, 1975) and to evaluate evidence about the validity of the test in a self-serving manner (Pyszczynski, Greenberg, & Holt, 1985). Attributions for success and failure also seem motivated by the desire to take credit for success and to avoid responsibility for failure. People are more likely to attribute success than failure to their ability; and failure is more likely to be attributed to others, to the circumstances, to a poor test, or to lack of effort—anything that avoids the implication that the person who failed is deficient (for reviews, see Blaine & Crocker, 1993; Bradley, 1978; Greenberg & Pyszczynski, 1985; Miller & Ross, 1975). People can also dismiss social or interpersonal threats. For example, people who are rejected by a group often say, after the fact, that they did not want to be accepted anyway (Leary, Tambor, Terdal, & Downs, 1995).

Compensating

Another response to threats to self-worth is to compensate by inflating the positivity of self-description on the threatened dimension (Gollwitzer & Wicklund, 1985; Gollwitzer, Wicklund, & Hilton, 1982; Wicklund, 1982) or inflating self-descriptions on another dimension (Baumeister & Jones, 1978; Greenberg & Pyszczynski, 1985). For example, people who are told that their personalities do not suit them for their chosen professions subsequently describe themselves in ways that indicate that they are, in fact, suited to that profession (Gollwitzer & Wicklund, 1985). And when compensating by inflating the self on the threatened do-

main is not possible, people will inflate themselves in other domains to compensate (Baumeister & Jones, 1978; Greenberg & Pyszczynski, 1985). These compensatory strategies are intended, first, to maintain positive self-views in domains in which self-definitions are at stake (i.e., self-esteem is contingent) and, second, to maintain global self-esteem when maintaining a specific positive self-view in a domain of contingency is not possible. This inflation of the self extends to actual performance; students committed to professional goals, such as becoming physicians or computer scientists, who failed on a task relevant to their professional goals showed enhanced performance on a subsequent task relevant to their goals, although they showed impaired performance on a later task that was irrelevant to their professional goal (Brunstein & Gollwitzer, 1996). This attempt to compensate for failure through enhanced performance on another, relevant task may be related to some problems with self-regulation. Attempts to compensate for failure can lead people to set inappropriately high goals and hence end up with fewer rewards (Baumeister, Heatherton, & Tice, 1993).

Abandoning Contingencies

One strategy to protect self-esteem following failure in a domain of contingency is to give up the contingency. James (1890) suggested that this strategy is quite ubiquitous: "To give up pretensions is as blessed a relief as to get them gratified; and where disappointment is incessant and the struggle unending, this is what men will always do" (p. 45). People may disengage self-esteem from specific experiences that are unlikely to satisfy a contingency of self-worth. For example, Major and her colleagues (Major & Schmader, 1998; Major, Spencer, Schmader, Wolfe, & Crocker, 1998) found that black students disengaged their self-worth from performance on a test when the possibility of racial bias in the test was raised. When people perform worse than close others in a domain that is relevant to their self-concept, they may protect self-esteem by diminishing the relevance of the domain (Major & Schmader, 1998; Major et al., 1998; see also Pyszczynski & Greenberg, 1987; Tesser, 1988, Chapter 14, this volume).

It is easier to abandon specific or subordinate contingencies (e.g., being good at engineering) than more encompassing or superordinate contingencies (e.g., being smart or good at school). A study conducted by Crocker and colleagues (in press) indicated that college seniors' contingencies remain largely unchanged across a 2-month period of time, and, notably, their endorsement of school competency as a contingency of self-worth was stable despite the fact that many participants received a preponderance of rejections from graduate programs. Despite the difficulty in revising superordinate contingencies of self-worth, they are not immutable. Abandoning contingencies may be particularly likely when a person is no longer able to satisfy a contingency of self-worth. An example of this can be seen in older adults. Despite losses in domains that are clearly prominent contingencies of self-worth among younger people (e.g., physical appearance, agility), older adults do not suffer from lower levels of self-esteem (Brandstadter & Greve, 1994). One explanation, consistent with research in the aging literature (Carstensen & Freund, 1994), is that as we age, we abandon those contingencies we are no longer able to satisfy.

Distancing from Others

A more interpersonal reaction to threats to self-esteem is the process of distancing the self from others. When a close other (e.g., a friend or family member) excels in a domain that is not central to the self-concept, people tend to bask in reflected glory, as if the credit for the other's outstanding performance extended to the self. However, when outperformed by a close other in a domain that is relevant to the self-concept, people either diminish the relevance of the domain or distance themselves from the other person (Tesser, 1988; Chapter 14, this volume). Thus people will sometimes cut themselves off from friends and family members whose superior performance constitutes a threat to self-esteem.

Downward Comparison

Another strategy for protecting self-esteem from threats is to focus on other people's shortcomings. Although this does not directly eliminate the threat, it can reduce it by suggesting that one is not really so bad in comparison with other people. For example, following threats in important domains, people are more likely to remember negative information about others, even information that is unrelated to the domain of the threat (Crocker, 1993). Indeed, people tend to seek out information about others who also did poorly (Pyszczynski, Greenberg, & Laprelle, 1985; Wood, Giordano-Beech, & Ducharme, 1999) and to compare themselves with worse-off others following failure (Beauregard & Dunning, 1998; Crocker, Thompson, McGraw, & Ingerman, 1987; Wills, 1981; Wood et al., 1999).

Prejudice and Derogation of Others

The tendency to focus on others' shortcomings following a threat to self-esteem extends to the derogation of outgroups and expression of ingroup favoritism (Aberson, Healy, & Romero, 2000; Crocker & Luhtanen, 1990; Crocker et al., 1987; Wills, 1981). When people have experienced a threat to the self-concept, they are more likely to evaluate another person stereotypically (Fein & Spencer, 1997) and automatically (Spencer, Fein, Wolfe, Fong, & Dunn, 1998). As a result, negative evaluations of those who belong to stereotyped groups can serve to restore self-esteem (Fein & Spencer, 1997).

Antagonism

In light of the evidence that people often distance themselves from close others, engage in downward comparison, seek out negative information about others, and derogate outgroup members, it is not surprising that people who fail in a domain of contingency tend to interact with others in an antagonistic manner (Heatherton & Vohs, 2000) that ultimately drives others away. Heatherton and Vohs (2000), for example, demonstrated that people with high self-esteem who receive a threat to the self-concept are liked less by interaction partners than people with high self-esteem who do not receive a threat to the self-concept.

Aggression and Violence

Finally, people who receive a threat to self-esteem may react with aggression and violence toward others (Baumeister et al., 1996). Based on an extensive review of several literatures, Baumeister and colleagues (1996) conclude that aggression is a response to "fragile egotism," or self-concepts that are positive but vulnerable (see also Bushman & Baumeister, 1998). In our terms, aggression represents a response to threats in domains in which self-esteem is highly contingent.

Why would people become surly or violent after a failure? This response would seem to increase the likelihood of being rejected by others and therefore seems particularly maladaptive. The answer may lie in research that demonstrates a link between frustration and aggression (e.g., Barker, Dembo, & Lewin, 1941). Failure or rejection in a domain on which self-esteem is staked may be particularly frustrating, especially if it is perceived to be unreasonable or unfair (Kulik & Brown, 1979), and may consequently trigger an aggressive response. At times, such aggression may be functional in the sense of removing an obstacle to a goal (Shaver, Schwarz, Kirson, & O'Connor, 1987), although the reactions it elicits from others may often lead to more frustration and more aggression.

Genuine or Defensive Self-Esteem?

Genuine self-esteem refers to a true sense of self-worth, self-respect, and acceptance of one's strengths and weaknesses (Rosenberg, 1979). The research we have reviewed suggests that people are typically defensive and unwilling to realistically acknowledge their flaws and shortcomings. The notion that people differ in their contingencies of self-worth provides an alternative way to think about the issue of defensive versus genuine self-esteem. According to this view, it is the potential loss of self-esteem in the face of self-threatening information that spurs defensiveness. Rather than focus on whether self-esteem is true or genuine, it may be more useful to focus on the bases of self-esteem and on whether those contingencies of self-worth are vulnerable to, or currently

subject to, attack. Self-esteem is relatively impervious to attack in domains in which it is noncontingent. That is, when confronted with negative information about the self, it may be easier to acknowledge nondefensively one's mistakes and failures and to take responsibility for them in noncontingent domains—domains in which self-worth is not on the line. Thus people are more likely to avoid self-threats in advance and react defensively to self-threats in domains in which their self-esteem is contingent. This is not the same as arguing that defensive self-esteem is ungenuine, untrue, or self-deceptive. The problem is not that this self-esteem is false, hiding inner feelings of worthlessness, but that it is fragile and consequently needs to be defended (Deci & Ryan, 1995; Kernis & Waschull, 1995).

Does Level of Self-Esteem Matter?

Although our analysis focuses on contingencies of self-worth, we recognize that level of self-esteem plays an important role in these processes. Many of the strategies people use to avoid self-threats are more characteristic of people who are low in self-esteem, and many of the reactions to unavoidable self-threats are more characteristic of people who are high in self-esteem (Baumeister, Tice, & Hutton, 1989). People high in trait self-esteem show a variety of defensive responses to threatening information, including dismissing the accuracy and validity of the feedback (Brockner, 1984; Brockner, Derr, & Laing, 1987; Shrauger, 1975), derogating the source of the feedback, derogating other people (e.g., Crocker et al., 1987; see Wills, 1981, for a review), dismissing the importance of the domain in which they did poorly (Brown, Dutton, & Cook, 2001), and attributing the negative outcome to external or temporary causes (see Blaine & Crocker, 1993; Bradley, 1978; Kernis & Waschull, 1995, for discussions). Because people with high trait self-esteem generally think more positively about themselves and have clearer and more certain self-concepts (Campbell & Lavallee, 1993), they may find it easier to disbelieve or discredit negative information about the self (Baumeister et al., 1989; Blaine & Crocker, 1993; Kernis & Waschull, 1995). People with high self-esteem also face potentially greater losses of self-esteem in the face of failure in contingent domains and therefore may be more motivated to avoid drops in self-esteem by discrediting self-threats in contingent domains.

Overall Contingency, or Specific Domains of Contingency?

Our analysis of contingencies of self-worth and their motivational consequences focuses on the domains on which people stake their self-worth. In contrast to this emphasis, other related perspectives have focused on differences between people in whether self-esteem is contingent or noncontingent. For example, Rogers (1951) emphasized the role of unconditional positive regard from others in producing noncontingent self-esteem in individuals. Deci and Ryan (1995) argue that self-esteem can be either contingent or "true," with true self-esteem developing naturally from autonomous, efficacious action in the context of supportive, authentic relationships. Kernis and Washull (1995) emphasize differences between people whose self-esteem tends to be stable and those whose self-esteem is unstable. Whereas these perspectives emphasize between-person differences in the overall quality of contingent self-esteem, our approach emphasizes a within-person perspective, examining the domains on which a person's self-esteem is contingent versus noncontingent.

There is, of course, no necessary incompatibility between these approaches. We emphasize within-person effects of domains of contingency and noncontingency because we believe that many of the most interesting and unexplored questions regarding contingencies of self-worth concern not whether a person has contingent or noncontingent self-esteem but what it is that he or she bases self-esteem on. Indeed, our data repeatedly show that different contingencies lead to different behaviors, vulnerabilities, and outcomes. A person whose self-esteem is based on being a good, moral person behaves very differently from a person whose self-esteem is based on being physically attractive or having power over others. Research that simply distinguishes between people with contingent versus noncontin-

gent self-esteem may obscure these important differences, to the point that the distinction seems irrelevant.

Seeking Self-Esteem: At What Cost?

In our view, the problem with self-esteem is not in *having* self-esteem but rather in *pursuing* self-esteem to the exclusion of other goals and needs. In particular, we argue that people's efforts to maintain, enhance, and protect self-esteem ultimately hinder them from attaining the things that they really need in life. And what is it that humans need? Many psychological human needs have been proposed (see Sheldon et al., 2001, for a discussion); we focus here on two psychological needs for which there is wide agreement across theories. One of the most important psychological needs may be to have a few close, mutually caring, and supportive relationships with others (Baumeister & Leary, 1995; Bowlby, 1969; E. M. Deci & Ryan, 2000). Close, mutually caring relationships provide a safe haven in times of distress (Collins & Feeney, 2000), which, in turn, contributes to more effective coping (Cohen, Sherrod, & Clark, 1986) and better mental and physical health (Ryff, 1995). In addition to the need for relatedness, humans have a need for competency—the ability to effect outcomes or to master the environment (E. M. Deci & Ryan, 2000; White, 1959). Mutually caring relationships and the ability to master one's environment both contribute to survival, the overarching and primary goal of humans (Pyszczynski, Greenberg, & Solomon, 1997). In our view, what people really need is true relatedness and competence, rather than illusory perceptions of relatedness and competence. Although positive illusions about the self are linked to positive affect, they do not enhance true competency and may incur long-term costs. For example, Robins and Beer (2001) found that college students with unrealistically positive views of their academic abilities were initially higher in self-esteem than students who appraised their abilities realistically but that over the course of their college experience they disengaged from academics, and their self-esteem declined. In the long run, people's attempts to maintain, enhance, and protect contingent self-esteem may detract from their ability to form and maintain mutually caring relationships and acquire mastery through learning experiences. In addition, seeking self-esteem may also exact a toll on people's mental and physical health.

Costs to Relationships

The ways in which people react to self-esteem threat interfere with forming and maintaining close, mutually caring relationships with others. Our review indicates that people tend to respond to threat with blame, excuses, anger, antagonism, aggression, avoidance, or withdrawal (Baumeister, 1998; Baumeister, Bushman, & Campbell, 2000; Baumeister et al., 1989, 1993, 1996; Heatherton & Vohs, 2000; Kernis & Waschull, 1995; Tice, 1993). These negative reactions reduce, rather than enhance, people's ability to fulfill their need for relatedness. In particular, seeking self-esteem may incur interpersonal costs because of the focus on maintaining and enhancing self-esteem rather than on attending to the needs and feelings of others. For example, people who fail in a domain of contingency may experience shame and a sense of worthlessness for not meeting their self-standards (Lewis, 2000). Shame, in turn, may lead to hostile intentions and maladaptive, aggressive responses (Tangney, Wagner, Hill-Barlow, Marschall, & Gramzow, 1996) that could strain interpersonal relationships. As another example, people with low self-esteem tend to react to self-doubts by questioning their partners' forgiveness, perceiving fewer positive qualities in their partners, and distancing themselves from their partners (Murray et al., 1998). This finding suggests that when people feel threatened, they may focus on repairing their self-esteem, even if it means devaluing or distancing themselves from close others. The evidence that people react to threats to the self with anger, hostility, and even violence also suggests that when people have the goal of maintaining and protecting self-esteem, they behave in ways that have high costs to their close relationships. Evidence that people who abuse spouses and children have fragile high self-esteem (Baumeister et al., 1996) is consistent with this view—when threatened, these people seem to completely lose sight of their goal to maintain their close and mutually caring relationships. Thus the crucial issue is not whether self-esteem is high or low but whether people feel their self-esteem is under assault and hence are attempting to restore it.

People who base their self-esteem on the approval of others may be particularly vulnerable to experiencing unstable relationships. In terms of attachment theory, those who are contingent on the approval of others may have an insecure (i.e., anxious–ambivalent) attachment style characterized by high levels of dependency and a need for constant reassurance (Bowlby, 1969). Whereas secures (i.e., those who have a safe haven) engage in more effective forms of support seeking and caregiving, insecures are less effective support seekers and caregivers (Collins & Feeney, 2000). Similarly, people with contingent self-esteem may be less effective at giving care to and receiving support from others. In the long run, this maladaptive style of interaction could weaken or even dissolve the relationships with close others on which people depend for their physical and emotional well-being.

Costs to Learning

When people experience a threat to self-esteem, they engage in defensive strategies in order to repair their self-esteem and maintain the belief that they have satisfied their contingencies. As we have seen, common strategies include dismissing the validity of the negative feedback, derogating the source of the information, or generating excuses for their behavior. These defensive responses, although temporarily alleviating distress, can drive away people who are trying to be helpful. Moreover, they detract from the ability to consider and incorporate feedback that might lead them to realistically evaluate and address their weaknesses. Thus seeking to maintain and enhance self-esteem by engaging in defensive behaviors—such as making external attributions for failure, derogating the source of the feedback, or discrediting a test—may ultimately impede learning and hinder the development of competence and mastery.

As noted, people tend to organize their lives around their contingencies in order to avoid increases in negative affect and maximize increases in positive affect. Although this strategy may protect self-esteem and affect in the short run, it may ultimately deter them from increasing their competence (Robins & Beer, 2001). Many achievement motivation theorists believe that basing self-esteem on academic achievement may increase students' susceptibility to academic difficulties (Burhans & Dweck, 1995; Covington, 1984). Basing self-esteem on competency, for example, may motivate people to demonstrate their competency to themselves and others. Because students who base their self-esteem on academic achievement wish to avoid the negative self-feelings that accompany poor performance, they may avoid challenges (Covington, 1984) and show learned helplessness in response to failure (Burhans & Dweck, 1995). The pressure they place on themselves may also lead them to underperform on academic tasks (Steele & Aronson, 1998; Stone, Lynch, Sjomeling, & Darley, 1999).

Self-determination theory (Deci, Nezlek, & Sheinman, 1981; E. M. Deci & Ryan, 2000; Ryan & Deci, 2000) also predicts that students whose self-worth depends on academic performance may experience pressure that undermines their motivation. According to self-determination theory (Deci & Ryan, 1991; Ryan & Deci, 2000), internally motivated behavior can be introjected or integrated. Introjected behavior is controlled by internally regulated sanctions and rewards, such as increases and decreases in self-esteem; on the other hand, integrated behavior is fully self-determined and performed for its own sake because of the intrinsic value of the activity. Because contingencies of self-worth are introjected, people may engage in tasks out of a feeling of obligation or a fear of loss of self-esteem rather than out of a sense of autonomy or genuine desire to learn. This attitude, in turn, may impair task performance and undermine intrinsic interest. Indeed, research has shown that, whereas introjection is associated with increased academic anxiety, maladaptive coping with failure, and decreased intrinsic motivation, integration is associated with school enjoyment and proactive coping (Deci, Vallerand, Pelletier, & Ryan, 1991). In addition, the negative affect associated with threats to the self in domains of contingency may undermine performance on cognitive tasks (Spencer & Quinn, 1995) and stifle creativity (Amabile, 1985). Again, the costs to learning come not from having self-esteem that is low (or high), but rather from reacting to events or feedback in ways that primarily serve to maintain, protect, and enhance self-esteem.

Costs to Mental Health

The repeated fluctuations in self-esteem due to events in domains of contingency may increase people's vulnerability to negative mental health outcomes. In particular, the instability of self-esteem associated with contingencies of self-worth may exacerbate the onset of depression (Crocker & Wolfe, 2001). Several models in the clinical literature suggest that people who are prone to depression also have self-esteem that is vulnerable, or contingent, in certain domains (Beck, 1983; Bibring, 1953; Blatt & Shichman, 1983; Higgins, 1987). Consistent with these models, we argue that it is the match between life events and contingencies of self-worth that contributes to increases in depression. However, it is the instability of self-esteem resulting from the fluctuation of positive and negative life events in domains of contingency that mediates the effects of contingencies on depression (Crocker & Wolfe, 2001). Instability of depression may derive from large drops in self-esteem (e.g., loss of a job, loss of a loved one), as well as more minor but repeated decreases in self-esteem (e.g., repeated rejections in a relationship). Recent research supports the hypothesis that contingencies, in concert with life events, lead to unstable self-esteem, which increases depressive symptoms (see Crocker & Wolfe, 2001, for a discussion; Kernis et al., 1998; Roberts & Gotlib, 1997; Roberts & Kassel, 1997; Roberts, Kassel, & Gotlib, 1995). Once again, level of self-esteem appears to be less important than whether self-esteem is contingent or vulnerable.

Costs to Physical Health

People's desire to maintain, enhance, and protect self-esteem may also lead them to engage in behaviors that are deleterious to their physical health. People may try to seek self-esteem by engaging in activities that are relevant to their contingencies. For instance, people who are concerned with how others perceive and evaluate them may be at greater risk for adopting negative health practices (Leary, Tchividjian, & Kraxberger, 1994), including drinking alcohol (Faber, Khavari, & Douglass, 1980), smoking (Camp, Klesges, & Relyea, 1993), sunbathing (Leary & Jones, 1993), using steroids (Schrof, 1992), driving recklessly (Jonah, 1990), and failing to engage in safe sex practices, such as using condoms (Schlenker & Leary, 1982).

Contingencies based on appearance and social approval may be particularly important in the case of eating disorders. Research has shown that anorexics tend to be highly motivated to live up to others' expectations (Bruch, 1978) and that bulimics tend to be concerned with pleasing others and avoiding rejection (Weinstein & Richman, 1984). Research directly examining the extent to which self-esteem is based on body image and appearance supports the view that this basis of self-esteem constitutes a risk factor for eating disorders (Geller, Johnston, & Madsen, 1997; Geller et al., 1998). Rather than disengaging self-esteem from appearance and the approval of others, people with eating disorders maladaptively persist in trying to achieve their unrealistically stringent self-standards. In the long run, this pattern of behavior may lead to depleted energy levels, malnutrition, lowered resistance to illness and infection, complications of the digestive system and heart, and, in extreme cases, even death (Brownell, 1991; Lissner et al., 1991).

Health outcomes may also be affected by the situations that people seek out based on their contingencies. Research has shown that the situation can exert powerful effects on behavior (Ross & Nisbett, 1991). People who are motivated to satisfy their contingencies may be drawn to situations that enable them to fulfill these needs.

In summary, seeking self-esteem can take a high toll on our relationships with others, our competency, and our mental and physical health. If we assume that people seek self-esteem because they think it will bring them love, respect, accomplishment, and happiness, then the pursuit of self-esteem is ironic because, ultimately, it gets us exactly what we don't want—loneliness, isolation, alienation, and illusory but not real competence.

What Is the Alternative?

Is there an alternative to seeking self-esteem? Given the high costs of pursuing self-esteem, is it possible to respond to self-threats in a way that is less destructive and more likely to satisfy the fundamental human needs for competence and relatedness? In this section, we consider three possibilities for exiting the vicious and costly cycle of seeking self-esteem: engaging in self-affirmation (Steele, 1988), developing noncontingent self-esteem (Deci & Ryan, 1995), and shifting goals from seeking self-esteem to more altruistic, compassionate, and other-oriented goals.

Self-Affirmation

One way that people can cope with a threat to the self is to affirm themselves in another domain (Steele, 1988). Self-affirmation involves recruiting and defending positive aspects of the self to maintain a phenomenal experience of the self as adaptively and morally adequate. Self-affirmation has been operationalized in a variety of ways—for example, by reminding people of their most central values, or by having people fill out a self-esteem scale (which presumably reminds people with high self-esteem of their many positive attributes). Self-affirmation restores the sense that the self has integrity and, consequently, reduces the need to defend against self-threat. For example, people who freely choose to write an essay that contradicts their beliefs tend to feel uncomfortable about their behavior (i.e., experience dissonance) and therefore respond by changing their beliefs to bring them in line with their behavior (Steele & Liu, 1983). Reminding people of their central values eliminates this shift in beliefs, presumably by restoring the phenomenal experience of the self as morally and adaptively adequate (see Steele, 1988, for a discussion). Self-affirmation may reduce defensiveness and increase openness to negative or threatening information, thus facilitating learning; for example, self-affirmation tends to increase receptiveness to self-threatening health messages (Sherman, Nelson, & Steele, 2000). However, because the goal of self-affirmation is to restore the integrity of the self, self-affirmation may also enable people to live with negative aspects of the self, such as smoking in spite of its health risks. In other words, self-affirmation allows people to dismiss critical and important feedback that could otherwise aid them in learning and growing from experience (Tesser, 2000). Self-affirmation has another drawback—it keeps people focused on the question of whether the self is worthy, moral, and adequate. That is, it keeps the focus on the self and fails to provide an exit from the constant need to defend and maintain self-worth. Consequently, although self-affirmation may temporarily relieve defensiveness, it does not provide a long-term solution to the problem of defending the self from threats.

Noncontingent Self-Esteem

Another alternative is what Deci and Ryan (1995) call "true" self-esteem. This type of self-esteem is noncontingent because it is not vulnerable to threat and therefore does not need to be defended. According to Deci and Ryan (1995), true self-esteem is rooted in autonomous, efficacious action that occurs in the context of authentic relationships characterized by unconditional positive regard (Rogers, 1951). We suspect that few people have noncontingent self-esteem, at least in our North American culture that emphasizes the importance of self-esteem and the relative worth or value of one person over another based on their accomplishments, appearance, athletic skills, net worth, or good works. Indeed, in our study of college freshmen, only 4% of students scored 3 or lower (on a 1–7 scale) on all seven contingencies of self-worth we assessed, and these 4% may well have contingencies of self-worth that are not captured by our measure (Crocker, 2002). It may be possible to arrive at a spiritual or philosophical understanding that all people have worth, and this understanding may form the basis of noncontingent self-esteem. Our own intuition is that this would be a desirable state, if one could achieve it. Yet giving up one's contingencies may be as difficult as it is relieving, because these contingencies tend to

be learned at a young age and are reinforced over a lifetime of social experience.

Shifting Goals

Is it possible to respond to self-threats in a way that is not focused on maintaining, enhancing, and protecting self-esteem? Perhaps the most promising alternative is to shift away from self-focused, self-centered goals of maintaining and protecting self-esteem toward goals that connect the self to others in an altruistic, compassionate, and meaningful way. This perspective is aligned with self-determination theory (Ryan & Deci, 2000), in which people consciously choose to engage in behaviors based on intrinsic, integrated motivation rather than extrinsic, introjected reasons. However, not all intrinsically motivated behaviors will suffice for shifting away from the goal of self-esteem maintenance and protection; we believe that these goals must connect the self to others in a benevolent, compassionate way. Goals focused on giving to others facilitate keeping attention off the self and self-worth and provide a reason to persist even if one faces difficulty. For example, the goal of writing a manuscript because one wants to share one's discoveries with others keeps the self out of the process more effectively than the goal of writing a manuscript to become famous (Ryan, Sheldon, Kasser, & Deci, 1996).

Conclusion

The pursuit of self-esteem has become a central preoccupation in our society (Pyszczynski et al., 1997; Sheldon et al., 2001). Schools have devoted aspects of their curriculum to raising children's self-esteem (Dawes, 1994; Seligman, 1998), and most people organize their lives, in part, around activities, situations, and people that help to protect, maintain, and enhance their self-esteem. The idea that our worth as people is contingent, that it depends on our accomplishments, appearance, and deeds, is pervasive in our culture (Greenberg et al., 1986). In this chapter, we have tried to articulate how these contingencies of self-worth operate in our daily lives. We noted the high costs of pursuing self-esteem on our relationships with others, on our ability to learn from experiences, and on our mental and physical health. In closing, we want to emphasize again that the problem is not in *having* self-esteem—whether one's trait self-esteem is high or low. Rather, the problem is in *seeking* self-esteem—in all the things we do, large and small, that have as their primary goal maintaining and protecting self-worth. Instead of seeking self-esteem, pursuing goals that connect oneself with others or with the world in caring and compassionate ways may not only avoid the costs of seeking self-esteem but also facilitate the development of authentic relationships that may, in the end, be more sustaining than self-esteem.

Appendix 15.1. Highest-Loading Items from Each Subscale of the Contingencies of Self-Worth Scale

1. I feel worthwhile when I have God's love. (God's Love)
2. It is important to my self-worth to feel loved by my family. (Love and Support from Family)
3. Doing better than others gives me a sense of self-respect. (Competition)
4. My self-esteem depends on whether or not I follow my moral/ethical principles. (Virtue)
5. I don't care what other people think of me. (Others' Approval)
6. My sense of self-worth suffers whenever I think I don't look good. (Appearance)
7. I feel better about myself when I know I'm doing well academically (Academic Competence)

Note: The total scale has 65 items; it can be obtained from Jennifer Crocker.

References

Aberson, C. L., Healy, M., & Romero, V. (2000). Ingroup bias and self-esteem: A meta-analysis. *Personality and Social Psychology Review, 4,* 157–173.

Amabile, T. M. (1985). Motivation and creativity: Effects of motivational orientation on creative writers. *Journal of Personality and Social Psychology, 48,* 393–397.

Bandura, A. (1986). *Social foundations of thought and action: A social cognitive theory.* Englewood Cliffs, NJ: Prentice Hall.

Bandura, A. (1991). Self-regulation of motivation through anticipatory and self-regulatory mechanisms. In R. A.

Dienstbier (Ed.), *Nebraska Symposium on Motivation: Vol. 38. Perspectives on motivation* (pp. 69–164). Lincoln: University of Nebraska Press.

Barker, R., Dembo, T., & Lewin, K. (1941). *Frustration and aggression: An experiment with young children* (Vol. 18, no. 1). Iowa City: University of Iowa Press.

Bartholomew, K. (1990). Avoidance of intimacy: An attachment perspective. *Journal of Social and Personal Relationships, 7,* 147–178.

Baumeister, R. F. (1998). The self. In D. T. Gilbert, S. T. Fiske, & G. Lindzey (Eds.), *Handbook of social psychology* (4th ed., Vol. 2, pp. 680–740). New York: McGraw-Hill.

Baumeister, R. F., Bushman, B. J., & Campbell, W. K. (2000). Self-esteem, narcissism, and aggression: Does violence result from low self-esteem or from threatened egotism? *Current Directions in Psychological Science, 9,* 141–156.

Baumeister, R. F., Heatherton, T. F., & Tice, D. M. (1993). When ego threats lead to self-regulation failure: Negative consequences of high self-esteem. *Journal of Personality and Social Psychology, 64,* 141–156.

Baumeister, R. F., & Jones, E. E. (1978). When self-presentation is constrained by the target's knowledge: Consistency and compensation. *Journal of Personality and Social Psychology, 36,* 608–618.

Baumeister, R. F., & Leary, M. R. (1995). The need to belong: Desire for interpersonal attachments as a fundamental human motivation. *Psychological Bulletin, 111,* 497–529.

Baumeister, R. F., Smart, L., & Boden, J. M. (1996). Relation of threatened egotism to violence and aggression: The dark side of high self-esteem. *Psychological Review, 103,* 5–33.

Baumeister, R. F., Tice, D. M., & Hutton, D. G. (1989). Self-presentational motivations and personality differences in self-esteem. *Journal of Personality, 57,* 547–579.

Beauregard, K. S., & Dunning, D. (1998). Turning up the contrast: Self-enhancement motives prompt egocentric contrast effects in social judgments. *Journal of Personality and Social Psychology, 74,* 606–621.

Beck, A. T. (1983). Cognitive therapy of depression: New perspectives. In P. J. Clayton & J. E. Barrett (Eds.), *Treatment of depression: Old controversies and new approaches* (pp. 265–284). New York: Raven Press.

Bibring, E. (1953). The mechanism of depression. In P. Greenacre (Ed.), *Affective disorders* (pp. 13–48). New York: International Universities Press.

Blaine, B., & Crocker, J. (1993). Self-esteem and self-serving biases in reactions to positive and negative events: An integrative review. In R. F. Baumeister (Ed.), *Self-esteem: The puzzle of low self-regard* (pp. 55–85). Hillsdale, NJ: Erlbaum.

Blankenstein, K. R., Flett, G. L., Hewitt, P. L., & Eng, A. (1993). Dimensions of perfectionism and irrational fears: An examination of the fear survey schedule. *Personality and Individual Differences, 15,* 323–328.

Blatt, S. J., & Shichman, S. (1983). Two primary configurations in psychopathology. *Psychoanalysis and Contemporary Thought, 6,* 187–254.

Bowlby, J. (1969). *Attachment and loss: Vol. 1. Attachment.* New York: Basic Books.

Bradley, G. W. (1978). Self-serving biases in the attribution process: A reexamination of the fact or fiction question. *Journal of Personality and Social Psychology, 36,* 56–71.

Brandstadter, J., & Greve, W. (1994). The aging self: Stabilizing and protective processes. *Developmental Review, 14,* 52–80.

Brockner, J. (1984). Low self-esteem and behavioral plasticity: Some implications of personality and social psychology. In L. Wheeler (Ed.), *Review of personality and social psychology* (Vol. 4, pp. 237–271). Beverly Hills, CA: Sage.

Brockner, J., Derr, W. R., & Laing, W. N. (1987). Self-esteem and reactions to negative feedback: Toward greater generalizability. *Journal of Research in Personality, 21,* 318–333.

Brown, J., Dutton, K. A., & Cook, K. E. (2001). From the top down: Self-esteem and self-evaluation. *Cognition and Emotion, 15,* 615–631.

Brownell, K. D. (1991). Dieting and the search for the perfect body: Where physiology and culture collide. *Behavior Therapy, 22,* 1–12.

Bruch, H. (1978). *The golden cage: The enigma of anorexia nervosa.* New York: Vintage.

Brunstein, J. C., & Gollwitzer, P. M. (1996). Effects of failure on subsequent performance: The importance of self-defining goals. *Journal of Personality and Social Psychology, 70,* 395–407.

Burhans, K. K., & Dweck, C. S. (1995). Helplessness in early childhood: The role of contingent worth. *Child Development, 66,* 1719–1738.

Bushman, B. J., & Baumeister, R. F. (1998). Threatened egotism, narcissism, self-esteem, and direct and displaced aggression: Does self-love or self-hate lead to violence? *Journal of Personality and Social Psychology, 75,* 219–229.

Camp, D. E., Klesges, R. C., & Relyea, G. (1993). The relationship between body weight concerns and adolescent smoking. *Health Psychology, 12,* 24–32.

Campbell, J. D., & Lavallee, L. F. (1993). Who am I? The role of self-concept confusion in understanding the behavior of people with low self-esteem. In R. F. Baumeister (Ed.), *Self-esteem: The puzzle of low self-regard* (pp. 3–20). New York: Plenum Press.

Cantor, N., & Norem, J. K. (1989). Defensive pessimism and stress and coping. *Social Cognition, 7,* 92–112.

Cantor, N., Norem, J. K., Langston, C., Zirkel, S., Fleeson, W., & Cook-Flannagan, C. (1991). Life tasks and daily life experience. *Journal of Personality, 59,* 425–451.

Carstensen, L. L., & Freund, A. M. (1994). The resilience of the aging self. *Developmental Review, 14,* 81–92.

Cohen, S., Sherrod, D. R., & Clark, M. S. (1986). Social skills and the stress-protective role of social support. *Journal of Personality and Social Psychology, 50,* 963–973.

Collins, N. L., & Feeney, B. (2000). A safe haven: An attachment theory perspective on support seeking and care giving in close relationships. *Journal of Personality and Social Psychology, 78,* 1053–1073.

Covington, M. V. (1984). The self-worth theory of achievement motivation: Findings and implications. *Elementary School Journal, 85,* 5–20.

Crocker, J. (1993). Memory for information about others: Effects of self-esteem and performance feedback. *Journal of Research in Personality, 27*(1), 35–48.

Crocker, J. (2002). Contingencies of self-worth: Implications for self-regulation and psychological vulnerability. *Self and Identity, 1,* 143–149.

Crocker, J., & Luhtanen, R. (1990). Collective self-esteem and ingroup bias. *Journal of Personality and Social Psychology, 58,* 60–67.

Crocker, J., & Luhtanen, R. K. (2002). *Level of self-esteem and contingencies of self-worth: Unique effects on academic, social, and financial problems in college freshmen.* Manuscript under review.

Crocker, J., Luhtanen, R. K., & Bouvrette, S. (2001). *Contingencies of self-worth in college students: The CSW-65 scale.* Manuscript under review.

Crocker, J., & Major, B. (1989). Social stigma and self-esteem: The self-protective properties of stigma. *Psychological Review, 96,* 608–630.

Crocker, J., Sommers, S. R., & Luhtanen, R. K. (in press). Hopes dashed and dreams fulfilled: Contingencies of self-worth and admissions to graduate school. *Personality and Social Psychology Bulletin.*

Crocker, J., Thompson, L., McGraw, K., & Ingerman, C. (1987). Downward comparison, prejudice, and evaluation of others: Effects of self-esteem and threat. *Journal of Personality and Social Psychology, 52,* 907–916.

Crocker, J., & Wolfe, C. T. (2001). Contingencies of self-worth. *Psychological Review, 108,* 593–623.

Dawes, R. M. (1994). *House of cards: Psychology and psychotherapy built on myth.* New York: Free Press.

Deci, E. L., Nezlek, J., & Sheinman, L. (1981). Characteristics of the rewarder and intrinsic motivation of the rewardee. *Journal of Personality and Social Psychology, 40,* 1–10.

Deci, E. L., & Ryan, R. M. (1991). A motivational approach to self: Integration in personality. In R. Dienstbier (Ed.), *Nebraska symposium on Motivation: Vol. 38. Perspectives on motivation* (pp. 237–288). Lincoln: University of Nebraska Press.

Deci, E. L., & Ryan, R. M. (1995). Human autonomy: The basis for true self-esteem. In M. H. Kernis (Ed.), *Efficacy, agency, and self-esteem* (pp. 31–49). New York: Plenum Press.

Deci, E. L., Vallerand, R. J., Pelletier, L. G., & Ryan, R. M. (1991). Motivation and education: The self-determination perspective. *Educational Psychologist, 26,* 325–346.

Deci, E. M., & Ryan, R. M. (2000). The "what" and "why" of goal pursuits: Human needs and the self-determination of behavior. *Psychological Inquiry, 11,* 227–268.

Emmons, R. A. (1991). Personal strivings, daily life events, and psychological and physical well-being. *Journal of Personality, 59,* 453–472.

Faber, P. D., Khavari, K. A., & Douglass, F. M. I. (1980). A factor analytic study of reasons for drinking: Empirical validation of positive and negative reinforcement dimensions. *Journal of Consulting and Clinical Psychology, 48,* 780–781.

Fein, S., & Spencer, S. J. (1997). Prejudice as self-image maintenance: Affirming the self through derogating others. *Journal of Personality and Social Psychology, 73,* 31–44.

Frey, D. (1978). Reactions to success and failure in public and private conditions. *Journal of Experimental Social Psychology, 14,* 172–179.

Frost, R. O., Marten, P., Lahart, C., & Rosenblate, R.

(1990). The dimensions of perfectionism. *Cognitive Therapy and Research, 14,* 449–468.

Geller, J., Johnston, C., & Madsen, K. (1997). The role of shape and weight in self-concept: The shape and weight based self-esteem inventory. *Cognitive Therapy and Research, 21,* 5–24.

Geller, J., Johnston, C., Madsen, K., Goldner, E. M., Remick, R. A., & Birmingham, C. L. (1998). Shape- and weight-based self-esteem and the eating disorders. *International Journal of Eating Disorders, 24,* 285–298.

Gollwitzer, P. M., & Wicklund, R. (1985). Self-symbolizing and the neglect of others' perspectives. *Journal of Personality and Social Psychology, 43,* 702–715.

Gollwitzer, P. M., Wicklund, R. A., & Hilton, J. L. (1982). Admission of failure and symbolic self-completion: Extending Lewinian theory. *Journal of Personality and Social Psychology, 43,* 358–371.

Greenberg, J., & Pyszczynski, T. (1985). Compensatory self-inflation: A response to the threat to self-regard of public failure. *Journal of Personality and Social Psychology, 49,* 273–280.

Greenberg, J., Pyszczynski, T., & Solomon, S. (1982). The self-serving attributional bias: Beyond self-presentation. *Journal of Experimental Social Psychology, 18,* 56–67.

Greenberg, J., Pyszczynski, T., & Solomon, S. (1986). The causes and consequences of the need for self-esteem: A terror management theory. In R. F. Baumeister (Ed.), *Public self and private self* (pp. 189–207). New York: Springer-Verlag.

Greenier, K. D., Kernis, M. H., McNamara, C. W., Waschull, S. B., Berry, A. J., Herlocker, C. E., & Abend, T. A. (1999). Individual differences in reactivity to daily events: Examining the roles of stability and level of self-esteem. *Journal of Personality, 67,* 185–208.

Heatherton, T. F., & Vohs, K. D. (2000). Interpersonal evaluations following threat to self. *Journal of Personality and Social Psychology, 78,* 725–736.

Heine, S. J., Lehman, D. R., Markus, H. R., & Kitayama, S. (1999). Is there a universal need for positive self-regard? *Psychological Review, 106,* 766–795.

Higgins, E. T. (1987). Self-discrepancy: A theory relating self to affect. *Psychological Review, 94,* 319–340.

Higgins, E. T. (1998). Promotion and prevention: Regulatory focus as a motivational principle. In M. P. Zanna (Ed.), *Advances in experimental social psychology* (Vol. 30, pp. 1–46). New York: Academic Press.

James, W. (1890). *The principles of psychology.* Cambridge, MA: Harvard University Press.

Jonah, B. A. (1990). Age differences in risky driving. *Health Education Research, 5,* 139–149.

Kernis, M. H., & Waschull, S. B. (1995). The interactive roles of stability and level of self-esteem: Research and theory. In M. P. Zanna (Ed.), *Advances in experimental social psychology* (Vol. 27, pp. 93–141). San Diego, CA: Academic Press.

Kernis, M. H., Whisenhunt, C. R., Waschull, S. B., Greenier, K. D., Berry, A. J., Herlocker, C. E., & Anderson, C. A. (1998). Multiple facets of self-esteem and their relations to depressive symptoms. *Personality and Social Psychology Bulletin, 24,* 657–668.

Kihlstrom, J. F., & Cantor, N. E. (1988). Information processing and the study of the self. In L. Berkowitz (Ed.), *Advances in experimental social psychology* (Vol. 21, pp. 145–178). San Diego, CA: Academic Press.

Kihlstrom, J. F., & Hastie, R. (1997). Mental representations of persons and personality. In L. Pervin (Ed.), *Handbook of personality psychology* (pp. 711–735). San Diego, CA: Academic Press.

Kolditz, T. A., & Arkin, R. M. (1982). An impression management interpretation of the self-handicapping strategy. *Journal of Personality and Social Psychology, 43,* 492–502.

Kulik, J., & Brown, R. (1979). Frustration, attribution of blame, and aggression. *Journal of Experimental Social Psychology, 15,* 183–194.

Larsen, R. J., & Diener, E. (1992). Promises and problems with the circumplex model of emotion. In M. S. Clark (Ed.), *Review of personality and social psychology: Emotion* (Vol. 13, pp. 25–59). Newbury Park, CA: Sage.

Lavallee, L. F., & Campbell, J. D. (1995). Impact of personal goals on self-regulation processes elicited by daily negative events. *Journal of Personality and Social Psychology, 69,* 341–352.

Leary, M. R., & Baumeister, R. F. (2000). The nature and function of self-esteem: Sociometer theory. In M. Zanna (Ed.), *Advances in experimental social psychology* (Vol. 32, pp. 1–62). San Diego, CA: Academic Press.

Leary, M. R., & Jones, J. L. (1993). The social psychology of tanning and sunscreen use: Self-presentational motives as a predictor of health risk. *Journal of Applied Social Psychology, 23,* 1390–1406.

Leary, M. R., Tambor, E. S., Terdal, S. K., & Downs, D. L. (1995). Self-esteem as an interpersonal monitor: The sociometer hypothesis. *Journal of Personality and Social Psychology, 68,* 518–530.

Leary, M. R., Tchividjian, L. R., & Kraxberger, B. E. (1994). Self-presentation can be hazardous to your health: Impression management and health risk. *Health Psychology, 13,* 461–470.

Levine, S. R., Wyer, R. S., Jr., & Schwarz, N. (1994). Are you what you feel? The affective and cognitive determinants of self-judgments. *European Journal of Social Psychology, 24,* 63–77.

Lewis, M. (2000). Self-conscious emotions: Embarrassment, pride, shame, and guilt. In M. Lewis & J. M. Haviland-Jones (Eds.), *Handbook of emotions* (2nd ed., pp. 623–636). New York: Guilford Press.

Lissner, L., Odell, P. M., D'Agostino, R. B., Stokes, J., Kreger, B. E., Belanger, A. J., & Brownell, K. D. (1991). Variability in body weight and health outcomes in Framingham population. *New England Journal of Medicine, 324,* 1839–1844.

Major, B., & Schmader, T. (1998). Coping with stigma through psychological disengagement. In J. Swim & C. Stangor (Eds.), *Prejudice: The target's perspective* (pp. 219–241). San Diego, CA: Academic Press.

Major, B., Spencer, S., Schmader, T., Wolfe, C., & Crocker, J. (1998). Coping with negative stereotypes about intellectual performance: The role of psychological disengagement. *Personality and Social Psychology Bulletin, 24,* 34–50.

McFarland, C., & Ross, M. (1982). Impact of causal attributions on affective reactions to success and failure. *Journal of Personality and Social Psychology, 43,* 937–946.

Merton, R. K. (1948). The self-fulfilling prophecy. *Antioch Review, 8,* 193–210.

Miller, D. T., & Ross, M. (1975). Self-serving biases in attribution of causality: Fact or fiction? *Psychological Bulletin, 82*, 213–225.

Moretti, M. M., & Higgins, E. T. (1990). The development of self-system vulnerabilities: Social and cognitive factors in developmental psychopathology. In R. J. Sternberg (Ed.), *Competence considered* (pp. 286–314). New Haven, CT: Yale University Press.

Murray, S. L., Holmes, J. G., & Griffin, D. W. (1996). The self-fulfilling nature of positive illusions in romantic relationships: Love is not blind, but prescient. *Journal of Personality and Social Psychology, 71*, 1155–1180.

Murray, S. L., Holmes, J. G., MacDonald, G., & Ellsworth, P. C. (1998). Through the looking glass darkly? When self-doubts turn into relationship insecurities. *Journal of Personality and Social Psychology, 75*(6), 1459–1480.

Norem, J. K., & Cantor, N. (1986a). Anticipatory and post hoc cushioning strategies: Optimism and defensive pessimism in "risky" situations. *Cognitive Therapy and Research, 10*, 347–362.

Norem, J. K., & Cantor, N. (1986b). Defensive pessimism: Harnessing anxiety as motivation. *Journal of Personality and Social Psychology, 51*, 1208–1217.

Pyszczynski, T. (1982). Cognitive strategies for coping with uncertain outcomes. *Journal of Research in Personality, 16*, 386–399.

Pyszczynski, T., & Greenberg, J. (1987). Self-regulatory perseveration and the depressive self-focusing style: A self-awareness theory of reactive depression. *Psychological Bulletin, 102*, 122–138.

Pyszczynski, T., Greenberg, J., & Holt, K. (1985). Maintaining consistency between self-serving beliefs and available data: A bias in information evaluation following success and failure. *Personality and Social Psychology Bulletin, 11*, 179–190.

Pyszczynski, T., Greenberg, J., & Laprelle, J. (1985). Social comparison after success and failure: Biased search for information consistent with a self-serving conclusion. *Journal of Experimental Social Psychology, 21*, 195–211.

Pyszczynski, T., Greenberg, J., & Solomon, S. (1997). Why do we need what we need? A terror management perspective on the roots of human social motivation. *Psychological Inquiry, 8*, 1–20.

Roberts, J. E., & Gotlib, I. H. (1997). Temporal variability in global self-esteem and specific self-evaluation as prospective predictors of emotional distress: Specificity in predictors and outcome. *Journal of Abnormal Psychology, 106*(4), 521–529.

Roberts, J. E., & Kassel, J. D. (1997). Labile self-esteem, life stress, and depressive symptoms: Prospective data testing a model of vulnerability. *Cognitive Therapy and Research, 21*, 569–589.

Roberts, J. E., Kassel, J. D., & Gotlib, I. H. (1995). Level and stability of self-esteem as predictors of depressive symptoms. *Personality and Individual Differences, 19*, 217–224.

Robins, R. W., & Beer, J. S. (2001). Positive illusions about the self: Short-term benefits and long-term costs. *Journal of Personality and Social Psychology, 80*, 340–352.

Rogers, C. R. (1951). *Client-centered therapy.* New York: Houghton Mifflin.

Rosenberg, M. (1965). *Society and the adolescent self-image.* Princeton, NJ: Princeton University Press.

Rosenberg, M. (1979). *Conceiving the self.* New York: Basic Books.

Ross, L., & Nisbett, R. E. (1991). *The person and the situation: Perspectives of social psychology.* Philadelphia: Temple University Press.

Ryan, R. M., & Deci, E. L. (2000). Self-determination theory and the facilitation of intrinsic motivation, social development, and well-being. *American Psychologist, 55*, 68–78.

Ryan, R. M., Sheldon, K. M., Kasser, T., & Deci, E. L. (1996). All goals are not created equal: An organismic perspective on the nature of goals and their regulation. In P. M. Gollwitzer & J. A. Bargh (Eds.), *The psychology of action: Linking cognition and motivation to behavior* (pp. 7–26). New York: Guilford Press.

Ryff, C. D. (1995). Psychological well-being in adult life. *Psychological Science, 4*, 99–104.

Schlenker, B. R., & Leary, M. R. (1982). Social anxiety and self-presentation: A conceptualization and model. *Psychological Bulletin, 92*, 641–669.

Schrof, J. M. (1992, June 1). Pumped up. *U. S. News and World Report*, pp. 55–63.

Seligman, M. E. P. (1998). The American way of blame. *APA Monitor, 29*, 4.

Shaver, P. R., Schwarz, J., Kirson, D., & O'Connor, C. (1987). Emotion knowledge: Further exploration of a prototype approach. *Journal of Personality and Social Psychology, 52*, 1061–1086.

Sheldon, K., Elliot, A. J., Kim, Y., & Kasser, T. (2001). What is satisfying about satisfying events? Testing 10 candidate psychological needs. *Journal of Personality and Social Psychology, 80*, 325–339.

Sherman, D. A., Nelson, L. D., & Steele, C. M. (2000). Do messages on health threaten the self? Increasing the acceptance of threatening health messages via self-affirmation. *Personality and Social Psychology Bulletin, 26*, 1046–1058.

Shrauger, J. S. (1975). Responses to evaluation as a function of initial self-perceptions. *Psychological Bulletin, 82*, 581–596.

Snyder, M. (1984). When belief creates reality. In L. Berkowitz (Ed.), *Advances in experimental social psychology* (Vol. 18, pp. 238–305). Orlando, FL: Academic Press.

Solomon, S., Greenberg, J., & Pyszczynski, T. (1991). Terror management theory of self-esteem. In C. R. Snyder & D. Forsyth (Eds.), *Handbook of social and clinical psychology: The health perspective* (pp. 21–40). New York: Pergamon.

Sommers, S., & Crocker, J. (2000, February). *The real world: How contingencies of self-esteem affect reactions to daily life.* Paper presented at the annual meeting of the Society for Personality and Social Psychology, Nashville, TN.

Spencer, S. J., Fein, S., Wolfe, C. T., Fong, C., & Dunn, M. A. (1998). Automatic activation of stereotypes: The role of self-image threat. *Personality and Social Psychology Bulletin, 24*, 1139–1152.

Spencer, S. J., & Quinn, D. M. (1995, August). *Stereotype threat and women's math performance: The mediating role of anxiety.* Paper presented at the annual meeting of the American Psychological Association, New York.

Steele, C. (1988). The psychology of self-affirmation: Sustaining the integrity of the self. In L. Berkowitz (Ed.),

Advances in experimental social psychology (Vol. 21, pp. 261–302). New York: Academic Press.

Steele, C. M. (1992, April). Race and the schooling of black Americans. *Atlantic, 269,* 68–78.

Steele, C. M. (1997). A threat in the air: How stereotypes shape intellectual identity and performance. *American Psychologist, 52,* 613–629.

Steele, C. M., & Aronson, J. (1998). Stereotype threat and the test performance of academically successful African Americans. In C. Jencks & M. Phillips (Eds.), *The Black–white test score gap* (pp. 401–427). Washington, DC: Brookings Institution.

Steele, C. M., & Liu, T. J. (1983). Dissonance processes as self-affirmation. *Journal of Personality and Social Psychology, 45,* 5–19.

Stone, J., Lynch, C. I., Sjomeling, M., & Darley, J. M. (1999). Stereotype threat effects on black and white athletic performance. *Journal of Personality and Social Psychology, 77,* 1213–1227.

Tangney, J. P., Wagner, P. E., Hill-Barlow, D., Marschall, D. E., & Gramzow, R. (1996). Relation of shame and guilt to constructive versus destructive responses to anger across the lifespan. *Journal of Personality and Social Psychology, 70,* 797–809.

Taylor, S. E., & Crocker, J. (1981). Schematic bases of social information processing. In E. T. Higgins, C. P. Herman, & M. P. Zanna (Ed.), *Social cognition* (pp. 89–134). Hillsdale, NJ: Erlbaum.

Tesser, A. (1988). Toward a self-evaluation maintenance model of social behavior. In L. Berkowitz (Ed.), *Advances in experimental social psychology* (Vol. 21, pp. 181–227). San Diego, CA: Academic Press.

Tesser, A. (2000). On the confluence of self-esteem maintenance mechanisms. *Personality and Social Psychology Review, 4,* 290–299.

Tice, D. M. (1991). Esteem protection or enhancement? Self-handicapping motives and attributions differ by trait self-esteem. *Journal of Personality and Social Psychology, 60,* 711–725.

Tice, D. M. (1993). The social motivations of people with low self-esteem. In R. Baumeister (Ed.), *Self-esteem: The puzzle of low self-regard* (pp. 37–54). Hillsdale, NJ: Erlbaum.

Weinstein, H. M., & Richman, A. (1984). The group treatment of bulimia. *Journal of American College Health, 32,* 208–215.

White, R. W. (1959). Motivation reconsidered: The concept of competence. *Psychological Review, 66,* 297–333.

Wicklund, R. A. (1982). *Symbolic self-completion.* Hillsdale, NJ: Erlbaum.

Wills, T. A. (1981). Downward comparison principles in social psychology. *Psychological Bulletin, 90,* 245–271.

Wolfe, C. T., & Crocker, J. (2002). What does the self want? A contingencies of self-worth perspective on motivation. In S. S. Z. Kunda (Ed.), *The Ontario Symposium: Goals and motivated cognition* (pp. 147–170). Hillsdale, NJ: Erlbaum.

Wood, J. V., Giordano-Beech, M., & Ducharme, M. J. (1999). Compensating for failure through social comparison. *Personality and Social Psychology Bulletin, 25,* 1370–1386.

16

Freedom versus Fear: On the Defense, Growth, and Expansion of the Self

TOM PYSZCZYNSKI
JEFF GREENBERG
JAMIE L. GOLDENBERG

This handbook is full of theories and research programs concerning the nature, operation, and defense of self and identity. This important work addresses questions such as how the self is constructed, how it changes, and how people defend aspects of self and identity. In this chapter, we focus more on *why* than *how*—why the self evolved, what functions it serves, why it must be defended, and how growth of the self is possible. To address these questions, we take an existential perspective that starts by positing that human beings are animals, living organisms in a seemingly purposeless universe, material transient beings struggling to eat, survive, and procreate, but fated to die, and, most importantly, painfully aware of this inevitable reality. This is equally true of Tiger Woods, Mother Teresa, Nelson Mandela, Julia Roberts, and Pope John Paul II; even we, the humble authors of this chapter; even you, the reader.

From this perspective, each individual's self and identity, goals and aspirations, occupations and titles, are humanly created adornments, disguises draped over an animal that is no more unique or significant than any individual cockroach, kangaroo, or kumquat. We suggest that the fundamental psychological motives that are served by this elaborate drapery of symbolic meaning are derived from even more fundamental animal motives. Perhaps the most basic of these motives are the evolved propensities for organismic preservation and for organismic expansion. These propensities are adaptive because they motivate animals both to defend against dangers, allowing them to stay alive long enough to procreate and pass on their genes, and to expand their capacities, facilitating development of skills to function effectively in their environments.

The history of psychological thinking about human motivation is replete with theories positing these two types of motives. Freud posited that humans were driven by a pleasure principle but also by a reality principle that protects the organism by steering it clear of displeasure (Freud, 1920/1950, 1930/1961). Maslow (1970) proposed deficit motives that serve survival and being motives that facilitate the expansion of the self. Rank explained how fears of life and death drive attachment and how a life force drives individuation and creativity (1930/1998, 1932/1989). Lewin (1935) wrote of approach and avoidance motives; his work is echoed in that of Higgins (1997) on prevention versus promotion regulatory focus. Atkinson (1964) proposed that two motives drive human achievement—a need for achievement and a fear of failure. For the most part, however, theorists and researchers have focused on one or the other of these motives without exploring their complex interplay. For example, theorists following the psychoanalytic tradition have focused primarily on defense of the self, and humanistic psychologists have focused primarily on expansion and actualization of the self.

We think that both traditions capture part of the truth concerning human motivation. In this chapter we explore the integration of these two motive systems—defense of the self and expansion of the self—building on the earlier work of Otto Rank (e.g., 1930/1998, 1936/1976), who influenced both traditions, and Ernest Becker (e.g., 1971, 1973), who was influenced by them. In contemporary social psychology, the two empirically based theories that most clearly follow in these traditions are terror management theory (psychoanalytic) and self-determination theory (humanistic). We lean heavily on these theories as the primary vehicles to achieve this integrated view of the basic motives of the self.

Terror management theory (TMT; Greenberg, Pyszczynski, & Solomon, 1986; Solomon, Greenberg, & Pyszczynski, 1991) views the self as an essentially defensive construction that functions to protect people from a deeply rooted fear of death that is an inherent by-product of the sophisticated cognitive abilities that make us human. Self-determination theory (SDT; Deci & Ryan, 1991, 2000) views the self as an inherently growth-oriented organismic structure that integrates new experiences with existing cognitive structures to produce an expanding repertoire of possibilities and potential. Although these theories may seem to paint dramatically different pictures of the role of self in human affairs, we believe that by specifying how the defensive motives emphasized by TMT and the acquisitive motives emphasized by SDT interact, a more comprehensive and well-rounded understanding of human behavior can be achieved.

Although these two motive systems operate according to very different principles, and sometimes (though not always) orient the individual toward very different goals, human behavior results from the dialectic interplay between them. To elucidate this interplay, we outline our conceptualization of the workings of these two systems, consider how each system can facilitate and interfere with the other, and discuss ways in which defensive needs can be served while allowing the individuals to optimize their creative potential and freedom.

Overview of Terror Management Theory and Research

Terror Management Theory

A wide array of theories and research programs (e.g., Adler, 1928; Allport, 1937; Horney, 1937; James, 1890; Maslow, 1970; Rank, 1959; Rogers, 1959; Rosenberg, 1965; Steele, 1988; Tesser, 1988; Wicklund & Gollwitzer, 1981) assert that the valuing and preservation of self are of great importance to people. TMT was developed to explain why these needs are so central and posits that they are an outgrowth of the desire for organismic preservation. Although one could argue that once the self evolved and became the individual's primary locus of concern, symbolic threats became more important than physical ones, the one ultimate and inevitable threat to the self, as well as the organism, is physical death. Indeed, George Kelly (1955) argued that death is the paradigmatic threat to the individual's construct (self) system. Evolutionary philosopher Suzanne K. Langer (1982, pp. 87, 90) put it this way:

> And with the rise and gradual conception of the "self" as the source of personal autonomy comes, of course, the knowledge of its limit—the ultimate prospect of death. The effect of this intellectual advance is momentous. Each

person's deepest emotional concern henceforth shifts to his own life, which he knows cannot be indefinitely preserved ... as a naked fact that realization is unacceptable.

TMT focuses on the defenses that humankind erected to cope with this most basic of all threats.

The ideas on which TMT builds reflect a long intellectual tradition that dates back at least to Plato, Aristotle, and other Greek philosophers and continues through the thinking of Pascal, Kierkegaard, Nietzsche, Freud, and Rank, in attempting to explain diverse forms of human behavior as resulting from the existential dilemma into which our species was born. The theory was most directly inspired by the work of cultural anthropologist Ernest Becker (e.g., 1971, 1973), whose life work focused on synthesizing ideas from the various social sciences and humanities to formulate what he hoped would become "a general science of man." Since its inception in 1986, TMT has been applied to a diverse array of social psychological phenomena, including altruism, aggression, attitude change, anxiety disorders, conformity, creativity, cultural pride and guilt, depression, ingroup favoritism, moral judgments, prejudice, reverence toward cultural icons, romantic relationships, risk taking, disgust, sexual ambivalence, objectification of women, and sports team affiliations (for reviews, see Goldenberg, Pyszczynski, Greenberg, & Solomon, 2000; Greenberg, Solomon, & Pyszczynski, 1997). Put simply, TMT argues that much human behavior is driven by the pursuit of meaning in life and value in oneself and that these two abstract psychological entities are sought because of the protection they provide against deeply rooted existential fears that are inherent in the human condition.

More specifically, TMT posits that the juxtaposition of an instinctive desire for life with the uniquely human awareness of the inevitability of death gave rise to the potential for paralyzing terror. Our species fashioned a partial solution to this problem by using the same sophisticated cognitive capacities that gave rise to existential terror to create cultural worldviews: shared symbolic conceptions of reality that (1) give meaning, order, and permanence to existence, (2) provide a set of standards for what is valuable, and (3) promise safety and either literal or symbolic immortality to those who believe in the cultural worldview and live up to its standards of value.

Literal immortality is provided by the explicitly religious aspects of cultural worldviews that directly address the problem of death by promising heaven, reincarnation, nirvana, or other forms of afterlife to those who live up to a particular religion's teachings and standards. Symbolic immortality is provided by cultural institutions and achievements that enable us to feel part of something larger, more significant, and more enduring than our own individual lives, such as families, nations, professions, or ideological groups. Our security is thus sustained by a cultural anxiety buffer that consists of faith in the validity of one's cultural worldview and belief that one is living up to the standards of value that are part of that worldview. Psychological equanimity results from the feeling that one is a valuable contributor to a meaningful universe—a sense that one's life has both meaning and value.

This implies that one's sense of personal value is highly dependent on the cultural worldview to which one subscribes. Thus, depending on the precepts of one's worldview, any given behavior could increase, decrease, or have no effect on self-esteem. The September 11, 2001, terrorist attacks on the World Trade Center and the Pentagon provided a particularly dramatic example. Most readers would probably view people who hijack airplanes and crash them into skyscrapers for the purpose of killing the thousands of people inside in the most negative terms imaginable. But how such behavior is viewed really depends entirely on the dictates of one's worldview; although most Americans saw these events as horrific, evil acts of cruelty committed by cowardly madmen, the terrorists and their supporters saw them as heroic acts in the service of a great cause that would ensure them certain death transcendence. From the perspective of TMT, self-esteem is inextricably tied to the cultural context within which the individual is acting.

Although we use the term "cultural worldview" to emphasize the cultural origins of the individual's security-providing conception of reality, TMT posits that each individual abstracts his or her own individualized worldview from the various conceptions of reality espoused by the many socializing influences to which he or she is exposed. Generally, these worldviews are derived from and sustained by parents, teachers, religious and spiritual authorities, and cultural institutions and rituals. Whereas some individuals absorb the core values of their mainstream culture in a seemingly wholesale fashion with little questioning or conflict, others creatively combine a broad range of diverse influences, sometimes with a great deal of inner turmoil and soul searching. Previous statements of TMT have not explicitly addressed the question of how individuals abstract their own individualized worldviews. The present chapter addresses this question by drawing heavily from SDT ideas and integrating them with TMT principles.

Empirical Evidence

To date, well over 130 separate experiments, conducted in nine different countries, have provided support for TMT hypotheses. Most of these studies have tested college students in North America and Europe, but others have examined Israeli soldiers and children, adults walking down city streets, municipal court judges, and members of traditional aboriginal culture in the Australian outback. Although a thorough review of this research would be beyond the scope of this chapter, we briefly summarize the most relevant evidence below.

Anxiety Buffer Hypothesis

Some of the earliest TMT research tested the hypothesis that self-esteem serves a general anxiety-buffering function. This hypothesis was first proposed by Becker (1962) and is a central derivation from this theoretical perspective. By adding ad hoc assumptions, it is conceivable that other views of self-esteem might be able to generate this hypothesis post hoc, but none of them ever considered this possibility except in reaction to the terror management research supporting it. In the initial test of this hypothesis, Greenberg and colleagues (1992) demonstrated that boosting self-esteem with positive feedback on a personality test led to lower levels of self-reported anxiety in response to graphic video depictions of death; two subsequent studies showed that success on a supposed IQ test led to lower levels of physiological arousal in response to the threat of painful electric shock.[1]

Additional support for this hypothesis was provided by Greenberg and colleagues (1993), who showed that both experimentally enhanced and dispositionally high levels of self-esteem led to lower levels of defensive distortions to deny one's vulnerability to an early death. Similarly, Sherman, Nelson, and Steele (2000) have shown that self-affirmations can reduce denial of one's vulnerability to serious health risks. Finally, Harmon-Jones, Simon, Greenberg, Pyszczynski, and Solomon (1997) and Arndt and Greenberg (1999) showed that dispositionally high or temporarily raised self-esteem more generally reduces defensive responses to reminders of death.

Mortality Salience Worldview Defense Hypothesis

The majority of TMT research has been focused on the hypothesis that reminders of mortality intensify defense of one's cultural worldview. To the extent that the worldview component of the cultural anxiety buffer is maintained through a process of social consensus, this implies that mortality salience should lead to especially positive reactions to anyone or anything that validates one's worldview and especially negative reactions to anyone or anything that challenges it. Consistent with this reasoning, research has shown that reminders of mortality lead to: (1) harsher judgments of moral transgressors and more favorable judgments of those who uphold moral principles (e.g., Florian & Mikulincer, 1997), (2) increased attraction to those who explicitly praise aspects of the cultural worldview and decreased attraction to those who criticize it (e.g., Greenberg et al., 1990), (3) ingroup favoritism, behavioral avoidance of outgroup members, stereotyping, and prejudice (e.g., Ochsmann & Reichelt, 1994), (4) discomfort when performing behavior that violates cultural standards (Greenberg, Simon, Porteus, Solomon, & Pyszczynski, 1995), (5) heightened conformity to cultural standards, especially those that have been recently primed (Greenberg, Simon, Pyszczynski, Solomon, & Chatel, 1992), (6) increased perceptions of social consensus for one's attitudes, especially when one is in the minority (e.g., Pyszczynski et al., 1996), and (7) aggression against those who challenge one's beliefs (H. McGregor et al., 1998).

Mortality Salience Self-Esteem Hypothesis

Other research has supported the hypothesis that reminders of mortality increase self-esteem striving and defense. Specifically, mortality salience has been found to: (1) increase identification with aspects of self that provide self-esteem and disidentification with aspects of self that threaten self-esteem (e.g., Goldenberg, McCoy, Pyszczynski, Greenberg, & Solomon, 2000); (2) increase the perception of oneself as similar to or different from others (cf., Brewer, 1991), depending on whether the view of self as unique or similar has recently been threatened (Simon et al., 1997); (3) increase identification with one's ingroup when positive aspects of the ingroup have been primed and decrease identification with one's ingroup when negative aspects of the ingroup have been primed (e.g., Dechesne, Greenberg, Arndt, & Schimel, 2000); (4) increase risk taking when riskiness is valued as a source of self-esteem (Taubman Ben-Ari, Florian, & Mikulincer, 1999); (5) increase romantic attraction among those with secure attachment styles and decrease romantic attachment among those with insecure styles (Mikulincer & Florian, 2000); and (6) increase helping for worldview-consistent causes (Jonas, Schimel, Greenberg, & Pyszczynski, in press).

Specificity to Death-Related Thought

TMT was designed to help explain why people defend their belief systems and reject those who espouse different belief systems and why people defend their self-esteem. Threats to cherished beliefs and self-worth should intensify defense of those structures, but if death concerns underlie these defenses, then mere reminders of mortality should do so as well, whereas the mere reminder of other aversive events should not. That is what most terror management research has

shown. In fact, in this research, thoughts of other aversive or anxiety-provoking events, including physical pain, failing an exam, giving a speech in front of a large audience, general worries, being socially excluded, or being paralyzed often do produce emotional reactions, but they do not produce parallel effects on behavior relevant to self-esteem or one's cultural worldview.[2] In these studies, death reminders have been operationalized in a variety of ways, including open-ended and true–false questions about death, films of gory automobile accidents, subliminal presentation of the words "dead" or "death," and proximity to a funeral home. The consistent findings across this wide variety of comparison conditions and operationalizations of mortality salience provide strong evidence for the unique psychological import of death-related thought. An additional body of work has documented that these effects are triggered specifically by the heightened accessibility of death-related thought outside of conscious awareness (for a review, see Pyszczynski, Greenberg, & Solomon, 1999).

Immortality Salience Hypothesis

Recent research has tested a new hypothesis concerning mortality and self-esteem. To the extent that increased pursuit of self-esteem and faith in one's cultural worldview in response to reminders of death function to quell concerns about one's mortality, defusing the threatening nature of death by convincing participants of the existence of some form of afterlife should reduce or eliminate such effects. Dechesne and colleagues (2001) tested this hypothesis as part of a series of studies investigating how belief in literal immortality affects mortality salience-induced self-esteem striving.

A preliminary study demonstrated that mortality salience leads to increased belief in an afterlife after reading a research summary that concluded that the "near-death experience" provides evidence of life after death. In two additional studies, participants read either this pro-afterlife research summary or one that concluded that reports of "so-called near-death experiences" are merely a by-product of a lack of oxygen to the brain as one approaches death. Participants were then exposed to mortality salience or various control conditions and given positive feedback on a personality inventory. Because previous research has shown that mortality salience increases ratings of the validity of positive personality feedback (Dechesne, Janssen, & van Knippenberg, 2000), Dechesne and colleagues (2001) used a similar assessment of perceptions of the validity of positive personality feedback as an indication of mortality-salience-induced self-esteem striving. Whereas participants who read a research summary debunking reports of near-death experiences and those who read an irrelevant control essay showed increased ratings of the validity of positive personality feedback after mortality salience, this effect was completely eliminated among participants who read that the near-death experience provides strong evidence of life after death. It is important to note that participants in this study were typically low in religiosity and skeptical about the existence of an afterlife prior to the study. By showing that increased belief in literal immortality decreases the need to bolster the self after being reminded of death, these studies provide further evidence of the importance of death-related concerns in the pursuit of self-esteem.

Death-Thought-Accessibility Hypothesis

The death-thought-accessibility hypothesis implies that if a psychological structure provides protection against death-related concerns, then threats to that structure should increase the accessibility of death-related thoughts, and strengthening it should reduce the accessibility of such thoughts. Consistent with this reasoning, Harmon-Jones and colleagues (1997) have shown that increasing participant's self-esteem eliminates the effect of reminders of mortality on death thought accessibility. Arndt, Greenberg, Solomon, Pyszczynski, and Simon (1997), Greenberg and colleagues (2001), and Mikulincer and Florian (2000) have shown that defending one's cultural worldview after it is threatened produces a similar decrease in death thought accessibility after a death-related prime. In a recent series of studies taking terror management research in a new direction (see Goldenberg, Pyszczynski, et al., 2000), conditions not directly related to death but that threaten symbolic conceptions of the self by reminding people of their basic animal nature (e.g., physical aspects of sex) also increase the accessibility of death-related thought; subsequent to such reminders, couching such animalistic behaviors and characteristics in symbolic terms (e.g., romantic love) eliminates such increases in death thought accessibility (Cox, Pyszczynski, Goldenberg, Greenberg, & Solomon, 2001; Goldenberg, Pyszczynski, McCoy, Greenberg, & Solomon, 1999; Goldenberg et al., 2001). It appears, then, that threats to the self that undermine self-esteem or faith in a meaningful cultural worldview produce theoretically predicted increases in the accessibility of death-related thoughts, both with and without previously priming the problem of death; but when self-esteem and a sense of meaning are strong, such effects are reduced or eliminated.

The Evolution of Self: Freedom and Terror

Now that we have reviewed the basics of the terror management literature, we can explore the implications of the theory for understanding the self. Becker (1962, 1973) argued that the emergence of the cognitive capacities that made pursuit of abstract linguistic self-goals (e.g., intelligence, creativity, kindness, greatness, toughness) possible was the critical evolutionary adaptation that provided the increased flexibility and relative freedom from fixed response patterns that is characteristic of our species. In any given situation, we have a level of freedom of reactivity that is unparalleled among animals on this planet. In other words, Becker (1962) argued that the volitional self evolved as a regulatory mechanism (a "software program") as our ancestors evolved toward increasing dependence on volitional control as opposed to rigid instinctive "hardware" programming and simple stimulus–response learning to guide behavior.

Unfortunately, the cognitive abilities that gave rise to this potential for freedom also made us aware of our ultimate vulnerability and mortality. By putting this capacity to pursue abstract linguistic goals into service as a means of providing meaning and personal value and thus managing our fear of death, humankind traded much of our potential for freedom for the protection from anxiety that meaning and value afford. Becker (1973) referred to this exchange of potential freedom for the security provided by cultural meaning as a "reinstinctivization" in which abstract cultural standards of value came to replace more concrete biological imperatives as forces governing our actions. As Rank (1936/1976, p. 13) put it, "we . . . create out of freedom, a prison." Because we humans pursue linguistic goals that exist only in the world of abstract meaning, we retain considerable flexibility in the ways in which these goals are pursued and also in the self-deceptions we can use to adjust our perceived standing relative to these goals. This is what makes it possible to defend our self-esteem in the absence of actually meeting our standards.

From the TMT perspective, the potential for anxiety inherent in our species' awareness of the inevitability of death provides the motivational impetus for the pursuit of these abstract meaning-filled goals. Viewing the pursuit of a positive conception of self as rooted in fear helps explain the "driven" and sometimes compulsive nature of self-esteem striving, the negative emotional reactions that result when one's sense of value has been threatened, and the panoply of defensive responses that have been documented to occur in response to threats to self-esteem (for reviews, see Greenberg et al., 1986; Crocker & Park, Chapter 15, Tesser, Chapter 14, Dunning, Chapter 21, and Rhodewalt & Sorrow, Chapter 26, this volume). Rather than enjoying the challenges that the pursuit of excellence might entail, the ego-involved individual is more often characterized as insecure, uptight, and anxious. But how does a newborn human develop into an adult driven to sustain and defend self-esteem?

The Development of the Anxiety Buffer

TMT follows a long theoretical tradition (e.g., Becker, 1973; Bowlby, 1969; Freud, 1930/1961; Horney, 1937; Mead, 1934) of tracing the emergence of the anxiety-buffering capacity of self-esteem through a developmental analysis that starts with the precarious situation into which the human infant is born. Because of the newborn infant's profound immaturity and helplessness, he or she is completely dependent on the parents for protection and fulfillment of basic needs. Based on Becker (1962), we suggest that the child's sense of vulnerability and consequent proneness to anxiety increases with the development of the increasingly sophisticated cognitive abilities that facilitate the awareness of mortality. Rather quickly, the child learns that his or her needs are fulfilled, and thus anxiety is attenuated, when he or she lives up to parental standards of goodness. In short, when the child does as the parents want and meets their standards of value, the child feels safe and secure. When the child does not do as the parents want, the child experiences a denial of that love and protection, if not in the form of overt punishment, then with a mild rebuke or a lessening of expressed affection. Thus the child's sense of security becomes increasingly contingent on meeting parental standards of value (cf. Rogers, 1959), which ultimately reflect the parents' internalized version of the prevailing cultural worldview. According to TMT, children learn that meeting these standards leads to feelings of significance and security and that failing to do so leads to feelings of inferiority, insecurity, and anxiety. In this fashion, self-esteem acquires its anxiety-buffering properties.

As the child's cognitive capacities increase, he or she begins to form an understanding of the world and how it works. This understanding is critical for the effective action needed for meeting the child's needs. With the emergence of language, the child becomes capable of forming linguistic representations of reality and, later, asking questions about how things work. The parents and primary caregivers supply ready answers to the child's questions, relying on their own version of the cultural worldview as the primary reference source for their answers. The parents express approval and anxiety-quelling affection as the child mimics their words and phrases and eventually more sophisticated explanations and expressions of belief and value back to them. Through the parents' expressions of anxiety-buffering affection, the child's acceptance of the parents' cultural worldview acquires its anxiety-buffering properties.

In the early stages of development, primitive self-evaluations and affirmations of the cultural worldview, which are probably a direct reflection of the parents' worldview, provide this anxiety-buffering function. The child's innate potential to respond with fear to threats to its continued existence is quelled by the parents' affection, quite often without the child fully understanding what it is that he or she fears. With the child's increasing cognitive capacities, fears of monsters and powerful malevolent others gradually give way to an understanding of the fragility of life and the inevitability of death. With this growing realization of mortality and the parents' limited ability to protect them from this and other threats, the primary basis of security shifts from the parents to a worldview ultimately derived from the culture at large. It is no longer good enough to be mom and dad's good little girl or boy; one has to be a valued player in a much grander framework—a doctor, lawyer, or lover, a good American, Christian, or Muslim. From the TMT perspective, self-esteem emerges out of the security provided by believing in and living up to internalized standards of value and is the feeling that one is "an object of primary value in a world of meaningful action" (Becker, 1971, p. 79).

The Contingent Nature of Self-Esteem Facilitates Self-Regulation

Because TMT defines self-esteem as the belief that one is living up to the standards of one's individualized version of the cultural worldview, it is clearly a model of contingent self-esteem. Control theory approaches to self-regulation (e.g., Carver & Scheier, 1981; Duval & Wicklund, 1972; Pyszczynski & Greenberg, 1987a) typically view the comparison of one's current state with standards on salient dimensions of self-worth as playing a critical role in self-regulation. Such comparisons are viewed as instigating behavior aimed at keeping the individual "on track" in his or her pursuit of important life goals. Specific concrete behavioral standards are linked to the more abstract values of self-esteem by means of a hierarchy of standards, ranging from specifications for levels of particular behaviors such as recycling newspapers, on the more concrete end of the hierarchy, to the goal of being a valuable person, on the more abstract end of the hierarchy (cf. Carver & Scheier, 1981). From a self-regulatory perspective, contingencies of self-esteem, which exist at an intermediate to high level of abstraction in the hierarchy, provide the standards that lend coherence to behavior and motivate the pursuit of more concrete self-relevant goals. TMT simply adds that the pursuit of self-esteem is ultimately subordinate to the even more abstract goal of controlling core existential fears (for a thorough discussion of the role of existential concerns in self-regulation, see Pyszczynski, Greenberg, & Solomon, 1998; Pyszczynski, Greenberg, Solomon, & Hamilton, 1990).

From the TMT perspective, contingencies of self-worth are necessary for ongoing regulation of most meaningful human behavior. Although Rogers (1961) and other humanistically oriented theorists have argued for the superiority of noncontingent self-esteem over contingency-based self-esteem, TMT implies that all self-esteem must be contingent on meeting standards of some sort. A sense of value that is completely indifferent to one's behavior and characteristics would essentially amount to a complete lack of concern with one's value. We suspect that what Rogers was referring to was really a sense of self-worth that reflects feedback from others that is contingent on thoroughly integrated abstract self-attributes rather than on specific behavior that is evaluated relative to specific concrete standards. Completely unconditional regard from others would not differentiate oneself from others and therefore would provide little information to support a sense of identity. As soon as the other shows a greater valuing of one person over another, that valuing becomes conditional on some constellation of characteristics that define the self and give the person a unique identity. People want to be accepted for who they feel they really are; they want their unique features as individuals to be recognized by others. We question the utility of regard from others that is truly unconditional and thus fails to differentiate self from others and argue that people are likely to function better when their self-esteem is based on core, abstract, unique features of self.

Summary

The terror management theoretical analysis and the research supporting it suggest that the pursuit of self-esteem and faith in one's cultural worldview function as a buffer against the potential for anxiety inherent in recognition of the inevitability of death in an animal strongly motivated to stay alive. Consequently, we are all imprisoned within this protective system of meaning and the contingencies by which we sustain our self-worth.

As Becker (1971, p. 86) notes:

> Children are trained to want to do as the society says they have to do. They have to earn their prestige in definitely fixed ways. The result is that people willingly propagate whole cultural systems that hold them in bondage, and since everyone plays the same hero-game, no one can see through the farce.

But is there any way out?

Beyond Terror

Maybe. As we noted at the outset of this chapter, when considered in conceptual isolation, TMT provides an incomplete picture of the human condition. By itself, it is unable to explain the human proclivities for growth, change, development, and exploration. A terror-stricken organism concerned only with shielding itself from its fears would never change and would avoid new information and experience at all costs, unless it was assured that such experience would do nothing to physically threaten it or undermine its prevailing view of self and world. This is clearly an incomplete picture of humankind. Indeed, a creature like that could never have developed Darwin's theory of evolution or any other worldview-challenging idea.

For this reason, we have been working to integrate the TMT perspective with other theories more capable of explaining the creative, growth-oriented, self-expansive side of the human condition (cf. Greenberg, Pyszczynski, & Solomon, 1995; Pyszczynski et al., 1998). In the following sections, we explore this theoretical interface and hope to show how a consideration of the interplay of expansive and defensive motives provides insights into the question of why, despite their potential for growth, people so rarely make the most of this opportunity.

A Motivational Theory of Human Growth

Humanistically oriented theories take a decidedly more optimistic perspective on the human condition than that portrayed by TMT. Rather than emphasizing the self-deceptive and socially destructive tactics that people use to hide from their deepest fears, the humanistic perspective emphasizes the human potential to grow and change, to move toward better, more fulfilling individual lives. As noted at the outset of this chapter, there is a long tradition within many branches of psychology of distinguishing between approach-oriented and avoidance-oriented motive systems (see, e.g., Higgins, 1997). There is also growing evidence that positive and negative emotions are two separate dimensions, driven by distinct motivational systems, produced by unique evolutionary pressures, rather than opposite ends of an affective continuum (e.g., Fredrickson & Branigan, 2001). Evidence at the neuroanatomical and neurochemical levels of analysis support these propositions (e.g., Ashby, Isen, & Turken, 1999).

All of this work points to a basic distinction between actions designed to avoid or minimize negative affect and those designed to provide experiences of positive affect. Many of our behavioral systems and action tendencies serve these hedonistic goals at a relatively physical level. Thus we withdraw our hand from a stove and seek out sensual pleasures of the tongue and other body parts. Although more symbolic self-concerns can contribute to such actions, they primarily serve circumscribed, concrete purposes of reducing unpleasant and increasing pleasant sensory experiences. Terror management and self-expansive motives operate analogously, serving the same underlying hedonistic goals of avoiding the unpleasant and seeking the pleasant, respectively, but at the more abstract, symbolic level of the self.

Whereas terror management motives entail the avoidance of negative affect through the pursuit of a conception of the world as meaningful and the self as valuable, self-expansive motives entail the pursuit of the positive affect that is generated by the optimal engagement of processes involved in the integration of new information and experiences with existing psychological structures. Because it is driven by the desire to avoid negative affect, defense of the self has a mandatory, driven character—meaning and value must be sustained. Growth and expansion of the self have more of an elective character; people can and often do go for extended periods of time with very little growth or stimulation and without experiencing the positive affect or exhilaration that growth can produce. Of course people want positive affect and will not be very happy without it, but the motivation to obtain it is generally less intense than the drive to avoid negative affect. There is a long tradition of viewing the avoidance of negative affect as a stronger and more compelling motive than the seeking of positive affect (e.g., Dollard & Miller, 1950; Lewin, 1935). Whereas an absence of positive affect is boring and unfulfilling, the experience or mere expectation of negative affect can be intolerable.

The Generation of Intrinsic Motivation

What provides the motivational impetus for the process of integrating new information and experiences with existing psychological structures? A long tradition of theorists, including Rank (1936/1976), Piaget (1952), White (1959), Rogers (1961), Maslow (1970), Csikszentmihalyi (1980), and Deci and Ryan (1991), have argued that people are intrinsically motivated to expand their understandings and capacities. Deci and Ryan (e.g., 1991, 2000) have integrated research on intrinsic motivation into the broader framework of self-determination theory (SDT). The premise of their theory is that intrinsic motivation is the "energizing basis for natural organismic activity" (1991, p. 244). Flow (Csikszentmihalyi, 1990), the subjective enjoyment felt when one is thoroughly engaged in an activity that is optimally challenging, can be viewed as a prototype of intrinsically motivated activity. From the perspective of SDT, intrinsic motivation instigates optimal self-development and more elaborate and extensive self-organization. If core organismic needs are met, over time, the self expands, becomes more integrated, and more and more behavior becomes self-determined.

Fredrickson (e.g., 2001) has recently developed the broaden-and-build theory of positive emotions, which we believe helps elucidate what it is that is so intrinsically motivating about intrinsic motivation and how this may produce the self-expansive effects proposed by SDT. Fredrickson (1998) calls the positive emotion that characterizes intrinsic motivation (and flow) *interest*. She views interest from a framework consistent with Izard (1971; Tomkins, 1962), who discovered that interest occurs in contexts that allow people to feel secure but that also offer novelty, change, and possibility. Fredrickson defines interest as similar to curiosity, intrigue, excitement, and wonder.

More specifically, Fredrickson suggests that positive emotions such as interest *broaden* people's momentary thought action repertoires, which helps *build* their physical, intellectual, social, and psychological resources. In contrast to negative emotions (including fear and anxiety) that narrow a person's thought–action repertoire by priming an urge to respond in a particular way, positive emotions have a broadening effect by increasing the range of thoughts and actions that one considers. She reviews empirical studies by Isen and colleagues that show that positive affect leads to thinking that is flexible (Isen & Daubman, 1984), creative (Isen, Daubman, & Nowicki, 1987), integrative (Isen, Rosenzweig, & Young, 1991), and open-minded (Estrada, Isen, & Young, 1997). Her own research shows that inducing positive emotions broadens the thought–action repertoire of students, as measured by the number things they listed as wanting to do at that moment (Fredrickson & Branigan, 2000). In this way, positive emotions stimulate growth, integration, and motivation.

Interest, in particular, has been found to promote exploration, and, as Fredrickson quotes Izard (1971), interest generates "a feeling of wanting to investigate, become involved, or extend or expand the self by incorporating new information and having new experiences with the person or object that has stimulated the interest" (Izard, 1971, p. 216). Consistent with this proposition, interest (or intrinsic motivation) has been shown to promote learning (Deci, Vallerand, Pelletier, & Ryan, 1991) and psychological complexity (Csikszentmihalyi & Rathunde, 1998).

Our attempts to integrate TMT with SDT have built on these ideas to suggest a simple motivational mechanism through which intrinsic motivation is generated (Greenberg, Pyszczynski, & Solomon, 1995). Intrinsic motivation is the sense of positive affect or exhilaration that results from the integrative processing of information that occurs when one engages in an activity that is just beyond one's current understandings or capacities (cf. Csikszentmihalyi, 1980). The slight lack of fit between one's current understandings or capacities and the task at hand leads to integrative processing, by which we mean a process of changing one's existing psychological structures to accommodate the new information or experience. Integrative processing is the mechanism through which growth, learning, and change within the individual occurs. A heightened level of integrative processing produces positive affect or a sense of exhilaration, which then acts as an incentive for one to approach challenging tasks in the future and as a reinforcer for such engagement once it has occurred. Thus it is through the *process* of integrative activity that occurs in challenging situations rather than the *products* or outcomes of such activity that intrinsic motivation is generated.

Although we view the affect that results from the process of integrative activity to be the basis for intrinsic motivation, this is not to say that the products of such activity play no role in motivating creative action or change. Most (but not all) cultures place a high value on creativity and the development of new capacities. The products of creative activity enable us to meet these standards and thus provide self-esteem. Of course, from the TMT perspective, the pursuit of self-esteem is defensive in nature and functions to control anxiety. We are arguing, then, that achievement-oriented behavior, creativity, exploration, and growth can be motivated both by the intrinsic sense of exhilaration that such activity can produce and by the extrinsic sense of personal value that success in such endeavors can produce. Interestingly, Stipek (2001) has observed that young children enjoy tasks for their own sake, but that as they mature, they focus more on pride over achievements. From this perspective, much human growth is viewed, at least in part, as motivated behavior that has both intrinsic and extrinsic elements that encourage the individual to engage in activities that will lead to change in his or her existing psychological structures. We are *not* arguing that the individual must

desire to change or develop; simply that the intrinsic exhilaration resulting from integrative activity coupled with the boost to self-esteem provided by success in such endeavors lies at the root of self-expansion.

The Potential for Self-Determination: The Self-Creation of Self

Deci and Ryan (2000) have argued that the human capacity for creatively integrating new information and experiences with existing aspects of self makes it possible for human beings to exert a measure of freedom and self-determination unheard of elsewhere in the animal kingdom. Whether it be through reading books, taking classes, talking with friends, or almost any other activity the individual undertakes, the individual is constantly faced with the potential for changing his or her existing psychological organization (standards, values, goals, etc.) in response to such experiences. The revised psychological structures that result are the product of the individual's own creative activity. In this sense the individual takes an active role in determining his or her behavior. Although not all changes in self that result from this integrative process necessarily produce increases in self-determination, it is this process of creatively reinventing the self that makes it reasonable to think of behavior as self-determined. Although behavior is far from random, capricious, or undetermined, it can be thought of as relatively free or self-determined in the sense that the person has created the standards that are used to regulate his or her actions.

SDT has elucidated the process by which activities that may initially be pursued for extrinsic reasons can become more or less self-determined by internalizing these external values and potentially integrating them into one's self. More specifically, SDT posits that motivation can entail (1) *external regulation,* by which a behavior is engaged in to satisfy an external demand; (2) *introjected regulation,* in which people are motivated to meet standards that have been accepted with little or no effort to integrate them with core aspects of self; (3) regulation through *identification,* in which there is a conscious valuing of the behavior; and (4) *integrated regulation,* in which the goals are fully incorporated into the individual's core self.

Unfortunately, there are powerful forces that often conspire to derail this potential for the self-creation of self and the freedom that this could produce. In the following sections, we discuss factors that inhibit the operation of this process and consider the potential of the development of a more self-determined regulatory system to provide greater creativity and openness to experience. We then use this analysis to explain how individuals create their own individualized versions of the cultural worldview and what leads to more and less self-determined integration of cultural beliefs and standards in this process.

Anxiety Inhibits Growth

Deci and Ryan (1991, 2000) argue that the integrative processing necessary for growth requires the meeting of three basic organismic psychological needs for belonging, competence, and autonomy. They posit that these needs provide required "nutriments" needed for the effective integration of new experiences necessary for self-determined behavior (identification and integration). We are not convinced that these are basic organismic needs. First, they seem to very greatly between individuals. There are loners and joiners. There are high achievers and those who would just as soon lie in the sun. And there are followers and leaders. Similarly, the valuing of these propensities varies considerably across cultures, with more collectivistic cultures probably emphasizing belonging more and autonomy less than more individualistic ones. We do not pretend to have a full understanding of precisely how these common human concerns fit within our dual motive system, but we do have some ideas on the matter.

First, we believe the desire for belonging or relatedness serves an important defensive terror management function. Other people, from our parents when we are children, to our romantic partners, friends, and colleagues in adult life, are the primary basis for helping us sustain our sense that the world is meaningful and that we are valuable. In fact, Rank (1932/1989) and Becker (1973) argued that romantic love has become a central basis of meaning and value for people in Western cultures as religion has become less so. Recent work by Mikulincer and Florian (2000) supports this idea by showing that mortality salience increases desire for and positive valuing of romantic relationships, particularly in securely attached individuals. Mikulincer, Florian, and Hirschberger (in press) suggest that attachments to others may serve as an anxiety buffer independent of their role in bolstering the symbolic constructs of the worldview and one's self-worth because of their role as the initial bases of security for the child. On the other hand, we view the pursuit of competence as partly stemming from the approach-oriented self-expansion system, which emerges out of a complex developmental process that unfolds gradually over the early years of life. The intrinsically motivating positive affect that results from actively pursuing a goal plays an important role in the instigation of activities that produce feelings of competence. We view the pursuit of autonomy as a more complex motive. Rather than viewing it as an innate need, we conceptualize the need for autonomy as an emergent process of the development of volitional control over one's behavior—what Rank referred to as the will. As the child's sense of control over his or her actions emerges and increases, he or she derives pleasure from the exertion of such control (because it entails an affect-producing process of integrating new information with existing structures) and responds negatively to forces that undermine the exertion of such control in the form of tantrums and increased striving to exert his or her autonomy (Brehm, 1966).

Of course, many cultures prescribe that a good person should belong, be competent, and be autonomous, and so accomplishing these things can provide self-esteem; thus pursuit of competence and autonomy can serve an anxiety-buffering defensive function, much as we argue belongingness does. This does not imply, however, that these psychological entities are sought *only* because they provide self-esteem or that we are convinced that there are not evolved proclivities in these directions that predate the need for self-esteem. Thus, although we view the meeting of cultural standards concerning these three goals as providing self-esteem, we do not believe that this is the only motivational force behind such needs; rather, strivings for competence and autonomy are a natural outgrowth of the positive affect inherently engendered by self-expansive and integrative experiences, and relatedness may serve a primitive anxiety-buffering function independent of its role in worldview and self-esteem validation. Thus, although we agree with Deci and Ryan (2000) that meeting defensive needs is a prerequisite for optimal growth, we view competence and autonomy primarily as components of the growth and self-expansion process rather than as needs that must be satisfied before this process can occur. Our analysis distinguishes between the intrinsic motivation inherent in the *process* of engagement in behavior and the self-esteem-conferring sense of meeting standards that results from the *products* of such pursuits.[3]

Based on Becker (1971), then, we posit that anxiety must be controlled via the symbolic anxiety buffer and perhaps basic attachments, as well, in order for unbiased integrative processing of new experiences to occur. Research by Deci and Ryan (2000) is consistent with our emphasis on the need to manage anxiety, in that they have shown that security is a prerequisite for integration. For example, findings that children who feel secure in their relationships with parents and teachers are more likely to internalize positive school attitudes (Ryan, Stiller, & Lynch, 1994), and similar findings related to autonomy and competence, all support the premise that security (meaning and value) fosters integration (e.g., Grolnick & Ryan, 1989). As Deci and Ryan note, "a secure relational base does seem to be important for the expression of intrinsic motivation to be in evidence" (p. 71).

Kasser and Ryan (1993, 1996) have conducted a series of studies examining correlates of intrinsic and extrinsic goals. Their research shows that putting high importance on intrinsic goals, such as affiliation, community feeling, physical fitness, and self-acceptance, correlates positively with a host of variables reflecting well-being and negatively with variables reflecting distress. On the other hand, striving to obtain the "American dream" of money, fame, and attractiveness (extrinsic goals) is associated with lower levels of well-being. Although this research was intended to provide support for the benefits of intrinsic motivation, as the authors themselves acknowledge, the

evidence is entirely correlational. Therefore, the alternative causal explanation that individuals with more distress and anxiety are more likely to be extrinsically motivated is just as feasible, and not inconsistent with SDT.

Other studies are consistent with the related idea that anxiety leads to defensiveness. Elliot, Sheldon, and Church (1997) showed that individuals high in neuroticism tend to pursue avoidance-oriented rather than approach-oriented goals. This is consistent with our proposition that if anxiety is not managed effectively, the pursuit of growth-oriented activities is unlikely, which is of course also consistent with Maslow's (1970) idea that deficit motives generally must be satisfied before being motives can be pursued. This research also provides evidence that individuals reporting avoidance-motivated striving exhibit less well-being over the course of a semester. This, too, is consistent with the perspectives offered by both TMT and SDT. In short, although we certainly agree with the proposition that intrinsic motivation has positive effects on well-being (Sheldon & Kasser, 1998), the evidence for this claim is equally consistent with our proposition that anxiety must be effectively managed in order for intrinsically motivated integrative activities to be pursued.

In our own experimental research, we have provided support for the idea that when security is undermined by priming thoughts of death, growth, creativity, and integration are hindered. For example, mortality salience has been shown to cause people to increase their reliance on cognitive heuristics (Landau, Johns, Goldenberg, Pyszczynski, Greenberg, & Solomon, 2002) and to respond more positively to information that is consistent with their preexisting schemas and stereotypes (Schimel et al., 1999). Similarly, Arndt, Greenberg, Solomon, Pyszczynski, and Schimel (1999) found that after mortality salience, creative action produced an increased desire to see oneself as similar to most others. Perhaps the most direct support for this proposition was provided recently by Koole (2001), who demonstrated that mortality salience reduces intrinsic motivation among those with low self-esteem but not among those with high self-esteem.

Diverse literatures on anxiety, learning, and creativity provide further support for the view that anxiety undermines the creative integration of new experiences with existing psychological structures. For example, following Harlow's classic work with primates (Harlow & Zimmerman, 1959), it has been shown that human infants cling to their caregiver when anxious and use her or him as a secure base from which to explore (Bowlby, 1988). Research on attachment styles in adulthood assumes that feelings of being protected from threat in infancy lead to styles of attachment in which people feel secure in their belief that others will be available in times of need. Attachment styles (secure, anxious–ambivalent, or avoidant; Ainsworth, Blehar, Waters, & Wall, 1978) have a predictable impact on adult interpersonal relationships (e.g., Hazen & Shaver, 1987). Of greater direct relevance to our argument, people with secure attachment styles have been shown to have less need for cognitive closure and to be more likely to rely on new information in making social judgments than either anxious–ambivalent or avoidant individuals (Mikulincer, 1997). Recently, the argument that security fosters creativity has been extended to the workplace (Obholzer, 2001). Of course, this evidence supports both SDT's need for relatedness proposition and the TMT proposition that an effective anxiety buffer is necessary for growth.

Construction of the Individualized Cultural Worldview

This analysis may provide insight into how each person's individualized version of the cultural worldview is constructed. The process of integrating new information and experience with existing psychological structures produces positive affect that is the impetus for growth (cf. Fredrickson, 2001). Thus, as Deci and Ryan (1991) have argued, there is intrinsic motivation to construct a more complete, complex, and differentiated conception of self and world. However, when one's emotional security is highly dependent on the approval of others or when one lacks emotional security because one's self-esteem or worldview is undermined in some way, one is unable to integrate new information in an open and unbiased manner. Rather, the integrative processing is biased toward either pleasing those on whom one is dependent or maintaining the existing organization on which one has been relying for protection. New information is either ignored or explained away so that beliefs and values that have been effective in controlling anxiety can be maintained. Our analysis thus implies that introjection of external influences or experience into the self with minimal integrative processing occurs when one is unable to control one's existential anxiety. Only when anxiety is adequately managed can one integrate new information and experiences in an open, relatively unbiased, and self-determined manner.

Young children, who are virtually entirely dependent on the good will of their parents for protection from anxiety and who furthermore lack the cognitive resources for seriously questioning what they are told, accept the parents' and other cultural agents' version of the worldview wholeheartedly with little integrative processing or consideration of alternatives. The child's initial understanding of the world and his or her role in it is a rather literal version of the views of those on whom he or she is most dependent for security, usually the parents. As the child matures, he or she becomes increasingly exposed to alternative viewpoints. This exposure to ideas that do not fit well with one's existing conception of world or self instigates integrative processing to varying degrees, depending on how discrepant the ideas are from one's own conception. This processing is most intense when the new information is at some optimal moderate level of discrepancy and thus produces the most affect and intrinsic motivation to reward such integrative activity (cf. Csikszentmihalyi, 1980).

Some people, especially those living in isolated areas or in past eras that offer little access to diverse belief systems and points of view, draw on a relatively homogeneous set of ideas, values, and rituals in constructing their worldviews. Such individuals are likely to have a relatively easy time finding a secure unchallenged sense of life's meaning. However, they are also likely have fewer opportunities for developing a self-determined worldview and self-concept because they lack the challenges to their existing conceptions that provide the impetus for integrative processing and the intrinsic motivation for future growth that such integrative activities produce. This is likely to be the case in relatively homogeneous cultures and in those in which the open exchange of ideas is discouraged, as exemplified by the Taliban regime in Afghanistan. However, these are now rare circumstances in contemporary Western cultures, which are characterized by mass communication, multicultural perspectives, widespread dissent about core beliefs and values, and minimal censorship. People in such cultures are routinely exposed to a panoply of ideas and values that challenge their existing conceptions and provide the instigation for integrative processing and the potential for intrinsic rewards that can motivate further integrative efforts and a greater potential for self-determination. The cost of our more complex world, with its multiple viewpoints and perspectives, is that it makes it more difficult to find meaning and solace in any given system of meaning (e.g., May, 1983; Schwartz, 1997). Thus, although exposure to diverse worldviews provides the opportunity and challenge that could lead to greater integrative processing and, ultimately, to a more self-determined conception of self and world, it makes it more difficult to find the security necessary for open integrative processing to occur.

The central point of our analysis is that the integrity of one's cultural anxiety buffer plays an important role in how people respond to information that challenges their existing conceptions of self and world. The more secure these structures, the more open and unbiased the integrative processing is likely to be. But there is a paradox here.

Although the security provided by self-esteem and faith in one's cultural worldview is needed for integrative processing to occur in an open and unbiased way, people typically control anxiety by clinging to their conceptions of self and world and defending them against threats. Such clinging to the status quo is, of course, antithetical to the integrative processing of new information and experiences through which growth occurs. Thus people are often left between the metaphorical "rock and a hard place," struggling to control their anxieties by clinging to their existing conceptions of self and

world; the protection provided by these conceptions could open the doors for creative growth and change, but by desperately clinging to them, slams those very doors shut. The more tentative one's basis of security, the more rigid and biased one's integrative processing is likely to be, and the more one is likely to reject new information in favor of early introjects. When there is extreme instability in one's existing world- or self-views, one may abandon the existing structures and introject new ideals and values with minimal integration. Dramatic cases of religious conversion, cult affiliation, or countercultural identification may be examples of this latter process (cf. Dein & Barlow, 1999; Kirkpatrick & Shaver, 1990; for a discussion of how dramatic changes in self can occur in the later years of life, see McCoy, Pyszczynski, Solomon, & Greenberg, 2000).

Ultimately, it is through this interaction of intrinsically motivated growth-producing integrative processing of new information and the defensive needs for security provided by our preexisting anxiety-buffering conceptions of self and world that the individual carves out his or her own individualized version of the cultural worldview. It is this individualized structure that provides him or her with protection from core existential fears. And it is this individualized structure that becomes the status quo that is subsequently defended and protected. Only when a sufficient level of security is provided by one's worldview to integrate new information in a relatively unbiased manner, or when so little security is provided by these structures that they are abandoned and other alternative conceptions are introjected with little or no integrative processing, does major change in these structures occur.

Growth and Expansion Can Undermine Security

We have previously argued that anxiety can undermine the potential for growth and expansion, but the converse is also true: When growth and changes *do* occur, security is often undermined. Stepping outside of one's security-providing worldview to grow and expand is risky because you never know what you might find. This is part of the meaning of the Biblical story of the Garden of Eden. By tasting the fruit of knowledge, the old security of everlasting life in paradise is shattered, and the vulnerabilities of mortal life and the concomitant capacities for anxiety, guilt, and shame come to the fore.

On a broad historical scale, one could view this theme as having been played out in Western culture over the last few centuries. Living in a culture with a Christian deistic worldview, Darwin and similarly curious scientists, presumably motivated by an acquisitive "thirst" for understanding, came to discoveries that threatened the prevailing worldview. Imagine the exhilaration as the logic of natural selection dawned on Darwin; and the likely terror as well, as he realized he was a product of a mindless process, a temporary link in a pointless chain. Imagine the feeling of foreboding that likely emerged as he prepared to reveal this new way of thinking to the rest of the world, a world full of people who would not take kindly to the implications of this new perspective on the genesis and nature of humankind. Reaching back to a far earlier epoch, one could speculate that, in a more collective sense, a similar sequence of events created the problem of existential terror in the first place. Indeed, Rank (1936/1976) proposed that the evolution of self-consciousness in our ancestors created the problem of awareness of mortality and that, consequently, the capacities for symbolic thought that led to this revelation had to be quickly utilized to manage this terrifying realization. We are still working out how to cope with this expansion of knowledge and cognitive capacity today, at the dawn of the 21st century.

And so, from both the broad cultural perspective and the individual developmental perspective, as we grow and think outside the confines of the security providing worldview, anxiety and guilt flood in and we must reconstruct our basis of meaning and value quickly (cf. Arndt et al., 1999). Ironically, then, a secure worldview and sense of self-worth allows us to venture forth to uncharted mental territory in which our discoveries may call into question those very security providing structures, requiring us to revise those structures to accommodate our self-expansions. Thus the need for anxiety control coupled with a desire for new experi-

ence and knowledge sets in play a dialectic spiral of meaning and value construction, threatened by expansions, and then requiring further internal revisions, which allow further expansions, and so forth.

Unfortunately, we often fail to allow this dialectical process to continue its forward momentum; rather, we cut off our potential for growth by clinging to our preexisting conceptions of self and the world because of the protection from anxiety that they provide. People so often stop growing and even actively resist change because they cling to the conceptions of the world and themselves that provided them maximum safety and security. People give up the potential pleasures of intrinsically motivated growth-promoting activity in exchange for the comfort and security that clinging to existing forms of psychological organization provide. We believe that this conflict between the human potentials for creativity and fear lies at the heart of what many refer to as the human dilemma: immense capacity for growth and change that is often thwarted by our slavish dependence on the existing psychological structures that protect us from our fears.

This conflict has been grappled with, in one way or another, by most of the major religions, ideologies, philosophies, and systems of psychotherapy throughout the history of our species. It has been depicted in countless myths, novels, paintings, films, and other works of art. The recent film *Chocolat* (2000) beautifully illustrates how terror management needs can stifle growth and self-expansion. The inhabitants of a Catholic village in France controlled by the local minister live with their desires for stimulation and self-expression all but completely stifled until a free-thinking individualistic chocolatier and her daughter move into town and open a shop full of *sinfully* tasty treats. Inspired by the orthodox priest's Sunday sermons continually reminding them of their mortality, the villagers' self-denials serve to keep them in the good graces of their God, thus helping them manage their terror. Despite great resistance, the chocolatier eventually wins over the people as their sensually liberating enjoyment of her chocolates generalizes to liberate their thoughts and lifestyle choices. Of course, that freedom may come at a price—will the people be able to sustain their terror-assuaging faith while also pursuing their restored desires for stimulation and self-expansion (and chocolate)? The film offers an answer by suggesting that the security-providing faith be expanded to accommodate personal growth and expansion as positive manifestations of the love and tolerance that have always been components of that (Christian) worldview.

The Delicate Balance

Thus for both individuals and societies, to adequately satisfy both defensive needs and acquisitive motives, a delicate dynamic balance must be sustained. But how? We propose that, with the sobering existential dilemma emphasized by TMT kept in mind, SDT provides at least a glimmer of hope.

> The problem of life is how to grow out of fetishism . . . continually broaden and expand one's horizons . . . the person's main task is to put his self-esteem as firmly as possible under his own control; he has to try to get individual and durable ways to earn self-esteem. (Becker, 1971, p. 191)

If the human capacity for creative integration of new information and experiences with existing psychological structures makes it possible to create a relatively self-determined self, perhaps such a self could function to provide standards for self-regulation and the control of core existential anxiety without detracting from our potential for creativity and growth. SDT (Deci & Ryan, 1995) and other humanistic perspectives (e.g., May, 1953; Rogers, 1961) suggest that the pursuit of self-esteem based on well-integrated intrinsic standards may have advantages over the pursuit of self-esteem based on introjected or extrinsic standards. As Deci and Ryan (1995) have argued, the pursuit of standards that are well integrated with the intrinsic self provides a subjective feeling of freedom, self-determination, and vitality. As literature on reactance theory has shown (Brehm, 1966; for a review, see Brehm & Brehm, 1981), people are highly motivated to perceive their behavior as free and self-determined, and they react to threats to their freedom in a variety of ways that function to restore their perceived freedom. And as a large body of studies inspired

by SDT has shown (for review, see Deci & Ryan, 2000), people are happier, more productive, and more creative when they feel they are the originators of their behavior. This evidence points to the possibility that self-esteem based on standards that have been integrated with core aspects of self in a relatively open and unbiased way, that provide a sense of value based on who one really is (as opposed to one based solely on culturally valued accomplishments), may provide a better means of opening the door to freedom and self-determination. We recently embarked on a series of studies to assess this possibility.

Intrinsic Self-Esteem and Defensiveness

Our first step was to determine if self-esteem based on a sense of who one really is produces less defensiveness in new situations than self-esteem based on living up to specific standards or achievements. We reasoned that defensiveness in new situations reflects a general reactivity to threat and a lack of openness to new information and experience. To make the point that it is general defensiveness and openness to experience that was being affected, we used a variety of different paradigms for assessing defensiveness, none of which bore any obvious relation to the domain used to manipulate intrinsic or extrinsic aspects of self. Because we view the self as requiring social validation from others but as also existing within the mind of the individual, we investigated both social interactions and relatively private priming of the individual's thoughts and memories as ways of activating intrinsic and extrinsic aspects of self. Although a great deal of additional research is needed, the results of our initial studies strongly suggest that self-esteem based on intrinsic factors requires less ongoing defense than self-esteem based on extrinsic factors, and that, whereas intrinsic self-esteem increases one's tendencies toward independence and self-determination, self-esteem based on extrinsic factors does not.

In our first study (Schimel, Arndt, Pyszczynski, & Greenberg, 2001, Study 2), we induced participants to disclose information to a supposed other participant that focused on either "who you really are as a person" or "your accomplishments and achievements." Participants were led to believe that the other participant would then give them feedback about their impressions. Half of the participants were then given positive feedback from the other participant and half were given no feedback, ostensibly because time had run out for that part of the study. Defensiveness was assessed using our distancing from an undesirable-other paradigm (cf. Pyszczynski et al., 1995) in which participants were first shown the personality profiles of an undesirable other (a depressed and highly dependent person) and then asked to rate themselves on the same set of traits. The absolute value of the difference between participants' self-ratings and those of the depressed other were used as a measure of defensive distancing. Whereas receiving positive feedback after a disclosure of one's intrinsic self reduced defensive distancing, identical positive feedback after a disclosure of one's achievements had no such effect. Interestingly, disclosing aspects of the intrinsic self without receiving positive feedback actually increased defensive distancing; this suggests that such disclosures are risky and may help explain why people often avoid disclosure of such core attributes. Such interactions put the self on the line and have the potential to undermine security if they are not validated.

In a follow-up study (Schimel et al., 2001, Study 3), participants revealed both "who they really are as a person" and their "most prized achievements" and then received a positive evaluation from another person based on one or the other aspect of their disclosure. Defensiveness was assessed as a relative preference for downward over upward counterfactual thinking; Roese and Olson (1993) have implicated a preference for downward counterfactual thinking as a form of defensiveness. Whereas positive evaluations from others based on intrinsic aspects of self led to reduced defensive counterfactual generation relative to a control condition, positive evaluations from others based on one's achievements did not.

Note that the effects of the self-esteem manipulations in these studies depended on feedback from another person. This is consistent with the general notion that the self is a social construction that is built on interactions with significant others over the course of one's life. Indeed, Rogers's (1959)

theory of self was based largely on the notion that whereas unconditional acceptance from others breeds security and a capacity for self-determination, acceptance that is contingent on meeting the others' conditions of worth breeds insecurity and undermines one's potential for self-determined action. Baldwin and Sinclair (1996) developed a procedure in which thoughts of either unconditionally accepting or conditionally accepting others is primed with a visualization exercise and demonstrated that priming conditionally accepting others increases the tendency to associate failure with rejection and success with acceptance. Baldwin's (1992) perspective on relational schemas implies that simply priming prior relationships with conditionally versus unconditionally accepting others would produce an effect on general defensiveness parallel to that of being accepted for intrinsic versus extrinsic aspects of self. Consistent with this reasoning, Schimel and colleagues (2001, Study 1) demonstrated that whereas priming thoughts of unconditionally accepting others reduces defensiveness in the form of downward social comparison seeking, priming thoughts of conditionally accepting others has no effect on such defensiveness. Arndt, Schimel, Greenberg, and Pyzczynski (2002) conceptually replicated this finding, demonstrating that priming thoughts of unconditionally accepting others reduces self-handicapping prior to an ego-relevant performance, whereas priming thoughts of conditionally accepting others does not. The fact that priming thoughts of past relationships can produce effects parallel to feedback in current social interactions attests to the importance of cognitive representations of past relationships in the ongoing functioning of the self.

Taken together, these four experiments demonstrate that whereas activation of intrinsic aspects of self can reduce general defensiveness, thereby making one more open to information and experience, activation of extrinsic aspects of self does not. These studies also demonstrate the social nature of self by illustrating the role of interactions with others in activating different aspects of self. However, although social interaction plays an important role in the validation of different self aspects, from our perspective, such validation should not be necessary at all times for individuals who have internalized an integrated sense of who they are as a means of feeling valuable. Perhaps social validation was necessary in the Schimel and colleagues (2001) studies because participants were led to expect feedback from others about their self-disclosures, thus activating concerns about social approval. Our reasoning implies that in situations in which no such evaluation is expected, simply activating thoughts about intrinsic aspects of self should be capable of reducing general defensiveness because intrinsic aspects of self are less dependent on continual social validation (although based on earlier experiences with such validation). Thus we examined the effect of simply priming intrinsic versus extrinsic aspects of self in a situation in which no feedback or validation was expected or possible (Arndt et al., 2002, Study 2). Would such thoughts have similar effects, even in the absence of explicit social validation?

An additional purpose of this study was to examine a type of behavior that gets closer to the essence of self-determination: susceptibility to conformity pressures. A failure to conform is a textbook example of self-determined action; such behavior reflects the individuals' own preferences in the face of pressure to behave otherwise. Thus in Arndt and colleagues (2002, Study 2), we primed participants to think about either "who they really are" (intrinsic self) or their "most treasured achievements" (extrinsic self) and then assessed the extent to which they conformed to the judgments of others when evaluating abstract art. Whereas both control and extrinsic-self participants were strongly influenced by the judgments of others, intrinsic-self participants were not. Thus priming intrinsic aspects of self reduced conformity and increased participants' tendencies to make aesthetic judgments based on their own personal preferences.

Although additional research will be needed to fully evaluate this position, the studies available to date clearly demonstrate that self-esteem based on intrinsic factors requires less defensiveness and leads to higher levels of self-determination than self-esteem based on extrinsic factors. Thus, whereas both types of self-esteem appear effective in buffering anxiety, extrinsic self-

esteem has the liability of requiring higher levels of vigilance and defense and thus interfering with creative integration of new experiences with existing psychological structures.

Implications and Issues

The present analysis and research raise a variety of interesting issues and have implications for understanding other phenomena that have recently received attention in the self literature. We turn now to a brief discussion of these implications and issues.

Stability of Self-Esteem

Kernis and colleagues (Kernis, Grannemann, & Barclay, 1989, 1992) have amassed a growing body of evidence indicating that people with stable high self-esteem are generally lower in defensiveness than those with unstable high self-esteem. Kernis and colleagues (e.g., Kernis & Waschull, 1995) propose that unstable high self-esteem results from two factors, a high dependency on everyday outcomes for self-esteem and an underdeveloped self-concept.

Our work suggests another possibility. We have consistently found that when people focus on achievements as a basis of self-worth, they tend to be highly defensive in response to situational threats, whereas when they focus on intrinsic aspects of self, they are much less defensive. This suggests a possible basis for stable high self-esteem; it may result from basing one's self-worth primarily on intrinsic self-aspects, whereas unstable high self-esteem may result from basing it primarily on extrinsic self-aspects. Intrinsic aspects of self—who you are—are unlikely to change, whereas performance in achievement domains is likely to fluctuate as new evaluative contexts arise. The intrinsic–extrinsic distinction helps explain why some people are highly dependent on specific outcomes for self-worth and thus have unstable self-worth.

Of course empirical work is needed to assess whether our findings for experimental manipulations of bases of self-worth extend to dispositional tendencies to base one's self-worth on intrinsic versus extrinsic sources. We would predict that if people with stable high self-esteem are those with primarily intrinsic bases of self-esteem, they would not only be less defensive but would also display a greater propensity for self-determination, self-expansion, and creativity. In fact, recent findings by Kernis, Paradise, Whitaker, Wheatman, and Goldman (2000) provide initial support for this idea. They found that highly stable self-esteem is associated with low external and introjected regulation and with high identified and intrinsic regulation. Using a general self-determination index, they found that stability of self-esteem correlated positively with self-determined self-regulation. This work suggests that further investigation of individual differences in use of intrinsic versus extrinsic bases of self-worth might be fruitful.

Self-Esteem and Aggression

In a widely cited article, Baumeister, Smart, and Boden (1996) suggested that, because of their propensities to defend against self-esteem threats, people with high self-esteem may be prone to violence. This proposition was based on their review of the literature on self-esteem and violence, from which they concluded that it is not people with explicitly low self-esteem who are likely to respond defensively to threat, but rather those who claim to hold a positive self-image. Although we question the inclusions of those who are exaggeratedly narcissistic and defensive in Baumeister and colleagues' conceptualization of high self-esteem, their point that some people who evaluate themselves highly are prone to defensiveness, hostility, and even aggression is an interesting and important one. This conclusion is highly consistent with Kernis's work on unstable self-esteem discussed previously, as well as with recent research on narcissism (Rhodewalt & Morf, 1998), bullying by young defensive egotists (Salmivalli, Kaukiainen, Kaistaniemi, & Lagerspetz, 1999), and the much earlier theorizing of Karen Horney about genuine self-esteem versus defensive self-inflation (e.g., Horney, 1937).

We suggest that considering the bases from which people derive self-worth might shed light on important distinctions among those who express high opinions of themselves. Based on their findings that self-esteem did not predict aggression in response to threat whereas narcissism did, Bushman and Baumeister (1998, p. 228) concluded that "it is not so much people who regard themselves as superior beings who are the most dangerous but, rather, those who have a strong desire to regard themselves as superior beings." Although we would not equate high self-esteem with viewing oneself as a superior being, their distinction is a good one. Our analysis and research adds the proposition that people who base their self-worth on intrinsic qualities should be much less susceptible to violence because their basis for self-worth is stable and less vulnerable to situational threats. Narcissists or those with unstable high self-esteem, on the other hand, probably lack a secure intrinsic base for their high self-evaluations.

Self-Affirmation

Steele and associates' (e.g., Steele, 1988; Steele & Liu, 1983) work on the effects of self-affirmation makes a related point—when people affirm important personal values, they have less need to defend against potential threats to self-worth in other domains. Their research shows that defensive responses to various types of threats to self can be averted by inducing individuals to affirm other, seemingly unrelated aspects of self. In their first set of studies, Steele and Liu (1983) showed that attitude change after freely chosen counterattitudinal behavior is averted if participants are able to affirm an important aspect of self. More recent work has found effects of self-affirmation that could be construed as not only reducing defensiveness but perhaps opening people up to growth and integration of new information as well. Sherman and colleagues (2000) and Reed and Aspinwall (1998) have found that self-affirmation allows people to be more open to potentially threatening health-relevant information. Similarly, Cohen, Aronson, and Steele (2000) have shown that self-affirmation can lead to less bias and more openness to attitude change when people are exposed to counterattitudinal information.

Steele (1988) interprets these findings as demonstrating the interrelatedness of various aspects of the self system and implying that affirmation of any important self-aspect can restore the damage to self produced by a threat in any other domain. However, to our knowledge, all of the self-affirmation inductions that have been shown to be effective in reducing defensiveness in other areas have entailed affirmation of what could be viewed as a core, intrinsic, or well-integrated aspect of self—who one thinks one really is. Most of these studies entailed affirming values that have been preselected as being central to the person. Our research on the defensiveness-reducing effects of activating the intrinsic self raises the question of whether affirmation of extrinsic aspects of self would produce similar defensiveness-reducing effects. Although not conducted with the explicit intention of assessing the generality of self-affirmation effects, the Schimel and colleagues (2001) and Arndt and colleagues (2002) studies suggest that activation of important but extrinsic aspects of self has little effect on later defensiveness. These findings may add an important qualification to the literature on self-affirmation: that only affirmation of intrinsic aspects of self reduces defensiveness in other domains.

Objectification of Self

Fredrickson and Roberts (1997) have recently argued that the tendency of our society to value women primarily for their appearance rather than for their unique characteristics as individuals produces a broad range of negative psychological consequences for women. They argue that our culture's preoccupation with appearance as the supremely important dimension on which women are evaluated puts women in a near constant state of self-evaluation of their appearance, which detracts from their performance in other domains, produces feelings of shame among those who do not meet our society's unrealistic standards of beauty, and interferes with their capacity for becoming maximally engaged in non-appearance-related activities, thus undermining their potential for flow experience and other aspects of intrinsic motivation. In support of their argument, they have shown that when women are wearing bathing suits (as opposed to baggy sweaters) in private,

they report lower self-esteem and increased feelings of shame and perform worse on a math test; men show none of these negative consequences of wearing a bathing suit (Fredrickson, Roberts, Noll, Quinn, & Twenge, 1998).

Fredrickson and Roberts (1997) argue that our culture's preoccupation with feminine beauty forces women to define their worth largely in terms of their physical appearance. This, of course, reduces the importance of other potential sources of self-worth and thus leads to a narrow sense of one's value among women. Their objectification theory analysis is highly consistent with our views of the impact of intrinsic versus extrinsic bases of self-worth advanced in this chapter. Although it may be theoretically possible for women to integrate a concern with physical appearance with other intrinsic aspects of self, the exaggerated concern with female appearance portrayed by the media and most other aspects of contemporary society to the virtual exclusion of other characteristics and the disdain that our society often expresses for women who do not meet such standards is likely to make such integration extremely difficult. It seems reasonable, then, to view self-esteem derived from one's physical appearance as relatively extrinsic in nature.

This chapter suggests a somewhat broader analysis of the objectification problem. It implies that virtually any narrow unidimensional aspect of self that a culture seizes on as the key to a person or group of people's value is likely to have similar objectifying consequences. People typically experience themselves as complex multidimensional beings whose value is based on a broad constellation of features, too complex to be reduced to one or a small set of easily observable factors. We like to think of ourselves as "deep," and we like to base our value on abstract features that are too complex for simple observation and easy evaluation. Although there is certainly self-esteem to be gained from praise on any given culturally valued dimension, such self-esteem often feels cheap and disingenuous. It may be that social validation is most effective in promoting intrinsic self-esteem when it is based on a very broad and abstract appraisal of oneself as opposed to when it is primarily linked to any specific and concrete culturally valued attribute.

Abstract versus Concrete Bases of Self-Esteem

Taking this point further, we suggest that the more abstract one's standards of self-worth, the less susceptible one's self-esteem is to failures to meet them. Although concrete standards can be met in relatively few ways, more abstract standards leave far greater latitude as to what represents a successful attainment of those standards. If a woman's basis of self-esteem is entirely tied up with narrow cultural conceptions of physical beauty, then a scarring accident, a couple of newly acquired pounds, or the natural consequences of aging can be undermining. Similarly, making one's self-esteem contingent on the very concrete standard of winning a gold medal in the Olympics is, for almost everyone, certain to lead to a loss of self-esteem after the games are concluded. However, making one's self-esteem contingent on more abstract standards, such as being a good spouse, parent, scientist, or athlete, leaves a great deal more latitude, both in terms of ways of actually satisfying that standard and ways of deceiving oneself that one has met these standards when one really has not. Therefore, abstract bases of self-worth may be more stable and therefore allow people to be less defensive and more open to new information and experiences.

Unfortunately, abstract standards of self-esteem also have several liabilities. Because of their abstractness, they provide less information as to exactly what needs to be done to meet them. Thus they are likely to be less useful when one is learning a skill or is relatively inexperienced in a given domain. In addition, because they entail a greater degree of ambiguity as to whether they are being satisfied, they are more susceptible to self-deception and defensive distortion. Although this susceptibility can be construed as an advantage in that it facilitates the maintenance of self-esteem, it can also interfere with learning and the accurate self-assessment needed to stay on track in the pursuit of important life goals. Thus, although abstract standards may facilitate more stable self-evaluation, they may also interfere with performance and goal attainment.

This trade-off between the value of a given form of self-organization for self-esteem and performance seems to be a recurring theme when thinking about motives for self-esteem protection versus accurate knowledge (e.g., Kruglanski, 1980; Pyszczynski & Greenberg, 1987b). One clear example is the phenomenon of self-handicapping, in which people create obstacles to their own success to protect self-esteem (Berglas & Jones, 1978). Research indicates that when self-esteem concerns are more salient, self-handicapping prevails, whereas when extrinsic incentives for success are more salient, self-handicapping is minimized (Greenberg, Pyszczynski, & Paisley, 1984). Analogously, perhaps when self-esteem is most needed, people try to focus on abstract bases of self-worth, whereas when specific performance goals are more salient, they focus more on concrete signifiers of successful performance. Similarly, when focused on abstract aspects of self, people may have less need to engage in self-esteem defense directed at defusing a specific threat than when they are focused on more concrete bases of self-evaluation.

Interestingly, Freitas, Salovey, and Liberman (2001) have recently reported the results of six studies that did indeed find that people engage in more self-esteem defense regarding a particular performance when they construed their action at relatively concrete levels rather than at more abstract levels. Although the authors explained these findings by suggesting that accuracy is a more abstract goal than self-esteem maintenance, we would argue that their results may instead have occurred because more abstract construals rendered their behaviors, and the evaluations of them, less threatening to global self-esteem. This may also be part of the reason that self-affirmations reduce defensiveness.

Escape from the Self

One last phenomenon that our analysis of the interplay between defense and growth motives may shed light on concerns self-awareness and escape from it. Self-awareness is typically regarded as an aversive state (Duval & Wicklund, 1972). Duval and Wicklund (1972) suggest that self-reflection automatically triggers a comparison between one's self and one's standards, which almost inevitably produces the perception of a negative discrepancy. Self-awareness has been posited to be so uncomfortable that people use alcohol, food, sexual masochism, television, and even suicide and spirituality as a means of escaping (e.g., Baumeister, 1991; Heatherton & Baumeister, 1991; Hull, Young, & Jouriles, 1986). We believe that our dual motive analysis suggests two useful points about self-awareness.

The first concerns the assumption that self-reflection is necessarily aversive. After its original introduction, self-awareness theory was revised to account for new data revealing that after a successful experience, self-awareness may be pleasurable (Wicklund, 1975; see also Carver & Scheier, 1981). Our analysis suggests, however, that if the basis of one's self-esteem is intrinsic and abstract, then perhaps self-awareness would not be so commonly aversive, as one might not compare the self to "standards" or only to very abstract standards; consequently, the person would be less likely to feel that he or she unequivocally falls short. A related possibility is that self-determined bases of meaning and value would be less extreme and unrealistic for the individual and thus would involve smaller discrepancies. For example, if one's goal is to work hard and do one's best, rather than to bring home the gold, self-awareness after finishing 15th in the Olympics could bring feelings of satisfaction rather than disappointment. And that 15th-place finisher would therefore be less in need of finding ways to escape self-awareness.

The second point is that, as many psychoanalytic, humanistic, and existential thinkers have suggested (e.g., Freud, 1930/1961; Nietzsche, 1911/1999; Rogers, 1961), self-awareness may be absolutely necessary in the quest for authenticity in one's life and in establishing and sustaining intrinsic paths to meaning and value. In our own research we have shown that when security is undermined by reminding participants of their own deaths, self-awareness is aversive and will be avoided (Arndt, Greenberg, Pyszczynski, Simon, & Solomon, 1998). However, perhaps when anxiety is at a minimum, either in the fleeting moments of an extrinsic success or by having relatively intrinsic or abstract bases for self-esteem, one can delve into self-awareness in a positive manner that serves growth and self-expansion without undermining defensive structures.

On the Limits of Self-Determined Bases of Meaning and Value

Self-determination of our worldviews and bases of self-worth may indeed be a useful path to less defensiveness and more freedom, but the reality of our inevitable mortality and our childhood introjections are still likely to limit us. At times, Becker (1971, 1973) and similar thinkers (e.g., Brown, 1959) have suggested that maximum self-reliance may require us to look at reality as it really is and strip away our drapery of meaning, identity, and self-worth. This is a noble goal, one also suggested by some forms of Buddhism; however, given the fears inherent in the human condition, we doubt that this is entirely possible, and so did Becker.

There are always likely to be difficulties in satisfying both growth and defensive motives in most domains of human action. Many, if not most, significant human pursuits can be guided by self-expansive motives, particularly if defensive needs are currently being satisfied. However, the pursuit of self-expansive motives often leads to additional defensive concerns, which then undermine their value for growth and enrichment. As Freud (1930/1961) noted, the two most important determinants of a "good life" are probably love and work. Thus we illustrate the problems that can arise from the interplay of the two motives, with one example from each of these domains (cf. Greenberg, Pyszczynski, & Solomon, 1995).

First, consider long-term relationships such as marriage. People often begin dating in the pursuit of new experiences, excitement, and sensual pleasure. Indeed, Aron, Paris, and Aron (1995) found that when people fall in love, their selves expand, as indicated by more complex self-descriptions. At the same time, as Rank (1936/1976), Becker (1973), and attachment theorists and researchers (e.g., Bowlby, 1969; Collins & Feeney, 2000) have long argued, romantic relationships also serve the very important function of providing security, becoming important bases of both meaning and value. Consistent with this idea, Aron and colleagues also found that when people fall in love, their self-esteem increases.

Over time, stable relationships continue to provide security, as the couple develops a shared life. Problems arise when the relationship begins to fall short in providing either security or self-expansion. The value of the relationship for security and terror management can be undermined if one's partner stops providing signs of love and appreciation, thereby failing to fulfill one's self-esteem needs, or if the stability of the relationship is called into question by the threat of a third party. The expansive value of the relationship is undermined if the partners come to know the other all too well and they settle into a routine that no longer provides the new experiences and stimulation that led them to commit to the relationship in the first place. In fact, the desire to sustain and enhance security can contribute to this problem by blocking the growth of one or both partners.

We suggest that this may be the greatest challenge for relationships over the long haul. Csikszentmihalyi (1980) suggested the continued growth of each partner as an individual as a solution to this problem; each partner's personal growth can keep the relationship stimulating for the other partner. Of course, the danger here is that one partner's growth may undermine the other partner's security. Another interesting possibility that illustrates the interplay of the two motives is that the best partner for keeping the excitement and challenge in a relationship may be one who is not all that stable, such as the anxious–ambivalent type, as conceptualized by Hazan and Shaver (1987). This idea was explored by Woody Allen in the films *Stardust Memories* (1980) and *Husbands and Wives* (1992). Of course, this is an example in which the best case for expansive purposes may be the worst case for security purposes. The married person who attempts to have a secret affair also illustrates this common tension between the two motives, for this person is dangerously trying to enhance his or her stimulation while trying to preserve the security provided by the primary relationship. Disaster commonly awaits.

As a brief work example, consider the pursuit of scientific ideas. When fascination with a phenomenon or question inspires research or conceptual developments, we have perhaps the purest example of seeking new experiences and the integration of them in the service of self-expansion. Undoubtedly, most of those reading this chapter can relate to this example. And yet you probably can also anticipate where we are going next—to what happens as one attempts to communicate one's ideas or findings to colleagues and tries to publish the work. One is either faced with intense criticism or praise or, perhaps worse, indifference. In all three cases, what was once a pursuit of knowledge now becomes an ego-involved struggle to defend and promote one's work to sustain or to enhance one's standing in the field and consequent sense of self-worth. Of course, this phenomenon is a specific example of the undermining of intrinsic interest, as focus is shifted from intrinsic to extrinsic reasons for one's actions (Deci, 1975; Lepper & Greene, 1975). As Plant and Ryan (1985) have shown, even increased self-awareness, which increases the ego-relevance of an activity, can kill intrinsic interest. Thus, we suggest that many of the pursuits initially begun for self-expansive purposes take on a defensive function over time and that this defensive function undermines the self-expansive value of the pursuit.

To summarize our general point, when defensive needs are adequately satisfied, accomplished best by pursuing largely self-determined bases of meaning and value, people can pursue self-expansive desires. When they do that, they often find new defensive concerns arising, and the impetus for the activity shifts to a defensive function, which tends to undermine its value for self-expansion. Thus many if not most domains of human activity involve a combination of defensive and self-expansive motives in an uneasy dialectic interplay in which an optimal balance is difficult to achieve and even more difficult to sustain.

Summary and Conclusions

Although TMT and SDT both attempt to explain how the self functions, they focus on very different aspects of self and very different types of motivation. Whereas TMT emphasizes the defensive aspects of self and the fundamental motive of anxiety control, SDT emphasizes the expansive aspects of self and the processes of intrinsic motivation and growth. Because we believe that both theories capture important aspects of the human condition but that neither provides a comprehensive picture of human motivation, we have been working toward an integration of these two perspectives. Complex human activity centered on the pursuit of meaning and value entails both defensive reliance on sources of meaning and value that have proven effective in controlling one's fears and anxieties and active integration of new experiences with existing psychological structures. In our analysis of the interplay between these two systems, we have argued that integrative processes work most effectively when anxiety is controlled and that, ironically, people typically control anxiety by clinging to their preexisting sources of meaning and value, which often undermines self-expansive pursuits.

We have also proposed, however, that the pursuit of well-integrated intrinsic sources of meaning and value requires less defensiveness and therefore may facilitate a more open and less biased mode of living and experiencing. We believe that clarifying the dialectic dynamics of these two motive systems is an extremely important priority for continued theory development and research. Understanding this interplay may hold the key to opening the door to both a better understanding of the human condition and a more free and self-determined mode of living.

Notes

1. Colleagues have sometimes wondered whether we are positing self-esteem as a general anxiety buffer or as a buffer only against death-related anxieties. Following Becker (1962, 1971) and the developmental analysis we present later in this chapter, we have proposed that it is a general anxiety buffer because it emerges out of the childhood link between being good and the love and protection provided by the apparently omnipotent parents. The parents protect us from all things negative, and the key for our analysis is that this sense of security provided by self-esteem

extends beyond direct threats to self-esteem or potentially controllable threats such as pain to the one uncontrollable ultimate threat, death. Empirically, the electric shock studies suggest support for this general view, but it is possible that what is really frightening about threat of shock is not the possibility of momentary pain but of death from the shock. Although self-esteem may protect us from a variety of threats, as described later, our mortality salience research indicates that mere reminders of other threats do not activate the same types of defenses as reminders of death, perhaps because death is the only negative future event that is inevitable and that threatens to undermine satisfaction of all needs and desires.

2. McGregor, Zanna, Holmes, and Spencer (2001) have recently reported an effect similar to that of mortality salience with a treatment designed to create "personal uncertainty." Specifically, they showed that a "temporal discontinuity" manipulation, in which participants were asked to think of an important event from their childhood and then imagine the setting where the event occurred 35 years in the future, produced the same effects on ingroup bias and polarization of personal attributes as a mortality salience manipulation consisting of open-ended questions about death. Although we have argued that the absence of effects parallel to mortality salience when participants contemplate other aversive events provides evidence for the role of death concerns in such effects, TMT in no way implies that threatening events that do not directly implicate death should never affect worldview or self-esteem defense. In fact, the theory was developed to explain such phenomena. McGregor and colleagues suggest, based on this single study, that "personal uncertainty" rather than mortality may be the key factor in the mortality salience treatment. However, they offer no explanation of how this notion can account for the evidence from studies using subliminal primes or proximity to a funeral home or for the wide variety of effects documented in the terror management literature, and we do not see how they could.

With regard to their one finding, to the extent that the protective shield provided by self-esteem and the worldview is damaged by an experience, this should lead to an increase in the accessibility of death-related thought, which in turn should lead to a shoring up of defenses. Although McGregor and colleagues (2001) cite an unpublished pilot study in which their temporal discontinuity manipulation (unfortunately, without the typically needed delay) purportedly did not produce increased death thought accessibility, we recently found a delayed increase in death thought accessibility in response to this temporal discontinuity manipulation in our own labs. To the extent that thoughts of temporal discontinuity produce increases in death thought accessibility, it seems likely that this manipulation does so by posing a threat to the cultural anxiety buffer and that its effects on worldview defense result from this increased accessibility. Indeed, it seems quite likely that their manipulation was threatening because it reminded people of the fleeting nature of existence and the ultimate temporal discontinuity, death.

3. Many cultures and individuals also place value on the process of engaging in learning or other self-expansive activity. In such cases, people may also acquire self-esteem from the process of pursuing a goal independent of the outcome or products. Acquiring self-esteem in this way is still a result of self-reflectively observing oneself living up to internalized cultural standards of value (in this case, engaging in potentially self-expansive activity), which we view as distinct from the intrinsic motivation that results directly from the process of integrating new information and experiences.

References

Adler, A. (1928). *Understanding human nature*. London: Allen & Unwin.

Ainsworth, M. D. S., Blehar, M. C., Waters, E., & Wall, T. (1978). *Patterns of attachment*. Hillsdale, NJ: Erlbaum.

Allport, G. W. (1937). *Personality: A psychological interpretation*. New York: Holt.

Arndt, J., & Greenberg, J. (1999). The effects of a self-esteem boost and mortality salience on responses to boost relevant and irrelevant worldview threats. *Personality and Social Psychology Bulletin, 25,* 1331–1341.

Arndt, J., Greenberg, J., Pyszczynski, T., Simon, L., & Solomon, S. (1998). Terror management and self-awareness: Evidence that mortality salience provokes avoidance of the self-focused state. *Personality and Social Psychology Bulletin, 24,* 1216–1227.

Arndt, J., Greenberg, J., Solomon, S., Pyszczynski, T., & Schimel, J. (1999). Creativity and terror management: The effects of creative activity on guilt and social projection following mortality salience. *Journal of Personality and Social Psychology, 77,* 19–32.

Arndt, J., Greenberg, J., Solomon, S., Pyszczynski, T., & Simon, L. (1997). Suppression, accessibility of death-related thoughts, and cultural worldview defense: Exploring the psychodynamics of terror management. *Journal of Personality and Social Psychology, 73,* 5–18.

Arndt, J., Schimel, J., Greenberg, J., & Pyszczynski, T. (2002). The intrinsic self and defensiveness: Evidence that activating the intrinsic self reduces self-handicapping and conformity. *Personality and Social Psychology Bulletin, 28,* 671–683.

Aron, A., Paris, M., & Aron, E. N. (1995). Falling in love: Prospective studies of self-concept change. *Journal of Personality and Social Psychology, 69,* 1102–1112.

Ashby, F. G., Isen, A. M., & Turken, A. U. (1999). A neuropsychological theory of positive affect and its influence on cognition. *Psychological Review, 106,* 529–550.

Atkinson, J. W. (1964). *An introduction to motivation*. Princeton, NJ: Van Nostrand.

Baldwin, M. W. (1992). Relational schemas and the processing of social information. *Psychological Bulletin, 112,* 461–484.

Baldwin, M. W., & Sinclair, L. (1996). Self-esteem and "if–then" contingencies of interpersonal acceptance. *Journal of Personality and Social Psychology, 71,* 1130–1141.

Baumeister, R. F. (1991). *Escaping the self: Alcoholism, spirituality, masochism, and other flights from the burden of selfhood*. New York: Basic Books.

Baumeister, R. F., Smart, L., & Boden, J. M. (1996). Relation of threatened egotism to violence and aggression. *Psychological Review, 111,* 497–529.

Becker, E. (1962). *The birth and death of meaning*. New York: Free Press.

Becker, E. (1971). *The birth and death of meaning* (2nd ed.). New York: Free Press.

Becker, E. (1973). *The denial of death*. New York: Free Press.

Berglas, S., & Jones, E. E. (1978). Drug choice as self-handicapping strategy in response to noncontingent success. *Journal of Personality and Social Psychology, 36,* 405–417.

Bowlby, J. (1969). *Attachment and Loss: Vol. 1. Attachment*. London: Hogarth Press.

Bowlby, J. (1988). *A secure base*. New York: Basic Books.

Bushman, B. J., & Baumeister, R. F. (1998). Threatened egotism, narcissism, self-esteem, and direct and displaced aggression: Does self-love or self-hate lead to violence? *Journal of Personality and Social Psychology, 75,* 219–229.

Brehm, J. W. (1966). *A theory of psychological reactance*. New York: Academic Press.

Brehm, S., & Brehm, J. W. (1981). *Psychological reactance and control: A theory of freedom and control*. New York: Academic Press.

Brewer, M. B. (1991). The social self: On being the same and different at the same time. *Personality and Social Psychology Bulletin, 17,* 475–482.

Brown, N. O. (1959). *Life against death: The psychoanalytical meaning of history*. Middletown, CT: Wesleyan University Press.

Carver, C., & Sheier, M. (1981). *Attention and self-regulation*. New York: Springer-Verlag.

Cohen, G. L., Aronson, J., & Steele, C. M. (2000). When beliefs yield to evidence: Reducing biased evaluation by affirming the self. *Personality and Social Psychology Bulletin, 26,* 1151–1164.

Collins, N. L., & Feeney, B. C. (2000). A safe haven: An attachment theory perspective on support seeking and caregiving in intimate relationships. *Journal of Personality and Social Psychology, 78,* 1053–1073.

Cox, C., Pyszczynski, T., Goldenberg, J., Greenberg, J., & Solomon, S. (2001). *Disgust, creatureliness and the accessibility of death-related thoughts*. Manuscript in preparation, University of Colorado, Colorado Springs, CO.

Csikszentmihalyi, M. (1990). *Flow: The psychology of optimal experience*. New York: Harper Perennial.

Csikszentmihalyi, M. (1980). Love and the dynamics of personal growth. In K. S. Pope (Ed.), *On love and loving* (pp. 306–326). San Francisco: Jossey-Bass.

Csikszentmihalyi, M., & Rathunde, K. (1998). The development of the person: An experiential perspective on the ontogenesis of psychological complexity. In W. Damon (Series Ed.) & R. M. Lerner (Vol. Ed.), *Handbook of child psychology: Vol. 1. Theoretical models of human development* (5th ed., pp. 635–684). New York: Wiley.

Dechesne, M., Greenberg, J., Arndt, J., & Schimel, J. (2000). Terror management and the vicissitudes of sports fan affiliation: The effects of mortality salience on optimism and fan identification. *European Journal of Social Psychology, 30*, 813–835.

Dechesne, M., Janssen, J., & Van Knippenberg, A. (2000). *Worldview allegiance vs. egotism in the face of existential threat: Need for closure as moderator of terror management strategies*. Unpublished manuscript, University of Nijmegen, Netherlands.

Dechesne, M., Pyszczynski, T., Arndt, J., Sheldon, K., van Knippenberg, A., & Janssen, J. (2001). *Literal and symbolic immortality: The effect of evidence of literal immortality on self-esteem striving in response to mortality salience*. Manuscript submitted for publication, University of Nijmegen, Netherlands.

Deci, E. L. (1975). *Intrinsic motivation*. New York: Plenum Press.

Deci, E. L., & Ryan, R. M. (1991). A motivational approach to self: Integration in personality. In R. Dienstbier (Ed.), *Nebraska Symposium on Motivation: Vol. 38. Perspectives on motivation* (pp. 237–288). Lincoln: University of Nebraska Press.

Deci, E. L., & Ryan, R. M. (1995). Human autonomy: The basis for true self-esteem. In M. Kernis (Ed.), *Efficacy, agency, and self-esteem* (pp. 31–49). New York: Plenum Press.

Deci, E. L., & Ryan, R. M. (2000). The "what" and "why" of goal pursuits: Human needs and the self-determination of behavior. *Psychological Inquiry, 11*, 227–268.

Deci, E. L., Vallerand, R. J., Pelletier, L. G., & Ryan, R. M. (1991). Motivation and education: The self-determination perspective. *Educational Psychologist, 26*, 325–346.

Dein, S., & Barlow, H. (1999). Why do people join the Hare Krishna movement? Deprivation theory revisited. *Mental Health, Religion, and Culture, 2*, 75–84.

Dollard, J., & Miller, N. E. (1950). *Personality and psychotherapy: An analysis in terms of learning, thinking, and culture*. New York: McGraw-Hill.

Duval, S., & Wicklund, R. A. (1972). *A theory of objective self-awareness*. New York: Academic Press.

Elliot, A. J., Sheldon, K. M., & Church, M. A. (1997). Avoidance personal goals and subjective well-being. *Personality and Social Psychology Bulletin, 23*, 915–927.

Estrada, C. A., Isen, A. M., & Young, M. J. (1997). Positive affect facilitates integration of information and decreases anchoring in reasoning among physicians. *Organizational Behavior and Human Decision Processes, 72*, 117–135.

Florian, V., & Mikulincer, M. (1997). Fear of personal death and the judgment of social transgressions: A multidimensional test of terror management theory. *Journal of Personality and Social Psychology, 73*, 369–380.

Fredrickson, B. L. (1998). What good are positive emotions? *Review of General Psychology, 2*, 300–319.

Fredrickson, B. L. (2001). The role of positive emotions in positive psychology: The broaden-and-build theory of positive emotions. *American Psychologist, 56*, 218–226.

Fredrickson, B. L., & Branigan, C. A. (2000). *Positive emotions broaden action urges and the scope of attention*. Manuscript in preparation.

Fredrickson, B. L., & Branigan, C. (2001). Positive emotions. In T. J. Mayne & G. A. Bonanno (Eds.), *Emotions: Current issues and future directions* (pp. 123–151). New York: Guilford Press.

Fredrickson, B. L., & Roberts, T. (1997). Objectification theory: Toward understanding women's lived experiences and mental health risks. *Psychology of Women Quarterly, 21*, 173–206.

Fredrickson, B. L., Roberts, T., Noll, S. M., Quinn, D. M., & Twenge, J. M. (1998). That swimsuit becomes you: Sex differences in self-objectification, restrained eating and math performance. *Journal of Personality and Social Psychology, 75*, 269–284.

Freitas, A. L., Salovey, P., & Liberman, N. (2001). Abstract and concrete self-evaluative goals. *Journal of Personality and Social Psychology, 80*, 410–424.

Freud, S. (1961). *Civilization and its discontents*. New York: Norton. (Original work published 1930)

Freud, S. (1950). *Beyond the pleasure principle*. New York: Liveright. (Original work published 1950)

Goldenberg, J., McCoy, S., Pyszczynski, T., Greenberg, J., & Solomon, S. (2000). The body as a source of self-esteem: The effect of mortality salience on appearance monitoring and identification with the body. *Journal of Personality and Social Psychology, 79*, 118–130.

Goldenberg, J. L., Pyszczynski, T. Greenberg, J., & Solomon, S. (2000). Fleeing the body: A terror management perspective on the problem of human corporeality. *Personality and Social Psychology Review, 4*, 200–218.

Goldenberg, J. L., Pyszczynski, T., Greenberg, J., Solomon, S., Kluck, B., & Cornwell, R. (2001). I am NOT an animal: Mortality salience, disgust, and the denial of human creatureliness. *Journal of Experimental Psychology: General, 130*, 427–435.

Goldenberg, J. L., Pyszczynski, T., McCoy, S. K., Greenberg, J., & Solomon, S. (1999). Death, sex, love, and neuroticism: Why is sex such a problem? *Journal of Personality and Social Psychology, 77*, 1173–1187.

Greenberg, J., Pyszczynski, T., & Paisley, C. (1984). Effect of extrinsic incentives on the use of test anxiety as an anticipatory attributional defense: Playing it cool when the stakes are high. *Journal of Personality and Social Psychology, 47*, 1136–1145.

Greenberg, J., Pyszczynski, T., & Solomon, S. (1986). The causes and consequences of a need for self-esteem: A terror management theory. In R. F. Baumeister (Ed.), *Public self and private self* (pp. 189–212). New York: Springer-Verlag.

Greenberg, J., Pyszczynski, T., & Solomon, S. (1995). Toward a dual motive depth psychology of self and social behavior. In M. Kernis (Ed.), *Efficacy, agency, and self* (pp. 73–99). New York: Plenum Press.

Greenberg, J., Pyszczynski, T., Solomon, S., Pinel, E., Simon, L., & Jordan, K. (1993). Effects of self-esteem on vulnerability-denying defensive distortions: Further evidence of an anxiety-buffering function of self-esteem. *Journal of Experimental Social Psychology, 28,* 229–251.

Greenberg, J., Pyszczynski, T., Solomon, S., Rosenblatt, A., Veeder, M., Kirkland, S., & Lyon, D. (1990). Evidence for terror management theory: II. The effects of mortality salience reactions to those who threaten or bolster the cultural worldview. *Journal of Personality and Social Psychology, 58,* 308–318.

Greenberg, J., Simon, L., Porteus, J., Solomon, S., & Pyszczynski, T. (1995). Evidence of a terror management function of cultural icons: The effects of mortality salience on reactions to the inappropriate use of cherished cultural symbols. *Personality and Social Psychology Bulletin, 21,* 1221–1228.

Greenberg, J., Simon, L., Pyszczynski, T., Solomon, S., & Chatel, D. (1992). Terror management and tolerance: Does mortality salience always intensify negative reactions to others who threaten one's worldview? *Journal of Personality and Social Psychology, 63,* 212–220.

Greenberg, J., Solomon, S., & Pyszczynski, T. (1997). Terror management theory of self-esteem and social behavior: Empirical assessments and conceptual refinements. In M. P. Zanna (Ed.), *Advances in experimental social psychology* (Vol. 29, pp. 61–139). New York: Academic Press.

Greenberg, J., Solomon, S., Pyszczynski, T., Rosenblatt, A., Burling, J., Lyon, D., & Simon, L. (1992). Assessing the terror management analysis of self-esteem: Converging evidence of an anxiety-buffering function. *Journal of Personality and Social Psychology, 63,* 913–922.

Grolnick, W. S., & Ryan, R. M. (1989). Parents styles associated with children's self-regulation and competence in school. *Journal of Educational Psychology, 81,* 143–154.

Harlow, H. F., & Zimmermann, R. R. (1959). Affectional responses in the infant monkey. *Science, 130,* 421.

Harmon-Jones, E., Simon, L., Greenberg, J., Pyszczynski, T., & Solomon, S. (1997). Support for the terror management view of self-esteem: Evidence that self-esteem attenuates mortality salience effects. *Journal of Personality and Social Psychology, 72,* 24–36.

Hazen, C., & Shaver, P. (1987). Romantic love conceptualized as an attachment process. *Journal of Personality and Social Psychology, 52,* 511–524.

Heatherton, T. F., & Baumeister, R. F. (1991). Binge eating as escape from self-awareness. *Psychological Bulletin, 110,* 86–108.

Higgins, E. T. (1997). Beyond pleasure and pain. *American Psychologist, 52,* 1280–1300.

Horney, K. (1937). *The neurotic personality of our time.* New York: Norton.

Hull, J. G., Young, R. D., & Jouriles, E. (1986). Applications of the self-awareness model of alcohol consumption: Predicting patterns of use and abuse. *Journal of Personality and Social Psychology, 51,* 790–796.

Isen, A. M., & Daubman, K. A. (1984). The influence of affect on categorization. *Journal of Personality and Social Psychology, 47,* 1206–1217.

Isen, A. M., Daubman, K. A., & Nowicki, G. P. (1987). Positive affect facilitates creative problem solving. *Journal of Personality and Social Psychology, 52,* 1122–1131.

Isen, A. M., Rosenzweig, A. S., & Young, M. J. (1991). The influence of positive affect on clinical problem solving. *Medical Decision Making, 11,* 221–227.

Izard, C. E. (1971). *The face of emotion.* New York: Appleton-Century-Crofts.

James, W. (1890). *The principles of psychology.* New York: Holt.

Jonas, E., Schimel, J., Greenberg, J., & Pyszczynski, T. (in press). The Scrooge Effect: Evidence that mortality salience increases prosocial attitudes and behavior. *Personality and Social Psychology Bulletin.*

Kasser, T., & Ryan, R. M. (1993). A dark side of the American dream: Correlates of financial success as a life aspiration. *Journal of Personality and Social Psychology, 65,* 410–422.

Kasser, T., & Ryan, R. M. (1996). Further examination of the American dream: Differential correlates of intrinsic and extrinsic goals. *Personality and Social Psychology Bulletin, 22,* 80–87.

Kelly, G. (1955). *The psychology of personal constructs.* New York: Norton.

Kernis, M. H., Grannemann, B. D., & Barclay, L. H. (1989). Stability and level of self-esteem as predictors of anger arousal and hostility. *Journal of Personality and Social Psychology, 56,* 1013–1022.

Kernis, M. H., Grannemann, B. D., & Barclay, L. C. (1992). Stability of self-esteem: Assessment, correlates, and excuse making. *Journal of Personality, 60,* 621–644.

Kernis, M. H., Paradise, A. W., Whitaker, D. J., Wheatman, S. R., Goldman, B. N. (2000). Master of one's psychological domain? Not likely if one's self-esteem is unstable. *Personality and Social Psychology Bulletin, 26,* 1297–1305.

Kernis, M. H., & Waschull, S. B. (1995). The interactive roles of stability and level of self-esteem: Research and theory. In M. R. Zanna (Ed.), *Advances in experimental social psychology* (Vol. 27, pp. 93–141). Hillsdale, NJ: Erlbaum.

Kirkpatrick, L. A., & Shaver, P. R. (1990). Attachment theory and religion: Childhood attachments, religious beliefs, and conversion. *Journal for the Scientific Study of Religion, 29,* 315–334.

Koole, S. (2001). *Mortality salience reduces intrinsic motivation.* Manuscript in preparation, Free University of Amsterdam, Netherlands.

Kruglanski, A. (1980). Lay epistemo-logic—process and contents: Another look at attribution theory. *Psychological Review, 87,* 70–87

Landau, M. J., Johns, M., Pyszczynski, T., Goldenberg, J., Greenberg, J., & Solomon, S. (2002). *Terror management and the need for nonspecific structure: Mortality and salience increases primacy, balance, and base-rate fallacy effects.* Unpublished manuscript, University of Colorado, Colorado Springs.

Langer, S. K. (1982). *Mind: An essay on human feeling* (Vol. 3). Baltimore: Johns Hopkins University Press.

Lepper, M. R., & Greene, D. (1975). Turning work into play: Effects of adult surveillance and extrinsic rewards on children's intrinsic motivation. *Journal of Personality and Social Psychology, 31,* 479–486.

Lewin, K. (1935). *A dynamic approach to personality.* New York: McGraw-Hill.

Maslow, A. (1970). *Motivation and personality* (2nd ed.). New York: Harper & Row.

May, R. (1953). *Man's search for self*. New York: Norton.

May, R. (1983). *The discovery of being*. New York: Norton.

McCoy, S. K., Pyszczynski, T., Solomon, S., & Greenberg, J. (2000). Transcending the self: A terror management perspective on successful aging. In A. Tomer & R. Neimeyer (Eds.), *The problem of death among older adults* (pp. 37–61). New York: Taylor & Francis.

McGregor, H., Lieberman, J. D., Solomon, S., Greenberg, T., Arndt, J., Simon, L., & Pyszczynski, T. (1998). Terror management and aggression: Evidence that mortality salience motivates aggression against worldview threatening others. *Journal of Personality and Social Psychology, 74,* 590–605.

McGregor, I., Zanna, M. P., Holmes, J. G., & Spencer, S. J. (2001). Conviction in the face of uncertainty: Going to extremes and being oneself. *Journal of Personality and Social Psychology, 80,* 472–488.

Mead, G. H. (1934). *Mind, self, and society*. Chicago: University of Chicago Press.

Mikulincer, M. (1997). Adult attachment style and information processing: Individual differences in curiosity and cognitive closure, *Journal of Personality and Social Psychology, 72,* 1217–1230.

Mikulincer, M., & Florian, V. (2000). Exploring individual differences in reactions to mortality salience: Does attachment style regulate terror management mechanisms? *Journal of Personality and Social Psychology, 79,* 260–273.

Mikulincer, M., Florian, V., & Hirschberger, G. (in press). The existential function of close relationships: Introducing death into the science of love. *Personality and Social Psychology Review*.

Nietzsche, F. (1999). *Thus spake zarathustra*. New York: Dover. (Original work published 1911)

Obholzer, A. (2001). *Security and creativity at work*. Philadelphia: Brunner-Routledge.

Ochsmann, R., & Reichelt, K. (1994). *Evaluation of moral and immoral behavior: Evidence for terror management theory*. Unpublished manuscript, University of Mainz, Germany.

Piaget, J. (1952). *The origins of intelligence in children*. New York: International Universities Press.

Plant, R. W., & Ryan, R. M. (1985). Intrinsic motivation and the effects of self-consciousness, self-awareness, and ego-involvement: An investigation of internally controlling styles. *Journal of Personality, 53,* 435–449.

Pyszczynski, T., & Greenberg, J. (1987a). Self-regulatory perseveration and the depressive self-focusing style: An integrative theory of reactive depression. *Psychological Bulletin, 102,* 122–138.

Pyszczynski, T., & Greenberg, J. (1987b). Toward an integration of cognitive and motivational perspectives on social inference: A biased hypothesis-testing model. In L. Berkowitz (Ed.), *Advances in experimental social psychology* (Vol. 20, pp. 297–340). San Diego, CA: Academic Press.

Pyszczynski, T., Greenberg, J., & Solomon, S. (1998). Controlling the uncontrollable: A terror management perspective on the psychology of control. In M. Kotta, G. Weary, & G. Sedek (Eds.), *Personal control in action: Cognitive and motivational mechanisms* (pp. 85–108). New York: Plenum Press.

Pyszczynski, T., Greenberg, J., & Solomon, S. (1999). A dual process model of defense against conscious and unconscious death-related thoughts: An extension of terror management theory. *Psychological Review, 106,* 835–845.

Pyszczynski, T., Greenberg, J., Solomon, S., Cather, C., Gat, I., & Sideris, J. (1995). Defensive distancing from victims of serious illness: The role of delay. *Personality and Social Psychology Bulletin, 21,* 13–20.

Pyszczynski, T., Greenberg, J., Solomon, S., & Hamilton, J. (1990). A terror management analysis of self-awareness and anxiety: The hierarchy of terror. *Anxiety Research, 2,* 177–195.

Pyszczynski, T., Wicklund, R. A., Floresku, S., Koch, H., Gauch, G., Solomon, S., & Greenberg, J. (1996). Whistling in the dark: Exaggerated consensus estimates in response to incidental reminders of mortality. *Psychological Science, 7*(6), 332–336.

Rank, O. (1959). *The myth of the birth of the hero, and other writings*. New York: Vintage Books.

Rank, O. (1976). *Will therapy and truth and reality*. New York: Knopf. (Original work published 1936)

Rank, O. (1989). *Art and artist*. New York: Norton. (Original work published 1932)

Rank, O. (1998). *Psychology and the soul* (G. C. Richter & E. J. Lieberman, Trans.). Baltimore: John Hopkins University Press. (Original work published 1930)

Reed, M. B., & Aspinwall, L. G. (1998). Self-affirmation reduces biased processing of health-risk information. *Motivation and Emotion, 22,* 99–132.

Rhodewalt, F., & Morf, C. C. (1998). On self-aggrandizement and anger: A temporal analysis of narcissism and affective reactions to success and failure. *Journal of Personality and Social Psychology, 74,* 672–685.

Roese, N. J., & Olson, J. M. (1993). Self-esteem and counterfactual thinking. *Journal of Personality and Social Psychology, 65,* 199–206.

Rogers, C. R. (1959). A theory of therapy, personality, and interpersonal relationships, as developed in the client-centered framework. In S. Koch (Ed.), *Psychology: A study of science* (Vol. 3). New York: McGraw-Hill.

Rogers, C. R. (1961). *On becoming a person*. Boston: Houghton Mifflin.

Rosenberg, M. (1965). *Society and adolescent self-image*. Princeton, NJ: Princeton University Press.

Ryan, R. M., Stiller, J., & Lynch, J. H. (1994). Representations of relationships to teachers, parents, and friends, as predictors of academic motivation and self-esteem. *Journal of Early Adolescence, 14,* 226–249.

Salmivalli, C., Kaukiainen, A., Kaistaniemi, L., & Lagerspetz, K. M. J. (1999). Self-evaluated self-esteem, peer-evaluated self-esteem, and defensive egotism as predictors of adolescents' participation in bullying situations. *Personality and Social Psychology Bulletin, 25,* 1268–1278.

Schimel, J., Arndt, J., Pyszczynski, T., & Greenberg, J. (2001). Being accepted for who we are: Evidence that social validation of the intrinsic self reduces general defensiveness. *Journal of Personality and Social Psychology, 80,* 35–52.

Schimel, J., Simon, L., Greenberg, J., Pyszczynski, T.,

Solomon, S., Waxmonsky, J., & Arndt, J. (1999). Stereotyping and terror management: Evidence that mortality salience increases stereotypic thinking and preferences. *Journal of Personality and Social Psychology, 77,* 905–926.

Schwartz, B. (1997). Self-determination: The tyranny of freedom. *American Psychologist, 55,* 79–88.

Sheldon, K. M., & Kasser, T. (1998). Pursuing personal goals: Skills enable progress, but not all progress is beneficial. *Personality and Social Psychology Bulletin, 24,* 1319–1331.

Sherman, D. A. K., Nelson, L. D., & Steele, C. M. (2000). Do messages about health risks threaten the self? Increasing the acceptance of threatening health messages via self-affirmation. *Personality and Social Psychology Bulletin, 26,* 1046–1058.

Simon, L., Greenberg, J., Arndt, J., Pyszczynski, T., Clement, R., & Solomon, J. (1997). Perceived consensus, uniqueness, and terror management: Compensatory responses to threats to inclusion and distinctiveness. *Personality and Social Psychology Bulletin, 23,* 1055–1065.

Solomon, S., Greenberg, J., & Pyszczynski, T. (1991). A terror management theory of social behavior: The psychological functions of self-esteem and cultural worldviews. In M. P. Zanna (Ed.), *Advances in experimental social psychology* (Vol. 24, pp. 93–159). New York: Academic Press.

Steele, C. M. (1988). The psychology of self-affirmation: Sustaining the integrity of the self. In L. Berkowitz (Ed.), *Advances in experimental social psychology* (Vol. 21, pp. 261–302). New York: Academic Press.

Steele, C. M., & Liu, T. J. (1983). Dissonance processes as self-affirmation. *Journal of Personality and Social Psychology, 45,* 5–19.

Stipek, D. J. (2001). Classroom context effects on young children's motivation. In F. Salili, C. Chiu, & Y. Hong (Eds.), *Student motivation: The culture and context of learning* (pp. 273–292). New York: Plenum Press.

Taubman Ben-Ari, O. T., Florian, V., & Mikulincer, M. (1999). The impact of mortality salience on reckless driving: A test of terror management mechanisms. *Journal of Personality and Social Psychology, 76,* 35–45.

Tesser, A. (1988). Towards a self-evaluation maintenance model of social behavior. In L. Berkowitz (Ed.), *Advances in experimental social psychology* (Vol. 21, pp. 181–227). New York: Academic Press.

Tompkins, S. S. (1962). *Affect, imagery, and consciousness. Vol. 1: The positive affects.* New York: Springer-Verlag.

White, R. W. (1959). Motivation reconsidered: The concept of competence. *Psychological Review, 66,* 297–333.

Wicklund, R. A. (1975). Objective self-awareness. In L. Berkowitz (Ed.), *Advances in experimental social psychology* (Vol. 8, pp. 233–275). New York: Academic Press.

Wicklund, R. A., & Gollwitzer, P. M. (1981). Symbolic self-completion, attempted influence, and self-deprecation. *Basic and Applied Social Psychology, 2,* 89–114.

17

How Important Is Social Comparison?

JOANNE V. WOOD
ANNE E. WILSON

People may compare themselves with others on all kinds of dimensions, such as physical appearance, abilities, and personal wealth. They may do so to serve a number of motives: They may wish to evaluate themselves, to improve themselves, to feel better about themselves, or to feel more connected with others (e.g., Helgeson & Taylor, 1993; Locke & Nekich, 2000; Wood, 1989). How important are such processes of social comparison?

To social psychologists, certainly, social comparison is highly important. A PsycLit search of 11 top journals in social, personality, and general psychology yielded 196 references to journal articles concerning social comparison published between 1991 and 2001. Two major volumes dedicated to social comparison have appeared since 1997 (Buunk & Gibbons, 1997; Suls & Wheeler, 2000). These come almost 50 years after Festinger (1954) published his theory of social comparison.

Researchers' interest in social comparison appears to stem from a widely held, heartfelt conviction that social comparison is of paramount significance to self-appraisal and to social life. Social comparison has been de-scribed as "a core aspect of human experi-ence" (Suls & Wheeler, 2000, p. 15) and as "a pervasive and fundamental feature of group life" (Hogg, 2000, p. 401). The liter-ature is replete with phrases such as, "peo-ple face information about others nearly constantly" (Wood, 1996, p. 523) and de-scriptions of social comparison as an "al-most inevitable element of social interac-tion" (Brickman & Bulman, 1977, p. 150). The word "ubiquitous" is ubiquitous (e.g., Buunk & Gibbons, 2000; Smith, 2000).

Are such views justified by empirical evi-dence? In this chapter, we evaluate the im-portance of social comparison. We admit at the outset, however, that the question as phrased, How important is social compari-son? is impossible to answer, for at least three reasons. The first is that one must ask, relative to what? The importance of social comparison can be judged only relative to something else. In this chapter, we focus pri-marily on the importance of social compari-son relative to two other sources of informa-tion about the self. First, we examine objective information, which Festinger (1954) claimed would be preferred over so-cial comparison. Second, we examine tem-

344

poral comparisons, which involve comparisons with one's own past standing or with one's imagined future standing (Albert, 1977). Although other sources of information about the self exist, such as feedback from others and current self-appraisal (e.g., Baumeister, 1998; Sedikedes & Skowronski, 1995), we focus on objective information and temporal comparisons because these are the ones with which social comparison has most often been compared, both theoretically and empirically. After reviewing the evidence concerning the importance of social comparison relative to objective information and temporal comparisons, we examine the evidence concerning how important lay people think social comparison is relative to these other standards. As is demonstrated, lay people's views are often discrepant from those of social comparison researchers.

A second stumbling block to answering the question, How important is social comparison? is that one's answer critically depends on one's operationalizations of social comparison and any other sources of information. If one is studying the relative importance of social and objective information, for example, and one's manipulation of social information is more potent or engaging than one's operationalization of objective information, one could draw an invalid conclusion about the primacy of social comparison. Only after researchers have accumulated many observations based on multiple operationalizations of each construct can they safely draw conclusions about relative importance. As this chapter makes clear, however, such systematic and thorough scrutiny of these issues has not been undertaken as yet.

A third reason that the simple question, How important is social comparison? is impossible to answer is that the answer almost certainly must be, "it depends." The importance of social comparison must vary under various conditions. In the final section of this chapter, we propose what we see as the most crucial moderators of the importance of social comparison. These moderators help to reconcile multiple inconsistencies in the literature.

Now that we have argued for the futility of answering the question, How important is social comparison? let us proceed to address it.

Objective Standards versus Social Comparisons

Festinger (1954) argued that when people want to evaluate an opinion or ability, they prefer to do so using objective information based in physical reality. His Hypothesis 2 reads, "To the extent that objective, nonsocial means are not available, people evaluate their opinions and abilities by comparison respectively with the opinions and abilities of others" (p. 118). In a corollary to Hypothesis 2, Festinger went so far as to say, "When an objective, non-social basis for the evaluation of one's ability or opinion is readily available persons will not evaluate their opinions or abilities by comparison with others" (p. 120).

According to Festinger (1954), then, social comparison is less valuable than objective information. Only when objective standards are unavailable will people compare themselves with other people.

Very little research has examined these crucial hypotheses. Rather, they have "generally been treated as axiomatic rather than hypothetical" (Miller, 1977, p. 343). Most journal articles and chapters in the social comparison literature that describe Festinger's (1954) theory in their introductory paragraphs refer to the preference for objective standards in passing without questioning it. The tone, if not exact wording, usually goes something like this: Festinger argued that people prefer to evaluate themselves against objective standards, but such standards are often nonexistent for the sorts of abilities and opinions that people evaluate; hence, they resort to comparing themselves with other people.

Although Festinger's (1954) belief in the primacy of objective, nonsocial bases for self-evaluation was challenged by several authors in the 1970s (Allen & Wilder, 1977; Brickman & Berman, 1971; Gastorf & Suls, 1978; Miller, 1977), these challenges have received little notice. Researchers still largely accept the idea that people prefer objective standards over social comparison, as evidenced by Suls and Wheeler's (2000) *Handbook of Social Comparison*, the most comprehensive book on social comparison to date. That volume includes seven chapters that refer to Festinger's objective-versus-social hypothesis, and virtually all of these (six) do so in the implicitly accepting manner illustrated here.

Is it true that people prefer to evaluate themselves against objective standards and use social comparisons only as a last resort? To answer this question, we must first consider what constitutes an "objective" basis of evaluation. Festinger provided examples involving immediate physical referents, such as testing the opinion that an object is fragile "by hitting it with a hammer" (1954, p. 118). Similarly, in an example of an ability evaluation, Festinger suggested that an objective way to test one's ability to jump across a particular brook is to attempt that very jump. However, in the single study Festinger cited concerning objective information, the operationalization of objective information was a far cry from such cut-and-dried physical referents. Specifically, as Festinger described it, half of the participants in a study by Hochbaum (1953) were provided an "objective basis for feeling that their opinion was likely to be correct" because they were "persuaded by the experimenter that they were extremely good at being able to make correct judgements" (Festinger, 1954, p. 120).

In this chapter, we do not restrict the term "objective" only to concrete referents such as the hammer test. However, we do reserve the term for information that, at a minimum, is unambiguous and that helps one to locate one's standing on an ordinal scale. In addition, we distinguish between objective information that constitutes a *standard* and objective information that does not. This distinction is captured in the following example provided by Bill Klein (personal communication, August 21, 2001): "If I get 15 questions out of 20 correct on a driver's license test, that is useful objective information, but I may need to get 18 to pass the test"—18 serves as the standard. It is possible, although not clear, that Festinger's (1954) hypothesis that people prefer objective to social comparison referred to objective standards and not simply objective information.

Complicating matters further is that whether a certain type of information constitutes an objective standard does not depend only on the features of the information itself but also on the question one is asking. If one's goal is not only to obtain the dri-

ver's license but also to become an excellent driver, then the standard may be 20, rather than 18. Festinger similarly implied that what constitutes a standard depends on the question one is asking:

> If the only use to which, say, jumping ability was put was to jump across a particular brook, it would be simple to obtain an accurate evaluation of one's ability in this respect. However, the unavailability of the opportunity for such clear testing and the vague and multipurpose use of various abilities generally make such a clear objective test not feasible or not useful. . . . One might find out how many seconds it takes a person to run a certain distance, but what does this mean with respect to his ability—is it adequate or not? (p. 119)

Certain types of information that would constitute an objective standard in some cases, then, may be insufficient for asking other self-evaluative questions.

With these complications in mind, we next examine the little research that exists that speaks to the question of whether people prefer objective to social standards of comparison. First we examine research concerning people's interest in objective and social information, and then we examine the influence of objective and social information on self-evaluations and behavior.

Selection of Objective versus Social Standards

In three studies that examined people's interest in various types of information, participants had access to objective information, although perhaps not objective standards. Specifically, participants had access to information about their own scores and the maximum possible score (Levine & Green, 1984; Miller, 1977) or their percentage of correct answers, which conveys the same information as the maximum possible score (Levin & Levin, 1973). One could view the maximum possible score as an objective standard against which participants could have compared their own scores (Gastorf & Suls, 1978). Or one could argue that the maximum possible score is an unlikely standard because people may see it as unattainable—as merely hypothetical.

In any case, in all three studies, participants showed a great deal of interest in receiving social comparison information—how their scores compared with those of other people—even though they had access to information about the maximum possible score (Levin & Levin, 1973; Levine & Green, 1984; Miller, 1977). For example, in the study that found the lowest level of interest in social comparison, Miller (1977) asked male military commanders attending a 1-week leadership course to choose between two modes of feedback regarding their final exam performance—their relative ranking in the class (social comparison) or their own scores out of the total possible points (objective). Overall, about 42% of the men chose the social comparison feedback. This preference was even higher in men who were highly attracted to their group (75%) and who viewed the army as their most important reference group (65%).

Although participants in these studies may not have viewed the available objective information to be objective *standards,* it is striking that, when two studies forced participants to choose between social and objective information, a sizable proportion of respondents preferred the social (Levin & Levin, 1973; Miller, 1977). Future outcomes did not appear to be contingent on participants' standing relative to others in either of these studies. Hence, one must ask why people wish to know how they stand relative to other people rather than how they stand relative to an absolute score.

In three other selection studies, participants received objective information that more clearly provided a useful standard. If Festinger (1954) was correct about the primacy of objective standards, these participants should have had no interest in social comparison. Yet they clearly did. Specifically, in two of these studies, university students were told not only their scores on an exam but also their letter grades, which presumably constitute the only objective standard students truly "need." Nonetheless, most students were very interested in seeing other students' exam scores (Brickman & Berman, 1971), as well as other information about the score distribution, such as the average score (Suls & Tesch, 1978). Similarly, Foddy and Crundall (1993) found that after students received graded assignments, about half of them reported making social comparisons concerning those assignments. Indeed, the students were especially likely to engage in social comparison when they already had the objective information about their performances.

These studies of participants' interest in information, then, appear to contradict Festinger's (1954) assertion that "when an objective, non-social basis for the evaluation . . . is readily available, persons will *not* evaluate [themselves] by comparison with others" (p. 120, italics added). Perhaps one could argue that students' interest in social comparisons despite their knowledge of their grades indicates that their question is different from the one we are assuming. For example, if the students are psychology majors, their question may not be, "How well did I do on this exam?" but "How strong am I in psychology?" or "How good a psychologist will I be?" In these cases, the letter grade on a particular exam may not serve as a sufficient standard. Yet we must then ask why other students' exam grades serve as a better standard for asking such questions than does one's own letter grade. Why does a person's strength as a psychologist depend on how many others received an A and not simply on whether he or she received an A? We return to this question after we review research concerning the impact of objective and social information.

Impact of Objective versus Social Standards

Festinger's hypotheses concerning the primacy of objective information also can be examined in studies of the impact of objective versus social standards. If Festinger (1954) was correct, social standards should have no impact when objective standards are available. However, one can cite vivid, "real life" examples in which social comparisons appear to have undue impact, despite the presence of objective criteria. The life-satisfaction and relative-deprivation literatures present many examples of how people's contentment with various domains of their lives is dependent not only on their objective circumstances (such as income) but also on how their circumstances compare with those of other people (e.g., Diener, 1984; Olson, Herman, & Zanna, 1986). Although such evidence has been challenged in various ways (e.g., Diener &

Fujita, 1997; Fox & Kahneman, 1992; Wood, 1996), recent research using new methods suggests that social comparisons do influence one's happiness. In several samples drawn from eight nations, Hagerty (2000) found that although happiness is predicted most strongly by absolute income, it is also predicted by the range and skew (inequality) of the income distribution in one's community.

Another real-life illustration of the impact of social comparisons stems from research on self-concept, especially academic self-concept. Marsh and Parker (1984) have presented evidence that students' views of their academic abilities depend on the average ability level of the school they attend; regardless of their objective ability, they evaluate their own academic ability more highly if the average ability in their school is low than if it is high (cf. Blanton, Buunk, Gibbons, & Kuyper, 1999). Even educational or career aspirations may depend less on one's objective qualifications than on one's relative standing among one's immediate peers (Tesser & Campbell, 1985). Thus an undergraduate who earns high grades at a college at which it is easy to do so tends to have higher career aspirations than an equally qualified student at a more competitive institution (Davis, 1966).

As compelling as these examples are, they do not derive from experimental studies that establish a causal role for social comparisons (Wood, 1996). However, a few experimental studies have been conducted that do speak to the question of whether social comparisons have impact when more objective comparisons are available, although they were not necessarily designed to. We again can distinguish between studies that provided objective information but perhaps not objective standards and studies that more clearly provided objective standards. Two studies that fall into the former category both found that participants' self-evaluations varied only with the type of social comparison they received, not with objective information (Gastorf & Suls, 1978; Klein, 1997). For example, Klein (1997, Study 2) found that when undergraduates participated in a bogus "esthetic judgment" task, their evaluations of their performances were not affected by the objective feedback that they were correct 40% or 60% of the

time. Instead, participants who were told that they were "above average" rated their esthetic-judgment ability higher and were happier with their performances than were participants who were told they were "below average," regardless of their absolute scores. People may be especially likely to weight social comparisons more heavily than objective information when the social comparison target is a friend rather than a stranger (Campbell, Fairey, & Fehr, 1986).

We have suggested that the types of objective information used in these studies, such as one's percentage of correct answers or the maximum possible score, may or may not serve as standards. A more clearly useful objective standard was provided by Boggiano and Ruble (1979), who gave children Hershey's Kisses if they obtained a certain score on a novel task. Later, the children had an opportunity to engage in the same task in a context in which they could expect no reward. Although preschool children's interest in the task depended on whether they had met the absolute criterion, schoolchildren's (ages 9–11) interest did not. These older children chose the task if they believed that they had performed better than other children. Although the "objective standard" no longer applied (participants could no longer receive chocolate), it is not clear why participants' task choices were guided more by the social comparisons they had made earlier than by whether they had met the objective standard earlier.

In the most forceful challenge to date of Festinger's (1954) belief in the primacy of objective standards, Klein (1997, Studies 2 and 3) similarly provided an objective standard in the form of a reward criterion. In this case the reward was still available when participants made judgments. Specifically, after completing the self-evaluation measure described previously, Klein's participants had a choice between two tasks, one of which involved new trials of the esthetic-judgment task. They were told that they would win $10 if their judgments were correct over 50% of the time (the objective standard). Participants did take the objective information into account: They were more likely to choose the esthetic-judgment task when they had scored 60% the first time than when they had scored 40%. At the same time, however, social comparison information also made a difference; participants who thought they had performed "above average" on the esthetic-judgment task were more likely than those who thought their performance was "below average" to choose that task again, regardless of their absolute level of performance the first time. These results suggest that people's (school-age and above) task selections are influenced by social comparison information, even when an objective standard is present.

A critic might argue, however, that in both the Boggiano and Ruble (1979) and the Klein (1997) studies, the reward criterion served as an absolute standard only for the question of whether participants would receive a reward, not for other questions that participants had in mind. If participants were asking, "What sorts of things am I good at?" and thought no objective standard was available to address this question, they had little choice but to consider the social comparison information. Again, however, one must ask why social comparisons answer that question better than do the reward criteria used in these studies. A reward criterion implies a relatively objective judgement about whether the participants' ability can be considered good. It is not clear why one's performance relative to other people serves as a better answer to that question.

Clearly, people often do measure their own abilities by how they measure up to those of other people. The question is why that is true. Festinger (1954) proposed that people use social comparisons only when there is no objective standard to help them self-evaluate. In contrast, we argue that social comparison is not merely a poor substitute for objective standards. The evidence that particularly persuades us of this point is that participants sometimes prefer social information to objective information (Levin & Levin, 1973; Miller, 1977) and that participants do pay attention to social comparison information even when a clear and useful objective criterion exists. Klein's (1997) participants' task choices were influenced by social comparisons even when their chances of winning a cash prize hinged only on whether they had met an objective standard. To our minds, such findings clearly

contradict Festinger's position.

We cannot completely refute the argument that the "real" questions that participants are asking in these studies are ones for which there are no objective standards and that therefore the participants must attend to social comparisons. However, this argument is weak on three counts: (1) it requires an explanation about why the objective information that is available is inferior to the social information, (2) its assumptions seem less parsimonious than the assumption that people simply prefer social comparisons, and (3) the overuse of this argument renders Festinger's hypothesis unfalsifiable. Whenever participants prefer social over objective information, one could argue that the objective information available does not serve as an objective standard for the question participants are asking.

It seems preferable to conclude that people value social comparisons because they convey some meaning that is not conferred by objective standards. We are inclined toward a conclusion that Foddy and Crundall (1993) drew. Observing that undergraduates were especially likely to seek social comparisons after receiving graded assignments, Foddy and Crundall said that people appear to "need to canvas a range of others to assess the meaning of objective feedback, and to establish their position relative to others in the group" (p. 302). This conclusion is the reverse of Festinger's belief that people seek social comparisons only when objective standards are not available. Apparently, people sometimes need to make social comparisons to "assess the meaning of objective feedback." Identifying precisely why people value social comparisons in such cases—what special meaning social comparisons have—is a topic for future research.

Conclusions

Only a handful of experimental studies address the selection of objective and social information. Even fewer studies address the impact of objective and social comparison information, and only a tiny subset of either type of study were explicitly designed to examine these issues. Only Klein's (1997) studies manipulated objective and social standards orthogonally. We interpret the evidence that does exist, however, as contradicting Festinger's (1954) hypotheses about the supremacy of objective standards. Given a choice, people often prefer social comparison information to objective information, and social comparisons have impact even when objective standards are available.

We would certainly not conclude from these studies that social comparisons always trump objective standards. Later we discuss in more detail the circumstances under which objective information may be more important than social comparison.

Temporal Comparisons versus Social Comparisons

How important are social comparisons relative to temporal comparisons—comparisons with one's own past standing or against one's imagined future standing? Two decades after Festinger's seminal paper, Stuart Albert (1977) proposed that people may use such "temporal comparisons" in their self-appraisals, particularly for the purpose of establishing a sense of self-identity over time. Just as Festinger expected social information to be the second choice after objective standards, Albert suggested that people would turn to temporal comparison only in the absence of *both* objective and social information. The second corollary of his Hypothesis 2 reads, "When objective evidence (and/or social evidence) providing a sense of self-identity over time is readily available, persons will not attempt to establish this sense by an internal and historical comparison of their present self-description with one from their past" (Albert, 1977, p. 490).

Note that even for the rather specific task of establishing a sense of *self-identity over time*, Albert held to Festinger's (1954) assumption of the primacy of objective standards. He also assumed that social comparison would be preferred over temporal comparison. Social comparison theorists have agreed with Albert's (1977) contention that temporal comparison processes are generally secondary to social comparison (e.g., Suls & Mullen, 1982). Are researchers correct? Next, we examine the evidence concerning the selection of social versus temporal information, and then we examine

research concerning the impact of such comparisons.

Selection of Social versus Temporal Standards

Given a choice between social and temporal comparison feedback, which would people prefer? The only selection study that we are aware of that examined relative interest in the two types of feedback was a clever study of schoolchildren by Ruble and Flett (1988). After completing two math tests and receiving no feedback on one and an ambiguous score on the other, participants had an opportunity to examine folders containing either (1) their own tests and the corresponding answer keys or (2) social information—the tests and scores of other children. Examining one's own tests might be considered a type of temporal comparison, in that participants could have compared their first test score with their second. However, participants completed these tests one after the other, so they were not very different temporally. In addition, Ruble and Flett did not distinguish between the time participants spent examining their most recent scores and their first scores, so it is possible that they focused on their most recent scores rather than on making temporal comparisons.

Results indicated that children whose school performances in general were low or average were more interested in the social information than in the information about their own tests; they spent approximately 60% of their feedback-seeking time with the social information. In contrast, children whose general school performances were high and who were in the higher school grades began to show a preference for information about their own test scores, spending more than 52% of their time examining this information. The authors argued that older children with high ability were more certain of their own standing, which, as Festinger (1954) would predict, decreased their interest in social comparison.

The Levine and Green (1984) study mentioned earlier also may be relevant here. After each of 10 trials, schoolchildren could choose to examine their objective task scores, scores of other children, or both. Children almost always chose to look at their own scores, but also chose to examine social comparisons over 90% of the time. Because participants were given feedback after each of 10 trials, those who examined their own scores were accessing temporal comparison information simultaneously. The meaning of choosing one's own score is unclear, however; it may reflect interest in objective, temporal, or even social comparison information, in that children needed to know their own scores to compare them with those of other children. Although the meaning of choosing one's own score may be ambiguous, Levine and Green's (1984) study does point to an impact of temporal comparisons on social comparisons: Children whose own performances were declining were especially interested in selecting downward social comparisons.

Impact of Social versus Temporal Standards

Level-of-aspiration research examined the influence of individuals' temporal performance (how they did from one trial to the next) and norms (how they did relative to others) on their feelings of success, satisfaction, and future expectations (Goethals, 1986b). Interestingly, the founder of social comparison theory had a hand in this early work on temporal comparison. For example, Festinger found, in his undergraduate thesis, that participants' level of aspiration was determined more by how others performed than by their own prior performances (Hertzman & Festinger, 1940). Indeed, because such level-of-aspiration research typically demonstrated that social norms had greater influence than personal progress, it may have helped to convince Festinger of the importance of social relative to temporal information (e.g., Goethals, 1986b).

Temporal comparisons also have been studied in the domain of subjective well-being and life satisfaction. Adaptation-level theorists (Brickman & Campbell, 1971) and relative-deprivation theorists (Runciman, 1966) have argued that satisfaction does not depend only on absolute levels of an outcome but also on whether one's current fortunes are better or worse than previously. Supporting these ideas is evidence that temporal comparison is associated with satisfaction in a variety of domains (e.g., Karney & Coombs, 2000; Sheeran, Abrams, & Orbell, 1995).

How important to subjective well-being is temporal information relative to social comparison? Three studies have examined this question. In two of these (Emmons & Diener, 1985; Fox & Kahneman, 1992), university students were asked about their life satisfaction, as well as how they compared with the average college student (how much better or worse off) and what recent changes had occurred in their lives (how much better or worse recently than before). In both studies, temporal change predicted satisfaction in several domains, but social comparison was by far the stronger predictor. However, as the researchers acknowledged, these results may not imply that social comparisons determine one's satisfaction; instead, one's global satisfaction may lead one to infer one's standing relative to others. Fox and Kahneman (1992) presented evidence that global satisfaction levels may have more influence on people's ratings of their relative standing than on their ratings of temporal change. Moreover, answers to the question, "How much worse off or better off are you than the average college student?" may not imply true social comparisons but may mean essentially the same thing as answers to the question, "How satisfied are you with your life?" (Wood, 1996).

Instead of using ratings of relative standing as the measure of social comparison, Dubé, Jodoin and Kairouz (1998) asked young adults and their middle-aged parents how much they used upward and downward social comparisons, as well as recent and distant past temporal comparisons, to evaluate their subjective well-being. They found that only social comparison frequency ratings predicted participants' reports of subjective well-being. Note, though, that the researchers assessed directional information for social comparisons (upward versus downward) but did not make that distinction for temporal comparisons. Had they done so, it is possible that they would have found, as they did for social comparison, that participants who reported more downward than upward temporal comparisons were more satisfied. In the research cited earlier for the association between temporal comparison and satisfaction, direction had been taken into account (e.g., Karney & Coombs, 2000; Sheeran et al., 1995).

Summary

In summary, very little research has examined people's preferences for social or temporal comparisons. Only one well-controlled study examined relative preferences for the two, and that study may have not have measured true temporal comparisons (Ruble & Flett, 1988). More research has examined the impact of temporal versus social comparisons, and all of that research has suggested that social comparisons have a stronger effect than temporal comparisons.

However, as was true for objective information, we would not conclude that social comparisons are always more influential than temporal comparisons. In these studies, temporal information was limited to very recent performance, and hence it may have been less useful than information about more distal previous performance. Moreover, in the subjective-well-being studies, questionable measures of social or of temporal comparisons were used. Later we propose other moderators of the relative impact of social and temporal comparisons.

How Important Do Lay People Think Social Comparison Is?

Next, we examine the views of lay people regarding the importance of social comparison, which may or may not differ from the actual importance of social comparison in their lives. Do lay people believe that they engage in it frequently or infrequently, and do they think that such comparisons are influential in serving their self-related motives? Do they regard them as being more important or less important than objective information or temporal comparisons? To address these questions, we first examine studies that have used a variety of self-report methods.

Respondents' Self-Reports

Open-Ended Questions

Several researchers have asked respondents open-ended questions about how they go about evaluating themselves or some aspect of their lives. For example, Sedikedes and Skowronski (1995, Study 1) asked under-graduate participants to list the ways or strategies they used to gain self-knowledge or increase self-understanding. Ross, Eyman, and Kishchuk (1986) asked participants not about how they evaluate themselves but about how they evaluate their life satisfaction or happiness. How often do people spontaneously mention social comparison when answering such questions?

These open-ended studies concerned two different domains (self-evaluation or life satisfaction), included six samples—three involving undergraduates and three involving community members who ranged between 20 and 77 years old—and employed a variety of methods, including interviews, questionnaires, and even a "think aloud" procedure (Ross et al., 1986; Schoeneman, 1981; Sedikedes & Skowronski, 1995). The coding schemes used to categorize participants' responses also varied widely between the studies, which presumably reflects either the answers that participants generated, the researchers' interests, or both. Hence, comparing some categories (e.g., temporal comparisons) across studies is difficult.

However, all of these researchers were interested in social comparison, and in terms of that category, the studies were remarkably consistent, given their diversity: Participants mentioned social comparison relatively infrequently. Indeed, in three of the six samples, participants referred to social comparisons least frequently of all the sources of information that they mentioned. For example, when participants answered questions about how they came to know that they possessed specific attributes, the relative rates at which they mentioned self-observation, feedback from others, and social comparison (collapsing across participants) were about 7:2:1, respectively (Schoeneman, 1981).

In all of the samples, respondents emphasized self-related, rather than social-comparison-based, sources of information. For example, when Ross and colleagues' (1986) respondents described how they decided how happy or satisfied they were with their lives, they referred most frequently to their general feelings (e.g., "The pleasant thoughts I have and the absence of negative emotions")—about half of the time.

Two sets of researchers categorized some of participants' responses involving self-observation into temporal comparisons. In Sedikedes and Skowronski's (1995) study, information about one's past and future selves (e.g., "remembering yourself in past interactions with other people"; "comparing yourself with the way you were in the past"; "imagining yourself in future interactions with other people") together made up 56% of the sources of self-knowledge that participants listed, compared with 16% for social comparison. (Note that the data were reported as frequencies of categories across participants, so we do not know whether these percentages represent a few or many participants.)

Temporal comparisons also were important to Ross and colleagues' (1986) participants, especially comparisons with future selves. One's future expectations and goals constituted the second most frequently mentioned source of information for evaluating one's life satisfaction (e.g., "So, I'm trying to learn them [new job skills] now so I can be in a healthy financial situation, eventually, instead of never"). Respondents referred to past comparisons much less frequently, less than social comparison in two of three samples.

Unfortunately, none of these researchers reported how many responses specifically involved objective information. It is possible that some of their categories—for example, Schoeneman's (1981) "feedback from others"—did include objective information. However, neither Sedikedes and Skowronski's (1995) nor Ross and colleagues' (1986) respondents appear to have mentioned objective sources at all. This result is especially surprising for Ross and colleagues' study, considering that objective indicators such as personal income would seem to be especially relevant to life satisfaction.

In summary, when participants respond to open-ended questions about how they evaluate themselves or their life satisfaction, they refer to social comparison relatively infrequently. Instead, they report that their own self-observations, often involving temporal comparisons, contribute much more to their self-knowledge. They also regard feedback from others as being very important for self-evaluation (Schoeneman, 1981; Sedikedes & Skowronski, 1995), but not for evaluation of life satisfaction (Ross et al., 1986). Although respondents tend to

mention social comparison least frequently, they also appear to regard it as more important than objective information, in that they appear to not mention objective information at all. We cannot trust this conclusion completely, however, without knowing for certain whether researchers sorted such mentions into other categories.

Rankings and Ratings

Researchers also have examined participants' self-reports by asking participants to rank-order or rate possible sources of information. For example, Schoeneman (1981) followed up his open-ended questions by asking participants to rank the importance of three sources of information. Participants' rankings followed the same order that their open-ended responses had yielded: self-observation, feedback from others, and social comparison.

Results of several additional studies have been strikingly consistent with these. People report that they call on self-observation, personal standards, or temporal comparisons most frequently (Dubé et al., 1998; Wayment & Campbell, 2000; Wayment & Taylor, 1995) and that such sources are most important (Schoeneman, 1981; Sedikedes & Skowronski, 1995), whereas they call on social comparisons least frequently (Dubé et al., 1998; Wayment & Campbell, 2000; Wayment & Taylor, 1995) and regard them as least important (Fox & Kahneman, 1992; Schoeneman, 1981; Sedikedes & Skowronski, 1995). This is true for respondents' evaluations of themselves (Schoeneman, 1981; Sedikedes & Skowronski, 1995; Wayment & Taylor, 1995), their relationships (Wayment & Campbell, 2000), and their subjective well-being and life satisfaction (Dubé et al., 1998; Fox & Kahneman, 1992). In addition, Wayment and Taylor (1995; see also Wayment & Campbell, 2000) asked participants to rate the usefulness of various sources of information not just for self-evaluation but also for meeting the goals of self-enhancement and self-improvement. Participants generally rated personal standards as most useful and social comparison as least useful for meeting all three motives.

When temporal comparisons have been examined specifically, they have emerged as highly important, just as they had for the open-ended questions. Participants typically rate temporal comparisons more highly than social comparisons (Dubé et al., 1998; Fox & Kahneman, 1992; Sedikedes & Skowronski, 1995), sometimes even attaching the most importance to comparisons with the self in the past, above all other sources of information (Sedikedes & Skowronski, 1995, Studies 2 and 3).

Fortunately, Wayment and Taylor (1995) and Wayment and Campbell (2000) specifically asked about objective information. Wayment and Taylor's definition of objective information for participants, in the case of the academic domain, was, "Sometimes when people are trying to assess their academic achievement, they look at objective information, such as their grade point average or their grades. How often do you assess your academic performance using objective information?" (p. 735).

In the academic domain, participants rated the frequency of using objective information as second to personal standards and ahead of social comparisons. In the social domain, objective information and social comparison tied for second. In addition, participants typically rated objective information as less useful than personal standards but more useful than social comparison for meeting all three motives (accuracy, self-enhancement, and self-improvement), in both academic and social domains (Wayment & Taylor, 1995). Similarly, people reported evaluating their relationships using objective information (e.g., number of disagreements) more frequently than either social standards or comparisons with past selves (Wayment & Campbell, 2000).

In fairness to social comparison, however, we should note that respondents' ratings suggest that they do not regard social comparison as trivial. Although participants typically assign their lowest ratings to social comparison, they tend to rate it at least near the midpoint or higher in terms of importance (Fox & Kahneman, 1992; Sedikedes & Skowronski, 1995, Study 3), frequency of use (Wayment & Taylor, 1995), and usefulness for meeting various self-relevant goals (but see Dubé et al., 1998; Wayment & Campbell, 2000; Wayment & Taylor, 1995).

Direct but General Questions

Several researchers have asked participants direct questions about their general social comparison activity. For example, Helgeson and Taylor (1993) asked cardiac patients, "Have you ever compared how you are doing with how other people with heart problems are doing?" (p. 1175). Forty percent of the patients responded "never." Similar questions asked of other patient groups also have yielded high numbers of respondents claiming not to have made social comparisons (Schulz & Decker, 1985; Wood, Taylor, & Lichtman, 1985).

Direct Questions about Specific Comparisons

Researchers also have asked participants to report specific social comparisons they made. Foddy and Crundall (1993) asked university students to report any social comparisons they made concerning important course assignments during the 2 weeks before they submitted the assignments and during the week following the return of their graded assignments. Students reported surprisingly few comparisons: The median was one comparison per recording period, and a sizable minority reported no social comparisons at all. In a study of women with fibromyalgia pain, researchers asked participants about an activity they called "downward comparison reminding" (Affleck, Tennen, Urrows, Higgins, & Abeles, 2000). Specifically, every night for 30 days, participants were asked to rate "how much they had reminded [themselves] 'that their pain was not as bad as it is for others (social comparison) and that their pain today was not as bad as it had been at one time' (temporal comparison)" (p. 505). On average, participants reported doing no social comparison reminding about 60% of the days and no temporal comparison reminding about 57% of the days.

Social Comparison Diaries

Wheeler and Miyake (1992) invented a measure to capture social comparisons as they occur in people's everyday lives. Wheeler and Miyake asked respondents to note the social comparisons that they made over a 2-week period and to record the dimension of comparison (e.g., academic, appearance), the direction of comparison (e.g., upward, downward), their relationship with the target person (e.g., stranger, close friend), and their moods before and after the comparison. Wood, Giordano, and Michela (2001) have collected data supporting the validity of various aspects of the measure. To date, Wheeler and Miyake's diary method (with some variations) has been used in published studies involving four different samples (Locke & Nekich, 2000; Olson & Evans, 1999; Wheeler & Miyake, 1992; Wood, Michela, & Giordano, 2000).

How many social comparisons would we expect respondents to report per day? If comparisons are "ubiquitous" or "almost constant," we might expect a few per waking hour. Perhaps as many as 10 to 20 per day? Consistently, the diary method has yielded far fewer comparisons. In the four samples in which the Wheeler and Miyake (1992) method has been used, participants typically have reported, on average, about 1.75 comparisons per day. Thus participants report between one and two social comparisons per day. This hardly seems "ubiquitous."

Although participants have recorded few comparisons in their diaries, they do report that comparisons have impact. For example, respondents typically report that their moods worsen after upward comparisons and improve after downward comparisons (e.g., Olson & Evans, 1999; Wheeler & Miyake, 1992).

Hypothetical Scenario Studies

In two studies, researchers have asked participants to imagine their reactions to hypothetical scenarios involving social comparisons. In stark contrast to the studies asking participants about their use of social comparison, these studies indicate that participants view social comparison as *highly* important. Goolsby and Chaplin (1988) asked students how they would feel if they obtained one of the best (or worst) scores in the class (social comparison) or one of their best (or worst) personal scores (temporal comparison). In one sample, they also provided objective information in the form of

grades (A, C, or F). Social comparisons had by far the strongest impact on hypothetical satisfaction ratings.

A study of objective information versus social comparison suggests that such effects are not limited to academic contexts (Klein, 1997, Study 1). Undergraduates imagined that they had a specific level of objective risk of experiencing a negative event (e.g., a car accident) and that this level of risk was either above average or below average in their peer group. Participants' judgments of how they would feel, how they would characterize their abilities (e.g., driving), and how likely they would be to change their behaviors (e.g., wearing seat belts) depended only on their risk relative to that of other people—not at all on their absolute risk.

Certainly, participants' responses to hypothetical scenarios may not reflect how people would truly respond to actual events. Yet these studies are interesting even if they reflect only participants' beliefs. These studies suggest that people *believe* that social comparisons are powerful (Klein, 1997) and that other sources of information are less powerful, whereas the studies reviewed earlier suggest that people regard social comparisons as much less important than other sources.

Summary of Self-Report Studies

The evidence that we have described thus far, then, is very consistent, with one exception. When participants respond to open-ended questions about how they go about evaluating themselves or their life satisfaction, they spontaneously mention social comparisons relatively infrequently. When asked to rank-order various sources of information, they typically rank social comparison as least important. When asked to rate the importance of sources of information, how frequently they have drawn on various sources, or how useful such sources are for meeting various goals, respondents typically give social comparisons their lowest ratings. When asked to report the social comparisons that occur in their everyday lives—even when they are asked to record them in diaries as they occur—participants report very few comparisons per day. Thus respondents from diverse samples (between them, the 16 articles cited included data from 23 samples) indicate that social comparison is unimportant to them—or, at least, unimportant relative to other sources of information.

The exception concerns two studies involving hypothetical scenarios, in which participants' estimates of how they would feel if they received certain types of information were more influenced by social comparisons than by objective or temporal information (Goolsby & Chaplin, 1988; Klein, 1997). Perhaps these studies contrast with the other self-report studies because participants' responses to hypothetical scenarios do not reflect their real responses to actual social comparisons. Alternatively, perhaps the other self-report studies do not reflect participants' true interest in social comparison. When participants are required to explicitly rate or rank their use of social comparison relative to other types of information, social desirability concerns may inhibit their true responses. Hypothetical scenario studies do not require such judgments; they only require admitting that social comparisons have impact, which may be much easier than saying that one relies on social comparison more than on other sources of information about the self. Or perhaps the key difference between the two types of studies is that the hypothetical-scenario studies focus on the impact of comparison, whereas the other self-report studies focus more on the frequency of comparison. Perhaps people recognize that social comparisons have impact more readily than they recognize how much they engage in social comparisons. As we show, however, another method not involving comparison impact reveals that people do recognize their use of social comparisons—at least under some conditions.

Self-Descriptions or Descriptions of Specific Incidents

Researchers have asked participants to describe themselves or their experiences in an open-ended manner and then have coded participants' responses for mentions of comparison standards. These studies involve self-report, but they differ from the other self-report studies in that they ask people to evaluate or simply to describe themselves or their experiences, rather than to reflect on how they go about evaluating themselves or their experiences.

One such study was conducted by Affleck and Tennen (1991). They examined descriptions of coping experiences provided by rheumatoid arthritis patients and by parents of medically fragile infants. In those descriptions, respondents of all ages were more likely to spontaneously compare their current status (or that of their child) with their past status (i.e., temporal comparisons) than to compare themselves (or their child) with other people. Similarly, Wilson and Ross (2000) investigated people's use of social and temporal comparisons in open-ended self-descriptions. In one study, they coded self-descriptions found in magazine interviews, a majority of which focused on well-known public figures. The interviewees showed an overwhelming preference for temporal comparison. For example, comments similar to Mary Tyler Moore's were quite common: "Of all the lives that I have lived, I would have to say that this one is my favorite. I have developed into a kinder person than I ever thought I would be" (Gerosa, 1997, p. 83). In contrast, social comparisons such as this one made by Elton John were more rare: "I've had a top 40 single on Billboard every year for the last 27 years.' He smiles slyly, 'I beat Elvis' record. He had 22 or 23 years'" (Bennetts, 1997, p. 147).

Because of the public nature of these self-descriptions and the unusually well-known population, these findings may be anomalous. Accordingly, in two other studies, Wilson and Ross (2000) asked university students to describe themselves privately. In one study, participants' self-descriptions contained more temporal than social comparisons, and in the other, they contained equal numbers of each type. The discrepancy may be due partly to the dimensions being described. In the first study, people were asked to "describe yourself as a person," whereas in Study 2, they described specific attributes. Results varied with the attribute. Respondents referred more often to social comparisons to describe their intelligence and temporal comparisons to appraise their self-confidence.

Attribute type has yet to be systematically investigated in the literature, but it may be an important determinant of comparison choice. For example, social comparisons might be preferred on dimensions for which outcome is determined by relative social rank (e.g., running a race, GRE scores) or in readily observable domains (e.g., height). In contrast, temporal comparisons may be preferred in domains in which personal progress is key (e.g., learning to play the piano) or for private, not easily observed information, such as one's self-confidence over time.

In another study of participants' descriptions, Taylor, Neter, and Wayment (1995) examined seven information sources: three types of social comparisons—namely, upward, downward, and lateral (i.e., comparisons that they had made with similar others); two types of temporal comparisons—namely, past behaviors and future selves; objective information; and feedback from others. Taylor and colleagues asked participants to recall incidents in which they felt each of four motives—self-enhancement (wanting to feel good about oneself), self-assessment (wanting an accurate assessment of oneself), self-verification (wanting to confirm one's self-view), and self-improvement (wanting to improve oneself)—and to describe them in detail. For example, for the incident involving self-enhancement motives, participants were asked to describe in detail the circumstances that had led them to be motivated to feel good about themselves. Then participants were asked whether they drew on objective sources of information, and if so, which ones; whether they drew on information from other people, and if so, what kind (e.g., feedback from others or social comparisons); and whether they drew on personal sources of information, such as their past behaviors or future goals (Taylor et al., 1995, p. 1280).

Across all four motives, sizable proportions of participants mentioned social comparisons. When they wrote about an incident involving the motive of self-assessment—the motive that most closely resembles the general self-knowledge or self-evaluation motives examined in most of the self-report studies—52% of the participants described lateral social comparisons (i.e., comparisons that they had made with similar others). This percentage appeared to be larger than that for any

other source of information, including feedback from others, mentioned by 40%; one's own past behaviors (31%); and objective sources (13%).[1] When the motive was self-improvement, 45% mentioned that they had made upward comparisons, whereas 40% mentioned feedback from others, 25% mentioned objective information, and 19% mentioned past behaviors. For the motives of self-enhancement and self-verification, close to one-third of the respondents mentioned at least one type of social comparison. Overall, more participants mentioned at least one type of social comparison than mentioned either objective information or temporal comparisons.

In summary, five studies that have asked participants to describe themselves or to describe specific incidents have yielded mixed results. In three of the four studies that pitted social comparisons against temporal comparisons, participants mentioned temporal comparisons more often; in the remaining study, they mentioned temporal and social comparisons equally often. In contrast, Taylor and colleagues (1995) examined social comparisons, temporal comparisons, and other sources, and, in general, social comparisons figured more prominently than other sources in participants' descriptions.

Overall, then, how important do people think social comparison is? Self-report, diary, and some description studies suggest that the answer is "not very." However, two hypothetical-scenario studies, one description study, and diary respondents' reports that comparisons influence their moods suggest that lay people view social comparisons as being highly important.

Reconciling the Inconsistent Evidence

Why have these studies yielded such discrepant results? And why do most of the self-report studies suggest that people think that social comparison is less important than other sources of information, whereas the evidence reviewed earlier suggests that social comparisons are often more important than objective information and temporal comparisons? We propose that these inconsistencies are due largely to two main factors: (1) the individual's motives and (2) the fit between the researcher's measure and certain characteristics of social comparison.

The Individual's Motives

Self-Appraisal Motives

Social comparison researchers have long accepted the idea that people may use social comparisons to serve multiple motives—not just the accurate self-evaluation that Festinger (1954) emphasized, but also such motives as self-improvement and self-enhancement (Wood, 1989). People's use of social comparisons may vary with motives. Taylor and colleagues' (1995) description study supports this possibility; for the motives of self-assessment and self-improvement, participants mentioned a type of social comparison more frequently than any other source of information, but this was not true for self-enhancement and self-verification.

Concern for Others' Reactions

Social comparisons may well elicit interpersonal discomfort. For example, if an individual outperforms a colleague, he or she might feel pleased but anxious at the same time about whether the comparison will strain the relationship, perhaps eliciting envy or resentment (Exline & Lobel, 1999). The "outperformed" colleague, in turn, may feel embarrassed and fear other people's rejection or pity (Brickman & Bulman, 1977). Such interpersonal concerns might cause people to avoid or hide their social comparisons, at least publicly (Brickman & Bulman, 1977).

Motives Aroused in the Study Context

When we emphasize the importance of motives, we also have in mind the motives that research participants experience in the context of their participation. For example, many of the studies that point to the importance of social comparisons involved probably competitive contexts. An example is a study by Tesser and Campbell (1980), in which university students were given a choice to continue with either of two tasks that they had engaged in earlier; on one task, their performance had been better

than that of a confederate, whereas on the other task, their performance had been worse than that of a confederate, but better than their own performance on the first task. Participants preferred the task on which they had surpassed a confederate, even though their own performance had been superior on the other task. This study may suggest that social comparisons have undue influence on task choices. However, participants may well have expected that they would perform in front of a confederate again, so their choice of task may have reflected some competitive or self-presentational concerns. Perhaps the feedback concerning their own relative strengths would have been more influential in a less competitive context or for private judgments.

Social Desirability

An especially important motive that may arise in the study context is social desirability. As many researchers who have used self-report measures of social comparison have acknowledged, respondents may not wish to admit, to others or to themselves, that they engage in social comparison (see Wood, 1996, for references). Relying on social comparison may make one appear to be insecure and spineless and may threaten such Western values as autonomy and individuality (Schoeneman, 1981; Sedikedes & Skowronski, 1995). Openly comparing oneself with others also can seem competitive, or, in the case of downward comparisons, to be taking pleasure in others' misfortune (Brickman & Bulman, 1977).

It is critical to note, however, that people's concerns about revealing their interest in social comparisons is likely to vary widely with a number of factors. One factor is domain of comparison. For example, academic grades are often based on students' relative standing, and such relative standings are often highly accessible (e.g., via postings on walls), so it is not surprising that students readily admit to making social comparisons in the academic domain (Gibbons & Buunk, 1999). People may be more reluctant to admit to comparisons involving physical beauty or wealth. A second factor that may affect social desirability concerns is the anonymity of the setting. In face-to-face interviews, many people may be reluctant to admit to making comparisons, whereas they may admit them more freely in anonymous questionnaires (cf. Schoeneman, 1981). A third factor is whether the researcher grants "permission" to respondents to admit to social comparisons. For example, the question, "How often do you compare yourself with other people?" is likely to elicit more admissions when it is preceded by a statement such as, "When students get test scores back or receive grades on a project or paper, they often like to find out how other people did . . ." (Gibbons & Buunk, 1999, p. 131).

Another factor that is likely to influence participants' degree of concern about social desirability involves how "close to home" the comparison is. When a colloquium speaker describes anecdotes involving social comparison, most audience members can chuckle in a tacit admission that they, too, sometimes engage in social comparison. It is something entirely different, however, for an audience member to admit to comparing himself or herself with a specific colleague down the hall.

If concerns about social desirability may awaken and dampen with a variety of factors, then associations between social desirability and self-reported social comparisons are likely to be inconsistent. They are. Sometimes researchers have found that their self-report measures are uncorrelated with measures of social desirability (Schoeneman, 1981, interview sample; Wayment & Campbell, 2000; Wayment & Taylor, 1995), yet other times they have found an association (Gibbons & Buunk, 1999; Schoeneman, 1981, questionnaire sample; Wilson & Ross, 1999).

Individual Differences

Motives may not only be aroused by the situation but may also stem from stable individual differences. Such individual differences, operating through motives, may influence one's overall interest in social comparison. For example, people's predominant motives, and hence their interest in social comparisons versus other standards, may vary with age (e.g., Suls & Mullen, 1982) and culture. Western cultures, which are considered to be more competitive than Eastern cultures, may encourage social com-

parisons (Klein, 1997). Greater interest in social comparison has been documented in people who have personality characteristics that are associated with heightened uncertainty, such as low self-esteem, depression, and neuroticism (see Gibbons & Buunk, 1999, for references). The more "interpersonally focused" one is, the more one is interested in social comparisons (Miller, 1977). Constructs involving the degree to which one pays attention to other people to decide how to act, such as self-monitoring and public self-consciousness, also may determine one's overall interest in social comparisons (see Gibbons & Buunk, 1999, for references).

It may be that the same people who tend to make social comparisons also tend to make temporal comparisons and comparisons with objective standards (see Affleck et al., 2000). Alternatively, individuals may vary in their characteristic preferences for social, temporal, or objective information. For example, children who have mastery goals (learning) rely more on temporal standards, whereas those who have performance goals (documenting skill level) rely more on social standards (Butler, 2000).

Fit between Measures and Features of Social Comparison

Our reconciliation of the inconsistent findings also revolves around certain features of social comparisons and how well researchers' measures accommodate those features.

Lack of Awareness

Several researchers have argued that social comparisons may occur automatically, without the individual's awareness (e.g., Goethals, 1986a; Wood, 1996). Supporting this idea is evidence that people attend to social comparisons automatically (Gilbert, Giesler, & Morris, 1995), that people are unaware of how they process comparative information about objects (Collins, 2000), and that participants in conformity research often lack awareness that their responses have been influenced by those of other people (Forsyth, 2000). If people sometimes lack awareness of their comparisons, any measure that depends on such awareness—

such as self-report measures—will yield distorted results.

Subtypes and Contexts of Social Comparison

Another feature of social comparison is that it is not a single, uniform entity, but has subtypes. Specific subtypes may be elicited in particular contexts. Global self-report questions about "social comparison" that fail to distinguish between types, such as upward and downward comparisons, may be difficult for participants to respond to, because their answers may well depend on the specific subtype of comparison. For example, in Wayment and Taylor's (1995) rating study, respondents rated general social comparison lowest in terms of frequency of use and usefulness for meeting goals, but when asked about subtypes of comparison, their answers were sometimes quite different. Participants reported, for example, that they used upward comparisons in particular almost as much, if not as much, as objective information and temporal comparisons and that downward comparisons and lateral comparisons were as useful for self-enhancement, if not more useful, than objective and personal standards.[2]

Perhaps participants are unable to "average" their directional comparisons (e.g., upward, downward) appropriately when they answer general social comparison questions. We suspect that the different pattern of responding is due to more than errors in averaging, however. When people are asked to report directional comparisons (e.g., a time when they compared with a better- or worse-off other), they may be likely to bring to mind important incidents involving novelty, uncertainty, or threat. Such incidents may be especially likely to elicit social comparisons (e.g., Taylor et al., 1995). In contrast, more general self-report questions probably do not remind respondents of such incidents, and hence respondents report fewer social comparisons.

Next, we apply these two ideas—the individual's motives and the fit between features of social comparison and operationalizations—to the evidence reviewed earlier concerning social comparisons versus objective standards, social comparisons versus temporal comparisons, and the importance of social comparisons to lay people.

Social Comparisons versus Objective Standards

Why did social comparison emerge as more important than objective standards in several studies? In part, this may be because virtually all of the studies involved contexts that seem likely to have aroused competitive motives. For example, some studies involved students who had taken an exam (e.g., Suls & Tesch, 1978). Even when students already know of their own letter grade on an exam, they may want to learn about other people's scores because, in academic contexts, information about relative standing is pivotal in determining one's own future outcomes. Settings that are less competitive may arouse less interest in social comparison.

More generally, people may adopt whichever standard best suits their motives. For example, if one wishes to self-enhance, one's choice of either objective standards or social comparisons may depend on which promises to yield the information that is most pleasing (Klein, 1997).

Social Comparisons versus Temporal Comparisons

Like the work that compares social and objective standards, much of the research examining social versus temporal comparisons, such as level-of-aspiration research, has been at least implicitly competitive (Hertzman & Festinger, 1940; Ruble & Flett, 1988). Such contexts may favor social comparisons because, typically, competitive outcomes depend more on social standing than on personal progress over time.

In addition, in these studies, participants may well have been uncertain about their performances on the experimental tasks. Consistent with Festinger's (1954) original formulation, social comparisons may be especially useful when a person's standing is uncertain and when the need for accurate assessment is strongest (e.g., Gibbons & Buunk, 1999). More generally, some theorists have proposed that the relative importance of different comparison standards may follow a time course (e.g., Ruble & Frey, 1991). In a novel situation or in the early stages of developing a new skill, uncertainty will be high, and hence people may measure themselves against others to assess their abilities or to improve them (e.g., Taylor et al., 1995). In contrast, once relative standing is more certain, people may focus on temporal comparisons to track finer shifts over time.

In other situations, people may be less interested in accuracy or improvement and more focused on self-enhancement motives. Wilson and Ross (2000) argued that young adults may prefer temporal comparisons for self-enhancement because they are most commonly downward and hence flattering: People tend to perceive steady improvement in almost all domains. To test this idea, Wilson and Ross manipulated accuracy and enhancement goals in two studies. For example, in one study young adult participants were simply primed with words such as "evaluate" and "accurate" or with words such as "worthy" and "praise." Although participants used both standards to meet both goals, they focused more on social comparisons to meet accuracy goals and more on temporal comparisons for self-enhancement. In most of the studies we reviewed, it is not clear which goal is primary, but it is possible that, like the priming manipulation, subtle differences in instructions (e.g., "evaluate yourself" versus simply "describe yourself") could have brought different goals to the forefront.

The relative importance of social and temporal comparisons also may change even if one's goal stays the same, because over time the standard that is best suited to meeting the goal may change. For example, temporal comparisons will not be enhancing when people perceive stability or decline, such as when they age. Generally, people should prefer whatever standards best meet their goals, given their perceived social standing and temporal trajectory (e.g., Ruble & Frey, 1991).

Importance of Social Comparison to Lay People

Open-Ended, Rating, and Ranking Measures

Global questions about how people go about evaluating themselves or their life satisfaction—the measures that yield the least interest in social comparisons—seem most susceptible to our concerns about motives and about the fit between features of social comparison and measures. Respondents

may not only worry about social desirability but they may also have difficulty synthesizing across multiple experiences and types of comparison. They may not even recall their social comparisons. Ross and colleagues (1986) have suggested a specific pathway by which people may fail to recognize the importance of social comparisons to their judgments of life satisfaction: "Social comparison may occur further back in the chain of inferences that ultimately yield life quality judgments (e.g., in the setting of goals). Conceivably, these more distant components are simply overlooked as our respondents focus on their more immediate affective reactions" (p. 91).

Even specific questions about social comparison are probably difficult for respondents to answer for the same reasons. For example, when asked how often they assess their academic performance using social comparison (Wayment & Taylor, 1995), respondents may fail to recall social comparisons, may have difficulty averaging across subtypes of social comparison, and may be inhibited by a concern for social desirability.

Self-report questions may favor standards other than social comparison in additional ways. Multiple sources of information (including social) may contribute to the ambiguous category of "personal standards," thereby inflating its importance. In addition, objective standards may be easier to report than social comparisons. Their salience and concreteness (e.g., clearly defined criteria) may make them especially noticeable and memorable. Also, students may make dozens of very different social comparisons but may have access to only a few objective determinants of course performance. Hence, they may report their use of objective standards with less ambiguity and greater accuracy.

Direct but General Questions

As in ranking and rating studies, direct questions about general social comparison activity burden participants' ability to recall comparison experiences and may well arouse social desirability concerns. Hence, respondents may claim that they do not make social comparisons (e.g., Helgeson & Taylor, 1993). Such claims are, however, difficult to reconcile with other evidence. For example, in an interview study, many breast cancer patients said, in response to a general question, that they rarely made social comparisons, but as they described their specific experiences, most respondents betrayed their interest in social comparisons by freely expressing comparisons that they had made (Wood et al., 1985).

Hypothetical-Scenario Studies

When participants are asked to imagine scenarios involving social comparison, they indicate that social comparisons have impact (Goolsby & Chaplin, 1988; Klein, 1997). Why are these responses so discrepant from most of the other self-report questions? One reason may be that hypothetical scenarios do not require participants to recall or summarize previous comparison experiences. In addition, they also involve specific subtypes of comparison rather than the general category of social comparison. Finally, hypothetical scenarios should not arouse social desirability concerns to the same degree as the other self-report measures because they do not require respondents to admit that they engage in social comparison frequently.

Description Studies

As we have seen, the apparent importance of social comparison varies across studies in which participants have been asked to describe themselves or their specific experiences. These discrepancies again may be disentangled by considering the motives aroused in various contexts and the match between comparisons and measures. First, in two studies (Affleck & Tennen, 1991; Wilson & Ross, 2000, Study 3) in which participants were interviewed face-to-face (in the latter study for national magazines), they mentioned temporal comparisons more than social comparisons, most dramatically in the case of the magazine interviews. This result may be due to self-presentation goals, which were likely to have been highly salient in these situations, and which may have been better served by temporal than social comparisons in this context. It is hard to imagine Madonna, for example, expressing aloud any thoughts she may have about her superiority to Britney Spears, but comparing herself with a teenage Madonna would not carry the same social risks.

The other three description studies were private, paper-and-pencil tasks, which may reduce (though not eliminate) self-presentation concerns. However, these three studies differed widely in terms of question specificity. In the first study by Wilson and Ross (2000), participants described themselves in general, and in the second study, respondents described particular attributes. In the Taylor and colleagues (1995) study, respondents described a specific incident in which they had a particular goal. The relative importance of social comparison standards increased across the three studies as specificity increased.[3] Again, people may be most attuned to their use of social comparisons when they can consider particular instances that do not require generalization and that do not imply frequent comparison. Whereas people may be reluctant to say that they frequently compare themselves with other people, they may be very willing to say that they specifically compare their singing voice with that of Barbra Streisand (an example provided by one of Taylor and colleagues' participants).

Taylor and colleagues' (1995) research approach also may have yielded more mentions of social comparison because of the types of events they elicited. Taylor and colleagues reported that the majority of goal-eliciting incidents involved either a threatening experience in the past or the anticipation of a significant future event. Such novel and threatening events may be especially likely to elicit social comparisons—much more so than the situations that participants may call to mind (if any) when asked to describe themselves in general (Wilson & Ross, 2000).

Questions about Specific Comparisons

If the key to revealing the importance of social comparisons is to inquire about specific subtypes of comparison and multiple goal-eliciting incidents, then researchers who ask participants about specific comparisons in their everyday lives would seem to be on the right track. This method should minimize the need for recall and synthesis of multiple comparisons. It also may alleviate participants' social desirability concerns, because questions about specific comparisons may imply that social comparisons are commonplace. Yet a sizable proportion of participants fail to report social comparisons in response to such methods (Affleck et al., 2000; Foddy & Crundall, 1993). Even diary methods, which should capture social comparisons as people make them in the actual situations in which they occur, tend to yield only one or two comparisons per day (e.g., Wood et al., 2000).

Were social comparison researchers simply wrong in regarding social comparison as "ubiquitous," "a nearly constant aspect" of everyday life? Before drawing that conclusion, we should keep in mind that some limitations of self-report measures still apply to direct questions about specific comparisons. Participants may be reluctant to admit to especially personal or unfavorable comparisons or to admit the extent to which they make comparisons. In addition, participants in diary studies have admitted that they have some difficulty being aware of their comparisons (Wood et al., 2001) and attending to comparisons (Wheeler & Miyake, 1992). Another issue is compliance; completing the diary forms is time consuming and intrusive (Wheeler & Miyake, 1992; Wood et al., 2001). In one sample, only 37% of participants stated that they had recorded their comparisons within an hour of their occurrence (Wood et al., 2001). Such compliance issues plague paper-and-pencil event-contingent recording methods in general, so researchers outside of social comparison have begun to use handheld computers (Feldman Barrett & Barrett, 2001), which can record the time of participants' recordings and perhaps boost compliance.

However, even after considering the potential barriers to accurate diary recording, the diary method still seems to be one of the more reliable ways of capturing comparison processes. Hence, it may be worth considering the possibility that social comparisons really do not occur constantly. Perhaps only novel, consequential, and uncertainty-evoking situations elicit social comparisons, and such situations do not happen every day, or at least not 10 to 20 times a day. Laboratory studies that capture social comparisons are modeled after these significant contexts, and the self-report studies that yield more evidence of reliance on social comparisons—namely, hypothetical-scenario studies and some description studies—seem to involve methods that bring such important circumstances to participants' minds.

In interpreting the diary studies, we should also consider the possibility that, although participants may record only one or two comparisons per day, those comparisons may be very psychologically significant (cf. Wheeler & Miyake, 1992). We should not gauge the importance of social comparison solely by the frequency with which participants record them. Indeed, perhaps one or two comparisons per day is not all that "infrequent." If a wife thinks of her love for her husband only one or two times a day, would we call that "infrequent"? One must ask, "infrequent compared with what"? In describing their result that fibromyalgia sufferers reported "downward comparison reminding" on 40% of the days, Affleck and colleagues (2000) noted that "these percentages approach or exceed the daily frequencies of some of the more common chronic pain coping strategies, such as using relaxation techniques, distracting oneself from the pain, and seeking spiritual comfort or emotional support" (p. 511).

Another issue is that the diary studies operationalize social comparisons as discrete activities, but social comparison processes may operate in a more subtle but pervasive schematic fashion—as ways of processing information about ourselves. Individuals' judgments about themselves may often implicitly refer to their standing relative to other people. People may call themselves "tall" only if they are tall relative to others in their social surround, yet this judgment may have long ago become divorced from the specific comparisons that led to it, and the judgment may not require discrete, obvious social comparisons to sustain itself.

In sum, although one or two comparisons per day may imply that social comparisons are not "ubiquitous," perhaps we should not call them "infrequent" either. And whether they are frequent or infrequent may say little about their psychological impact.

Conclusion

How important is social comparison? Social comparison researchers have displayed contradictory attitudes toward social comparison: On the one hand, they have regarded it as being a highly frequent activity that profoundly influences people's feelings about themselves and about their personal outcomes; on the other hand, researchers have typically simply accepted Festinger's (1954) assumption that objective standards are more desirable and more influential than social comparisons. Our review of the small body of evidence addressing this issue suggests that uncritical acceptance of Festinger's assumption is unwarranted; people often prefer social comparisons over objective standards, and social comparisons often may have more impact. In addition, a few studies suggest that social comparisons have stronger effects than do temporal comparisons.

The evidence that social comparison is of paramount importance stands in stark contrast to the views of lay people. They do not often mention social comparison in response to open-ended questions about their self-appraisals; they typically rate and rank social comparison as occurring less frequently and as being less influential than other sources of information; and they report very few social comparisons per day. Yet respondents' self-reports of social comparison may be inhibited by a lack of awareness of their comparisons and by social desirability concerns. Self-report methods that minimize these factors (namely, hypothetical-scenario studies and some description studies) have yielded somewhat more evidence that lay people regard social comparison as being important.

Still, the overall impression left by the self-reports of lay people is humbling. We must consider the possibility that social comparisons are less important to ordinary people than we think. Perhaps our methods have exaggerated our views of social comparison's importance. We create powerful situations in the laboratory in which we force powerful social comparisons on participants or in which we allow participants to select salient, accessible social comparison information. In everyday life, social comparison is only one of many information sources competing for people's attention.

More generally, we have proposed that the importance of social comparison will vary relative to that of other sources of information and that two main factors—participants' motives and the fit between the researcher's operationalizations and features of social comparison—largely determine its relative importance. Although these two main factors help us to reconcile the inconsistencies in the existing literature, strong confidence in this reconciliation must await future research in which these factors are measured and manipulated.

Acknowledgments

We thank several people who offered helpful comments on earlier versions of this chapter: Mark Leary, Mike Ross, June Price Tangney, Ladd Wheeler, and especially, Bill Klein.

Notes

1. We say "appeared to be" because Taylor and colleagues (1995) did not report analyses comparing sources within motives, probably because participants were free to mention more than one source.
2. Wayment and Taylor (1995) did not report analyses comparing subtypes of social comparison with other categories of information, so these statements are based simply on a look at the reported means.
3. Ross and colleagues' (1986) research also illustrates differences in reporting for general versus specific questions. Respondents rarely mentioned social comparisons in response to open-ended questions, but when Ross and colleagues followed up the open-ended questions by asking participants with whom they compared themselves, 92% and 79% of the two samples named at least one person or group with whom they compared.

References

Affleck, G., & Tennen, H. (1991). Social comparison and coping with major medical problems. In J. M. Suls & R. L. Miller (Eds.), *Social comparison processes: Theoretical and empirical perspectives* (pp. 369–393). Washington, DC: Hemisphere.

Affleck, G., Tennen, H., Urrows, S., Higgins, P., & Abeles, M. (2000). Downward comparisons in daily life with chronic pain: Dynamic relations with pain intensity and mood. *Journal of Social and Clinical Psychology, 19,* 499–518.

Albert, S. (1977). Temporal comparison theory. *Psychological Review, 84,* 485–503.

Allen, V. L., & Wilder, D. A. (1977). Social comparison, self-evaluation, and conformity to the group. In J. M. Suls & R. L. Miller (Eds.), *Social comparison processes: Theoretical and empirical perspectives* (pp. 187–208). Washington, DC: Hemisphere.

Baumeister, R. F. (1998). The self. In D. T. Gilbert, S. T. Fiske, & G. Lindzey (Eds.), *The handbook of social psy-*

chology (4th ed., Vol. 2., pp. 680–740). New York: Mc-Graw-Hill.

Bennetts, L. (1997, November). Still Captain Fantastic. *Vanity Fair*, pp. 134–156.

Blanton, H., Buunk, B. P., Gibbons, F. X., & Kuyper, H. (1999). When better-than-others compare upward: Choice of comparison and comparative evaluation as independent predictors of academic performance. *Journal of Personality and Social Psychology, 76*, 420–430.

Boggiano, A. K., & Ruble, D. N. (1979). Competence and the overjustification effect: A developmental study. *Journal of Personality and Social Psychology, 37*, 1462–1468.

Brickman, P., & Berman, J. J. (1971). Effects of performance expectancy and outcome certainty on interest in social comparison. *Journal of Experimental Social Psychology, 7*, 600–609.

Brickman, P., & Bulman, R. J. (1977). Pleasure and pain in social comparison. In J. M. Suls & R. L. Miller (Eds.), *Social comparison processes: Theoretical and empirical perspectives* (pp. 149–186). Washington, DC: Hemisphere.

Brickman, P., & Campbell, D. T. (1971). Hedonic relativism and planning the good society. In M. H. Appley (Ed.), *Adaptation-level theory* (pp. 278–302). New York: Academic Press.

Butler, R. (2000). Making judgments about ability: The role of implicit theories of ability in moderating inferences from temporal and social comparison information. *Journal of Personality and Social Psychology, 78*, 965–978.

Buunk, B. P., & Gibbons, F. X. (Eds.). (1997). *Health, coping, and well-being: Perspectives from social comparison theory*. Mahwah, NJ: Erlbaum.

Buunk, B. P., & Gibbons, F. X. (2000). Toward an enlightenment in social comparison theory: Moving beyond classic and renaissance approaches. In J. Suls & L. Wheeler (Eds.), *Handbook of social comparison: Theory and research* (pp. 487–499). New York: Kluwer Academic/Plenum Press.

Campbell, J. D., Fairey, P. J., & Fehr, B. (1986). Better than me or better than thee? Reactions to intrapersonal and interpersonal performance feedback. *Journal of Personality, 54*, 480–493.

Collins, R. L. (2000). Among the better ones: Upward assimilation in social comparison. In J. Suls & L. Wheeler (Eds.), *Handbook of social comparison: Theory and research* (pp. 159–171). New York: Kluwer Academic/Plenum Press.

Davis, J. A. (1966). The campus as a frog pond: An application of the theory of relative deprivation to career decisions of college men. *American Journal of Sociology, 72*, 17–31.

Diener, E. (1984). Subjective well-being. *Psychological Bulletin, 95*, 542–575.

Diener, E., & Fujita, F. (1997). Social comparisons and subjective well-being. In B. P. Buunk & F. X. Gibbons (Eds.), *Health, coping, and well-being: Perspectives from social comparison theory* (pp. 329–358). Mahwah, NJ: Erlbaum.

Dubé, L., Jodoin, M., & Kairouz, S. (1998). On the cognitive basis of subjective well-being analysis: What do individuals have to say about it? *Canadian Journal of Behavioral Science, 30*, 1–13.

Emmons, R. A., & Diener, E. (1985). Personality correlates of subjective well-being. *Personality and Social Psychology Bulletin, 11*, 89–97.

Exline, J. J., & Lobel, M. (1999). The perils of outperformance: Sensitivity about being the target of a threatening upward comparison. *Psychological Bulletin, 125*, 307–337.

Feldman Barrett, L., & Barrett, D. J. (2001). An introduction to computerized experience sampling in psychology. *Social Science Computer Review, 19*, 175–185.

Festinger, L. (1954). A theory of social comparison processes. *Human Relations, 7*, 117–140.

Foddy, M., & Crundall, I. (1993). A field study of social comparison processes in ability evaluation. *British Journal of Social Psychology, 32*, 287–305.

Forsyth, D. R. (2000). Social comparison and influence in groups. In J. Suls & L. Wheeler (Eds.), *Handbook of social comparison: Theory and research* (pp. 81–103). New York: Kluwer Academic/Plenum Press.

Fox, C. R., & Kahneman, D. (1992). Correlations, causes and heuristics in surveys of life satisfaction. *Social Indicators Research, 27*, 221–234.

Gastorf, J. W., & Suls, J. (1978). Performance evaluation via social comparison: Performance similarity versus related-attribute similarity. *Social Psychology, 41*, 297–305.

Gerosa, M. (1997, Fall). Moore than ever. *More: Smart Talk for Smart Women*, pp. 79–83.

Gibbons, F. X., & Buunk, B. P. (1999). Individual differences in social comparison: Development of a scale of social comparison orientation. *Journal of Personality and Social Psychology, 76*, 129–142.

Gilbert, D. T., Giesler, R. B., & Morris, K. A. (1995). When comparisons arise. *Journal of Personality and Social Psychology, 69*, 227–236.

Goethals, G. R. (1986a). Fabricating and ignoring social reality: Self-serving estimates of consensus. In J. M. Olson, C. P. Herman, & M. P. Zanna (Eds.), *Relative deprivation and social comparison: The Ontario Symposium* (Vol. 4, pp. 135–158). Hillsdale, NJ: Erlbaum.

Goethals, G. R. (1986b). Social comparison theory: Psychology from the lost and found. *Personality and Social Psychology Bulletin, 12*, 261–278.

Goolsby, L. L., & Chaplin, W. F. (1988). The impact of normative, ipsative, and idiothetic information on feelings about academic performance. *Journal of Research in Personality, 22*, 445–464.

Hagerty, M. R. (2000). Social comparisons of income in one's community: Evidence from national surveys of income and happiness. *Journal of Personality and Social Psychology, 78*, 764–771.

Helgeson, V. S., & Taylor, S. E. (1993). Social comparisons and adjustment among cardiac patients. *Journal of Applied Social Psychology, 23*, 1171–1195.

Hertzman, M., & Festinger, L. (1940). Shifts in explicit goals in a level of aspiration experiment. *Journal of Experimental Psychology, 27*, 439–452.

Hochbaum, G. M. (1953). *Certain personality aspects and pressures to uniformity in groups*. Unpublished doctoral dissertation, University of Minnesota. (Described in Festinger, L. [1954]. A theory of social comparison processes. *Human Relations, 7*, 117–140.)

Hogg, M. A. (2000). Social identity and social comparison. In J. Suls & L. Wheeler (Eds.), *Handbook of social comparison: Theory and research* (pp. 401–421). New York: Kluwer Academic/Plenum Press.

Karney, B. R., & Coombs, R. H. (2000). Memory bias in long-term close relationships: Consistency or improvement? *Personality and Social Psychology Bulletin, 26,* 959–970.

Klein, W. M. (1997). Objective standards are not enough: Affective, self-evaluative, and behavioral responses to social comparison information. *Journal of Personality and Social Psychology, 72,* 763–774.

Levin, W. C., & Levin, J. (1973). Social comparison of grades: The influence of mode of comparison and Machiavellianism. *Journal of Social Psychology, 91,* 67–72.

Levine, J. M., & Green, S. M. (1984). Acquisition of relative performance information: The roles of intrapersonal and interpersonal comparison. *Personality and Social Psychology Bulletin, 10,* 385–393.

Locke, K. D., & Nekich, J. C. (2000). Agency and communion in naturalistic social comparison. *Personality and Social Psychology Bulletin, 26,* 864–874.

Marsh, H. W., & Parker, J. W. (1984). Determinants of student self-concept: Is it better to be a relatively large fish in a small pond even if you don't learn to swim as well? *Journal of Personality and Social Psychology, 47,* 213–231.

Miller, R. L. (1977). Preferences for social vs. non-social comparison as a means of self-evaluation. *Journal of Personality, 45,* 343–355.

Olson, B. D., & Evans, D. L. (1999). The role of the big five personality dimensions in the direction of affective consequences of everyday social comparisons. *Personality and Social Psychology Bulletin, 25,* 1498–1508.

Olson, J. M., Herman, C. P., & Zanna, M. P. (Eds.). (1986). *Relative deprivation and social comparison: The Ontario Symposium* (Vol. 4). Hillsdale, NJ: Erlbaum.

Ross, M., Eyman, A., & Kishchuk, N. (1986). Determinants of subjective well-being. In J. M. Olson, C. P. Herman, & M. P. Zanna (Eds.), *Relative deprivation and social comparison: The Ontario Symposium* (Vol. 4, pp. 79–93). Hillsdale, NJ: Erlbaum.

Ruble, D. N., & Flett, G. L. (1988). Conflicting goals in self-evaluative information seeking: Developmental and ability level analyses. *Child Development, 59,* 97–106.

Ruble, D. N., & Frey, K. S. (1991). Changing patterns of comparative behavior as skills are acquired: A functional model of self-evaluation. In J. Suls & T. A. Wills (Eds.), *Social Comparison: Contemporary theory and research* (pp. 79–116). Hillsdale, NJ: Erlbaum.

Runciman, W. G. (1966). *Relative deprivation and social justice: A study of attitudes to social inequality in twentieth-century England.* Berkeley: University of California Press.

Schoeneman, T. J. (1981). Reports of the sources of self-knowledge. *Journal of Personality, 49,* 284–294.

Schulz, R., & Decker, S. (1985). Long-term adjustment to physical disability: The role of social support, perceived control, and self-blame. *Journal of Personality and Social Psychology, 48,* 1162–1172.

Sedikedes, C., & Skowronski, J. J. (1995). On the sources of self-knowledge: The perceived primacy of self-reflection. *Journal of Social and Clinical Psychology, 14,* 244–270.

Sheeran, P., Abrams, D., & Orbell, S. (1995). Unemployment, self-esteem, and depression: A social comparison theory approach. *Basic and Applied Social Psychology, 17,* 65–82.

Smith, R. H. (2000). Assimilative and contrastive emotional reactions to upward and downward social comparisons. In J. Suls & L. Wheeler (Eds.), *Handbook of social comparison: Theory and research* (pp. 173–200). New York: Kluwer Academic/Plenum Press.

Suls, J., & Mullen, B. (1982). From the cradle to the grave: Comparison and self-evaluation across the life-span. In J. Suls (Ed.), *Psychological perspectives on the self* (pp. 97–125). Hillsdale, NJ: Erlbaum.

Suls, J., & Tesch, F. (1978). Students' preferences for information about their test performance: A social comparison study. *Journal of Applied Social Psychology, 8,* 189–197.

Suls, J., & Wheeler, L. (2000). *Handbook of social comparison: Theory and research.* New York: Kluwer Academic/Plenum Press.

Taylor, S. E., Neter, E., & Wayment, H. A. (1995). Self-evaluation processes. *Personality and Social Psychology Bulletin, 21,* 1278–1287.

Tesser, A., & Campbell, J. (1980). Self-definition: The impact of relative performance and similarity of others. *Social Psychology Quarterly, 43,* 341–347.

Tesser, A., & Campbell, J. (1985). A self-evaluation maintenance model of student motivation. In C. Ames & R. Ames (Eds.), *Research on motivation in education: The classroom milieu* (pp. 217–247). New York: Academic Press.

Wayment, H. A., & Campbell, S. (2000). How are we doing? The impact of motives and information use on the evaluation of romantic relationships. *Journal of Social and Personal Relationships, 17,* 31–52.

Wayment, H. A., & Taylor, S. E. (1995). Self-evaluation processes: Motives, information use, and self-esteem. *Journal of Personality, 63,* 729–757.

Wheeler, L., & Miyake, K. (1992). Social comparison in everyday life. *Journal of Personality and Social Psychology, 62,* 760–773.

Wilson, A. E., & Ross, M. (1999). [Individual differences in social and temporal comparison orientation]. Unpublished raw data.

Wilson, A. E., & Ross, M. (2000). The frequency of temporal-self and social comparisons in people's personal appraisals. *Journal of Personality and Social Psychology, 78,* 928–942.

Wood, J. V. (1989). Theory and research concerning social comparisons of personal attributes. *Psychological Bulletin, 106,* 231–248.

Wood, J. V. (1996). What is social comparison and how should we study it? *Personality and Social Psychology Bulletin, 22,* 520–537.

Wood, J. V., Giordano, C., & Michela, J. L. (2001). *Effects of social comparisons in everyday life: Moderators and validation of the diary method.* Unpublished manuscript.

Wood, J. V., Michela, J. L., & Giordano, C. (2000). Downward comparison in everyday life: Reconciling self-enhancement models with the mood-cognition priming model. *Journal of Personality and Social Psychology, 79,* 563–579.

Wood, J. V., Taylor, S. E., & Lichtman, R. R. (1985). Social comparison in adjustment to breast cancer. *Journal of Personality and Social Psychology, 49,* 1169–1183.

18

Self-Verification: The Search for Coherence

WILLIAM B. SWANN, JR.
PETER J. RENTFROW
JENNIFER S. GUINN

> Old patterns, no matter how negative and painful they may be, have
> an incredible magnetic power—because they do feel like home.
> —STEINEM (1992, p. 38)

Why do some people find that hurtful, humiliating relationships have an "incredible magnetic power"? And why do these same people sometimes wander from one miserable relationship to the next? We suggest that the answer to these and related questions can be found in the construct of psychological coherence. Furthermore, we suggest that understanding the allure of coherence will lay bare a host of phenomena that have heretofore remained rather baffling and mysterious, including the tendency for people to enter into and maintain relationships that seem punitive or even abusive.

Our argument rests on three key assumptions. First, once patterns of living have been established and maintained for some time, they come to provide people with a powerful sense of coherence. Second, because these patterns are summarized by people's self-views, stable self-views become intimately tied to feelings of coherence. Third,

these feelings of coherence are so alluring that people will fight to maintain them even if it means enduring pain and discomfort. For example, when people's life experiences lead them to develop negative self-views, these negative self-views will provide them with a sense of coherence that they will work to maintain by seeking and creating confirming (i.e., negative) feedback. This points to an important qualifier to the widely held belief that people have a strong preference for positive evaluations (Jones, 1973).

The first section of this chapter focuses on the nature and origin of coherence strivings, with a distinction made between coherence and its cousin construct, self-consistency. The second section reviews research on how people translate their coherence strivings into efforts to verify their self-views. The third and final section examines the interplay between people's desire for self-verification and other important social psychological phenomena, including the desire for objectively accurate information, self-enhancement, and strategic self-presentation.

Coherence Strivings and Why Leon Overlooked Prescott

Philosophers tell us that the desire for coherence is so essential for survival that even children possess it, albeit in rudimentary form (e.g., Guidano & Liotti, 1983). As soon as children begin to form generalizations about the world, they start looking for information that confirms those generalizations. Popper (1963) discussed this process in terms of a search for regularities: "Every organism has inborn reactions or responses. . . . The newborn baby "expects" . . . to be fed (and, one could even argue, to be protected and loved). . . . One of the most important of these expectations is the expectation of finding a regularity" (p. 47).

As people mature, they acquire vast amounts of information about the world, and they organize this information into an elaborate set of theories. At the heart of this theoretical system reside people's views of themselves. People's self-views represent the lens through which they perceive reality, lending meaning to all experience. Should people's self-views flounder, they will no longer have a secure basis for understanding and responding to the world because they will have been stripped of their fundamental means of knowing the world. Murphy (1947) likened self-views to a map or chart: "Indeed, the self-picture has all the strength of other perceptual stereotypes, and in addition serves as the chart by which the individual navigates. If it is lost, he can make only impulsive runs in fair weather; the ship drifts helplessly whenever storms arise" (p. 715).

Evidence for the critical role of the self in providing people with a source of coherence comes from a case study of a man who drowned his self-views in a sea of alcohol. Chronic alcohol abuse led William Thompson to develop Korsakoff syndrome, a brain disease marked by profound memory loss. According to his physician, Oliver Sacks (1985), the memory loss was so severe that Thompson had essentially "erased himself."

Able to remember only scattered fragments from his past, he constantly confused fantasy and reality. The case was particularly poignant because he desperately wanted to recover the self that constantly eluded his grasp. When Thompson encountered other people, he launched into a whirlwind of activity designed to determine his own identity. Frantically, he would develop hypotheses about who he was and then test these hypotheses on whoever happened to be present ("I am a grocer and you are my customer, right? Well now, what'll it be—Nova or Virginia? But wait; why are you wearing that white coat? You must be Hymie, the Kosher butcher next door. Yes, that's it. But why are there no bloodstains on your coat?"). Sadly, he could never remember the results of the latest test for more than a few seconds. Sacks (1985) concludes that Thompson was "continually creating a world and self, to replace what was continually being forgotten and lost . . . such a patient must literally make himself (and his world) up every moment. . . . The world keeps disappearing, losing meaning, vanishing—and he must seek meaning [by] throwing bridges of meaning over abysses of meaninglessness" (pp. 110–111).

Desperately seeking an elusive self that kept disappearing like the Cheshire cat, Thompson was cast adrift in a world that was devoid of meaning. Thompson's case not only shows that a stable sense of self is essential to feelings of coherence but also provides some hints about how people try to find coherence as they move from one situation to the next. Thompson repeatedly generated hypotheses about who he was and then proceeded to test them by seeking supportive evidence. It turns out that this is essentially what most people do. That is, people perceive evidence that confirms their hypotheses and beliefs to be especially trustworthy, diagnostic, and easy to process (e.g., Bruner, Goodnow & Austin, 1956; Klayman & Ha, 1987). And when people test the validity of their propositions and beliefs, they are especially likely to seek hypothesis-confirmatory evidence (e.g., Snyder & Swann, 1978; Wason & Johnson-Laird, 1972).

This preference for coherent information appears functional in that people seem to be better off when their worlds seem coherent to them. For example, Rentfrow, Swann, and Keough (2002) had participants write about either positive or negative life experiences several times over a period of 4 weeks. At the end of each week participants indicated the extent to which their essays told a coherent story. Overall, the more coherence participants perceived in their essays, the less likely they were to report symptoms of physical illness or to visit the student health center. Thus those who "saw" a great deal of coherence in their lives were more apt to enjoy psychological and even physical health later on. Furthermore, perceptions of coherence were unrelated to self-esteem measured at the beginning of the semester, indicating that it was not simply that people who felt worthless experienced a lack of coherence and fell ill.

In addition to demonstrating the health implications of coherence, Rentfrow et al.'s (2002) findings point to an important difference between psychological coherence and a related construct, psychological consistency. Perceptions of coherence grow out of the ability of participants to integrate their experiences into their evolving theory of self. Although theories of self could, in principle, contribute to people's feelings of cognitive consistency, most consistency theories have excluded the self (for exceptions, see Aronson, 1969; Lecky, 1945; Secord & Backman, 1965). For example, in the most influential exposition of consistency theory, Festinger (1957) suggested that a man would experience dissonance if, after discovering that he had a flat tire but no jack, he proceeded to remove the lug nuts from his wheel. Theoretically, dissonance would grow out of the pointlessness of removing the wheel because, without a jack, he could not replace the wheel. The source of the dissonance, then, was the inconsistency between the man's knowledge of what needed to be done and what he did—his enduring sense of self was largely irrelevant.

No wonder, then, that in his 1957 classic on dissonance, Festinger failed to cite Prescott Lecky's 1945 book, *Self-Consistency: A Theory of Personality*. Whereas Festinger studiously avoided implicating the self in his dissonance processes, Lecky placed people's enduring sense of self at center stage.[1] Despite the title of his book, then, Lecky's theory actually said more about the allure of psychological coherence than

about consistency. He thus laid the groundwork for self-verification theory.

Self-Verification Theory

Self-verification theory (Swann, 1983, 1987, 1990, 1999) assumes that stable self-views provide people with a crucial source of coherence, an invaluable means of defining their existence, organizing experience, predicting future events, and guiding social interaction (cf. Cooley, 1902; Lecky, 1945; Mead, 1934; Secord & Backman, 1965). Moreover, by stabilizing behavior, stable self-views make people more predictable to *others* (Goffman, 1959). This added predictability will, in turn, stabilize the way others respond to people. In this way, stable self-views foster a coherent social environment, which, in turn, further stabilizes their self-views.

This reasoning suggests that people may seek self-verification for one or both of two reasons: to bolster their feelings of psychological coherence ("epistemic" concerns) or to ensure that their interactions proceed smoothly ("pragmatic" concerns). For this reason, just as being perceived in a self-congruent manner may bolster feelings of existential security and calm the waters of social interaction, being perceived in an incongruent manner may produce the epistemic and pragmatic equivalents of a tidal wave. People strive to avoid such disasters by entering into and creating social worlds that confirm their self-views.

Which statement brings us back to the topic with which we began this chapter: close relationships. Because we infer who we are by observing how others react to us (Cooley, 1902; Mead, 1934), our close relationships play a prominent role in nurturing and sustaining a coherent sense of self. Specifically, we can maintain stable self-views only insofar as we receive—or at least think that we have received—a steady supply of self-verifying feedback from others. In this section, we discuss some of the ways that people pursue this objective.

How Self-Verification Maintains Coherence

People may enlist two classes of self-verification activities in their search for self-veri-

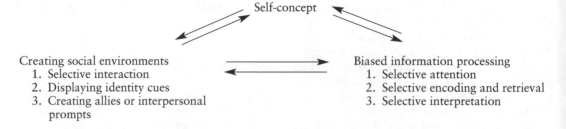

FIGURE 18.1. Self-verification processes.

fying evaluations. As shown in Figure 18.1, the first such class of activities involves their overt behaviors. Specifically, people work to create social environments that reinforce their self-views (e.g., McCall & Simmons, 1966). The second class of self-verification activities is cognitive. Through biased information processing, people develop perceptions of reality that are more compatible with their self-views than is warranted by the objective evidence.

Developing a Self-Confirmatory Social Environment

All living organisms inhabit "niches" that routinely satisfy their basic needs (e.g., Clark, 1954). Human beings satisfy their need for self-verification by attempting (consciously or not) to construct self-confirmatory social environments (McCall & Simmons, 1966). To this end, they employ three distinct activities: They strategically choose interaction partners and social settings; they display identity cues; and they adopt interaction strategies that evoke self-confirmatory responses. We consider each of these strategies in turn.

Selective Interaction

The notion that people seek social contexts that provide them with self-confirmatory feedback has been around for several decades (e.g., Secord & Backman, 1965; Wachtel, 1977). Until recently, the evidence for this hypothesis was anecdotal or based on field studies. For instance, Pervin and Rubin (1967) reported that students tended to drop out of school if they found themselves in colleges that were incompatible with their self-views (see also Backman &

Secord, 1962; Broxton, 1963; Newcomb, 1956).

Recent laboratory investigations have complemented earlier evidence by showing that people prefer interaction partners who see them as they see themselves. Swann, Pelham, and Krull (1989), for example, told participants that two evaluators had evaluated them on performance dimensions that participants had previously identified as their "best" or "worst" attribute (e.g., athletic ability, physical appearance, etc.). One evaluator offered an unfavorable evaluation; the other offered a favorable evaluation. Targets chose to interact with the congruent evaluator. Most surprisingly, as displayed in Figure 18.2, targets with negative self-views preferred the unfavorable self-verifying evaluator to the favorable nonverifying one.

In a similar vein, Swann, Stein-Seroussi and Giesler (1992) asked participants with positive and negative self-views whether they would prefer to interact with evaluators who had favorable or unfavorable impressions of them. Just as those with positive self-views preferred favorable partners, those with negative self-views preferred unfavorable partners. More than a dozen replications of this effect using diverse methodologies have confirmed that people prefer self-verifying evaluations and interaction partners, even if their self-views happen to be negative (e.g., Hixon & Swann, 1993; Robinson & Smith-Lovin, 1992; Swann, Hixon, Stein-Seroussi, & Gilbert, 1990; Swann et al., 1989; Swann, Wenzlaff, Krull, & Pelham, 1992). Both men and women display this propensity, whether the self-views are or are not easily changed and whether the self-views are associated with specific qualities (intelligence, sociability,

Preferred interaction partners

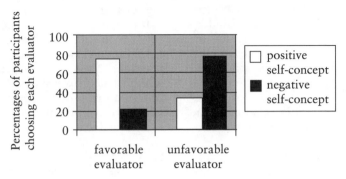

FIGURE 18.2. Preferred interaction partners.

dominance) or with global self-worth (self-esteem, depression). Similarly, people prefer to interact with self-verifying partners even if given the alternative of taking part in a different experiment (Swann, Wenzlaff, & Tafarodi, 1992).[2] Finally, people are particularly likely to seek self-verifying evaluations if their self-views are confidently held (e.g., Pelham & Swann, 1994; Swann & Ely, 1984; Swann, Pelham, & Chidester, 1988), important (Swann & Pelham, 2000), or extreme (Giesler, Josephs, & Swann, 1996).

There is also evidence that the self-verification strivings of people with low self-esteem and depression are not masochistic, for rather than savoring unfavorable evaluations, they feel torn and ambivalent about them. In choosing a negative evaluator, one person with low self-esteem noted: "I like the [favorable] evaluation but I am not sure that it is, ah, correct, maybe. It *sounds* good, but [the unfavorable evaluator] . . . seems to know more about me. So, I'll choose [the unfavorable evaluator]" (Swann, Stein-Seroussi, & Gielser, 1992).

Field studies reveal a parallel phenomenon. For example, if people wind up in marriages in which their spouses perceive them more (or less) favorably than they perceive themselves, they become less intimate with those spouses (Burke & Stets, 1999; De La Ronde & Swann, 1998; Katz, Beach, & Anderson, 1996; Ritts & Stein, 1995; Schafer, Wickram, & Keith, 1996; Swann, De La Ronde, & Hixon, 1994). A prospective study of MBA students revealed a similar phenomenon. Swann, Milton, and Polzer

(2000) found that members of groups felt more connected to their group insofar as the other members brought their appraisals into line with the members' own self-views. In addition, they discovered that the groups in which the most self-verification occurred were also the groups with the highest grades at the end of the semester. Presumably the increased feelings of connectedness that grow out of self-verification would encourage members of self-verifying groups to work together more often, thereby ensuring that people are associated with self-verifying partners not only in their intimate relationships but also in the classroom and workplace.

Considered together, these data offer clear evidence that people gravitate toward relationships that provide them with self-confirmatory feedback. An important characteristic of such selective interaction strategies is that once people enter particular social relationships, legal contracts and social pressures encourage them to remain there. The power of such contractual arrangements is obvious in the case of marriage, but friendships, collaborations, and dating relationships are also characterized by a good deal of inertia. Thus people who choose self-verifying interaction partners may discover that their choices are self-sustaining, as well as self-verifying.

Displaying Identity Cues

People can also ensure that they receive self-verifying reactions by "looking the part." Ideally, identity cues will be readily controlled and will predictably evoke desired responses from others. Physical appearances represent a particularly salient class of identity cues. The clothes one wears, for instance, can advertise one's political leanings, income level, sexual preference, and so on. Even body posture and demeanor communicate identities to others. Take, for example, the teenager who radiates anomie, the "punk" who projects danger, or the neophyte who exudes naiveté.

People may even alter their bodies to convey various identities to others. Whereas self-perceived athletes may diet and lift weights to keep their muscles bulging, self-proclaimed rock stars may cover themselves in tattoos and piercings to convey an image of rebelliousness. Those who are squeamish about surgery may rely on titles or material possessions to convey their identities to others. The cars people drive, the homes they live in, and the bumper stickers they display may all be used to tell others who they are and how they expect to be treated (Goffman, 1959; Schlenker, 1980).

It is noteworthy that people display identity cues to communicate negative, as well as positive, identities. Some highly visible examples include skinheads and members of the Ku Klux Klan. Furthermore, Gosling, Ko, Mannarelli and Morris (2002) have shown that people structure their personal environments (e.g., bedrooms, offices) to communicate negative, as well as positive, identities to others. For example, observers were as adept in recognizing people who saw themselves as "closed" and "messy" as they were in recognizing those who saw themselves as "open" and "tidy."

Interpersonal Prompts

Even if people fail to gain self-verifying evaluations by selective interaction and displaying identity cues, they still may acquire such feedback. Swann, Wenzlaff, Krull, and Pelham (1990), for example, found that mildly depressed college students were more likely to solicit unfavorable feedback from their roommates than were nondepressed students. Moreover, students' efforts to acquire unfavorable feedback apparently bore fruit: The more unfavorable feedback they solicited in the middle of the semester, the more their roommates derogated them and

planned to find another roommate at the semester's end.

If people are motivated to bring others to verify their self-conceptions, they should *intensify* their efforts to elicit self-confirmatory reactions when they suspect that they are misconstrued. Swann and Read (1981, Study 2) tested this idea by informing participants who perceived themselves as either likeable or dislikeable that they would be interacting with evaluators who had evaluated them. Some learned that the evaluators probably found them likeable; others learned that the evaluators probably found them dislikeable; still others learned nothing of the evaluators' appraisals. Participants tended to elicit reactions that confirmed their self-views. More important, this tendency was especially pronounced when participants suspected that evaluators' appraisals might *disconfirm* their self-conceptions. Participants who thought of themselves as likeable elicited particularly favorable reactions when they thought their evaluators disliked them, and participants who thought of themselves as dislikeable elicited particularly unfavorable reactions when they suspected that their evaluators liked them. Participants therefore displayed increased interest in self-verification when they suspected that evaluators' appraisals challenged their self-views.

Swann and Hill (1982) obtained similar findings using a different procedure and a different dimension of the self-concept (dominance). Participants began by playing a game (with a confederate) in which each player alternately assumed the dominant "leader" role or the submissive "assistant" role. During a break in the game, the experimenter asked the players to decide who should be the leader for the next set of games. This was the confederate's cue to give participants self-relevant feedback. In some conditions, the confederate said the participant seemed dominant; in others, the confederate said the participant seemed submissive. If the feedback confirmed participants' self-conceptions, they passively accepted the confederate's appraisal. If the feedback *dis*confirmed their self-conceptions, however, participants vehemently resisted the feedback and sought to demonstrate that they were not the persons the confederate made them out to be. Furthermore, having the opportunity to resist the discrepant feedback insulated participants against changes in their self-views.

Not surprisingly, in these studies of responses to discrepant feedback, some people resisted the discrepant feedback more than others. Swann and Ely (1984) theorized that high self-concept certainty was associated with heightened interest in self-verification and thus heightened resistance in the face of disconfirmation. To test this hypothesis, Swann and Ely had evaluators interview participants who were either certain or uncertain of their self-conceived extraversion. When evaluators were highly certain of their expectancies, participants who were low in self-certainty generally answered in ways that confirmed evaluators' expectancies, thus disconfirming their own self-conceptions but providing behavioral confirmation for the expectancies of evaluators. In contrast, participants who were high in self-certainty actively resisted the questions—regardless of the evaluators' level of certainty. Thus, as long as participants were high in self-certainty, self-verification overrode behavioral confirmation.

The tendency for self-verification to triumph over behavioral confirmation seems to generalize to naturally occurring situations. For example, McNulty and Swann (1994) studied college students over a semester. They discovered that students were more likely to bring their roommates to see them as they saw themselves than to conform their self-views to their roommates' initial impressions of them. Similarly, in an investigation of MBA students in study groups, Swann, Milton, and Polzer (2000) found that the tendency of individual members of each group to bring the appraisals of other group members into agreement with their self-views was stronger than the countervailing tendency for the group members to shape the self-views of individuals in the group.

In summary, the research literature suggests that people enlist several distinct strategies for bringing their evaluators to see them as they see themselves. In so doing, they may, in effect, enlist accomplices who will assist them in their efforts to create coherent, self-verifying worlds. Evidence for this possibility comes from research by De La Ronde and Swann (1998). These researchers brought married couples into the laboratory, asked both to rate themselves

and their partners on a number of personality attributes, and presented one of the partners with a bogus evaluation of his or her spouse. The evaluation was designed to be inconsistent with the ratings participants had made of their spouses earlier in the session. Participants responded to the inconsistent evaluations by rushing to refute them—even if this meant undermining a positive evaluation of their spouses.

Furthermore, other research suggests that merely *seeing* a self-verifying partner after receiving discrepant feedback may exert a similar stabilizing effect on people's self-views (Swann & Predmore, 1985). Such evidence of "partner verification" suggests that when people find partners who see them congruently, they will position themselves to receive a steady supply of self-verifying feedback in the future.

As effective as such behavioral self-verification strivings may be, people sometimes fail to create fully self-confirmatory relationships. When this happens, several cognitive biases may step in to rescue the self-view in question. In particular, people may misperceive and misremember social experiences in ways that are more compatible with their existing self-views than those experiences actually are, thereby preserving coherent views of themselves.

Seeing More Self-Confirmatory Evidence than Actually Exists

Researchers have shown that expectancies (including self-conceptions) exert a powerful channeling influence on information processing (e.g., Higgins & Bargh, 1987). As such, self-conceptions may guide the processing of social feedback so as to promote their own survival (Shrauger & Schoeneman, 1979; Story, 1998).

Selective Attention

To the extent that people are motivated to acquire self-confirmatory feedback, they should be especially attentive to it. Swann and Read (1981, Study 1) tested this proposition. Participants who perceived themselves as either likeable or dislikeable were led to suspect that an evaluator had either a favorable or an unfavorable impression of them. All participants were then given an opportunity to examine some remarks that the evaluator had ostensibly made about them. These remarks were sufficiently vague as to apply to anyone.

The results showed that participants spent longer scrutinizing evaluations when they anticipated that the evaluations would confirm their self-conceptions. That is, just as self-perceived likeables spent the most time reading when they expected the remarks would be favorable, self-perceived dislikeables spent the most time reading when they expected the remarks would be unfavorable. In short, people are more attentive to social feedback when they suspect that it will confirm their chronic self-views.

Selective Encoding and Retrieval

Just as people may selectively attend to self-confirmatory feedback, they also may selectively remember it. Crary (1966) and Silverman (1964), for example, reported that people recalled more incidental information about experimental tasks in which they received self-confirmatory rather than self-discrepant feedback. Moreover, other research suggests that self-conceptions channel the *type*, as well as the *amount*, of feedback people recall. In particular, Swann and Read (1981, Study 3) had participants who saw themselves as likeable or dislikeable listen to an evaluator make a series of positive and negative statements about them. Some participants expected that the statements would be generally positive; others expected that the statements would be generally negative. After a brief delay, participants attempted to recall as many of the statements as possible. Participants who perceived themselves as likeable remembered more positive than negative statements, and those who perceived themselves as dislikeable remembered more negative than positive statements. In addition, this tendency to recall self-confirmatory statements was greatest when participants had anticipated that the evaluators' statements would confirm their self-conceptions.

Selective Interpretation

On being evaluated, people may ask, "How trustworthy is the source of feedback? What does the feedback tell me about myself?"

They may answer these questions in ways that promote the survival of their self-views.

Researchers have reported clear evidence that people endorse the validity of feedback only if it fits with their self-conceptions (Markus, 1977). Similarly, Shrauger and Lund (1975) reported that people expressed greater confidence in the perceptiveness of an evaluator when his impression confirmed their self-conceptions. Swann, Griffin, Predmore, and Gaines (1987) replicated Shrauger and Lund's effect and also found that people tended to attribute self-confirmatory feedback to characteristics of themselves and self-disconfirmatory feedback to the source of the feedback. Finally, Story (1998) reported that people with high self-esteem remembered feedback as being more favorable than it actually was, whereas people with low self-esteem remembered it as being more negative than it actually was.

Together, the attentional, encoding, retrieval, and interpretational processes described in this section may prove formidable adversaries for self-discrepant feedback. This may be one reason why people's self-conceptions sometimes conflict with the actual appraisals of others and, more specifically, why people overestimate the extent to which the appraisals of their friends and acquaintances confirm their self-conceptions (Shrauger & Schoeneman, 1979). Yet there is another reason that people's self-views sometimes conflict with the appraisals of others: People do not always self-verify. In the next section, we identify some of the boundary conditions of self-verification.

Self-Verification and Self-Assessment

Sedikides and Strube (1997) have suggested that people are motivated to obtain objectively accurate or "diagnostic" information and that this motive reflects a self-assessment motive (e.g., Trope, 1975) that is distinct from self-verification. We certainly agree that people value information that seems accurate; in fact, we believe that this is what motivates self-verification strivings. From our vantage point, the two motives often represent complementary means through which people search for truth. Insofar as a given self-view is firmly held, people will usually feel no need to assess its "objective" accuracy but will instead accept it as a proxy for truth (e.g., Kruglanski, 1990). After all, firmly held self-views will generally be based on considerable evidence (Pelham, 1991) and should thus offer a reasonably accurate rendering of reality. On the other hand, when the self-view is weakly held or when people have good reason to question its accuracy (e.g., when they are making an important decision or when they have received contradictory information that is difficult to refute), they will seek diagnostic information pertaining to its objective accuracy (i.e., engage in self-assessment).

Two studies have attempted to distinguish the desire for self-verification from the desire for objective accuracy. Swann, Stein-Seroussi, and Giesler (1992) had students think aloud as they chose interaction partners. When objective raters coded these think-aloud protocols, they discovered that there were three major reasons why people self-verified. The most prominent reason was epistemic. For example, a person with negative self-views said, "I think the unfavorable evaluator is a better choice because . . . he sums up basically how I feel." A person with positive self-views said, "the positive evaluator better reflects my own view of myself, from experience." The second reason was pragmatic. A person with negative self-views said, "the unfavorable evaluator seems like a person I could sort of really get along with . . . if I choose the unfavorable evaluator it seems to me that he'll be more prepared for my anxiety about being around people I don't know. Seeing as he knows what he's dealing with we might get along better." This evidence of epistemic and pragmatic concerns, then, supported the idea that participants were interested in obtaining self-verification. Independent of these self-verification strivings, however, participants also mentioned a desire for objective accuracy. Specifically, some students voiced a concern with their partners' perceptiveness. Participants with positive self-views said things such as "I'd like to meet with the favorable evaluator because obviously they're more intelligent . . . are more able to see the truth"; "Well, actually the favorable evaluator . . . hits me right on the point . . . someone who could see that just by the answers is pretty astute" (Swann, Stein-Seroussi, & Giesler, 1992, p. 401).

Swann, Stein-Seroussi, and Giesler's (1992) findings, then, suggest that when people choose relationship partners who see them as they see themselves, they may do so because they are interested in obtaining self-verification or because they suspect that a self-verifying partner is highly perceptive (and thus likely to give them information that is objectively accurate). Although we suspect that the two concerns frequently overlap, the results of a later study by Swann and colleagues (1994) seem to be driven by self-verification strivings alone. As noted previously, participants displayed more intimacy toward spouses who saw them as they saw themselves. Consistent with self-verification theory, married persons expressed more intimacy insofar as they believed that their spouses' appraisals made them feel that they really knew themselves. Contrary to the idea that self-assessment strivings might influence intimacy, the extent to which participants believed that their partners were highly perceptive was unrelated to intimacy.

In general, then, it appears that although self-assessment strivings cannot explain the evidence that researchers have amassed for self-verification processes, people are in fact sensitive to the truth-likeness of the evaluations they receive. We suspect that this sensitivity extends to the truth-likeness of self-views themselves and that it could perpetuate some of the compensatory reactions observed in narcissists (e.g., Colvin, Block & Funder, 1995; John & Robbins, 1994). Presumably, at some level narcissists are aware of the disjunction between their self-views on the one hand and their objective accomplishments and reputation on the other. Their awareness of this disjunction may be associated with their tendency to seek exalted evaluations from others and to overreact to criticism (Brown, Bosson, & Swann, 2000).

Self-Verification and Self-Enhancement

Of the explanatory tools in the social psychological literature, none has been used as extensively as the desire for self-enhancement (Jones, 1973). Self-enhancement strivings, which we prefer to call positivity strivings,[3] are theoretically manifested in people's efforts to obtain positive evaluations. The appeal of positivity strivings is their apparent versatility; in his widely cited treatise, Baumeister (1998) enlisted self-enhancement's help in explaining virtually every phenomenon that self researchers have studied over the past five decades. In the wake of such imperialism, our assertion that people will strive to confirm their self-views "even if these self-views happen to be negative" is provocative, because it not only implies that there exists a self-related motive other than the desire for positivity, but it also suggests that this motive will sometimes override positivity strivings. In what follows, we first explain why it is appropriate to maintain a distinction between positivity versus self-verification strivings. We then focus on the conditions under which each desire will prevail.

Why Positivity Strivings Cannot Subsume Self-Verification Strivings

In the interests of parsimony, it would be useful to bring self-verification strivings into the positivity-strivings family. One strategy for accomplishing this goal is to suggest that the feeling of coherence produced by stable beliefs is nothing more than a sense of competence and that people's efforts to shore up their feelings of coherence are thus merely a manifestation of the more general desire to feel good about themselves. Unfortunately, this approach overlooks the fact that the feelings of coherence produced by self-verification are unlike any other form of competence. Whereas most competences are localized to particular tasks or domains (social, athletic, etc.), the sense of coherence emanating from self-verification is associated with people's core sense of who they are—indeed, their fundamental ability to understand reality and themselves. As a result, when people's desire for self-verification is frustrated, they will not merely feel incompetent; they will suffer the severe disorientation and psychological anarchy that occurs when people recognize that their very existence is threatened.

Alternatively, one might argue that, in some ultimate sense, people strive for self-verification for precisely the same reason that they strive for positivity—because it is reinforcing in the long run. Although self-verification surely is reinforcing in some ultimate sense, this does not mean that the desire for self-verification can be subsumed by the desire for positivity. That is, in the here and now, positivity theory assumes that people strive for favorable feedback, and self-verification theory assumes that people strive for self-confirmatory feedback. In the case of people with negative self-views, the two approaches thus make competing predictions.

And what if one expands positivity theory to include instances in which people seek negative evaluations in the service of obtaining positive evaluations later on (e.g., Sedikides & Strube, 1997)? For this position to be viable, one must determine whether people do indeed self-verify in an effort to obtain favorable evaluations down the road (otherwise, the position is not falsifiable). Unfortunately for this temporally expanded version of positivity theory, the research literature has offered it little support. For example, in two independent studies of people who thought out loud as they chose interaction partners (Swann, Bosson, & Pelham, in press; Swann, Stein-Seroussi, & Geisler, 1992), self-verifying participants with negative self-views specifically mentioned a desire for self-confirming reactions but said nothing about choosing a partner who would help them obtain positive evaluations later on.

Related research tested the idea that people with negative self-views chose the negative evaluator over the positive one because they feared that the positive evaluator might soon "find them out" and reject them with righteous indignation. If so, their choice of a negative evaluator was designed to avoid the wrath of an initially positive evaluator who later became disappointed (i.e., they were engaging in positivity strivings). To test this idea, Swann, Wenzlaff, & Tafarodi (1992) had people choose between interacting with an evaluator or being in a different experiment. People with positive self-views chose to interact with the favorable evaluator over participating in another experiment, and they chose being in a different experiment over interacting with an unfavorable evaluator. In contrast, people with negative self-views chose to interact with the unfavorable evaluator over participating in another experiment, and they chose being in a different experiment over interacting with a favorable evaluator. Therefore, people with negative self-views not only preferred to interact with someone who thought poorly of them, they actually preferred being in a different experiment over interacting with someone who thought well of them. People with negative self-views thus seem to be truly drawn to self-verifying interaction partners rather than simply avoiding nonverifying ones.

Numerous demonstrations also indicate that people with negative self-views seek negative feedback in settings in which it is clear that there will be no opportunity to obtain positive evaluations later on. First, people with negative self-views seek negative feedback when they have no prospect of receiving additional feedback in the future (e.g., Bosson & Swann, 1999; Giesler, Josephs, & Swann, 1996; Hixon & Swann, 1993; Pelham & Swann, 1994; Robinson & Smith-Lovin, 1992; Swann et al., 1989, 1990; Swann, Wenzlaff, Krull, & Pelham, 1992). Finally, among Swann and colleagues' (1994) self-verifying married couples, there was no evidence that people with negative self-views were more intimate with spouses who thought poorly of them because they wanted to improve themselves, or as a means of obtaining negative specific appraisals coupled with global acceptance, or because they believed that negative spouses were more perceptive than positive spouses.

In short, there is now considerable evidence that self-verification strivings are distinct from positivity strivings both conceptually and empirically. It thus becomes important to identify the boundary conditions of the two motives.

The Conditions under which Self-Verification and Positivity Strivings Will Prevail

We believe that the interplay between self-verification and positivity strivings can be best understood in terms of three principles: accessibility, investment, and idiosyncratic worlds.

The Accessibility Principle

Logically, for people to strive to verify a self-view, they must possess the mental resources needed to access that self-view. To test this idea, Swann and colleagues (1990)

deprived some participants of cognitive resources by having them rush their choice of an interaction partner. Participants who were rushed chose the positive evaluator even if they had negative self-views. In contrast, participants with negative self-views who were not rushed chose the negative evaluator, presumably because they had time to realize that the negative evaluator knew them and was thus preferable.

Just as depriving people of cognitive resources can lower the accessibility of self-views, asking participants questions that encourage them to consider their self-views can raise it. For example, when experimenters provide participants with an evaluation and ask them to indicate how self-descriptive it is, participants will typically compare the evaluation with relevant self-views and respond accordingly. In light of this, it is not surprising that researchers have repeatedly found evidence of self-verification when they have studied "cognitive responses" such as rating the accuracy of feedback (e.g., Moreland & Sweeney, 1984; Swann et al., 1987). In contrast, when experimenters give participants feedback and then ask them how they feel, participants have no reason to consider their self-views, and they thus say that they are in a better mood when the feedback is positive, even when it clashes with their negative self-views. An exception to this result may arise when discrepant feedback comes from a highly credible evaluator, for a credible evaluator should have accurate knowledge of who they are. In support of this reasoning, Pinel and Swann (1999) found that when positive feedback came from a highly credible evaluator, participants with negative self-views grew anxious on receiving it (on the other hand, when feedback was low in credibility, participants' self-views had no impact on their reactions to it: The more positive the feedback, the better they felt).

The nature of the relationship may also influence how likely people are to access their self-views and translate them into behavior. For example, Tice, Butler, Muraven, and Stillwell (1995) found that people exaggerated their positive qualities when presenting themselves to a stranger but presented themselves in a relatively accurate manner to a friend. Presumably, within a friendship relationship, it is important to be known and understood, and this makes exaggeration of one's positive qualities a liability. In contrast, with strangers people have much to gain and little to lose by presenting themselves in a highly favorable light (e.g., Leary & Kowalski, 1990).

In a similar vein, Swann and colleagues (1994) discovered that married people were most intimate with spouses who saw them as they saw themselves, even if they had negative self-views. In contrast, dating partners felt most intimate with their partners to the extent that their partners viewed them favorably. Swann and colleagues explained this finding by suggesting that, having made the decision to stay together for the long haul, married people switch their attentions to the goal of carrying out the day-to-day activities of married life as smoothly as possible. Because this goal is best facilitated if both partners are in agreement about one another's relative strengths and weaknesses, people access their self-views and consider them in reacting to their spouses' evaluations. In contrast, a central goal of dating relationships is to ensure that the partner is fond of oneself, and one's self-view has little bearing on this issue.

The Investment Principle

We suggest that as the investment involved in a set of behaviors increases (e.g., getting to know a potential spouse), people will be more apt to self-verify. One way to increase investment in a behavior is to increase the investment in self-views associated with the behavior. Thus, for example, to the extent that self-views are firmly held, people will be more inclined to rely on them in organizing their perceptions of the world and their social relationships. As a result, people should be more inclined to access highly certain, important self-views when deciding how to behave. Support for this proposition comes from evidence that people are most inclined to act on self-views that are high in certainty (e.g., Pelham, 1991; Pelham & Swann, 1994; Swann & Ely, 1984; Swann et al., 1988).[4] Similarly, people are more inclined to remain in relationships with roommates who support their important rather than unimportant self-views (e.g., Swann & Pelham, in press). Furthermore, certainty and importance have the effect of intensify-

ing self-verification even if the relevant self-views are negative.

People will also be more inclined to behave in line with their self-views if the behavior itself is highly consequential. Hixon and Swann (1993) gave participants with negative self-views a choice of interacting with a relatively positive or negative evaluator under low or high consequences. In the low-consequences condition, the experimenter indicated that the evaluator was not particularly credible (thus minimizing the epistemic consequences of the evaluation) and that the interaction would be quite brief (thus minimizing the pragmatic consequences of the evaluation). In the high-consequences condition, the experimenter indicated that the evaluator was credible and that the interaction would be lengthy (2 hours long).[5] When participants had adequate time to reflect, those in the low-consequences condition preferred the positive evaluator and those in the high-consequences condition preferred the negative evaluator. Apparently, then, when the epistemic and pragmatic stakes are high, people are more inclined to access their self-views and seek self-verification.

The Idiosyncratic-Worlds Principle

The idiosyncratic-worlds principle suggests that people can structure their personal and interpersonal worlds so that they can satisfy their positivity and self-verification strivings simultaneously. Dunning, Meyerowitz, and Holzberg (1989), for example, showed that people assign more importance to their own positive than negative qualities. Thus, for example, just as a gymnast might define athleticism in terms of balance and flexibility, a long-distance runner might emphasize stamina. Because both definitions are entirely legitimate, the ability to use these idiosyncratic self-definitions allows people to satisfy their desires for positivity and subjective accuracy simultaneously. Campbell (1986) showed that people in general, and people with high self-esteem in particular, exploit this principle by perceiving the abilities of others in ways that preserve their positive self-views.

There is also an interpersonal version of this process: People may create idiosyncratic worlds that selectively reinforce their positive self-views. Swann, Bosson, and Pelham (in press), for example, found not only that participants wanted their dating partners to see them as much more attractive than they saw themselves but also that they actually were seen this way by their partners. Apparently, people with negative self-views recognize that for their relationships to "work," they must be perceived in a fairly positive manner on relationship-relevant dimensions. They accordingly structure their interactions so that their partners actually develop such positive evaluations.

Swann and colleagues' (in press) findings are important because they provide an empirical foundation for a reconciliation of self-presentation and self-verification theories. As self-presentation approaches (e.g., Schlenker, 1980, 1984) would suggest, on dimensions that were critical to the survival of the relationship, participants desired evaluations that were considerably more positive than their self-views. Consistent with self-verification theory, on dimensions that were critical to the survival of the relationship, dating participants apparently succeeded in either locating relationship partners who viewed them quite positively or brought their partners to see them this way. Moreover, participants felt that being seen highly positively on these high-relationship-relevant dimensions was verifying even though these evaluations far exceeded their self-views. Presumably, they felt the evaluations were verifying because they had behaved in ways that made them feel deserving of such evaluations. In this instance, people appeared to be seeking verification of their highly circumscribed ideal selves rather than of their "typical" selves—a phenomenon that Swann and Schroeder (1995) dubbed "strategic self-verification." In contrast, on dimensions that were personally important to participants but not of paramount importance to the survival of the relationship, dating participants preferred and elicited evaluations that were much more congruent with their self-views.

At first blush, Swann and colleagues' (in press) findings may seem to support an assertion of Murray and her colleagues (Murray, Holmes, & Griffin, 1996) that people want to create positive illusions in their relationships. Our position is distinct, however. Although our participants anticipated

that their performances in their romantic lives would outstrip their chronic self-views, they actually elicited highly positive reactions. Therefore, rather than illusions, our participants created idiosyncratically skewed realities that validated their highly positive desired selves.

Our suggestion that people work to verify idealized self-views may seem incompatible with Swann and colleagues' (1994) claim that married people strive to attain verification for their *characteristic* self-views such that people with negative self-views are less committed to marriages in which they are perceived positively (e.g., De La Ronde & Swann, 1998; Ritts & Stein, 1995; Swann, De La Ronde, & Hixon, 1994; Swann & Pelham, 2000). Note, however, that these researchers examined how people with negative self-views react to positive reactions *on several dimensions*, only some of which were high in relationship relevance. This is critical because the results of Swann and colleagues' (in press) research suggest that people did *not* present themselves in an exceptionally positive manner on traits low in relationship relevance. If so, favorable evaluations on these dimensions would have felt underserved, incoherent, and unpleasant.

This reasoning may also explain why Murray and her colleagues (1996) found that people with negative self-views embraced positive evaluations. An examination of the items in the self-concept scale (Interpersonal Qualities Scale) used by Murray and colleagues reveals a strong focus on qualities related to the success of the relationship (e.g., "emotional," "moody," "patient," "tolerant," "complaining," "open"). In contrast, with one exception (physical attractiveness), the Self-Attributes Questionnaire (SAQ) items used in the Swann, Bosson, and Pelham (in press) study refer to competences (intellectual, artistic, sociable, athletic) that are largely independent of the person's activities within the relationship. Conceivably, people prefer highly positive evaluations on relationship-relevant dimensions because they can (and do) behave in ways that they believe merit such evaluations. In contrast, because four of the five SAQ attributes refer to relatively "objective" qualities that are expressed in multiple contexts, people may be reluctant to seek highly positive evaluations on these dimensions. Consistent with this reasoning, when judges rated the IQS and SAQ items, they indicated that the IQS qualities were less specific, more difficult to judge, required more behavioral referents to make a judgment (i.e., more vague), and were more desirable (Swann & Rentfrow, 2000). From this perspective, people may strive to keep their relationships alive by cultivating highly positive perceptions of themselves in dimensions that are high in relationship relevance and low in specificity while seeking self-verification of their chronic self-views on dimensions that are low in relationship relevance and high in specificity.

But if the notion of idiosyncratic worlds is compatible with previous research generated by self-verification theory, it is inconsistent with the theory's assumption that people strive to negotiate identities that match their characteristic self-views (Swann, 1983). Apparently, people's relationship goals cause them to enact idealized, relationship-specific selves, and they thus come to prefer having these idealized selves verified. This revised version of self-verification theory goes beyond the original idea that people want verification for the selves that they negotiate by positing that, because people care most about the behavior of relationship partners in their own presence, people may be primarily concerned with verifying situation-specific selves. This new emphasis, then, departs from the assumptions of classical trait and self theory. Instead, it draws on Swann's (1984) suggestion that people strive for circumscribed accuracy and on Shoda and Mischel's (1996) notion that people strive for intraindividual consistency.

Conclusions

Recently, reviewers of the literature on the self (Baumeister, 1998; Sedikides & Strube, 1997) have made it their business to compare the power of the three major motives (self-assessment, positivity, self-verification) and to declare positivity the "victor." We believe that this is unfortunate, because the vast majority of the studies that have been presented as evidence for the pervasiveness of positivity strivings do not even include measures of self-views. For example, the centerpiece of Baumeister's (1998) discussion of the major motives was a study by Sedikides (1993). Because Sedikides failed to measure self-views, his findings say nothing about the pervasiveness of positivity versus self-verification strivings. That is, although the fact that his participants regarded positive traits as more self-descriptive than negative traits could have reflected positivity strivings, it could just as easily be understood to reflect the self-verification strivings of people with positive self-views, who are overrepresented in most samples (Swann, 1987). In addition, of those studies that do include measures of self-views, many are quite low on the dimensions of self-view accessibility and investment. For example, because role-playing studies (Morling & Epstein, 1997) are quite low on the accessibility and investment dimensions, participants may have little reason to self-verify. Due to these and related limitations in the relevant research literature, much work remains to be done before anyone is positioned to declare which of the three motives is most important.

However this debate is ultimately resolved, recent work on idiosyncratic worlds suggests that the conflict may exist more in the minds of researchers than in the hearts of their participants. Perhaps it is time to move away from attempting to identify the "winner" of the three-motives sweepstakes and concentrate instead on more nuanced questions, such as, How do people engineer social worlds that simultaneously satisfy their desires for accuracy, positivity and self-verification?

Acknowledgments

This research was supported by Grant No. MH57455-01A2 from the National Institute of Mental Health to William B. Swann, Jr. We thank Constantine Sedikides for comments on portions of a draft of this chapter.

Notes

1. Although we suspect that Festinger's failure to cite Lecky reflected this conceptual distinction, we will probably never know the real reason. When we asked Elliot Aronson, one of Festinger's most distinguished former students, he chalked it up to Lecky's low visibili-

ty: "I'm not 100% certain as to why not. My best guess is that, at that time, Lecky was hardly a household name. I think that Lecky's book on self-consistency was his only publication and, as you know, it was originally published by 'The Shoestring Press' in the 1940s. I don't think many people (aside from a few of his students) ever read it in the '40s and '50s. I had certainly never heard of him in grad school" (E. Aronson, personal communication, April 15, 2002)

2. The nature of the different experiment was not specified. Nevertheless, the overall pattern of data suggested that it was quite unlikely that participants assumed that it was apt to be a dreadful experience. That is, people with positive self-views chose the different experiment when the alternative was a negative partner, and people with negative self-views chose the different experiment when the alternative was a positive partner.

3. Our reservation about the term "self-enhancement" is that inconsistent usage has rendered it ambiguous. For example, sometimes it has been used to refer to processes that improve one's self-evaluation, at other times to refer to processes that maintain one's self-evaluation, and at still other times to processes that have little to do with the self.

4. In principle, a person who is *extremely* high in self-certainty may simply dismiss discrepant feedback out of hand. Thus far, however, we have not encountered participants who are sufficiently certain of their self-views to do this.

5. The conceptual focus of the Hixon and Swann (1983) study (i.e., the effectiveness of introspection) led them to emphasize the results of the low-epistemic–low-pragmatic-consequences condition and merely allude to the results of the high-epistemic–high-pragmatic-consequences condition in a footnote.

References

Aronson, E. (1969). A theory of cognitive dissonance: A current perspective. In L. Berkowitz (Ed.), *Advances in experimental social psychology* (Vol. 4, pp. 1–34). New York: Academic Press.

Backman, C. W., & Secord, P. F. (1962). Liking, selective interaction, and misperception in congruent interpersonal relations. *Sociometry, 25,* 321–335.

Baumeister, R. F. (1998). The self. In D. Gilbert & S. Fiske (Eds.), *Handbook of social psychology* (pp. 680–740). Boston: McGraw-Hill.

Bosson, J., & Swann, W. B., Jr. (1999). Self-liking, self-competence, and the quest for self-verification. *Personality and Social Psychology Bulletin, 25,* 1230–1241.

Brown, R., Bosson, J., & Swann, W. B., Jr. (2000). *How do*

I love me: Assessing self-love and -loathing in the narcissist. Unpublished manuscript.

Broxton, J. A. (1963). A test of interpersonal attraction predictions derived from balance theory. *Journal of Abnormal and Social Psychology, 66,* 394–397.

Bruner, J. S., Goodnow, J. J., & Austin, G. A. (1956). *A study of thinking.* New York: Wiley.

Burke, P. J., & Stets, J. E. (1999). Trust and commitment through self-verification. *Social Psychology Quarterly, 62,* 347–366.

Campbell, J. D. (1986). Similarity and uniqueness: The effects of attribute type, relevance, and individual differences in self-esteem and depression. *Journal of Personality and Social Psychology, 50,* 281–294.

Clark, G. L. (1954). *Elements of ecology.* New York: Wiley.

Colvin, C. R., Block J., & Funder, D. C. (1995). Overly positive self-evaluations and personality: Negative implications for mental health. *Journal of Personality and Social Psychology, 68,* 1152–1162.

Cooley, C. S. (1902). *Human nature and the social order.* New York: Scribner's.

Crary, W. G. (1966). Reactions to incongruent self-experiences. *Journal of Consulting Psychology, 30,* 246–252.

De La Ronde, C., & Swann, W. B., Jr. (1998). Partner verification: Restoring shattered images of our intimates. *Journal of Personality and Social Psychology, 75,* 374–382.

Dunning, D., Meyerowitz, J. A., & Holzberg, A. D. (1989). Ambiguity and self-evaluation: The role of idiosyncratic trait definitions in self-serving assessments of ability. *Journal of Personality and Social Psychology, 57,* 1082–1090.

Festinger, L. (1957). *A theory of cognitive dissonance.* Evanston, IL: Row, Peterson.

Giesler, R. B., Josephs, R. A., & Swann, W. B., Jr. (1996). Self-verification in clinical depression: The desire for negative evaluation. *Journal of Abnormal Psychology, 105,* 358–368.

Goffman, E. (1959). *The presentation of self in everyday life.* Garden City, NY: Doubleday-Anchor.

Gosling, S. D., Ko, S. J., Mannarelli, T., & Morris, M. E. (2002). A room with a cue: Personality judgments based on offices and bedrooms. *Journal of Personality and Social Psychology, 82,* 379–398.

Guidano, V. F., & Liotti, G. (1983). *Cognitive processes and emotional disorders: A structural approach to psychotherapy.* New York: Guilford Press.

Higgins, E. T., & Bargh, J. A. (1987). Social cognition and social perception. In M. R. Rosenzweig & L. W. Porter (Eds.), *Annual Review of Psychology, 38,* 369–425.

Hixon, J. G., & Swann, W. B., Jr. (1993). When does introspection bear fruit? Self-reflection, self-insight, and interpersonal choices. *Journal of Personality and Social Psychology, 64,* 35–43.

John, O. P., & Robbins, R. W. (1994). Accuracy and bias in self-perception: Individual differences in self-enhancement and the role of narcissism. *Journal of Personality and Social Psychology, 66,* 206–219.

Jones, S. C. (1973). Self and interpersonal evaluations: Esteem theories versus consistency theories. *Psychological Bulletin, 79,* 185–199.

Katz, J., Beach, S. R. H, & Anderson, P. (1996). Self-enhancement versus self-verification: Does spousal support always help? *Cognitive Therapy and Research, 20,* 345–360.

Klayman, J., & Ha, Y. W. (1987). Confirmation, disconfirmation, and information in hypothesis testing. *Psychological Review, 94,* 211–228.

Kruglanski, A. W. (1990). Lay epistemic theory in social–cognitive psychology. *Psychological Inquiry, 1,* 181–197.

Leary, M. R., & Kowalski, R. M. (1990). Impression management: A literature review and two-component model. *Psychological Bulletin, 107,* 34–47.

Lecky, P. (1945). *Self-consistency: A theory of personality.* New York: Island Press.

Markus, H. (1977). Self-schemas and processing information about the self. *Journal of Personality and Social Psychology, 35,* 63–78.

McCall, G. J., & Simmons, J. L. (1966). *Identities and interactions: An examination of human associations in everyday life.* New York: Free Press.

McNulty, S. E., & Swann, W. B., Jr. (1994). Identity negotiation in roommate relationships: The self as architect and consequence of social reality. *Journal of Personality and Social Psychology, 67,* 1012–1023.

Mead, G. H. (1934). *Mind, self and society.* Chicago: University of Chicago Press.

Moreland, R. L., & Sweeney, P. D. (1984). Self-expectancies and reaction to evaluations of personal performance. *Journal of Personality, 52,* 156–176.

Morling, B., & Epstein, S. (1997). Compromises produced by the dialectic between self-verification and self-enhancement. *Journal of Personality and Social Psychology, 73,* 1268–1283.

Murphy, G. (1947). *Personality: A biosocial approach to origins and structure.* New York: Harper & Brothers.

Murray, S. L., Holmes, J. G., & Griffin, D. W. (1996). The benefits of positive illusions: Idealization and the construction of satisfaction in close relationships. *Journal of Personality and Social Psychology, 70,* 79–98.

Newcomb, T. M. (1956). The prediction of interpersonal attraction. *American Psychologist, 11,* 575–586.

Pelham, B. W. (1991). On confidence and consequence: The certainty and importance of self-knowledge. *Journal of Personality and Social Psychology, 60,* 518–530.

Pelham, B. W., & Swann, W. B., Jr. (1994). The juncture of intrapersonal and interpersonal knowledge: Self-certainty and interpersonal congruence. *Personality and Social Psychology Bulletin, 20,* 349–357.

Pervin, L. A., & Rubin, D. B. (1967). Student dissatisfaction with college and the college dropout: A transactional approach. *Journal of Social Psychology, 72,* 285–295.

Pinel, E. C., & Swann, W. B., Jr. (1999). *The cognitive–affective crossfire revisited: Affective reactions to self-discrepant evaluations.* Unpublished manuscript, University of Texas at Austin.

Popper, K. R. (1963). *Conjectures and refutations.* London: Routledge.

Rentfrow, P. J., Swann, W. B., Jr., & Keough, K. A. (2002). *The interplay between psychological coherence and health.* Manuscript in preparation.

Ritts, V., & Stein, J. R. (1995). Verification and commitment in marital relationships: An exploration of self-verification theory in community college students. *Psychological Reports, 76,* 383–386.

Robinson, D. T., & Smith-Lovin, L. (1992). Selective inter-

action as a strategy for identity maintenance: An affect control model. *Social Psychology Quarterly, 55,* 12–28.

Sacks, O. (1985). *The man who mistook his wife for a hat.* New York: Simon & Schuster.

Schafer, R. B., Wickram, K. A. S., & Keith, P. M. (1996). Self-concept disconfirmation, psychological distress, and marital happiness. *Journal of Marriage and the Family, 58,* 167–177.

Schlenker, B. R. (1980). *Impression management.* Monterey, CA: Brooks/Cole.

Schlenker, B. R. (1984). Identities, identifications and relationships. In V. Derlega (Ed.), *Communication, intimacy and close relationships* (pp. 71–104). New York: Academic Press.

Secord, P. F., & Backman, C. W. (1965). An interpersonal approach to personality. In B. Maher (Ed.), *Progress in experimental personality research* (Vol. 2, pp. 91–125). New York: Academic Press.

Sedikides, C. (1993). Assessment, enhancement, and verification determinants of the self-evaluation process. *Journal of Personality and Social Psychology, 65,* 317–338.

Sedikides, C., & Strube, M. J. (1997). Self evaluation: To thine own self be good, to thine own self be sure, to thine own self be true, and to thine own self be better. In M. P. Zanna (Ed.), *Advances in experimental social psychology* (Vol. 29, pp. 209–269). New York: Academic Press.

Shoda, Y., & Mischel, W., (1996). Toward a unified, intraindividual dynamic conception of personality. *Journal of Research in Personality, 30,* 414–428.

Shrauger, J. S., & Lund, A. (1975). Self-evaluation and reactions to evaluations from others. *Journal of Personality, 43,* 94–108.

Shrauger, J. S., & Schoeneman, T. J. (1979). Symbolic interactionist view of self-concept: Through the looking glass darkly. *Psychological Bulletin, 86,* 549–573.

Silverman, I. (1964). Self-esteem and differential responsiveness to success and failure. *Journal of Social Psychology, 69,* 115–119.

Snyder, M., & Swann, W. B., Jr. (1978). Hypothesis testing processes in social interaction. *Journal of Personality and Social Psychology, 36,* 1202–1212.

Steinem, G. (1992). *Revolution from within: A book of self-esteem.* Boston: Little, Brown.

Story, A. L. (1998). Self-esteem and memory for favorable and unfavorable personality feedback. *Personality and Social Psychology Bulletin, 24,* 51–64.

Swann, W. B., Jr. (1983). Self-verification: Bringing social reality into harmony with the self. In J. Suls & A. G. Greenwald (Eds.), *Psychological perspectives on the self* (Vol. 2, pp. 33–66). Hillsdale, NJ: Erlbaum.

Swann, W. B., Jr. (1984). The quest for accuracy in person perception: A matter of pragmatics. *Psychological Review, 91,* 457–477.

Swann, W. B., Jr. (1987). Identity negotiation: Where two roads meet. *Journal of Personality and Social Psychology, 53,* 1038–1051.

Swann, W. B., Jr. (1990). To be adored or to be known?: The interplay of self-enhancement and self-verification. In E. T. Higgins & R. M. Sorrentino (Eds.), *Handbook of motivation and cognition: Foundations of social behavior* (Vol. 2, 408–448). New York: Guilford Press.

Swann, W. B., Jr. (1999). *Resilient identities: Self, rela-*

tionships, and the construction of social reality. New York: Basic Books.

Swann, W. B., Jr., Bosson, J., & Pelham, B. W. (in press). Different partners, different selves: Strategic verification of circumscribed identities. *Personality and Social Psychology Bulletin.*

Swann, W. B., Jr., De La Ronde, C., & Hixon, J. G. (1994). Authenticity and positivity strivings in marriage and courtship. *Journal of Personality and Social Psychology, 66,* 857–869.

Swann, W. B., Jr., & Ely, R. J. (1984). A battle of wills: Self-verification versus behavioral confirmation. *Journal of Personality and Social Psychology, 46,* 1287–1302.

Swann, W. B., Jr., Griffin, J. J., Predmore, S., & Gaines, B. (1987). The cognitive–affective crossfire: When self-consistency confronts self-enhancement. *Journal of Personality and Social Psychology, 52,* 881–889.

Swann, W. B., Jr., & Hill, C. A. (1982). When our identities are mistaken: Reaffirming self-conceptions through social interaction. *Journal of Personality and Social Psychology, 43,* 59–66.

Swann, W. B., Jr., Hixon, J. G., Stein-Seroussi, A., & Gilbert, D. T. (1990). The fleeting gleam of praise: Behavioral reactions to self-relevant feedback. *Journal of Personality and Social Psychology, 59,* 17–26.

Swann, W. B., Jr., Milton, L., & Polzer, J. (2000). Creating a niche or falling in line: Identity negotiation and small group effectiveness. *Journal of Personality and Social Psychology, 79,* 238–250.

Swann, W. B., Jr., & Pelham, B. W. (in press). Who wants out when the going gets good? Psychological investment and preference for self-verifying college roommates. *Journal of Self and Identity.*

Swann, W. B., Jr., & Pelham, B. W. (2002). The truth about illusions: Authenticity and positivity in social relationships. In C. R. Snyder & S. J. Lopez (Eds.), *Handbook of positive psychology* (pp. 366–381). New York: Oxford University Press.

Swann, W. B., Jr., Pelham, B. W., & Chidester, T. (1988). Change through paradox: Using self-verification to alter beliefs. *Journal of Personality and Social Psychology, 54,* 268–273.

Swann, W. B., Jr., Pelham, B. W., & Krull, D. S. (1989). Agreeable fancy or disagreeable truth? Reconciling self-enhancement and self-verification. *Journal of Personality and Social Psychology, 57,* 782–791.

Swann, W. B., Jr., & Predmore, S. C. (1985). Intimates as agents of social support: Sources of consolation or despair? *Journal of Personality and Social Psychology, 49,* 1609–1617.

Swann, W. B., Jr., & Read, S. J. (1981). Self-verification processes: How we sustain our self-conceptions. *Journal of Experimental Social Psychology, 17,* 351–372.

Swann, W. B., Jr., & Rentfrow, P. J. (2000). [A comparison of the properties of the SAQ and IQS]. Unpublished raw data.

Swann, W. B., Jr., & Schroeder, D. G. (1995). The search for beauty and truth: A framework for understanding reactions to evaluative feedback. *Personality and Social Psychology Bulletin, 21,* 1307–1318.

Swann, W. B., Jr., Stein-Seroussi, A., & Giesler, B. (1992). Why people self-verify. *Journal of Personality and Social Psychology, 62,* 392–401.

Swann, W. B., Jr., Wenzlaff, R. M., Krull, D. S., & Pelham, B. W. (1992). The allure of negative feedback: Self-verification strivings among depressed persons. *Journal of Abnormal Psychology, 101,* 293–306.

Swann, W. B., Jr., Wenzlaff, R. M., & Tafarodi, R. W. (1992). Depression and the search for negative evaluations: More evidence of the role of self-verification strivings. *Journal of Abnormal Psychology, 101,* 314–371.

Tice, D. M, Butler, J. L., Muraven, M. B., & Stillwell, A. M. (1995). When modesty prevails: Differential favorability of self-presentation to friends and strangers. *Journal of Personality and Social Psychology, 69,* 1120–1138.

Trope, Y. (1975). Seeking information about one's own ability as a determinant of choice among tasks. *Journal of Personality and Social Psychology, 32,* 1004–1113.

Wachtel, P. L. (1977). *Psychoanalysis and behavior therapy: Toward an integration.* New York: Basic Books.

Wason, P. C., & Johnson-Laird, P. N. (1972). *Psychology of reasoning: Structure and content.* London: Batsford.

19

Self-Relevant Emotions

JUNE PRICE TANGNEY

All human emotions are, in a loose sense, "self-relevant." Emotions arise when something self-relevant happens or is about to happen. In the language of appraisal theory (Lazarus, 1966), we experience emotions when we judge that events have positive or negative significance for our well-being. The specific type of emotional response is shaped both by primary appraisals of the positive versus negative implications of the event for the individual and by secondary appraisals (e.g., of one's ability to cope with the events). But all emotions arise from events that in some way have relevance for oneself. There is, however, a special class of human emotions that are even more immediately self-relevant. This chapter focuses on the "self-conscious" emotions, which directly involve self-reflection and self-evaluation.

Self-Conscious Emotions

Shame, guilt, embarrassment, and pride are members of a family of "self-conscious emotions" that are evoked by self-reflection and self-evaluation. This self-evaluation may be implicit or explicit, consciously experienced or transpiring beyond our awareness. But in one way or another, these emotions are fun-

damentally about the self. For example, when good things happen, we may feel a range of positive emotions—joy, happiness, satisfaction, or contentment. But we feel pride in our *own* positive attributes or actions. By the same token, when bad things happen, many different types of negative emotions are possible—for example, sadness, disappointment, frustration, or anger. But feelings of shame and guilt typically arise from a recognition of one's *own* negative attributes or negative behaviors. We feel ashamed of ourself, guilty over our behavior, and embarrassed by our pratfalls. Even when we feel shame due to another person's behavior, that person is almost invariably someone with whom we are closely affiliated or identified (e.g., a family member, friend, or colleague closely associated with the self). We experience shame because that person is part of our self-definition.

Self-Conscious Emotions Are Emotions of Self-Regulation

The self-conscious emotions are fundamentally emotions of self-regulation. Shame, guilt, embarrassment, and pride serve an important self-regulatory function by providing critical feedback to the self about the self's thoughts, intentions, and behavior. In the face of triumph, transgression, or error, the self turns toward the self—evaluating and rendering judgment in reference to moral standards, personal expectations, and social conventions. When we violate (or anticipate violating) important standards, we are inclined to experience negative self-conscious emotions, such as shame, guilt, and embarrassment. When we meet or exceed standards, we are inclined to experience pride and attendant increases in self-esteem. In this way, shame, guilt, embarrassment, and pride function as an emotional moral barometer, providing immediate and salient feedback on our social and moral acceptability—and our worth as human beings. These self-conscious emotions play an important role in guiding our behavior, motivating us to adhere to moral and social standards and to respond appropriately (e.g., with contrition and reparation) when we don't.

"Emotions of Morality" Form Part of a Triad of Morally Relevant Processes

Although long neglected in the behavioral sciences, the class of "self-conscious" emotions lies at the heart of a triad of morally relevant processes (see Figure 19.1). According to this model, moral decisions and moral behavior are guided by three broad classes of factors—moral standards, moral reasoning, and moral affect.

Moral standards represent the individual's knowledge of culturally defined moral norms and conventions. As Blasi (1980) pointed out, there are very small individual differences in knowledge of accepted rules and norms beyond the early age of 7 or 8. For example, most people know that, barring extenuating circumstances, it is wrong to lie, cheat, or steal.

Naturally, people do, on occasion, lie, cheat, and steal, even though they know such behavior is wrong, according to moral and societal norms. Individual differences in both moral reasoning and moral emotion likely play a key role in determining people's actual moral choices and behavior in real-life contexts.

Moral reasoning involves thinking through the implications of alternative behaviors in terms of moral principles. Not infrequently, people are faced with competing moral considerations, and it is here that individual differences in moral developmental level presumably come into play. Most notable among theories of moral thought or reasoning is Kohlberg's (1969) cognitive-developmental theory. Kohlberg proposed that people's thinking about moral issues progresses in stages, paralleling Piaget's

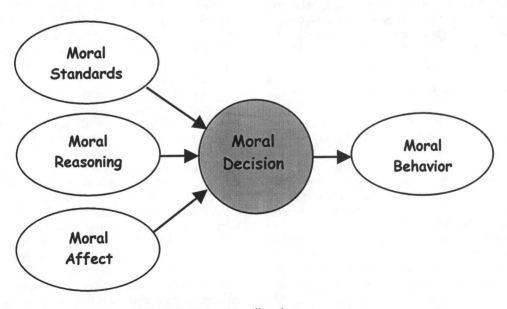

FIGURE 19.1. Morally relevant processes.

(1952) more general theory of cognitive development. At the lowest levels of moral reasoning, people focus on concrete ideas of right and wrong (e.g., "that's the rule") and consequences for oneself (e.g., "getting in trouble"). At successively higher levels of moral reasoning, the arguments become more complex and less egocentric, incorporating notions of community, justice, and reciprocity (e.g., "fairness for the common good"). Kohlberg and his colleagues use a series of moral "dilemmas" to assess people's level of moral reasoning. For example, there's the classic dilemma faced by "Heinz," who must decide whether or not to steal a prohibitively expensive drug to save his dying wife. The issue isn't *what* people decide (steal vs. not steal) but *how* they decide. At lower levels of moral reasoning, a person might emphasize that stealing is against the rules, or that Heinz might get caught and go to jail. At higher levels of moral reasoning, a person might also argue against stealing but draw on notions of fairness (someone else equally deserving would be deprived of the drug) or the need for order and justice in society.

How does level of moral reasoning relate to people's behavior? The very strong assumption among moral developmentalists is that people who reason at more sophisticated levels behave better. In the vast literature on moral reasoning, remarkably few studies have actually examined people's *behavior*, but the available evidence suggests only a modest link between moral thinking and moral action (Arnold, 1989; Blasi, 1980). Level of moral reasoning does not account for the lion's share of variance in people's choices to engage in moral or immoral behavior.

This modest relationship between moral reasoning and moral behavior is not so surprising when one takes a closer look at the nature of moral reasoning, á la Kohlberg. As Blasi (1980) pointed out, in many instances there is no obvious correspondence between a given mode of moral reasoning and a particular behavioral choice. For example, altruistic behavior may result from reasoning at any level. A person might choose to help because "it's the rule" or out of appreciation for the needs of human society. By the same token, two individuals operating from the same moral cognitive level may behave in radically different ways, depending on the manner in which a situation is construed. It is possible to reason in a simple concrete fashion both that Heinz should steal and that he should not.

A second factor that may further contribute to the modest relationship between moral reasoning and moral behavior is that cognitive theories of moral development lack any systematic consideration of moral emotion. Researchers interested in moral reasoning focus on how people *think* rather than how they *feel* in the face of moral dilemmas. But perhaps more important is people's capacity for moral emotions.

Moral affect represents a third key element of the moral psychological process that determines moral choice and moral behavior. Moral emotions provide the motivational force—the power and energy—to do good and to avoid doing bad. As the self reflects on the self, moral "self-conscious" emotions provide immediate punishment (or reinforcement) of behavior. When we sin, transgress, or err, aversive feelings of shame, guilt, or embarrassment are likely to ensue. When we "do the right thing" to meet or exceed important standards, positive feelings of pride and self-approval result. Moreover, actual behavior is not necessary for the press of moral emotions to have impact. People can *anticipate* their likely emotional reactions (e.g., guilt vs. pride/self-approval) as they consider behavioral alternatives. Thus the "self-conscious," moral emotions can exert a strong influence on moral choice and behavior by providing critical feedback regarding both anticipated and actual outcomes.

Of the three elements that compose our human moral apparatus, moral affect has received the least empirical attention. Until recently, remarkably little research has been devoted to these moral, self-conscious emotions. The past 15 years, however, have brought a profusion of basic research on the nature and implications of the negative self-conscious emotions—shame, guilt, and embarrassment. Far less attention has been devoted to pride, the positive self-conscious emotion. But even here, important inroads have been made in the empirical literature. The remainder of this chapter summarizes current theory and research on these most self-relevant human emotions.

Shame and Guilt

To many, shame and guilt are the quintessential "moral emotions"—woven inextricably in our imagery of the repentant sinner. Shame and guilt are typically mentioned in the same breath, as moral emotions that inhibit antisocial, morally objectionable behavior. But an extensive theoretical and empirical literature underscores striking differences in the phenomenology of these emotions (H. B. Lewis, 1971; Lindsay-Hartz, 1984; Tangney, 1989, 1993; Tangney & Dearing, 2002; Weiner, 1985; Wicker, Payne, & Morgan, 1983)—differences that have important and very different implications for subsequent motivation and behavior. Most notably, a decade of research now indicates that shame and guilt are not equally "moral" or adaptive emotions. Evidence suggests that, whereas guilt consistently motivates people in positive directions (Baumeister et al., 1994; Eisenberg, 1986; Tangney, 1991, 1995a, 1995b), shame is a moral emotion that can easily go awry (Tangney, 1991, 1995a, 1995b, 1996).

What Is the Difference between Shame and Guilt?

Most people use the terms "shame" and "guilt" interchangeably. It's not uncommon, for example, to hear people refer to "feelings of shame and guilt" or "the effects of shame and guilt" without making any distinction between the two. Nonetheless, there have been a number of attempts over the years to differentiate between shame and guilt. Two bases for distinguishing between shame and guilt stand out as especially influential—the anthropologists' focus on public versus private transgressions (e.g., Benedict, 1946), and Helen Block Lewis's (1971) focus on self versus behavior.

In distinguishing between shame and guilt, anthropologists focused on differences in the content or structure of events that elicit these emotions. The notion is that certain *kinds of situations* lead to shame, whereas other *kinds of situations* lead to guilt. More specifically, shame is viewed as a more "public" emotion than guilt (Benedict, 1946), arising from public exposure and disapproval of some shortcoming or transgression. Guilt, on the other hand, is conceived as a more "private" experience arising from self-generated pangs of conscience. As it turns out, empirical research has failed to support this public–private distinction (Tangney, Marschall, Rosenberg, Barlow, & Wagner, 1994; Tangney, Miller, Flicker, & Barlow, 1996). For example, we conducted a systematic analysis of the social context of personal shame- and guilt-eliciting events, described by several hundred children and adults (Tangney et al., 1994). Results indicated that shame and guilt are equally likely to be experienced in the presence of others. "Solitary" shame experiences were about as common as "solitary" guilt experiences. Even more to the point, the frequency with which others were *aware* of the respondents' behavior did not vary as a function of shame and guilt, in direct contradiction to the anthropologists' conceptualization.

We have also assessed whether shame and guilt might differ in terms of the *types* of the transgressions or failures that elicit them. Analyses of personal shame and guilt experiences provided by children and adults revealed few, if any, "classic" shame-inducing or guilt-inducing situations (Tangney, 1992; Tangney et al., 1994). Most types of events (e.g., lying, cheating, stealing, failing to help another, disobeying parents, etc.) are cited by some people in connection with feelings of shame and by other people in connection with guilt. Similarly, Keltner and Buswell (1996) reported a high degree of overlap in the types of events that cause shame and guilt.

How do shame and guilt differ, if not in terms of the types of situations that elicit them? Empirical research has been much more supportive of Helen Block Lewis's (1971) emphasis on self versus behavior. According to Lewis, shame involves a negative evaluation of the global self; guilt involves a negative evaluation of a specific behavior. Although this distinction may, at first glance, appear rather subtle, this differential emphasis on self ("*I* did that horrible thing") versus behavior ("I *did* that horrible *thing*") sets the stage for very different emotional experiences and very different patterns of motivations and subsequent behavior.

Shame is an acutely painful emotion that is typically accompanied by a sense of shrinking or of "being small" and by a sense of worthlessness and powerlessness. Shamed people also feel exposed. Although shame does not necessarily involve the presence of an actual observing audience to witness one's shortcomings, a person often has an image of how his or her defective self would appear to others. H. B. Lewis (1971) described a split in self-functioning in which the self is both agent and object of observation and disapproval. An observing self witnesses and denigrates the observed self as unworthy and reprehensible. Not surprisingly, shame often leads to a desire to escape or to hide—to sink into the floor and disappear.

Guilt, in contrast, is typically a less painful, less devastating experience because the object of condemnation is a specific behavior, not the entire self. One's core identity or self-concept is less at stake. Rather than feeling a need to defend a vulnerable self under attack, people experiencing guilt are focused on the offense and its consequences, feeling tension, remorse, and regret over the "bad thing done." People feeling guilt often report a nagging focus or preoccupation with the transgression—thinking of it over and over, wishing they had behaved differently or could somehow undo the harm that was done. Rather than motivating avoidance and defense, guilt motivates reparative behavior—confession, apology, and attempts to fix the situation.

Shame and Guilt Are Not Equally "Moral" Emotions

One of the consistent themes emerging from empirical research is that shame and guilt are not equally "moral" emotions. On balance, guilt appears to be the more adaptive emotion, benefiting individuals and their relationships in a variety of ways (Baumeister, Stillwell, & Heatherton, 1994, 1995a, 1995b; Tangney, 1991, 1995b). Five sets of findings illustrate the adaptive functions of guilt, in contrast to the hidden costs of shame.

Hiding versus Amending

First, research consistently shows that shame and guilt lead to contrasting motivations or "action tendencies" (Ferguson, Stegge, &

Damhuis, 1991; H. B. Lewis, 1971; Lindsay-Hartz, 1984; Tangney, 1993; Tangney, Miller, et al., 1996; Wallbott & Scherer, 1995; Wicker et al., 1983). In the face of failure or transgression, shame typically leads to attempts to deny, hide, or escape the shame-inducing situation; guilt typically leads to reparative action—confessing, apologizing, undoing. For example, when people are asked to anonymously describe and rate personal shame and guilt experiences along a number of phenomenological dimensions (Tangney, 1993; Tangney, Miller, et al., 1996), their ratings indicate that they feel more compelled to hide from others and less inclined to admit what they had done when feeling shame as opposed to guilt. Taken together, findings across studies suggest that guilt motivates people in a constructive, proactive, future-oriented direction, whereas shame motivates people toward separation, distance, and defense.

Other-Oriented Empathy

Second, there appears to be a special link between guilt and empathy. Empathy is a highly valued, prosocial emotional process. Empirical research has shown that empathy motivates altruistic, helping behavior; that it fosters warm, close interpersonal relationships; and that it inhibits antisocial behavior and interpersonal aggression (Eisenberg, 1986; Eisenberg & Miller, 1987; Feshbach, 1978, 1984, 1987; Feshbach & Feshbach, 1969, 1982, 1986). Research also indicates that guilt and empathy go hand in hand, whereas feelings of shame often interfere with an empathic connection. This differential relationship of shame and guilt to empathy has been observed at the levels of both emotion dispositions and emotion states.

Studies of affective dispositions focus on *individual differences*. When faced with a failure or transgression, to what degree is a person likely to feel shame, guilt, or both? To assess proneness to shame and proneness to guilt, we make use of a scenario-based method in which respondents are presented with a series of situations often encountered in daily life. Each scenario is followed by responses that capture phenomenological aspects of shame, guilt, and other theoretically relevant experiences (e.g., externalization, pride). For example, in the adult version of our Test of Self-Conscious Affect (TOSCA; Tangney, Wagner, & Gramzow, 1989), participants are asked to imagine that "You make a big mistake on an important project at work. People were depending on you and your boss criticizes you." People then rate their likelihood of reacting with a shame response ("You would feel like you wanted to hide"), a guilt response ("You would think 'I should have recognized the problem and done a better job'") and so forth. Responses across the scenarios capture affective, cognitive, and motivational features associated with shame and guilt, respectively, as described in the theoretical, phenomenological, and empirical literature. (See Tangney, 1996, and Tangney & Dearing, 2002, for a summary of research supporting the reliability and validity of the TOSCA.)

Using the TOSCA, researchers have examined the relationship of shame-proneness and guilt-proneness to a dispositional capacity for interpersonal empathy (Leith & Baumeister, 1998; Tangney, 1991, 1994, 1995b; Tangney, Wagner, Burggraf, Gramzow, & Fletcher, 1991; Tangney & Dearing, 2002). Across numerous independent studies of people from all walks of life, the results are remarkably consistent. Guilt-prone individuals are generally empathic individuals. Proneness to guilt consistently correlates with measures of perspective taking and empathic concern. In contrast, shame-proneness has been associated with an impaired capacity for other-oriented empathy and a propensity for problematic, "self-oriented" personal distress responses.

Individual differences aside, similar findings are obtained when considering emotion states—feelings of shame and guilt "in the moment." When people describe personal guilt experiences, they convey greater empathy for others involved in the situation, compared with their descriptions of personal shame experiences (Leith & Baumeister, 1998; Tangney et al., 1994). Moreover, when people are experimentally induced to feel shame, they exhibit less empathy than nonshamed controls (Marschall, 1996). Marschall (1996) manipulated feelings of shame using false negative feedback on a purported intelligence test. After making a public estimate of their test scores, participants in the shame condition were told that

they scored substantially below their guess by experimenters who exchanged expressions of shock and surprise.[1] Marschall found that people induced to feel shame subsequently reported less empathy for a disabled student. The effect was most pronounced among low-shame-prone individuals. Consistent with the dispositional findings (Tangney, 1991, 1995b), shame-prone participants were fairly unempathic across conditions (i.e., regardless of whether they had just been shamed in the laboratory). But among low-shame-prone participants—who have a higher capacity for empathy in general—the shame induction had an effect, apparently serving to short-circuit an empathic response. In short, as a result of the shame induction, low-shame-prone people were rendered relatively unempathic—more like their shame-prone peers.

Why does shame, but not guilt, interfere with other-oriented empathy? In focusing on a bad behavior (as opposed to a bad self), people experiencing guilt are relatively free of the egocentric, self-involved process of shame. Instead, their focus on a specific behavior is likely to highlight the consequences of that behavior for distressed others, further facilitating an empathic response (Tangney, 1991, 1995b). In contrast, the painful self-focus of shame is apt to derail the empathic process. As indicated by content analyses of autobiographical accounts of shame and guilt experiences, the shamed individual is inclined to focus on himself or herself, as opposed to the harmed other (Tangney et al., 1994).

Anger and Aggression

Third, research has shown that there is a special link between shame and anger, again observed at both the dispositional and state levels. Helen Block Lewis (1971) first speculated on the dynamics between shame and anger (or humiliated fury) based on her clinical case studies, noting that clients' feelings of shame often precede expressions of anger and hostility in the therapy room. In years since, numerous empirical studies of children, adolescents, college students, and diverse samples of adults have shown a consistent positive correlation between proneness to shame and feelings of anger and hostility (Tangney, 1994, 1995b;

Tangney, Wagner, Fletcher, & Gramzow, 1992; Tangney et al., 1991).

What accounts for this rather counterintuitive link between shame and anger? When feeling shame, people initially direct hostility inward ("*I'm* such a bad person"). But not infrequently, this hostility may be redirected outward, in a defensive attempt to protect the self, by "turning the tables" to shift the blame elsewhere. In fact, the positive correlation between proneness to shame and externalization of blame is one of the most robust findings in our research. Without exception, across some 20 independent studies of children, adolescents, college students, and noncollege adults, using various versions of our scenario-based TOSCA measure, we have found that people who are inclined to experience shame are also significantly more likely to blame the situation and other people for the very same set of failures and transgressions (Tangney, 1994; Tangney & Dearing, 2002; Tangney, Wagner, Fletcher, & Gramzow, 1992).

Shame-prone individuals are not just more prone to externalization of blame and anger than their non-shame-prone peers. Once angered, they are also more likely to manage and express their anger in a destructive fashion. For example, in a cross-sectional developmental study of children, adolescents, college students, and adults (Tangney, Wagner, et al., 1996), proneness to shame was consistently correlated with malevolent intentions and a propensity to engage in direct physical, verbal, and symbolic aggression, indirect aggression (e.g., harming something important to the target, talking behind the target's back), all manner of displaced aggression, self-directed aggression, and anger held in (a ruminative unexpressed anger). Not surprisingly, shame-prone individuals reported that their anger typically results in negative long-term consequences—for themselves and for their relationships with others. In contrast, guilt-proneness was generally associated with more constructive means of handling anger. Proneness to "shame-free" guilt was positively correlated with constructive intentions and negatively correlated with direct, indirect, and displaced aggression. Instead, relative to non-guilt-prone persons, guilt-

prone individuals are inclined to engage in constructive behavior, such as nonhostile discussion with the target of their anger and direct corrective action. Moreover, guilt-prone individuals reported that their anger typically results in positive long-term consequences. The relationship of shame and guilt to these anger-related dimensions appears remarkably robust. For example, the findings are largely independent of the influence of social desirability.

A similar link between shame and anger has been observed at the situational level, too. For example, Wicker and colleagues (1983) found that college students reported a greater desire to punish others involved in personal shame rather than guilt experiences. Tangney, Miller, and colleagues (1996) found a similar trend among college students who reported more feelings of anger in connection with narrative accounts of shame than of guilt experiences. Finally, in a study of specific real-life episodes of anger among romantically involved couples, shamed partners were significantly more angry, more likely to engage in aggressive behavior, and less likely to elicit conciliatory behavior from their perpetrating significant other (Tangney, 1995b). Specifically, when faced with an angry, shamed, hostile partner, perpetrating boyfriends and girlfriends responded in turn with anger, resentment, defiance, and denial—rather than, for example, apologies and attempts to fix the situation. Not surprisingly, on balance, couples reported more negative long-term consequences for anger episodes involving partner shame compared with those not involving shame.

These findings regarding situation-specific feelings of shame in the midst of couples' real-life episodes of anger converge with results from dispositional studies linking trait shame with trait anger and characteristic maladaptive responses to anger. And these data provide a powerful empirical example of the shame–rage spiral described by H. B. Lewis (1971) and Scheff (1987), with (1) partner shame leading to feelings of rage and (2) destructive retaliation, which then (3) sets into motion anger and resentment in the perpetrator, as well as (4) expressions of blame and retaliation in kind, which is then (5) likely to further shame the initially shamed partner, and so forth—without any constructive resolution in sight.

Psychological Symptoms

The research reviewed thus far suggests that guilt is, on balance, the more "moral" or adaptive emotion—at least when considering social behavior and interpersonal adjustment. But is there a trade-off vis-à-vis individual psychological adjustment? Does the tendency to experience guilt over one's transgressions ultimately lead to increases in anxiety and depression or to decreases in self-esteem? Is shame perhaps less problematic for intrapersonal as opposed to interpersonal adjustment?

Researchers consistently report a relationship between proneness to shame and whole host of psychological symptoms, including depression, anxiety, eating disorder symptoms, subclinical sociopathy, and low self-esteem (Allan, Gilbert, & Goss, 1994; Brodie, 1995; Cook, 1988, 1991; Gramzow & Tangney, 1992; Harder, 1995; Harder, Cutler, & Rockart, 1992; Harder & Lewis, 1987; Hoblitzelle, 1987; Sanftner, Barlow, Marschall, & Tangney, 1995; Tangney, 1993; Tangney, Burggraf, & Wagner, 1995; Tangney & Dearing, 2002; Tangney et al., 1991; Tangney, Wagner, & Gramzow, 1992). This relationship appears to be robust across a range of measurement methods and across diverse age groups and populations. Moreover, the link between shame-proneness and depression is robust, even after controlling for attributional style (Tangney et al., 1992). Shame is frequently part of the clinical picture when considering psychological maladjustment. People who frequently experience feelings of shame about the self seem vulnerable to a range of psychological symptoms.

There is less consensus regarding the implications of guilt for psychopathology. The traditional view is that guilt plays a significant role in psychological symptoms. Clinical theory and case studies make frequent reference to a maladaptive guilt characterized by chronic self-blame and obsessive rumination over one's transgressions (e.g., Blatt, 1974; Blatt, D'Afflitti, & Quinlin, 1976; Bush, 1989; Ellis, 1962; Freud, 1909/1955, 1917/1957, 1923/1961c,

1924/1961a; Hartmann & Loewenstein, 1962; Piers & Singer, 1953; Rodin, Silberstein, & Striegel-Moore, 1985; Weiss, 1993; Zahn-Waxler, Kochanska, Krupnick, & McKnew, 1990). In contrast, recent theory and research has emphasized the adaptive functions of guilt, particularly for interpersonal behavior (Baumeister, Stillwell, & Heatherton, 1994, 1995a; Hoffman, 1982; Tangney, 1991, 1994, 1995b; Tangney et al., 1992).

Attempting to reconcile these perspectives, Tangney and colleagues (1995) argued that once one makes the critical distinction between shame and guilt, there is no compelling reason to expect guilt over specific behaviors to be associated with poor psychological adjustment. Rather, guilt is most likely to be maladaptive when it becomes fused with shame. When a person begins with a guilt experience ("Oh, look at what a horrible *thing* I have *done*") but then magnifies and generalizes the event to the self ("and aren't I a horrible *person*"), many of the advantages of guilt are lost. Not only is a person faced with tension and remorse over a specific behavior that needs to be fixed, but he or she is also saddled with feelings of contempt and disgust for a bad, defective self. And it is the shame component of this sequence—not the guilt component—that poses the problem. Often, an objectionable behavior can be altered and the negative effects repaired, or at least one can offer a heartfelt apology. Even in cases in which direct reparation or apology is not possible, one can resolve to do better in the future. In contrast, a self that is defective at its core is much more difficult to transform or amend. Shame—and, in turn, shame-fused guilt—offers little opportunity for redemption. Thus it is guilt *with an overlay of shame* that most likely leads to the interminable painful rumination and self-castigation so often described in the clinical literature.

The empirical results are quite consistent with this view. Studies employing adjective-checklist-type (and other globally worded) measures of shame and guilt have found that both shame-prone and guilt-prone styles are associated with psychological symptoms (Harder, 1995; Harder, Cutler, & Rockart, 1992; Harder & Lewis, 1987; Jones & Kugler, 1993; Meehan et al., 1996).

On the other hand, when measures are used that are sensitive to H. B. Lewis's (1971) distinction between shame about the self and guilt about a specific behavior (e.g., scenario-based methods, such as the TOSCA, assessing shame-proneness and guilt-proneness with respect to specific situations), the tendency to experience "shame-free" guilt is essentially unrelated to psychological symptoms. Numerous independent studies converge: guilt-prone children, adolescents, and adults are not at increased risk for depression, anxiety, low self-esteem, and so forth (Burggraf & Tangney, 1990; Gramzow & Tangney, 1992; Tangney, 1994; Tangney, Burggraf, & Wagner, 1995; Tangney & Dearing, 2002; Tangney et al., 1991, 1992).

Deterring Transgression and Socially Undesirable Behavior

Shame may be very painful; it may interfere with other-oriented empathy; it may render us vulnerable to anxiety and depression. But there is the widely held assumption that because shame is so painful, at least it motivates people to avoid "doing wrong," decreasing the likelihood of transgression and impropriety (Barrett, 1995; Ferguson & Stegge, 1995; Kahan, 1997; Zahn-Waxler & Robinson, 1995). As it turns out, there is virtually no direct evidence supporting this presumed adaptive function of shame. To the contrary, research suggests that shame may even make things worse.

In a study of college undergraduates, self-reported moral behaviors (assessed by the Conventional Morality Scale; Tooke & Ickes, 1988) were substantially positively correlated with proneness to guilt but unrelated to proneness to shame (Tangney, 1994). For example, compared with their less guilt-prone peers, guilt-prone individuals were more likely to endorse such items as, "I would not steal something I needed, even if I were sure I could get away with it," "I will not take advantage of other people, even when it's clear that they are trying to take advantage of me," and "Morality and ethics don't really concern me" (reversed). In other words, results from this study suggest that guilt, *but not shame,* motivates people to choose the "moral paths" in life.

The most direct evidence linking moral emotions with moral behavior comes from our ongoing longitudinal family study of moral emotions (see Tagney & Dearing, 2002). In this study, 380 children, their parents, and their grandparents were initially studied when children were in the fifth grade. Children were recruited from public schools in an ethnically and socioeconomically diverse suburb of Washington, D.C. (Sixty percent of the sample is white, 31% black, and 9% other. Most children generally came from low- to moderate-income families. The typical parents had attained a high school education.) The sample was followed up 8 years later. Index children, at that point ages 18–19, participated in an in-depth social and clinical history interview assessing their emotional and behavioral adjustment across all major life domains. Initial analyses of these extensive interviews show that moral emotional style in the fifth grade predicts critical "bottom line" behaviors in young adulthood, including drug and alcohol use, risky sexual behavior, involvement with the criminal justice system (arrests, convictions, incarceration), suicide attempts, high school suspension, and community service involvement.

More specifically, shame-proneness assessed in the fifth grade predicted later high school suspension, drug use of various kinds (amphetamines, depressants, hallucinogens, heroin), and suicide attempts. Relative to their less shame-prone peers, shame-prone children were less likely to apply to college or engage in community service. In contrast, guilt-proneness in the fifth grade was positively associated with later applying to college and doing community service. Guilt-prone fifth-graders were less likely to make suicide attempts, to use heroin, and to drive under the influence, and they began drinking at a later age. Compared with peers who experienced guilt infrequently in fifth grade, these guilt-prone children were, in adolescence, less likely to be arrested, convicted, and incarcerated. Furthermore, they had fewer sexual partners and were more likely to practice "safe sex" and use birth control.

These links between early moral emotional style and subsequent behavioral adjustment held when controlling for family income and mothers' education. Thus this is not simply an SES effect. Equally important, the effects remained even when controlling for children's anger in fifth grade. The robustness with respect to initial levels of anger is especially impressive, given that early indices of anger and aggression are one of the most important predictors of later criminal activity and other behavioral maladjustment (Huesmann, Eron, Lefkowitz, & Walder, 1984). Thus these findings do not simply reflect the fact that badly behaved children are inclined to become badly behaved adults.

Why Do We Have the Capacity to Experience Shame?

The research summarized throughout this chapter underscores the dark side of shame. Empirical findings in five areas illustrate the adaptive functions of guilt, in contrast to the hidden costs of shame, when considering both interpersonal adjustment and psychological well-being. An obvious question, then, is, Why do we have the capacity to experience this emotion? What adaptive purpose does it serve? Is it a moral emotion after all?

Certainly a characterological propensity to experience shame on a daily basis is maladaptive. Common sense tells us that the vast majority of people's quotidian transgressions and errors do not warrant a shameful, global condemnation of the self. It is overkill—rather like sending people to prison for a minor traffic violation. In the case of shame, the self-inflicted punishment often does not fit the crime.

Although a generalized proneness to shame is problematic, it is possible that state-specific feelings of shame can, in certain special circumstances, be useful. No doubt, there *are* occasional instances when individuals are faced with fundamental shortcomings of the self (moral or otherwise) that would best be corrected. The acute pain of shame may, in some cases, motivate productive soul-searching and revisions to one's priorities and values. The challenge, then, is to engage in such introspection and self-repair without becoming sidetracked by defensive reactions (e.g., denial, externalization, and anger) so often provoked by shame. Perhaps non-shame-prone, high "ego-strength" individuals with a solid sense of self may occasionally use

shame constructively in the privacy of their own thoughts. Such adaptive uses of shame may be especially likely in the case of private, self-generated experiences of shame, as opposed to public, other-generated shame episodes. But for most people, the debilitating, ego-threatening nature of shame makes such constructive outcomes difficult, if not impossible.

The more relevant question may not be, What adaptive purpose might shame serve now? but rather, What purpose might it have served at earlier stages of evolution? Shame may represent a relatively primitive emotion that more clearly served adaptive functions in the distant past, among ancestors whose cognitive processes were less sophisticated in the context of a much simpler human society. This notion is consistent with the sociobiological approach, taken by Gilbert (1997), Fessler (1999), and others. Fessler, for example, describes a primitive form of shame—protoshame—as an early mechanism for communicating submission, thus affirming relative rank in the dominance hierarchy of early humans. Similarly, Gilbert has discussed the appeasement functions of shame and humiliation displays, noting continuities across human and nonhuman primates (see also Keltner, 1995; and Leary's [1989; Leary, Landel, & Patton, 1996] analysis of the appeasement functions of blushing and embarrassment). This perspective emphasizes the role of shame (and embarrassment) as a means of communicating one's acknowledgment of wrongdoing, thus diffusing anger and aggression. In a related fashion, the motivation to withdraw—so often a component of the shame experience—may be a useful response, interrupting potentially threatening social interactions until the shamed individual has a chance to regroup or the situation has blown over.

Humankind, however, has evolved not only in terms of physical characteristics but also in terms of emotional and cognitive complexity. With increasingly complex perspective taking and attributional abilities, modern human beings have the capacity to distinguish between oneself and one's behavior, to take another person's perspective, and to empathize with others' distress. Whereas early moral goals centered on reducing potentially lethal aggression, clarifying social rank, and enhancing conformity to social norms, modern morality centers on the ability to acknowledge one's wrongdoing, accept responsibility, and take reparative action. In this sense, guilt may be the more modern, adaptive moral emotion.

Embarrassment and Pride: Other Self-Conscious Emotions of Self-Regulation

Early in this chapter, I suggested that self-conscious emotions are, by their very nature, emotions of self-regulation. As the self reflects on the self, feelings of shame, guilt, embarrassment, and pride serve as an emotional moral barometer, providing immediate feedback on the social and moral acceptability of our thoughts, feelings, behaviors, and core selves. Thus far, I've focused exclusively on the moral, self-regulatory functions of shame and guilt—the two self-conscious emotions that have received the most empirical attention to date and about which I know the most. Although a comprehensive analysis of the self-regulatory functions of embarrassment and pride are beyond the scope of this chapter, some initial observations can be offered.

Embarrassment may have less direct implications for morality than do shame and guilt. But it is clearly an important component of our self-regulatory apparatus. Miller (1995a) defines embarrassment as "an aversive state of mortification, abashment, and chagrin that follows public social predicaments" (p. 322). Analyzing personal accounts of embarrassment from hundreds of high school students and adults, Miller (1992) found that the most common causes of embarrassment were "normative public deficiencies"—situations in which the individual behaved in a clumsy, absentminded, or hapless way (tripping in front of a large class, forgetting someone's name, unintended bodily induced noises). Other common types of embarrassing situations included awkward social interactions and just being conspicuous.

Some theorists believe that the crux of embarrassment is negative evaluation by others (Edelmann, 1981; Miller, 1996; Miller & Leary, 1992; Semin & Manstead, 1981) or transient drops in self-esteem secondary to negative evaluation by others (Modigliani, 1968). Other theorists subscribe to the "dramaturgic" account of embarrassment (Goffman, 1956; Gross & Stone, 1964; Silver, Sabini, & Parrott, 1987), surmising that embarrassment occurs when implicit social roles and scripts are disrupted. But in any event, these events signal that something is amiss—some aspect of the self or one's behavior needs to be carefully monitored, hidden, or changed. Not surprisingly, empirical research shows that when embarrassed, people are inclined to behave in conciliatory ways designed to win approval and (re)inclusion from others (Cupach & Metts, 1990, 1992; Leary, Landel, & Patton, 1996; R. S. Miller, 1996, personal communication, January 19, 2002; Sharkey & Stafford, 1990).

Embarrassment apparently is less centrally relevant to the regulation of behavior in the moral domain. Whereas embarrassment often ensues in response to normative social faux pas and transgressions (a forgotten name, an open fly, a flubbed performance), shame is more likely the response to serious failures and moral transgressions that reflect badly on global and enduring attributes of the self. Consistent with this view, a comparison of adults' ratings of personal shame and embarrassment experiences indicated that shame is a more intense, painful emotion that involves a greater sense of moral transgression (Tangney, Miller, et al., 1996).

As with shame and guilt, there are individual differences in the degree to which people are prone to experience embarrassment. Research has shown that embarrassability is associated with neuroticism, high levels of negative affect, self-consciousness, and a fear of negative evaluation from others (Edelmann & McCusker, 1986; Leary & Meadows, 1991; Miller, 1995b). Miller's (1996) research indicates that this fear of negative evaluation is not due to poor social skills but rather to a sensitivity to social norms. Importantly with regard to self-regulation, people who are prone to embarrassment tend to be highly aware of and concerned with social rules and standards. Consistent with the notion that embarrassment serves a self-regulatory function, Keltner, Moffitt, and Stouthamer-Loeber (1995) found that aggressive and delinquent boys showed less embarrassment on a cognitive task than well-adjusted boys.

Of the self-conscious emotions, pride is the neglected sibling, having received the least attention by far. Mascolo and Fischer (1995) define pride as an emotion "generated by appraisals that one is responsible for a socially valued outcome or for being a socially valued person" (p. 66). From their perspective, pride serves to enhance people's self-worth and, perhaps more important, to encourage future behavior that conforms to social standards of worth or merit (see also Barrett, 1995).

Paralleling the self-versus-behavior distinction of guilt and shame, it may be useful to distinguish between two types of pride— what I term "alpha" pride (pride in self) and "beta" pride (pride in behavior). Along similar lines, M. Lewis (1992) has distinguished between pride and hubris. According to Lewis, pride is experienced when one's success is attributed to a specific action or behavior. Hubris (pridefulness) arises when success is attributed to the global self. Most of his discussions appear to focus on hubris as a trait (tendencies to experience hubris frequently across multiple situations) rather than as a state (e.g., momentary feelings of pride in self). Lewis views hubris as largely maladaptive, noting that hubristic individuals are inclined to distort and invent situations to enhance the self, which can lead to interpersonal problems.

Little empirical research has been conducted to examine individual differences in proneness to pride in self (or pride in behavior, for that matter). The TOSCA (e.g., Tangney et al., 1989) and its forerunners, the Self-Conscious Affect and Attribution Inventories (SCAAI; e.g., Tangney, Burggraf, Hamme, & Domingos, 1988; see Tangney & Dearing, 2002, for details), each contain measures of the propensity to experience alpha pride and beta pride, respectively. These scales, however, have very modest reliabilities, owing to the fact that they draw on a rather small subset of SCAAI and TOSCA scenarios. Thus we and other investigators have made little use of these ancillary scales. It remains to be seen how individual differences in pride or hubris relate to the capacity to self-regulate

or to choose the moral path in life. One possibility is that pride and hubris represent the flip side of guilt and shame—one the "modern," adaptive moral emotion and the other its "evil twin."

Directions for Future Research

In this chapter, I've summarized current theory and research on the self-conscious emotions, emphasizing their moral, self-regulatory functions. The self-conscious emotions—shame, guilt, embarrassment, and pride—are an important, but long neglected, component of morally relevant processes that guide moral decisions and moral behavior. In recent years, a profusion of research has emerged on the negative self-conscious emotions—shame, guilt, and embarrassment. But in a very real sense, we have only scratched the surface, and much work remains.

Here I mention just a few of the promising directions for future research. The first concerns the dynamics involved in people's attempts to use self-conscious emotions (particularly shame, guilt, and embarrassment) as a form of interpersonal control. Sharkey (1991, 1992, 1993) has made important inroads in our understanding of "intentional embarrassment"—efforts to intentionally cause feelings of embarrassment in others. Based on data from more than 1,000 adult respondents, Sharkey concluded that fully half of people's efforts to induce embarrassment are motivated by benign, friendly intentions—as a sign of affection. To date, only a handful of studies have explicitly examined the phenomena of guilt induction (Baumeister, Stillwell, & Heatherton, 1995a; Tangney & Yerington, 1998; Vangelisti, Daly, & Rudnick, 1991). These initial studies indicate that conscious attempts to induce guilt occur relatively frequently, particularly in the context of close relationships, and especially in response to real or perceived periods of neglect. But other questions remain. For example, do people use different methods to induce shame versus guilt versus embarrassment, and with what results? What are the relative costs and benefits of inducing shame, guilt, and embarrassment? How do those costs and benefits vary as a function of transgression, type of relationship, and personality characteristics of the inductee? Are some people more vulnerable than others to guilt (or shame or embarrassment) inductions?

A related phenomenon of interest is the vicarious experience of self-conscious emotions—people's experience of shame, guilt, embarrassment, or pride owing to the actions of *other* individuals. Although some research has examined the causes and consequences of "empathic" or vicarious embarrassment (Miller, 1996), empirical work on shame, guilt, and pride has focused almost exclusively on reaction to one's *own* misdeeds or accomplishments. Virtually no research has examined feelings of shame and guilt in response to others' transgressions and failures. Recently, Schmader, Lickel, and Ames (2002) have embarked on an exciting series of studies to examine the antecedents and motivational and behavioral consequences of vicarious shame and guilt experiences. Perhaps more than other emotions, the assessment of self-conscious emotions poses some real challenges—not least because these emotions are not marked by unique, clearly definable facial expressions. Although quite a number of measurement methods have been developed in recent years, the coming decade will no doubt see improvements in our ability to capture these self-conscious emotions. Two especially promising developments concern the assessment of *state* shame and guilt (feelings of shame and guilt "in the moment") and the propensity to experience shame and guilt in specific domains. Recently, Turner (1998) developed the Experiential Shame Scale (ESS), an inventive measure of state shame explicitly intended to circumvent the inevitable defensive biases inherent in experiencing shame. Recognizing that people are often unable or reluctant to directly acknowledge feelings of shame, Turner attempted to develop a more "opaque" measure of state shame, purposely reducing the "face validity" of her measure. The ESS is composed of 10 bipolar items tapping physical (e.g., "Physically, I feel: 1, *pale,* to 7, *flushed*"), emotional (e.g., "Emotionally, I feel: 1, *content,* to 7, *distressed*), and social/interpersonal (e.g., "Socially, I feel like: 1, *hiding,* to 7, *being sociable* [reversed]) dimensions of the shame experience. Initial

data on the reliability and validity of the ESS are encouraging (Turner, 1998), opening the door to more precise examinations of the implications of shame "in the moment," in specific, observable contexts. Regarding domain-specific self-conscious emotions, Andrews (1998) has underscored the long-ignored distinction between generalized proneness to shame and proneness to shame in specific domains. Virtually all of the extant literature on shame-prone dispositions focuses exclusively on generalized shame-proneness—that is, people's propensity to experience shame across a wide variety of frequently experienced situations. Andrews incisively observes that, in addition to a generalized tendency to experience shame, people differ in their propensity to experience shame in specific domains—emotional "hot spots," as it were (e.g., eating, sexual abuse, etc.). This distinction (and the corresponding shift in measurement strategy) ushers in important new avenues for theory and research, in areas that are especially likely to have clear and immediate implications for clinical intervention.

As emphasized several times in this chapter, pride is a topic wide open for empirical inquiry. In particular, very little work has addressed individual differences in the tendency to take pride in one's self or one's accomplishments. What are the implications of such individual differences for achievement motivation and behavior as people negotiate the challenges of education and career, as well as the moral dilemmas of daily life? Is the proposed distinction between global and specific pride empirically useful? The next decade will surely see exciting advances in our understanding of this long-neglected, but very important, self-conscious emotion.

Finally, there is a rich universe of questions—virtually untapped—concerning culture and the self-conscious emotions. Researchers have just begun to examine how the nature, functions, and psychosocial implications of self-conscious emotions might vary across cultural groups (Bierbrauer, 1992; Chiang & Barrett, 1989; Johnson et al., 1987; Kitayama, Markus, & Matsumoto, 1995; Lebra, 1973; Shaver, Schwartz, Kirson, & O'Connor, 1987; Wallbott & Scherer, 1988, 1995). Kitayama and colleagues (1995) make the compelling argument that because there are cultural variations in the construction of the *self* (e.g., independent vs. interdependent selves; cf. Markus & Kitayama, 1991), *self*-conscious emotions may show especially marked variations across cultural contexts.

Cross-cultural questions about the self-conscious emotions can be asked at several levels. Do people from different cultures vary in their propensity to experience shame, guilt, embarrassment, behavioral pride, or self-pride? Are there cultural differences in the *quality* of these emotions? In their valence or intensity? Or in the kinds of situations that give rise to them? Regarding individual differences within each cultural group, are there cultural differences in the types of parenting styles or other early experiences that foster the propensity to experience shame, guilt, embarrassment, or pride? And are there cultural differences in the implications of those individual differences? Is proneness to shame less maladaptive, a more effective self-regulatory mechanism, in interdependent cultures? These are just a sampling of the kinds of questions about self-conscious emotions and culture that can be examined—and they no doubt will substantially influence the shape of our field to come.

Note

1. The experiment was immediately followed by extensive "process" debriefing procedures, conducted by carefully trained, closely supervised senior research assistants.

References

Allan, S., Gilbert, P., & Goss, K. (1994). An exploration of shame measures: 2. Psychopathology. *Personality and Individual Differences, 17,* 719–722.

Andrews, B. (1998). Shame and childhood abuse. In P. Gilbert & B. Andrews (Eds.), *Shame: Interpersonal behavior, psychopathology, and culture* (pp. 176–190). New York: Oxford University Press.

Arnold, M. L. (1989, April). *Moral cognition and conduct: A qualitative review of the literature.* Poster presented at the meeting of the Society for Research in Child Development, Kansas City, MO.

Barrett, K. C. (1995). A functionalist approach to shame and guilt. In J. P. Tangney & K. W. Fischer (Eds.), *Self-conscious emotions: The psychology of shame, guilt, embarrassment, and pride* (pp. 25–63). New York: Guilford Press.

Baumeister, R. F., Stillwell, A. M., & Heatherton, T. F. (1994). Guilt: An interpersonal approach. *Psychological Bulletin, 115,* 243–267.

Baumeister, R. F., Stillwell, A. M., & Heatherton, T. F. (1995a). Interpersonal aspects of guilt: Evidence from narrative studies. In J. P. Tangney & K. W. Fischer (Eds.), *Self-conscious emotions: The psychology of shame, guilt, embarrassment, and pride* (pp. 255–273). New York: Guilford Press.

Baumeister, R. F., Stillwell, A. M., & Heatherton, T. F. (1995b). Personal narratives about guilt: Role in action control and interpersonal relationships. *Basic and Applied Social Psychology, 17,* 173–198.

Benedict, R. (1946). *The chrysanthemum and the sword.* Boston: Houghton Mifflin.

Bierbrauer, G. (1992). Reactions to violation of normative standards: A cross-cultural analysis of shame and guilt. *International Journal of Psychology, 27,* 181–193.

Blasi, A. (1980). Bridging moral cognition and moral action: A critical review of the literature. *Psychological Bulletin, 88,* 1–45.

Blatt, S. (1974). Levels of object representation in anaclitic and introjective depression. *Psychoanalytic Study of the Child, 29,* 107–157.

Blatt, S. J., D'Afflitti, J. P., & Quinlin, D. M. (1976). Experiences of depression in normal young adults. *Journal of Abnormal Psychology, 86,* 203–223.

Brodie, P. (1995). *How sociopaths love: Sociopathy and interpersonal relationships.* Unpublished doctoral dissertation, George Mason University, Fairfax, VA.

Burggraf, S. A., & Tangney, J. P. (1990, June). *Shame-proneness, guilt-proneness, and attributional style related to children's depression.* Poster presented at the meeting of the American Psychological Society, Dallas, TX.

Bush, M. (1989). The role of unconscious guilt in psychopathology and psychotherapy. *Bulletin of the Menninger Clinic, 53,* 97–107.

Chiang, T., & Barrett, K. C. (1989, April). *A cross-cultural comparison of toddlers' reactions to the infraction of a standard: A guilt culture vs. a shame culture.* Paper presented at the meeting of the Society for Research in Child Development, Kansas City, MO.

Cook, D. R. (1988, August). *The measurement of shame: The Internalized Shame Scale.* Paper presented at the annual meeting of the American Psychological Association, Atlanta, GA.

Cook, D. R. (1991). Shame, attachment, and addictions: Implications for family therapists. *Contemporary Family Therapy, 13,* 405–419.

Cupach, W. R., & Metts, S. (1990). Remedial processes in embarrassing predicaments. In J. Anderson (Ed.), *Communication yearbook* (Vol. 13, pp. 323–352). Newbury Park, CA: Sage.

Cupach, W. R., & Metts, S. (1992). The effects of type of predicament and embarrassability on remedial responses to embarrassing situations. *Communications Quarterly, 40,* 149–161.

Edelmann, R. J. (1981). Embarrassment: The state of research. *Current Psychological Reviews, 1,* 125–138.

Edelmann, R. J., & McCusker, G. (1986). Introversion, neuroticism, empathy, and embarrassability. *Personality and Individual Differences, 7,* 133–140.

Eisenberg, N. (1986). *Altruistic cognition, emotion, and behavior.* Hillsdale, NJ: Erlbaum.

Eisenberg, N., & Miller, P. A. (1987). Empathy, sympathy, and altruism: Empirical and conceptual links. In N. Eisenberg & J. Strayer (Eds.), *Empathy and its development* (pp. 292–316). New York: Cambridge University Press.

Ellis, A. (1962). *Reason and emotion in psychotherapy.* New York: Stuart.

Ferguson, T. J., & Stegge, H. (1995). Emotional states and traits in children: The case of guilt and shame. In J. P. Tangney & K. W. Fischer (Eds.), *Self-conscious emotions: The psychology of shame, guilt, embarrassment, and pride* (pp. 174–197). New York: Guilford Press.

Ferguson, T. J., Stegge, H., & Damhuis, I. (1991). Children's understanding of guilt and shame. *Child Development, 62,* 827–839.

Feshbach, N. D. (1978). Studies of empathic behavior in children. In B. A. Maher (Ed.), *Progress in experimental personality research* (Vol. 8, pp. 1–47). New York: Academic Press.

Feshbach, N. D. (1984). Empathy, empathy training, and the regulation of aggression in elementary school children. In R. M. Kaplan, V. J. Konenci, & R. Novoco (Eds.), *Aggression in children and youth* (pp. 198–208). The Hague, Netherlands: Nijhoff.

Feshbach, N. D. (1987). Parental empathy and child adjustment/maladjustment. In N. Eisenberg & J. Strayer (Eds.), *Empathy and its development* (pp. 271–291). New York: Cambridge University Press.

Feshbach, N. D., & Feshbach, S. (1969). The relationship between empathy and aggression in two age groups. *Developmental Psychology, 1,* 102–107.

Feshbach, N. D., & Feshbach, S. (1982). Empathy training and the regulation of aggression: Potentialities and limitations. *Academic Psychology Bulletin, 4,* 399–413.

Feshbach, N. D., & Feshbach, S. (1986). Aggression and altruism: A personality perspective. In C. Zahn-Waxler, E. M. Cummings, & R. Iannotti (Eds.), *Altruism and aggression: Biological and social origins* (pp. 189–217). Cambridge, UK: Cambridge University Press.

Fessler, D. M. T. (1999). Toward an understanding of the universality of second order emotions. In A. L. Hinton (Ed.), *Biocultural approaches to the emotions* (pp. 75–116). New York: Cambridge University Press.

Freud, S. (1955). Notes upon a case of obsessional neurosis. In J. Strachey (Ed. & Trans.), *The standard edition of the complete psychological works of Sigmund Freud* (Vol. 10, pp. 155–318). London: Hogarth Press. (Original work published 1909)

Freud, S. (1957). Mourning and melancholia. In J. Strachey (Ed. & Trans.), *The standard edition of the complete psychological works of Sigmund Freud* (Vol. 14, pp. 243–258). London: Hogarth Press. (Original work published 1917)

Freud, S. (1961a). The dissolution of the Oedipus Complex. In J. Strachey (Ed. & Trans.), *The standard edition of the complete psychological works of Sigmund Freud* (Vol. 19, pp. 173–182). London: Hogarth Press. (Original work published 1924)

Freud, S. (1961b). The economic problem of masochism. In J. Strachey (Ed. & Trans.), *The standard edition of the complete psychological works of Sigmund Freud* (Vol. 19, pp. 159–170). London: Hogarth Press. (Original work published 1924)

Freud, S. (1961c). The ego and the id. In J. Strachey (Ed. &

Trans.), *The standard edition of the complete psychological works of Sigmund Freud* (Vol. 19, pp. 1–66). London: Hogarth Press. (Original work published 1923)

Gilbert, P. (1997). The evolution of social attractiveness and its role in shame, humiliation, guilt, and therapy. *British Journal of Medical Psychology, 70,* 113–147.

Goffman, E. (1956). Embarrassment and social organization. *American Journal of Sociology, 62,* 264–271.

Gramzow, R., & Tangney, J. P. (1992). Proneness to shame and the narcissistic personality. *Personality and Social Psychology Bulletin, 18,* 369–376.

Gross, E., & Stone, G. P. (1964). Embarrassment and the analysis of role requirements. *American Journal of Sociology, 70,* 1–15.

Harder, D. W. (1995). Shame and guilt assessment, and relationships of shame- and guilt-proneness to psychopathology. In J. P. Tangney & K. W. Fischer (Eds.), *Self-conscious emotions: The psychology of shame, guilt, embarrassment, and pride* (pp. 368–392). New York: Guilford Press.

Harder, D. W., Cutler, L., & Rockart, L. (1992). Assessment of shame and guilt and their relationship to psychopathology. *Journal of Personality Assessment, 59,* 584–604.

Harder, D. W., & Lewis, S. J. (1987). The assessment of shame and guilt. In J. N. Butcher & C. D. Spielberger (Eds.), *Advances in personality assessment* (Vol. 6, pp. 89–114). Hillsdale, NJ: Erlbaum.

Hartmann, E., & Loewenstein, R. (1962). Notes on the superego. *Psychoanalytic Study of the Child, 17,* 42–81.

Hoblitzelle, W. (1987). Attempts to measure and differentiate shame and guilt: The relation between shame and depression. In H. B. Lewis (Ed.), *The role of shame in symptom formation* (pp. 207–235). Hillsdale, NJ: Erlbaum.

Hoffman, M. L. (1982). Development of prosocial motivation: Empathy and guilt. In N. Eisenberg-Berg (Ed.), *Development of prosocial behavior* (pp. 281–313). New York: Academic Press.

Huesmann, L. R., Eron, L. D., Lefkowitz, M. M., & Walder, L. O. (1984). Stability of aggression over time and generations. *Developmental Psychology, 20,* 1120–1134.

Johnson, R. C., Danko, G. P., Huang, Y. H., Park, J. Y., Johnson, S. B., & Nagoshi, C. T. (1987). Guilt, shame and adjustment in three cultures. *Personality and Individual Differences, 8,* 357–364.

Jones, W. H., & Kugler, K. (1993). Interpersonal correlates of the Guilt Inventory. *Journal of Personality Assessment, 61,* 246–258.

Kahan, D. M. (1997). Ignorance of law is an excuse—But only for the virtuous. *Michigan Law Review, 96,* 127–154.

Keltner, D. (1995). Signs of appeasement: Evidence for the distinct displays of embarrassment, amusement, and shame. *Journal of Personality and Social Psychology, 68,* 441–454.

Keltner, D., & Buswell, B. N. (1996). Evidence for the distinctness of embarrassment, shame, and guilt: A study of recalled antecedents and facial expressions of emotion. *Cognition and Emotion, 10,* 155–171.

Keltner, D., Moffitt, T., & Stouthamer-Loeber, M. (1995). Facial expressions of emotion and psychopathology in adolescent boys. *Journal of Abnormal Psychology, 104,* 644–652.

Kitayama, S., Markus, H. R., & Matsumoto, H. (1995). Culture, self, and emotion: A cultural perspective on "self-conscious" emotion. In J. P. Tangney & K. W. Fischer (Eds.), *Self-conscious emotions: The psychology of shame, guilt, embarrassment, and pride* (pp. 439–464). New York: Guilford Press.

Kohlberg, L. (1969). Stage and sequence: The cognitive developmental approach to socialization. In D. A. Goslin (Ed.), *Handbook of socialization theory and research* (pp. 347–480). Chicago: Rand McNally.

Lazarus, R. S. (1966). *Psychological stress and the coping process.* New York: McGraw-Hill.

Leary, M. R. (1989, August). Fear of exclusion and appeasement behaviors: The case of blushing. In R. F. Baumeister (Chair), *The need to belong.* Symposium conducted at the meeting of the American Psychological Association, New Orleans, LA.

Leary, M. R., Landel, J. L., & Patton, K. M. (1996). The motivated expression of embarrassment following a self-presentational predicament. *Journal of Personality, 64,* 619–637.

Leary, M. R., & Meadows, S. (1991). Predictors, elicitors, and concomitants of social blushing. *Journal of Personality and Social Psychology, 60,* 254–262.

Lebra, T. S. (1973). The social mechanism of guilt and shame: The Japanese case. *Anthropological Quarterly, 44,* 241–255.

Leith, K. P., & Baumeister, R. F. (1998). Empathy, shame, guilt, and narratives of interpersonal conflicts: Guilt-prone people are better at perspective taking. *Journal of Personality, 66,* 1–37.

Lewis, H. B. (1971). *Shame and guilt in neurosis.* New York: International Universities Press.

Lewis, M. (1992). *Shame: The exposed self.* New York: Free Press.

Lindsay-Hartz, J. (1984). Contrasting experiences of shame and guilt. *American Behavioral Scientist, 27,* 689–704.

Markus, H. R., & Kitayama, S. (1991). Culture and the self: Implications for cognition, emotion, and motivation. *Psychological Review, 98,* 224–253.

Marschall, D. E. (1996). *Effects of induced shame on subsequent empathy and altruistic behavior.* Unpublished master's thesis, George Mason University, Fairfax, VA.

Mascolo, M. F., & Fischer, K. W. (1995). Developmental transformations in appraisals of pride, shame, and guilt. In J. P. Tangney & K. W. Fischer (Eds.), *Self-conscious emotions: The psychology of shame, guilt, embarrassment, and pride* (pp. 64–113). New York: Guilford Press.

Meehan, M. A., O'Connor, L. E., Berry, J. W., Weiss, J., Morrison, A., & Acampora, A. (1996). Guilt, shame, and depression in clients in recovery from addiction. *Journal of Psychoactive Drugs, 28,* 125–134.

Miller, R. S. (1992). The nature and severity of self-reported embarrassing circumstances. *Personality and Social Psychology Bulletin, 18,* 190–198.

Miller, R. S. (1995a). Embarrassment and social behavior. In J. P. Tangney & K. W. Fischer (Eds.), *Self-conscious emotions: The psychology of shame, guilt, embarrassment, and pride* (pp. 322–339). New York: Guilford Press.

Miller, R. S. (1995b). On the nature of embarrassability: Shyness, social-evaluation, and social skill. *Journal of Personality, 63,* 315–339.

Miller, R. S. (1996). *Embarrassment: Poise and peril in everyday life.* New York: Guilford Press.

Miller, R. S., & Leary, M. R. (1992). Social sources and interactive functions of emotion: The case of embarrassment. In M. Clark (Ed.), *Review of personality and social psychology* (Vol. 14, pp. 202–221). Newbury Park, CA: Sage.

Modigliani, A. (1968). Embarrassment and embarrassability. *Sociometry, 31,* 313–326.

Piaget, J. (1952). *The origins of intelligence in children.* New York: International Universities Press.

Piers, G., & Singer, A. (1953). *Shame and guilt.* Springfield, IL: Thomas

Rodin, J., Silberstein, L., & Striegel-Moore, R. (1985). Women and weight: A normative discontent. In T. B. Sondregger (Ed.), *Nebraska Symposium on Motivation: Vol. 32. Psychology and gender* (pp. 267–307). Lincoln: University of Nebraska Press.

Sanftner, J. L., Barlow, D. H., Marschall, D. E., & Tangney, J. P. (1995). The relation of shame and guilt to eating disorders symptomatology. *Journal of Social and Clinical Psychology, 14,* 315–324.

Scheff, T. J. (1987). The shame–rage spiral: A case study of an interminable quarrel. In H. B. Lewis (Ed.), *The role of shame in symptom formation* (pp. 109–149). Hillsdale, NJ: Erlbaum.

Schmader, T., Lickel, B., & Ames, D. R. (2002). *Vicarious shame and guilt.* Unpublished manuscript.

Semin, G. R., & Manstead, A. S. R. (1981). The beholder beheld: A study of social emotionality. *European Journal of Social Psychology, 11,* 253–265.

Sharkey, W. F. (1991). Intentional embarrassment: Goals, tactics, and consequences. In W. R. Cupach & S. Metts (Eds.), *Advances in interpersonal communication research—1991* (pp. 105–128). Normal, IL: Personal Relationships Interest Group.

Sharkey, W. F. (1992). Uses of and responses to intentional embarrassment. *Communication Studies, 43,* 257–275.

Sharkey, W. F. (1993). Who embarrasses whom? Relational and sex differences in the use of intentional embarrassment. In P. J. Kalbfleisch (Ed.), *Interpersonal communication: Evolving interpersonal relationships* (pp. 147–168). Hillsdale, NJ: Erlbaum.

Sharkey, W. F., & Stafford, L. (1990). Responses to embarrassment. *Human Communication Research, 17,* 315–342.

Shaver, P., Schwartz, J., Kirson, D., & O'Connor, C. (1987). Emotional knowledge: Further exploration of a prototype approach. *Journal of Personality and Social Psychology, 52,* 1061–1086.

Silver, M., Sabini, J., & Parrott, W. G. (1987). Embarrassment: A dramaturgic account. *Journal for the Theory of Social Behaviour, 17,* 47–61.

Tangney, J. P. (1989, August). *A quantitative assessment of phenomenological differences between shame and guilt.* Poster session presented at the meeting of the American Psychological Association, New Orleans, LA.

Tangney, J. P. (1991). Moral affect: The good, the bad, and the ugly. *Journal of Personality and Social Psychology, 61,* 598–607.

Tangney, J. P. (1992). Situational determinants of shame and guilt in young adulthood. *Personality and Social Psychology Bulletin, 18,* 199–206.

Tangney, J. P. (1993). Shame and guilt. In C. G. Costello

(Ed.), *Symptoms of depression* (pp. 161–180). New York: Wiley.

Tangney, J. P. (1994). The mixed legacy of the super-ego: Adaptive and maladaptive aspects of shame and guilt. In J. M. Masling & R. F. Bornstein (Eds.), *Empirical perspectives on object relations theory* (pp. 1–28). Washington, DC: American Psychological Association.

Tangney, J. P. (1995a). Recent advances in the empirical study of shame and guilt. *American Behavioral Scientist, 38,* 1132–1145.

Tangney, J. P. (1995b). Shame and guilt in interpersonal relationships. In J. P. Tangney & K. W. Fischer (Eds.), *Self-conscious emotions: The psychology of shame, guilt, embarrassment, and pride* (pp. 114–139). New York: Guilford Press.

Tangney, J. P. (1996). Conceptual and methodological issues in the assessment of shame and guilt. *Behaviour Research and Therapy, 34,* 741–754.

Tangney, J. P., Burggraf, S. A., Hamme, H., & Domingos, B. (1988). *The Self-Conscious Affect and Attribution Inventory (SCAAI).* Bryn Mawr, PA: Bryn Mawr College.

Tangney, J. P., Burggraf, S. A., & Wagner, P. E. (1995). Shame-proneness, guilt-proneness, and psychological symptoms. In J. P. Tangney & K. W. Fischer (Eds.), *Self-conscious emotions: The psychology of shame, guilt, embarrassment, and pride* (pp. 343–367). New York: Guilford Press.

Tangney, J. P., & Dearing, R. L. (2002). *Shame and guilt.* New York: Guilford Press.

Tangney, J. P., Marschall, D. E., Rosenberg, K., Barlow, D. H., & Wagner, P. E. (1994). *Children's and adults' autobiographical accounts of shame, guilt and pride experiences: An analysis of situational determinants and interpersonal concerns.* Unpublished manuscript.

Tangney, J. P., Miller, R. S., Flicker, L., & Barlow, D. H. (1996). Are shame, guilt and embarrassment distinct emotions? *Journal of Personality and Social Psychology, 70,* 1256–1269.

Tangney, J. P., Wagner, P. E., Barlow, D. H., Marschall, D. E., & Gramzow, R. (1996). The relation of shame and guilt to constructive vs. destructive responses to anger across the lifespan. *Journal of Personality and Social Psychology, 70,* 797–809.

Tangney, J. P., Wagner, P. E., Burggraf, S. A., Gramzow, R., & Fletcher, C. (1991, June). *Children's shame-proneness, but not guilt-proneness, is related to emotional and behavioral maladjustment.* Poster session presented at the meeting of the American Psychological Society, Washington, DC.

Tangney, J. P., Wagner, P. E., Fletcher, C., & Gramzow, R. (1992). Shamed into anger? The relation of shame and

guilt to anger and self-reported aggression. *Journal of Personality and Social Psychology, 62,* 669–675.

Tangney, J. P., Wagner, P., & Gramzow, R. (1989). *The Test of Self-Conscious Affect (TOSCA).* Fairfax, VA: George Mason University.

Tangney, J. P., Wagner, P. E., & Gramzow, R. (1992). Proneness to shame, proneness to guilt, and psychopathology. *Journal of Abnormal Psychology, 103,* 469–478.

Tangney, J. P., & Yerington, T. (1998, August). Shaming and guilt-tripping in everyday life: Motivations, methods, and consequences. In R. F. Baumeister (Chair), *Guilt and shame as interpersonal communications and regulators.* Symposium conducted at the meeting of the American Psychological Association, San Francisco.

Tooke, W. S., & Ickes, W. (1988). A measure of adherence to conventional morality. *Journal of Social and Clinical Psychology, 6,* 310–334.

Turner, J. E. (1998). *An investigation of shame reactions, motivation, and achievement in a difficult college course.* Unpublished doctoral dissertation, University of Texas, Austin.

Vangelisti, A. L., Daly, J. A., & Rudnick, J. R. (1991). Making people feel guilty in conversations: Techniques and correlates. *Human Communication Research, 18,* 3–39.

Wallbott, H. G., & Scherer, K. R. (1988). How universal and specific is emotional experience? Evidence from 27 countries and five continents. In K. R. Scherer (Ed.), *Facets of emotion: Recent research* (pp. 31–56). Hillsdale, NJ: Erlbaum.

Wallbott, H. G., & Scherer, K. R. (1995). Cultural determinants in experiencing shame and guilt. In J. P. Tangney & K. W. Fischer (Eds.), *Self-conscious emotions: The psychology of shame, guilt, embarrassment, and pride* (pp. 465–487). New York: Guilford Press.

Weiner, B. (1985). An attributional theory of achievement motivation and emotion. *Psychological Review, 92,* 548–573.

Weiss, J. (1993). *How psychotherapy works: Process and technique.* New York: Guilford Press.

Wicker, F. W., Payne, G. C., & Morgan, R. D. (1983). Participant descriptions of guilt and shame. *Motivation and Emotion, 7,* 25–39.

Zahn-Waxler, C., Kochanska, G., Krupnick, J., & McKnew, D. (1990). Patterns of guilt in children of depressed and well mothers. *Developmental Psychology, 26,* 51–59.

Zahn-Waxler, C., & Robinson, J. (1995). Empathy and guilt: Early origins of feelings of responsibility. In J. P. Tangney & K. W. Fischer (Eds.), *Self-conscious emotions: The psychology of shame, guilt, embarrassment, and pride* (pp. 143–173). New York: Guilford Press.

20

Individual Differences in Self-Esteem: A Review and Theoretical Integration

MARK R. LEARY
GEOFF MacDONALD

Trait self-esteem ranks among the most widely investigated yet least understood constructs in behavioral science. Despite the fact that thousands of studies have examined individual differences in self-esteem, the area has lacked an overriding theoretical framework that parsimoniously accounts for the relationships between self-esteem and other psychological constructs and explains why self-esteem seems to be such an important psychological entity. As a result, the literature on trait self-esteem resembles an indexed catalogue of empirical findings rather than an integrated body of research. Our goal in this chapter is to review what is known about trait self-esteem, using the framework provided by sociometer theory. To begin, we will clarify what we mean by "trait self-esteem," then provide a brief overview of sociometer theory. After describing how the theory explains the empirical correlates of self-esteem, we review six areas in which interest in trait self-esteem has been particularly intense: emotions, interpersonal behavior, relationships, person-

ality, maladaptive behavior and psychopathology, and self-esteem development.

The Concept and Measurement of Trait Self-Esteem

Self-esteem is an affectively laden self-evaluation. It is, at heart, how a person feels about him- or herself. Just as people have positive or negative feelings about other people and inanimate objects, they also have valenced feelings about themselves. *State self-esteem* refers to how a person feels about him- or herself at a particular moment in time, whereas *trait self-esteem* refers to how a person generally or most typically feels about him- or herself.

Most researchers have been interested in global trait self-esteem—how people feel about themselves overall. However, people may have different levels of self-esteem with respect to particular dimensions or domains, such as their intellect, physical appearance, social skill, and athletic ability.

Two individuals with the same level of global trait self-esteem may differ greatly in how they feel about themselves with respect to particular attributes. Although domain-specific self-esteem is important in some contexts, for reasons that will become clear as we proceed, global self-esteem can tell us things about a person that domain-specific self-esteem cannot.

Many measures of trait self-esteem have been developed, but most researchers have relied on only a few. (See Blascovich and Tomaka's, 1991, excellent review for detailed descriptions of the most commonly used measures.) By far, the most frequently used measure has been Rosenberg's (1965) Self-Esteem Inventory. Indeed, Rosenberg's publication of his scale seems to have stimulated the rapid growth of research on trait self-esteem in the late 1960s. Earlier, Janis and Field (1959) had developed a Feelings of Inadequacy Scale that received relatively little attention until it was revised by Fleming and Courtney (1984). Fleming and Courtney's 33-item scale contains both a measure of global trait self-esteem (which they called "general self-regard") that correlates in excess of .90 with Rosenberg's scale and subscales that measure self-esteem pertaining to social confidence, school abilities, physical appearance, and physical ability. To measure self-esteem in children, researchers have traditionally used Coopersmith's (1967) Self-Esteem Inventory, but the Piers–Harris Children's Self-Concept Scale (Piers, 1984) and the Self-Perception Profile for Children (Harter, 1985) have been increasingly used in recent years.

In general, scores on various measures of trait self-esteem correlate very highly with one another and, aside from assuring that the items are age-appropriate, the choice of which scale to use is generally not consequential. However, inspection of the item content of the commonly used scales shows that they all tend to assess primarily beliefs about one's ability, efficacy, popularity, and worth and only secondarily (if at all) the affective reactions that are central to the conceptualization of self-esteem. Of course, believing that one possesses socially valued characteristics is typically associated with positive self-feelings, and vice versa, so it may not matter that self-evaluative feelings are rarely assessed directly. Even so, some such measures run the risk of confounding the assessment of self-esteem with the measurement of people's self-concepts, self-efficacy, or self-confidence, all of which deal with people's beliefs about themselves or about their ability to produce certain outcomes.

Trait Self-Esteem as an Index of Relational Evaluation

The thousands of studies that have included measures of trait self-esteem have revealed that self-esteem relates to a wide array of cognitive, emotional, and behavioral phenomena. As we explore in detail, compared with people who score low on measures of trait self-esteem, people who score higher tend to be happier and less depressed, to have more friends, to be more satisfied with their interpersonal relationships, to worry less about being rejected, to conform less, to work harder on difficult tasks, to feel less lonely, to be less likely to abuse alcohol, and to be less prone to a variety of psychological problems. Individual differences in self-esteem predict a good deal of human behavior, typically (but by no means always) in the direction of higher self-esteem being associated with indices of psychological well-being. Our goal is to offer an overriding conceptualization that helps to explain why trait self-esteem correlates with the outcomes with which it does.

We must acknowledge up front an assumption (some might call it a bias) that pervades our review. Many researchers who have attempted to explain the relationship between trait self-esteem and other psychological variables have assumed that self-esteem *causes* people to think, feel, or behave in particular ways. Many articles in the literature suggest that high or low self-esteem "influences," "determines," "affects," or otherwise causes outcomes such as depression, teenage pregnancy, shyness, drug abuse, and academic achievement. We see two serious problems with interpretations that attribute causality to trait self-esteem.

First, researchers who assert that trait self-esteem influences behavior disregard the admonition that one cannot infer from a correlation that one variable causes another. Studies that measure trait self-esteem are invariably correlational in nature and, even when trait self-esteem is included as a factor in an experimental design, one cannot draw causal conclusions from the fact that self-esteem moderates the effects of the manipulated independent variable. Not only can we not know the direction of causal influence (if there is one), but unidentified extraneous variables may create a spurious relationship between self-esteem and other variables.

Second, those who conclude that self-esteem causes particular thoughts, emotions, or behaviors are at a loss to explain the nature of the causal process. Some writers have assumed that the effects occur because people with high self-esteem are more self-confident than those with low self-esteem. So, for example, their self-confidence makes them less likely to conform and more likely to persevere in the face of obstacles. However, explanations that invoke self-confidence confuse self-esteem with perceptions of one's self-efficacy or ability. As noted, self-esteem involves evaluative affect and thus is more akin to liking or feeling good about oneself than to having self-confidence (Brown, 1993). Although self-efficacy may correlate with self-esteem, they are not the same, and they are not necessarily related. Just as we may like other people even though we have little confidence in their ability, we may like ourselves despite our various shortcomings. Researchers have found it difficult to explain why *feeling good* about oneself results in the myriad outcomes that have been explained by trait self-esteem. Looking at the literature critically, one finds virtually no direct evidence that trait self-esteem causes any of the phenomena that have been attributed to it, although the existing correlational data do not eliminate this possibility.

Although the notion that self-esteem has a causal influence on people's feelings and behavior is pervasive, at least a few theories have largely avoided the causal fallacy. Dominance theory (Barkow, 1980), terror management theory (Greenberg et al., 1992), and self-determination theory (Deci & Ryan, 1995), for example, all offer explanations that attribute self-esteem's effects to other, more basic psychological processes (such as maintaining social dominance, reducing existential anxiety, or fostering autonomy). Space does not permit us to review these approaches nor to discuss how they explain the relationships between trait self-esteem and other psychological variables. Instead, our review focuses on sociometer theory, which suggests that the cognitive, emotional, and behavioral concomitants of self-esteem may be explained by reference to the fact that self-esteem reflects the degree to which an individual believes that other people regard their relationships with him or her to be valuable or important.

According to sociometer theory (Leary & Baumeister, 2000; Leary & Downs, 1995), the self-esteem system is an evolutionary adaptation that emerged to monitor one's relational value to other people. Being valued as a relational partner (whether as a friend, group member, mating partner, or other) is important because it increases the likelihood that others will be available for practical, social, and emotional support, thereby enhancing one's reproductive success. Particularly in the ancestral environment in which human evolution occurred, it would have been vitally important to maintain strong connections with other people (Baumeister & Leary, 1995). Thus having a mechanism that automatically monitors one's relational value on an ongoing basis would have been an asset. The subjective feelings that are associated with changes in self-esteem provide feedback regarding one's relational value in other people's eyes and motivate behaviors that help to maintain or enhance one's relational value. High self-esteem is associated with perceiving that one has high relational value, whereas low self-esteem is related to perceiving that one has low or declining relational value.

Sociometer theory was proposed initially as a theory of state self-esteem and self-esteem motivation (Leary & Downs, 1995), but it is relevant to understanding trait self-esteem as well. To thrive interpersonally, people must monitor their relational value to other people on two fronts. On one hand, they must monitor how they are being regarded in the immediate interpersonal context. According to the theory, state self-esteem provides feedback regarding one's current relational value. People experience surges or downturns in state self-esteem when they perceive increases or decreases in the degree to which other people value them.

In addition, however, people must monitor their general acceptability to other people across situations and over time. They must know not only how relationally valued they are at present but also what their prospects for relationships and memberships are in the future. Just as a savvy investor must monitor both the current price and long-term prospects of a stock, people must monitor both short-term fluctuations in their relational value (state self-esteem) and their relational value in the long run (trait self-esteem). How people respond to their current interpersonal circumstances is influenced by their long-term prospects (as reflected in trait self-esteem), just as how investors react to daily stock prices depends on their perception of the long-term value of a stock.

Furthermore, people cannot always assess their current relational value with confidence, either because other people are not present (and, thus, there are no cues from which to judge others' appraisals) or because circumstances prevent them from ascertaining how they are being perceived and evaluated at present (as when others purposefully hide their reactions, for example). Even when information about their relational value is not currently available, people nonetheless often need to have an idea of how they are faring interpersonally. In such cases, they may rely on their trait self-esteem to help them infer their standing.

According to sociometer theory, people's trait self-esteem develops from their history of relational evaluation or, more concretely, the degree to which they have been accepted and rejected by other people over time. Many studies show that a developmental history of rejection, neglect, and abuse (all of which imply low relational evaluation) strongly predict low self-esteem (Briere, 1992; Harter, Chapter 30, this volume). Furthermore, trait self-esteem correlates highly with people's current beliefs about the degree to which they are generally accepted, valued, and supported by other people (Lakey, Tardiff, & Drew, 1994; Leary, Cottrell, & Phillips, 2001; Leary, Tambor, Terdal, & Downs, 1995). People with high trait self-esteem feel generally accepted by other people, whereas people with low trait self-esteem feel less accepted, if not rejected.[1]

People often bring rejection on themselves, evoking disinterest, disapproval, or devaluation because their own characteristics or behavior are objectionable to others. However, people may also be devalued and rejected for reasons that have little to do with their personal characteristics, as when children are neglected or abused by maladjusted parents or people are rejected by their peers simply for being different. Such individuals typically have lower self-esteem than those who are raised by loving parents or who are warmly embraced by their peer groups. Thus, from the standpoint of sociometer theory, trait self-esteem does not necessarily reflect on a person's true value, worth, or desirability.

In brief, self-esteem is intimately related to how people perceive they are accepted and rejected by others, because the self-esteem system monitors relational evaluation. Particular responses, traits, and patterns of behavior relate to trait self-esteem, not because self-esteem has any direct causal effect on them but rather because, like self-esteem, those particular responses, traits, and patterns of behavior are the result of real, imagined, or anticipated acceptance and rejection. Rather than causing these outcomes, as many have assumed, trait self-esteem reflects the perceived state of the individual's relationships with others.

In the sections that follow, we briefly review research that examines the relationships between trait self-esteem and emotion, interpersonal behavior, relationships, personality, maladaptive behavior and psychopathology, and the development of self-esteem. In each case, we show that these relationships can be explained by reference to the role of the self-esteem system in monitoring the quality of people's interpersonal relationships. Given the extent of the self-esteem literature and the fact that many findings have been replicated by several studies, we must necessarily be selective, and even arbitrary, in the references that we cite to support various conclusions.

Self-Esteem and Emotion

One finding that has stimulated a great deal of interest in self-esteem is that people with lower trait self-esteem tend to experience virtually every aversive emotion more frequently than people with higher self-esteem. Trait self-esteem correlates negatively with scores on measures of anxiety (Battle, Jarratt, Smit, & Precht, 1988; Rawson, 1992), sadness and depression (Hammen, 1988; Ouellet & Joshi, 1986; Smart & Walsh, 1993), hostility and anger (Dreman, Spielberger, & Darzi, 1997), social anxiety (Leary & Kowalski, 1995; Santee & Maslach, 1982; Sharp & Getz, 1996), shame and guilt (Tangney & Dearing, 2002), embarrassability (Leary & Meadows, 1991; Maltby & Day, 2000; Miller, 1995), and loneliness (Haines, Scalise, & Ginter, 1993; Vaux, 1988), as well as general negative affectivity and neuroticism (Watson & Clark, 1984). Clearly, people with low self-esteem live less affectively pleasant lives than those with high self-esteem. But why?

Many writers have implied that these negative emotions are caused by low self-esteem, suggesting that feeling badly about oneself naturally makes people feel anxious, sad, angry, ashamed, and so on. Others have offered the tautological suggestion that low self-esteem causes dysphoric emotions because people need high self-esteem in order to feel good, although they do not explain why self-feelings should have such emotional potency. Sociometer theory provides an alternative answer to the question of why self-esteem correlates with negative affect by suggesting that, like self-esteem, these emotions are typically responses to real, imagined, or anticipated interpersonal rejection (Leary, 1990; Leary, Koch, & Hechenbleikner, 2001). We offer just a few examples to show how the link between emotion and self-esteem may be explained by the fact that low perceived relational evaluation underlies both.

Baumeister and Tice (1990) made the compelling argument that anxiety always results from expectations of either physical harm or social exclusion. Because of the severe consequences of being abandoned or ostracized, especially in the ancestral environment, the prospect of interpersonal rejection causes the same sorts of emotional reactions as physical threats. Thus people who have experienced a history of rejection and, as a result, expect to be rejected in the future are prone to anxiety. Viewed in this fashion, anxiety and low self-esteem are co-effects of believing that one is insufficiently valued and accepted and that one's interpersonal prospects for the future are not bright. So, for example, perceiving that one is not adequately accepted predicts trait anxiety (Lakey et al., 1994; Spivey, 1990), and people who generally expect that others will not accept them score higher on measures of trait anxiety and neuroticism (Downey & Feldman, 1996).

Likewise, low self-esteem is strongly associated with the tendency to feel sad, if not depressed (Tarlow & Haaga, 1996), leading some theorists to propose that a negative self-evaluation lies at the heart of depression (Beck, Steer, Epstein, & Brown, 1990). Again, sociometer theory suggests that depression and low self-esteem are coeffects of low perceived relational evaluation rather than directly related. A great deal of research shows that people who are neglected, rejected, or abandoned suffer marked losses of self-esteem and are also particularly prone to be sad or depressed (Baumeister, Wotman, & Stillwell, 1993; Leary et al., 1995). When Shaver, Schwartz, Kirson, and O'Connor (1987) asked participants to write about a typical instance in which people feel sad, 63% of the descriptions involved the loss of a relationship or separation from a loved one, and over one-fourth of them dealt specifically with rejection. Furthermore, people's general perceptions of social acceptance are inversely related to scores on standard depression inventories (Spivey, 1990). Kupersmidt and Patterson (1991) found that low peer acceptance was the best single predictor of depression in preadolescent girls, and Panak and Garber (1992) found that perceived social acceptance predicted childhood depression one year later.

Although anger arises for many reasons having nothing to do with rejection, people often become angry when they are ignored, shunned, rejected, or ostracized by other people (Bourgeois & Leary, 2001; Buckley, Winkel, & Leary, 2002; Cohen, Nisbett, Bowdle, & Schwarz, 1996; Williams, 1997; Williams & Zadro, 2001). Jealousy, which occurs when people attribute relational devaluation by another person to the presence or intrusion of a third party, also tends to be accompanied by anger. Not only do the same kinds of rejecting episodes that make people angry also lower their self-esteem (Bourgeois & Leary, 2001; Williams & Zadro, 2001), but also lower self-esteem has generally been found to be related to greater jealousy (Salovey & Rodin, 1992; White & Mullen, 1989). Importantly, the link between self-esteem and jealousy seems to have less to do with ego threats per se than with the mere prospect of losing the other person (Salovey & Rodin, 1992). Participants in one study indicated they would feel as much of a blow to their self-esteem if their partner simply rejected them as if they lost their partner to a rival (Mathes, Adams, & Davies, 1985), suggesting that the effects of jealousy-provoking incidents on self-esteem may be a result of relational devaluation.

Many of the so-called self-conscious emotions—social anxiety, embarrassment, and shame, for example—involve concerns with how one's behavior or characteristics are perceived and evaluated by others (Leary & Kowalski, 1995; Miller, 1995, 1996; Tangney & Dearing, 2002). People who are prone to self-conscious emotions worry a great deal about how others view them, believing that their personal failures, shortcomings, and misdeeds will lead others to evaluate them negatively and possibly reject them. Given their doubts about their social value and acceptability, people with low self-esteem are particularly likely to worry about other people's evaluations and, thus, are more likely to feel socially anxious, embarrassed, and ashamed. Again, these emotions are caused not by low self-esteem per se but rather by the perceived prospect of low relational evaluation (Leary, Koch, & Hechenbleikner, 2001).

Loneliness is more straightforwardly related to feeling inadequately valued than any other emotion. Loneliness arises when people feel that their social contacts have dropped below some minimum level, and chronically lonely people go through life feeling that they are not adequately included in other people's lives (Russell, Cutrona, Rose, & Yurko, 1984). Again, loneliness correlates negatively with self-esteem because both arise from perceived low relational evaluation.

Given that all of these negative emotions are related to low self-esteem, it is not surprising that self-esteem is also inversely correlated with general negative affectivity (Miller, 1995; Stokes & Levin, 1990; Whitley & Gridley, 1993). Again, the relationship may stem from perceived relational evaluation. In fact, Watson and Clark (1984) suggested that negative affectivity includes "a sense of rejection" (p. 465). We would state it differently, noting that feeling inadequately accepted by others predisposes people to experience negative rejection-related affect.

Interpersonal Behavior

Trait self-esteem predicts many features of interpersonal behavior. To demonstrate how the relationship between self-esteem and certain behaviors may be explained by sociometer theory, we discuss four of these features: social confidence, conformity, self-presentation, and prosocial behavior.

Social Confidence

People with high self-esteem exude greater confidence in social situations than people with low self-esteem. They are more sociable, outgoing, and assertive, as well as less shy (Cheek & Buss, 1981; Halamandaris & Power, 1997; Schmidt & Fox, 1995). From the standpoint of sociometer theory, the confidence that individuals with high self-esteem have in interpersonal situations stems from their perception that other people respond positively to them (Baldwin & Keelan, 1999). People are able to interact with greater confidence and spontaneity when they are not worried about whether others are likely to accept or reject them.

Conformity

Likewise, high self-esteem frees people from rigid adherence to social norms. Observing that self-esteem is related to being autonomous, some theorists have suggested that self-esteem is high when people respond in an autonomous, self-directed manner (Deci & Ryan, 1995). Although this is sometimes true, we believe that people with high self-esteem feel freer to be themselves than people with low self-esteem because they already feel adequately valued by other people. People with low self-esteem, often sensing that their social value in other people's eyes is tenuous, are more careful not to behave in ways that might lead others to reject them. As a result, their behavior is sometimes guided more by social pressures than by their inner compass.

This may explain why people with low self-esteem are more malleable in social encounters (Brockner, 1983). They are more likely to conform (Heaven, 1988; Janis, 1954; Romer, 1981) and less likely to dissent (Santee & Maslach, 1982) than people with high self-esteem. Typically, their conformity takes the form of compliance—attitude change at the public level without a change in private attitudes (Romer, 1981)—suggesting that it is driven by interpersonal concerns rather than merely a lack of confidence in their own judgments. As Santee and Maslach (1982) observed, "the aspect of self-esteem that is relevant for conformity and dissent is the absence of worry and discomfort over what others think about oneself, rather than the presence of a sense of personal worth" (p. 698).

Similarly, people who score low in self-esteem are more likely to behave in line with others' expectations than people with high self-esteem (Baumeister, 1982; Briggs & Cheek, 1988). Furthermore, Baumeister (1982) showed that people with low versus high self-esteem differ in how they live up to others' expectations. In one study, individuals with low and high self-esteem received false feedback indicating that they were either competitive or cooperative. Participants with low self-esteem behaved consistently with their randomly assigned descriptions if they thought their partners had seen it, too. Apparently, people with low self-esteem are worried about the interpersonal consequences of violating others' expectations.

Self-Presentation

Almost by definition, people with high self-esteem generally describe themselves more positively than people with low self-esteem (Baumeister, Tice, & Hutton, 1989). In fact, evidence suggests that people who have high self-esteem sometimes go overboard with their positive self-descriptions (Raskin, Novacek, & Hogan, 1991; Roth, Harris, &

Snyder, 1988). Similarly, research has shown that high self-esteem is associated with "acquisitive" self-presentational strategies that allow people to enhance social approval and acceptance, whereas low self-esteem is associated with "protective" self-presentational strategies that allow people to avoid losses in approval and acceptance (Baumeister, Tice, & Hutton, 1989; Tice, 1991; Wolfe, Lennox, & Cutler, 1986).

These findings raise the question of why people with high self-esteem try to present themselves positively if they already feel relationally valued and why people with low self-esteem, who presumably lack acceptance, are not more motivated to seek approval through self-presentation. The answer may be that there is often an advantage to increasing one's acceptance and standing in a group even when one already feels accepted. However, such self-presentational tactics involve a risk of losing acceptance and status, which may seem too great for people who are uncertain of their acceptance. Thus people with high self-esteem can capitalize on their social acceptance by enhancing their public images even further, whereas people with low self-esteem fear losing whatever little relational value they have accrued. As a result, they are reluctant to try to convey self-enhancing images that they may be unable to sustain or that may backfire (Leary, 1995), finding it safer to protect their current evaluations rather than to enhance them. These tendencies also help to explain why people with low self-esteem seem concerned with fitting in, whereas people with high self-esteem concern themselves with standing out (Wolfe et al., 1986). Having largely satisfied their belongingness needs, individuals with high self-esteem seem to take opportunities to enhance their relational value even further.

Prosocial Behavior

Overall, high trait self-esteem is related to a higher inclination to behave in prosocial ways toward others and, possibly, to a lower likelihood of antisocial behavior. Several studies have shown that self-esteem correlates positively with prosocial behavior and negatively with antisocial behavior (Rigby & Slee, 1993; Simons, Paternite, & Shore,

2001). Furthermore, personal failure seems to increase prosocial behavior for people with high self-esteem but lower it for people with low self-esteem (Brown & Smart, 1991), and interventions that increase self-esteem also heighten cooperativeness (Aronson & Osherow, 1980).

In some ways, these patterns are paradoxical, because one might expect people with low self-esteem to try to ingratiate themselves with others by being helpful. However, like positive self-presentations, prosocial behavior may involve a certain degree of social risk. For example, one's efforts to help may be rebuffed or botched, and people with low self-esteem may be unwilling to take these risks. Furthermore, given that negative affect is associated with a lower willingness to help, people with low self-esteem (who, as we saw, are more prone to unpleasant emotions) may be less inclined to extend themselves on other's behalf than are people with high self-esteem.

Relationships

Trait self-esteem is related to people's feelings about and their actions in their relationships with other people. High trait self-esteem is related to higher levels of satisfaction in dating and marriage relationships (Fincham & Bradbury, 1993; Murray, Holmes, & Griffin, 2000) and to higher quality same-sex friendships (Shechtman, 1993; Voss, Markiewicz, & Doyle, 1999). In the case of romantic relationships, Murray and colleagues (2000) showed that the link between trait self-esteem and relationship perceptions (such as satisfaction) is nearly completely mediated by the extent to which people feel valued by their partners. That is, self-esteem is related to relationship satisfaction because people with lower self-esteem worry more about how much their partners accept and love them, making it difficult for them to be satisfied with the state of the relationship. This chronic concern with rejection on the part of people with low self-esteem makes their views of their relationships more tenuous (Baldwin & Sinclair, 1996). To make matters worse, people with low self-esteem become even more concerned about how much they are valued by their partners after being given either negative *or* positive feedback about themselves (Murray, Holmes, MacDonald, & Ellsworth, 1998), and threats to reflected appraisals result in angry reactions from people with low self-esteem (MacDonald, Zanna, & Holmes, 2000). Apparently, anything that makes their personal qualities salient reminds people with low self-esteem that their relationships are fragile and that they may be rejected at any time.

Other studies have linked low self-esteem to mania (Hendrick & Hendrick, 1986; Mallandain & Davies, 1994), a jealous style of love that involves being demanding and possessive toward the loved one. Given the link between self-esteem and possessiveness, it should not be surprising that low self-esteem has been linked to violence in relationships (Murphy, Meyer, & O'Leary, 1994; Russell & Hulson, 1992). This evidence stands in contrast to suggestions that people with high self-esteem are responsible for a wide range of aggressive acts, including domestic violence (Baumeister, Smart, & Boden, 1996). Pointing out that much domestic violence involves an abuser who is of lower status than the abused, Baumeister and colleagues (1996) concluded that abuse reflects an attempt to reestablish a feeling of lost dominance. However, another interpretation that can reconcile this observation with the link between low self-esteem and relationship violence is that the status differences typically observed between abusers and their victims represent a threat to the existence of the relationship in the abuser's eyes. Specifically, a higher status partner is likely to have more alternatives to the present relationship and more resources for leaving it. Thus relationship violence can be seen as an attempt by abusers to keep their partners from leaving. Furthermore, experimental work by MacDonald, Zanna, and Holmes (2000) showed that when men with low self-esteem both experience a strong threat to their sense of being valued by their partners and have narrowed attentional focus because of alcohol intoxication, they indicate an increased likelihood of aggressing against their partners. Murphy and colleagues (1994) found not only that low self-esteem predicted relationship violence but also that the more people relied on their relationships (dependence) and were concerned about acceptance by others (low self-esteem), the more likely violence was to occur.

Research on the link between trait self-esteem and attachment styles is also relevant here. Securely attached individuals have higher trait self-esteem than those with either preoccupied (Collins & Read, 1990; Feeney & Noller, 1990) or fearful (Bartholomew & Horowitz, 1991; Brennan & Morris, 1997) styles of attachment. Again, such patterns are consistent with the idea that trait self-esteem reflects the perception that other people value their relationships with the individual.

Interestingly, people with a dismissing attachment style, whose lack of trust in others leads to an emphasis on independence, have self-esteem that is as high as those with a secure attachment style (Bartholomew & Horowitz, 1991; Brennan & Morris, 1997; Bylsma, Cozzarelli, & Sumer, 1997). On the surface, this finding appears inconsistent with sociometer theory, because dismissively attached people expect rejection more than securely attached people and thus might be expected to have lower self-esteem. However, as noted, sociometer theory posits that trait self-esteem reflects chronic feelings of relational value rather than acute acceptance per se. As Bartholomew and Horowitz (1991) observed, dismissiveness "indicates a sense of loveworthiness combined with a negative disposition toward other people" (p. 227). Thus dismissively attached people seem to be less concerned about being rejected and more concerned that they will not be appreciated should they allow themselves to become close to another person. This sort of stance is evidenced by that fact that dismissives' high self-esteem is accompanied by interpersonal coldness and low sociability (Bartholomew & Horowitz, 1991; Duggan & Brennan, 1994).

If trait self-esteem serves as an indicator of one's relational value, the sociometer should have no more important role than monitoring acceptance (and rejection) in close relationships, and self-esteem should be acutely sensitive to the state of people's relationships with close others. The evidence suggests that self-esteem is strongly associated with outcomes in close relationships.

Personality

Many of the personality characteristics that are most strongly related to low self-esteem involve a sensitivity to rejection and negative evaluation. For example, trait self-esteem correlates negatively with rejection sensitivity and fear of negative evaluation (Downey & Feldman, 1996; Watson & Friend, 1969). These correlations make a great deal of sense if trait self-esteem is conceptualized as a monitor of relational value. People whose monitor registers low or declining relational value are understandably worried about disapproval and rejection.

Low self-esteem has also been consistently linked with higher levels of neuroticism (Halamandaris & Power, 1997; Kwan, Bond, & Singelis, 1997). In fact, neuroticism correlates more strongly with self-esteem than any other of the Big Five personality traits, with correlations around .60 often reported (e.g., Kwan et al., 1997). One study suggests that self-esteem is a facet of the neuroticism or emotional stability factor of the Big Five (Whitley & Gridley, 1993). As previously discussed, people with low self-esteem tend to be more anxious and experience less secure attachment than people with high self-esteem. Further, people with low self-esteem tend to report experiencing more negative emotions than people with high self-esteem (Halamandaris & Power, 1997; Miller, 1995). Importantly, researchers have consistently found that high neuroticism is viewed less positively than low neuroticism (Fleeson & Heckhausen, 1997) and that neuroticism is related to the dissolution of close relationships (Karney & Bradbury, 1995; Kelly & Conley, 1987; Kurdek, 1997). Thus neuroticism may relate to self-esteem, in part, because people who are highly neurotic are less positively evaluated and accepted.

In contrast, self-esteem is associated with higher extraversion (Halamandaris & Power, 1997; Kwan et al., 1997). People with high self-esteem are not only more sociable and outgoing but also report experiencing more positive affect than people with low self-esteem, both of which are characteristics of extraverts (Halamandaris & Power, 1997; Miller, 1995). People with high self-esteem are also higher in dispositional optimism than people with low self-esteem (Chemers, Watson, & May, 2000; Lucas, Diener, & Suh, 1996). Not only is extraversion more highly valued than introversion (Fleeson & Heckhausen, 1997) but also the sociotropic and optimistic interpersonal style of extraverts does appear to lead to greater liking and interpersonal acceptance (Aron, Melinat, Aron, Vallone, & Bator, 1997; Berry & Miller, 2001). Even introverted people generally prefer extraverts over introverts (Hendrick & Brown, 1971).

Trait self-esteem is weakly, if at all, linked to the personality trait of agreeableness (Amirkhan, Risinger, & Swickert, 1995; Kwan et al., 1997; Pullmann & Allik, 2000). One might expect that people's feelings about their own acceptability ought to be related to traits that facilitate interpersonal interactions and endear them to other people, such as friendliness, cooperativeness, and helpfulness, which are all aspects of agreeableness (Jensen-Campbell, Graziano, & West, 1995). Surprisingly, however, the limited available research suggests that agreeableness may not strongly predict being accepted (Berry & Miller, 2001; Graziano, Jensen-Campbell, & Hair, 1996). One possible explanation is that mere agreeableness, in the absence of other valued attributes, is related to relational value only tangentially. All other things being equal, we may prefer people who are agreeable rather than disagreeable, yet unless they also have something else to offer, agreeable people are not sought out simply for their agreeableness.

Self-esteem is also largely unrelated to openness to experience (Cramer, 2000; Kwan et al., 1997; Pullmann & Allik, 2000), even though, as noted earlier, people with low self-esteem are more prone to conform (e.g., Heaven, 1988). Thus people with low self-esteem may be more likely to conform in certain situations (for example, when they are seeking social approval), but they do not demonstrate a general tendency toward conventional behavior. Along these lines, authoritarianism is also unrelated to trait self-esteem (Feather, 1993; Heaven, 1986).

Self-esteem is positively related to conscientiousness (Kwan et al., 1997; Pullmann & Allik, 2000), possibly because conscientious people gain approval and acceptance for fulfilling their obligations to others. A good deal of conscientiousness involves meeting commitments made to other people, pulling one's weight in cooperative efforts, setting aside personal goals to attend to others' needs, and not inconveniencing other people. All other things being equal, a conscientious person is arguably a better friend, group member, or mate than a nonconscientious one. In addition, conscientiousness often leads to outcomes, such as success, that increase social approval and acceptance and, thus, heighten self-esteem. Indeed, other variables that are related to agency and accomplishment, such as the masculine gender role (or instrumentality) and desire for control, also correlate with trait self-esteem (Burger, 1995; Marsh, Antill, & Cunningham, 1989; Whitley, 1983). Conscientiousness is a valued characteristic (Fleeson & Heckhausen, 1997), both because conscientious people are more highly valued as relational partners and group members than nonconscientious people and because conscientiousness facilitates the achievement of socially valued outcomes, such as success.

The relationship between agency and success on one hand and self-esteem on the other has led some researchers to posit that "healthy" self-esteem arises from personal achievement rather than social approval (e.g., Deci & Ryan, 1995). However, it is difficult to separate the effects of personal feelings of efficacy and accomplishment from the effects of approval from others in a domain that is as highly valued as achievement. Nevertheless, MacDonald, Saltzman, and Leary (in press) demonstrated that high achievers who do not believe that achievement is strongly tied to approval and acceptance have levels of self-esteem that differ little from low achievers. In contrast, high achievers who believe that achievement is valued by others have higher self-esteem.

Although we have reviewed only a few of the hundreds of traits that have been correlated with trait self-esteem, the patterns can be explained in reference to the link between self-esteem and perceived relational value. People whose personalities facilitate interpersonal acceptance will have higher self-esteem than people whose personalities have no effect on acceptance or, worse, lead others to reject them.

Maladaptive Behavior and Psychopathology

Psychologists have often viewed high self-esteem as an important part of psychological well-being (Taylor & Brown, 1988) and low self-esteem as a culprit in a variety of emotional and behavioral problems. Although high self-esteem is not always more adaptive than low self-esteem (Baumeister et al., 1996), it is nonetheless true that self-esteem correlates negatively with dysfunctional behavior, deviance, and psychopathology.

Alcohol and Drug Use

Several studies have shown that people who abuse alcohol and drugs tend to have lower self-esteem than those who do not (Cookson, 1994; Griffin-Shelley, Sandler, & Lees, 1990; Vega, Zimmerman, Warheit, & Apospori, 1993). However, the relation between self-esteem and alcohol consumption may depend to an extent on the gender of the individual. The data for men have been inconsistent, with some studies suggesting either a small negative or no relationship between trait self-esteem and consumption of alcohol (Beckman, 1978; Pandina & Schuele, 1983) and other studies supporting a positive relationship (Corbin, McNair, & Carter, 1996; Konovsky & Wilsnack, 1982). The data for women are more clear-cut, with lower trait self-esteem consistently related to higher levels of drinking (Beckman, 1978; Corbin et al., 1996; Konovsky & Wilsnack, 1982). In fact, alcoholic women have lower self-esteem than either nonalcoholic women or alcoholic men (Beckman, 1978).

Some research on the link between self-esteem and alcohol use suggests that concerns over social acceptability may lie at the heart of this relationship. In an experimental study, Konovsky and Wilsnack (1982) showed that people with low self-esteem consumed more alcohol than people with high self-esteem during a party at which they interacted with strangers. Furthermore, after consuming alcohol, women who scored high in femininity (i.e., endorsement of female gender roles) experienced a decline in self-esteem. The authors interpreted this finding by suggesting that, because traditional sex roles define heavy drinking as less appropriate for women than for men, being intoxicated makes sex-typed women feel less acceptable when they drink. Along these lines, Beckman (1978) suggested that a core feature of alcoholism for women is "a sense of futility about being able to fulfill the female role" (p. 491), which certainly connotes the possibility of not being valued as a relational partner. In contrast, many men perceive that heavy drinking is occasionally encouraged, if not expected, for them. As Corbin and colleagues (1996) noted, "heavier drinking males may have higher self-esteem due to the social acceptability and rewards of such behavior" (p. 3).

The use of illegal drugs also correlates with lower self-esteem (Cookson, 1994; Guiterres & Reich, 1988). Interestingly, however, one longitudinal study found that the use of hard drugs actually predicted increases in some aspects of self-esteem, particularly in feelings of social attractiveness (Stein, Newcomb, & Bentler, 1987). From the standpoint of sociometer theory, people with low self-esteem should be more likely than people with high self-esteem to use drugs either to dampen the negative emotions associated with rejection or as a means of being included in a drug-using group (Leary, Schreindorfer, & Haupt, 1995). Thus people with low self-esteem may be drawn to drugs but then experience increased self-esteem after they feel included by other members of the drug subculture.

Delinquency and Crime

Research into juvenile delinquency suggests a similar reciprocal relationship between self-esteem and antisocial behavior. Juvenile delinquency typically correlates with lower levels of self-esteem (Peiser & Heaven, 1996; Rigby & Cox, 1996), although this relation is not universally found (Oyserman & Markus, 1990). Longitudinal research has also produced mixed results, with some studies linking low self-esteem to higher rates of delinquency (Kaplan, 1980; Rosenberg, Schooler, & Schoenbach, 1989) but others finding no relationship (Jang & Thornberry, 1998).

At present, the best conclusion is that feelings of unacceptability predict increased involvement in delinquent behavior but that becoming involved in a delinquent group may raise the person's self-esteem. Feeling undervalued predisposes people to seek social acceptance in relatively extreme ways, including delinquency, if doing so brings them respect or permits them to join a delinquent group. Then, if the delinquent behavior does, in fact, increase their social value in peers' eyes, their self-esteem may rise. This interpretation is supported by the consistent finding that becoming involved in delinquency can increase self-esteem (Kaplan, 1980; Latkin, 1990; Rosenberg et al., 1989). Vigil's (1988, p. 88) explanation of this effect is consistent with sociometer theory: "often youths feel loved, respected, and supported for the first time as a result of joining a gang."

Rosenberg and colleagues (1989) found that the self-esteem boost associated with delinquent behavior was greatest for individuals who were low in socioeconomic status. That is, the most disenfranchised individuals in their study experienced the largest benefit to their self-esteem as a result of antisocial behavior. Jang and Thornberry (1998) did not find that delinquent behavior per se was associated with high self-esteem but that associations with delinquent peers was. Again, this increase in self-esteem from association with "renegade" peers was strongest for disenfranchised groups, specifically girls and African Americans. As with drug use, evidence suggests that antisocial behavior can serve as a tonic for the self-esteem of individuals with concerns about their social acceptability.

Psychopathology

Although the relationships are often weak, virtually every clinically recognized variety of emotional and behavioral problem is more common among people with low than high self-esteem. Low self-esteem is associated with dysthymic disorder, major depression, anxiety disorder, eating disorders, sexual dysfunction, pathological shame, suicide attempts, and an array of personality disorders in both children and adults (Beck et al., 1990; Cicchetti, Rogosch, Lynch, & Holt, 1993; Frankel & Myatt,

1996; Masi, Favilla, Mucci, Poli, & Romano, 2001; O'Connor, Berry, & Weiss, 1999; Plutchik, Botsis, & Van Praag, 1995; Schweitzer, Seth-Smith, & Callan, 1992; Shisslak, Pazda, & Crago, 1990; Yang & Clum, 1996; see also Westen & Heim, Chapter 31, this volume).

Two primary mechanisms may underlie these relationships. First, considerable evidence suggests that ostracism, abandonment, and other forms of rejection create emotional and behavioral problems. The incidence of virtually every form of psychopathology is higher among people who have experienced a life history of rejection. Not only do children not develop optimally when rejected, but also feeling rejected sometimes leads people to engage in dysfunctional means of obtaining approval and support. Thus self-esteem itself is not the cause of maladjustment but rather a coeffect of rejection (Leary et al., 1995).

Second, people who have psychological difficulties are often avoided and stigmatized, if not outright rejected, by other people (Farina, 1982). As we have seen, being devalued and unaccepted causes low self-esteem, so that people who feel stigmatized, disliked, or avoided will tend to have low self-esteem. In such cases, low self-esteem is an indirect effect of having psychological problems.

Summary

The prevailing view among the public, as well as among many mental health professionals, is that low self-esteem is the root of much, if not all, personal and social evil. Indeed, it was this belief that led the California State Assembly to create the California Task Force to Promote Self-Esteem and Personal and Social Responsibility. The goal of this initiative was to attack problems such as teen pregnancy, delinquency, welfare dependency, drug abuse, and violence by raising the self-esteem of the citizens of California. However, as the program's advocates themselves admitted, research findings supporting a link between self-esteem and problem behaviors were scattered and weak. In spite of the empirical evidence, however, they continued to maintain that self-esteem "is simultaneously one of the most central and one of the most elusive factors in understanding and explaining the behaviors that constitute major social problems" (Smelser, 1989, p. 18). No one seems to have considered the possibility that its elusiveness might suggest that self-esteem is not really so central after all.

We do not find its elusiveness surprising. Not only are all human behaviors, adaptive and maladaptive, multiply determined, but, according to sociometer theory, self-esteem is only spuriously associated with them. If our analysis of these problems in terms of sociometer theory is correct, the problem is not that people have too little self-esteem but rather that they feel inadequately valued as members of relationships and social groups. Low perceived relational evaluation then undermines adaptive development and promotes risky, desperate behaviors, such as gang membership, promiscuity, and association with the drug culture, all of which enhance feelings of social acceptance albeit at a personal price (Leary et al., 1995).

The Development of Self-Esteem

From the beginnings of behavioral science, theorists have recognized that how people feel about themselves depends in large part on how they think other people feel about them. The symbolic interactionist perspective advocated by Cooley (1902) and Mead (1934) traced self-perceptions and self-esteem to reflected appraisals—people's perceptions of how other people perceived them. Since then, researchers in many areas of behavioral science have studied the interpersonal origins of self-esteem.

Research has supported the insight of the symbolic interactionists that children adopt the opinions that other people, particularly caregivers and other significant adults, appear to have of them. Thus parents who are approving, nurturant, and responsive tend to produce children with higher self-esteem than parents who are disapproving, uninterested, and unresponsive (Coopersmith, 1967; Harter, 1999; Chapter 30, this volume). Not surprisingly, abusive and rejecting parents have children with the lowest self-esteem (Westen & Heim, Chapter 31, this volume). Although the link between parental regard and self-esteem weakens during adolescence, the relationship is still

quite strong, even as peer acceptance exerts a growing influence on the adolescent's self-esteem. In adolescence, peer approval is the strongest predictor of self-worth (Harter, Whitesell, & Junkin, 1998), but the self-esteem of a significant number of children and adolescents is also affected by relationships with special, nonparental adults—such as teachers, coaches, neighbors, and grandparents—who provide support, guidance, and acceptance. Such findings are consistent with the notion that self-esteem reflects the degree to which people believe they are valued by other people.

Not all sources of trait self-esteem involve explicit approval and acceptance. High self-esteem is also associated with the belief that one possesses valued attributes, such as being a good student, physically attractive, or skilled athletically, artistically, or musically. Although most writers have assumed that these self-assessments of one's abilities and attributes contribute directly to a personal sense of self-worth, we argue that the relationship is mediated by perceived relational value. Possessing certain positive attributes or being successful in particular domains contribute to self-esteem because they lead the person to believe that others value him or her as a friend, group member, or relational partner. Indeed, believing that one possesses desirable attributes (such as competence, social skill, or physical attractiveness) predicts trait self-esteem to the extent that the person believes that these characteristics promote social acceptance or are important to other people (MacDonald et al., in press).

Conclusions

Trait self-esteem regularly emerges as a potent predictor of psychological outcomes in research on a wide array of phenomena. These findings have led researchers to conclude that self-esteem is an exceptionally important entity that underlies a great deal of human emotion and behavior. From the standpoint of sociometer theory, self-esteem is intertwined with such a variety of emotions and behaviors because it mirrors one of the most powerful influences on human behavior—a person's sense that he or she is valued and accepted rather than devalued and rejected by other people (Baumeister & Leary, 1995; Leary, 2001).

Conceptualizing self-esteem in this manner might suggest that most research on self-esteem has focused on the wrong variable—self-esteem rather than perceived relational value or social acceptance. We view the issue a bit differently, however. It is not that self-esteem is the "wrong" variable but rather that most research on trait self-esteem stopped prematurely with the conclusion that self-esteem predicts particular responses or traits without considering precisely why self-esteem relates to other variables as it does. Self-esteem is by no means irrelevant to the story. As part of the individual's subjective representation of his or her interpersonal world, it plays an important role. However, to fully understand how and why self-esteem relates to behavior, we must realize that the distal causes of both trait self-esteem and the outcomes with which it correlates involve the degree to which people believe they are valued and accepted by other people.

Notes

1. Although we refer loosely in this chapter to "low" versus "high" self-esteem, it is essential to stress that very few individuals have self-esteem that can be characterized as truly "low." People who are identified as having low self-esteem on standard measures are more accurately characterized as having moderate self-esteem (Baumeister, Tice, & Hutton, 1989). They either feel neutrally about themselves or else have an ambivalent mixture of positive and negative self-feelings. Given that virtually everybody feels relationally valued by at least a few individuals, it is quite rare for people chronically to feel unequivocally unacceptable.

References

Amirkhan, J. H., Risinger, R. T., & Swickert, R. J. (1995). Extraversion: A "hidden" personality factor in coping? *Journal of Personality, 63,* 189–212.

Aron, A., Melinat, E., Aron, E., Vallone, R., & Bator, R. J. (1997). The experimental generation of interpersonal closeness: A procedure and some preliminary findings. *Personality and Social Psychology Bulletin, 23,* 363–377.

Aronson, E., & Osherow, N. (1980). Cooperation, prosocial behavior, and academic performance: Experiments in the desegregated classroom. *Applied Social Psychology Annual, 1,* 163–196.

Baldwin, M. W., & Keelan, J. P. R. (1999). Interpersonal expectations as a function of self-esteem and sex. *Journal of Social and Personal Relationships, 16,* 822–833.

Baldwin, M. W., & Sinclair, L. (1996). Self-esteem and "if . . . then" contingencies of interpersonal acceptance. *Journal of Personality and Social Psychology, 71,* 1130–1141.

Barkow, J. (1980). Prestige and self-esteem: A biosocial interpretation. In D. R. Omark, F. F. Strayer, & D. G. Freedman (Eds.), *Dominance relations* (pp. 319–332). New York: Garland.

Bartholomew, K., & Horowitz, L. M. (1991). Attachment styles among young adults: A test of a four-category model. *Journal of Personality and Social Psychology, 61,* 226–244.

Battle, J., Jarratt, L., Smit, S., & Precht, D. (1988). Relations among self-esteem, depression, and anxiety of children. *Psychological Reports, 62,* 999–1005.

Baumeister, R. F. (1982). Self-esteem, self-presentation, and future interaction: A dilemma of reputation. *Journal of Personality, 50,* 29–45.

Baumeister, R. F., & Leary, M. R. (1995). The need to belong: Desire for interpersonal attachments as a fundamental human motivation. *Psychological Bulletin, 117,* 497–529.

Baumeister, R. F., Smart, L., & Boden, J. M. (1996). Relation of threatened egotism to violence and aggression: The dark side of high self-esteem. *Psychological Review, 103,* 5–33.

Baumeister, R. F., & Tice, D. M. (1990). Anxiety and social exclusion. *Journal of Social and Clinical Psychology, 9,* 165–196.

Baumeister, R. F., Wotman, S. R., & Stillwell, A. M. (1993). Unrequited love: On heartbreak, anger, guilt, scriptlessness, and humiliation. *Journal of Personality and Social Psychology, 64,* 377–394.

Baumeister, R. F., Tice, D. M., & Hutton, D. G. (1989). Self-presentational motivations and personality differences in self-esteem. *Journal of Personality, 57,* 547–579.

Beck, A. T., Steer, R. A., Epstein, N., & Brown, G. (1990). Beck Self-Concept Test. *Psychological Assessment, 2,* 191–197.

Beckman, L. J. (1978). Self-esteem of women alcoholics. *Journal of Studies on Alcohol, 39,* 491–498.

Berry, D. S., & Miller, K. M. (2001). When boy meets girl: Attractiveness and the five-factor model in opposite-sex interactions. *Journal of Research in Personality, 35,* 62–77.

Blascovich, J., & Tomaka, J. (1991). Measures of self-esteem. In J. P. Robinson, P. R. Shaver, & L. S. Wrightsman (Eds.), *Measures of personality and social psychological attitudes* (pp. 115–160). San Diego, CA: Academic Press.

Bourgeois, K. S., & Leary, M. R. (2001). Coping with rejection: Derogating those who choose us last. *Motivation and Emotion, 25,* 101–111.

Brennan, K. A., & Morris, K. A. (1997). Attachment styles, self-esteem, and patterns of seeking feedback from romantic partners. *Personality and Social Psychology Bulletin, 23,* 23–31.

Briere, J. (1992). *Child abuse traumas: Theory and treatment of the lasting effects.* Newbury Park, CA: Sage.

Briggs, S. R., & Cheek, J. M. (1988). On the nature of self-monitoring: Problems with assessment, problems with validity. *Journal of Personality and Social Psychology, 54,* 663–678.

Brockner, J. (1983). Low self-esteem and behavioral plasticity: Some implications. In L. Wheeler & P. Shaver (Eds.), *Review of personality and social psychology* (Vol. 4, pp. 237–271). Beverly Hills, CA: Sage.

Brown, J. D. (1993). Self-esteem and self-evaluations: Feeling is believing. In J. Suls (Ed.), *Psychological perspectives on the self* (Vol. 4, pp. 27–58). Hillsdale, NJ: Erlbaum.

Brown, J. D., & Smart, S. A. (1991). The self and social conduct: Linking self-representations to prosocial behavior. *Journal of Personality and Social Psychology, 60,* 368–375.

Buckley, K. E., Winkel, R. E., & Leary, M. R. (2002). *Emotional and behavioral responses to interpersonal rejection: Anger, sadness, hurt, and aggression.* Manuscript submitted for publication.

Burger, J. M. (1995). Need for control and self-esteem: Two routes to a high desire for control. In M. H. Kernis (Ed.), *Efficacy, agency and self-esteem* (pp. 217–233). New York: Plenum Press.

Bylsma, W. H., Cozzarelli, C., & Sumer, N. (1997). Relation between adult attachment styles and global self-esteem. *Basic and Applied Social Psychology, 19,* 1–16.

Cheek, J. M., & Buss, A. H. (1981). Shyness and sociability. *Journal of Personality and Social Psychology, 41,* 330–339.

Chemers, M. M., Watson, C. B., & May, S. T. (2000). Dispositional affect and leadership effectiveness: A comparison of self-esteem, optimism, and efficacy. *Personality and Social Psychology Bulletin, 26,* 267–277.

Cicchetti, D., Rogosch, F. A., Lynch, M., & Holt, K. D. (1993). Resilience in maltreated children: Processes leading to adaptive outcome. *Development and Psychopathology, 5,* 629–647.

Cohen, D., Nisbett, R. E., Bowdle, B. F., & Schwarz, N. (1996). Insult, aggression, and the southern culture of honor: An "experimental ethnography." *Journal of Personality and Social Psychology, 70,* 945–960.

Collins, N. L., & Read, S. J. (1990). Adult attachment, working models, and relationship quality in dating couples. *Journal of Personality and Social Psychology, 58,* 644–663.

Cookson, H. (1994). Personality variables associated with alcohol use in young offenders. *Personality and Individual Differences, 16,* 179–182.

Cooley, C. H. (1902). *Human nature and the social order.* New York: Scribner's.

Coopersmith, S. (1967). *The antecedents of self-esteem.* San Francisco: W. H. Freeman.

Corbin, W. R., McNair, L. D., & Carter, J. (1996). Self-esteem and problem drinking among male and female college students. *Journal of Alcohol and Drug Education, 42,* 1–14.

Cramer, P. (2000). Development of identity: Gender makes a difference. *Journal of Research in Personality, 34,* 42–72.

Deci, E. L., & Ryan, R. M. (1995). Human agency: The basis for true self-esteem. In M. H. Kernis (Ed.), *Efficacy, agency, and self-esteem* (pp. 31–50). New York: Plenum Press.

Downey, G., & Feldman, S. I. (1996). Implications of rejection sensitivity for intimate relationships. *Journal of Personality and Social Psychology, 70,* 1327–1343.

Dreman, S., Spielberger, C., & Darzi, O. (1997). The relation of state-anger to self-esteem, perceptions of family structure and attributions of responsibility for divorce of custodial mothers in the stabilization phase of the divorce process. *Journal of Divorce and Remarriage, 28,* 157–170.

Duggan, S. E., & Brennan, K. A. (1994). Social avoidance and its relation to Bartholomew's adult attachment typology. *Journal of Social and Personal Relationships, 11,* 147–153.

Farina, A. (1982). The stigma of mental disorders. In A. Miller (Ed.), *In the eye of the beholder: Contemporary issues in stereotyping* (pp. 305–363). New York: Praeger.

Feather, N. T. (1993). Authoritarianism and attitudes toward high achievers. *Journal of Personality and Social Psychology, 65,* 152–164.

Feeney, J. A., & Noller, P. (1990). Attachment style as a predictor of adult romantic relationships. *Journal of Personality and Social Psychology, 58,* 281–291.

Fincham, F. D., & Bradbury, T. N. (1993). Marital satisfaction, depression, and attributions: A longitudinal analysis. *Journal of Personality and Social Psychology, 64,* 442–452.

Fleeson, W., & Heckhausen, J. (1997). More or less "me" in past, present, and future: Perceived lifetime personality during adulthood. *Psychology and Aging, 12,* 125–136.

Fleming, J. S., & Courtney, B. E. (1984). The dimensionality of self-esteem: II. Hierarchical facet model for revised measurement scales. *Journal of Personality and Social Psychology, 46,* 404–421.

Frankel, F., & Myatt, R. (1996). Self-esteem, social competence, and psychopathology in boys without friends. *Personality and Individual Differences, 20,* 401–407.

Graziano, W. G., Jensen-Campbell, L. A., & Hair, E. L. (1996). Perceiving interpersonal conflict and reacting to it: The case for agreeableness. *Journal of Personality and Social Psychology, 70,* 820–835.

Greenberg, J., Solomon, S., Pyszczynski, T., Rosenblatt, A., Burling, J., Lyon, D., Simon, L., & Pinel, E. (1992). Why do people need self-esteem? Converging evidence that self-esteem serves an anxiety-buffering function. *Journal of Personality and Social Psychology, 63,* 913–922.

Griffin-Shelley, E., Sandler, K. R., & Lees, C. (1990). Sex-role perceptions in chemically dependent subjects: Adults versus adolescents. *International Journal of the Addictions, 25,* 1383–1391.

Guiterres, S. E., & Reich, J. W. (1988). Attributional analysis of drug abuse and gender: Effects of treatment and relationship to rehabilitation. *Journal of Social and Clinical Psychology, 7,* 176–191.

Haines, D. A., Scalise, J. J., & Ginter, E. J. (1993). Relationship of loneliness and its affective elements to self-esteem. *Psychological Reports, 73,* 479–482.

Halamandaris, K. F., & Power, K. G. (1997). Individual differences, dysfunctional attitudes, and social support: A study of the psychosocial adjustment to university life of home students. *Personality and Individual Differences, 22,* 93–104.

Hammen, C. (1988). Self-cognitions, stressful events, and the prediction of depression in children of depressed mothers. *Journal of Abnormal Child Psychology, 16,* 347–360.

Harter, S. (1985). *The Self-Perception Profile for Children.* Unpublished manual, University of Denver, Denver, CO.

Harter, S. (1993). Causes and consequences of low self-esteem in children and adolescents. In R. F. Baumeister (Ed.), *Self-esteem: The puzzle of low self-regard* (pp. 87–116). New York: Plenum Press.

Harter, S. (1999). *The construction of the self: A developmental perspective.* New York: Guilford Press.

Harter, S., Whitesell, N. R., & Junkin, L. J. (1998). Similarities and differences in domain-specific and global self-evaluations of learning-disabled, behaviorally disordered, and normally achieving adolescents. *American Educational Research Journal, 35,* 653–682.

Heaven, P. C. (1988). Correlates of conformity in three cultures. *Journal of Personality and Social Psychology, 54,* 883–887.

Hendrick, C., & Brown, S. R. (1971). Introversion, extraversion, and interpersonal attraction. *Journal of Personality and Social Psychology, 20,* 31–35.

Hendrick, C., & Hendrick, S. S. (1986). A theory and method of love. *Journal of Personality and Social Psychology, 54,* 980–988.

Jang, S. J., & Thornberry, T. P. (1998). Self-esteem, delinquent peers, and delinquency: A test of the self-enhancement thesis. *American Sociological Review, 63,* 586–598.

Janis, I. L. (1954). Personality correlates of susceptibility to persuasion. *Journal of Personality, 22,* 504–518.

Janis, I. L., & Field, P. B. (1959). A behavioral assessment of persuasibility: Consistency of individual differences. In C. I. Hovland & I. L. Janis (Eds.), *Personality and persuasibility* (pp. 55–68). New Haven, CT: Yale University Press.

Jensen-Campbell, L. A., Graziano, W. G., & West, S. G. (1995). Dominance, prosocial orientation, and female preferences: Do nice guys really finish last? *Journal of Personality and Social Psychology, 68,* 427–440.

Kaplan, H. B. (1980). *Deviant behavior in defense of self.* New York: Academic Press.

Karney, B. R., & Bradbury, T. N. (1995). The longitudinal course of marital quality and stability: A review of theory, methods, and research. *Psychological Bulletin, 118,* 3–34.

Kelly, E. L., & Conley, J. J. (1987). Personality and compatibility: A prospective analysis of marital stability and marital satisfaction. *Journal of Personality and Social Psychology, 52,* 27–40.

Konovsky, M., & Wilsnack, S. C. (1982). Social drinking and self-esteem in married couples. *Journal of Studies on Alcohol, 43,* 319–333.

Kupersmidt, J. B., & Patterson, C. J. (1991). Childhood peer rejection, aggression, withdrawal, and perceived competence as predictors of self-reported behavior problems in preadolescence. *Journal of Abnormal Child Psychology, 19,* 427–449.

Kurdek, L. A. (1997). Relation between neuroticism and dimensions of relationship commitment: Evidence from gay, lesbian, and heterosexual couples. *Journal of Family Psychology, 11,* 109–124.

Kwan, V. S. Y., Bond, M. H., & Singelis, T. M. (1997). Pancultural explanations for life satisfaction: Adding relationship harmony to self-esteem. *Journal of Personality and Social Psychology, 73,* 1038–1051.

Lakey, B., Tardiff, T. A., & Drew, J. B. (1994). Negative social interactions: Assessment and relations to social support, cognition, and psychological distress. *Journal of Social and Clinical Psychology, 13,* 42–62.

Latkin, C. A. (1990). The self-concept of Rajneeshpuram commune members. *Journal for the Scientific Study of Religion, 29,* 91–98.

Leary, M. R. (1990). Responses to social exclusion: Social anxiety, jealousy, loneliness, depression, and low self-esteem. *Journal of Social and Clinical Psychology, 9,* 221–229.

Leary, M. R. (1995). *Self-presentation: Impression management and interpersonal behavior.* Boulder, CO: Westview Press.

Leary, M. R. (2001). Toward a conceptualization of interpersonal rejection. In M. R. Leary (Ed.), *Interpersonal rejection* (pp. 3–20). New York: Oxford University Press.

Leary, M. R., & Baumeister, R. F. (2000). The nature and function of self-esteem: Sociometer theory. In M. P. Zanna (Ed.), *Advances in experimental social psychology* (Vol. 32, pp. 1–62). San Diego, CA: Academic Press.

Leary, M. R., Cottrell, C. A., & Phillips, M. (2001). Deconfounding the effects of dominance and social acceptance on self-esteem. *Journal of Personality and Social Psychology, 81,* 898–909.

Leary, M. R., & Downs, D. L. (1995). Interpersonal functions of the self-esteem motive: The self-esteem system as a sociometer. In M. Kernis (Ed.), *Efficacy, agency, and self-esteem* (pp. 123–144). New York: Plenum Press.

Leary, M. R., Koch, E. J., & Hechenbleikner, N. R. (2001). Emotional responses to interpersonal rejection. In M. R. Leary (Ed.), *Interpersonal rejection* (pp. 145–166). New York: Oxford University Press.

Leary, M. R., & Kowalski, R. M. (1995). *Social anxiety.* New York: Guilford Press.

Leary, M. R., & Meadows, S. (1991). Predictors, elicitors, and concomitants of social blushing. *Journal of Personality and Social Psychology, 60,* 254–262.

Leary, M. R., Schreindorfer, L. S., & Haupt, A. L. (1995). The role of low self-esteem in emotional and behavioral problems: Why is low self-esteem dysfunctional? *Journal of Social and Clinical Psychology, 14,* 297–314.

Leary, M. R., Tambor, E., Terdal, S., & Downs, D. L. (1995). Self-esteem as an interpersonal monitor: The sociometer hypothesis. *Journal of Personality and Social Psychology, 68,* 518–530.

Lucas, R. E., Diener, E., & Suh, E. (1996). Discriminant validity of well-being measures. *Journal of Personality and Social Psychology, 71,* 616–628.

MacDonald, G., Saltzman, J. L., & Leary, M. R. (in press). Social approval and trait self-esteem. *Journal of Research in Personality.*

MacDonald, G., Zanna, M. P., & Holmes, J. G. (2000). An experimental test of the role of alcohol in relationship conflict. *Journal of Experimental Social Psychology, 36,* 182–193.

Mallandain, I., & Davies, M. F. (1994). The colors of love: Personality correlates of love styles. *Personality and Individual Differences, 17,* 557–560.

Maltby, J., & Day, L. (2000). The reliability and validity of a susceptibility to embarrassment scale among adults. *Personality and Individual Differences, 29,* 749–756.

Marsh, H. W., Antill, J. K., & Cunningham, J. D. (1989). Masculinity and femininity: A bipolar construct and independent constructs. *Journal of Personality, 57,* 625–663.

Masi, G., Favilla, L., Mucci, M., Poli, P., & Romano, R. (2001). Depressive symptoms in children and adolescents with dysthymic disorder. *Psychopathology, 34,* 29–35.

Mathes, E. W., Adams, H. E., & Davies, R. M. (1985). Jealousy: Loss of relationship rewards, loss of self-esteem, depression, anxiety, and anger. *Journal of Personality and Social Psychology, 48,* 1552–1561.

Mead, G. H. (1934). *Mind, self, and society.* Chicago: University of Chicago Press.

Miller, R. S. (1995). On the nature of embarrassability: Shyness, social evaluation, and social skill. *Journal of Personality, 63,* 315–339.

Miller, R. S. (1996). *Embarrassment: Poise and peril in everyday life.* New York: Guilford Press.

Mookherjee, H. N. (1986). Comparison of some personality characteristics of male problem drinkers in rural Tennessee. *Journal of Alcohol and Drug Education, 31,* 23–28.

Murphy, C. M., Meyer, S. L., & O'Leary, D. K (1994). Dependency characteristics of partner assaultive men. *Journal of Abnormal Psychology, 103,* 729–735.

Murray, S. L., Holmes, J. G., & Griffin, D. W. (2000). Self-esteem and the quest for felt security: How perceived regard regulates attachment processes. *Journal of Personality and Social Psychology, 78,* 478–498.

Murray, S. L., Holmes, J. G., & Griffin, D. W. (1996). The benefits of positive illusions: Idealization and the construction of satisfaction in close relationships. *Journal of Personality and Social Psychology, 70,* 79–98.

Murray, S. L., Holmes, J. G., MacDonald, G., & Ellsworth, P. C. (1998). Through the looking glass darkly? When self-doubts turn into relationship insecurities. *Journal of Personality and Social Psychology, 75,* 1459–1480.

O'Connor, L. E., Berry, J. W., & Weiss, J. (1999). Interpersonal guilt, shame, and psychological problems. *Journal of Social and Clinical Psychology, 18,* 181–203.

Ouellet, R., & Joshi, P. (1986). Loneliness in relation to depression and self-esteem. *Psychological Reports, 58,* 821–822.

Orlofsky, J. L., & O'Heron, C. A. (1987). Stereotypic and nonstereotypic sex role trait and behavior orientations: Implications for personal adjustment. *Journal of Personality and Social Psychology, 52,* 1034–1042.

Oyserman, D., & Markus, H. R. (1990). Possible selves and delinquency. *Journal of Personality and Social Psychology, 59,* 112–125.

Panak, W. F., & Garber, J. (1992). Role of aggression, rejection, and attributions in the prediction of depression in children. *Development and Psychopathology, 4,* 145–165.

Pandina, R. J., & Schuele, J. A. (1983). Psychosocial correlates of alcohol and drug use of adolescent students and adolescents in treatment. *Journal of Studies on Alcohol, 44,* 950–973.

Peiser, N. C., & Heaven, P. C. (1996). Family influences on self-reported delinquency among high school students. *Journal of Adolescence, 19,* 557–568.

Piers, E. V. (1984). *Piers–Harris Self-Concept Scale: Revised manual.* Los Angeles: Western Psychological Services.

Plutchik, R., Botsis, A. J., & Van Praag, H. M. (1995). Psychopathology, self-esteem, and ego functions as correlates of suicide and violence risk. *Archives of Suicide Research, 1,* 27–38.

Pullmann, H., & Allik, J. (2000). The Rosenberg Self-Esteem Scale: Its dimensionality, stability and personality correlates in Estonian. *Personality and Individual Differences, 28,* 701–715.

Raskin, R., Novacek, J., & Hogan, R. (1991). Narcissism, self-esteem, and defensive self-enhancement. *Journal of Personality, 59,* 19–38.

Rawson, H. E. (1992). The interrelationship of measures of manifest anxiety, self-esteem, locus of control, and depression in children with behavior problems. *Journal of Psychoeducational Assessment, 10,* 319–329.

Rigby, K., & Cox, I. (1996). The contribution of bullying at school and low self-esteem to acts of delinquency among Australian teenagers. *Personality and Individual Differences, 21,* 609–612.

Rigby, K., & Slee, P. T. (1993). Dimensions of interpersonal relation among Australian children and implications for psychological well-being. *Journal of Social Psychology, 133,* 33–42.

Romer, D. (1981). A person–situation causal analysis of self-reports of attitudes. *Journal of Personality and Social Psychology, 41,* 562–576.

Rosenberg, M. (1965). *Society and the adolescent self-image.* Princeton, NJ: Princeton University Press.

Rosenberg, M., Schooler, C., & Schoenbach, C. (1989). Self-esteem and adolescent problems: Modeling reciprocal effects. *American Sociological Review, 54,* 1004–1018.

Roth, D. L., Harris, R. N., & Snider, C. R. (1988). An individual differences measure of attributive and repudiative tactics of favorable self-presentation. *Journal of Social and Clinical Psychology, 6,* 159–170.

Russell, D., Cutrona, C., Rose, J., & Yurko, K. (1984). Social and emotional loneliness: An examination of Weiss' typology of loneliness. *Journal of Personality and Social Psychology, 46,* 1313–1321.

Russell, R. J., & Hulson, R. (1992). Physical and psychological abuse of heterosexual partners. *Personality and Individual Differences, 13,* 457–473.

Salovey, P., & Rodin, J. (1992). Provoking jealousy and envy: Domain relevance and self-esteem threat. *Journal of Social and Clinical Psychology, 10,* 395–413.

Santee, R. T., & Maslach, C. (1982). To agree or not to agree: Personal dissent amid social pressure to conform. *Journal of Personality and Social Psychology, 42,* 690–700.

Schlesinger, S., Susman, M., & Koenigsberg, J. (1990). Self-esteem and purpose in life: A comparative study of women alcoholics. *Journal of Alcohol and Drug Education, 36,* 127–141.

Schmidt, L. A., & Fox, N. A. (1995). Individual differences in young adults' shyness and sociability: Personality and health correlates. *Personality and Individual Differences, 19,* 455–462.

Schweitzer, R. D., Seth-Smith, M., & Callan, V. J. (1992). The relationship between self-esteem and psychological adjustment in young adolescents. *Journal of Adolescence, 15,* 83–97.

Sharp, M. J., & Getz, G. J. (1996). Substance use as impression management. *Personality and Social Psychology Bulletin, 22,* 60–67.

Shaver, P., Schwartz, J., Kirson, D., & O'Connor, C. (1987). Emotion knowledge: Further exploration of a prototype approach. *Journal of Personality and Social Psychology, 52,* 1061–1086.

Shechtman, Z. (1993). Group psychotherapy for the enhancement of intimate friendship and self-esteem among troubled elementary-school children. *Journal of Social and Personal Relationships, 10,* 483–494.

Shisslak, C. M., Pazda, S., & Crago, M. (1990). Body weight and bulimia as discriminators of psychological characteristics among anorexic, bulimic, and obese women. *Journal of Abnormal Psychology, 99,* 380–384.

Simons, K. J., Paternite, C. E., & Shore, C. (2001). Quality of parent/adolescent attachment and aggression in young adolescents. *Journal of Early Adolescence, 21,* 182–203.

Smart, R. G., & Walsh, G. W. (1993). Predictors of depression in street youth. *Adolescence, 28,* 41–53.

Smelser, N. J. (1989). Self-esteem and social problems: An introduction. In A. M. Mecca, N. J. Smelser, & J. Vasconcellos (Eds.), *The social importance of self-esteem* (pp. 1–23). Berkeley: University of California Press.

Spivey, E. (1990). *Social exclusion as a common factor in social anxiety, loneliness, jealousy, and social depression: Testing an integrative model.* Unpublished master's thesis, Wake Forest University, Winston-Salem, NC.

Stein, J. A., Newcomb, M. D., & Bentler, P. M. (1987). Personality and drug use: Reciprocal effects across four years. *Personality and Individual Differences, 8,* 419–430.

Stokes, J. P., & Levin, I. M. (1990). The development and validation of a measure of negative affectivity. *Journal of Social Behavior and Personality, 5,* 173–186.

Tangney, J. P., & Dearing, R. L. (2002). *Shame and guilt.* New York: Guilford Press.

Tarlow, E. M., & Haaga, D. A. F. (1996). Negative self-concept: Specificity to depressive symptoms and relation to positive and negative affectivity. *Journal of Research in Personality, 30,* 120–127.

Taylor, S. E., & Brown, J. D. (1988). Illusion and well-being: A social psychological perspective on mental health. *Psychological Bulletin, 103,* 193–210.

Tice, D. M. (1991). Esteem protection or enhancement? Self-handicapping motives and attributions differ by trait self-esteem. *Journal of Personality and Social Psychology, 60,* 711–725.

Vaux, A. (1988). Social and emotional loneliness: The role of social and personal characteristics. *Personality and Social Psychology Bulletin, 14,* 722–735.

Vega, W. A., Zimmerman, R. S., Warheit, G. J., & Apospori, E. (1993). Risk factors for early adolescent drug use in four ethnic and racial groups. *American Journal of Public Health, 83,* 185–189.

Vigil, J. D. (1988). *Barrio gangs: Street life and identity in southern California.* Austin: University of Texas Press.

Voss, K., Markiewicz, D., & Doyle, A. B. (1999). Friendship, marriage and self-esteem. *Journal of Social and Personal Relationships, 16,* 103–122.

Watson, D., & Clark, L. A. (1984). Negative affectivity: The disposition to experience aversive emotional states. *Psychological Bulletin, 96,* 465–490.

Watson, D., & Friend, R. (1969). Measurement of social–evaluative anxiety. *Journal of Consulting and Clinical Psychology, 33,* 448–457.

White, G. L., & Mullen, P. E. (1989). *Jealousy: Theory, research, and clinical strategies.* New York: Guilford Press.

Whitley, B. E. (1983). Sex role orientation and self-esteem: A critical meta-analytic review. *Journal of Personality and Social Psychology, 44,* 765–778.

Whitley, B. E., & Gridley, B. E. (1993). Sex role orientation, self-esteem, and depression: A latent variable analysis. *Personality and Social Psychology Bulletin, 19,* 363–369.

Williams, K. D. (1997). Social ostracism. In R. M. Kowalski (Ed.), *Aversive interpersonal behaviors* (pp. 133–170). New York: Plenum Press.

Williams, K. D., & Zadro, L. (2001). Ostracism: On being ignored, excluded and rejected. In M. R. Leary (Ed.), *Interpersonal rejection* (pp. 21–53). New York: Oxford University Press.

Wolfe, R. N., Lennox, R. D., & Cutler, B. L. (1986). Getting along and getting ahead: Empirical support for a theory of protective and acquisitive self-presentation. *Journal of Personality and Social Psychology, 50,* 356–361.

Yang, B., & Clum, G. A. (1996). Effects of early negative life experiences on cognitive functioning and risk for suicide: A review. *Clinical Psychology Review, 16,* 177–195.

PART V

INTERPERSONAL ASPECTS
OF THE SELF

21

The Relation of Self to Social Perception

DAVID DUNNING

When one begins a close and careful examination of the judgments people reach about other people, one is introduced quickly to a curious fact. People disagree, sometimes vehemently. If given a target to judge and exactly the same information about that target, two people can differ dramatically in the attributions they make for the target's behavior, the conclusions they reach about the target's character, and the predictions they make about how that target will behave in the future. Such disagreements are obvious to the researcher as he or she goes over the numerical ratings that participants provide on 7-point Likert scales in a psychological experiment. It is also obvious to the researcher when he or she returns home to discuss the latest escapade or policy pronouncement of whatever political candidate is on television.

In this chapter, I focus on one important source—or at least a significant predictor—of these disagreements in social judgment. That source is the self. Over the past century, psychological researchers and scholars have kept running into the fact that people's judgments of their peers and familiars seem to contain a heavy dose of the self. Such an observation came easily to the earliest mod-

ern scholars in psychology, writers coming from such diverse perspectives as James (1915), McDougall (1921), Mead (1934), Rogers (1951), and Sullivan (1947). Both Freuds (Anna and Sigmund) noted that people's judgments of others seemed designed to explain, excuse, or minimize certain feelings and beliefs about the self (A. Freud, 1936; S. Freud, 1924/1956). Combs and Snygg (1959) observed that the "self provides the frame of reference from which all else is observed. People are not really fat unless they are fatter than we" (p. 145). James (1915) remarked that self-understanding often involved watching others closely, to see "my own lusts in the mirror of the lusts of others" (p. 314). Krech, Crutchfield, and Ballachey (1962) professed that the "nature of the relationships of the self to other parts of the [psychological] field—to other objects, to people, to groups, to social organizations—is of critical importance" (p. 69).

Beyond broad theoretical generalizations, researchers in their data have found evidence, sometimes inadvertent, that social judgments are systematically and pervasively related to the perceiver's self-concept. For example, Hovland and Sherif (1952), while working on methods for measuring attitudes, began to notice a pervasive tendency for a person's own attitudes to influence his or her perceptions of the attitudes of others. Ross, Greene, and House (1977), while working on studies on causal attribution, stumbled on the pervasive tendency for people to overestimate the commonness of their own attitudes, dispositions, and responses in the general population.

However, even though research has established repeatedly that the self is in some way connected to how people perceive and evaluate others, researchers have yet to attack systematically two tasks that must be done to better understand the link between self and social judgment. The first task is to collate a far-flung collection of research phenomena strewn across many decades and research traditions and to organize it into a taxonomy of the ways the self is related to social judgment. The second is to see if there are any overall guiding principles that explain why people's self-views are so often implicated in their views of other people.

Thus, in this chapter, I set myself a twofold task. The first is to distill the miscellany of the self-related judgmental patterns into an initial classification scheme of the ways the self is linked to social judgment. In doing so, I categorize the literature into three different families of effects. First, the self produces *similarity effects* in social judgment. People assume that others are like them if they have no information or ambiguous information about those others. Second, the self produces *emphasis effects* in social judgment. People emphasize their own particular strengths and talents in their judgments of others. Third, the self produces *comparative effects* in social judgment. People compare the performances of others with their own to produce judgments of others.

The second task is to identify any general themes that would explain why the self is so often implicated in evaluations, predictions, and attributions of others. There are many candidate explanations for why the self looms over social perception so pervasively. For example, some scholars have suggested that one's own characteristics, habits, and attitudes tend to be *accessible* to the individual. They are easily brought to mind, and as a consequence they are easily applied to

other people and, once invoked, bring other aspects of the self to mind to bear on social judgment (Holyoak & Gordon, 1983; Prentice, 1990). Other scholars have suggested that the presence of the self in social judgment is a matter of *expertise*. People become experts in the traits and abilities they possess. They develop a sophisticated and complex understanding of what those traits signify. They become able to make many fine-grained evaluations about the trait and can do so quickly and efficiently (see, e.g., Markus, Crane, Bernstein, & Siladi, 1982). Thus it is not a surprise that people lean on this expertise when it comes time to judge others.

However, throughout the decades in which the relation of self to social judgment has been studied, one explanation has received continual and consistent empirical support. As a consequence, I emphasize it in my treatment of the links between the self and social judgment. That explanation focuses on the *symbolic functions* that social judgments are designed to serve (Dunning, 1999, 2000, in press). When people judge others, they act as though they are also implicitly judging themselves, that the conclusions they reach about other people imply certain conclusions about themselves. As a consequence, they tailor those judgments to ensure that those judgments comment favorably on themselves, making sure that those judgments are symbols that reaffirm positive images of self. They ensure that their pronouncements of others keep faith with the notion that they are wonderful, capable, and lovable human beings. As a consequence, it is inevitable that what they think about themselves becomes entwined in what they believe about others.

In this chapter, I begin by describing the three patterns of phenomena—similarity, emphasis, and comparative effects—that have implicated the self in social perception. I also discuss mechanisms that have been proposed to account for these patterns. I emphasize the symbolic functions that these patterns may serve, because that account has received the most consistent support across the relevant research, although I note some instances in which other psychological mechanisms have been supported by empirical evidence. I conclude by discussing possible avenues for future research.

Similarity Effects

When information about another person or a collection of other people is missing or ambiguous, people tend to assume that those others are similar to the self. This is true in their generalizations about peer groups and single individuals, as well as the abstract categories they use to judge themselves and other people. This observation is supported by work on the *false consensus effect, attributive projection,* and *self-serving trait definitions* in social judgment.

False Consensus

The false consensus effect refers to the tendency of people to overestimate the commonness of their own responses, attitudes, behaviors, and habits within the general population (Ross, Greene, & House, 1977; see G. Marks & Miller, 1987, for a review). Relative to their more honest peers, children who say they would cheat if given the chance predict that a greater number of their peers would cheat (Katz & Allport, 1931). College students who are willing to wear a sandwich board around campus beseeching others to "Repent" state that a greater proportion of their peers would do likewise than do students who refuse to wear the sign (Ross et al., 1977). Indeed, the false consensus has become one of the most documented phenomena in social psychological research (G. Marks & Miller, 1987), although (as I soon show) the phenomenon tellingly does not appear in all circumstances.

In some sense, basing one's estimate of how the general population will react to a situation on one's own reaction is quite sensible. One's own response is a datum, and hence may be a diagnostic and valuable indicator of how others would behave. However, a good deal of work on the false consensus effect has shown that false consensus does not arise simply because of the datum that one's own behavior provides. People tend to generalize from their own behavior to the general population much more than they are willing to generalize from the behavior of any single other individual. That is, the self is not just a useful data point but seems to be *a special* data point, one that is especially more diagnostic about how oth-

ers will behave than anyone else's behavior. In fact, the self is so special that when Krueger and Clement (1994) confronted participants with data showing that 20 of their peers would unanimously react the same way to a situation, people still primarily relied on their own reactions when they estimated how people in general would behave. To be sure, their estimates were swayed by the data about those 20 individuals, but those data failed to diminish in any way their reliance on their own reactions in estimating how the general population would behave.

What psychological mechanisms produce this reliance on the self to predict what others will do, thus giving rise to the false consensus effect? Many potential mechanisms have been proposed, and it is likely that they all conspire to bring the effect about. One such mechanism is *selective exposure* to similar others. People tend to surround themselves with like-minded folk. As a consequence, if they base their impressions of the general population on the behaviors and opinions of their acquaintances, they will overestimate how much people in general share their characteristics and opinions. Another mechanism consists of the logical fallout from the act of causal attribution. To the extent that people attribute their behavior to some feature of the choice or situation they confront (e.g., "I laughed because the movie was funny"), they believe that others will act similarly (see G. Marks & Miller, 1987, for a review of empirical evidence about these mechanisms).

One last mechanism, however, has received a good deal of empirical support. This mechanism centers on the desire people have to maintain positive impressions of the self. People overestimate how common their behaviors are because they wish to think favorably of themselves. At first blush, it may be difficult to see how seeing one's own response as relatively common would help maintain one's own self-worth. After all, would that not suggest that one is a rather typical, ordinary, or nondescript individual?

That conclusion would be correct, except that people are selective in their expression of false consensus. People express false consensus more enthusiastically on traits that they consider to be undesirable than they do on traits that they consider to be desirable.

Indeed, it is often difficult to observe people generalizing their own desirable traits onto the general population at all. One can see how this pattern of perception would aid the maintenance of self-esteem. By generalizing one's own shortcomings onto others, one can lessen the importance of those shortcomings. By refusing to generalize one's strengths to the general population, one can maintain the sense that one is uniquely skilled and competent.

Perhaps the most direct example of this selectivity in perceptions of consensus comes from Sherman, Presson, and Chassin (1984). They asked college undergraduates to look over two suicide notes, one real and one fake. In one condition, students were asked to select which note they believed to be the real one, after which they were told (based on a random schedule) that their choice had been correct or incorrect. In another condition, students read both notes, were told that one note was authentic and the other fabricated, and were told which note a previous student had chosen as real. They were then informed (again, according to a random schedule) that the other student had chosen correctly or incorrectly. Regardless of whether they chose a note or just heard about another student choosing a note, participants estimated the percentage of students who would choose the same note that they or the other student had.

Sherman and colleagues (1984) were interested in how choosing correctly (the desirable attribute) or incorrectly (the undesirable attribute) would influence participants' expression of false consensus relative to the second condition, in which another student had chosen correctly or incorrectly. They found that participants generalized their own behavior to other students more than they did the behavior of the second student—but only when the participant had chosen incorrectly. When participants had chosen incorrectly, they estimated that 57% of their peers would also choose the wrong note. However, when told only that another student had chosen incorrectly, they estimated that only 42% of their peers would do the same. Participants who were told they chose correctly showed no such evidence of generalizing their own responses to others more than they did that of the other student. When they themselves had chosen

the right suicide note, they estimated that 70% of their peers would do likewise, the exact same figure given when they were told that the second student had chosen the right note. In short, one's own choice was especially diagnostic of the general population only when one had chosen the undesirable response, not the desirable one.

Similar patterns of data that compare consensus estimates with actual prevalence rates have been reported by other researchers: Respondents who possess undesirable traits tend to overestimate the commonness of those traits among their peers. Respondents possessing desirable traits tend to underestimate the commonness of their desired traits among their peers, thus showing no false consensus whatsoever—and sometimes the opposite (Agostinelli, Sherman, Presson, & Chassin, 1992; Campbell, 1986; Goethals, 1986; Sherman, Presson, Chassin, Corty, & Olshavsky, 1983; Suls, Wan, & Sanders, 1988). Indeed, Mullen and Goethals (1990) conducted a meta-analysis of 134 tests of false consensus, splitting the tests into those focusing on negative, neutral, or positive attributes. Among negative attributes, they found robust tendencies toward false consensus. However, among positive attributes, they found a significant tendency for the opposite, an *under*estimation of one's own attributes among one's peers. In short, people tend to exhibit false consensus in a way that is congenial to the self: One's own shortcomings are common, and one's strengths unique.

Other empirical evidence, focusing on attitudes toward social issues rather than on personal attributes, shows a similar pattern. Campbell (1986) found that people perceived less false consensus for the attitudes that were important to them than for attitudes they did not feel were important. Similarly, Bosveld, Koomen, and van der Pligt (1996) found that committed Christians in the Netherlands estimated that their nation contained fewer Christians than did less committed Christians or "nonbelievers." This pattern of perception makes sense from a self-esteem point of view: Important attitudes best represent significant aspects of a person's self-concept, aspects that a person may wish to emphasize. As well, people like to think of themselves as morally righteous and intellectually superior to their peers. Often this requires people to think that they uniquely have the correct position on attitude issues and that people who think differently fail to share the same attitudes or the same moral stature.

Other research provides convergent evidence for this self-esteem account of the false consensus effect by examining consensus estimates when self-esteem in threatened. In one such study, Pyszczynski and colleagues (1996) showed that the magnitude of the false consensus effect is increased when people's mastery over their own fates is brought into doubt. Respondents were approached in two different locations. One location was directly in front of a funeral home, which Psyzynski and colleagues hypothesized would prompt participants to consider their own mortality and, thus, their fragile mastery over the future. Other respondents were approached either 100 meters before or 100 meters after they had passed a funeral home. As predicted, in front of the funeral home, respondents who were in the minority side of a number of social issues (e.g., the teaching of Christian values in schools) perceived higher consensus for their positions than they did elsewhere.[1]

Other research points to the motivated and managed nature of consensus estimates but suggests that the motivation need not necessarily be a desire for self-esteem. As pointed out by Brewer (1991, Chapter 24, this volume) in her optimal distinctiveness analysis, people possess two contradictory motivations that govern their perceptions of similarity to others. On the one hand, people like to be included in social groups and thus are motivated to emphasize the similarity between themselves and others. On the other hand, people also like to be distinct human beings and so also like to emphasize their differences from others.

According to Brewer (1991), people strive to keep perceptions of inclusion and distinctiveness in balance. When that balance is upset, people may emphasize perceptions of similarity or difference to regain a sense of equilibrium. Empirical evidence supports this analysis. In one experiment, participants were putatively given a personality test that categorized them as either a rather common type or as a rare one (Brewer & Weber, 1994). The researchers presupposed that participants placed in the common group would have their needs for inclusion met but would still have needs for distinctiveness. In contrast, participants placed in the rare group would have their desires for distinctness met but would still possess desires for inclusion. Participants' descriptions of another person in their personality type group were consistent with these presuppositions. Participants in the common group described an ingroup target as rather dissimilar from themselves, thus fulfilling a need for distinctiveness. Participants in the rare group, with their needs for distinctiveness quenched, rated an ingroup target as rather similar, thus fulfilling inclusion needs.

Attributive Projection

Whereas false consensus focuses on the relationship between the self and perceptions of the general population, attributive projection refers to the tendency for people to project their attitudes and attributes to specific other individuals (Holmes, 1968, 1978). This tendency has been documented in various forms. When people are asked to describe their acquaintances in open-ended formats, the traits that appear early and often in their descriptions tend to be the same ones that people use to describe themselves (Dornbusch, Hastorf, Richardson, Muzzy, & Vreeland, 1965; Lemon & Warren, 1974; Shrauger & Patterson, 1974). People who think of themselves as happy rate photographs of other people as happy relative to their unhappy peers (Goldings, 1954). Students filling out an inventory of interpersonal motives overestimate the extent to which an acquaintance will fill out the inventory in the same way (Bender & Hastorf, 1950). People playing prisoner's dilemma games are likely to assume that their playing partners will choose the same moves, cooperation or defection, as they do themselves (Messe & Sivacek, 1979). The social psychological literature is replete with demonstrations that people assume that other people, whether they be friends or individuals they just met, will possess the same traits, emotions, and motivations as they do themselves (for reviews, see Holmes, 1968, 1978).

But, again, this tendency is selective in ways that appear tailored to bolster self-esteem. People do not project their attributes onto just any other person. Instead, they generalize their attributes only to others whom they look on with some favor. In doing so, people reaffirm the desirability of their own personal attributes—their attributes must be desirable if they are shared with skilled, competent, or high-status others. For example, G. Marks and Miller (1982) showed that people project important, self-defining attributes only to those they consider desirable. They asked college students to indicate their attitudes on a series of important or trivial issues. They then presented these students with photographs of other college students, some of whom had been previously rated as physically attractive and some as unattractive. For each photograph, participants were asked to estimate the person's opinions on the same attitude issues. Students projected their attitudes on unimportant issues to both attractive and unattractive people. However, when it came to more important issues, students projected their attitudes onto only attractive others, indicating that people would project important self-attributes only to those they considered desirable (see Mashman, 1978, for similar findings).

Similar effects have been shown for impressions of political candidates. People assume that those candidates that they like share their attitudes on social issues (Judd, Kenny, & Krosnick, 1983). Importantly, longitudinal analyses suggest that it is attraction to the candidate that produces perceived similarity, not the other way around (Brent & Granberg, 1982). Indeed, Moreland and Zajonc (1982) presented experimental evidence that liking another individual prompted projection of one's own traits onto that other person. They manipulated the number of times that participants were exposed to differing photographs. Participants grew to like the photographs they had seen numerous times more than they did the photographs they had seen rarely. They were also more likely to imbue the people contained in those photographs with their own attitudes and values than they did the people depicted in rarely seen photos. Importantly, this tendency to project their own attributes onto frequently seen photographs was mediated by measures of attraction toward these photos.

Other experiments have also revealed the selective nature of attributive projection. Inspired by the clinical implications of the notion, several researchers in the 1960s and 1970s explored whether people would project their own stigmatized or undesirable traits onto others. In these studies, they did—but again only to people viewed favorably. For example, Sherwood (1979) presented nurses with personality test feedback that indicated that they were neurotic. When convinced by the evidence, nurses attributed more neuroticism to an individual they liked but not to an individual they disliked. Similarly, Secord, Backman, and Eachus (1964) told students that they possessed a trait that they had previously rated as undesirable. Presented with this information, students attributed more of the undesirable trait to their friends, but not to someone they disliked. Bramel (1963) showed male college students photographs of male nudes and informed them that they had shown signs of homosexual arousal (at that time a stigmatized characteristic). In response, participants who had high self-esteem perceived another college student, a favorable target, as displaying more homosexual arousal than they perceived a criminal, an undesirable target, doing.

Consistent with a self-esteem account, Lewicki (1984) found that attributive projection toward well-regarded others is exacerbated by esteem threat. He asked students at a Polish university to complete a questionnaire of "general psychological abilities" (actually, the Marlowe–Crowne Social Desirability Scale) and to help the experimenter to calculate their own scores on the test. In an esteem-bolstering condition, participants were told that they had scored a "276" on the test, and a surprised experimenter questioned the score because no one had ever scored that well. In an esteem-threatening condition, the participant scored the same "276," but the experimenter rather ominously began to console the participant for scoring so low. In this second condition, participants later showed more enthusiasm for projecting their positive strengths onto well-liked others, thus affirming the worth of the positive attributes. Participants in the esteem-bolstering condition showed less, if any, tendency toward attributive projection.

In short, the studies examining how people deal with feedback concerning undesirable attributes shows that they tend to project those attributes onto others, but only others that they hold in some esteem. The implications of this tendency for one's own self-esteem are clear. If other highly regarded individuals also share these negative traits, then those traits cannot be so bad. With this inference in place, the threat of these traits to one's esteem is deftly handled.

Given the theoretical impetus for studies on attributive projection, it is surprising that researchers failed to study another way in which such projective tendencies might be selective. If people project attributes onto others in order to enhance esteem, then they should be more enthusiastic about projecting negative attributes than positive ones onto other individuals. That is, much as has been found in studies on false consensus, people should minimize the importance of their negative traits by viewing them as common and maximize the importance of their positive traits by seeing them as unique.

However, one extant study can be construed as the selective projection of negative attributes over positive ones. Tesser and Campbell (1982) brought students into the laboratory and asked them to complete tests of "social sensitivity" and "aesthetic judgment." For each item on each test, experimenters gave participants feedback (according to random schedules) on whether they had responded correctly or incorrectly. Participants were then asked to predict whether a friend or a stranger would respond correctly. Estimates on this last measure showed evidence of selective projection. For the specific test the participant viewed as more important, participants predicted that their friends would do less well than a stranger. In short, when the ability in question was significant to the participant, he or she was more willing to project undesirable responses onto friends than onto strangers.[2]

Self-Serving Trait Definitions

Finally, people tend to project their own characteristics onto their definitions of the concepts and categories they use in their judgments of others. Ask people about the habits and skills necessary to be a leader, and the attributes they list may look a lot like their own. Whether people believe a leader should be extraverted or independent or ambitious or pleasant depends, in part, on whether they believe that they possess these traits themselves. Whether people think that an intelligent person can do math depends in part on whether that person feels he or she is mathematically skilled (Beauregard & Dunning, 2001; Dunning, Perie, & Story, 1991).

This projection of self on definitions of social traits and categories prompts people to make inferences about others that tend to reflect quite favorably on the self. For example, people judge others who have similar traits as more likely to be good leaders, intelligent, and outgoing than they do people possessing different attributes (Dunning et al., 1991; see also Beauregard & Dunning, 2001; McElwee, Dunning, Tan, & Hollman, 2001). People can also infer the reverse: that others who display high levels of skill must be similar to the self. For example, McElwee and colleagues (2001) asked college students to describe the personalities of four individuals overwhelmingly nominated as the best leaders they had ever heard of (e.g., Martin Luther King, Jr., Mahatma Gandhi). Students disagreed quite a bit in how they described these venerable individuals—and these disagreements tended to be systematically related to how students described themselves. People-oriented students described the leaders in more socially oriented terms than did their more task-oriented peers, who instead tended to emphasize such task skills as persistence and independence in their descriptions.

Kunda (1987) found a similar pattern in a study focusing on attributions for success versus failure. She asked college students to read over a case study of a person who had either succeeded or failed at a maintaining a twenty-five-year marriage. She then asked students which attributes of the person had been most crucial in creating that success or failure. When dealing with a successful individual, students tended to emphasize attributes that they shared with the target. For example, if the successfully married person was a firstborn child, participants who were themselves firstborn stated that birth order was a more important determinant of success than did those participants who were not firstborn. However, when dealing with a failure, students were disinclined to emphasize those shared attributes.

Again, there are many theoretical explanations for why people construct self-serving definitions of traits. For example, Story and Dunning (1998) found that people may come to possess self-serving trait definitions because life experiences lead them to conclude that they uniquely have the skills to succeed. For example, students receiving A's or B's in an introductory psychology based their definitions of the successful psychology student more on themselves than did those who received lackluster grades.

But, importantly, the theoretical explanation receiving the most empirical support once again focuses on the implications of these definitions for images of self. People are, again, selective in projecting themselves onto their definitions of social traits and abilities. This projection is constrained to desirable social concepts. When people consider undesirable concepts, they reverse the tendency to see themselves in that concept. Ask people whether letting other people choose the night's movie is submissive, and one finds that the answer depends on what the people believe they would do. Those who frequently let others decide the night's entertainment do not see this deference as submissive. People who assert that they keep the choice to themselves do label such deference as submissive (Dunning et al., 1991).

The construction of self-serving trait definitions is also sensitive to self-esteem concerns. It becomes more pronounced when self-esteem is threatened and evaporates after self-esteem is bolstered. In one study that examined this tendency, participants were brought into the laboratory and informed them that they would complete two tests that assessed their level of "integrative orientation" ability (Dunning, Leuenberger, & Sherman, 1995, Study 2). They were also informed that the ability was quite important and that students hoping to go to graduate or professional school would have their integrative orientation ability tested on standardized exams (e.g., the Graduate Record Exam) central to the application process. Participants then completed either a very difficult version of a test (the failure condition) or a very easy one (the success condition).

While waiting to take a second version of the test, participants were asked to complete a social judgment questionnaire unrelated to the test-taking study. The questionnaire presented participants with a description of a person who purportedly had taken part in longitudinal study on success in marriage. The character had enjoyed a long and happy marriage, and participants read over a brief description of the attributes and habits of the character. Participants were asked to relate the importance of several attributes, some of which they shared with the character and some of which they did not, for achieving that success in marriage. As to be expected, participants described attributes they shared with the character as being more important than the ones they did not—but only in the failure condition, that is, when their self-esteem was in need of some repair. Participants in the success condition, their self-esteem concerns presumably satiated, showed no evidence of such a self-aggrandizing tendency.

Emphasis Effects

The second major way in which the self is linked to social judgment is in matters of emphasis. People tend to emphasize their own particular strengths and proficiencies in their judgments of others. If a person believes they have a positive trait (e.g., sociability, intelligence, independence), they give that trait more weight in their judgments of others than if they think they have the complementary negative trait (e.g., unsociability, lack of intelligence, dependence). This tendency manifests itself in two different ways. First, people make more extreme judgments of others along favorable traits that they consider self-descriptive. Second, once they are given information about another person's standing along a favorable trait that they consider self-descriptive, they make more inferences about that person's other dispositions than when they are given information about a trait that they do not consider self-descriptive. In each case, the patterning of the emphasis of self-descriptive traits follows a symbolic logic of self-enhancement.

Polarized Judgments

People who believe they possess positive traits make more extreme evaluative judgments of others in those trait domains than do people who do not believe they possess the trait. For example, people who consider themselves "sociable" judge another person who exhibits outgoing behavior (e.g., tries to go to at least one party per week) as more sociable than do people who do not consider themselves to be sociable. The former group also rate people who show introverted behaviors (e.g., do not try to get acquainted with many of the neighbors at the dorm) as less sociable than the latter group (Lambert & Wedell, 1991). Such judgmental polarization effects have been seen in a variety of trait domains (Cromwell & Caldwell, 1962; Lambert & Wedell, 1991; Markus & Smith, 1981; Sedikides & Skowronski, 1993).

A similar phenomenon has been found in people's reactions to the classic prisoner's dilemma game. Those who are predisposed to cooperate (the socially desirable option) in the game, relative to those who would defect, tend to evaluate others more extremely based on whether they cooperate (good) or defect (bad; Beggan, Messick, & Allison, 1988). Similar polarization effects have been observed in attitude domains (Selltiz, Edrich, & Cook, 1965). For example, Judd and Johnson (1981) found that feminists committed to the cause tended to see the world in polarized terms, perceiving others as either feminist or antifeminist, with few people falling in between. Other researchers have noted that people make more confident judgments of others in trait domains in which they have positive impressions of themselves (Fong & Markus, 1982; Markus, Smith, & Moreland, 1985).

Two underlying mechanisms can be implicated in explaining this polarized pattern. The first mechanism involves, again, the management of social judgment for the protection of self-esteem. For people who view themselves positively in a trait domain, judging others in a polarized fashion bolsters their self-image. Others who are like them are seen as possessing the positive trait

in abundance. Others who are not like them are viewed as inferior to the self. For people who evaluate themselves more negatively in a given trait domain, muted judgments of others also serve self-esteem purposes. The unsociable person who learns that another person is a "party animal" need not view himself or herself as particularly less socially skilled than the other person. The unsociable person who hears that another does not like social occasions need not label that person (and the self) as socially deficient.

However, it could be argued that this pattern of polarized judgment need not be produced by the desire to think well of oneself. Instead, people who possess positive traits may become "expert" or "schematic" on those traits. That is, they develop richly organized and elaborated cognitive schemata that they apply to their social judgments (Kelly, 1955; Markus et al., 1982, 1985). This expertise in self-descriptive trait domains might prompt people to make more fine-grained distinctions in their judgments of other people's behavior. Because of this expertise, people might make more meaningful, and thus more extreme, judgments of others.

Both this self-image maintenance and the expertise account explain the pattern of judgmental polarization previously described. However, additional data suggest that the self-esteem explanation is a more successful account of this pattern. In particular, consider what happens when a positive behavior is turned into a negative. People who at first provided polarized evaluations of the behavior suddenly become more muted in their evaluations. For example, Eiser and Mower White (1974, 1975) presented teenagers with statements that took either "proauthority" or "antiauthority" stances. They found that their participants provided polarized judgments of the statements, but only when the particular scale on which they judged the statements portrayed their own position in favorable terms. Proauthority students, for instance, made extreme judgments on a scale that suggested that proauthority positions were "obedient," a favorable term, and antiauthority opinions were "disobedient," an unfavorable term. They enthusiastically labeled obedient behaviors as obedient and disobedient actions as disobedient. However, when presented with a scale that cast negative aspersions on proauthority positions, such as "unadventurous–adventurous," proauthority participants provided much more muted judgments. That is, they were much less likely to describe obedient behaviors as "unadventurous" and disobedient ones as "adventurous," although their antiauthority peers enthusiastically labeled obedience as "unadventurous" and disobedient actions as "adventurous" (see Eiser & van der Pligt, 1984, for a review).

Inference Effects

Beyond these extremity effects, people also make a broader range of inferences about other people when they receive information about traits they consider their own. For example, people with computer skills, relative to those without, give those skills greater weight when assessing another person's analytical ability (Hill, Smith, & Hoffman, 1988). Extraverted college students are more likely than their introverted peers to give great weight to social competence when predicting whether another person will achieve a successful college grade point average (Carpenter, 1988). Committed feminists make more inferences about the attitudes and attributes of others based on whether they share the same commitment (Judd & Johnson, 1981). A variety of studies in a number of domains have shown the same pattern: People make personality inferences about others based on whether those others share or fail to share the same strengths and abilities as the self (Alicke, 1993; Catambone & Markus, 1987; Crocker, Thompson, McGraw, & Ingerman, 1987; Markus et al., 1985; van der Pligt, 1984).

Indeed, this pattern of inference has led Lewicki (1983; see also Hill, Smith, & Lewicki, 1989) to propose that the self influences social judgment via a *self-image bias*. This bias refers to the fact that if people think they possess a desirable trait, then that trait becomes more central in their impressions of others. By central, Lewicki means that judgments along that trait dimension are more highly correlated with that person's judgments along all other trait dimensions. For example, if the trait *even-tempered* is central to the individual, then if

he or she considers another person to be even-tempered, he or she is likely to presume that that other person also possesses a good number of positive traits.

Although many researchers have documented inference effects in social judgment, this is one area in which there is little, if any, research on underlying mechanisms, although there are many candidates. For example, it may be the case that self-attributes, because they are cognitively accessible, are just more likely to evoke other accessible thoughts and beliefs (Dunning & Hayes, 1996). Or it may be the case that people develop expertise on self-relevant traits, and so when they judge others on these traits, they have a number of well-developed ideas and hypotheses to go beyond the information that they have been given (Markus et al., 1985). Or, consistent with a self-esteem account, when people conclude that another individual has a large number of desirable traits because they share the same strengths as the self, then people might be implicitly reinforcing the idea that their personal strengths are important for social life. Conversely, when people make relatively few inferences about another person in those domains representing their shortcomings, then they implicitly deny the importance of those shortcomings.

To date, only one psychological mechanism other than the ones just described, has received empirical study and support. That mechanism focuses on the lessons people learn as they succeed in life. As they succeed, they begin to conclude that they must have skills that are important. As a consequence, those skills become central in their impressions of others. Lewicki (1983) first demonstrated this in a study in which he gave participants personality feedback before examining whether they exhibited the self-image bias. Participants to whom he gave glowing and admiring feedback displayed the self-image bias much more than did those receiving lackluster and unfavorable feedback. In a different study conducted in a more real-world setting, college students doing well in a math class began to think of math skills as more central than did their counterparts who were doing rather poorly (Hill, Smith, & Lewicki, 1983). In short, the tendency toward these self-image effects, as well as inference effects more generally, are learned. People decide that their traits are central ones as they achieve success and decide on the lesson to draw from those successes.

However, this is only one extant study, and thus other potential explanatory accounts (e.g., availability, self-esteem maintenance) still remain plausible and untested. As a consequence, future research could profitably focus more squarely on the mechanisms that underlie inference effects in social judgment.

Comparative Effects

The final way in which the self connects to social judgment is through comparative effects. The self influences social judgment by being a common reference point against which to judge others. For example, is a person who plays pickup basketball 2 hours a week an athletic person? People tend to disagree to a surprising degree, with their judgments related to their own behavior. Those who do not participate in any athletic activity tend to see the basketball player as rather athletic. Those who devote a large chunk of their week to athletic pursuits tend to rate the individual as far less athletic. Such *contrast effects* in judgments of traits and abilities have been observed in a number of domains, such as math skill, intelligence, punctuality, and studiousness (Beauregard & Dunning, 1998; Dunning & Cohen, 1992; Dunning & Hayes, 1996).

Indeed, such contrast effects are some of the oldest documented phenomena implicating the self in social judgment. In the early 1950s, Hovland and Sherif (1952) noticed that whether participants saw statements about the civil rights movement as being *pro-* or *anti*-African American depended on their own attitudes toward civil rights. Those who favored civil rights saw moderate statements on the issue as anti-African American. Those who opposed civil rights viewed the exact same statements as more pro-African American. Such contrast effects in judgments of attitude were demonstrated for a number of social issues, such as prohibition (Hovland, Harvey, & Sherif, 1957), abortion (Corenblum & Corfield, 1976), the Arab–Israeli conflict (Prothro, 1955), and environmentalism (Bruvold, 1975). Still

older data reveal such contrast effects in people's judgments concerning the physical characteristics of others, such as height (Hinckley & Rethlingshafer, 1951) and skin color (Marks, 1943).

What produces these contrast effects? To be sure, one answer has been clearly articulated and supported by data. Sherif and Hovland (1961) suggested that the self serves as an anchor for social judgment. Indeed, Dunning and Hayes (1996) found evidence that people explicitly compare other people's behavior with their own as they reach social judgments. In one study, people admitted that they compared others to themselves when judging their peers. Participants were given a description of a target to judge along a number of trait and performance dimensions. Afterward, they were vaguely asked if they had compared the target with "anyone or anything" as they made their judgments. A full 70% of participants stated that they compared the target with themselves (the next most frequently comparison object was "acquaintances," at 38%). Another study revealed more unobtrusive evidence of this comparison process. Participants were asked either to judge another person (e.g., one who tended to be late to class one time per week) or to perform some other, filler task. Later, participants were asked to report on their own behavior in the same domain (e.g., are you late to class more than once a week?). Participants who had judged another person along a relevant trait reported their own behavior more quickly, indicating that they had thought about themselves as they judged that other person.

But why, of all the comparison points that one could use in social judgment, do people so commonly choose to use their own behavior? One answer is that one's own behavior can be quickly brought to mind when attempting to evaluate the actions of others. However, the explanation that has received the most support is one that focuses on concerns over self-esteem. People exhibit comparative effects to ensure that whatever judgment they make implies favorable conclusions about the self. If one looks at contrast effects, and specifically the conditions that increase and decrease the magnitude of these effects, one sees that the effect takes on a self-serving nature.

This is most evident in Study 4 by Dunning and Cohen (1992). In that study, paticipants evaluated targets who exhibited a high level of performance (e.g., spent 12 hours per week in athletic pursuits), a moderate level (e.g., spent 5 hours per week in athletic activities), or a low level (e.g., spent only 1 hour each week in such activities) elicited the strongest contrast effects. In all, participants judged behaviors that fell in the domains of athleticism, math skill, and studiousness.

Figure 21.1 offers a schematic of how evaluations of high-, medium-, and low-performing targets were related to the participant's own performance. As seen in the figure, evaluations tended to take on a self-serving cast. This is evident when one looks at the judgments provided by low- and high-performing participants separately. As seen in the figure, low-performing participants tended to rate all targets— regardless of their performance—rather positively. In doing so, they gave themselves permission to rate themselves positively as

well. In comparison, high-performing participants distinguished among the high-, medium-, and low-performing target a good deal, rating those targets they outperformed much more negatively. This pattern, too, can serve a self-esteem function. High-performing participants knew they possessed the relevant trait, and thus they could gain no self-esteem boost by rating everyone else highly, too. Instead, their self-esteem needs were better served by derogating the inferior performances of others to the extent that those performances allowed. In doing so, they could heighten the distinctiveness of their own achievements and habits.[3]

Further implicating self-esteem concerns in comparative effects, the appearance of contrast effects are also sensitive to momentary self-esteem issues. People show the contrast effect when their self-esteem is threatened, but not so much after their self-esteem is bolstered. In two studies, Beauregard and Dunning (1998) had participants either fail or succeed at a test of an intellectual ability. While waiting to take a second version of

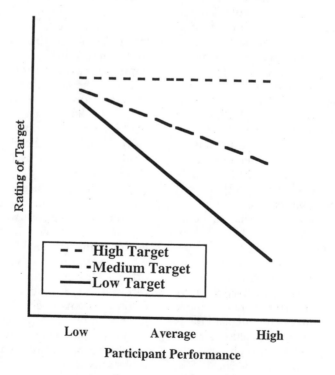

FIGURE 21.1. A schematic representation of how participants judge high-, medium-, and low-performing targets as a function of their own performance. Based on data from Dunning and Cohen (1992, p. 349).

the test, participants were asked to evaluate the intelligence of a character who had achieved a combined score of 1320 on his SAT. After failure, participants showed strong contrast effects. Participants with low SAT scores rated the target to be very intelligent (so that they could claim to be intelligent themselves; see Alicke, LoShiavo, Zerbst, & Zhang, 1997, for similar data). Participants with high SAT scores rated the target as rather unintelligent (affirming their own intelligence relative to other people). After success, no such difference between low-scoring and high-scoring SAT participants emerged. Regardless of their own SAT scores, they rated the target as rather intelligent.

Directions for Future Research

Although there has been a good deal of research demonstrating that the self is often involved in social judgment, one might have noted that the research has rarely been theoretically or empirically organized. The research is ad hoc and far-flung. Researchers note in their data that the self is correlated with and seems to influence how people evaluate others, but then they move on to other topics. To be sure, some specific phenomena have received exhaustive and systematic study, such as the contrast effect (Sherif & Hovland, 1961) and false consensus (Ross et al., 1977), but much of the work has not (e.g., inference effects). In addition, researchers have yet to take care to examine commonalities and differences in all the self-related effects that have arisen in the literature to see if there are any underlying themes or theoretical models that could link all these phenomena together. This chapter can be considered a start in that direction, but it is, of course, one very small step.

One direction for future research would be to continue to examine the breadth of self-effects to examine underlying mechanisms that may explain all of them in common. I have outlined one here—the desire to maintain and bolster a positive self-image via one's judgments of others—but there may be other mechanisms responsible, in part, for many of the phenomena enumerated herein. Thus future research could prof-

itably return to the many candidate mechanisms that researchers have more often proposed than empirically verified (e.g., accessibility, expertise, learning) to see if they also help to account for the imprint of the self on social judgment.

But besides further study of the underlying themes and mechanisms that account for all the relations of the self to social judgment, the review in this chapter suggests three further, perhaps more constrained, avenues for thought and effort.

The Interpersonal Self

Looking over the research that has been reviewed in this chapter, one sees that it has concentrated on only a specific type of "self" for study. That self is the *intrapersonal* self, the one defined by one's inborn characteristics—the internal dispositions, abilities, and attitudes that define who a person is. There are other ways to define the self. For example, one can consider an *interpersonal* self, one that is defined by one's social relations with other people, as well as their interpersonal niche in the overall social world. Does one have the right friends? Does one have status? Does one garner respect among others?

That is, each individual finds himself or herself in a web of complex social relations. It is likely that people's thoughts about where they fit in this web has a significant effect on their judgments of others. In particular, people might be motivated to believe that their place in their particular web is a favorable, or at least an appropriate, one. Similar to observations about the intrapersonal self, people may be eager to maintain a positive image of the interpersonal self.

In particular, in any web of social relations, some people have more status than others and some have more power over the behavior and fates of others. It is likely that people want to believe that their niche in any status hierarchy is a fair and correct one and thus manage their social judgments accordingly. The notion that concerns over one's own status has an impact on their perceptions of others is not a new one, at least in one area of social psychological inquiry. In the area of intergroup relations, Lippman (1922) noted several decades ago that people form stereotypes of other groups as "defenses of [their] position in society" (p. 95). Other theorists have noted how stereotypes of groups who are "second-class" citizens have grown from their position of low status in society. For example, contemporary stereotypes of African Americans in the United States can be traced to their former status as slaves. A major part of the stereotype, such as the notion that slaves were childlike and unreliable, served to justify the constant supervision that overseers and slaveowners provided (Sunar, 1978). Similarly, stereotypes of women as emotional and nurturing can be traced to the role to which they have been traditionally constrained in Western society (Hoffman & Hurst, 1990; Jost & Banaji, 1994; Sunar, 1978).

Further evidence ties the nature of these stereotypes to concerns over status. Ashmore and McConahay (1975), for example, found that individuals had more negative stereotypes of the poor to the extent that they themselves were high on the socioeconomic ladder. Presumably, those with high status had more status to preserve and justify, and they justified their place in society implicitly through their explicit attitudes toward those lacking in that status. More telling, Sidanius, Pratto, and Bobo (1996) found that negative attitudes toward African Americans were more prevalent among European American respondents who reported high levels of "social dominance orientation," that is, a concern over the status of one's group relative to others. Presumably, those concerned with their own group's maintaining higher status over others were willing to adopt negative attitudes toward lower status groups.

However, evidence about concerns of status and reports of negative stereotypes carries two weaknesses. First, virtually all of it is correlational, and so it is unclear whether the desires to maintain status play a causal role in social stereotypes and interpersonal judgments. Many other explanations of the link between status and stereotyping can be offered that do not invoke a need to maintain one's status in the social world (Sunar, 1978). Second, the preceding data fail to show whether concerns over status and power in the personal realm, rather than at the societal level, lead people to manage their judgments of others. Does a boss, for example, tailor his or her judgments of employees to bolster the belief that his or her authority over them is appropriate?

One research program suggests that concerns over power and status in the personal realm can influence social judgment, often leading people to denigrate those they have power over. Kipnis (1972) examined the impact of giving power to an individual on his or her judgments of others. Participants were all assigned the role of supervisor, overlooking the efforts of four high school students working in the next building. Some participants were given little power to control the behavior of those students. Others were given a good deal of power over the students. For example, they could communicate with the students over an intercom and revise the pay schedule they used to reward the high schoolers. In actuality, the high school students did not exist, and so Kipnis could arrange for the "students" in each condition to perform at equivalent levels. Participants who thought they had a high level of power relative to their low-power counterparts disparaged their underlings, rating their performance and motivation more negatively. This result can be read as an attempt by participants to justify their own status and performance in the experiment. In follow-up research conducted in the field, Kipnis and colleagues found that marriage partners who perceived themselves as having a high degree of influence over their partners rated themselves as superior to their partners. Housewives who viewed themselves as having influence over housemaids described their employees as less motivated than did those who thought they had little influence (Kipnis, Castell, Gergen, & Mauch, 1976).

Boundaries

Another avenue of future research could profitably explore the boundary conditions constraining the relationship of self to social judgment. Consider, for example, the issue of individual differences. Who is more likely to invoke thoughts of self in judgments of others, and who is more likely to avoid doing so?

One possible individual difference that might predict the presence of self in social judgment is suggested by the pervasive presence of self-esteem concerns. If people involve the self to judge others because they are protecting their self-esteem, then such activity should be present only when people have self-esteem to protect. When self-esteem is low, one should see much smaller doses of the self in judgments of others.

Thus a straightforward prediction would be that low self-esteem would serve as a boundary condition for the impact of self on social judgment. People with low self-esteem should show less, or perhaps even none, of the previously documented self-serving tendencies in their social judgments. Indeed, in ongoing work in my laboratory, we have found evidence that the impact of self on social judgment is reduced for people with low self-esteem (Beauregard & Dunning, 2001). Individuals with low self-esteem articulate fewer self-serving trait definitions than their peers with high self-esteem do. For example, Figure 21.2 shows the degree to which participants with high and low self-esteem defined traits in self-serving ways. As seen in the figure, participants with high esteem tended to emphasize their behaviors and attributes when defining positive traits but to deemphasize them when defining negative ones. Participants with low esteem showed much less tendency to follow this pattern. Their definitions of positive and negative traits were still somewhat self-serving, but they were not as self-serving as their peers, who presumably had

positive self-images to protect. Further research focusing on reaction-time data and judgments of others affirmed this diminished tendency for individuals with low esteem to construct self-serving trait definitions. Individuals with high self-esteem tend to rate others who have similar attributes more favorably than they do individuals who possess dissimilar attributes. Individuals with low self-esteem show this tendency to a markedly less degree.

In another study, we found that people with negative self-views also fail to show comparative contrast effects in social judgment (Dunning & Beauregard, 2000). In that study, we selected college students who had either high or low opinions of their social skills. We then gave them a test that purportedly evaluated those skills. People with high self-views tended to use their own performances—in self-serving ways—as reference points when they judged others. When they performed poorly, they rated the performances of others favorably, regardless of whether those others had done horribly or quite well. However, when participants with positive self-views performed well, they denigrated the performances of people they had outperformed. Participants with low opinions of their social skills showed no such evidence of using their own performance as a reference point against which to judge others. Whether they did well or not had no effect on their evaluations of others.

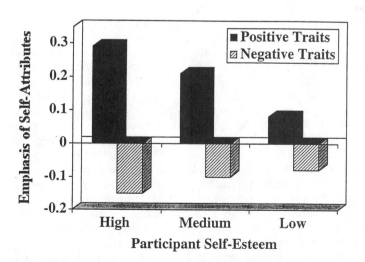

FIGURE 21.2. Emphasis of self-attributes in definitions of positive and negative traits as a function of the participant's self-esteem. Based on data from Beauregard and Dunning (2001).

To be sure, they were paying attention, in that their judgments were influenced by whether the target had performed well or poorly, but data about the self did not influence what they thought about those performances.

Costs and Benefits

Other avenues of research could profitably explore the costs and benefits of the connection between self and social judgment. Are people better or worse off because they engage in such practices, or does it depend on the circumstances? Such a question is probably best answered by focusing separately on the short and the long term.

In the short term, the key question is whether the presence of the self in social judgment ultimately bolsters what it appears designed to bolster—namely, positive images of self. Does managing judgments of others leave people with more favorable self-esteem? Does it reduce the anxiety associated with questions about one's abilities and proficiencies?

There are some studies that have explored this issue, although their number is small. Bennett and Holmes (1978) exposed participants to failure on a putatively important test. One group was then asked to predict how three of their friends would have done on the test, whereas another group provided no such predictions. On subsequent measures of anxiety, the first group expressed significantly less anxiety than did the second.

In similar research, Alicke and colleagues (1997) allowed participants to evaluate the performance of another individual who had outperformed them on a task. When given a chance to evaluate that other individual, participants tended to rate that person rather highly (a contrast effect). Subsequently, when compared with a group who provided no ratings, participants who had evaluated the other person also tended to rate themselves as rather more intelligent. That is, in labeling the person who outperformed them as a "genius," people gave themselves the opportunity to think of themselves as rather intelligent. However, other research has suggested that such effects may be inconsistent (see the debate between Holmes, 1978, 1981, and Sherwood,

1981, 1982). As such, the question of whether the management of social judgment leads to short-term benefits is an open one requiring more data.

For the long term, the benefit that symbolic management processes would provide is straightforward. If one shapes judgment after judgment of other people in order to bolster positive images of self, then one should be left with a rather favorable impression of oneself. And, indeed, that is what the literature shows: People tend to have favorable views of themselves, their abilities, and their achievements. Indeed, their impressions tend to be too favorable when compared with objective criteria (Alicke, 1985; Brown, 1986; Dunning, Meyerowitz, & Holzberg, 1989; Epley & Dunning, 2000; Kruger & Dunning, 1999; Weinstein, 1980) or the impressions of their peers (Hayes & Dunning, 1997).

Dunning and colleagues (1989) directly showed how the management of the definitions of social traits and categories led to rather favorable impressions of self. When people evaluate themselves on trait dimensions that allow for self-serving trait definitions, they tend to provide self-evaluations that are far too favorable to be possible. For example, on ambiguous traits, such as *disciplined, idealistic,* and *sophisticated,* that allow respondents to construct self-serving trait definitions, a large number of them rate themselves as "above average" among their peers, whereas very few rate themselves as "below average." Of course, it is objectively impossible for so many people to possess above-average impressions when so few people rate themselves as below average. Such logically indefensible evaluations are not observed for traits that have clear-cut, unambiguous definitions (e.g., *punctual, thrifty, wordy, sarcastic*) that people cannot rearrange to their own benefit (Dunning et al., 1989; Hayes & Dunning, 1997). For these traits, the average rating among respondents converges on "average," where it logically and statistically should.

However, one caveat: I have described people's rather positive self-impressions as a "benefit," but could they also be considered a cost? Researchers disagree on the ultimate payoff, positive or negative, of these unrealistically favorable impressions of self. Taylor and Brown (1988) have argued that a little positive illusion can go a long way toward providing the individual with happiness and good psychological adjustment. Other researchers disagree (Colvin & Block, 1994; Colvin, Block, & Funder, 1995). As such, the question of whether the self-serving management of social judgment is, in the long run, a benefit or a detriment to the individual will probably reside in the resolution of this current controversy about benefits and costs of unrealistic self-assessments.

But beyond that discussion, I think there is one cost prompted by the management of social judgment that is more self-evident. This cost comes not from examining the consequences for the individual but rather for any collection of individuals committed to working together toward some goal, even if the goal is just "getting along." The impact of self on social judgment causes people to disagree in their assessments of others (Dunning, 1999, in press; Dunning & Cohen, 1992; Dunning & Hayes, 1996; Dunning & McElwee, 1995; Dunning et al., 1991; Hayes & Dunning, 1997). These disagreements, at times, could be the source of much interpersonal conflict and disengagement. If people fail or refuse to recognize that concerns over self-image can be the source of these disagreements, then the resolution of these differences may be difficult if not impossible to achieve. As such, whereas the issue of costs and benefits may be controversial when examined at the level of the individual, it is clearer at the level of the collective.

Conclusions

In sum, the research reviewed herein has revealed that the self is linked to social judgment in a myriad of ways. However, after reviewing the literature, it appears that the diversity and abundance of these findings can be safely grouped into three families of phenomena. First, given little or no information about others, people assume similarity between themselves and others. Second, if given specific and concrete information about another individual, they emphasize that information if they think it falls into a trait domain they feel particularly proficient in. In such cases, they will make extreme

and confident evaluations and will make many inferences about the personality of the other individual, and they hold their evaluation of the individual in that domain as central in their overall impression. If they do not feel proficient, they will be less likely to make confident evaluations and personality inferences. Finally, people compare the performances of others with their own, using their own behavior as a benchmark against which to judge the behavior of others.

But beyond this classification of self-effects on social judgment, I explored the mechanisms that might underlie all these self-effects. Many have been proposed (e.g., accessibility, expertise, learning), but one mechanism has received more attention, and more consistent empirical documentation, than the others. That mechanism centers on the symbolic functions of social judgment. The self is so commonly implicated in social judgment because of a "hidden agenda" that people possess. Social judgment is a symbolic act, one that holds tacit implications for the self. As such, people treat evaluations of others as evaluations of themselves, even when the self is not being explicitly judged, and thus manage their judgments of others to affirm and retain flattering self-images. In support of this proposal, I noted how many phenomena—false consensus, attributive projection, self-serving trait definitions, polarized appraisals of others, inference effects, and egocentric contrast effects—tend to reflect favorably on the self. Further tying the operation of these phenomena to the agenda of esteem maintenance, I found that the degree of many of these phenomena was greater when esteem was threatened than when that esteem was bolstered.

But any careful reading of the chapter will quickly reveal that much work—theoretical and empirical—has yet to be done to completely describe all the ways in which the relation of self to social judgment reveals itself. Many plausible mechanisms that could explain the link have not been completely studied. Researchers have yet to consider all the possible boundary conditions that might limit conditions under which the self has its influence. As well, researchers have focused on the impact of an intrapersonal self on social judgment while ignoring potential ideas that may be inspired by thinking about the self as an interpersonal being. Scholars have yet to think through the many ways in which "self thinking" in social judgment might provide benefits or produce costs. As such, although it has been an issue that researchers have returned to throughout the past century, the relation of self to social judgment still remains a potentially fruitful topic of research for many years ahead.

Notes

1. Careful readers will note that an esteem-maintaining account of the false consensus effects in the Pyszczynski and colleagues (1996) study contradicts the findings of Campbell (1986) and Bosveld and colleagues (1996), in which self-esteem concerns produce *less* false consensus, not more. A reconciliation can be proposed between these contradictory statements. Worries about self-esteem might cause less false consensus when people consider their abilities or their most self-defining attitudes (as was the case in both the Campbell and Bosveld and colleagues studies). Self-esteem worries, however, may cause more false consensus when people consider their attitudes and opinions more generally, including ones they consider not so important (e.g., Pyszczynski et al., 1996). However, this is a speculation, and future empirical work could be devoted to delineating the complexities and nuances undoubtedly linked to a symbolic management account of social judgment.

2. Some attentive readers, knowledgeable about the intellectual history of psychology, might be surprised by this discussion of projection. As originally described by S. Freud (1924/1956), projection was not about seeing one's own characteristics in others but rather seeing in others the characteristics one *denied* in oneself. That is, if a person denied being selfish, he or she was prone to see selfishness in others. If people wanted to deny being anxious, they were driven to see anxiety in others. To be sure, this type of projection, termed *classical* or *defensive* projection, has been studied, although not as much as has its attributive cousin (for a review, see Holmes, 1978), and the empirical support for the phenomenon is problematic (see exchanges by Holmes, 1981; Sherwood, 1981, 1982). One recent research stream, however, has suggested a way in which defensive projection arises. When people wish to deny a trait in themselves, they begin to monitor themselves for any sign of the trait. If they see that sign, they suppress it. However, because they keep the trait in mind, it becomes cognitively available for them to apply to others, and they do so with greater frequency (Newman, Duff, & Baumeister, 1997). As a consequence, not only do people attribute to others traits that they believe they possess, but they also see in others traits that they wish to disown in themselves.

3. In this regard, two points must be made about contrast effects in social judgment. First, the pattern of responses depicted in Figure 21.1 looks much like a polarization effect in disguise. People whose performances are on the desirable end of the scale make more extreme judgments of others, particularly in the negative direction, than do people on the undesirable end of the scale (a point also made by Eiser & van der Pligt, 1984). As such, comparative effects may actually be an emphasis effect by another name, or, alternatively, polarized judgments might be produced by comparative mechanisms.

Acknowledgments

Preparation of this chapter was facilitated by National Institute of Mental Health Grant No. R01 56072. I thank Bill Klein and Keith Beauregard for their comments on an earlier version of the manuscript. Mark Stalnaker is commended for his legwork in tracking down many of the articles cited.

References

Agostinelli, G., Sherman, S. J., Presson, C. C., & Chassin, L. (1992). Self-protection and self-enhancement biases in estimates of population prevalence. *Personality and Social Psychology Bulletin, 18,* 631–642.

Alicke, M. D. (1985). Global self-evaluation as determined by the desirability and controllability of trait adjectives. *Journal of Personality and Social Psychology, 49,* 1621–1630.

Alicke, M. D. (1993). Egocentric standards of conduct evaluation. *Basic and Applied Social Psychology, 14,* 171–192.

Alicke, M. D., LoSchiavo, F. M., Zerbst, J., & Zhang, S. (1997). The person who outperforms me is a genius: Maintaining perceived competence in upward social comparison. *Journal of Personality and Social Psychology, 72,* 781–789.

Ashmore, R. D., & McConahay, J. B. (1975). *Psychology and American's urban dilemmas.* New York: McGraw-Hill.

Beauregard, K. S., & Dunning, D. (1998). Turning up the contrast: Self-enhancement motives prompt egocentric contrast effects in social judgments. *Journal of Personality and Social Psychology, 74,* 606–621.

Beauregard, K. S., & Dunning, D. (2001). Defining self-worth: Trait self-esteem moderates the use of self-serving social definitions in social judgment. *Motivation and Emotion, 25,* 132–165.

Beggan, J. K., Messick, D. M., & Allison, S. T. (1988). Social values and egocentric bias: Two tests of the might over morality hypothesis. *Journal of Personality and Social Psychology, 55,* 606–611.

Bender, I. E., & Hastorf, A. H. (1950). The perception of persons: Forecasting another person's responses on three personality scales. *Journal of Abnormal and Social Psychology, 45,* 566–561.

Bennett, D. H., & Holmes, D. S. (1978). Influence of denial (situational redefinition) and projection on anxiety associated with threat to self-esteem. *Journal of Personality and Social Psychology, 32,* 915–921.

Bosveld, W., Koomen, W., & van der Pligt, J. (1996). Estimating group size: Effects of category membership, differential construal and selective exposure. *European Journal of Social Psychology, 26,* 523–535.

Bramel, D. A. (1963). Selection of a target for defensive projection. *Journal of Abnormal and Social Psychology, 66,* 318–324.

Brent, E., & Granberg, D. (1982). Subjective agreement with the presidential candidates of 1976 and 1980. *Journal of Personality and Social Psychology, 42,* 393–403.

Brewer, M. B. (1991). The social self: On being the same and different at the same time. *Personality and Social Psychology Bulletin, 17,* 474–482.

Brewer, M. B., & Weber, J. G. (1994). Self-evaluation effects of interpersonal versus intergroup social comparison. *Journal of Personality and Social Psychology, 66,* 268–275.

Brown, J. D. (1986). Evaluations of self and others: Self-enhancement biases in social judgment. *Social Cognition, 4,* 353–376.

Bruvold, W. H. (1975). Judgmental bias in the rating of attitude statements. *Educational and Psychological Measurement, 35,* 605–611.

Campbell, J. D. (1986). Similarity and uniqueness: The effects of attribute type, relevance, and individual differences in self-esteem and depression. *Journal of Personality and Social Psychology, 50,* 281–294.

Carpenter, S. L. (1988). Self-relevance and goal-directed processing in the recall of weighting of information about others. *Journal of Experimental Social Psychology, 24,* 310–322.

Catambone, R., & Markus, H. (1987). The role of self-schemas in going beyond the information given. *Social Cognition, 5,* 349–368.

Colvin, C. R., & Block, J. (1994). Do positive illusions foster mental health? An examination of the Taylor and Brown formulation. *Psychological Bulletin, 116,* 3–20.

Colvin, C. R., Block, J., & Funder, D. (1995). Overly positive self-evaluations and personality: Negative implications for mental health. *Journal of Personality and Social Psychology, 68,* 1152–1162.

Combs, A. W., & Snygg, D. (1959). *Individual behavior: A perceptual approach to behavior.* New York: Harper.

Corenblum, B., & Corfield, V. K. (1976). The effect of attitude and statement of favorability upon the judgment of attitude statements. *Social Behavior and Personality, 4,* 249–256.

Crocker, J., Thompson, L., McGraw, K., & Ingerman, C. (1987). Downward comparison, prejudice, and evalua-

tions of others: Effects of self-esteem and threat. *Journal of Personality and Social Psychology, 52,* 907–916.

Cromwell, R. L., & Caldwell, D. F. (1962). A comparison of ratings based on personal constructs of self and others. *Journal of Clinical Psychology, 1,* 43–46.

Dornbusch, S. M., Hastorf, A. J., Richardson, S. A., Muzzy, R. E., & Vreeland (1965). The perceiver and the perceived: Their relative influence on the categories of interpersonal cognition. *Journal of Personality and Social Psychology, 1,* 671–684.

Dunning, D. (1999). A newer look: Motivated social cognition and the schematic representation of social concepts. *Psychological Inquiry, 10,* 1–11.

Dunning, D. (2000). Social judgment as implicit social comparison. In J. Suls & L. Wheeler (Eds.), *Handbook of social comparison: Theory and research* (pp. 353–378). New York: Kluwer Academic/Plenum Press.

Dunning, D. (in press). The zealous self-affirmer: How and why the self lurks so pervasively behind social judgment. In. S. Spencer & S. Fein (Eds.), *Motivated social perception: The ninth Ontario Symposium.* Mahwah, NJ: Erlbaum.

Dunning, D., & Beauregard, K. S. (2000). Regulating others to affirm images of the self. *Social Cognition, 18,* 198–222.

Dunning, D., & Cohen, G. L. (1992). Egocentric definitions of traits and abilities in social judgment. *Journal of Personality and Social Psychology, 63,* 341–355.

Dunning, D., & Hayes, A. F. (1996). Evidence for egocentric comparison in social judgment. *Journal of Personality and Social Psychology, 71,* 213–229.

Dunning, D., Leuenberger, A., & Sherman, D. A. (1995). A new look at motivated inference: Are self-serving theories of success a product of motivational forces? *Journal of Personality and Social Psychology, 69,* 58–68.

Dunning, D., & McElwee, R. O. (1995). Idiosyncratic trait definitions: Implications for self-description and social judgment. *Journal of Personality and Social Psychology, 68,* 936–946.

Dunning, D., Meyerowitz, J. A., & Holzberg, A. D. (1989). Ambiguity and self-evaluation: The role of idiosyncratic trait definitions in self-serving assessments of ability. *Journal of Personality and Social Psychology, 57,* 1082–1090.

Dunning, D., Perie, M., & Story, A. L. (1991). Self-serving prototypes of social categories. *Journal of Personality and Social Psychology, 61,* 957–968.

Eiser, J. R., & Mower White, C. J. (1974). Evaluative consistency and social judgment. *Journal of Personality and Social Psychology, 30,* 349–359.

Eiser, J. R., & Mower White, C. J. (1975). Categorization and congruity in attitudinal judgment. *Journal of Personality and Social Psychology, 31,* 769–775.

Eiser, J. R., & van der Pligt, J. (1984). Accentuation theory, polarization, and the judgment of attitude statements. In J. R. Eiser (Ed.), *Attitudinal judgment* (pp. 43–63). New York: Springer-Verlag.

Epley, N., & Dunning, D. (2000). Feeling "holier than thou": Are self-serving assessments produced by errors in self or social prediction? *Journal of Personality and Social Psychology, 79,* 861–875.

Fong, G., & Markus, H. (1982). Self-schemas and judgments about others. *Social Cognition, 3,* 191–204.

Freud, A. (1936). *The ego and the mechanisms of defence.* New York: International Universities Press.

Freud, S. (1956). Further remarks on the defense neuropsychoses. In P. Rieff (Ed.), *Collected papers of Sigmund Freud* (Vol. 1, pp. 155–182). London: Hogarth Press. (Original work published 1924)

Goethals, G. R. (1986). Fabricating and ignoring social reality: Self-serving estimates of consensus. In J. M. Olson, C. P. Herman, & M. P. Zanna (Eds.), *Social comparison and relative deprivation: The Ontario Symposium* (Vol. 4, pp. 135–157). Hillsdale, NJ: Erlbaum.

Goldings, H. J. (1954). On the avowal and projection of happiness. *Journal of Personality, 23,* 30–47.

Hayes, A. F., & Dunning, D. (1997). Construal processes and trait ambiguity: Implications for self–peer agreement in personality judgment. *Journal of Personality and Social Psychology, 72,* 664–677.

Hill, T., Smith, N. D., & Hoffman, H. (1988). Self-image bias and the perception of other persons' skills. *European Journal of Social Psychology, 18,* 293–297.

Hill, T., Smith, N. D., & Lewicki, P. (1989). The development of self-image bias: A real-world demonstration. *Personality and Social Psychology Bulletin, 15,* 205–211.

Hinckley, E., & Rethlingshafer, D. (1951). Value judgments of heights of men by college students. *Journal of Psychology, 31,* 257–296.

Hoffman, C., & Hurst, N. (1990). Gender stereotypes: Perception or rationalization? *Journal of Personality and Social Psychology, 58,* 197–208.

Holmes, D. S. (1968). Dimensions of projection. *Psychological Bulletin, 69,* 248–268.

Holmes, D. S. (1978). Projection as a defense mechanism. *Psychological Bulletin, 83,* 677–688.

Holmes, D. S. (1981). Existence of classical projection and the stress-reducing function of attributive projection: A reply to Sherwood. *Psychological Bulletin, 90,* 460–466.

Holyoak, K. J., & Gordon, P. C. (1983). Social reference points. *Journal of Personality and Social Psychology, 44,* 881–887.

Hovland, C. I., Harvey, O. J., & Sherif, M. (1957). Assimilation and contrast effects in reactions to communications and attitude change. *Journal of Abnormal and Social Psychology, 55,* 244–252.

Hovland, C. I., & Sherif, M. (1952). Judgmental phenomena and scales of attitude measurement: Item displacement in Thurstone scales. *Journal of Abnormal and Social Psychology, 47,* 822–832.

James, W. (1915). *Psychology: Briefer course.* New York: Holt.

Jost, J. T., & Banaji, M. R. (1994). The role of stereotyping in system-justification and the production of the false consciousness. *British Journal of Social Psychology, 33,* 1–27.

Judd, C. M., & Johnson, J. T. (1981). Attitudes, polarization, and diagnosticity. *Journal of Personality and Social Psychology, 41,* 26–36.

Judd, C. M., Kenny, D. A., & Krosnick, J. A. (1983). Judging the positions of political candidates: Models of assimilation and contrast. *Journal of Personality and Social Psychology, 44,* 952–963.

Katz, D., & Allport, F. (1931). *Student attitudes.* Syracuse, NY: Craftsman Press.

Kelly, G. A. (1955). *The psychology of personal constructs* (Vol. 1). New York: Norton.

Kipnis, D. (1972). Does power corrupt? *Journal of Personality and Social Psychology, 27,* 33–41.

Kipnis, D., Castell, P. J., Gergen, M., & Mauch, D. (1976). Metamorphic effects of power. *Journal of Applied Psychology, 61,* 127–135.

Krech, D., Crutchfield, R. S., & Ballachey, E. L. (1962). *Theory and problems of social psychology.* New York: McGraw-Hill.

Krueger, J., & Clement, R. W. (1994). The truly false consensus effect: An ineradicable and egocentric bias in social perception. *Journal of Personality and Social Psychology, 67,* 596–610.

Kruger, J. M., & Dunning, D. (1999). Unskilled and unaware of it: How difficulties in recognizing one's own incompetence lead to inflated self-assessments. *Journal of Personality and Social Psychology, 77,* 1121–1134.

Kunda, Z. (1987). Motivated inference: Self-serving generation and evaluation of causal theories. *Journal of Personality and Social Psychology, 53,* 37–54.

Lambert, A. J., & Wedell, D. H. (1991). The self and social judgment: Effects of affective reaction and "own position" on judgments of unambiguous and ambiguous information about others. *Journal of Personality and Social Psychology, 61,* 884–898.

Lemon, N., & Warren, N. (1974). Salience, centrality, and self-relevance of traits in construing others. *British Journal of Social and Clinical Psychology, 13,* 119–124.

Lewicki, P. (1983). Self-image bias in person perception. *Journal of Personality and Social Psychology, 45,* 384–393.

Lewicki, P. (1984). Self-schema and social information processing. *Journal of Personality and Social Psychology, 47,* 1177–1190.

Lippman, W. (1922). *Public opinion.* New York: Macmillan.

Marks, E. (1943). Skin color judgments of Negro college students. *Journal of Abnormal and Social Psychology, 388,* 370–376.

Marks, G., & Miller, N. (1982). Target attractiveness as a mediator of assumed attitude similarity. *Personality and Social Psychology Bulletin, 8,* 728–735.

Marks, G., & Miller, N. (1987). Ten years of research on the false-consensus effect: An empirical and theoretical review. *Psychological Bulletin, 102,* 72–90.

Markus, H., Crane, M., Bernstein, S., & Siladi, M. (1982). Self-schemas and gender. *Journal of Personality and Social Psychology, 42,* 38–50.

Markus, H., & Smith, J. (1981). The influence of self-schemas on the perception of others. In N. Cantor & J. F. Kihlstrom (Eds.), *Personality, cognition, and social interaction* (pp. 233–262). Hillsdale, NJ: Erlbaum.

Markus, H., Smith, J., & Moreland, R. L. (1985). Role of the self-concept in the social perception of others. *Journal of Personality and Social Psychology, 49,* 1494–1512.

Mashman, R. C. (1978). The effect of physical attractiveness on perception of attitude similarity. *Journal of Social Psychology, 106,* 103–110.

McDougall, W. (1921). *An introduction to social psychology.* Boston: Luce.

McElwee, R. O., Dunning, D., Tan, P., & Hollman, S. (2001). The role of the self and self-serving trait definitions in social judgment. *Basic and Applied Social Psychology, 23,* 123–136.

Mead, G. H. (1934). *Mind, self and society.* Chicago: University of Chicago Press.

Messe, L. A., & Sivacek, J. M. (1979). Predictions of others' responses in a mixed-motive game: Self-justification or false consensus? *Journal of Personality and Social Psychology, 37,* 602–607.

Moreland, R. L., & Zajonc, R. B. (1982). Exposure effects in person perception: Familiarity, similarity, and attraction. *Journal of Experimental Social Psychology, 18,* 395–415.

Mullen, B., & Goethals, G. R. (1990). Social projection, actual consensus and valence. *British Journal of Social Psychology, 29,* 279–282.

Newman, L. S., Duff, K. J., & Baumeister, R. F. (1997). A new look at defensive projection: Thought suppression, accessibility, and biased person perception. *Journal of Personality and Social Psychology, 72,* 980–1001.

Prentice, D. (1990). Familiarity and differences in self-and other-representations. *Journal of Personality and Social Psychology, 59,* 369–383.

Prothro, E. T. (1955). The effect of strong negative affect on the placement of items in a Thurstone scale. *Journal of Social Psychology, 41,* 11–17.

Pyszczynski, T., Wicklund, R. A., Floresku, S., Koch, H., Gauch, G., Solomon, S., & Greenberg, J. (1996). Exaggerated consensus estimates in response to incidental reminders of mortality. *Psychological Science, 7,* 332–336.

Rogers, C. P. (1951). *Client-centered therapy.* Boston: Houghton-Mifflin.

Ross, L., Greene, D., & House, P. (1977). The "false consensus effect": An egocentric bias in social perception and attribution processes. *Journal of Experimental Social Psychology, 13,* 279–301.

Secord, P. F., Backman, C. W., & Eachus, H. T. (1964). Effects of imbalance in the self concept on the perception of persons. *Journal of Abnormal and Social Psychology, 68,* 442–446.

Sedikides, C., & Skowronski, J. J. (1993). The self in impression formation: Trait centrality and social perception. *Journal of Experiental Social Psychology, 29,* 347–457.

Selltiz, C., Edrich, H., & Cook, S. W. (1965). Ratings of favorableness about a social group as an indication of attitude toward the group. *Journal of Personality and Social Psychology, 2,* 403–415.

Sherif, M., & Hovland, C. I. (1961). *Social-judgment: Assimilation and contrast effects in communication of attitude change.* New Haven, CT: Yale University Press.

Sherman, S. J., Presson, C. C., & Chassin, L. (1984).

Mechanisms underlying the false consensus effect: The special role of threats to the self. *Personality and Social Psychology Bulletin, 10,* 127–138.

Sherman, S. J., Presson, C. C., Chassin, L., Corty, E., & Olshavsky, R. (1983). The false consensus effect in estimates of smoking prevalence: Underlying mechanisms. *Personality and Social Psychology Bulletin, 82,* 581–596.

Sherwood, G. G. (1979). Classical and attributive projection: Some new evidence. *Journal of Abnormal Psychology, 88,* 635–640.

Sherwood, G. G. (1981). Self-serving biases in person perception: A reexamination of projection as a mechanism of defense. *Psychological Bulletin, 90,* 445–459.

Sherwood, G. G. (1982). Consciousness and stress reduction in defensive projection: A reply to Holmes. *Psychological Bulletin, 91,* 372–375.

Shrauger, S. J., & Patterson, M. B. (1974). Self-evaluation and the selection of dimensions for evaluating others. *Journal of Personality, 42,* 569–585.

Sidanius, J., Pratto, F., & Bobo, L. (1996). Racism, conservatism, affirmative action, and intellectual sophistication: A matter of principled conservatism or group dominance? *Journal of Personality and Social Psychology, 70,* 476–491.

Story, A. L., & Dunning, D. (1998). The more rational side of self-serving prototypes: The effects of success and failure performance feedback. *Journal of Experimental Social Psychology, 34,* 513–529.

Sullivan, H. S. (1947). *Conceptions of modern psychiatry.* Washington, DC: William Alanson White Psychiatry Foundation.

Suls, J., Wan, C. K., & Sanders, G. S. (1988). False consensus and false uniqueness in estimating the prevalence of health-protective behaviors. *Journal of Applied Social Psychology, 18,* 66–79.

Sunar, D. (1978). Stereotypes of the powerless: A social psychological analysis. *Psychological Reports, 43,* 511–528.

Taylor, S. E., & Brown, J. D. (1988). Illusions and well-being: A social psychological perspective on mental health. *Psychological Bulletin, 103,* 193–210.

Tesser, A., & Campbell, J. (1982). Self-evaluation maintenance and the perception of friends and strangers. *Journal of Personality, 50,* 261–279.

van der Pligt, J. (1984). Attributions, false consensus, and valence: Two field studies. *Journal of Personality and Social Psychology, 46,* 57–68.

Weinstein, N. D. (1980). Unrealistic optimism about future life events. *Journal of Personality and Social Psychology, 58,* 806–820.

22

Self and Close Relationships

ARTHUR ARON

This chapter reviews several major themes in the social and personality psychology research and theory on the self and close relationships. I make occasional reference to related work in clinical and developmental psychology, sociology, and other fields as it is directly relevant to these themes. Yet even within personality and social psychology, some important topics are inevitably left out, such as self and culture (e.g., Kwan, Bond, & Singelis, 1997) and self-focused emotions (e.g., Tangney, 2002). Also, I have not attempted to review the massive relevant developmental literature on the link of the self to close relationships of children with parents and peers (e.g., Maccoby, 2000).

In this chapter, I focus on the self in terms of those processes that involve self-reflection or that relate to the person's overall individuality as distinguished from others. Loosely speaking, this includes most topics in social and personality psychology that include the words "self" or "identity." Close, or personal, relationships refer to ongoing patterns of interactions that involve affectively strong bonds between individuals and considerable interdependence, such as romantic and marital relationships, friend-

ships, and parent–child relationships. Typically, such ongoing patterns of dyadic interactions function so that relationship pairs become meaningful social units in their own right (Kelley et al., 1983). However, from the subjective perspective that characterizes most research and thinking on the self, the focus is typically on each individual's experience: "the processes on which relationships depend go on, by-and-large, in the head of each participant with partial independence from what is going on in the head of the other ... therefore ... we should think also of A's relationship with B and B's relationship with A" (Hinde, Finkenauer, & Auhagen, 2001). Also, before proceeding I want to note that the development of the overall chapter owes much to four recent literature reviews on the same or closely related overall topics (Berscheid & Reis, 1998; Hinde et al., 2001; Holmes, 2000; Leary, 2002).

This chapter covers five main topics: effects of close relationships on the self; effects of the self on close relationships; self-related relational cognitive structures; self-disclosure and self–other connectedness; and self-relevant motivations and close relationships.

Effects of Close Relationships on the Self

Even as adults, what we are and what we see ourselves as being seems to be constantly under construction and reconstruction, with the architects and remodeling contractors largely being those with whom we have close interactions. To use Cooley's (1902) metaphor, to some extent who we are is a reflection of those to whom we are close— our self is a "looking glass self" (see also Cook & Douglas, 1998; Felson, 1989; Kenny & DePaulo, 1993). Taking this idea very literally, there is evidence that married couples come to look more similar over time. That is, judges were significantly less accurate in matching photos of just-married spouses than in matching photos of the same spouses taken 25 years later (Zajonc, Adelmann, Murphy, & Niedenthal, 1987). A quite different approach has focused on the effect of relationships on self-presentation. For example, Tice, Butler, Muraven, and Stillwell (1995) showed that people employ more self-enhancing self-presentation strategies with strangers than with friends (see also Bornstein, Riggs, Hill, & Calabrese, 1996).

For the same reasons that relationships shape one's conceptions of the self in general, they presumably also shape how positively or negatively one feels about oneself. Leary (1999; Leary & Downs, 1995) has argued that a particularly important source of self-esteem is the perceived opinions others hold of us—that self-esteem represents a kind of "sociometer." That is, self-esteem serves as a kind of meter that tells you how much you are socially accepted or rejected. In support of this model, in a series of five studies, Leary, Tambor, Terdal, and Downs (1995) showed that people feel worse about themselves when they believe others have excluded or rejected them. Further, Leary and Baumeister (2000) systematically lay out how this idea is consistent with a great deal of data showing that people are highly responsive to rejection and acceptance. They also argue that most of the factors that affect self-esteem and that are not themselves directly social nevertheless have implications for how one believes one is perceived by others as a desirable relationship partner. More specifically, Elliott (1996) reported an analysis from a large U.S. national sample of women tested in 1980 when they were between 15 and 23 years old and again in 1987 when they were between 22 and 30. After controlling for various background characteristics (age, education level, mother's education, etc.), Elliott found a small but significantly greater increase in self-esteem for those who married and for those who became mothers. A related view, based on an evolutionary perspective that self-esteem is a kind of meter of one's mate value and of reproductively related costs (such as partner infidelity) has also received some support (Shackelford, 2001).

Behavioral Confirmation

A key mechanism by which relationships seem to affect the self, behavioral confirmation (sometimes called "self-fulfilling prophecy"), refers to a process by which people act to confirm the expectations of others (Darley & Fazio, 1980; Harris & Rosenthal, 1985; Merton, 1948). Several experimental studies that have manipulated interaction partners' expectations have shown reliable effects on a person's behavior. For example, Rosenthal and Jacobson's (1968) study showed improvement in the performance of pupils whose teachers were randomly told that these pupils would be "academic spurters." Similarly, Snyder, Tanke, and Berscheid (1977) set up male–female getting-acquainted conversations over an intercom in which the male participants, unknown to their partners, were given a photograph of either an attractive or unattractive woman whom he was told was his partner. Perhaps not surprisingly, ratings of the man's half of the conversation were quite different between the two photograph conditions. However, the key point from the behavioral confirmation point of view is that raters listening to just the *woman's* half of the conversations, with no knowledge of what condition she was in, rated women as more attractive who were interacting with a man who believed she was attractive. That is, the man's expectations spontaneously created a quite different pattern of behavior (and perhaps an at least temporarily different self-conception) on the part of the woman partner.

Berk and Andersen (2000) conducted a behavioral confirmation study that is especially relevant to close relationships. In this study, participants had a getting-acquainted conversation with someone they were led to believe had a particular set of characteristics. In one of the conditions, participants were led to believe that their interaction partner had the characteristics of a person with whom the participant had had a significant and positive relationship earlier in life. In this condition, as compared with various controls, participants expressed more positive affect to the partner. More important, *the partners of such participants* expressed more positive affect in the interaction. Thus this study shows the usual behavioral confirmation effect in which a person's behavior (and perhaps self-conception) is shaped by an interaction partner's expectations. In addition, it shows that a prior relationship can shape how we expect new interaction partners to behave (a result consistent with a number of previous studies; for a review, see Andersen & Berensen, 2001). In addition, the Berk and Andersen findings suggest that the now-reconfigured self affects future relationships. Similarly, Riggs and Cantor (1984) showed that participants' self-concepts shaped their behavior toward partners, which, in turn, via the usual behavioral confirmation effect, shaped the partners' behavior to the participants.

As emphasized by Drigotas, Rusbult, Wieselquist, and Whitton (1999), in the context of behavioral confirmation (as in the more general context), it seems likely that the influences of others would be especially important in ongoing close relationships. The reason is that people are likely to be especially sensitive to a close partners' expectations and that in such relationships there is substantial and ongoing opportunity to be exposed to those expectations. Indeed, given these normal conditions of a close relationship, one might expect changes not only in behavior in a particular situation but also in the person's ongoing characteristics (and, ultimately, in self-conception). Following up this idea in a series of longitudinal studies with dating and married couples, Drigotas and colleagues reported results supporting each stage of a process in which partner *A*'s holding a view of partner *B* that is specifically consistent with *B*'s ideal self specifically leads to *B*'s becoming more like *B*'s ideal self. (Also, the extent to which this occurs leads to *B*'s being more satisfied with the relationship.) The researchers labeled this process the "Michelangelo phenomenon," in light of the sculptor's idea that he was simply chipping away the stone to reveal the ideal figure lying within. (Of course the same data also suggest that a partner's expectations that are incongruent with one's ideal self can undermine one's development of that ideal self.) In addition, Drigotas and colleagues provided substantial evidence consistent with a causal process in which the effect of *A*'s expectations about *B* on *B*'s movement toward *B*'s ideal self is mediated by *A*'s performing behaviors in relation to *B* that imply those expectations. That is, it is not enough for the sculptor to envision the ideal; the sculptor must also actually chip away at the stone.

Including the Other in the Self

Another mechanism by which relationships affect the self, in which close others shape and reshape the self, is based on the notion that in a close relationship, the other is "included in the self." The idea here is that in close relationships, cognitive representations of self and other overlap (Aron, Aron, & Norman, 2001). According to this model, who we are is to some extent who our partners are—that is, in a close relationship, we incorporate into ourselves the others' social and material resources, the others' perspectives, and the others' identities.

Much of this work emerged out of research on the self-reference effect, a reliable difference in memory and response time between making judgments regarding oneself and making judgments regarding other persons (Symons & Johnson, 1997). More important in the present context, the degree to which self-referent and other-referent judgments differ seems to depend on the nature of one's relationship to the other person being referenced; that is, judgments relevant to close others versus less close others are recalled more similarly to judgments relevant to oneself (Symons & Johnson, 1997).

Presuming that judgments regarding close others versus less close others are in fact processed more similarly to judgments regarding oneself, *why* is this so? One model says that it is so in part because the knowledge structures of close others actually share elements (or activation potentials) with the knowledge structures of the self (Aron, Aron, Tudor, & Nelson, 1991; Aron & Fraley, 1999; Smith, Coats, & Walling, 1999).[1] For example, one's own and a close other's traits may actually be confused or interfere with each other.

To test this idea, Aron and colleagues (1991) evaluated the patterns of response latencies in making "me–not me" decisions (that is, Does the trait describe me?) about traits previously rated for their descriptiveness of self and of spouse. These researchers found that for traits on which the self matched the partner (the trait was true of both or false of both), responses were faster than when a trait was mismatched for self and partner (was true for one but false for the other). Further, Aron and Fraley (1999) found that this match–mismatch reaction-time index (serving as a measure of overlap of self and other) goes beyond simply distinguishing between a close and nonclose relationship partner; the magnitude of the effect correlates substantially with self-report measures of relationship quality, including predicting increases in subjective closeness over a 3-month period. Using this same match–mismatch reaction-time paradigm, Smith and colleagues (1999) replicated both the overall difference between close and nonclose others and the correlation with the magnitude of self-reported closeness to the close other. Smith and colleagues eloquently articulated why such patterns may result: "if mental representations of two persons . . . overlap so that they are effectively a single representation, reports on attributes of one will be facilitated or inhibited by matches and mismatches with the second" (p. 873).

Taking another approach, Mashek, Aron, and Boncimino (2002) had participants rate one set of traits for self, a different set of traits for a close other, and still other traits for one or more nonclose others, such as media personalities. Then the researchers gave a surprise recognition task in which participants were presented each trait and asked to indicate for which person they had rated it. The focus of the analysis was on confusions—traits on which the participant remembered having rated the trait for one person when the participant had actually rated the trait for a different person. Results were consistent with predictions. For example, if participants did not correctly recognize a trait as having been originally rated for the self, they were significantly more likely to remember it as having been rated for the partner than as having been rated for the media personality. Similarly, if the participant did not correctly recognize a trait as having been originally rated for the partner, he or she was significantly more likely to remember it as having been rated for the self than as having been rated for the media personality. These results were replicated in two follow-up studies and held up after controlling for a variety of potential confounds, such as a greater tendency to see traits in general as having been rated for self, valence and extremity of ratings, and similarity to the close other.[2]

Finally, focusing on the issue of the perceived overlap of oneself with a relationship partner, Aron, Aron, and Smollan (1992) asked participants to describe their closest relationship using the Inclusion of Other in the Self (IOS) Scale. This IOS scale consists of seven pairs of circles overlapping to different degrees from which the respondent selects the pair (the degree of overlap) that best describes his or her relationship with a particular person. The scale appears to have levels of reliability, as well as of discriminant, convergent, and predictive validity, that match or exceed other measures of closeness—measures that are typically more complex and lengthy. Since its development, the scale has been used effectively in a number of studies of relationships (e.g., Agnew, Van Lange, Rusbult, & Langston, 1998; Aron, Melinat, Aron, Vallone, & Bator, 1997; Cross, Bacon, & Morris, 2000; Knee, 1998). It seems plausible that this measure has been so successful because the metaphor of overlapping circles representing self and other corresponds to how people actually process information about self and other in relationships.

In sum, these various data suggest that one way in which close others may shape the self is that these others become part of the self, with the cognitive representations of the partner overlapping with the self-representations and thus becoming part of the self-representations. Furthermore, the extent to which the other's resources and perspectives are taken on to ourselves, not just how we think of ourselves—but who we actually are—may be strongly shaped by our close others.[3]

Summary of Effect of Relationships on the Self

Even as adults, close relationships shape and reshape the self, including even one's appearance and how one presents oneself to others, and seem to be a particularly fundamental element in regulating one's self-esteem. Two processes by which others shape the self that have received considerable attention are behavioral confirmation, by which one comes to behave according to the way one's partner expects one to behave, and inclusion of other in the self, in which to some extent one incorporates into oneself close others' resources, perspectives, and identities.

Effects of the Self on Close Relationships

How we understand our own traits and motivations inevitably shapes how we relate to the world, including how we relate to close others. The reason is that our self-understandings structure the attributions we make for our own behavior and experience, the expectations we have for our own future actions and responses to others, and the evaluations we make of our similarities to and differences from relationship partners and potential relationship partners. Indeed, regarding the latter, we tend to assume that others will be like ourselves (e.g., Kenny, 1994).

Two specific aspects of self-conceptions that shape relationships have received significant research attention: relational self-concepts and self-esteem.

Relational Self-Concepts

Individuals appear to differ in their general tendency for relationships to be central or peripheral to who they are, and this difference has important implications for their relationships. Cross and colleagues (2000) developed a measure of "relational-interdependent self-construal," which they define as "the tendency to think of oneself in

terms of relationships with close others" (p. 791). Those who score high on this measure have relationships that are closer and more committed, they are more likely to consider their partners' needs, and they are perceived as closer, more committed, and considerate of partners' needs, even by previously unacquainted laboratory interaction partners.

Similarly, Acitelli, Rogers, and Knee (1999) found that among dating couples the well-documented link between thinking about a relationship and satisfaction in that relationship (e.g., Acitelli & Antonucci, 1994) was stronger for those with a high level of "relational identity, or the tendency to see oneself in relation to others in general" (p. 591). This general notion may also relate to Clark, Ouellette, Powell, and Milberg's (1987) notion of individual differences in "communal orientation" (a tendency to adopt a norm of attending to the needs of close others) and to the attachment theory (Bowlby, 1969) concept of positive working models of self in relationships, both of which I consider in more detail later in this chapter.

Effects of Self-Esteem on Close Relationships

Self-esteem seems to have small to moderate positive correlations with the quality of close relationships such as marriages and friendships (e.g., Voss, Markiewicz, & Doyle, 1999). There are also some longitudinal data on married couples that support there being a small but consistent positive causal effect of self-esteem on relationship satisfaction and stability over time (Aube & Koestner, 1992; Doherty, Su, & Needle, 1989; Karney & Bradbury, 1995; Larson, Anderson, Holman, & Niemann, 1998; Steinberg & Silverberg, 1987). Similarly, with dating couples, Murray, Holmes, and Griffin (1996b) found that self-esteem predicted increases in an individual's seeing the partner in a more positive light, and Hendrick, Hendrick, and Adler (1988) found that those with low self-esteem were more likely to break up 2 months later.

If low self-esteem does have a negative effect on relationships, why? Murray, Holmes, and Griffin (2000) provide strong data from multiple studies that support each step in a complex scenario in which people with low self-esteem fail to appreciate their partners' typical idealized regard for them, instead assuming that their partners see them as they see themselves (as not so consistently positive). They thus pull away and devalue their partners to protect themselves, ultimately undermining their partners' actual regard for them.

There appear, however, to be some exceptions to the generally positive effect of self-esteem on relationships. First, in a series of laboratory experiments, Heatherington and Vohs (2000) showed that under neutral conditions, people with high and low self-esteem are about equally likeable; but under ego threat (such as failing at something important), people with high self-esteem become *less* likeable and people with low self-esteem become *more* likeable. Subsequently, Vohs and Heatherington (2000) demonstrated that this effect occurs because, under ego threat, people with low self-esteem become more interdependent and people with high self-esteem become more independent. Consistent with this interpretation, in a study of married couples reporting on their reactions to a recent ego threat from their partners, Schutz (1998a) found that those with high self-esteem focused more on the problem and less on their partners. And in part of yet another study, Schutz (1998b) had participants recount an experience of being hurt by someone. The pattern of findings was that "high self-esteem subjects aim at being admired for their abilities and low self-esteem subjects aim at being liked for being nice" (p. 466).

The other possible limitation to the general principle that more self-esteem is better for relationships is narcissism. Narcissism is a personality style involving a seemingly damaged sense of self that often shows itself as kind of high self-esteem but that leads to poor relationship outcomes (W. Campbell, 1999; W. Campbell, Reeder, Sedikides, & Elliot, 2000; Morf & Rhodewalt, 1993, 2001; Sedikides, Campbell, Reeder, Elliot, & Gregg, 2002)—"A grandiose yet vulnerable self-concept" (Morf & Rhodewalt, 2001, p. 177). Basically, narcissists use relationships as opportunities to receive admiration or to bask in the reflected glory of a socially admired partner—in each case largely ignoring the needs of those partners, even at the cost of losing the relationship.

Summary of Effects of the Self on Relationships

Relationships, like all domains of life, are affected by the people in them and how these people understand themselves. However, there are also some special senses in which aspects of self shape relationships that have received significant research attention. First, those who understand themselves as centrally relationally oriented, those whose identity is deeply rooted in their relationships, behave in relationships and experience their relationships accordingly. Second, those with higher self-esteem seem to have better relationships, possibly because those with low self-esteem presume that they are seen by their partners as they see themselves. However, there are also a couple of possible exceptions to the general principle that more self-esteem is better for relationships—(1) when people with high self-esteem are threatened, they become less relationally oriented; and (2) narcissism, though not exactly high self-esteem, does involve a highly positive self-conception and is consistently dysfunctional for relationships.

Self-Related Relational Cognitive Structures

The past decade has seen considerable integration of social cognition approaches into the study of close relationships (Reis & Downey, 1999). One major line of work in this domain, on "including other in the self" (Aron et al., 2001), was considered in some detail earlier. Much of the other work of this kind has focused on cognitive structures that seem related to both self and partner. These include partner representations, relational schemas, working models of self and other in relationships, and prototypes of cardinal relationship concepts.

Partner Representations

Gurung, Sarason, and Sarason (2001) assessed "clarity" of participants' "significant-others concepts," by which they mean the degree to which one's mental representation of the other is "confidently defined, internally consistent, and temporally stable" (a conceptualization they adapted from J.

Campbell et al.'s, 1996, work on the clarity of the self-concept). Gurung and colleagues found that clarity of a person's significant-other concept predicted relationship quality even after controlling for self-concept clarity, positivity of the significant-other concept, and perceived connectedness of self and other. Showers and Kevlyn (1999) focused on the extent to which a person's representation of a close partner is integrated or compartmentalized. (This approach applies to the partner-concept work Showers and her colleagues have done on integration versus compartmentalization of the self-concept; e.g., Showers & Kling, 1996.) Integrated partner representations are ones in which the person has spontaneously organized partner traits into clusters that include mixtures of positive and negative; compartmentalized organizations are ones in which some clusters are all positive and others are all negative. Showers and Kevlyn found that relationship quality is highest with compartmentalized organization in new relationships, in which negative information is relatively peripheral. But integrative organization becomes better as relationships proceed, as people are inevitably forced to confront moderate to high levels of negative information about their partners. That is, if a person is not forced to see the negatives, then compartmentalized structures keep the negatives from coming up; but if a person is going to be forced to deal with the negatives, it is better if they also bring to mind positives.

Murray and Holmes (1999), in a somewhat similar study, showed that those whose partner representations had an integrated structure spontaneously minimized partner faults and tended to find virtues in the faults they recognized. In their study, even after controlling for amount of overall negative content in the representation of the other, integrative organization predicted relationship satisfaction and whether a relationship stayed stable over time. These findings are consistent with Showers and Kevlyn's (1999) findings for ongoing relationships.

Relational Schemas

Representations of self-with-other also seem to play a substantial role in shaping rela-

tionships. The most influential idea here is the relational schema, originally introduced by Planalp (1987). Elaborating on the concept in some detail, Baldwin (1992, 1997) describes it as a mental representation that includes expectations about oneself in interaction with others, a partner representation, and a set of "if–then" scripts (e.g., "if I do X, then my partner will do Y"). In support of this notion, Baldwin and his colleagues have shown that priming a particular relationship (even with subliminal primes) leads to responses consistent with what is expected in that relationship (Baldwin, 1994; Baldwin, Carrell, & Lopez, 1990; Baldwin, Fehr, Keedian, Seidel, & Thompson, 1993; Baldwin & Holmes, 1987; Baldwin & Sinclair, 1996; see also Pierce & Lydon, 1998). For example, in one study, students who had visualized their parents rated a sexual passage as less enjoyable 10 minutes later, in a different context, than did those who had instead visualized their friends. The idea here is that most students would believe that their parents, compared with their friends, were less approving of the enjoyment of sexual material. Recently, Beer and Kihlstrom (2000) explored relational schemas in terms of the memory systems involved in the trait knowledge they embody. They found that recalling trait knowledge of how one acts with dating partners was facilitated by having recalled a relevant autobiographical event, implying that such relational schemas are at least somewhat dependent on autobiographical memory. However, there was little facilitation of this kind for trait knowledge of how one acts with parents or friends, suggesting that such knowledge is well abstracted.

Working Models of Self and Other in Relationships

Working models of self and other are a core idea in Bowlby's (1969) highly influential attachment theory. Shaver, Collins, and Clark (1996) present a detailed, deeply considered analysis of the concept (see also Pietremonico & Barrett, 2000). They begin by explaining that "working models are cognitive representations of self and others that evolve out of experiences with attachment figures and are concerned with the regulation and fulfillment of attachment needs. . . . What begin as representations of specific relationships and specific partners result in the formation of more abstract, generalized representations of self and social world" (p. 39). Shaver and colleagues go on to explain that working models have much in common with cognitive representations more generally but that they also tend to be more multidimensional, to involve more elements of motivation and emotion, and to include content that is not easily available to conscious awareness. Most important, from the point of view of this chapter, individual differences in working models are thought to explain the multitude of findings that those with different attachment styles behave in and experience relationships differently (Shaver & Hazan, 1993).

Other Relationship-Relevant Cognitive Structures

Several researchers have demonstrated that people hold prototypes of key relationship constructs that influence how people recognize, experience, and evaluate partners and relationships. These prototypes, which tend to have both a consensual (at least within cultures) and individual-difference component, include prototypes of commitment (Fehr, 1988); intimacy (Helgeson, Shaver, & Dyer, 1987); love (Aron & Westbay, 1996; Fehr, 1988; Fehr & Russell, 1991; Shaver, Schwartz, Kirson, & O'Connor, 1987); beliefs about ideal partners and relationships (e.g., Fletcher & Kininmouth, 1992; Fletcher, Simpson, Thomas, & Giles, 1999); mental models of ideal romantic relationships (Rusbult, Onizuka, & Lipkus, 1993); and the prototype of a "good relationship" (Hassebrauck, 1997; Hassebrauck & Aron, 2001). Similarly, Knee (1998; Knee, Nanayakkara, Vietor, Neighbors, & Patrick, 2001) has demonstrated that relationships are influenced by the "implicit theories" the partners hold as to whether good relationships are developed over time ("growth beliefs") or whether people simply are or are not meant for each other ("destiny beliefs"). For example, those who hold destiny beliefs (versus those with growth beliefs) have shorter relationships when there are problems at the outset but longer relationships when things go well at the outset. In the few cases in which studies have examined the issue, individual differences in these various cognitive structures have shown surprisingly little linkage with individual differences in attachment models (e.g., Aron & Westbay, 1996).

Summary of Self-Related Relational Cognitive Structures

The integration of social cognition approaches into the study of close relationships has led, among other things, to the identification of central cognitive structures that seem related to both self and partner. In addition to the idea of including other in the self, discussed earlier, four main kinds of such representations have been studied: (1) partner representations, the clarity and organization of which seem to have effects on relationships to partners similar to the effects of clarity and organization of self-representations; (2) relational schemas, which include expectations about self in interaction with others, a partner representation, and a set of "if–then" scripts, have been shown to shape relationship-relevant cognition and action; (3) working models of self and other in relationships, a concept emerging out of attachment theory, are very general, emotionally laden expectations of what to expect in close relationships that emerge out of early experience with caregivers; (4) prototypes of key relationship constructs, such as love, ideal partner, and a good relationship, influence how people recognize, experience, and evaluate partners and relationships.

Self-Disclosure and Self–Other Connectedness

Self-disclosure is one of the oldest topics in the modern study of relationships, and it is usually seen as associated with (or leading to) intimacy, closeness, connectedness, or even a merging of self and other.

Self-Disclosure

Self-disclosure refers to "revealing information about oneself to another" (Collins & Miller, 1994). In their meta-analysis, Collins and Miller found that we are more likely to disclose intimate information to those we like initially; also, after disclosing intimate information, we like more and are more liked by those to whom we disclose. Another set of generally well-established findings suggests that relationships tend to develop by a process of gradually escalating reciprocated self-disclosure (Aron et al., 1997; Derlega, Metts, Petronio, & Margulis, 1993). Self-disclosure may also play a central role in other self-related processes. For example, self-disclosure of intimate information may mediate the link between attachment working models and relationship quality (Keelan, Dion, & Dion, 1998).

Reis and Shaver (1988; see also Reis & Patrick, 1996), integrating much of the self-disclosure literature, proposed that there are two conditions necessary for self-disclosure to create intimacy: (1) that the self-disclosure is emotional, as opposed to merely factual; and (2) that the partner is responsive to the self-disclosure, making one feel understood, validated, and cared for. This model has received overall support in three studies focusing on the relation of these variables to intimacy using a method in which participants kept diaries for 1 to 2 weeks of every social interaction of 10 minutes or longer, recording their responses to the interaction as soon after as possible (Laurenceau, Barrett, & Pietromonaco, 1998, Studies 1 and 2; Lin, 1992). Thus, in the context of self-disclosure, what seems to matter in the development of intimacy is that the partners reveal core, emotional information about themselves to which the other is responsive.

Self–Other Connectedness

The very nature of a "close" or "personal" relationship usually refers to some kind of significant connection between self and other. Kelley and colleagues (1983) focused on the pattern of ongoing mutual influence. Berscheid, Snyder, and Omoto (1989) developed and validated the Relationship Closeness Inventory (RCI) as a measure of this kind of closeness. The RCI assesses the amount of time spent together, the diversity of shared activities, and perceived influence of the other on one's decisions. It is internally consistent and has solid discriminant and convergent validity in relation to other relevant measures of relationship experience

and behavior. Other approaches to self–other interconnectedness have focused on subjectively experienced sense of intimacy or feeling of knowing and caring for one another (e.g., Erikson, 1950; Helgeson et al., 1987; McAdams, 1989; Reis & Patrick, 1996; Sternberg, 1986; Waring, 1988). In a series of exploratory and confirmatory factor analyses, Aron and colleagues (1992) showed that these two notions of closeness represent related but clearly not identical constructs, which they labeled "behaving close" and "feeling close." They also showed that their overlapping-circles measure of perceived inclusion of other in the self (the IOS Scale, which Aron et al. found that respondents explicitly interpret in terms of self–other connectedness) had significant paths from latent variables representing both kinds of closeness and that the IOS Scale is associated with relationship quality and stability.

However, too much connectedness may exist in a relationship, so that people feel controlled or that they are losing their identity (Mashek, in press). For example, Brewer (1993; see also Brewer & Pickett, 1999) has shown that people seek an optimal level of distinctiveness from others. As another example, family systems theories (e.g., Olson, Russell, & Sprenkle, 1983) propose that clinically disruptive patterns in which partners are "enmeshed" are due to overidentification with relationship partners.

Summary of Self-Disclosure and Self–Other Connectedness

Some key findings regarding self-disclosure are that people are more likely to disclose intimate information to those they like initially, and, after disclosing intimate information, they like more and are more liked by those to whom they disclose. Further, relationships often develop by a process of gradually escalating reciprocated self-disclosure. The Reis and Shaver (1988) model of the development of intimacy, which has received substantial empirical support, posits that what is most important is that each partner reveals core, emotional information about him- or herself to which the other is responsive. The actual nature of the closeness that develops in a relationship is linked with both behaving close (frequent and diverse interactions and mutual influence) and feeling close (sense of knowing and caring about each other); both of which are represented to some extent in people's sense of including other in the self, or self–other connectedness. However, there is also evidence that it may be possible for there to be too much connectedness, so that people feel controlled or that they are losing their identity.

Self-Relevant Motivations and Close Relationships

Close relationships are a major arena for the display and influence of self-related motivations. In this section I consider the links of close relationships to four topics: self-evaluation maintenance, self-verification motives, self-serving and self-sacrificing behavior, and self-expansion motivation. Chapters in this volume are devoted to the first two (Tesser, Chapter 14; Swann, Rentfrow, & Guinn, Chapter 18); thus, my review of them here is brief and focused specifically on the implications for close relationships.

Self-Evaluation Maintenance

Tesser's (1988) self-evaluation maintenance model is about how we maintain our self-esteem in the face of another person outperforming us. Specifically, Tesser theorized that if an interpersonally close other outperforms us in an area that is of low relevance to the self, we are likely to "reflect" his or her success, "basking in reflected glory" (Cialdini et al., 1976). However, when the area of performance is highly self-relevant, and especially if the one who outperforms us is similar to us or interpersonally close, then we are more likely to experience comparison, a negative reaction. This model, which has received substantial support in studies with strangers and friends (e.g., Tesser, 1988; Tesser, Millar, & Moore, 1988), demonstrates one way in which self-esteem and relationship variables, at least at the level of friendships, systematically interact.

Recent extensions of the model also consider more long-term, committed relationships such as marriage (Beach & Tesser, 1993). Beach and colleagues (1996, Studies 1 and 2) showed that self-evaluation maintenance mechanisms influence recall of relationship events—participants had more negative reminiscences of their relationship history after participation in performance situations experimentally manipulated to produce comparison (vs. reflection). In another study reported in the same article (Beach et al., 1996), self-evaluation maintenance mechanisms seemed to account for the distribution of activities within the marriage—specifically, married individuals participated in relatively more activities that were either (1) of high relevance to the self in which the participant typically outperformed the partner, or (2) of low relevance to the self in which the partner typically outperformed the participant. Perhaps most interesting are findings that in committed relationships, partners appear to be motivated not only to maintain their own self-esteem but also, to some extent, to protect the self-esteem of their partners. Beach and colleagues (Study 3) found that married individuals systematically distorted perceptions of their partners' needs so as to maximize perceived partner reflection and minimize perceived partner comparison. Similarly, in a series of four experiments, Beach and colleagues (1998) showed that married and dating partner's affective reactions to outperforming their partners, as compared with outperforming a stranger, were more influenced by the perceived relevance of the performance domain to the other person. Finally, Mendolia, Beach, and Tesser (1996) showed that the extent to which affective reactions were linked to partners' needs was associated with more positive interactions in 20-minute videotaped discussions.

Self-Verification

Another motivation relevant to relationships is a self-verification motive, a desire to seek out information that verifies one's own preexisting understanding of oneself, even when those views are negative (Swann, 1990). Such information reassures people about the stability and coherence of the self so that the self can serve as a more solid foundation for experience and planning. Further, self-verification, by fostering a more stable and coherent self, facilitates social interaction by making the person more predictable to others. A large number of studies support this model (see Swann et al., Chapter 18, this volume).[4] Most relevant to close relationships are studies showing that married individuals whose partners see them *either* less or more positively than they see themselves become less intimate (e.g., Swann, De La Ronde, & Hixon, 1994).

However, in this particular domain of close relationships, Murray, Holmes, and Griffin (1996a) found a seemingly opposite result—greater marital satisfaction was associated with perceiving oneself as being seen more positively by one's partner, regardless of how one sees oneself. Reis and Patrick (1996) suggested that this apparent discrepancy may arise because what really matters is not how positively or accurately the other sees one but rather how well one feels understood and appreciated. Yet another possibility is that self-verification operates when the characteristics being rated are relatively objective, as in Swann's studies, but the desire to be seen as positively as possible (called "self-enhancement" in Swann's terms) operates when what is being rated is less concrete, as in the Murray and colleagues study.

Ultimately, it seems likely that, under some conditions, people are primarily motivated to be seen as they assume they are and that, under other conditions, they are motivated to be seen as positively as possible. That is, both motives probably operate (see Sedikides & Strube, 1995, for a discussion of these and related motives). The question that remains is under which conditions does each predominate, and why? For example, Katz, Anderson, and Beach (1997) found effects for both self-verification and the desire to see oneself as positively as possible in promoting attraction to potential romantic partners.

Self-Serving and Self-Sacrificing Behavior in Close Relationships

A third major set of self-related motivational issues to which close relationships are relevant has to do with self-serving versus self-sacrificing actions. There is some evidence that people's gut-level initial response when facing a motivational dilemma in a relationship is selfish—a placing of one's own needs ahead of those of others (e.g., Yovetich & Rusbult, 1994). However, particularly in the context of close relationships, there also appears to be considerable caring and compassionate behavior that seems anything but selfish. Several models of close relationship functioning have attempted to address how this seeming unselfishness comes about.

Transformation of Motivation

Interdependence theory (e.g., Kelley & Thibaut, 1978) describes a "transformation of motivation" such that close relationship partners come to value outcomes that benefit the partner and the relationship even at the expense of oneself. One reason people make such transformations from immediate, pure self-interest, according to this model, is that they are dependent on the relationship; another reason (among several) is that they expect to be in the relationship for some time and take into account long-term costs and benefits. Consistent with this idea of transformation of motivation, Rusbult and her colleagues emphasize the impact of interdependence on the development of commitment (e.g., Rusbult & Arriaga, 2000), which centrally involves long-term orientation to the relationship. Using this concept, they have demonstrated that commitment promotes partner-oriented acts such as willingness to ignore partner's bad behavior (Rusbult, Verette, Whitney, Slovik, & Lipkus, 1991) and willingness to sacrifice self-interest for the needs of the partner (Van Lange et al., 1997). Consistent with the specific idea of selfish gut feelings being transformed in the context of commitment, Yovetich and Rusbult (1994) demonstrated that when participants were presented with scenarios of a partner's destructive behavior, they chose less accommodating responses when they had limited time to respond versus when they had plentiful time to respond. Further, the magnitude of this effect was strongly moderated by the degree of commitment to the relationship. Testing a conceptually related idea with a similar experimental paradigm, Finkel and Campbell (2001) showed lesser tendencies for accommodative (nonselfish) responses to destructive behavior among those who had low levels of dispositional self-control. They also showed more accommodative responses to destructive behavior among participants whose self-control had been temporarily lowered by a standard "ego-depletion" manipulation (from Baumeister, Bratslavsky, Muraven, & Tice, 1998) in which they had to try not to feel anything while watching a highly emotional film. That is, these various findings suggest that people are less able to carry out the transformation of motivation when they do not have either time (Yovetich & Rusbult, 1994) or adequate self-control (Finkel & Campbell, 2001).

Communal Norms

Clark and Mills (1993) have shown that there are distinct normative bases for giving benefits to others. Specifically, they argue that in "communal relationships" people assume responsibility for the needs of others and therefore give benefits, noncontingently, in response to those needs. The norms that operate in a communal relationship are contrasted in their model with the norms that operate in an exchange (in which reciprocity is emphasized) or purely self-serving relationship. In this regard, it is notable that Campbell, Sedikides, Reeder, and Elliot (2000; see also Sedikides et al., 2002) showed that close others, compared with strangers, spontaneously make less self-serving attributions for their own success or failure in relation to their partners. These researchers interpret this result as due to the adoption of a communal norm with close others (an interpretation also consistent with studies by McCall [1995; McCall, Reno, Jalbert, & West, 2000] showing that even in a stranger-interaction situation similar to that used by Campbell and colleagues those with a more communal orientation are less likely to make self-serving attributions).

One of several factors that may lead to the adoption of communal norms in a given relationship is empathy with the partner (e.g., Williamson & Clark, 1992), which may be biologically or culturally driven. One of the more interesting implications of this model is that when a communal norm is in place in a relationship, partners pay less attention to who contributed what and more attention to each other's needs (e.g., Clark, Mills, & Powell, 1986). Similarly, communal orientation, an individual-difference variable discussed earlier, seems to be associated with greater likelihood of attending to the needs of others (Clark et al., 1986).

Including Other in the Self

As noted earlier, Aron and his colleagues (e.g., 2001) argue that close partners "include the other in their self" in the sense that cognitive representations of the partner overlap with those of the self. Thus people sometimes spontaneously act for the benefit of a close other because, to some extent, acting for the benefit of the close other is also acting for one's own benefit. For example, Aron and colleagues (1991) found that, in an allocation game involving real money and in which the partner would not be able to know one's allocations, participants distributed money about equally to themselves and close others; but they distributed more to themselves when the other was a mere acquaintance. Similarly, Medvene, Teal, and Slavich (2000) found the usual equity effect of greatest satisfaction for those who are neither under- nor overbenefited in a romantic relationship; however, this pattern was much weaker for those who perceived their relationship as having high levels of interconnectedness. Finally, Cialdini, Brown, Lewis, Luce, and Neuberg (1997) asked participants to respond to a variety of scenarios involving a person in need (most of whom had various degrees of closeness to the participant). The extent to which a person indicated that he or she would help the other was mediated by measures of both empathic feeling and including other in the self; however, when they included both in the equation, empathic feeling dropped out, and the measure of including other in the self turned out to be the key mediator. (However, see Batson et al., 1997, for an alternative interpretation of this finding.)

Comparison of These Three Mechanisms

Probably all three of these processes operate (along with others). Indeed, each of the theoretical models behind these different mechanisms explicitly acknowledges one or more of the others. It may be in fact that, instead of or in addition to these being alternative routes through which apparently non-self-oriented behavior may occur, they may be linked as part of a causal sequence in which one leads to the other. For example, communal norms would motivate a transformation of motivation; the result of a transformation of motivation could be a perception that the other is part of the self; and perceiving other as part of the self could spontaneously lead to attention to the other's needs in a communal relationship.

Self-Expansion Motivation and Close Relationships

Aron and colleagues (2001; see also Aron, Norman, & Aron, 1998) argue that a central human motivation is the desire to expand the self—to acquire social and material resources, perspectives, and identities that enhance one's ability to accomplish goals. The basic idea is linked to longstanding models of competence motivation, self-efficacy, and intrinsic motivation; most recently Taylor, Neter, and Wayment (1995) proposed that self-improvement, an idea much like self-expansion, may be an important self-related motive. The self-expansion motive is also specifically relevant to major relationship theories in that it specifies one basis for evaluating ultimate benefits and costs in interdependence approaches and that it seems to describe well the exploratory motive that plays an important, though mainly implicit, role in attachment theories.

There have also been a number of relationship studies involving self-expansion motivation. Aron, Paris, and Aron (1995), in two prospective longitudinal studies, showed that entering a new relationship (operationalized as falling in love) expands the self in the sense that one's spontaneous self-description increases in diversity and in the sense of an increase in perceived self-efficacy. Other studies have focused on the implication of the model that rapid self-expansion creates positive affect and thus that people are motivated to experience rapid self-expansion in order to experience this positive affect—an idea consistent with a proposal by Carver and Scheier (1990) that strong positive affect is associated with rapid progress toward goals. For example, in both a 10-week field experiment and in a series of laboratory experiments, couples randomly assigned to participate together in self-expanding (novel and challenging) activities showed increased relationship quality compared with couples assigned to merely pleasant activities (Aron, Norman, Aron, McKenna, & Heyman, 2000; Reissmann, Aron, & Bergen, 1993).

Further, this motivation suggests key attraction mechanisms. That is, according to this model, people enter and maintain relationships because in a relationship one includes the other in the self—and thus expands the self by gaining access to the other's resources, perspectives, and identities (Aron & Aron, 1986). In this context, Aron, Steele, and Kashdan (2002) found a predicted greater attractiveness for those with *different* interests than one's own (permitting maximum self-expansion) under conditions in which participants believed a relationship was likely if one desired it, but not under the more usual conditions in which the possibility of a relationship was ambiguous (so that similar interests functioned as an important cue that a relationship—and thus some degree of self-expansion—was possible). Following a quite different prediction from the same model, Amodio and Showers (2002) found greater attraction to partners perceived to have dissimilar personalities in the context of relationships involving low degrees of commitment (so that long-term compatibility was less important than short-term benefits of new experiences).

Summary of Self-Related Motivations and Close Relationships

A number of self-related motives play an important role in relationships. First, people attempt to maintain their self-esteem in the face of another person's outperforming them by basking in the glory of their success if they can; but if the other's success is in an area in which one is also trying to achieve, one may have a more negative reaction. Research in this area shows that, in the context of a close relationship, we also try to some extent to maintain the self-esteem of the partner. Second, a desire for consistency motivates people to prefer information (and the people that provide such information) that verifies their own preexisting understanding of themselves, even when those views are negative. However, at least in the context of close relationships, it seems that people may be influenced by both the desire to be seen as they actually are and the desire to be seen as positively as possible.

Another major set of self-related motivational issues relevant to relationships has to do with how it is that in close relationships people often act in ways that benefit the partner even at the apparent expense of self-interest. One line of work supports the notion that in committed relationships people transform gut-level selfish responses into more relationship-promotive ones in the interest of enhancing their long-term outcomes. Another line of work has shown that in close relationships people often adopt, in part out of empathy, communal norms in which they spontaneously attend to the needs of the other. A third line of work has shown that when partners feel interconnected, they act more equally for the benefit of themselves and the other, presumably because the other is part of self, so that benefiting other is benefiting oneself.

A final self-related motivation I considered is a desire to expand the self by acquiring social and material resources, perspectives, and identities that enhance one's ability to accomplish goals. Relationship-relevant studies involving self-expansion motivation have found that entering a new relationship expands the self in the sense that one's spontaneous self-description increases in diversity and in perceived self-efficacy; that couples who participate together in self-expanding (novel and challenging) activities show increased relationship quality; and that self-expansion motives seem to explain the dialectical role of similarity and difference in initial attraction.

Conclusions

Relationships play a central role, probably *the* central role, in shaping and reshaping the self; and the self plays a central role, perhaps *the* central role, in shaping and reshaping relationships. Much of the process, perhaps most of the process, of becoming close has to do with disclosing the self and linking self and other. Finally, much, if not most, self-related cognitive processing and much, if not most, self-related motivation is in the context of close relationships.

My informal sense of the field is that relationship researchers well recognize the crucial role of the self in understanding what they are studying. However, I hope this review has pointed out even to relationship researchers some of the very broad array of possibilities here, particularly possibilities of taking well-constructed theoretical models or research paradigms from other areas and applying them in creative ways to deepen our understanding of relationships. At the same time, my informal sense of the field is that self researchers do not adequately appreciate the centrality of relationships to their enterprise. Thus I especially hope that this review will bring home to them the importance and great opportunities for deepening understanding of the self that lie in explicitly taking into account close relationship phenomena.

Notes

1. Niedenthal and Beike (1997) developed an interesting related idea in which they adapt Goldstone's (1996) distinction between interrelated and isolated concepts to the self-concept. An interrelated concept is one whose meaning depends on links with other concepts at the same level of abstraction. In the case of a self-concept, this is usually a similarity or difference with another person. (Niedenthal & Beike do not emphasize any special role for close others, but their examples are mainly of siblings, parents, and spouses.) An isolated concept is one whose meaning does not depend on its link with other concepts at the same level of abstraction—it is a kind of primitive, fundamental-level concept usually based on direct experience. In three studies, Niedenthal and Beike showed that interrelated and isolated self-concepts functioned in parallel ways to those in which interrelated and isolated concepts more generally have been shown to function. For example, in one study, participants either (1) thought about ways in which they were different from a sibling (thus emphasizing the relation of the self-concept to the sibling concept) or (2) just thought about what they were like and what their sibling was like (thus not linking the two). As predicted from the model, in the interrelated-focus condition, participants made ratings of themselves and their siblings that were less abstract.

2. A possible interpretation of these various results showing smaller (or absent) self–other

differences for close others is that close others are more familiar and thus share with the self greater elaboration and organization (Symons & Johnson, 1997). Closeness and familiarity are confounded in most real-life situations, and it seems quite plausible that both operate to at least some extent. However, there are at least three reasons to consider a closeness interpretation as one major mechanism in this process. First, the response-time match–mismatch effect for partners has consistent large correlations with subjectively reported closeness (Aron et al., 1991; Aron & Fraley, 1999; Smith et al., 1999); but it has near zero correlations with reported familiarity and with variables that would seem to be relatively objective indicators of familiarity, such as number of different activities shared with other, amount of time spent with other, and relationship length (Aron et al., 1991; Aron & Fraley, 1999). Second, Symons and Johnson (1997) coded the other-referent in all 65 of the relevant self-reference studies for degree of familiarity and degree of intimacy. The mean difference between effect sizes in studies in which other was familiar and studies in which the other was not familiar was not significant and near zero; the mean difference between studies in which the other was intimate and studies in which the other was not intimate was significant and substantial. Finally, Mashek and colleagues (2002, Studies 2 and 3), attempted to pit the two explanations against each other. They employed samples of individuals who were closer to their closest friend than they were to their closest parent— but more familiar with the closest parent in the sense of having known the parent substantially longer and in substantially more different contexts. The results in both studies showed significantly more confusions between self and one's closest friend than between self and one's closest parent.

3. This line of thinking is closely related to ideas (and substantial supporting data) put forward by social identity (e.g., Tajfel, 1981) and social categorization (e.g., Turner, Hogg, Oakes, Reicher, & Wetherell, 1987) theorists, mainly in the context of group processes. In particular, they argue that we take on the identities of groups of which we are part—in principle including families and even dyads. This approach and that of the inclusion of other in the self, however, may well be closely linked. For example, Smith (Smith & Henry, 1996; Smith et al., 1999), applying a modified version of the Aron and colleagues (1991) match–mismatch response-time paradigm, showed that we include ingroups in the self in the same way as we include close others. Further, the magnitude of this effect correlates strongly with self-reported ingroup identification (Coats, Smith, Claypool, & Banner, 1999; Tropp & Wright, 2001).

4. In a related line of work, Weisz and Wood (in press) found that students were more likely to maintain closeness and contact with friends who provided more support for their social identities (such as athlete).

References

Acitelli, L. K., & Antonucci, T. C. (1994). Gender differences in the link between marital support and satisfaction in older couples. *Journal of Personality and Social Psychology, 67,* 688–698.

Acitelli, L. K., Rogers, S., & Knee, C. R. (1999). The role of identity in the link between relationship thinking and relationship satisfaction. *Journal of Social and Personal Relationships, 16*(5), 591–618.

Agnew, C. R., Van Lange, P. A. M., Rusbult, C. E., & Langston, C. A. (1998). Cognitive interdependence: Commitment and the mental representation of close relationships. *Journal of Personality and Social Psychology, 74,* 939–954.

Amodio, D. M., & Showers, C. J. (2002). *Romantic styles: Similarity, self-expansion, and the role of commitment.* Manuscript submitted for publication.

Andersen, S. M., & Berensen, K. (2001). Perceiving, feeling, and wanting: Motivation and affect deriving from significant other representations and transference. In J. P. Forgas, K. D. Williams, & L. Wheeler (Eds.), *The social mind: Cognitive and motivational aspects of interpersonal behavior* (pp. 231–256). New York: Cambridge University Press.

Aron, A., & Aron, E. (1986). *Love as the expansion of self: Understanding attraction and satisfaction.* New York: Hemisphere.

Aron, A., Aron, E., & Smollan, D. (1992). Inclusion of Other in the Self Scale and the structure of interpersonal closeness. *Journal of Personality and Social Psychology, 63,* 596–612.

Aron, A., Aron, E. N., & Norman, C. (2001). Self-expansion model of motivation and cognition in close relationships and beyond. In M. Clark & G. Fletcher (Eds.), *Blackwell's handbook of social psychology: Vol. 2. Interpersonal processes* (pp. 478–501). Oxford, UK: Blackwell.

Aron, A., Aron, E. N., Tudor, M., & Nelson, G. (1991). Close relationships as including other in the self. *Journal of Personality and Social Psychology, 60,* 241–253.

Aron, A., & Fraley, B. (1999). Relationship closeness as including other in the self: Cognitive underpinnings and measures. *Social Cognition, 17*(2), 140–160.

Aron, A., Melinat, E., Aron, E. N., Vallone, R., & Bator, R. (1997). The experimental generation of interpersonal closeness: A procedure and some preliminary findings. *Personality and Social Psychology Bulletin, 23,* 363–377.

Aron, A., Norman, C. C., & Aron, E. N. (1998). The self-expansion model and motivation. *Representative Research in Social Psychology, 22,* 1–13.

Aron, A., Norman, C. C., & Aron, E. N., McKenna, C., &

Heyman, R. (2000). Couple's shared participation in novel and arousing activities and experienced relationship quality. *Journal of Personality and Social Psychology, 78,* 273–284.

Aron, A., Paris, M., & Aron, E. N. (1995). Falling in love: Prospective studies of self-concept change. *Journal of Personality and Social Psychology, 69*(6), 1102–1112.

Aron, A., Steele, J., & Kashdan, T. (2002). *Attraction to others with similar interests as moderated by perceived opportunity for a relationship.* Manuscript in preparation.

Aron, A., & Westbay, L. (1996). Dimensions of the prototype of love. *Journal of Personality and Social Psychology, 70,* 535–551.

Aube, J., & Koestner, R. (1992). Gender characteristics and adjustment: A longitudinal study. *Journal of Personality and Social Psychology, 63,* 274–285.

Baldwin, M. W. (1992). Relational schemas and the processing of social information. *Psychological Bulletin, 112,* 461–484.

Baldwin, M. W. (1994). Primed relational schemas as a source of self-evaluative reactions. *Journal of Social and Clinical Psychology, 13,* 380–403.

Baldwin, M. W. (1997). Relational schemas as a source of if–then self-inference procedures. *Review of General Psychology, 1,* 326–335.

Baldwin, M. W., Carrell, S. E., & Lopez, D. F. (1990). Priming relationship schemas: My advisor and the Pope are watching me from the back of my mind. *Journal of Experimental Social Psychology, 26,* 434–454.

Baldwin, M. W., Fehr, B., Keedian, W., Seidel, M., & Thompson, D. W. (1993). An exploration of the relational schemas underlying attachment styles: Self-report and lexical decision approaches. *Personality and Social Psychology Bulletin, 19,* 746–754.

Baldwin, M. W., & Holmes, J. G. (1987). Salient private audiences and awareness of the self. *Journal of Personality and Social Psychology, 53,* 1087–1098.

Baldwin, M. W., & Sinclair, L. (1996). Self-esteem and "if . . . then" contingencies of interpersonal acceptance. *Journal of Personality and Social Psychology, 71,* 1130–1141.

Batson, C. D., Sager, K., Garst, E., Kang, M., Rubchinsky, K., & Dawson, K. (1997). Is empathy-induced helping due to self–other merging? *Journal of Personality and Social Psychology, 73,* 495–509.

Baumeister, R. F., Bratslavsky, E., Muraven, M., & Tice, D. M. (1998). Ego depletion: Is the active self a limited resource? *Journal of Personality and Social Psychology, 74,* 1252–1265.

Beach, S. R. H., & Tesser, A. (1993). Decision making power and marital satisfaction: A self-evaluation maintenance perspective. *Journal of Social and Clinical Psychology, 12,* 471–494.

Beach, S. R. H., Tesser, A., Fincham, F. D., Jones, D. J., Johnson, D., & Whitaker, D. J. (1998). Pleasure and pain in doing well, together: An investigation of performance-related affect in close relationships. *Journal of Personality and Social Psychology, 74*(4), 923–938.

Beach, S. R. H., Tesser, A., Mendolia, M., Anderson, P., Crelia, R., Whitaker, D., & Fincham, F. D. (1996). Self-evaluation maintenance in marriage: Toward a performance ecology of the marital relationship. *Journal of Family Psychology, 10*(4), 379–396.

Beer, J. S., & Kihlstrom, J. F. (2000). *The relational self: Representations of self-with-others in close relationships.* Manuscript submitted for publication.

Berk, M. S., & Andersen, S. M. (2000). The impact of past relationships on interpersonal behavior: Behavioral confirmation in the social-cognitive process of transference. *Journal of Personality and Social Psychology, 79*(4), 546–562.

Berscheid, E., & Reis, H. T. (1998). Attraction and close relationships. In S. Fiske, D. Gilbert, & G. Lindzey (Eds.), *The handbook of social psychology* (4th ed., pp. 193–281). Boston: McGraw-Hill.

Berscheid, E., Snyder, M., & Omoto, A. M. (1989). The Relationship Closeness Inventory: Assessing the closeness of interpersonal relationships. *Journal of Personality and Social Psychology, 57,* 792–807.

Bornstein, R. F., Riggs, J. M., Hill, E. L., & Calabrese, C. (1996). Activity, passivity, self-denigration, and self-promotion: Toward an interactionist model of interpersonal dependency. *Journal of Personality, 64*(3), 638–673.

Bowlby, J. (1969). *Attachment and loss: Vol. 1. Attachment.* New York: Basic Books.

Brewer, M. B. (1993). Social identity, distinctiveness, and in-group homogeneity. *Social Cognition, 11,* 150–164.

Brewer, M. B., & Pickett, C. L. (1999). Distinctiveness motives as a source of the social self. In T. Tyler, R. Kramer, & O. John (Eds.), *The psychology of the social self: Applied social research* (pp. 71–87). Mahwah, NJ: Erlbaum.

Campbell, J. D., Trapnell, P. D., Heine, S. J., Katz, I. M., Lavellee, L. F., & Lehman, D. R. (1996). Self-concept clarity: Measurement, personality correlates, and cultural boundaries. *Journal of Personality and Social Psychology, 70,* 141–156.

Campbell, W. K. (1999). Narcissism and romantic attraction. *Journal of Personality and Social Psychology, 77*(6), 1254–1270.

Campbell, W. K., Reeder, G. D., Sedikides, C., & Elliot, A. J. (2000). Narcissism and comparative self-enhancement strategies. *Journal of Research in Personality, 34,* 329–347.

Campbell, W., Sedikides, C., Reeder, G. D., & Elliot, A. J. (2000). Among friends? An examination of friendship and the self-serving bias. *British Journal of Social Psychology, 39*(2), 229–239.

Carver, C. S., & Scheier, M. F. (1990). Principles of self-regulation: Action and emotion. In E. T. Higgins & R. M. Sorrentino (Eds.), *Handbook of motivation and cognition: Foundations of social behavior* (Vol. 2, pp. 3–52). New York: Guilford Press.

Cialdini, R. B., Borden, R. J., Thorne, A., Walker, M. R., Freeman, S., & Sloan, L. R. (1976). Basking in reflected glory: Three (football) field studies. *Journal of Personality and Social Psychology, 34,* 366–375.

Cialdini, R. B., Brown, S. L., Lewis, B. P., Luce, C., & Neuberg, S. L. (1997). Reinterpreting the empathy–altruism relationships: When one into one equals oneness. *Journal of Personality and Social Psychology, 73,* 481–494.

Clark, M. S., & Mills, J. (1993). The difference between communal and exchange relationships: What it is and is not. *Personality and Social Psychology Bulletin, 19,* 684–691.

Clark, M. S., Mills, J., & Powell, M. (1986). Keeping track of needs in two types of relationships. *Journal of Personality and Social Psychology, 51,* 333–338.

Clark, M. S., Ouellette, R., Powell, M. C., & Milberg, S. (1987). Recipient's mood, relationship type, and helping. *Journal of Personality and Social Psychology, 53,* 94–103.

Coats, S., Smith, E. R., Claypool, H. M., & Banner, M. J. (1999). Overlapping mental representations of self and in-group: Reaction time evidence and its relationship with explicit measures of group identification. *Journal of Experimental Social Psychology, 36,* 304–315.

Collins, N. L., & Miller, L. C. (1994). Self-disclosure and liking: A meta-analytic review. *Psychological Bulletin, 116*(3), 457–475.

Cook, W. L., & Douglas, E. M. (1998). The looking-glass self in family context: A social relations analysis. *Journal of Family Psychology, 3,* 299–309.

Cooley, C. H. (1902). *Human nature and the social order.* New York: Scribner's.

Cross, S. E., Bacon, P. L., & Morris, M. L. (2000). The relational-interdependent self-construal and relationships. *Journal of Personality and Social Psychology, 78*(4), 791–808.

Darley, J. M., & Fazio, R. H. (1980). Expectancy confirmation processes arising in the social interaction sequence. *American Psychologist, 35,* 867–881.

Derlega, V. J., Metts, S., Petronio, S., & Margulis, S. T. (1993). *Self-disclosure.* Newbury Park, CA: Sage.

Doherty, W. J., Su, S., & Needle, R. (1989). Marital disruption and psychological well-being. *Journal of Family Issues, 10,* 72–85.

Drigotas, S. M., Rusbult, C. E., Wieselquist, J., & Whitton, S. W. (1999). Close partner as sculptor of the ideal self: Behavioral affirmation and the Michelangelo phenomenon. *Journal of Personality and Social Psychology, 77*(2), 293–323.

Elliott, M. (1996). Impact of work, family, and welfare receipt on women's self-esteem in young adulthood. *Social Psychology Quarterly, 59*(1), 80–95.

Erikson, E. (1950). *Childhood and society.* New York: Norton.

Fehr, B. (1988). Prototype analysis of the concepts of love and commitment. *Journal of Personality and Social Psychology, 55,* 557–579.

Fehr, B., & Russell, J. A. (1991). The concept of love viewed from a prototype perspective. *Journal of Personality and Social Psychology, 60,* 425–438.

Felson, R. B. (1989). Parents and the reflected appraisal process: A longitudinal analysis. *Journal of Personality and Social Psychology, 56,* 965–971.

Finkel, E. J., & Campbell, W. K. (2001). Self-control and accommodation in close relationships: An interdependence analysis. *Journal of Personality and Social Psychology, 81,* 263–277.

Fletcher, G. J. O., & Kininmouth, L. (1992). Measuring relationship beliefs: An individual differences scale. *Journal of Research in Personality, 26,* 371–397.

Fletcher, G. J. O., Simpson, J. A., Thomas, G., & Giles, L. (1999). Ideals in intimate relationships. *Journal of Personality and Social Psychology, 76,* 72–89.

Goldstone, R. L. (1996). Isolated and interrelated concepts. *Memory and Cognition, 24,* 608–628.

Gurung, R. A. R., Sarason, B. R., & Sarason, I. G. (2001).

Predicting relationship quality and emotional reactions to stress from significant-other concept clarity. *Personality and Social Psychology Bulletin, 27,* 1267–1276.

Harris, M. J., & Rosenthal, R. (1985). Mediation of interpersonal expectation effects: 31 meta-analyses. *Psychological Bulletin, 97,* 363–386.

Hassebrauck, M. (1997). Cognitions of relationship quality: A prototype analysis of their structure and consequences. *Personal Relationships, 4,* 163–185.

Hassebrauck, M., & Aron, A. (2001). Prototype matching in close relationships. *Personality and Social Psychology Bulletin, 27,* 1111–1122.

Heatherington, T. F., & Vohs, K. D. (2000). Interpersonal evaluations following threats to self: Role of self-esteem. *Journal of Personality and Social Psychology, 78,* 725–736.

Helgeson, V. S., Shaver, P., & Dyer, M. (1987). Prototypes of intimacy and distance in same-sex and opposite-sex relationships. *Journal of Social and Personal Relationships, 4,* 195–233.

Hendrick, S. S., Hendrick, C., & Adler, N. L. (1988). Romantic relationships: Love, satisfaction, and staying together. *Journal of Personality and Social Psychology, 54,* 980–988.

Hinde, R. A., Finkenauer, C., & Auhagen, A. E. (2001). Relationships and the self-concept. *Personal Relationships, 8,* 187–204.

Holmes, J. G. (2000). Social relationships: The nature and function of relational schemas. *European Journal of Social Psychology, 30,* 447–455.

Karney, B. R., & Bradbury, T. N. (1995). The longitudinal course of marital quality and stability: A review of theory, method, and research. *Psychological Bulletin, 118*(1), 3–34.

Katz, J., Anderson, P., & Beach, S. R. H. (1997). Dating relationship quality: Effects of global self-verification and self-enhancement. *Journal of Social and Personal Relationships, 14*(6), 829–842.

Keelan, J. P. R., Dion, K. K., & Dion, K. L. (1998). Attachment style and relationship satisfaction: Test of a self-disclosure explanation. *Canadian Journal of Behavioural Science, 30*(1), 24–35.

Kelley, H. H., Berscheid, E., Christensen, A., Harvey, J. H., Huston, T. L., Levinger, G., McClintock, E., Peplau, L. A., & Peterson, D. R. (1983). *Close relationships.* San Francisco: Freeman.

Kelley, H. H., & Thibaut, J. W. (1978). *Interpersonal relationships: A theory of interdependence.* New York: Wiley.

Kenny, D. A. (1994). *Interpersonal perception: A social relations analysis.* New York: Guilford Press.

Kenny, D. A., & DePaulo, B. M. (1993). Do people know how others view them? An empirical and theoretical account. *Psychological Bulletin, 114,* 145–161.

Knee, C. R. (1998). Implicit theories of relationships: Assessment and prediction of romantic relationship initiation, coping, and longevity. *Journal of Personality and Social Psychology, 74*(2), 360–370.

Knee, C. R., Nanayakkara, A., Vietor, N. A., Neighbors, C., & Patrick, H. (2001). Implicit theories of relationships: Who cares if romantic partners are less than ideal? *Personality and Social Psychology Bulletin, 27,* 808–819.

Kwan, V. S. Y., Bond, M. H., & Singelis, T. M. (1997).

Pancultural explanations for life satisfaction: Adding relationship harmony to self-esteem. *Journal of Personality and Social Psychology, 73*(5), 1038–1051.

Larson, J. H., Anderson, S. M., Holman, T. B., & Niemann, B. K. (1998). A longitudinal study of the effects of premarital communication, relationship stability, and self-esteem on sexual satisfaction in the first year of marriage. *Journal of Sex and Marital Therapy, 24*(3), 193–206.

Laurenceau, J.P., Barrett, L. F., & Pietromonaco, P. R. (1998). Intimacy as an interpersonal process: The importance of self-disclosure, partner disclosure, and perceived partner responsiveness in interpersonal exchanges. *Journal of Personality and Social Psychology, 74*(5), 1238–1251.

Leary, M. R. (1999). The social and psychological importance of self-esteem. In R. M. Kowalski & M. R. Leary (Eds.), *The social psychology of emotional and behavioral problems: Interfaces of social and clinical psychology* (pp. 197–221). Washington, DC: American Psychological Association.

Leary, M. R. (2002). When selves collide: The nature of the self and the dynamics of interpersonal relationships. In A. Tesser, D. Stapel, & J. V. Wood (Eds.), *Self and motivation: Emerging psychological perspectives.* Washington, DC: American Psychological Association.

Leary, M. R., & Baumeister, R. F. (2000). The nature and function of self-esteem: Sociometer theory. In M. Zanna (Ed.), *Advances in experimental social psychology* (Vol. 32, pp. 1–62). San Diego, CA: Academic Press.

Leary, M. R., & Downs, D. L. (1995). Interpersonal functions of the self-esteem motive: The self-esteem system as a sociometer. In M. Kernis (Ed.), *Efficacy, agency, and self-esteem* (pp. 123–144). New York: Plenum Press.

Leary, M. R., Tambor, E. S., Terdal, S. K., & Downs, D. L. (1995). Self-esteem as an interpersonal monitor: The sociometer hypothesis. *Journal of Personality and Social Psychology, 68*(3), 518–530.

Lin, Y. C. (1992). *The construction of the sense of intimacy from everyday social interaction.* Unpublished doctoral dissertation, University of Rochester.

Maccoby, E. E. (2000). Parenting and its effects on children: On reading and misreading behavior genetics. *Annual Review of Psychology, 51,* 1–27.

Mashek, D. J., Aron, A., & Boncimino, M. (2002). *Confusions of self and close others.* Manuscript submitted for publication.

Mashek, D. J. (in press). Too much of a good thing? The experience of feeling too close to intimate others. In D. J. Mashek & A. Aron (Eds.), *Handbook of closeness and intimacy.* Mahwah, NJ: Erlbaum.

McAdams, D. P. (1989). *Intimacy: The need to be close.* New York: Doubleday.

McCall, M. (1995). Orientation, outcome, and other-serving attributions. *Basic and Applied Social Psychology, 17*(1–2), 49–64.

McCall, M., Reno, R. R., Jalbert, N., & West, S. G. (2000). Communal orientation and attributions between the self and other. *Basic and Applied Social Psychology, 22*(4), 301–308.

Medvene, L. J., Teal, C. R., & Slavich, S. (2000). Including the other in self: Implications for judgments of equity

and satisfaction in close relationships. *Journal of Social and Clinical Psychology, 19,* 396–419.

Mendolia, M., Beach, S. R. H., & Tesser, A. (1996). The relationship between marital interaction behaviors and affective reactions to one's own and one's spouse's self-evaluation needs. *Personal Relationships, 3,* 279–292.

Merton, R. K. (1948). The self-fulfilling prophecy. *Antioch Review, 8,* 193–210.

Morf, C. C., & Rhodewalt, F. (1993). Narcissism and self-evaluation maintenance: Explorations in object relations. *Personality and Social Psychology Bulletin, 19,* 668–676.

Morf, C. C., & Rhodewalt, F. (2001). Unraveling the paradoxes of narcissism: A dynamic self-regulatory processing model. *Psychological Inquiry, 12,* 177–196.

Murray, S. L., & Holmes, J. G. (1999) The (mental) ties that bind: Cognitive structures that predict relationship resilience. *Journal of Personality and Social Psychology, 77,* 1228–1244.

Murray, S. L., Holmes, J. G., & Griffin, D. W. (1996a). The benefits of positive illusions: Idealization and the construction of satisfaction in close relationships. *Journal of Personality and Social Psychology, 70,* 79–98.

Murray, S. L., Holmes, J. G., & Griffin, D. W. (1996b). The self-fulfilling nature of positive illusions in romantic relationships: Love is not blind but prescient. *Journal of Personality and Social Psychology, 71,* 1155–1180.

Murray, S. L., & Holmes, J. G., & Griffin, D. W. (2000). Self-esteem and the quest for felt security: How perceived regard regulates attachment processes. *Journal of Personality and Social Psychology, 78,* 478–498.

Niedenthal, P. M., & Beike, D. R. (1997). Interrelated and isolated self-concepts. *Personality and Social Psychology Review, 1,* 106–128.

Olson, D. H., Russell, C. S., & Sprenkle, D. H. (1983). Circumplex model of marital and family systems: 6. Theoretical update. *Family Process, 22,* 69–83.

Pierce, T., & Lydon, J. (1998). Priming relational schemas: Effects of contextually activated and chronically accessible interpersonal expectations on responses to a stressful event. *Journal of Personality and Social Psychology, 75,* 1441–1448.

Pietromonaco, P. R., & Barrett, L. F. (2000). Attachment theory as an organizing framework: A view from different levels of analysis. *Review of General Psychology, 4*(2), 107–110.

Planalp, S. (1987). Interplay between relational knowledge and events. In R. Burnet, P. McGhee, & D. D. Clarke (Eds.), *Accounting for relationships: Explanation, representation, and knowledge* (pp. 175–191). London: Methuen.

Reis, H. T., & Downey, G. (1999). Social cognition in relationships: Building essential bridges between two literatures. *Social Cognition, 17,* 97–117.

Reis, H. T., & Patrick, B. C. (1996). Attachment and intimacy: Component processes. In E. T. Higgins & A. W. Kruglanski (Eds.), *Social psychology: Handbook of basic principles* (pp. 523–563). New York: Guilford Press.

Reis, H. T., & Shaver, P. (1988). Intimacy as interpersonal process. In S. Duck (Ed.), *Handbook of personal relationships: Theory, research and interventions* (pp. 367–389). Chichester, UK: Wiley.

Reissmann, C., Aron, A., & Bergen, M. R. (1993). Shared activities and marital satisfaction: Causal direction and self-expansion versus boredom. *Journal of Social and Personal Relationships, 10,* 243–254.

Riggs, J. M., & Cantor, N. (1984). Getting acquainted: The role of the self-concept and preconceptions. *Personality and Social Psychology Bulletin, 10,* 432–445.

Rosenthal, R., & Jacobson, L. F. (1968). Teacher expectations for the disadvantaged. *Scientific American, 218,* 19–23.

Rusbult, C. E., & Arriaga, X. B. (2000). Interdependence in personal relationships. In W. Ickes & S. Duck (Eds.), *The social psychology of personal relationships* (pp. 79–108). Chichester, UK: Wiley.

Rusbult, C. E., Onizuka, R. K., & Lipkus, I. (1993). What do we really want? Mental models of ideal romantic involvement explored through multidimensional scaling. *Journal of Experimental Social Psychology, 29,* 493–527.

Rusbult, C. E., Verette, J., Whitney, G. A., Slovik, L. F., & Lipkus, I. (1991). Accommodation processes in close relationships: Theory and preliminary empirical evidence. *Journal of Personality and Social Psychology, 60,* 53–78.

Schutz, A. (1998a). Autobiographical narratives of good and bad needs: Defensive and favorable self-description moderated by trait self-esteem. *Journal of Social and Clinical Psychology, 17*(4), 466–475.

Schutz, A. (1998b). Coping with threats to self-esteem: The differing patterns of subjects with high versus low trait self-esteem in first-person accounts. *European Journal of Personality, 12,* 169–186.

Sedikides, C., Campbell, W. K., Reeder, G. D., & Elliot, A. J. (2002). The self in relationships: Whether, how and when close others put the self "in its place." *European Review of Social Psychology, 12,* 237–265.

Sedikides, C., Campbell, W. K., Reeder, G. D., Elliot, A. J., & Gregg, A. P. (2002). Do others bring out the worst in narcissists? The "other exist for me" illusion. In Y. Kashima, M. Foddy, & M. Platow (Eds.), *Self and identity: Personal, social, and symbolic* (pp. 103–123). Mahwah, NJ: Erlbaum.

Sedikides, C., & Strube, M. J. (1995). The multiply motivated self. *Personality and Social Psychology Bulletin, 21*(12), 1330–1335.

Shackelford, T. K. (2001). Self-esteem in marriage. *Personality and Individual Differences, 30,* 371–390.

Shaver, P. R., Collins, N., & Clark, C. L. (1996). Attachment styles and internal working models of self and relationship partners. In G. J. O. Fletcher & J. Fitness (Eds.), *Knowledge structures in close relationships: A social psychological approach* (pp. 25–61). Mahwah, NJ: Erlbaum.

Shaver, P. R., & Hazan, C. (1993). Adult romantic attachment: Theory and evidence. In D. Perlman & W. Jones (Eds.), *Advances in personal relationships* (Vol. 4, pp. 29–70). London: Kingsley.

Shaver, P. R., Schwartz, J., Kirson, D., & O'Connor, C. (1987). Emotional knowledge: Further explorations of a prototype approach. *Journal of Personality and Social Psychology, 52,* 1061–1086.

Showers, C. J., & Kevlyn, S. B. (1999). Organization of knowledge about a relationship partner: Implications for liking and loving. *Journal of Personality and Social Psychology, 76,* 958–971.

Showers, C. J., & Kling, K. C. (1996). The organization of

self-knowledge: Implications for mood regulation. In L. L. Martin & A. Tesser (Eds.), *Striving and feeling: Interactions among goals, affect, and self-regulation* (pp. 151–174). Mahwah, NJ: Erlbaum.

Smith, E., & Henry, S. (1996). An in-group becomes part of the self: Response time evaluation. *Personality and Social Psychology Bulletin, 22,* 635–642.

Smith, E. R., Coats, S., & Walling, D. (1999). Overlapping mental representations of self, in-group, and partner: Further response time evidence for a connectionist model. *Personality and Social Psychology Bulletin, 25*(7), 873–882.

Snyder, M., Tanke, E. D., & Berscheid, E. (1977). Social perception and interpersonal behavior: The self-fulfilling nature of social stereotypes. *Journal of Personality and Social Psychology, 35,* 656–666.

Steinberg, L., & Silverberg, S. B. (1987). Influences on marital satisfaction during the middle stages of the family life cycle. *Journal of Marriage and the Family, 49,* 751–760.

Sternberg, R. (1986). A triangular theory of love. *Psychological Review, 93,* 119–135.

Swann, W. B., Jr. (1990). To be adored or to be known?: The interplay of self-enhancement and self-verification. In E. T. Higgins & R. Sorrentino (Eds.), *Handbook of motivation and cognition* (Vol. 2, pp. 408–448). New York: Guilford Press.

Swann, W. B., Jr., De La Ronde, C., & Hixon, J. G. (1994). Authenticity and positive strivings in marriage and courtship. *Journal of Personality and Social Psychology, 66,* 857–869.

Symons, C. S., & Johnson, B. T. (1997). The self-reference effect in memory: A meta-analysis. *Psychological Bulletin, 121*(3), 371–394.

Tajfel, H. (1981). *Human groups and social categories: Studies in social psychology.* Cambridge, UK: Cambridge University Press.

Tangney, J. P. (2002). Self-conscious emotions: The self as a moral guide. In A. Tesser, D. I. Stapel, & J. V. Wood (Eds.). *Self and motivation: Emerging psychological perspectives* (pp. 97–117). Washington, DC: American Psychological Association.

Taylor, S. E., Neter, E., & Wayment, H. A. (1995). Self-evaluative processes. *Personality and Social Psychology Bulletin, 21,* 1278–1287.

Tesser, A. (1988). Toward a self-evaluation maintenance model of social behavior. In L. Berkowitz (Ed.), *Advances in experimental social psychology* (Vol. 11, pp. 288–338). San Diego, CA: Academic Press.

Tesser, A., Millar, M., & Moore, J. (1988). Some affective consequences of social comparison and reflection processes: The pain and pleasure of being close. *Journal of Personality and Social Psychology, 54,* 49–61.

Tice, D. M., Butler, J. L., Muraven, M. B., & Stillwell, A. M. (1995). When modesty prevails: Differential favorability of self-presentation to friends and strangers. *Journal of Personality and Social Psychology, 69*(6), 1120–1138.

Tropp, L. R., & Wright, S. C. (2001). Ingroup identification as the inclusion of ingroup in the self. *Personality and Social Psychology Bulletin, 27,* 585–600.

Turner, J. C., Hogg, M. A., Oakes, P. J., Reicher, S. D., & Wetherell, M. S. (1987). *Rediscovering the social group: A self-categorization theory.* Oxford, UK: Blackwell.

Van Lange, P. A. M., Rusbult, C. E., Drigotas, S. M., Arriaga, X. B., Witcher, B. S., & Cox, C. L. (1997). Willingness to sacrifice in close relationships. *Journal of Personality and Social Psychology, 72,* 1373–1395.

Vohs, K. D., & Heatherington, T. F. (2000). *Self-esteem and threats to self: Implications for self-construals and interpersonal perceptions.* Manuscript submitted for publication.

Voss, K., Markiewicz, D., & Doyle, A. B. (1999). Friendship, marriage and self-esteem. *Journal of Social and Personal Relationships, 16*(1), 103–122.

Waring, E. M. (1988). *Enhancing marital intimacy through facilitating cognitive self disclosure.* New York: Brunner/Mazel.

Weisz, C., & Wood, L. F. (in press). Social identities and friendships: A longitudinal study of support for social identities. *Journal of Social Behavior and Personality.*

Williamson, G. M., & Clark, M. S. (1992). Impact of desired relationship type on affective reactions to choosing and being required to help. *Personality and Social Psychology Bulletin, 18,* 10–18.

Yovetich, N. A., & Rusbult, C. E. (1994). Accommodative behavior in close relationships: Exploring transformation of motivation. *Journal of Experimental Social Psychology, 30,* 138–164.

Zajonc, R. B., Adelmann, R. K., Murphy, S. B., & Niedenthal, R. N. (1987). Convergence in the physical appearances of spouses. *Motivation and Emotion, 11,* 335–346.

23

Social Identity

MICHAEL A. HOGG

Human groups lie at the heart of social life. We are brought up in families, we are educated in classes, we affiliate with peer groups, we play team games, we work in organizations, and we make decisions in committees. We also belong to professional groups, and we identify with gender, ethnic, political, and national groups. Groups vary enormously in size, longevity, function, entitativity, and cohesiveness. They can range from small, interactive, and transitory groups, such as a committee in an organization, to large-scale, enduring social categories, such as an ethnic group.

The groups we belong to profoundly influence how others know us—they are the lens through which people view us. Groups also profoundly influence how we view ourselves; they influence the type of people we are, the things we do, the attitudes and values we hold, and the way we perceive and react to people around us. Groups furnish us with an identity, a way of locating ourselves in relation to other people. Indeed, our sense of self derives from the groups and categories we belong to, and in many ways individuality may "merely" be the unique combination of distinct groups and categories that define who we are. The enduring centrality of groups in human life may even have had an evolutionary impact on our species (Caporael, 2001; Hogg, 2001e).

This chapter focuses on the relationship between group life and self-conception. How do groups and categories influence self and identity, and in turn how does self-conception in group terms (i.e., the collective self) influence processes within and between groups? These questions revolve around the nature of social identity.

Social identity has been defined by Tajfel as "the individual's knowledge that he belongs to certain social groups together with some emotional and value significance to him of his group membership" (1972, p. 292). For Tajfel, social identity is knowledge of being a group member and thus of what attributes define membership in the group, but it is also an emotional attachment to the group and knowledge of the social standing of the group in relation to other groups (i.e., its status). Since this early definition, the concept of social identity has been the unifying principle at the core of the social identity perspective in social psychology—a perspective that has become one of the main theoretical frameworks in social psychology for the analysis of the relationship between collective self, group membership, group processes, and intergroup relations. As such, a discussion of social identity is, inevitably, a discussion of the social identity perspective.

A great deal has been published over the past 30 years on social identity. Some of the more recent major sources include: Abrams and Hogg (1990b, 1999, 2001), Ellemers, Spears, and Doosje (1999), Hogg (2001c), Hogg and Abrams (1988), Oakes, Haslam, and Turner (1994), Robinson (1996), Turner, Hogg, Oakes, Reicher, and Wetherell (1987), and Worchel, Morales, Páez, and Deschamps (1998). Unsurprisingly, there are differing interpretations of social identity theory and the social identity perspective. The position taken in this chapter is that the social identity perspective is an umbrella conceptual framework that contains a number of compatible and interrelated conceptual components or subtheories that emphasize different aspects of the perspective (e.g., Abrams & Hogg, 2001; Hogg, 2001c; Hogg & Abrams, 1988; Hogg & McGarty, 1990; Turner, 1999). In recent years the social identity perspective has made a significant impact on social psychology and has helped reenergize interest in groups (e.g., Abrams & Hogg, 1998; Hogg & Abrams, 1999; Moreland, Hogg, & Hains, 1994).

In this chapter I provide an integrative review of the social identity perspective. The chapter is organized in a relatively historical progression according to what I consider to be some of the key conceptual components of the approach and some of the key areas of research: collective self and the social group; categorization and accentuation; categorization and discrimination; social comparison; self-enhancement and self-esteem; intergroup relations and social beliefs; self-categorization and depersonalization; salience; conformity and influence; structural differentiation within groups; and uncertainty reduction. I close with some brief comments on social identity research in neighboring disciplines—specifically, social cognition, the social psychology of language, organizational psychology, and sociology.

Collective Self and the Social Group

Social identity theory is a theory of the self. It rests on a fundamental distinction between the collective self (social identity), which is associated with group membership, group processes, and intergroup behavior, and the individual self (personal identity), which is associated with close personal relationships and idiosyncratic attributes of self (e.g., Tajfel & Turner, 1979; Turner, 1982; also see Hogg & Abrams, 1988). More specifically, social identity referred to commonalities among people within a group and differences between people in different groups and was associated with group behaviors (e.g., ethnocentrism, ingroup bias, intergroup discrimination, conformity, normative behavior, stereotyping, cohesion, collective self-definition). Personal identity referred to self as distinct from other people or self as defined in terms of specific relationships with other individuals and was not associated with group behaviors. Both forms of self-conceptualization were socially constructed and grounded, but social identity theory, as a theory of intergroup relations and group membership, did not explore personal identity.

This sharp discontinuity between social identity and group phenomena on the one hand and personal identity and interpersonal/individual phenomena on the other was intended to avoid the reduction of group and intergroup phenomena to an aggregation of individual and interpersonal processes—group phenomena and the collective self require a different level of explanation. Social identity theorists have long believed that the social psychology of collective phenomena is limited by reductionism (e.g., Hogg, 1993; Taylor & Brown, 1979; Turner & Oakes, 1986) and that levels of explanation need to be differentiated and then articulated (e.g., Doise, 1986). It should be recognized that social identity theory developed in Europe as an integral part of the wider development of post-World War II European social psychology. It is thus framed by a European metatheory that has systematically promoted nonreductionist approaches in social psychology (e.g., Tajfel, Jaspars, & Fraser, 1984).

More recent research in the broad social identity–social categorization tradition has provided a more textured classification of self. For example, Brewer and Gardner (1996) distinguish between three aspects of the self: the individual self (defined by personal traits that differentiate self from all others), the relational self (defined by dyadic relationships that assimilate self to significant other persons), and the collective self (defined by group membership that differentiates "us" from "them"). Elsewhere (Hogg, 2001e; Hogg & Williams, 2000) I have suggested that, in social identity terms, although the distinction between relational and individual self is valid, these two forms of self may nonetheless be different aspects of personal identity rather than of social identity—and, furthermore, that relational and individual self may gain their meanings within the parameters of the collective self.

Other distinctions between collective and individual selves have been made by, for example, Deaux (1996; Deaux, Reid, Mizrahi, & Cotting, 1999), Greenwald and Pratkanis (1984), Luhtanen and Crocker (1992), and Triandis (1989). Reid and Deaux (1996) acknowledge a basic difference between collective and individual selves (they use the terms [social] "identities" and [personal] "attributes" rather than "social identity" and "personal identity") but suggest that the cognitive organization of self-structure involves a significant amount of linkage between certain identities and certain attributes. Deaux, Reid, Mizrahi, and Ethier (1995) have also suggested that although social and personal identities differ qualitatively from one another, there are also important qualitative differences among types of social identity (e.g., ethnicity, religion, stigma, political).

This last point is also taken up by Brewer (2001), who integrates social psychological, sociological, and political science literatures to identify four general types of, or perspectives on, social identity: (1) *person-based social identities* emphasize the way in which properties of groups are internalized by individual group members as part of the self-concept; (2) *relational social identities* define self in relation to specific other people with whom one interacts in a group context; this definition corresponds closely to Brewer and Gardner's (1996) "relational self," described previously, and to Markus and Kitayama's (1991) "interdependent self"; (3) *group-based social identities* are equivalent to the collective self or social identity as defined in this chapter; and (4) *collective identities* refer to a process where-

by group members do not just share self-defining attributes but also engage in social action to forge an image of what the group stands for and how it is represented and viewed by others. The view that the interpersonal self should be counted as a form of social identity is again different from the view proposed by social identity theory that it should be considered part of individual or personal identity.

Categorization and Accentuation

Social identity theory distinguishes between collective and individual self because of evidence for qualitatively different behaviors in group and interpersonal contexts. One early perceptual finding was that the categorization of physical or social stimuli produced an accentuation effect. When people believed that a judgment dimension (e.g., line length) was correlated with a categorization (e.g., lines labeled X and lines labeled Y), they perceptually accentuated similarities among stimuli falling within the same category and differences between stimuli from different categories (e.g., Tajfel, 1959; Tajfel & Wilkes, 1963). Tajfel believed that the effect would be amplified under four conditions: (1) the judgment dimension was subjectively important (e.g., intelligence), (2) the categorization was subjectively important (e.g., ethnic groups), (3) self was a member of one of the categories, and (4) the perceiver had few other category memberships or few other favorable category memberships (e.g., ethnicity was the single most important and self-enhancing identity for the perceiver). Programs of research have broadly confirmed the accentuation principle as it applies to both physical stimuli and to people (e.g., Eiser & Stroebe, 1972; Taylor, Fiske, Etcoff, & Ruderman, 1978).

The accentuation effect provides a rather nice, purely cognitive–perceptual, analysis of stereotyping. Indeed, Tajfel's interest in the effect was precisely to explore the cognitive dimension of stereotyping and prejudice (Tajfel, 1969). Assuming that a stereotype is a belief that an attribute is correlated with a social category (e.g., Hamilton, 1979; Hamilton & Gifford, 1976; Hamilton & Sherman, 1989), then the process of social categorization perceptually accentuates stereotypical similarities within the category and differences between categories—people are viewed stereotypically. In a later publication, Tajfel warned that a complete account of stereotyping would need to incorporate a full analysis of how stereotypes are widely shared by members of a particular group and of the various functions that stereotypes serve for groups—for example, stereotypes (e.g., men are violent, women are emotional) can justify actions committed or planned against an outgroup (Tajfel, 1981; also see Oakes, Haslam & Turner, 1994).

Categorization and Discrimination

The accentuation principle focuses on the effect of social categorization on the perception of others, but it does not elaborate the involvement of self in the categorization process. What happens when self is also explicitly categorized? To answer this broader question, the minimal group paradigm, which has now assumed near-legendary status in the social identity literature, was devised. Building on earlier studies by Rabbie (e.g., Rabbie & Horwitz, 1969), Tajfel and his colleagues (e.g., Tajfel, Billig, Bundy & Flament, 1971) devised a paradigm in which experimental participants are explicitly categorized on an ostensibly random basis (e.g., X-group vs. Y-group) or on the basis of a trivial criterion such as over- or underestimation of dots. There is no interaction, the groups have no history or future, and participants are anonymous, identified only by code numbers and category labels. The groups are minimal because they are minimally defined, being designated only by a self-inclusive category label. The main task that participants perform is the allocation of points on distribution matrices between anonymous ingroup and outgroup members, not including self. The robust finding from literally thousands of replications and variants of the paradigm is that people who are categorized discriminate in favor of the ingroup, whereas people who are not categorized do not (e.g., Bourhis, Sachdev, & Gagnon, 1994; Diehl, 1990).

Why do people who are categorized discriminate? One explanation that has been

suggested by Rabbie (e.g., Rabbie, Schot, & Visser, 1989) is that people discriminate because they assume positive interdependence among ingroup members and negative interdependence between groups. The alternative, and now more widely accepted, explanation is that proposed by social identity theory (Turner & Bourhis, 1996; but see L. Gaertner & Insko, 2000)—that people discriminate because they identify with the minimal group and that discrimination is generated by identification as a means of differentiating between groups (see the following section).

But the question remains as to *why* people bother to identify with a minimal group in the first place. Probably the most plausible explanation to date is a relatively recent one based on the motivational role of uncertainty reduction in social identity processes (Hogg, 2000b, 2001b; Hogg & Mullin, 1999; see "Uncertainty Reduction"). Minimal group situations are relatively strange, and they may make participants feel uncertain about the sort of people they are in that situation. To resolve their feelings of uncertainty, they use the explicit categorization to define themselves in the experimental context. A number of experiments show that minimal intergroup discrimination and associated identification occur only when people are categorized under uncertainty. When uncertainty is reduced, the minimal intergroup discrimination effect disappears.

It is also important to recognize that the link between categorization and discrimination is far from mechanical. For example, there is a positive–negative asymmetry effect (e.g., Otten, Mummendey, & Blanz, 1996), in which people who are categorized are more likely to display ingroup favoritism and intergroup discrimination when they are allocating "rewards" (positive resources) rather than "punishments" (negative resources). People give the ingroup greater rewards than the outgroup, but they do not give the ingroup fewer penalties or punishments than the outgroup. The positive–negative asymmetry effect disappears when people feel their group is under threat; they now give the ingroup greater rewards and fewer penalties than the outgroup.

More generally, moving away from minimal groups, whether a "real" group decides to engage in intergroup discrimination and what form of discrimination is chosen will be influenced by a range of relatively strategic considerations having to do with the perceived consequence of discriminating (e.g., Ellemers, 1993; Hogg & Abrams, 1988; Tajfel & Turner, 1979; see "Intergroup Relations and Social Beliefs"). In addition, discrimination violates one's sense of justice. According to Tyler's relational model (e.g., Tyler, 1997; Tyler & Lind, 1992), people tolerate intergroup injustice and intragroup distributive injustice but fight against intragroup procedural injustice. Presumably, if an outgroup is considered in a particular context to be an ingroup, then intergroup discrimination may be dampened by procedural justice considerations.

Social Comparison

Social categorization-based intergroup discrimination involves a process of comparison between ingroup and outgroup—people in groups make comparisons between people in their group and people who are not in their group or who are in a specific outgroup. Social categorization entails social comparison.

Not surprisingly, social comparison theory (Festinger, 1954; see Suls & Wheeler, 2000) played a key role in the early development of social identity theory—it allowed Tajfel to link self-conception to social categorization and group behavior (Tajfel, 1972; Turner, 1975; see Hogg, 2000a). Festinger (1954) had proposed that in the absence of physical reality checks, people confirm their attitudes and perceptions through interpersonal comparisons with the attitudes and perceptions of similar other people. This process produces movement toward uniformity and assimilation among people.

Tajfel extended and modified social comparison theory. He believed that almost all nontrivial evaluations rest on social comparisons and that the scope of nonsocial means of acquiring knowledge is tiny. Even the most apparently nonsocial physical judgments acquire meaning, and therefore validity, socially. Social comparison processes may be much more widespread than Festinger (1954) supposed; they may underpin

virtually all evaluations of opinions and abilities (Moscovici, 1976) and thus underpin one's self-conception.

Tajfel recognized that Festinger was mainly concerned with individuals comparing themselves with other individuals in order to evaluate their own personal characteristics and, therefore, that Festinger's notion of similarity, both as a precursor and an outcome of comparison, was interpersonal similarity (see Wheeler, 1991). Tajfel believed that Festinger focused on within-group effects of social comparison, and thus on pressures toward uniformity among individuals within groups, and that comparisons between groups might have an entirely different dynamic. Groups and thus social identity acquire meaning because ingroups are different from outgroups; logically it cannot be otherwise, because it is differentiation that delineates categories. Thus intergroup comparisons seek to evaluate or confirm differences, not similarities: 'social comparisons between groups are focused on the establishment of distinctiveness between one's own and other groups' (Tajfel, 1972, p. 296). Furthermore, because social identity is self-evaluative and derives its evaluation from the evaluative properties of one's own group relative to other groups, the intergroup social comparison process strives to accentuate differences that evaluatively favor the ingroup; that is, it strives to achieve evaluatively positive intergroup differentiation.

If we tie this together, collective self-conception (social identity) is anchored in valence-sensitive social comparisons that strive for similarity within groups and differentiation between groups.

Self-Enhancement and Self-Esteem

The intergroup social comparison process is oriented toward positive distinctiveness for one's ingroup and, thus, the maintenance and achievement of evaluatively positive social identity. The group's striving for positive distinctiveness is predicated on people's motivation for self-enhancement. Indeed, the self-enhancement motivation underlying intergroup comparisons is, it is assumed, underpinned by a fundamental individual need for positive self-esteem that influences social identity processes (e.g., Turner, 1978, 1982).

The implication is that low self-esteem motivates social identification and intergroup behavior and that social identification elevates self-esteem—the self-esteem hypothesis (Abrams & Hogg, 1988). Reviews of research on the self-esteem hypothesis reveal inconsistent and unreliable findings that suggest a distinction between individual and group membership-based self-esteem and that the relationship between self-esteem and group behavior may be affected by other variables, such as the extremity of self-esteem, the degree to which people identify with the group, and the extent to which groups and their members may feel under threat (e.g., Abrams & Hogg, 1988; Hogg & Abrams, 1990, 1993; Long & Spears, 1997; Rubin & Hewstone, 1998). Crocker and her colleagues have addressed some of these issues and have developed a collective self-esteem scale (e.g., Crocker, Blaine, & Luhtanen, 1993; Luhtanen & Crocker, 1992) that many researchers employ to measure social identity, thus equating social identity with collective self-esteem. It should also be noted that many researchers believe that self-esteem does not motivate behavior at all but rather acts as an internal monitor of how well one is doing in satisfying other motivations, such as maintaining rewarding interpersonal relationships (e.g. Leary, Tambor, Terdal, & Downs, 1995).

Despite the problematic relationship between self-esteem motivation and intergroup behavior, there is little doubt that self-enhancement through positive social identity plays a key role in intergroup behavior and social identity processes. After all, research suggests that self-enhancement is one of the most basic of human motivations (e.g., Sedikides, 1993; Sedikides & Strube, 1997).

Intergroup Relations and Social Beliefs

Although unfavorable social identity mediates low self-esteem, groups and their members are, not surprisingly, extremely adept at avoiding these negative self-evaluative consequences (Crocker & Major, 1989; Crocker, Major, & Steele, 1998). People

have a formidable repertoire of strategies to protect self-esteem and to pursue self-enhancement (Baumeister, 1998).

Subjective Belief Structures

In the context of social identity and intergroup relations, the strategies that groups and their members adopt to protect or promote positive social identity are determined by people's beliefs about the nature of relations between groups—their subjective belief structures (see Ellemers, 1993; Hogg & Abrams, 1988; Tajfel & Turner, 1979; Taylor & McKirnan, 1984). These beliefs (which are not necessarily accurate reflections of reality, as they can be, and often are, ideological constructs) concern the stability and legitimacy of intergroup status relations and the possibility of social mobility (psychologically passing from one group to another) or social change (psychologically changing the self-evaluative consequences of existing ingroup membership). Subjective belief structures influence the specific behaviors that group members adopt in the pursuit of self-enhancement through positive social identity.

For example, a group that believes its lower status position is relatively legitimate and stable but that it is quite possible to pass psychologically into the dominant group (i.e., to acquire a social identity as a member of the higher status group) will be unlikely to show much solidarity or engage in much direct intergroup competition—instead, members will attempt, as individuals, to disidentify and to gain psychological entry to the dominant group. This strategy of social mobility is often unsuccessful, leaving people marginalized by both their original group and the group they are seeking to enter.

People who recognize that intergroup boundaries are impermeable have a social-change belief structure. They adopt relatively creative group strategies to improve the evaluative consequences of their existing group membership. They may try to compare themselves with the dominant group on dimensions that are less unfavorable to their own group; they may try to reverse the evaluative polarity of existing social comparison dimensions; or they may avoid upward comparisons altogether and make downward comparisons with groups that have even lower standing than their own. When groups believe that their lower status position is illegitimate and unstable, that passing is not viable, and that a different social order is achievable, they show marked solidarity and engage in direct collective action and intergroup competition to change the status quo.

System Justification, Social Dominance, and Social Orientation

Other factors may prevent minority groups from taking social action to address status concerns. For example, people often believe that other members of their group are discriminated against and disadvantaged more than they are themselves, and so they feel diminished personal motivation to act (e.g., Crosby, Cordova, & Jaskar, 1993). Social competition and collective action can be an uncertain and risky path to follow, and so groups may develop belief systems that justify the status quo and thus make it easier to acquiesce (e.g., Jost, 1995; Jost & Banaji, 1994).

An additional possibility is that some people may be more inclined than others to accept legitimizing belief systems. According to social dominance theory (e.g., Pratto, 1999; Pratto, Sidanius, Stallworth, & Malle, 1994; Sidanius & Pratto, 1999), people differ in the extent to which they accept or reject societal ideologies or myths that legitimize hierarchy and discrimination or that legitimize equality and fairness. People who desire their own group to be dominant and superior to outgroups have a high social dominance orientation that encourages them to reject egalitarian ideologies and to accept myths that legitimize hierarchy and discrimination. These kinds of people are more inclined to be prejudiced than are people who have a low social dominance orientation, and they may be more likely to engage in intergroup competition.

Finally, Hinkle and Brown (1990) suggest that groups can vary in terms of their social orientations (from collectivist to individualist) and in their orientations toward defining themselves through comparisons or not (from a comparative ideology to a noncomparative ideology). Groups that are both collectivist and have a comparative ideology are more likely to engage in intergroup competition.

Self-Categorization and Depersonalization

In response to the gathering momentum of social cognition (Devine, Hamilton, & Ostrom, 1994), Turner and his colleagues set out in the early 1980s to specify the cognitive underpinnings of social identity processes in greater detail, thus producing self-categorization theory (Turner, 1985; Turner et al., 1987; see also Hogg, 2001c).

Social categorization of self and others into ingroup and outgroup accentuates the perceived similarity of the target to the relevant ingroup or outgroup prototype (cognitive representation of features that describe and prescribe attributes of the group). People are no longer represented as unique individuals but rather as embodiments of the relevant prototype; a process of *depersonalization* occurs. Social categorization of self, self-categorization, cognitively assimilates self to the ingroup prototype and thus depersonalizes self-conception. This transformation of self is the fundamental process underlying group phenomena, because it brings self-perception and behavior in line with the contextually relevant ingroup prototype. It produces, for instance, normative behavior, stereotyping, ethnocentrism, positive ingroup attitudes and cohesion, cooperation and altruism, emotional contagion and empathy, collective behavior, shared norms, and mutual influence. "Depersonalization" refers simply to a change in self-conceptualization and the basis of perception of others; it is not intended to have the negative connotations of terms such as "deindividuation" or "dehumanization."

The notion of prototypes, which is not part of the earlier intergroup focus of social identity theory, is central to self-categorization theory. People cognitively represent the defining and stereotypical attributes of groups in the form of prototypes. Prototypes are typically not checklists of attributes but are fuzzy sets that capture the context-dependent features of group membership, often in the form of representations of exemplary members (actual group members who best embody the group) or ideal types (an abstraction of group features). For example, Americans might cognitively represent Australians in terms of an exemplar (e.g., Paul Hogan) or an ideal type (e.g., a fuzzy set of features including friendly, straightforward, sporty, bronzed, and so forth).

Of course, not all 20 million Australians are like Paul Hogan, nor are they all friendly or bronzed or sporty; but prototypes focus on features that people believe make a group distinctive. Prototypes embody all attributes that people believe characterize groups and distinguish them from other groups, including beliefs, attitudes, feelings, and behaviors. A critical feature of prototypes is that they maximize similarities within and differences between groups and thus define groups as distinct entities. Prototypes focus on distinctive features that also capture similarities among people within the same group. Prototypes form according to the principle of metacontrast: maximization of the ratio of intergroup differences to intragroup differences. For example, students often think of law students as being argumentative and engineering students as being boring because they believe that these attributes capture within-group properties and differentiate between the groups; the attribute *intelligent* does not have these properties and so does not form part of the prototype tied to a law-student versus engineering-student categorization. Finally, because members of the same group are exposed to similar social information, their prototypes will usually be similar and thus shared.

Prototypes are stored in memory but are constructed, maintained, and modified by features of the immediate or more enduring social interactive context. They are context dependent and are particularly influenced by which outgroup is contextually salient. Enduring changes in prototypes and thus changes in self-conception can therefore arise if the relevant comparison outgroup changes over time; for instance, French Canadian autoprototypes will change if the relevant outgroup changes from Anglo-Canadians to French people. Such changes are also transitory in that they are tied to whatever outgroup is salient in the immediate social context. For instance, a psychology department may experience a contextual change in self-definition if it compares itself

with a management school rather than with a history department. Thus social identity is dynamic—it changes as a consequence of what outgroup one is comparing oneself against. The changes can be quite profound (a change in the entire representation of the ingroup) or more subtle (a change in emphasis on ingroup defining features).

A slightly different, but generally compatible, emphasis on depersonalization has been proposed by Wright and his associates (Tropp & Wright, 2001; Wright, Aron, & Tropp, in press). Drawing on the ideas that people can internalize the properties of other people as part of themselves (e.g., Aron, Aron, Tudor, & Nelson, 1991) and that people can include the ingroup as part of the self (e.g., Smith, Coats, & Walling, 1999; Smith & Henry, 1996), Wright and his colleagues propose that strength of identification is a function of the degree to which the group is included in the self.

Salience

When does a particular self-categorization (social identity) become the psychologically salient basis for self-construal, behavior, and social perception? Self-categorization theory has generated a set of principles that govern the contextual salience of social identity or of specific social identities. Building on early work by Bruner (1957), Oakes (1987; Oakes, Haslam, & Turner, 1994; Oakes & Turner, 1990) proposes that salience is a function of category accessibility and category fit.

People draw on readily available social categorizations—ones that are valued, important, and frequently employed aspects of the self-concept (i.e., they are chronically accessible in memory) because they are self-evident and perceptually salient in the immediate situation (i.e., they are situationally accessible). For many people in the United States, social categorization based on race is chronically and situationally accessible in a mixed-race context. People use available categories to try to make sense of the social context in terms of people's attitudes, behaviors, and so forth. They investigate the extent to which the categorization accounts for similarities and differences among people (called structural or comparative fit) and the extent to which the stereotypical properties of the categorization account for why people behave as they do (called normative fit). If the fit of the category to the social field is poor, people cycle through other available categorizations until an optimal level of fit is achieved. Optimal fit identifies and locks in the psychologically salient categorization that acts as the basis of depersonalization and self-categorization in that context. The salient categorization perceptually accentuates intragroup similarities and intergroup differences in order to construct situationally adjusted ingroup and outgroup prototypes that maximize entitativity and intergroup separateness and clarity.

Although I have described this process in terms of people deliberatively using categorizations, the process is largely an automatic function of the human cognitive system. However, salience is not always a mechanical product of accessibility and fit (see Hogg, 1996). Social interaction involves the motivated manipulation of symbols (e.g., through speech, appearance, behavior) by people who are strategically competing with one another to influence the frame of reference within which accessibility and fit interact. People are not content to have their identity determined by the social–cognitive context. On the contrary, they say and do things to try to change the parameters so that a subjectively more meaningful and self-favoring identity becomes salient.

Conformity and Influence

The previous point recognizes that social interaction overwhelmingly involves attempts at influence, and invites the question of what form such influence takes within and between groups. One of the most obvious characteristics of groups is the pressure toward uniformity—people in groups tend to converge in their attitudes and behaviors (e.g., Festinger, 1954). Furthermore, interaction in groups tends to create norms that can influence new members (e.g., Sherif, 1936), and indeed normative discontinuities delineate the boundaries of groups. From a social identity perspective, the social influence process associated with group membership is referent informational influence (e.g., Turner, 1982, 1985). When group

membership is salient, people learn the context-specific group norms from prototype-consistent behavior of prototypical members. Self-categorization depersonalizes self-conception in terms of the relevant norm and thus transforms behavior so that it is normative. The influence process represents true cognitive change rather than mere behavioral compliance. There is good evidence for this process from studies of conformity, self-stereotyping, and group polarization (for overviews, see Abrams & Hogg, 1990a; Turner, 1991; Turner & Oakes, 1989).

Collective Behavior

Reicher (1984) has used this analysis to explain crowd behavior (see also Reicher, 2001; Reicher, Spears, & Postmes, 1995). Reicher argues that, far from crowd behavior representing loss of identity and self-awareness and regression to deep-seated aggressive instincts (i.e. deindividuation), crowd events are situations of highly salient social identity. Crowd behavior has clear limits set by the parameters of the social identity that the crowd represents (a crowd of "grey power" activists will probably behave differently from a crowd of AC/DC fans). Within these limits referent informational influence and depersonalization occur to produce context-specific normative behavior.

Attitudes, Norms, and Behavior

From a social identity perspective, group norms are not merely surface descriptions of regularities within groups. They are internalized cognitive structures (prototypes) that define and prescribe perceptual, affective, attitudinal, and behavioral attributes of group membership. Therefore, to the extent that an attitude or a behavior is normative of a salient ingroup, the depersonalization process will ensure that group members behave in ways that are consistent with such attitudes. This idea speaks to the relationship between people's attitudes and their behavior—the attitude–behavior relationship.

Conventional attitude–behavior research has tended to find that norms do not greatly improve attitude–behavior correspondence (e.g., Farley, Lehmann, & Ryan, 1981);

however, this research has generally not viewed norms as group membership-defining attributes. In contrast, social identity research by Terry and her associates (e.g., Terry & Hogg, 1996; Terry, Hogg, & White, 2000) has shown that behavior is more likely to correspond with attitudes if the attitudes define membership in an important and contextually salient ingroup with which people identify. For example, people are more likely to take physical exercise if a proexercise attitude defines membership in an important group to which they belong.

Structural Differentiation within Groups

The social identity perspective is generally associated with the analysis of intergroup behavior and with an emphasis on intergroup differentiation and intragroup homogeneity. However, we are all well aware that groups are internally differentiated—they are highly textured entities. A social identity analysis of intragroup structural differentiation rests on the fact that within a group some people are more prototypical than others and that, because prototypicality is the critical and highly salient yardstick of group life, people are highly attuned to the relative prototypicality of fellow members (Hogg, 1996, 2001c). A perceived prototypicality gradient emerges within groups.

Prototypicality, Social Attraction, and Deviance

People who are highly prototypical are liked more than those who are less prototypical (e.g., Hogg, 1993; Hogg & Hains, 1996). This is group membership-based liking (depersonalized social attraction) that rests on how prototypical an ingroup member is considered to be, not interpersonal liking based on close relationships and idiosyncratic preferences. If a consensual prototype exists, then the most prototypical group members are consensually socially attractive—they are popular, in group membership terms. In contrast, people who are very unprototypical can be marginalized and rejected as deviants or "black sheep" (e.g., Marques & Páez, 1994; see also Marques, Abrams, Páez, & Hogg, 2001).

One reason that ingroup deviants may attract particularly negative reactions from fellow ingroupers is that they threaten the integrity and distinctiveness of the ingroup (e.g., Branscombe, Wann, Noel, & Coleman, 1993; Jetten, Spears, Hogg, & Manstead, 2000). Research also shows that peripheral members may try to reestablish their membership credentials by acting in a markedly derogatory manner toward an outgroup, particularly when this behavior is publicly observable by an ingroup audience (Noel, Wann, & Branscombe, 1995). Core members act in this way only when the group's position as a whole is under threat (Jetten, Spears & Manstead, 1997).

The process of evaluative marginalization by the group of deviants may target not only isolated peripheral individuals but also peripheral subgroups. In these circumstances an intergroup dynamic may come into play between the dominant majority subgroup and the deviant minority subgroup. The minority subgroup may adopt classic minority influence tactics (e.g., promulgating a consistent and consensual message) in order to reinstate itself or to convert the majority to its own position (Mugny, 1982; see Martin & Hewstone, 2001). This sort of process is often seen in political maneuvering; for example, the British Labour party has long tried to marginalize its left wing, which in turn has promulgated a consistent and consensual message in order to try to reinstate itself as the true British Labour party or to convert the majority to its own position.

Leadership

One of the key structural features of almost all groups is the existence of leaders and followers. Effective leaders are people who are able to be innovative and to motivate others to work toward group goals (Chemers, 2001). Typically, leadership effectiveness and endorsement is influenced by the extent to which the group considers the leader to have the right leadership qualities for effective leadership. However, in highly salient groups with which people identify very strongly, perceptions of prototypicality become a significant basis for person perception and evaluation and thus for leadership endorsement (Hogg, 2001a, 2001d, 2001f; Hogg & van Knippenberg, in press). Under these conditions, highly prototypical members, even if they do not possess general leadership skills, will become influential and will be endorsed and viewed as effective leaders. A number of recent studies supports this analysis (for a review, see Hogg, 2001f; Hogg & van Knippenberg, in press).

Roles, Subgroups, and Cross-Cutting Categories

Another obvious structural feature of groups is the existence of different roles within the group. Although roles are distinct from one another, they are promotively interdependent in the life of the group. Roles can be very specific in circumscribing behaviors; for example, pilot, navigator, and cabin crew in an airplane. Other roles can be more generic, such as newcomer, full member, oldtimer, or marginal member (e.g., Levine & Moreland, 1994; Moreland & Levine, 1982). Identification with and commitment to the group as a whole is influenced by generic role position (different roles prescribe different prototypes for the same group) and by role transition processes (e.g., initiation rites) that vary in terms of the strength of commitment to the group that they elicit. Research in organizational psychology suggests that people actually identify more strongly with roles or work groups within the organization than with the organization as a whole (e.g., Pratt, 1998)—perhaps such groups are, in Brewer's terms (e.g., Brewer, 1991), optimally distinctive.

Roles are rarely of equal status. According to expectation states theory, or status characteristics theory (e.g., Berger, Fisek, Norman, & Zelditch, 1977; Berger, Wagner, & Zelditch, 1985; Ridgeway, 2001), roles acquire their status within the group partly from the extent to which role occupants have qualities and skills that are very specifically related to the group's purpose (called specific status characteristics) but also from role occupants' general social status outside the group (called diffuse status characteristics). Diffuse status creates favorable expectations that the person is also valuable to the group, when in fact diffuse status may have little relevance to the group. This analysis of category differentiation within groups is useful for understanding the dy-

namics of power and influence within groups in a way that incorporates a consideration of power and influence in the wider society within which groups are located.

Another way to approach category structure within groups is in terms of sociodemographic diversity. Groups are often a face-to-face arena (e.g., an organization) in which people from different sociodemographic groups (e.g., based on gender, race, ethnicity) interact with one another. Because sociodemographic intergroup relations are often polarized and emotionally charged, conflict, disadvantage, marginalization, and minority victimization can characterize life within the face-to-face group. The problem is particularly acute when sociodemographic intergroup boundaries correspond with role differentiation within the group (Brewer, 1996; Brewer, von Hippel, & Gooden, 1999)—for example, in an organization in which all the men are in sales and all the women are in customer service. One way to dampen the effect is to have demographic categorization and role assignment cross-cut or uncorrelated within the group (see Vescio, Hewstone, Crisp, & Rubin, 1999).

The general issue here is of how subgroups relate to one another when they are nested within or cross-cut with a superordinate group. Social identity theory, and more general social categorization perspectives, make predictions about the nature of relations between subgroups as a function of the nature of their relationship to the superordinate group (e.g., Brown, 1996; S. Gaertner, Dovidio, Anastasio, Bachman, & Rust, 1993; Hewstone, 1996; Hornsey & Hogg, 2000; Pettigrew, 1998).

Subgroups often resist attempts by a superordinate group to dissolve subgroup boundaries and merge them into one large group. This resistance can be quite marked if the superordinate group is very large, amorphous, and impersonal. Thus assimilationist strategies within nations or organizations can produce fierce subgroup loyalty and intersubgroup competition. Subgroup members derive social identity from their groups and thus view externally imposed assimilation as an identity threat. The threat may be stronger in large superordinate groups due to optimal distinctiveness considerations (Brewer, 1991). People strive for a balance between conflicting motives for inclusion/sameness (satisfied by group membership) and for distinctiveness/uniqueness (satisfied by individuality). So, in very large organizations, people feel overincluded and strive for distinctiveness, often by identifying with distinctive subunits or departments.

Some research (see Hornsey & Hogg, 2000) suggests that an effective strategy for managing intersubgroup relations within a larger group is to make both subgroup and superordinate group identity simultaneously salient. This arrangement reduces subgroup distinctiveness and identity threat at the same time as it reconfigures intersubgroup relations so that they resemble promotively interdependent role relations rather than competitively interdependent intergroup relations. A focus on subgroup distinctiveness within a salient superordinate identity that emphasizes subgroup complementarity is a social arrangement that may capture the policy of multiculturalism adopted by some countries to manage ethnic diversity at a national level (see Prentice & Miller, 1999).

Uncertainty Reduction

Social identity provides one with a self-definition that prescribes attitudes, perceptions, feelings, behaviors, and so forth and also evaluates one's attributes and thus one's self-concept. Much of the motivational emphasis in the social identity perspective has been on the roles of self-enhancement and positive distinctiveness and their relationship to mechanisms of social change. We should not, however, lose sight of the fact that, above all, social categorization imposes order on and ascribes meaning to a potentially bewilderingly complex social field. This idea has been revisited and elaborated in the proposal that a key motivation for social identity processes is subjective uncertainty reduction (e.g., Hogg, 2000b, 2001b; Hogg & Mullin, 1999).

In addition to self-enhancement, social identity processes are also motivated by a need to reduce subjective uncertainty about one's perceptions, attitudes, feelings, behaviors, and ultimately one's self-concept and place within the social world. Uncertainty reduction, particularly about subjectively important matters that are generally self-

conceptually relevant, is a core human motivation. Certainty renders existence meaningful and confers confidence in how to behave and what to expect from the physical and social environment within which one finds oneself. Self-categorization reduces uncertainty by transforming self-conception and assimilating self to a prototype that describes and prescribes perceptions, attitudes, feelings, and behaviors. Because prototypes are relatively consensual, they also furnish moral support and consensual validation for one's self-concept and attendant cognitions and behaviors.

It is the prototype that actually reduces uncertainty. Hence, uncertainty is better reduced by prototypes that are simple, clear, highly focused, and consensual and that, therefore, describe groups that have pronounced entitativity (Campbell, 1958; see also Brewer & Harasty, 1996; Hamilton & Sherman, 1996), are very cohesive (e.g., Hogg, 1993), and provide a powerful social identity. Such groups and prototypes will be attractive to individuals who are contextually or more enduringly highly uncertain or during times of or in situations characterized by great uncertainty. Such groups may also tend to be relatively orthodox, extreme, and homogenous in their attitudes, intolerant of diversity, harsh on deviance, and hierarchically organized with a powerful leader or leadership clique (e.g., Hogg, 2001a).

Uncertainty reduction and self-enhancement are probably independent motivations for social identity processes, with self-esteem quite probably acting as a psychological monitor of satisfaction of these motives (e.g., Leary et al., 1995). Together these motives may underpin the human need to belong (cf. Baumeister & Leary, 1995)—people feel a need to belong to groups when they are self-conceptually uncertain and/or when the valence of their self-concept is assailed. In some circumstances it may be more urgent to reduce uncertainty than to pursue self-enhancement (e.g., when group entitativity is threatened), whereas in others it may be the opposite (e.g., when group prestige is threatened). However, uncertainty reduction may be more fundamentally adaptive because it constructs a self-concept that defines who we are and prescribes what we should perceive, think, feel, and do.

The Wider Context of Social Identity Research

Because the social identity perspective is a wide-ranging perspective on the relationship between collective self and group phenomena, it has increasingly acted as a conceptual bridge to neighboring disciplines. For example, it played a key role in the genesis and early development during the 1970s and 1980s of the social psychology of language. Language and speech style are defining or normative features of membership in certain groups—for example, ethnolinguistic groups. Thus, whether a language dies out or thrives, whether people become fully proficient or not in another language, whether people accommodate their speech style to someone who speaks a different language or has a different speech style, and so forth, is largely a matter of social identity dynamics (e.g., Giles, Bourhis, & Taylor, 1977; Giles & Johnson, 1987; Giles & Robinson, 1993).

More recently, building on Ashforth and Mael's (1989) introduction of social identity theory to organizational psychologists, there has been a growing integration of social and organizational psychological research on social identity processes in organizational contexts—after all, organizations are groups (e.g., Haslam, 2000; Hogg & Terry, 2000, 2001). There has also been a growing engagement between psychological and sociological social psychologists who seek to explore differences, similarities, and complementarity between social identity theory on the one hand and role identity theory and expectation states theory on the other (e.g., Hogg, Terry, & White, 1995; Ridgeway, 2001; Thoits & Virshup, 1997). Finally, there is a growing integration or engagement between social identity research and traditional social cognition research (e.g., Abrams & Hogg, 1999; Leyens, Yzerbyt, & Schadron, 1994; Oakes, Haslam, & Turner, 1994).

Conclusion

Social identity is that aspect of the self-concept that derives from group membership and is associated with cognitive, motivational, and social processes that are associated with group and intergroup behaviors.

The concept of social identity lies at the core of the social identity perspective, and so this chapter has largely been an overview of the social identity perspective. I have discussed the various conceptual components of the approach, some of the main research foci, and some of the ways in which the approach reaches out to neighboring disciplines.

Social identity phenomena are associated with the operation of the social categorization process, which depersonalizes perception in terms of context-specific ingroup or outgroup prototypes. When applied to self, self-categorization depersonalizes self, transforms self-conception to correspond to the relevant ingroup identity, and generates typical group and intergroup behaviors, such as ethnocentrism, intergroup differentiation, social attraction, normative behavior, self-stereotyping, conformity to norms, and so forth. The process operates within parameters set by people's motivation to reduce subjective uncertainty and to pursue an evaluatively positive social identity that services self-enhancement and self-esteem needs. Behavior is, however, influenced by people's beliefs about the nature of relations between groups and about the efficacy of particular behavioral strategies.

This perspective contributes to our understanding of conformity, normative conduct, collective behavior, stereotyping, group solidarity and cohesion, intergroup relations, prejudice, prejudice reduction, multiculturalism, leadership, roles, deviance, group decision making, the correspondence between attitudes and behavior, and many other group and intergroup phenomena and their relationship to the collective self.

References

Abrams, D., & Hogg, M. A. (1988). Comments on the motivational status of self-esteem in social identity and intergroup discrimination. *European Journal of Social Psychology, 18,* 317–334.

Abrams, D., & Hogg, M. A. (1990a). Social identification, self-categorization and social influence. *European Review of Social Psychology, 1,* 195–228.

Abrams, D., & Hogg, M. A. (Eds.). (1990b). *Social identity theory: Constructive and critical advances.* New York: Springer-Verlag.

Abrams, D., & Hogg, M. A. (1998). Prospects for research in group processes and intergroup relations. *Group Processes and Intergroup Relations, 1,* 7–20.

Abrams, D., & Hogg, M. A. (Eds.). (1999). *Social identity and social cognition*. Oxford, UK: Blackwell.

Abrams, D., & Hogg, M. A. (2001). Collective identity: Group membership and self-conception. In M. A. Hogg & R. S. Tindale (Eds.), *Blackwell handbook of social psychology: Group processes* (pp. 425–460). Oxford, UK: Blackwell.

Aron, A., Aron, E. N., Tudor, M., & Nelson, G. (1991). Close relationships as including other in the self. *Journal of Personality and Social Psychology, 60,* 241–253.

Ashforth, B. E., & Mael, F. A. (1989). Social identity theory and the organization. *Academy of Management Review, 14,* 20–39.

Baumeister, R. F. (1998). The self. In D. T. Gilbert, S. T. Fiske, & G. Lindzey (Eds.), *Handbook of social psychology* (4th ed., Vol. 1, pp. 680–740). New York: McGraw-Hill.

Baumeister, R. F., & Leary, M. R. (1995). The need to belong: Desire for interpersonal attachments as a fundamental human motivation. *Psychological Bulletin, 117,* 497–529.

Berger, J., Fisek, M. H., Norman, R. Z., & Zelditch, M., Jr. (1977). *Status characteristics and social interaction.* New York: Elsevier.

Berger, J., Wagner, D., & Zelditch, M., Jr. (1985). Expectation states theory: Review and assessment. In J. Berger & M. Zelditch, Jr. (Eds), *Status, rewards and influence* (pp. 1–72). San Francisco, CA: Jossey-Bass.

Bourhis, R. Y., Sachdev, I., & Gagnon, A. (1994). Intergroup research with the Tajfel matrices: Methodological notes. In M. Zanna & J. Olson (Eds.), *The psychology of prejudice: The Ontario Symposium* (Vol. 7, pp. 209–232). Hillsdale, NJ: Erlbaum.

Branscombe, N. R., Wann, D. L., Noel, J. G., & Coleman, J. (1993). In-group or out-group extremity: Importance of the threatened social identity. *Personality and Social Psychology Bulletin, 19,* 381–388.

Brewer, M. B. (1991). The social self: On being the same and different at the same time. *Personality and Social Psychology Bulletin, 17,* 475–482.

Brewer, M. B. (1996). Managing diversity: The role of social identities. In S. Jackson & M. Ruderman (Eds.), *Diversity in work teams* (pp. 47–68). Washington, DC: American Psychological Association.

Brewer, M. B. (2001). The many faces of social identity: Implications for political psychology. *Political Psychology, 22,* 115–125.

Brewer, M. B., & Gardner, W. (1996). Who is this "we"? Levels of collective identity and self representation. *Journal of Personality and Social Psychology, 71,* 83–93.

Brewer, M. B., & Harasty, A. S. (1996). Seeing groups as entities: The role of perceiver motivation. In R. M. Sorrentino & E. T. Higgins (Eds.), *Handbook of motivation and cognition: Vol. 3. The interpersonal context* (pp. 347–370). New York: Guilford Press.

Brewer, M. B., von Hippel, W., & Gooden, M. P. (1999). Diversity and organizational identity: The problem of entrée after entry. In D.A. Prentice & D.T. Miller (Eds.), *Cultural divides: Understanding and overcoming group conflict* (pp. 337–363). New York: Russell Sage Foundation.

Brown, R. J. (1996). Tajfel's contribution to the reduction of intergroup conflict. In W. P. Robinson (Ed.), *Social groups and identities: Developing the legacy of Henri Tajfel* (pp.169–189). Oxford, UK: Butterworth-Heinemann.

Bruner, J. S. (1957). On perceptual readiness. *Psychological Review, 64,* 123–152.

Campbell, D. T. (1958). Common fate, similarity, and other indices of the status of aggregates of persons as social entities. *Behavioral Science, 3,* 14–25.

Caporael, L. R. (2001). Parts and wholes: The evolutionary importance of groups. In C. Sedikides & M. B. Brewer (Eds.), *Individual self, relational self, collective self* (pp. 241–258). Philadelphia: Psychology Press.

Chemers, M. M. (2001). Leadership effectiveness: An integrative review. In M. A. Hogg & R. S. Tindale (Eds.), *Blackwell handbook of social psychology: Group processes* (pp. 376–399). Oxford, UK: Blackwell.

Crocker, J., Blaine, B., & Luhtanen, R. (1993). Prejudice, intergroup behaviour and self-esteem: Enhancement and protection motives. In M. A. Hogg & D. Abrams (Eds.), *Group motivation: Social psychological perspectives* (pp. 52–67). London: Harvester Wheatsheaf.

Crocker, J., & Major, B. (1989). Social stigma and self-esteem: The self-protective properties of stigma. *Psychological Review, 96,* 608–630.

Crocker, J., Major, B., & Steele, C. (1998). Social stigma. In D. T. Gilbert, S. T. Fiske, & G. Lindzey (Eds.), *The handbook of social psychology* (4th ed., Vol. 2, pp. 504–553). New York: McGraw-Hill.

Crosby, F., Cordova, D., & Jaskar, K. (1993). On the failure to see oneself as disadvantaged: Cognitive and emotional components. In M. A. Hogg & D. Abrams (Eds.), *Group motivation: Social psychological perspectives* (pp. 87–104). London: Harvester Wheatsheaf.

Deaux, K. (1996). Social identification. In E. T. Higgins & A. W. Kruglanski (Eds.), *Social psychology: Handbook of basic principles* (pp. 777–798). New York: Guilford Press.

Deaux, K., Reid, A., Mizrahi, K., & Cotting, D. (1999). Connecting the person to the social: The functions of social identification. In T. R. Tyler & R. M. Kramer (Eds.), *The psychology of the social self: Applied social research* (pp. 91–113). Mahwah, NJ: Erlbaum.

Deaux, K., Reid, A., Mizrahi, K., & Ethier, K. A. (1995). Parameters of social identity. *Journal of Personality and Social Psychology, 68,* 280–291.

Devine, P. G., Hamilton, D. L., & Ostrom, T. M. (Eds.). (1994). *Social cognition: Impact on social psychology.* San Diego, CA: Academic Press.

Diehl, M. (1990). The minimal group paradigm: Theoretical explanations and empirical findings. *European Review of Social Psychology, 1,* 263–292.

Doise, W. (1986). *Levels of explanation in social psychology.* Cambridge, UK: Cambridge University Press.

Eiser, J. R., & Stroebe, W. (1972). *Categorization and social judgement.* London: Academic Press.

Ellemers, N. (1993). The influence of socio-structural variables on identity management strategies. *European Review of Social Psychology, 4,* 27–57.

Ellemers, N., Spears, R., & Doosje, B. (Eds.). (1999). *Social identity.* Oxford, UK: Blackwell.

Farley, J. U., Lehmann, D. R., & Ryan, M. J. (1981). Generalizing from "imperfect" replication. *Journal of Business, 54,* 597–610.

Festinger, L. (1954). A theory of social comparison processes. *Human Relations, 7,* 117–140.

Gaertner, L., & Insko, C. A. (2000). Intergroup discrimination in the minimal group paradigm: Categorization, reciprocation, or fear? *Journal of Personality and Social Psychology, 79,* 77–94.

Gaertner, S. L., Dovidio, J. F., Anastasio, P. A., Bachman, B. A., & Rust, M. C. (1993). Reducing intergroup bias: The common ingroup identity model. *European Review of Social Psychology, 4,* 1–26.

Giles, H., Bourhis, R. Y., & Taylor, D. M. (1977). Towards a theory of language in ethnic group relations. In H. Giles (Ed.), *Language, ethnicity, and intergroup relations* (pp. 307–348). London: Academic Press.

Giles, H., & Johnson, P. (1987). Ethnolinguistic identity theory: A social psychological approach to language maintenance. *International Journal of the Sociology of Language, 68,* 66–99.

Giles, H., & Robinson, W. P. (Eds.). (1993). *Handbook of language and social psychology.* Oxford, UK: Pergamon.

Greenwald, A. G., & Pratkanis A. R. (1984). The self. In R. S. Wyer & T. K. Srull (Eds.), *Handbook of social cognition* (Vol. 3, pp. 129–178). Hillsdale, NJ: Erlbaum.

Hamilton, D. L. (1979). A cognitive attributional analysis of stereotyping. In L. Berkowitz (Ed.), *Advances in experimental social psychology* (Vol. 12, pp. 53–84). New York: Academic Press.

Hamilton, D. L., & Gifford, R. K. (1976). Illusory correlation in interpersonal perception: A cognitive basis of stereotypic judgments. *Journal of Experimental Social Psychology, 12,* 392–407.

Hamilton, D. L., & Sherman, J. W. (1989). Illusory correlations: Implications for stereotype theory and research. In D. Bar-Tal, C.F. Graumann, A.W. Kruglanski, & W. Stroebe (Eds.), *Stereotyping and prejudice: Changing conceptions* (pp. 59–82). New York: Springer.

Hamilton, D. L., & Sherman, S. J. (1996). Perceiving persons and groups. *Psychological Review, 103,* 336–355.

Haslam, S. A. (2000). *Psychology in organisations: The social identity approach.* London: Sage.

Hewstone, M. (1996). Contact and categorization: Social psychological interventions to change intergroup relations. In C. N. Macrae, C. Stangor, & M. Hewstone (Eds.), *Stereotypes and stereotyping* (pp. 323–368). New York: Guilford Press.

Hinkle, S., & Brown, J. J. (1990). Intergroup comparisons and social identity: Some links and lacunae. In D. Abrams & M. A. Hogg (Eds.), *Social identity theory: Constructive and critical advances* (pp. 48–70). New York: Springer-Verlag.

Hogg, M. A. (1993). Group cohesiveness: A critical review and some new directions. *European Review of Social Psychology, 4,* 85–111.

Hogg, M. A. (1996). Intragroup processes, group structure and social identity. In W. P. Robinson (Ed.). *Social groups and identities: Developing the legacy of Henri Tajfel* (pp. 65–93). Oxford, UK: Butterworth-Heinemann.

Hogg, M. A. (2000a). Social identity and social comparison. In J. Suls & L. Wheeler (Eds.), *Handbook of social comparison: Theory and research* (pp. 401–421). New York: Kluwer Academic/Plenum Press.

Hogg, M. A. (2000b). Subjective uncertainty reduction through self-categorization: A motivational theory of social identity processes. *European Review of Social Psychology, 11,* 223–255.

Hogg, M. A. (2001a). From prototypicality to power: A social identity analysis of leadership. In S. R. Thye, E. J. Lawler, M. W. Macy, & H. A. Walker (Eds.), *Advances in group processes* (Vol. 18, pp. 1–30). Oxford, UK: Elsevier.

Hogg, M. A. (2001b). Self-categorization and subjective uncertainty resolution: Cognitive and motivational facets of social identity and group membership. In J. P. Forgas, K. D. Williams, & L. Wheeler (Eds.), *The social mind: Cognitive and motivational aspects of interpersonal behavior* (pp. 323–349). New York: Cambridge University Press.

Hogg, M. A. (2001c). Social categorization, depersonalization, and group behavior. In M. A. Hogg & R. S. Tindale (Eds.), *Blackwell handbook of social psychology: Group processes* (pp. 56–85). Oxford, UK: Blackwell.

Hogg, M. A. (2001d). Social identification, group prototypicality, and emergent leadership. In M. A. Hogg & D. J. Terry (Eds.), *Social identity processes in organizational contexts* (pp. 197–212). Philadelphia: Psychology Press.

Hogg, M. A. (2001e). Social identity and the sovereignty of the group: A psychology of belonging. In C. Sedikides & M. B. Brewer (Eds.), *Individual self, relational self, collective self* (pp. 123–143). Philadelphia: Psychology Press.

Hogg, M. A. (2001f). A social identity theory of leadership. *Personality and Social Psychology Review, 5,* 184–200.

Hogg, M. A., & Abrams, D. (1988). *Social identifications: A social psychology of intergroup relations and group processes.* London: Routledge.

Hogg, M. A., & Abrams, D. (1990). Social motivation, self-esteem and social identity. In D. Abrams & M. A. Hogg (Eds.), *Social identity theory: Constructive and critical advances* (pp. 28–47). London: Harvester Wheatsheaf.

Hogg, M. A., & Abrams, D. (1993). Towards a single-process uncertainty-reduction model of social motivation in groups. In M. A. Hogg & D. Abrams (Eds.), *Group motivation: Social psychological perspectives* (pp. 173–190). London: Harvester Wheatsheaf.

Hogg, M. A., & Abrams, D. (1999). Social identity and social cognition: Historical background and current trends. In D. Abrams & M. A. Hogg (Eds.), *Social identity and social cognition* (pp. 1–25). Oxford, UK: Blackwell.

Hogg, M. A., & Hains, S. C. (1996). Intergroup relations and group solidarity: Effects of group identification and social beliefs on depersonalized attraction. *Journal of Personality and Social Psychology, 70,* 295–309.

Hogg, M. A., & McGarty, C. (1990). Self-categorization and social identity. In D. Abrams & M. A. Hogg (Eds.), *Social identity theory: Constructive and critical advances* (pp. 10–27). New York: Springer-Verlag.

Hogg, M. A., & Mullin, B.-A. (1999). Joining groups to reduce uncertainty: Subjective uncertainty reduction and group identification. In D. Abrams & M. A. Hogg (Eds.), *Social identity and social cognition* (pp. 249–279). Oxford, UK: Blackwell.

Hogg, M. A., & Terry, D. J. (2000). Social identity and self-categorization processes in organizational contexts. *Academy of Management Review, 25,* 121–140.

Hogg, M. A., & Terry, D. J. (Eds.). (2001). *Social identity processes in organizational contexts*. Philadelphia: Psychology Press.

Hogg, M. A., Terry, D. J., & White, K. M. (1995). A tale of two theories: A critical comparison of identity theory with social identity theory. *Social Psychology Quarterly, 58,* 255–269.

Hogg, M. A., & van Knippenberg, D. (in press). Social identity and leadership processes in groups. In M. P. Zanna (Ed.), *Advances in experimental social psychology* (Vol. 35). San Diego, CA: Academic Press.

Hogg, M. A., & Williams, K. D. (2000). From I to we: Social identity and the collective self. *Group Dynamics: Theory, Research, and Practice, 4,* 81–97.

Hornsey, M. J., & Hogg, M. A. (2000). Assimilation and diversity: An integrative model of subgroup relations. *Personality and Social Psychology Review, 4,* 143–156.

Jetten, J., Spears, R., Hogg, M. A., & Manstead, A. S. R. (2000). Discrimination constrained and justified: Variable effects of group variability and ingroup identification. *Journal of Experimental Social Psychology, 36,* 329–356.

Jetten, J., Spears, R., & Manstead, A. S. R. (1997). Identity threat and prototypicality: Combined effects on intergroup discrimination and collective self-esteem. *European Journal of Social Psychology, 27,* 635–657.

Jost, J. T. (1995). Negative illusions: Conceptual clarification and psychological evidence concerning false consciousness. *Political Psychology, 16,* 397–424.

Jost, J. T., & Banaji, M. R. (1994). The role of stereotyping in system-justification and the production of false consciousness. *British Journal of Social Psychology, 33,* 1–27.

Leary, M. R., Tambor, E. S., Terdal, S. K., & Downs, D. L. (1995). Self-esteem as an interpersonal monitor: The sociometer hypothesis. *Journal of Personality and Social Psychology, 68,* 518–530.

Levine, J. M., & Moreland, R. L. (1994). Group socialization: Theory and research. *European Review of Social Psychology, 5,* 305–336.

Leyens, J.-P., Yzerbyt, V., & Schadron, G. (1994). *Stereotypes and social cognition*. London: Sage.

Long, K., & Spears, R. (1997). The self-esteem hypothesis revisited: Differentiation and the disaffected. In R. Spears, P. J. Oakes, N. Ellemers, & S. A. Haslam (Eds.), *The social psychology of stereotyping and group life* (pp. 296–317). Oxford, UK: Blackwell.

Luhtanen, R., & Crocker, J. (1992). A collective self-esteem scale: Self-evaluation of one's social identity. *Personality and Social Psychology Bulletin, 18,* 302–318.

Markus, H., & Kitayama, S. (1991). Culture and the self: Implications for cognition, emotion and motivation. *Psychological Review, 98,* 224–253.

Marques, J. M., Abrams, D., Páez, D., & Hogg, M. A. (2001). Social categorization, social identification, and rejection of deviant group members. In M. A. Hogg & R. S. Tindale (Eds.), *Blackwell handbook of social psychology: Group processes* (pp. 400–424). Oxford, UK: Blackwell.

Marques, J. M., & Páez, D. (1994). The "black sheep effect": Social categorization, rejection of ingroup deviates and perception of group variability. *European Review of Social Psychology, 5,* 37–68.

Martin, R., & Hewstone, M. (2001). Conformity and independence in groups: Majorities and minorities. In M. A. Hogg & R. S. Tindale (Eds.), *Blackwell handbook of social psychology: Group processes* (pp. 209–234). Oxford, UK: Blackwell.

Moreland, R. L., Hogg, M. A., & Hains, S. C. (1994). Back to the future: Social psychological research on groups. *Journal of Experimental Social Psychology, 30,* 527–555.

Moreland, R. L., & Levine, J. M. (1982) Socialization in small groups: Temporal changes in individual-group relations. In L. Berkowitz (Ed.), *Advances in experimental social psychology* (Vol. 15, pp. 137–192). New York: Academic Press.

Moscovici, S. (1976). *Social influence and social change.* London: Academic Press.

Mugny, G. (1982). *The power of minorities.* London: Academic Press.

Noel, J. G., Wann, D. L., & Branscombe, N. R. (1995). Peripheral in-group membership status and public negativity toward out-group. *Journal of Personality and Social Psychology, 68,* 127–137.

Oakes, P. J. (1987). The salience of social categories. In J. C. Turner, M. A. Hogg, P. J. Oakes, S. D. Reicher, & M. S. Wetherell, *Rediscovering the social group: A self(categorization theory* (pp. 117–141). Oxford, UK: Blackwell.

Oakes, P. J., Haslam, S. A., & Turner, J. C. (1994). *Stereotyping and social reality.* Oxford, UK: Blackwell.

Oakes, P. J., & Turner, J. C. (1990). Is limited information processing the cause of social stereotyping? *European Review of Social Psychology, 1,* 111–135.

Otten, S., Mummendey, A., & Blanz, M. (1996). Intergroup discrimination in positive and negative outcome allocations: Impact of stimulus valence, relative group status, and relative group size. *Personality and Social Psychology Bulletin, 22,* 568–581.

Pettigrew, T. F. (1998). Intergroup contact theory. *Annual Review of Psychology, 49,* 65–85.

Pratt, M. G. (1998). To be or not to be: Central questions in organizational identification. In D. Whetten & P. Godfrey (Eds.), *Identity in organizations: Developing theory through conversations* (pp. 171–207). Thousand Oaks, CA: Sage.

Pratto, F. (1999). The puzzle of continuing group inequality: Piecing together psychological, social and cultural forces in social dominance theory. In M. P. Zanna (Ed.), *Advances in experimental social psychology* (Vol. 31, pp. 191–263). New York: Academic Press.

Pratto, F., Sidanius, J., Stallworth, L. M., & Malle, B. F. (1994). Social dominance orientation: A personality variable predicting social and political attitudes. *Journal of Personality and Social Psychology, 67,* 741–763.

Prentice, D. A., & Miller, D. T. (Eds.). (1999). *Cultural divides: Understanding and overcoming group conflict.* New York: Russell Sage Foundation.

Rabbie, J. M., & Horwitz, M. (1969). Arousal of ingroup–outgroup bias by a chance win or loss. *Journal of Personality and Social Psychology, 13,* 269–277.

Rabbie, J. M., Schot, J. C., & Visser, L. (1989). Social identity theory: A conceptual and empirical critique from the perspective of a behavioural interaction model. *European Journal of Social Psychology, 19,* 171–202.

Reicher, S. D. (1984). The St. Pauls' riot: An explanation of the limits of crowd action in terms of a social identity model. *European Journal of Social Psychology, 14,* 1–21.

Reicher, S. D. (2001). The psychology of crowd dynamics. In M. A. Hogg & R. S. Tindale (Eds.), *Blackwell handbook of social psychology: Group processes* (pp. 182–207). Oxford, UK: Blackwell.

Reicher, S. D., Spears, R., & Postmes, T. (1995). A social identity model of deindividuation phenomena. *European Review of Social Psychology, 6,* 161–198.

Reid, A., & Deaux, K. (1996). Relationship between social and personal identities: Segregation or integration. *Journal of Personality and Social Psychology, 71,* 1084–1091.

Ridgeway, C. L. (2001). Social status and group structure. In M. A. Hogg & R. S. Tindale (Eds.), *Blackwell handbook of social psychology: Group processes* (pp. 352–375). Oxford, UK: Blackwell.

Robinson, W. P. (Ed.). (1996). *Social groups and identities: Developing the legacy of Henri Tajfel.* Oxford, UK: Butterworth-Heinemann.

Rubin, M., & Hewstone, M. (1998). Social identity theory's self-esteem hypothesis: A review and some suggestions for clarification. *Personality and Social Psychology Review, 2,* 40–62.

Sedikides, C. (1993). Assessment, enhancement, and verification determinants of the self-evaluation process. *Journal of Personality and Social Psychology, 65,* 317–338.

Sedikides, C., & Strube, M. J. (1997). Self-evaluation: To thine own self be good, to thine own self be sure, to thine own self be true, and to thine own self be better. In M. P. Zanna (Ed.), *Advances in experimental social psychology* (Vol. 29, pp. 209–296). New York: Academic Press.

Sherif, M. (1936). *The psychology of social norms.* New York: Harper.

Sidanius, J., & Pratto, F. (1999). *Social dominance: An intergroup theory of social hierarchy and oppression.* New York: Cambridge University Press.

Smith, E., & Henry, S. (1996). An in-group becomes part of the self: Response time evaluation. *Personality and Social Psychology Bulletin, 22,* 635–642.

Smith, E. R., Coats, S., & Walling, D. (1999). Overlapping mental representations of self, in-group, and partner: Further response time evidence and a connectionist model. *Personality and Social Psychology Bulletin, 25,* 873–882.

Suls, J., & Wheeler, L. (Eds.). (2000). *Handbook of social comparison: Theory and research.* New York: Kluwer Academic/Plenum Press.

Tajfel, H. (1959). Quantitative judgement in social perception. *British Journal of Psychology, 50,* 16–29.

Tajfel, H. (1969). Cognitive aspects of prejudice. *Journal of Social Issues, 25,* 79–97.

Tajfel, H. (1972). Social categorization. In S. Moscovici (Ed.), *Introduction à la psychologie sociale* (Vol. 1, pp. 272–302). Paris: Larousse.

Tajfel, H. (1981). Social stereotypes and social groups. In J. C. Turner & H. Giles (Eds.), *Intergroup behaviour* (pp. 144–167). Oxford, UK: Blackwell.

Tajfel, H., Billig, M., Bundy R. P., & Flament, C. (1971). Social categorization and intergroup behaviour. *European Journal of Social Psychology, 1,* 149–177.

Tajfel, H., Jaspars, J. M. F., & Fraser, C. (1984). The social dimension in European social psychology. In H. Tajfel (Ed.), *The social dimension: European developments in social psychology* (Vol. 1, pp. 1–5). Cambridge, UK: Cambridge University Press.

Tajfel, H., & Turner, J. C. (1979). An integrative theory of intergroup conflict. In W. G. Austin & S. Worchel (Eds.), *The social psychology of intergroup relations* (pp. 33–47). Monterey, CA: Brooks/Cole.

Tajfel, H., & Wilkes, A. L. (1963). Classification and quantitative judgement. *British Journal of Psychology, 54,* 101–114.

Taylor, D. M., & Brown, R. J. (1979). Towards a more social social psychology? *British Journal of Social and Clinical Psychology, 18,* 173–179.

Taylor, D. M., & McKirnan, D. J. (1984). A five-stage model of intergroup relations. *British Journal of Social Psychology, 23,* 291–300.

Taylor, S. E., Fiske, S. T., Etcoff, N. L., & Ruderman, A. J. (1978). Categorical and contextual bases of person memory and stereotyping. *Journal of Personality and Social Psychology, 36,* 778–793.

Terry, D. J., & Hogg, M. A. (1996). Group norms and the attitude–behavior relationship: A role for group identification. *Personality and Social Psychology Bulletin, 22,* 776–793.

Terry, D. J., Hogg, M. A., & White, K. M. (2000). Attitude-behavior relations: Social identity and group membership. In D. J. Terry & M. A. Hogg (Eds.), *Attitudes, behavior, and social context: The role of norms and group membership* (pp. 67–93). Mahwah, NJ: Erlbaum.

Thoits, P. A., & Virshup, L. K. (1997). Me's and we's: Forms and functions of social identities. In R. D. Ashmore & L. J. Jussim (Eds.), *Rutgers series on self and social identity: Vol. 1. Self and identity: Fundamental issues* (pp. 106–133). New York: Oxford University Press.

Triandis, H. C. (1989). The self and social behavior in differing cultural contexts. *Psychological Review, 96,* 506–520.

Tropp, L. R., & Wright, S. C. (2001). Ingroup identification as inclusion of ingroup in the self. *Personality and Social Psychology Bulletin, 27,* 585–600.

Turner, J. C. (1975). Social comparison and social identity: Some prospects for intergroup behaviour. *European Journal of Social Psychology, 5,* 5–34.

Turner, J. C. (1978). Social categorization and social discrimination in the minimal group paradigm. In H. Tajfel (Ed.), *Differentiation between social groups: Studies in the social psychology of intergroup relations* (pp. 101–140). London: Academic Press.

Turner, J. C. (1982). Towards a cognitive redefinition of the social group. In H. Tajfel (Ed.), *Social identity and intergroup relations* (pp. 15–40). Cambridge, UK: Cambridge University Press.

Turner, J. C. (1985). Social categorization and the self-concept: A social cognitive theory of group behavior. In E. J. Lawler (Ed.), *Advances in group processes: Vol. 2. Theory and research* (pp. 77–122). Greenwich, CT: JAI Press.

Turner, J. C. (1991). *Social influence.* Milton Keynes, UK: Open University Press.

Turner, J. C. (1999). Some current issues in research on social identity and self-categorization theories. In N. Ellemers, R. Spears, & B. Doosje (Eds.), *Social identity* (pp. 6–34). Oxford, UK: Blackwell.

Turner, J. C., & Bourhis, R. Y. (1996). Social identity, interdependence and the social group: A reply to Rabbie et al. In W. P. Robinson (Ed.), *Social groups and identities: Developing the legacy of Henri Tajfel* (pp. 25–63). Oxford, UK: Butterworth-Heinemann.

Turner, J. C., Hogg, M. A., Oakes, P. J., Reicher, S. D., & Wetherell, M. S. (1987). *Rediscovering the social group: A self-categorization theory.* Oxford, UK: Blackwell.

Turner, J. C., & Oakes, P. J. (1986). The significance of the social identity concept for social psychology with reference to individualism, interactionism and social influence. *British Journal of Social Psychology, 25,* 237–239.

Turner, J. C., & Oakes, P. J. (1989). Self-categorization and social influence. In P. B. Paulus (Ed.), *The psychology of group influence* (2nd ed., pp. 233–275). Hillsdale, NJ: Erlbaum.

Tyler, T. R. (1997). The psychology of legitimacy: A relational perspective on voluntary deference to authorities. *Personality and Social Psychology Review, 1,* 323–345.

Tyler, T. R., & Lind, E. A. (1992). A relational model of authority in groups. In M. P. Zanna (Ed.), *Advances in experimental social psychology* (Vol. 25, pp. 115–191). New York: Academic Press.

Vescio, T. K., Hewstone, M., Crisp, R. J., & Rubin, M. J. (1999). Perceiving and responding to multiply categorizable individuals: Cognitive processes and affective intergroup bias. In D. Abrams & M. A. Hogg (Eds.), *Social identity and social cognition* (pp. 111–140). Oxford, UK: Blackwell.

Wheeler, L. (1991). A brief history of social comparison theory. In J. Suls & T. A. Wills (Eds.), *Social comparison: Contemporary theory and research* (pp. 3–21). Hillsdale, NJ: Erlbaum.

Worchel, S., Morales, J. F., Páez, D., & Deschamps, J.-C. (Eds.). (1998). *Social identity: International perspectives.* London: Sage.

Wright, S. C., Aron, A., & Tropp, L. R. (in press). Including others (and groups) in the self: Self-expansion and intergroup relations. In J. P. Forgas & K. Williams (Eds.), *The social self: Cognitive, interpersonal and intergroup perspectives.* Philadelphia: Psychology Press.

24

Optimal Distinctiveness, Social Identity, and the Self

MARILYNN B. BREWER

The concept of "social identity" provides a link between the psychology of the individual—the representation of self—and the structure and process of social groups within which the self is embedded. Because it serves this critical function in connecting individual and group levels of analysis, the social identity concept has been invented and reinvented in a wide variety of theoretical frameworks and across all the social and behavioral science disciplines. As a consequence, the term has acquired multiple different meanings in different disciplinary contexts (Brewer, 2001). Within social psychology, however, the concept is most associated with social identity theory as articulated by Tajfel and Turner (Tajfel, 1981; Tajfel & Turner, 1986). In this theoretical framework, social identity is an extension of the self-concept that entails a shift in the level of self-representation from that of the individual self to that of the collective self (Brewer & Gardner, 1996; Turner, Hogg, Oakes, Reicher, & Wetherell, 1987). When social identities are activated, significant group memberships are not simply a component of the individual's self concept; the individual perceives the self as *part of* the larger collective unit.

Social identity as self-embedded-in-groups makes salient the fact that social identities are not simply individual cognitive constructions; they are based on collective beliefs about shared attributes, values, and experiences that constitute the content of specific social identities. A given social identity determines who is seen as sharing common ingroup membership with the self and what attributes and values are presumed to be self-defining. Thus, when a particular social identity is engaged, both the structure and the content of the self-concept are changed. Different social identities are associated with transformations in the definition of self and the basis for self-evaluation (Brewer, 1991; Brewer & Gardner, 1996).

The shift in level of self-representation from personal identity to social identity has cognitive, affective, and motivational consequences. When a particular social identity is made salient, individuals are likely to think of themselves as having characteristics that are representative of that social category (Hogg & Turner, 1987; Simon & Hamilton,

1994; Smith & Henry, 1996). Consistent with this perspective, experimental research has demonstrated that retrieval cues that activate the "private" self-representation generate self-cognitions that are quite different from the self-cognitions retrieved when the "collective" self-aspect is activated (Trafimow, Triandis, & Goto, 1991). Further, when a collective social identity is activated, self-evaluations are based on intergroup social comparisons rather than on interpersonal comparisons (Brewer & Weber, 1994). Finally, the shift from personal to social identity entails a concomitant shift from self-interest to group interest as the basic motivation for behavior (Brewer, 1991; Kramer & Brewer, 1986).

Motivational Theories of Social Identification

Because group identity sometimes entails self-sacrifice in the interests of group welfare and solidarity, understanding why and when individuals are willing to relegate their sense of self to significant group identities requires motivational, as well as cognitive, analysis. Motivational explanations are also needed to account for why group membership does not always lead to identification and why individuals are more chronically identified with some ingroups than with others.

Self-Esteem

The motivational concept most associated with social identity theory is that of self-esteem enhancement. And it is true that initial development of social identity theory (e.g., Turner, 1975; Tajfel & Turner, 1986) implicated self-esteem in postulating a need for "positive distinctiveness" in ingroup–outgroup comparisons. However, it is not clear from these writings whether positive self-esteem was being invoked as a motive for social identity itself or as a motive for ingroup favoritism, given that social identity had been engaged. Whatever the original intent, subsequent research on the role of self-esteem in ingroup bias has generally supported the idea that enhanced self-esteem may be a consequence of achieving a positively distinct social identity, but there is little evidence that the need to increase self-

esteem motivates social identification in the first place (Rubin & Hewstone, 1998). To the contrary, there is considerable evidence that individuals often identify strongly with groups that are disadvantaged, stigmatized, or otherwise suffer from negative intergroup comparison (e.g., Crocker, Luhtanen, Blaine, & Broadnax, 1994; Doosje, Ellemers, & Spears, 1995; Turner, Hogg, Turner, & Smith, 1984).

Cognitive Motives: Uncertainty Reduction

Given the inadequacy of self-esteem as an explanation for why social identity is engaged, other motives have been proposed that do not require positive ingroup status as a basis for attachment to groups and self-definition as a group member. One proposal is that group identity meets fundamental needs for reducing uncertainty and achieving meaning and clarity in social contexts (Hogg & Abrams, 1993; Hogg & Mullin, 1999; see Hogg, Chapter 23, this volume). In support of this hypothesis, Hogg and his colleagues (Grieve & Hogg, 1999; Mullin & Hogg, 1998) have generated compelling evidence that identification and ingroup bias are increased under conditions of high cognitive uncertainty and reduced or eliminated when uncertainty is low. And it is undoubtedly true that one function that group memberships and identities serve for individuals is that of providing self-definition and guidance for behavior in otherwise ambiguous social situations (Deaux, Reid, Mizrahi, & Cotting, 1999; Vignoles, Chryssochoou, & Breakwell, 2000). However, group identity is only one of many possible modes of reducing social uncertainty. Roles, values, laws, and so forth, serve a similar function without necessitating social identification processes. Thus uncertainty reduction alone cannot account for the pervasiveness of group identification as a fundamental aspect of human life.

Uncertainty reduction as a theory of social identity places the explanation for group identification in a system of cognitive motives that includes needs for meaning, certainty, and structure. An alternative perspective is that the motivation for social identification arises from even more fundamental needs for security and safety. Consistent with this idea, Baumeister and Leary

(1995) postulate a universal need for *belonging* as an aspect of human nature derived from our vulnerability as lone individuals who require connection with others in order to survive. But belonging alone cannot account for the selectivity of social identification, as any and all group memberships should satisfy the belonging motive. My own theory (Brewer, 1991) postulates that the need for belonging and inclusion is paired with an opposing motive—the need for differentiation—that together regulate the individual's social identity and attachment to social groups.

Optimal Distinctiveness Theory: Basic Premises

Optimal distinctiveness theory (Brewer, 1991) is an extension of social identity theory, developed to account for individuals' seeking identification with social groups and to explain the role of social identities in achieving and maintaining a stable self-concept. Briefly, the theory is based on the thesis that distinctiveness per se is a factor underlying the selection and strength of social identities because distinct social groups satisfy basic psychological needs derived from our evolutionary history as a social species.

The theory has its origins in the premise that group living represents the fundamental survival strategy that characterizes the human species. In the course of our evolutionary history, humans lost most of the physical characteristics and instincts that make possible survival and reproduction as isolated individuals or pairs of individuals, in favor of other advantages that require cooperative interdependence with others in order to survive in a broad range of physical environments. In other words, as a species we have evolved to rely on cooperation rather than strength and on social learning rather than instinct as basic adaptations. The result is that, as a species, human beings are characterized by *obligatory interdependence* (Brewer, 1997; Caporael, 1997). For long-term survival, we must be willing to rely on others for information, aid, and shared resources, and we must be willing to give information and aid and to share resources with others.

For individual humans, the potential benefits (receiving resources from others) and

costs (giving resources to others) of mutual cooperation go hand in hand and set natural limits on cooperative interdependence. The decision to cooperate (to expend resources to another's benefit) is a dilemma of trust, as the ultimate benefits depend on everyone else's willingness to do the same. A cooperative system requires that trust dominate over distrust. But indiscriminate trust (or indiscriminate altruism) is not an effective individual strategy; altruism must be contingent on the probability that others will cooperate as well.

Social differentiation and clear group boundaries provide one mechanism for achieving the benefits of cooperative interdependence without the risk of excessive costs. Shared ingroup membership provides a basis for contingent altruism. By limiting aid to mutually acknowledged ingroup members, total costs and risks of nonreciprocation can be contained. Thus ingroups can be defined as bounded communities of mutual trust and obligation that delimit mutual interdependence and cooperation. An important aspect of this mutual trust is that it is *depersonalized* (Brewer, 1981), extended to any member of the ingroup, whether personally related or not. Psychologically, expectations of cooperation and security promote positive attraction toward other ingroup members and motivate adherence to ingroup norms of appearance and behavior that assure that one will be recognized as a good or legitimate ingroup member. Symbols and behaviors that differentiate the ingroup from local outgroups become particularly important here, to reduce the risk that ingroup benefits will be inadvertently extended to outgroup members and to ensure that ingroup members will recognize one's own entitlement to receive benefits. Assimilation within and differentiation between groups is thus mutually reinforcing, along with ethnocentric preference for ingroup interactions and institutions (Brewer, 1999).

If social differentiation and intergroup boundaries are functional for social cooperation, and if social cooperation is essential for human survival, then there should be psychological mechanisms at the individual level that motivate and sustain ingroup identification and differentiation. The optimal distinctiveness model postulates just such motivational mechanisms. According to the model, social identities derive from a fundamental tension between human needs for validation and similarity to others (on the one hand) and a countervailing need for uniqueness and individuation (on the other) (Brewer, 1991). More specifically, it is proposed that social identities are selected and activated to the extent that they help to achieve a balance between needs for inclusion and for differentiation in a given social context.

The basic premise of the optimal distinctiveness model is that the two identity needs (inclusion/assimilation and differentiation/distinctiveness) are independent and work in opposition to motivate group identification. Individuals seek social inclusion in order to alleviate or avoid the isolation or stigmatization that may arise from being highly individuated. In a recent review of the literature on social attachment, Baumeister and Leary (1995) conclude that "existing evidence supports the hypothesis that the need to belong is a powerful, fundamental, and extremely pervasive motivation" (p. 497). And researchers studying the effects of tokenism and solo status have generally found that individuals are both uncomfortable and cognitively disadvantaged in situations in which they feel too dissimilar to others. On the other hand, too much similarity or excessive deindividuation provides no basis for comparative appraisal or self-definition, and hence individuals are also uncomfortable in situations in which they lack distinctiveness (Fromkin, 1972). Arousal of either motive will be associated with negative affect and should motivate change in level of self identification.

One dimension along which self-representations can vary is the degree of inclusiveness of the social category in which one is classified. Some categorizations refer to broadly inclusive social groupings that include a large number of individuals with only a few characteristics held in common (e.g., gender, racial categories, national groups); other categories are relatively exclusive, based on highly distinctive characteristics or multiple shared features (e.g., deaf persons, Mensa members, Baptist Korean Americans). Within any social context, categories at different levels of inclusiveness can be identified, either hierarchically (e.g.,

in a gathering of academics, subgroups are differentiated in terms of academic discipline) or orthogonally (e.g., among social psychologists, those who are sailing enthusiasts constitute a cross-cutting category membership). The question is, at what level of inclusion are social identities most likely to be established?

The theory of optimal distinctiveness takes into account the role of the relative distinctiveness or inclusiveness of a social category as a factor in social identification. Within a given social context, or frame of reference, an individual can be categorized (by self or others) along a dimension of social distinctiveness–inclusiveness that ranges from uniqueness (i.e., features that distinguish the individual from any other persons in the social context) at one extreme to total submersion in the social context at the other. Satisfaction of the drive toward social assimilation is directly related to level of inclusiveness, whereas satisfaction of self-differentiation needs is inversely related to level of inclusiveness.

Optimal identities are those that satisfy the need for inclusion *within* the ingroup and simultaneously serve the need for differentiation through distinctions *between* the ingroup and outgroups. In effect, optimal social identities involve *shared distinctiveness*. Individuals will resist being identified with social categorizations that are either too inclusive or too differentiating but will define themselves in terms of social identities that are optimally distinctive. To satisfy the needs simultaneously, individuals will select group identities that are inclusive enough so that they have a sense of being part of a larger collective but exclusive enough that they provide some basis for distinctiveness from others. Equilibrium is maintained by correcting for deviations from optimality. A situation in which a person is overly individuated will excite the need for assimilation, motivating the person to adopt a more inclusive social identity. Conversely, situations that arouse feelings of deindividuation will activate the need for differentiation, resulting in a search for more exclusive or distinct identities. Thus the theory holds that individuals will actively seek to achieve and maintain identification with groups that are optimally distinctive within a given social context.

Optimal Social Identities and the Self-Concept

The motivational assumptions of the optimal distinctiveness model of social identity have direct implications for the structure and content of an individual's self-concept. If individuals are motivated to sustain identification with optimally distinct social groups, then the self-concept should be adapted to fit the normative requirements of such group memberships. Achieving optimal social identities should be associated with a secure and stable self-concept in which individual characteristics are congruent with representation as a good and typical group member. Conversely, if optimal identity is challenged or threatened, the individual should react to restore congruence between the self-concept and the group representation. Optimal identity can be restored either by adjusting individual self-construals to be more consistent with the ingroup prototype or by shifting social identification to a group that is more congruent with the self. In recent research on the optimal distinctiveness model, we have focused on the former—alterations of self-concept in response to threats to specific group identities.

Effects on Self-Stereotyping

Self-stereotyping is one mechanism for matching the self-concept to characteristics that are distinctively representative of particular group memberships. According to self-categorization theory, when people adopt a social identity, "there is a perceptual accentuation of intragroup similarities and intergroup differences on relevant correlated dimensions. People stereotype themselves and others in terms of salient social categorizations, and this stereotyping leads to an enhanced perceptual identity between self and ingroup members and an enhanced perceptual contrast between ingroup and outgroup members" (Turner & Onorato, 1999, p. 21). Consistent with the assumptions of optimal distinctiveness theory, Simon and Hamilton (1994) found that members of distinctive minority groups exhibited more self-stereotyping than members of large majority groups. This finding supports the idea that self-stereotyping occurs in the service of establishing and maintaining optimally distinct social identities, as small distinctive groups motivated more self-stereotyping than did large nondistinctive ingroups.

If these assumptions about the role of self-stereotyping in maintaining optimal distinctiveness are correct, then threats to the optimality of an ingroup should lead to motivated self-stereotyping. Optimal identity can be threatened either by challenging the individual's inclusion within a distinctive social category (arousing the assimilation motive) or by challenging the distinctiveness of that social category vis à vis a larger, more inclusive grouping (arousing the differentiation motive; see also Branscombe, Ellemers, Spears, & Doosje, 1999). Previous research (Jetten, Spears, & Manstead, 1997, 1999, 2001) has demonstrated that threats to group distinctiveness result in attempts to restore intergroup differentiation through means such as ingroup favoritism, negative evaluations of the outgroup, and stereotypic group differentiation. In addition, threats to group status and group distinctiveness have been shown to affect individuals' perceptions of typicality. In two studies, Spears, Doosje, and Ellemers (1997) found that in response to threatened group distinctiveness, low identifiers perceived themselves as being less like the average ingroup member, whereas high identifiers tended to see themselves as being more like the average ingroup member. This work provides support for the hypothesis that enhanced differentiation need results in heightened levels of content-specific self-stereotyping.

Self-stereotyping has the effect of enhancing both intragroup similarity and intergroup differentiation. Thus self-stereotyping provides one mechanism through which individuals can maintain or restore an optimal social identity when inclusion or differentiation needs are aroused.

Because of this hypothesized relationship between self-stereotyping and the satisfaction of inclusion and differentiation needs, optimal distinctiveness theory predicts that threats to optimal identities will lead to *increases* in self-stereotyping. Self-stereotyping enhances the perceptual closeness of the self to the ingroup. The more a person sees group stereotype traits as being descriptive of the self, the more intragroup assimilation this person should be able to achieve. Thus, when assimilation needs are heightened, individuals should be motivated to self-stereotype more in relation to that ingroup. By the same logic, arousal of the need for differentiation should have a parallel effect on self-stereotyping. The more that group members perceive themselves (and other group members) in a stereotypical fashion, the more intergroup differentiation they can achieve. To the extent that all group members conform to their respective group stereotypes, there should be less overlap between the ingroup and corresponding outgroups. Thus, in order to satisfy their need for differentiation, individuals should be motivated to self-stereotype in relation to that group in order to achieve greater intergroup differentiation.

Pickett, Bonner, and Coleman (2002) conducted a series of experiments to test this hypothesis. In each study, need activation was experimentally manipulated through threats to existing optimal social identities. In different conditions, the need for assimilation or differentiation was aroused by providing participants with false feedback regarding their scores on a previously administered personality test (the Self-Attributes Questionnaire; SAQ). Participants were also given false feedback regarding the group averages for the ingroup on the same test.[1]

In the *control condition* (no need arousal/optimal distinctiveness), participants were told that the mean for ingroup students on the SAQ is 62 and that past studies have shown that one of the areas in which their group differs from other groups is in their scores on the SAQ. The mean for outgroups was said to be 34. Below this written information were two curves (containing approximately 20% overlap) that represented the distribution of ingroup students and outgroup students. Participants' own score was written in as 61, which placed the participant at the mean of the ingroup distribution. It was predicted that participants in this condition would feel fairly satisfied and nonthreatened by this feedback. Their inclusion need would be met by knowing that they are typical of other ingroup members, and their differentiation motive would be met by the clear intergroup distinction between ingroup and outgroups.

The information given to participants in the *inclusion motive condition* was identical to the information provided to control participants, except that participants' *own* scores on the SAQ were written in as 48. This was designed to make participants feel that they were in the peripheral position within the ingroup, part of a small subgroup at the tail of the ingroup distribution. This feedback was expected to arouse the motive for inclusion and assimilation.

Similar to the control condition, participants assigned to the *differentiation motive condition* were told that they scored a 61 on the SAQ. However, in the differentiation motive condition, the distance between ingroup and outgroup students on the SAQ was dramatically reduced. The mean for the ingroup was set at 58 (close to the outgroup mean of 61), and the curves that represented the distribution of SAQ scores for the two groups overlapped by approximately 80%. Participants were also told that "one of the areas in which ingroup students and other students *do not* differ is in their scores on the SAQ." This feedback was intended to threaten intergroup differentiation and was expected to excite participants' need for differentiation and distinctiveness.

Following this motivational manipulation, self-stereotyping was assessed by asking participants to rate themselves on a long list of personality traits and dispositions, which included traits previously identified as stereotypic of the target ingroup and many filler items that were stereotype irrelevant. The critical measure was the extremity of self-ratings on the stereotypic traits in particular.

For the inclusion need arousal manipulation, the predicted increase in self-stereotyping is particularly counterintuitive. Generally, one would assume that being made aware of one's difference from other group members (as the manipulation in this condition entails) would result in feeling *less* like the prototypical group member and the belief that the traits typical of the group are less descriptive of oneself. However, because of the relationship proposed by ODT between extreme individuation and the arousal of assimilation needs, we predicted that individuals would react to this feedback by perceiving stereotypical traits of the ingroup as being *more* descriptive of the self. Consistent with optimal distinctiveness predictions, participants in all three studies (involving three different ingroups and diverse stereotypic traits) exhibited heightened self-stereotyping when either the need for inclusion *or* the need for differentiation had been activated. (See Table 24.1 for summary of findings.) In Study 1, the target ingroup was college honors students, and the outgroup was "other Ohio State University students." All participants recruited for the study were highly identified with this ingroup membership. Nonetheless, self-stereotyping on ingroup-relevant traits was significantly greater when this optimal identity had been threatened (assimilation or differentiation need arousal) than in the control condition. Because traits characteristic of honors students are generally positive (e.g., intelligent, hardworking), it was important to demonstrate that the elevated ratings were specific to stereotypic traits. On ratings of other positive trait characteristics that were not associated with the honors-student stereotype (e.g., likeable, honest), there were no significant mean differences across conditions in self-ratings.

In Study 2, identity as OSU students defined the target ingroup, and the outgroup was "other U.S. college students." Because initial level of identification with the specific ingroup is expected to moderate responses to identity threat, participants were classified as either high or low identifiers based on a pretest measure of their group identification. Only those initially classified as high in identification with the university showed

effects of identity threat on self-stereotyping, consistent with the idea that self-stereotyping serves to restore optimal identities and is not a response to the personality feedback per se. Finally, results of Study 3 demonstrated specifically that participants who were high in prior social identification with the target group (sororities) showed increased self-stereotyping on both positive (e.g., popular, attractive, fun-loving) *and* negative (e.g., snobbish, materialistic, spoiled) ingroup traits (Pickett et al., 2002). The fact that we were able to observe negative self-stereotyping under need arousal conditions testifies to the fundamental nature of inclusion and differentiation needs above and beyond self-enhancement motives.

Effects on Self-Worth

According to the theory, optimal social identities serve to meet basic needs for security and belonging and also provide a basis for a stable self-concept. Because clarity and certainty of self-concept are generally associated with positive self-esteem (Baumgardner, 1990; Campbell, 1990), there are a number of grounds for predicting that achieving an optimal social identity should enhance or maintain a sense of positive self-worth.

In making this prediction, I draw a distinction between the specific concept of self-esteem and the more general concept of self-worth. Specific self-esteem is the valuation that is attached to the traits and characteris-

TABLE 24.1. Mean Self-Stereotyping Ratings

		Motive condition		
		Need inclusion	Control	Need differentiation
Experiment 1 Ingroup: Honors students		5.58$_a$	5.10$_b$	5.50$_a$
Experiment 2 Ingroup: University (high identifiers)		5.44$_a$	4.92$_b$	5.23$_a$
Experiment 3 Ingroup: Sorority (high identifiers)	Positive Negative	5.61$_a$ 3.56$_a$	5.07$_b$ 2.68$_b$	5.71$_a$ 4.31$_c$

Note. Higher numbers reflect greater self-stereotyping. Cell means within the same row that do not share a common subscript differ significantly from each other at the $p < .05$ level. Data from Pickett, Bonner, & Coleman (2002).

tics associated with the self, and it has been further differentiated into *personal* self-esteem and *collective* self-esteem. Personal self-esteem is derived from the evaluation of traits attributed to the individual self in comparison with others. Measures such as the Coopersmith Self-Esteem Inventory (Coopersmith, 1967) or the SAQ (Pelham & Swann, 1989), in which respondents rate their standing on positive and negative personality traits and abilities, are representative of this conceptualization of self-esteem. Collective self-esteem is the evaluation of the social groups associated with the self, as measured by the private and membership subscales of the Collective Self-Esteem Scale[2] (Luhtanen & Crocker, 1992) with items such as, "I feel good about the social group I belong to," and "I am a cooperative participant in the social group I belong to." Research indicates that these two levels of specific self-esteem are only moderately correlated (Luhtanen & Crocker, 1992).

Other conceptualizations of self-esteem appear to reflect a more global sense of self-worth, as represented by the Rosenberg (1965) Self-Esteem Scale (e.g., items such as "I feel I am a person of worth, at least on an equal basis with others"; I often feel like a failure"). Although the Rosenberg scale is often referred to as a measure of *personal* self-esteem, self-worth is more like a summary index of self-satisfaction or general well-being, which could be derived *either* from personal characteristics, group memberships, or both.

Optimal social identity could be expected to have some impact on all three types of self-esteem. The connection between optimal identity and collective self-esteem is most straightforward. Secure membership in optimally distinctive groups should be associated with high positive collective self-esteem, particularly on the private and membership esteem subscales. To the extent that collective self-esteem contributes to overall self-worth, there should also be a positive relationship between optimal social identity and global self-esteem. Generalizing yet further, global self-worth may spill over to personal self-esteem as part of a positive feedback loop whereby general feelings of self-satisfaction translate into positive evaluations on specific trait characteristics.

A relationship between collective identi-

ties (or collective self-esteem) and general self-worth or well-being has been demonstrated in a number of contexts (e.g., Bettencourt, Charleton, Eubanks, Kernahan, & Fuller, 1999; Bettencourt & Dorr, 1997; Crocker & Luhtanen, 1990). There is reason to believe that group identity may play a particularly important role in enhancing self-worth and subjective well-being for individuals who have stigmatizing characteristics or belong to disadvantaged social categories. In the original presentation of optimal distinctiveness theory (Brewer, 1991), I speculated about the effects of redefining a personal stigma as a source of shared distinctiveness:

> excessive individuation is undesirable—having any salient feature that distinguishes oneself from everyone else in a social context . . . is at least uncomfortable and at worst devastating to self-esteem. One way to combat the nonoptimality of stigmatization is to convert the stigma from a *personal identity* to a basis of a *social identity*. . . . What is painful at the individual level becomes a source of pride at the group level—a badge of distinction rather than a mark of shame . . . (p. 481; italics in original)

The implications of this idea find some support in research on the functions of support groups for individuals with physical or psychological disabilities (Coates & Winston, 1983; Fine & Asch, 1988) and on the relationship between strength of ethnic identity and self-worth among minority group members (e.g., Branscombe, Schmitt, & Harvey, 1999; Crocker et al., 1994; Kernahan, Bettencourt, & Dorr, 2000). In each of these domains, focus on a collective self, or shared identity, is associated with more positive self-worth or subjective well-being than is the case when collective identification is low or absent.

In order to test experimentally the causal relationship between optimal social identities (shared distinctiveness) and collective self-esteem, Leonardelli and Brewer (2001) conducted a series of studies in which participants were experimentally classified into one of two perceptual categories. Participants were told that one of the categories contained a large proportion of people (around 80%), whereas the other category was a distinctive minority. Participants' identification with their assigned category was then reinforced by inducing them to think of ways in which they were typical of the category. The presumption of the studies was that being an identified member of a large majority category would be nonoptimal compared with identification with a relatively smaller, more distinct social group. Thus it was predicted that, although participants in both categories would be identified with their ingroups, those classified in the minority category would be more satisfied and have higher collective self-esteem than those in the majority category.

In the Leonardelli and Brewer (2001) experiments, participants were randomly categorized into groups in accord with the procedures of the minimal group paradigm (Tajfel, Billig, Bundy, & Flament, 1971). A dot estimation exercise was used as the vehicle for categorization into two social groups, and the ingroup size manipulation was embedded in the participants' dot estimation performance feedback. The experimenter and an assistant explained that the study investigated dot estimation as an indicator of perceptual acuity and preconscious style. A brief description of the estimation task was provided, and the students then made estimates for a total of ten dot trials. A sheet was prepared for each participant that contained an estimation task "score" (all participants received a score of 43) and a description of their classification. All participants who were categorized as *minority* group members read the following description:

"The test you just took examined one's abilities underlying dot estimation. Dot estimation has been related to perceptual acuity and preconscious style, two important abilities of the mind which are used to classify people as overestimators and underestimators. *Your test results indicate that you are an underestimator, and that you are part of a minority portion of the population. Most people are overestimators; in fact, 75–80% of them are. You fall into a group that represents 20–25% of the population.* We don't have time right now, but we will be glad to spend time discussing your score with you after the session. For purposes of identifying your category membership for the rest of the study, we have attached the letter 'U' to your identification number.

Please use this full designation on all remaining forms."

Those categorized as members of a *majority* read the same paragraph, but with the following sentences in place of the italicized sentences:

"*Your test results indicate that you are an overestimator, and that you are part of the majority portion of the population. Few people are underestimators; in fact only 20–25% of them are. You fall into a group that represents 75–80% of the population.*"

Following the categorization phase of the experiment, all participants completed questionnaires assessing their level of identification with their category and their satisfaction with their category membership. The identification measure was essentially a check on the effectiveness of the identity induction and included items such as: "This group's characteristics mirror my characteristics"; "I feel that I am a part of this group"; "I feel ties to people in this group"; and "I do not belong to this group" (reverse scored). The ingroup satisfaction scale was essentially equivalent to items from the private Collective Self-Esteem Scale of Luhtanen and Crocker (1992). Participants rated their level of agreement (on a 6-point scale) with the following four items with reference to their ingroup: "I am pleased to be a member of this group"; "This group is not satisfying to me" (reverse scored); "I am unhappy with this group" (reverse scored); and "I am satisfied with this group." Across two experiments, minority group participants reported somewhat higher identification with their ingroup than did majority group participants, but, more important, they expressed significantly higher collective self-esteem on the 24-point satisfaction scale ($M = 17.42$ vs. 16.05, respectively). Consistent with predictions from optimal identity theory, belonging to a smaller, more distinctive minority ingroup (which meets both inclusion and differentiation needs) proved to be a more optimal collective identity than belonging to a larger, less distinctive ingroup (Leonardelli & Brewer, 2001).

In another study (Leonardelli, 1998) we explored the generalized effects of classification into majority (nonoptimal) and minority (optimal) categories on *personal* self-esteem, above and beyond collective esteem. In addition, this experiment tested predictions derived from optimal distinctiveness about the self-esteem effects of placement in a nonoptimal, overly distinctive category. Excessive distinctiveness was manipulated by exclusion from membership in either one of the relevant social categories. According to optimal distinctiveness theory, unclassified individuals, like individuals classified in a majority category, should experience a decrease in self-esteem associated with nonoptimal identity.

In this experiment, participants were either randomly assigned to a majority or minority dot estimation category, as described previously, or were placed in the "unclassified" condition. Unclassified participants received a description with a similar outline to the classified group members but were told that their scores did not fall into either category:

"You, however, scored as an exception; we were unable to classify you as an overestimator or an underestimator. Considering that your score is unique, we decided to classify you as an underestimator because fewer people fall into that category."

Before participants received their category assignments, the experimenter discussed the dot estimation task as it related to group size, emphasizing that one of the categories was much larger than the other. To make the "unclassifiable" condition feedback more convincing, an interruption was staged; the assistant came into the room, explained that she was having trouble categorizing "one of the forms," and asked the experimenter for help. The planned interruption was intended to reinforce the idea that not falling into one of the categories was an unusual event.

Following the categorization, ratings of self-esteem were collected using a 10-item version of a state self-esteem scale (Heatherton & Polivy, 1991). Participants responded to the items on a 5-point scale (1 = *not at all*; 5 = *extremely*). A measure of change in self-esteem following categorization to minority, majority, or unclassified status was generated by regressing the postcategorization self-esteem scores onto pretested Rosenberg Self-Esteem Scale scores and computing the unstandardized residual as a measure of self-esteem change for each individual.

Consistent with optimal distinctiveness predictions, participants in the classified minority condition experienced an increase in self-esteem ($M = 0.95$), whereas those in the classified majority condition experienced the greatest decrease in self-esteem ($M = -1.21$). The mean for the unclassified participants was also negative ($M = -0.24$), but closer to zero than for the majority nonoptimal categorization. Although the difference between the means for the unclassified participants and the optimal minority participants was only marginally significant, the overall pattern of relationship between inclusiveness of categorization and self-esteem showed the curvilinear (inverted-U) function predicted by optimal distinctiveness theory (Leonardelli, 1998).

Conclusions

The optimal distinctiveness model is a theory of self that assigns primacy to the role of group memberships and collective identity in defining the self-concept and maintaining positive self-worth. This model counteracts the highly individualized representation of the self that dominates much of American psychology and acknowledges the importance of social interdependence as a characteristic of human beings. Sedikides and Gaertner (2001; Gaertner, Sedikides, & Graetz, 1999) have argued that this shift of emphasis from the individual to the collective self is misplaced, but I doubt that the concept of the personal self is going to get lost in the shuffle. Certainly, both levels of self-representation exist and serve critical functions for individual thriving. I have argued elsewhere (Brewer & Roccas, 2001) that the individual self and the collective self can be thought of as two different self-maintenance systems. The function of the personal self is to monitor and maintain individual integrity and continuity; the function of the collective self is to monitor and maintain connectedness to social groups and security. Both are necessary to, and neither is sufficient for, survival and well-being.

Notes

1. Across three different experiments, the target ingroup from which participants were selected varied, but the basic procedures of the experimental manipulation remained the same.
2. The Collective Self-Esteem Scale (Luhtanen & Crocker, 1992) also contains a "public esteem" subscale, which is a measure of how the ingroup is valued by society in general. This is effectively a measure of ingroup status and is not necessarily correlated with private esteem or membership esteem.

References

Baumeister, R. F., & Leary, M. R. (1995). The need to belong: Desire for interpersonal attachments as a fundamental human motivation. *Psychological Bulletin, 117,* 497–529.

Baumgardner, A. H. (1990). To know oneself is to like oneself: Self-certainty and self-affect. *Journal of Personality and Social Psychology, 58,* 1062–1072.

Bettencourt, B. A., Charlton, K., Eubanks, J., Kernahan, C., & Fuller, B. (1999). Development of collective self-esteem among students: Predicting adjustment to college. *Basic and Applied Social Psychology, 21,* 213–222.

Bettencourt, B. A., & Dorr, N. (1997). Collective self-esteem as a mediator of the relationship between allocentrism and subjective well-being. *Personality and Social Psychology Bulletin, 23,* 955–964.

Branscombe, N. R., Ellemers, N., Spears, R., & Doosje, B. (1999). The context and content of social identity threat. In N. Ellemers, R. Spears, & B. Doosje (Eds.), *Social identity: Context, commitment, content* (pp. 35–58). Oxford, UK: Blackwell Science.

Branscombe, N. R., Schmitt, M. T., & Harvey, R. D. (1999). Perceiving pervasive discrimination among African-Americans: Implications for group identification and well-being. *Journal of Personality and Social Psychology, 77,* 135–149.

Brewer, M. B. (1981). Ethnocentrism and its role in intergroup trust. In M. Brewer & B. Collins (Eds.), *Scientific inquiry in the social sciences* (pp. 214–231). San Francisco: Jossey-Bass.

Brewer, M. B. (1991). The social self: On being the same and different at the same time. *Personality and Social Psychology Bulletin, 17,* 475–482.

Brewer, M. B. (1997). On the social origins of human nature. In C. McGarty & S. A. Haslam (Eds.), *The message of social psychology* (pp. 54–62). Oxford, UK: Blackwell.

Brewer, M. B. (1999). The psychology of prejudice: Ingroup love or outgroup hate? *Journal of Social Issues, 55,* 429–444.

Brewer, M. B. (2001). The many faces of social identity: Implications for political psychology. *Political Psychology, 22,* 115–125.

Brewer, M. B., & Gardner, W. (1996). Who is this "we"? Levels of collective identity and self representation. *Journal of Personality and Social Psychology, 71,* 83–93.

Brewer, M. B., & Roccas, S. (2001). Individual values, social identity, and optimal distinctiveness. In C. Sedikides & M. Brewer (Eds.), *Individual self, relational self, collective self* (pp. 219–237). Philadelphia: Psychology Press.

Brewer, M. B., & Weber, J. G. (1994). Self-evaluation effects of interpersonal versus intergroup social comparison. *Journal of Personality and Social Psychology, 66,* 268–275.

Campbell, J. D. (1990). Self-esteem and clarity of the self-concept. *Journal of Personality and Social Psychology, 59,* 538–549.

Caporael, L. R. (1997). The evolution of truly social cognition: The core configurations model. *Personality and Social Psychology Review, 1,* 276–298.

Coates, D., & Winston, T. (1983). Counteracting the deviance of depression: Peer support groups for victims. *Journal of Social Issues, 39,* 169–194.

Coopersmith, S. (1967). *The antecedents of self-esteem.* New York: Freeman.

Crocker, J., & Luhtanen, R. (1990). Collective self-esteem and ingroup bias. *Journal of Personality and Social Psychology, 58,* 60–67.

Crocker, J., Luhtanen, R., Blaine, B., & Broadnax, S. (1994). Collective self-esteem and psychological well-being among white, black, and Asian college students. *Personality and Social Psychology Bulletin, 20,* 503–513.

Deaux, K., Reid, A., Mizrahi, K., & Cotting, D. (1999). Connecting the person to the social: The functions of social identification. In T. Tyler, R. Kramer, & O. John (Eds.), *The psychology of the social self* (pp. 91–113). Mahwah, NJ: Erlbaum.

Doosje, B., Ellemers, N., & Spears, R. (1995). Perceived intragroup variability as a function of group status and identification. *Journal of Experimental and Social Psychology, 31,* 410–436.

Fine, M., & Asch, A. (1988). Disability beyond stigma: Social interaction, discrimination, and activism. *Journal of Social Issues, 44,* 3–21.

Fromkin, H. L. (1972). Feelings of interpersonal undistinctiveness: An unpleasant affective state. *Journal of Experimental Research in Personality, 6,* 178–182.

Gaertner, L., Sedikides, C., & Graetz, K. (1999). In search of self-definition: Motivational primacy of the individual self, motivational primacy of the collective self, or contextual primacy? *Journal of Personality and Social Psychology, 76,* 5–18.

Grieve, P. G., & Hogg, M. A. (1999). Subjective uncertainty and intergroup discrimination in the minimal group situation. *Personality and Social Psychology Bulletin, 25,* 926–940.

Heatherton, T. F., & Polivy, J. (1991). Development and validation of a scale for measuring state self-esteem. *Journal of Personality and Social Psychology, 60,* 895–910.

Hogg, M. A., & Abrams, D. (1993). Towards a single-process uncertainty-reduction model of social motivation in groups. In M. Hogg & D. Abrams (Eds.), *Group motivation: Social psychological perspectives* (pp. 173–190). Hemel Hempstead, UK: Harvester Wheatsheaf.

Hogg, M. A., & Mullin, B.-A. (1999). Joining groups to reduce uncertainty: Subjective uncertainty reduction and group identification. In D. Abrams & M. A. Hogg (Eds.), *Social identity and social cognition* (pp. 249–279). Oxford, UK: Blackwell.

Hogg, M. A., & Turner, J. C. (1987). Intergroup behaviour, self-stereotyping and the salience of social categories. *British Journal of Social Psychology, 26,* 325–340.

Jetten, J., Spears, R., & Manstead, A. S. R. (1997). Distinctiveness threat and prototypicality: Combined effects on intergroup discrimination and collective self-esteem. *European Journal of Social Psychology, 27,* 635–657.

Jetten, J., Spears, R., & Manstead, A. S. R. (1999). Group distinctiveness and intergroup discrimination. In N. Ellemers, R. Spears, & B. Doosje (Eds.), *Social identity: Context, commitment, content* (pp. 107–126). Oxford, UK: Blackwell Science.

Jetten, J., Spears, R., & Manstead, A. S. R. (2001). Similarity as a source of differentiation: The role of group identification. *European Journal of Social Psychology, 31,* 621–640.

Kernahan, C., Bettencourt, B. A., & Dorr, N. (2000). Benefits of allocentrism for the subjective well-being of African-Americans. *Journal of Black Psychology, 26,* 181–193.

Kramer, R. M., & Brewer, M. B. (1986). Social group identity and the emergence of cooperation in resource conservation dilemmas. In H. Wilke, D. Messick, & C. Rutte (Eds.), *Psychology of decisions and conflict: Vol. 3. Experimental social dilemmas* (pp. 205–230). Frankfurt, Germany: Verlag Peter Lang.

Leonardelli, G. (1998). *The motivational underpinnings of social discrimination: A test of the self-esteem hypothesis.* Unpublished master's thesis, Ohio State University.

Leonardelli, G., & Brewer, M. B. (2001). Minority and majority discrimination: When and why. *Journal of Experimental Social Psychology, 37,* 468–485.

Luhtanen, R., & Crocker, J. (1992). A collective self-esteem scale: Self-evaluation of one's social identity. *Personality and Social Psychology Bulletin, 18,* 302–318.

Mullin, B.-A., & Hogg, M. A. (1998). Dimensions of subjective uncertainty in social identification and minimal intergroup discrimination. *British Journal of Social Psychology, 37,* 345–365.

Pelham, B. W., & Swann, W. B. (1989). From self-conceptions to self-worth: On the sources and structure of global self-esteem. *Journal of Personality and Social Psychology, 57,* 672–680.

Pickett, C. L., Bonner, B. L., & Coleman, J. M. (2002). Motivated self-stereotyping: Heightened assimilation and differentiation needs result in increased levels of positive and negative self-stereotyping. *Journal of Personality and Social Psychology, 82,* 543–562.

Rosenberg, M. (1965). *Society and the adolescent self-image.* Princeton, NJ: Princeton University Press.

Rubin, M., & Hewstone, M. (1998). Social identity theory's self-esteem hypothesis: A review and some suggestions for clarification. *Personality and Social Psychology Review, 2,* 40–62.

Sedikides, C., & Gaertner, L. (2001). A homecoming to the individual self: Emotional and motivational primacy. In C. Sedikides & M. Brewer (Eds.), *Individual self, relational self, collective self* (pp. 7–23). Philadelphia: Psychology Press.

Simon, B., & Hamilton, D. L. (1994). Social identity and self-stereotyping: The effects of relative group size and group status. *Journal of Personality and Social Psychology, 66,* 699–711.

Smith, E. R., & Henry, S. (1996). An in-group becomes part of the self: Response time evidence. *Personality and Social Psychology Bulletin, 22,* 635–642.

Spears, R., Doosje, B., & Ellemers, N. (1997). Self-stereotyping in the face of threats to group status and distinctiveness: The role of group identification. *Personality and Social Psychology Bulletin, 23,* 538–553.

Tajfel, H. (1981). *Human groups and social categories.* Cambridge, UK: Cambridge University Press.

Tajfel, H., Billig, M., Bundy, R., & Flament, C. (1971). Social categorization and intergroup behaviour. *European Journal of Social Psychology, 1,* 149–178.

Tajfel, H., & Turner, J. C. (1986). The social identity theory of intergroup behavior. In S. Worchel & W. G. Austin (Eds.), *Psychology of intergroup relations* (pp. 7–24). Chicago: Nelson-Hall.

Trafimow, D., Triandis, H. C., & Goto, S. G. (1991). Some tests of the distinction between the private and the collective self. *Journal of Personality and Social Psychology, 60,* 649–655.

Turner, J. C. (1975). Social comparison and social identity: Some prospects for intergroup behaviour. *European Journal of Social Psychology, 5,* 5–34.

Turner, J. C., Hogg, M., Oakes, P., Reicher, S., & Wetherell, M. (1987). *Rediscovering the social group: A self-categorization theory.* Oxford, UK: Blackwell.

Turner, J. C., Hogg, M., Turner, P., & Smith, P. (1984). Failure and defeat as determinants of group cohesiveness. *British Journal of Social Psychology, 23,* 97–111.

Turner, J. C., & Onorato, R. (1999). Social identity, personality and the self-concept: A self-categorization perspective. In T. R. Tyler, R. Kramer, & O. John (Eds.), *The psychology of the social self* (pp. 11–46). Hillsdale, NJ: Erlbaum.

Vignoles, V. L., Chryssochoou, Z., & Breakwell, G. M. (2000). The distinctiveness principle: Identity, meaning, and the bounds of cultural relativity. *Personality and Social Psychology Review, 4,* 337–354.

25

Self-Presentation

BARRY R. SCHLENKER

> When an individual appears in the presence of others, there will usually be some reason for him to mobilize his activity so that it will convey an impression to others which it is in his interests to convey.
>
> —GOFFMAN (1959, p. 4)

> You never get a second chance to make a first impression. Never let them see you sweat.
>
> —MEDIA ADVICE

Impression management is the goal-directed activity of controlling information in order to influence the impressions formed by an audience. Through impression management, people try to shape an audience's impressions of a person (e.g., self, friends, enemies), a group (e.g., a club, a business organization), an object (e.g., a gift, a car), an event (e.g., a transgression, a task performance), or an idea (e.g., prolife versus prochoice policies, capitalism versus socialism). When people try to control impressions of themselves, as opposed to other people or entities, the activity is called *self-presentation*. The study of self-presentation involves examining (1) how people, as agents, try to shape the attitudes and behaviors of audiences through the presentation of self-relevant information and (2) how people, as targets, respond to the self-presentation activities of others.

Research on self-presentation has exploded in the past 25 years. Twenty-five years ago, the term "self-presentation" could not be found in the index of social psychology texts. Today, self-presentation has emerged as an important topic in social psychology, as well as in counseling and clinical psychology (Friedlander & Schwartz, 1985; Kelly, 2000; Schuetz, Richter, Koehler, & Schiepek, 1997), developmental psychology (Aloise-Young, 1993; Bennett & Yeeles, 1990a, 1990b; Emler & Reicher, 1995; Hatch, 1987), sports psychology (B. James & Collins, 1997; Leary, 1992), organizational behavior and management (Bozeman & Kacmar, 1997; Judge & Bretz, 1994; Rosenfeld, Giacalone, & Riordan, 1995), marketing (Wooten & Reed, 2000), and political science (McGraw, 1991). In sociology, self-presentation has a venerable history (e.g., Brissett & Edgley, 1990), after being popularized by Erving Goffman (1959) in his classic, *The Presentation of Self in Everyday Life*. Given the sheer volume of research on the topic, no single chapter can hope to cover it all. Instead, I explore some of the major themes and directions that have generated much of the research.

Gamesmanship and Authenticity

Self-presentation evokes images of gamesmanship, with people jockeying for position in the social world by trying to convey a particular image of self to others. Examples that come readily to mind are the politician whose appearance, mannerisms, and opinions conform to what each constituency prefers; the salesperson who smiles warmly and flatters a customer to make the sale; the social chameleon who tries to impress others by wearing the latest designer outfits and shows the world a face and body that have been improved by the marvels of cosmetic surgery; or nearly anyone who has an important date or job interview and describes personal information in ways that might impress the other person. These examples illustrate a meaningful class of social behavior, in which people are concerned about how they appear to others and regulate their behavior in order to create a preferred impression. Whether the objective is to gain friends, increase psychological and material well-being, or secure a preferred public identity, self-presentation can be used to accomplish interpersonal goals that can be realized only by influencing the responses of others to oneself.

This view of self-presentation tells only part of the story, however. Self-presentation is not just superficial, deceptive, or manipulative activity. It can also involve attempts to convey to audiences an "accurate" portrait of oneself (Baumeister, 1982; Cheek & Hogan, 1983; Leary, 1995; Schlenker, 1980, 1985; Schlenker & Pontari, 2000). Usually, this portrait reflects a slightly polished and glorified conception of self, but one that is genuinely believed by the actor to be true (J. D. Brown, 1998; Greenwald & Breckler, 1985). The objective may be to ensure that others view one appropriately (i.e., in ways that secure the desired regard and treatment associated with one's identity), to receive validating feedback that might minimize personal doubts about what one is really like, or even to follow the principle that "honesty is the best policy" and thereby feel

authentic while minimizing the hazards of deceit. Furthermore, it appears to take as much self-presentation skill to communicate an accurate, "truthful" impression of self as it does to convey a false one. People with better acting skills, for instance, show smaller discrepancies between their own self-ratings and their friends' ratings of them (Cheek, 1982). People with poor self-presentation skills, who are subpar in expressive ability and the empathic tendency to gauge the reactions of others, are ineffective at convincing others of what they are feeling even when they are telling the truth (DePaulo, 1992). Thus self-presentation can be guided by truthful motives, as well as duplicitous ones, and valid information must be presented with as much self-presentation skill as invalid information if it is to have the desired impact on the audience.

An analogy is the conduct of an award-winning college lecturer. This lecturer considers the ability and experience of the audience, makes sure that the take-home messages are salient, the organization flows, the examples are relevant and memorable, the facts are correct, and the presentation is delivered in an enthusiastic, attention-capturing fashion. Compare this to the bad lecturer who seems oblivious to the students' capabilities, ignores nonverbal feedback during the lecture, never seems to get to the point, "dumps" information in a disorganized fashion as it comes to mind, makes frequent factual errors because of the failure to refresh memory on the details beforehand, and drones on as the audience's attention shifts to more pleasing pursuits. The former is packaging information in order to create a desired impact on the audience. Yet, just because it is "packaged," this superior performance would not be considered more superficial, inauthentic, deceptive, or self-centered than that of the bad lecturer. Indeed, the attention to the audience and careful packaging increase the likelihood that the good teacher's goal—communicating truthful, meaningful information to the class—will be accomplished. In contrast, spontaneity and expressiveness often involve nothing more than self-centeredness and a lack of concern for others. Thus, although self-presentation involves the packaging of information in order to accomplish goals, the goals can include conveying an authentic portrayal of self (as perceived by the actor at the time), not just a deceptive one (see Schlenker & Pontari, 2000).

Self-presentation thus includes a range of activities that are united by the central idea that social behavior is a performance that symbolically communicates information about self to others. The real or anticipated reactions of others to this information influences the timing, form, and content of self-presentational activity. Symbolic interactionists such as Mead (1934) and Cooley (1902) were among the first to emphasize that actions carry symbolic meanings that influence the responses of others to self. Goffman (1959) elaborated the theme when he described social life as a series of performances in which people project their identities or "faces" to others and engage in mutual activities that are governed by social rules and rituals. Goffman's dramaturgical approach provided an intricately detailed exposition of the Shakespearean theme that "All the world's a stage, and all the men and women merely players."

Self-presentation is distinguished from other behaviors because of the importance of these real or anticipated reactions in influencing the communication of information about the self. Self-presentations have their own interpersonal ends and effects and are not purely expressive of feelings or descriptive of facts and beliefs about the self. Children as young as six years of age are able to identify the interpersonal functions of self-presentations (e.g., they can indicate that ingratiating actions are designed to obtain approval) and appreciate that such actions are not just descriptions of private feelings and psychological states (Banerjee & Yuill, 1999; Bennett & Yeeles, 1990a, 1990b).

Self-presentation is sometimes characterized as having additional features, including behavior that is self-conscious, pretentious, and formal (Buss & Briggs, 1984) or that is guided by power-augmenting motives (Jones & Pittman, 1982) or by the audience's values and beliefs rather than the actor's own (Carver & Scheier, 1985; Snyder, 1987). These characterizations reflect attempts to distinguish between what might be called self-expression—which is authentic and spontaneous and originates from within the actor—from self-presentation—which is in-

authentic, labored, and influenced by social pressures outside the actor. Although there are differences between these categories, they seem to distinguish between types of self-presentations, not between situations in which self-presentation does or does not occur. Researchers have expanded the range of social behaviors that seem to have self-presentational properties and the range of situations in which self-presentation occurs (Schlenker & Weigold, 1992). In my view, self-presentation is guided by a variety of motives, not just power; it occurs among friends, even in familiar situations; it occurs even in long-standing relationships such as marriage; and it does not necessarily involve conscious attention and control.

Automatic and Controlled Processes in Self-Presentation

Like most social behaviors, self-presentation can vary in the extent to which it involves automatic versus controlled cognitive processes. Automatic processes are characterized as ones that (1) occur outside of *conscious awareness,* in that the actor is unaware of the initiation, flow, or impact of the activity; (2) involve relatively little *cognitive effort,* in that the actor does not expend valuable and limited cognitive resources on the activity; (3) are *autonomous,* in that the activities do not have to be consciously monitored once initiated; and (4) are *involuntary,* in that the activities are initiated by certain cues or prompts in the situation (Bargh, 1989, 1996). These components are somewhat independent, so any particular behavior may include only some of them. Automatic processes also can be intentional (Bargh, 1989). Bargh (1989) suggested that most well-learned social scripts and social action sequences are guided by intended, goal-dependent automaticity. In fact, self-presentational activities that involve familiar others, well-learned scripts, and overlearned behavior patterns seem to be examples of intended, goal-dependent automaticity.

Acting Naturally

In everyday life, self-presentations are frequently automatic in nature. They reflect modulated units of action that eventually "settle in" to become habits. At one time, some of these behaviors may have been arduously practiced, as in the case of the child who practices different facial expressions and gestures in front of a mirror until perfecting favorites. Other behaviors become routine because they are so frequently rewarded, as when people smile, listen attentively, and nod, and then receive approval and friendship in return. Schlenker (1980, 1985; Schlenker, Britt, & Pennington, 1996) suggested that such patterns form self-presentation scripts that guide action, often unthinkingly, in relevant situations. These self-scripts are embedded in larger cognitive scripts (Abelson, 1976) that help people negotiate social situations.

Self-presentation scripts can be cued automatically by specific features of the audience and situation, and actors are often unaware of the extent to which such behavior is influenced by the social context and their own interpersonal goals (Jones, 1990; Schlenker, 1980, 1985; Tetlock & Manstead, 1985). An interesting example is the chameleon effect, which refers to nonconscious mimicry of interaction partners' mannerisms and expressions (Chartrand & Bargh, 1999). The chameleon effect occurs automatically, is exhibited more by people who are high in empathy, and increases liking between the interaction partners. Research also shows that people will match the self-presentations of others, becoming more positive when interacting with egotistical others and more modest when interacting with self-deprecating others, and that these shifts occur without apparent awareness of the contingencies (Baumeister, Hutton, & Tice, 1989; Jones, Rhodewalt, Berglas, & Skelton, 1981). People tend to underestimate the extent to which their own self-presentations both are influenced by the other and will influence the other (Baumeister et al., 1989).

In general, automatic processes are more likely to occur in routine, frequently encountered situations in which there is low motivation to switch to more effortful processing or in which there is information overload or time pressure that interferes with more effortful processing (Bargh, 1996). In the realm of self-presentation, automaticity seems most likely to prevail when actors are in routine, unstructured situations in which tasks are relatively trivial or unimportant and in which they are with people they know well and in whose positive regard they feel secure. Relaxing at home among friends is a prototypic case. Indeed, college students report thinking less about how others are perceiving or evaluating them and being less nervous when they interact with familiar, same-sex friends, as compared with interacting with unfamiliar individuals or even familiar members of the opposite sex (Leary, Nezlek, et al., 1994). In such comfortable situations, automaticity of self-presentation prevails, unless or until something happens that threatens the actors' image.

In the mind of an actor in automatic mode, there is no self-conscious attempt to control the impression made on others. Yet the goal-directed activity of constructing and protecting a desired identity takes place. To illustrate the point, Schlenker and his colleagues (Schlenker et al., 1996; Schlenker & Pontari, 2000) used the analogy of computer programs running in either visible or minimized windows on a screen. Programs the operator wants to monitor closely because of their importance are left open and visible on the screen. In contrast, other programs can be minimized and run in the background, because they are more familiar and no problems are anticipated during operation. The programs running in the background still have a specific goal and are actively working toward goal accomplishment, but they are not salient to the operator as they run. Only if problems arise, such as when program checking for viruses detects an intruder, does an alarm go off and the program again become salient to the operator.

Even when people interact in comfortable settings with familiar friends, a desired self-presentation script—or self-program—contains instructions about important features of self that are relevant and how they are symbolically communicated through actions. If events threaten the identity that actors want to portray, the discrepancy between the events and their script triggers the alarm—analogous to the intruding virus being detected on the system—and actors focus their attention on image repair. The idea that a self-presentation script is operating automatically helps to explain why people "stay in character" during social interactions and why they become upset if audiences, even friends, seem to "get the wrong impression." If feedback indicates that an undesired impression has been created, controlled processes are activated, and people take corrective action to restore the desired impression.

Self-presentation is also likely to involve controlled processes when the situation or audience is significant or the actor is uncertain about the type of impression that might be created (Schlenker et al., 1996; Schlenker & Pontari, 2000). Under these conditions, people are likely to focus, often self-consciously, on the impression they might make and to plan and rehearse their performances. An important date, a job interview, and a business presentation are occasions on which making a good impression is important, but the outcome is not assured. These are the times at which people are most likely to report being self-conscious, "on stage," and concerned about the evaluations of others.

Investigating Automatic and Controlled Self-Presentation

People's cognitive resources are limited and it is difficult to deal with more than one cognitively demanding task at a time (Bargh, 1996). This limited cognitive capacity provides researchers with an opportunity to investigate empirically the differences between automatic and controlled self-presentations. If a process is automatic, introducing a second, cognitively demanding task should produce relatively little disruption of ongoing activities. However, if a process is controlled, introducing a second demanding task should disrupt ongoing activities.

Automatic Egotism

Paulhus and his colleagues (Paulhus, 1988, 1993; Paulhus, Graf, & van Selst, 1989; Paulhus & Levitt, 1987) manipulated cognitive load and found that people's self-descriptions became more positive and socially desirable when they occurred automatically. For instance, Paulhus and colleagues (1989) asked participants to describe themselves by responding "me" or "not me" to positive and negative trait adjectives (e.g., "cheerful," "defensive") that appeared on a computer screen. Participants described themselves more positively if they were given a second, effortful task to perform (monitoring numbers on the screen) than if they could simply focus on their self-descriptions.

Paulhus (1988) proposed that the default mode for self-descriptions is highly positive. This favorable judgment is tempered primarily when people have the cognitive resources to perform a more thorough search through memory for relevant information and then find less positive data. It might also be the case that cognitive resources permit people to consider more fully how their actions will appear to others; they then temper their self-descriptions to seem humble and avoid the appearance of being a braggart. People's descriptions of their successes are more self-glorifying when done privately than publicly (Baumeister & Ilko, 1995), which suggests that people prefer to avoid the public appearance of egotism.

Paulhus (1988) also suggested that if people are highly motivated to make a positive impression, as during a job interview in which it is important to appear competent and to stand out from others, they might be even more self-glorifying than they are when responding automatically. They thus risk seeming egotistical, because humility might be misinterpreted as incompetence (Schlenker & Leary, 1982a). Public self-presentations, on the one hand, thereby offer possible opportunities to impress others, but on the other hand, they pose a risk of appearing egotistical or even being discredited if the audience knows of publicly available, contradictory information. These competing pressures explain why public performances sometimes produce more, sometimes less, and sometimes about the same levels of self-glorification as private responding (see Schlenker & Weigold, 1992).

Automaticity and Audiences

Different self-presentation strategies are associated with different types of audiences. People generally are more self-enhancing with strangers and more modest with friends (Tice, Butler, Muraven, & Stillwell, 1995). Tice and colleagues (1995) suggested that with strangers, self-enhancement is the more automatic style; it routinely occurs to impress others who may have no other independent knowledge of the actor. With friends, modesty is the more automatic style, because people are relatively secure in their friends' regard and need not brag. Tice and colleagues reasoned that if people are induced to present themselves in a way that differs from the automatic style, it will require greater cognitive effort and interfere with the capacity to accomplish other cognitive tasks, such as remembering information about the interaction.

As hypothesized, Tice and colleagues (1995) found that participants who interacted with strangers remembered less about their interaction if they had been instructed to present themselves modestly rather than self-enhancingly (Baumeister et al., 1989, found similar results). Also as hypothesized, participants who interacted with friends remembered less if they had been instructed to be self-enhancing rather than modest. Certain self-presentation scripts thus seem to be more appropriate and automatic with some audiences than with others. If the self-presentation and social context match, self-presentation seems effortless and undemanding. If they do not match, cognitive resources are consumed.

Automaticity and Personality

Self-presentation also should be more automatic when it involves qualities that are consistent with existing self-images and personality characteristics. If people are induced to present themselves in out-of-character ways, as when they are tempted to misrepresent themselves to impress an audience, the behavior should require greater cognitive resources and be more likely to be disrupted by a second demanding cognitive task. To test these ideas, Pontari and Schlenker (2000) preselected highly extraverted or highly introverted participants and induced them to play an extraverted or introverted role during an interview. Half of the participants were asked to rehearse an 8-digit number during the interview, supposedly simulating situations in which people had to keep extra information, such as addresses or phone numbers, in mind during interviews.

As hypothesized, Pontari and Schlenker (2000) found that participants who played the familiar role were unaffected by the extra cognitive load. Extraverts who played extraverts and introverts who played introverts created the impression they desired on the interviewer and did it equally well regardless of cognitive load. In contrast, participants who played the unfamiliar role were significantly affected by cognitive load. Extraverts were less effective in playing the introverted role when they were cognitively busy, as the interviewer perceived the busy extraverts as less introverted than the nonbusy ones. This finding supports the idea that controlled performances, such as unfamiliar self-presentations, are disrupted by the addition of a demanding cognitive task.

However, introverts did just the reverse of what the cognitive busyness literature suggests should happen. Introverts who played the extraverted role actually were more effective in getting the interviewer to see them as extraverted if they were cognitively busy than not. Pontari and Schlenker (2000) thought that effect may have been due to the fact that their highly introverted participants also scored high in social anxiety. Prior research shows that socially anxious people actually perform better when they are distracted. Distracting tasks lower arousal level by directing attention toward the distraction and away from disruptive feelings of anxiety (Carver & Scheier, 1982) and provide an excuse for poor social performance (Brodt & Zimbardo, 1981; Leary, 1986). Rehearsing the number may have been just the sort of distracting task that could benefit socially anxious people in challenging social situations. In a second study, Pontari and Schlenker confirmed that highly introverted people are benefited by distracting tasks because such tasks reduce their public self-consciousness and negative ruminations about themselves.

These findings support the idea that self-presentations can reflect either automatic or controlled processes, depending on the familiarity of the self-presentation in the particular social context. When confronting challenging self-presentation situations, the availability of cognitive resources can be an advantage or a disadvantage, depending on how those resources might otherwise be used. To the extent that cognitive resources can be devoted to controlling the self-presentation, say by planning and monitoring one's own actions and the feedback from the audience, then greater resources yield better performance. To the extent that available cognitive resources might actually interfere with task performance because individuals are filled with self-conscious doubts about a public appearance, then the addition of an otherwise neutral distracting task actually can improve performance.

Configuring Self-Presentations: Drawing from Self, Audience, and Situation

Self-presentation is an *activity* that is shaped by a combination of personality, situational, and audience factors (Schlenker, 1985; Schlenker & Pontari, 2000). It reflects the *transaction* between self and audience in a particular social context. It is not purely an expression of self, purely a role-played response to situational pressures, or purely conformity to the identity expectations of salient others. It is a combination and reflection of all of these. Self-presentations incorporate features of the actor's self-concept, personality style, salient social roles, and beliefs about their audience's preferences.

Although much of the incorporated information may be relatively truthful, there also may be exaggerations or distortions of personal experiences and qualities, and even fabrications. From mass media, books, and personal experience, people acquire extensive knowledge of a variety of prototypical people who are exemplars of particular identity types (e.g., Clint Eastwood, the tough, principled loner; Bill Clinton, the gregarious, empathetic leader), personality styles (e.g., extraversion versus introversion), and social roles (e.g., man or woman, banker or hairdresser). Even if people do not usually see themselves as having a specific set of attributes, they can readily imagine exemplars and social scripts for how particular types of people should behave. They can then try to portray specific identities, regardless of whether these are usually part of their self-conception and public identity. In other words, people have knowledge of a vast array of identity types and

roles and can piece together self-presentations that comprise a mix of information from their self-conceptions, including prior personal experiences, and their knowledge of identity types and roles that may not usually be included in their self-conceptions. In social situations, people draw from or sample this knowledge to construct their self-presentations to others.

The aspects of self that become accessible in memory and therefore are more likely to be expressed in self-presentations seem to be determined by the relevance and importance of the knowledge, given the actors' goals, the particular audience, and the nature of the situation (see Jones, 1990; Schlenker, 1986). Features of self that are usually more important to the actor's identity, that have been recently activated (e.g., expressed in recent self-presentations), that are associated with current interpersonal goals, and that seem to be relevant to the situation or audience (e.g., because they correspond to situational norms or audience preferences) are more likely to become salient and accessible (e.g., Leary, 1995; Leary & Kowalski, 1990; Schlenker, 1986; Schlenker & Pontari, 2000). Further, people reconstruct past experiences from their memories by organizing stories and remembering (even making up) details that are compatible with their current goals and experiences (Baumeister & Newman, 1994; J. D. Brown, 1998; Gergen & Gergen, 1988; Singer & Salovey, 1993). Thus information about self is brought to mind and hence becomes available for self-presentations, based not just on the content of the self-concept but on the actors' social goals, salient audience, and social situation.

Constructing a Desired Identity

Researchers on the self have suggested two broad answers to the question, How do people want others to see them? One approach focuses on self-glorification: People want others to see them as having positive, socially desirable qualities. The idea that people want to view themselves positively and prefer others to share this opinion is a fundamental motivational principle in theories of self that emphasize self-esteem enhancement (e.g., J. D. Brown, 1998; Hoyle, Kernis, Leary, & Baldwin, 1999; Leary &

Baumeister, 2000). A second approach focuses on self-consistency: People want others to see them in ways that will confirm how they see themselves. Swann (1983; Swann, Stein-Seroussi, & Giesler, 1992) argued that people have a cognitive need for order and predictability, which is fulfilled by receiving feedback that confirms important self-beliefs. He proposed that people try to verify their existing self-conceptions, including by presenting themselves in ways that increase the likelihood of receiving self-verifying feedback.

These approaches have been highly productive and have generated volumes of research. Each approach focuses on a specific motive and assumes that the motive applies broadly. Data that support the opposite motive are explained by adding qualifiers, as when (1) self-esteem advocates suggest that consistency is sometimes obtained because it is self-esteem deflating to make claims that are contradicted by salient information, or (2) self-consistency advocates suggest that self-enhancement is sometimes obtained because the relevant belief is not held with sufficient certainty to motivate a verification process. In either case, though, theoretical attention is focused on the individual and his or her self-concept and self-evaluation.

Alternatively, self-presentations can be seen as goal-directed activities that occur in a social context consisting of an actor, an audience, and a social situation (Schlenker, 1985; Schlenker & Weigold, 1992). When self-presentation is viewed as a transaction rather than an expression of self, theoretical attention shifts from the individual to the relationship between actor and audience. What is desirable in this social context depends on factors relevant to the actor (e.g., self-concept, goals), the audience (e.g., perceived preferences, power to mediate valued outcomes), and the situation (e.g., relevant social roles, opportunities for valued outcomes).

According to this transactional view, two features define the desirability of a self-presentation for the individual. First, a desirable self-presentation is perceived as *beneficial* in that the actor regards it as facilitating his or her goals and values relative to alternative claims. Second, it is perceived as *believable*, that is, it should be regarded as a reasonably accurate construal of the salient evidence that can be credibly presented to the audience. Desirable self-presentations thus reflect the integration of what people would like to be and think they can be in a given social context (Schlenker, 1985). Research (see Schlenker & Weigold, 1989) is consistent with the proposition that a particular self-presentation is more likely to occur when factors (1) increase the expected beneficial consequences if the self-presentation is believed (e.g., it becomes more rewarding to present oneself consistently with an employer's preferences, such as immediately before promotions decisions), (2) decrease the expected detrimental consequences if the self-presentation is disbelieved or backfires (e.g., it becomes less embarrassing or punitive even if a self-presentation is disbelieved by the audience), and (3) increase the perceived likelihood that the audience will believe the self-presentation (e.g., the audience is seen as supportive and accepting of the actor's claims).

Beneficial Self-Presentations

The self-presentation literature provides strong support for the general principle that people's self-presentations shift in ways that improve the likelihood of achieving desired outcomes (see Baumeister, 1982; Jones & Wortman, 1973; Leary, 1995; Leary & Kowalski, 1990; Rosenfeld et al., 1995; Schlenker, 1980; Schlenker & Weigold, 1989, 1992; Tedeschi, 1981; Tedeschi & Norman, 1985). In his pioneering research on ingratiation, Jones (1964) showed that people's self-presentations are more likely to conform to the preferences of the target when actors are dependent on the target for desired outcomes. Furthermore, people will try to camouflage their strategic objectives by balancing self-serving information on the preferred dimensions with negative information on irrelevant dimensions, thus appearing more credible in their claims.

In organizational settings, self-presentation strategies are relatively routine components of job procurement and career advancement (Fandt & Ferris, 1990; Gould & Penley, 1984; Judge & Bretz, 1994; Kacmar, Delery, & Ferris, 1992; Rosenfeld et al., 1995; Stevens & Kristof, 1995). During actual job interviews, the use of self-presentation tactics such as self-promotion and ingratiation predicted interviewers' evaluations of applicants and whether applicants later were invited for site visits (Stevens & Kristoff, 1995). Self-enhancing and ingratiatory communications enhance subordinates' performance appraisals by supervisors (Wayne & Kacmar, 1991; Wayne, Kacmar, & Ferris, 1995) and have been related to career success (Gould & Penley, 1984; Kacmar et al., 1992). However, seeming to be too self-absorbed and self-promoting can also backfire. Although displays of competence and accomplishment often work (e.g., Gould & Penley, 1984; Kacmar et al., 1992), they also have been shown to generate negative reactions in onlookers (Godfrey, Jones, & Lord, 1986; Schlenker & Leary, 1982a), particularly if the actor volunteers such information without a specific request from the audience (Holtgraves & Srull, 1989). Furthermore, Judge and Bretz (1994) found that career success was positively related to supervisor-focused tactics such as ingratiation and negatively related to job-focused tactics such as self-promotion. This suggests that it may be easier to try to increase the positive regard in which one is held by complimenting others than by single-mindedly promoting oneself, an idea that is consistent with Dale Carnegie's (1940) advice on how to win friends and influence people. Self-promotion may be especially likely to backfire when it is not fully matched by corresponding accomplishments and makes the actor appear to be self-absorbed to the detriment of others (Schlenker, Pontari, & Christopher, 2001). Even ingratiation can backfire if it is perceived as insincere and self-serving, as when people ingratiate to superiors but are harsh and nasty to subordinates (Vonk, 1998). It also can backfire and make an opponent less conciliatory if an ingratiator appears overly friendly and nice during tough negotiations (Baron, Fortin, Frei, Hauver, & Shack, 1990).

People claim desirable images both directly—through verbal and nonverbal activities that communicate information about their own attributes and accomplishments—and indirectly—by communicating information about the qualities and accomplishments of their associates and enemies (Cialdini,

Finch, & DeNicholas, 1990). Cialdini and his colleagues found that people will bask in the reflected glory of the accomplishments of others, distance themselves from unattractive people, blast the accomplishments of rivals, and boost their evaluations of otherwise unattractive people with whom they are already associated. This indirect self-presentation takes advantage of the evaluative generalization that occurs when two concepts are linked in the minds of perceivers (Cialdini et al., 1990). By linking themselves to successful, admirable others, people thereby look better to others and feel better about themselves.

The association of self with others who are known for their accomplishments can boomerang, however, and make the actor look worse by comparison. Tesser's (1988) self-evaluation maintenance model indicates that boosting others does not occur if emphasizing the superior qualities of the other threatens people's own self-evaluation, as in cases in which the superior performance is by a close other (e.g., friend, sibling) on a dimension of high personal relevance. For example, if the other is psychologically close and performs well on a dimension that is irrelevant to the pretensions of the actor (e.g., the other is a great musician, whereas the actor prefers to be seen as an athlete and has no musical pretensions), the actor will bask in the reflected glory of the other's accomplishments. However, if the other is close and performs well on a dimension on which the actor also has pretensions (e.g., the actor also wants to be seen as a great musician), the comparison is threatening, and the actor will take steps to avoid it or harm the standing of the comparison other. Lockwood and Kunda (2000) similarly examined the impact of stellar role models known for their accomplishments. They found that when people compare themselves to relevant "star" models, they react positively if they think the role model's success is personally attainable and negatively if they think the role model's success is personally unattainable.

Beneficial images are ones that are perceived by the actor to facilitate goals; they are not necessarily socially desirable or positive images. Much of the time, people prefer to project socially desirable images because these are associated with valued interpersonal goals. However, people will present themselves in socially undesirable or negative ways if doing so facilitates their goals. For example, people will present themselves as irrational and intimidating if they want to generate fear, or as weak and helpless if they want to be cared for by others (Jones & Pittman, 1982; Schlenker, 1980). In addition, people will be self-deprecating if (1) they believe that well-adjusted people will be assigned to perform an embarrassing task (Kowalski & Leary, 1990); (2) the audience seems to admire lower levels of competence (Zanna & Pack, 1975); (3) they think claims of competence will threaten the audience (Jones & Wortman, 1973); (4) they confront unrealistically high public expectations by others and want to lower them to levels that are more attainable (Baumeister, Hamilton, & Tice, 1985; Baumgardner & Brownlee, 1987; Gibson & Sachau, 2000), and (5) they want to coax competitors into underestimating them (Gibson & Sachau, 2000; Shepperd & Socherman, 1997). Thus many different types of self-presentations can be beneficial depending on the actor's goals, resources, audience, and social context.

Believable Self-Presentations

People cannot simply claim anything that might facilitate their goals, regardless of its accuracy. In any social group, general well-being depends on people being able to count on one another to do what they say they will do and to be what they claim to be. From the group's perspective, people who routinely lie, mislead others for personal profit, or exaggerate to the point at which they cannot fulfill the expectations that are created pose a threat to those who might otherwise need to depend on them. Untrustworthy individuals cannot be counted on for cooperative ventures. Social norms thus prescribe being reliable, sincere, and trustworthy. From the actors' perspective, failing to appear in these ways produces personal and interpersonal problems. Unbounded self-glorification, for example, can create the impression that the actor is narcissistically self-absorbed (perhaps to the detriment of others), can lead onlookers to conclude that the actor is deceitful or foolish, and can condemn the actor to failure if un-

realistically high public expectations are not fulfilled (Schlenker et al., 2001).

Self-presentations produce obligations for people to be what they say they are or risk personal and interpersonal sanctions (Goffman, 1959, 1967; Schlenker, 1980; Schlenker et al., 2001). People prefer others whose claims are consistent with their accomplishments; in general, the greater the discrepancy between claims and accomplishments, the less the actor is liked (Schlenker & Leary, 1982a). Appreciating this relationship, people will try to match their self-presentations to publicly known information about them (Baumeister & Jones, 1978; Schlenker, 1975). If contradictory information can be hidden from public view, people tend to be self-enhancing, but if contradictory information has or will become public knowledge, people shift their self-presentations to be consistent with the information (Baumeister & Jones, 1978; Schlenker, 1975). Although people routinely exaggerate their skills, accomplishments, and past salaries on job applications, they are much less likely to do so if it could be readily verified by previous employers (Cascio, 1975).

When negative information is publicly known, people try to compensate for it by elevating their self-presentations on other dimensions (Baumeister & Jones, 1978). People usually present themselves in ways that they expect to be able to substantiate to onlookers, and they will go so far as to be self-deprecating or even fail in order to lower public expectations that they regard as too high (Baumeister, Hamilton, & Tice, 1985; Baumgardner & Brownlee, 1987) and avoid the appearance of inconsistency.

Desired Self-Presentations: Synopsis

The desirability of a particular image of self is not a constant, fixed by properties of the self-concept. Desirability is multiply determined by factors in the social context, including not only the actor's preferences but also the audience's preferences and the roles appropriate in the social situation. Depending on who the audience is (e.g., Are they significant by virtue of being powerful or attractive?) and what they know (e.g., Are they aware of potentially contradictory information?), different images of self become more or less desirable to the actor. Desirability thus reflects information that is beneficial but believable.

The Public Becomes Private

Self-presentations that are initiated and guided by their anticipated impact on others can also produce a change in the private self. Symbolic interactionists such as Mead (1934) and Cooley (1902) emphasized the interplay between the public and private sides of self. They proposed that the self is constructed through social interaction, as people come to view themselves through the roles they play and the reactions of others to them. Research shows that people's strategic self-presentations can influence how they privately characterize themselves later. People will shift their global self-evaluations (Gergen, 1965; Jones et al., 1981; Rhodewalt & Agustsdottir, 1986) and the specific contents of their self-beliefs (McKillop, Berzonsky, & Schlenker, 1992; Schlenker, Dlugolecki, & Doherty, 1994; Schlenker & Trudeau, 1990; Tice, 1992) in the direction of their public behavior. Changes produced by public self-presentations carry over to new settings with different audiences, as people who portray a particular role will continue to behave consistently with that role even after they leave the situation in which it was initially induced (Schlenker et al., 1994; Tice, 1992).

Public self-presentations are most likely to generate changes in private self-beliefs when they occur in contexts that make the public images appear to be representative of self. The appearance of representativeness is produced when people freely choose to engage in the self-presentation rather than being required to do so or are free to draw on their own personal experiences during the performance rather than being forced to use nonpersonal examples (Jones et al., 1981; Rhodewalt & Agustsdottir, 1986; Schlenker & Trudeau, 1990; Tice, 1992). Representativeness also is produced by public commitment to the role. Self-presentations that carry a public commitment, such as ones that are performed publicly or are expected to be performed publicly, produce more change in self-beliefs than ones that are privately performed with no public ramifications (Schlenker et al., 1994; Tice, 1992).

Simply rehearsing a role privately for an upcoming interview produces a change in self-beliefs if people anticipate that they will actually perform the role shortly, but it produces no change if people believe that they will not have to go through with the interview because it was canceled (Schlenker et al., 1994). People also regard their self-presentations as more representative if they can be easily assimilated into existing self-schemas. If self-presentations are greatly discrepant from clear prior self-beliefs, people reject them as "not me" and do not internalize them. However, if self-presentations are only moderately discrepant from clear prior self-beliefs or if prior self-beliefs are weak, people will shift their private self-beliefs to bring them in line with their public performances (Schlenker & Trudeau, 1990). Finally, audience feedback can convince people that their self-presentations are representative. People are more likely to bring their beliefs in line with self-presentations that produce approval and acceptance from others (Gergen, 1965). Such audience acceptance helps substantiate the new view of self.

From a practical perspective, public performances are an important vehicle for self-concept change. Act the part and it becomes incorporated into the self-concept, provided the performance appears to be representative and the actor comes to regard the image as personally beneficial.

Audiences for the Performance

Social behavior takes place in the context of real or imagined audiences whose existence and reactions (real or anticipated) influence actors' thoughts, feelings, and conduct. Symbolic interactionists (Cooley, 1902; Mead, 1934) proposed that self-regulation is not a personal or private matter but must take into account an audience. Mead (1934) went so far as to argue that thought itself is social in character and takes the form of an inner dialogue, in which self alternates between the roles of speaker and audience, and not a monologue. Self-regulation involves taking the role of others, anticipating their likely reactions to one's own possible actions, and selecting one's conduct accordingly. The ability to put oneself in the place of others and imagine how they are likely to interpret and respond to information is the basis for effective communication (Hardin & Higgins, 1996; E. T. Higgins, 1992).

Most research on self-presentation has examined people's behavior in the presence of real others, whose qualities are varied to make them seem more or less powerful, attractive, and expert (see Baumeister, 1982; Leary, 1995; Schlenker, 1980; Schlenker & Weigold, 1992; Tedeschi & Norman, 1985; Tetlock & Manstead, 1985). Social impact theory (Nowak, Szamrej, & Latané, 1990) indicates that the impact of an audience on an individual's thoughts, feelings, and conduct is a function of the audience's significance, size, and psychological immediacy. Audiences create greater impact when they are more powerful and attractive, have a greater number of members, and are psychologically proximal rather than distant. Consistent with these factors, people's self-presentations tend to conform to the expectations and preferences of audiences who are more significant (e.g., attractive, powerful), have more members, and are either present or about to be encountered (see Baumeister, 1982; Jones & Wortman, 1973; Leary, 1995; Leary & Kowalski, 1990; Schlenker, 1980; Schlenker & Weigold, 1992; Tedeschi & Norman, 1985). Such audiences provide actors with opportunities to obtain desired outcomes, such as approval, respect, social validation, and material rewards, and to avoid their undesired opposites. Audiences thus can influence actors' self-presentations by shifting the reward–cost ratios that are associated with particular self-descriptions.

Many researchers think of self-presentation primarily in the context of immediate real audiences, situations in which people have something to gain (or avoid) by creating desired impressions. However, audiences can influence self-presentations in at least two other ways: as targets of communication and as sources of information that cue or prime desired identities (Schlenker & Weigold, 1992).

In order to communicate, people must put themselves in the place of others, take into account the others' knowledge and value systems, and package information using ideas, examples, and evidence that are comprehensible to those others. People change their verbal and nonverbal communications

to take into account the particular characteristics of the audience (DePaulo, 1992; Hardin & Higgins, 1996; E. T. Higgins, 1992). For instance, they talk differently to adults than to children or to those who have backgrounds similar to or different from themselves (DePaulo, 1992). People also tune their messages to create different impacts on different audiences, as when they confront several audiences simultaneously and embed information in their communications that can be decoded accurately by one but not another (Fleming, Darley, Hilton, & Kojetin, 1990). E. T. Higgins (1992) described how people's communications create a shared reality that is sometimes different from the actual reality that was the basis for the messages. For example, people shift their descriptions of the behaviors of an individual depending on whether they are talking to someone who likes or dislikes that individual. These descriptions then have a greater impact on their memory of that individual than the original information itself has. Thus people's conceptions of reality are shaped by a social validation process. People's descriptions of self and events are influenced by the knowledge and preferences of the audience, and these descriptions, rather than the actual event itself, become reality (Hardin & Higgins, 1996; E. T. Higgins, 1992). Indeed, people's self-presentations, which reflect in part exaggerations and omissions designed to create a particular impression on others, can carry over to new situations and become internalized as part of the self-concept (Schlenker et al., 1994; Tice, 1992).

Audiences also can prime or activate relevant personal goals and identity images, which then guide people's subsequent self-presentations. For instance, seeing an attractive member of the opposite sex may bring to mind a romantic-quest script and a set of roles that the actor associates with impressing potential dates. Different audiences will trigger different goals and relevant identity images. Further, the audience does not even have to be present for such effects to occur. People often bring to mind imagined audiences who can serve as significant positive or negative reference groups for conduct. For instance, a soldier during World War II may have imagined how John Wayne would act, and thereby activated a script for what should be done, how it should be done, and how well it should be done. Or, as Christmas approaches, children imagine the types of behaviors that will be approved or disapproved by Santa. Such imagined exemplars provide relevant goals, scripts, and evaluative standards for conduct.

Research has demonstrated the power of imagined audiences to influence people's behavior. Doherty, Van Wegenen, and Schlenker (1991) asked people to visualize a variety of stimuli, such as bright red apples and balls of cotton, supposedly so that the physiological correlates of mental imagery could be assessed. During this task, they imagined either a parent, a best friend, or a romantic partner. Later, in the context of a different task, they provided self-descriptions. Participants rated themselves as less independent (e.g., more obedient, cooperative, respectful) and as less sexual (e.g., sexy, passionate) after they had previously imagined a parent than a close peer. As these results illustrate, an audience does not even have to be present for it to shape how people think about and present themselves. As William James (1890) noted, people seem to have as many social selves as there are audiences they encounter. By making a particular audience salient, the relevant facet of self becomes salient, too.

Baldwin (1992) proposed that people store information about themselves and others in relationship schemas. These schemas contain three components: a self-schema, a significant-other schema, and a script pertaining to expected patterns of behavior in this relationship. The components are seen as structurally associated in memory, so that priming one element can activate others. Baldwin showed that priming particular audiences changes people's evaluative orientation. Baldwin and Holmes (1987) showed that women evaluated a sexually permissive piece of fiction more negatively after they visualized a parent, who might be expected to disapprove, than a friend. Baldwin, Carrell, and Lopez (1990) asked students to evaluate themselves or their ideas after unconscious exposure to pictures of approving or disapproving others. Evaluations were more negative after exposure to disapproving others. Priming salient audiences also can change people's current inter-

action patterns. Chen and Anderson (1999) found that aspects of past relationships with significant individuals can reemerge in present relationships with other people if the prior schemas are activated in memory.

Inner and Outer Self-Presentation Orientations

Self-presentations sometimes appear to be guided largely by pressures from audiences and situations and at other times largely by internal values and beliefs. This distinction between inner and outer orientations has been frequently discussed in the self-presentation literature as both an individual difference variable and a situational variable (Carver & Scheier, 1985; Cheek, 1989; Gangestad & Snyder, 2000; Hogan & Cheek, 1983). More broadly, the inner–outer metaphor runs through writings in psychology, sociology, and philosophy (Hogan & Cheek, 1983). Hogan and Cheek proposed that the dimensions of inner versus outer orientation are relatively independent, such that both orientations can be salient simultaneously (e.g., the individual who is aware of both public pressures and private principles and tries to work out some resolution when there is a conflict), that one can be salient while the other is not, or that neither might be salient (e.g., the individual who is indifferent to immediate others but also does not have a clear set of internal principles as guides for conduct in the situation). Data are consistent with the idea that the dimensions are positively correlated yet distinct (e.g., Carver & Scheier, 1985; Cheek, 1989; Hogan & Cheek, 1983).

Analyses of individual differences in self-presentation have focused largely on variables that reflect the distinction between inner versus outer orientations. Personality measures of self-monitoring (Gangestad & Snyder, 2000; M. Snyder, 1987), private versus public self-consciousness (Carver & Scheier, 1985), personal and social identity (Cheek, 1989; Hogan & Cheek, 1983), and the need for social approval (Paulhus, 1991) all assess aspects of differences in inner and outer orientations. Despite their common emphasis, the measures do differ. The Self-Consciousness Scale (Fenigstein, Scheier, & Buss, 1979) was designed to assess differences in how much attention is focused on the private and public sides of self. The Aspects of Identity Scale (Cheek, 1989) was designed to assess the importance people attach to the personal and social sides of their identity. The Need for Approval Scale (see Paulhus, 1991) assesses people's willingness to distort information about themselves in order to make a positive impression on others and to feel good about themselves. The Self-Monitoring Scale (M. Snyder, 1987) was designed to assess people's sensitivity to social cues regarding appropriate behavior and their willingness to engage in such behavior. More recently, Gangestad and Snyder (2000) suggested that high self-monitors seem to be motivated to enhance their social status. Their chameleon-like behavior to different audiences may primarily reflect status enhancement strategies of impression management. Further, high self-monitors do not seem to display the "close attention and responsiveness to other people" that was originally a core component of the concept (Gangestad & Snyder, 2000, p. 545). However, they are high on expressive control and nonverbal decoding skills, which contribute to their strong acting skills.

At one time, researchers entertained the idea that people who were inner oriented, such as those low in self-monitoring or high in private self-consciousness, were able to tune out social pressures, remain oblivious to audience expectations, and be guided exclusively by inner values and beliefs (Buss & Briggs, 1984; Carver & Scheier, 1985; M. Snyder, 1987). Increasingly, though, researchers are recognizing the power of audiences to shape the self-presentations of those who are inner oriented. In their recent analysis of self-monitoring, Gangestad and Snyder (2000) questioned the original view that low self-monitors are oblivious to social pressure and raised the possibility that low self-monitors are concerned about their "reputations of being genuine and sincere people who act on their beliefs" (p. 547).

Schlenker and Weigold (1990) showed that privately self-conscious people are concerned with their reputations to audiences. Privately self-conscious people describe themselves as independent, autonomous, and somewhat unique, whereas publicly self-conscious people describe themselves as being cooperative team players who are able to get along well. Schlenker and Weigold found that both publicly and privately self-

conscious people changed their publicly expressed beliefs based on audience feedback, but for different reasons. Publicly self-conscious people conformed to the expectations of their partners—they presented themselves consistently with the type of identity the partners thought they should have. Privately self-conscious people, however, presented themselves in ways that were designed to convey an image of autonomy to the audience. They shifted their behavior just as much as publicly self-conscious participants, but for a different purpose. These results indicate that inner and outer orientations, at least as represented by private and public self-consciousness, do not seem to be distinguished by whether self-presentations are influenced by audiences but rather by how they are influenced. People who are publicly self-conscious look to audiences to tell them who to be; they then present themselves in these ways. In contrast, privately self-conscious people look to audiences to tell them if they are coming across as they want to; they present themselves in ways that make them appear autonomous and change their behavior if feedback suggests they are not effectively creating that impression.

Focusing on Immediate Audiences: Self-Presentation Problems

Many problems in social life arise from a single-minded focus on gaining the approval and acceptance of immediate audiences. Outer orientations are associated with social trepidations. Public self-consciousness, for example, is positively related to social anxiety, shyness, and fear of negative evaluation (Schlenker & Weigold, 1990) and produces conformity designed to please immediate audiences (Carver & Scheier, 1985). When people look to immediate audiences to help them define who they should be, how they should look, and what they should do, they are in danger of acting in ways that compromise their integrity and may even endanger their health.

In their analysis of self-presentational hazards, Leary, Tchividjian, and Kraxberger (1994) reviewed literature indicating that self-presentational concerns are related to numerous health problems, including HIV infection, skin cancer, eating disorders, alcohol and drug abuse, accidental death, and even acne. For example, concerns about how one might appear to a partner reduce condom use and increase the likelihood of contracting sexually transmitted diseases. The desire to cultivate the appearance of being bronzed and beautiful causes people to tan excessively and risk skin cancer and to overuse makeup and risk acne. Eating disorders are due in part to concerns about body appearance. Alcohol and drug use are related to peer pressure and acceptance, and accidents are often caused by people showing off to friends in order to be seen as brave, adventuresome, and reckless. Despite the potential hazards of drinking from a stranger's water bottle, people will do so if they previously experienced a threat to their social image and were challenged by the stranger (Martin & Leary, 1999). Thus, attempts to look good to immediate audiences can increase health risk.

It is worth noting that these problems are not really self-presentation problems; they are outer orientation problems. They arise because people are focused on gaining the approval and acceptance of immediate others and will do whatever is necessary, including often ignoring their own principles and good judgment, in order to impress the immediate audience. Everyone cares about acceptance and approval. Not everyone, though, needs approval from whatever audience happens to be around nor needs approval to the point at which personal principles are abandoned. Hogan and Cheek (1983) proposed that maturity involves being able to recognize and deal with both inner (e.g., personal principles) and outer concerns (e.g., the expectations and preferences of others). To be oriented exclusively toward outer concerns is to allow others to dictate one's life. Conversely, to be oriented exclusively toward inner concerns often amounts to being egocentric, eccentric, and unable to deal effectively with others (Hogan & Cheek, 1983). Balancing inner and outer concerns evidences more mature social functioning.

How Effectively Can People Control Their Self-Presentations?

As noted earlier, people have extensive knowledge about different identity types and roles and can draw from this information even if they do not normally view themselves as having the particular set of personal attributes. How effectively are people able to portray someone they are not? Are most people, like actors on a stage, able to step into new roles and perform them competently, at least enough to convince an audience?

People are able to express attitudes and emotions, describe prior personal experiences, play social roles, and fulfill audience expectations, even when these are inconsistent with their own self-conceptions, feelings, and personal experiences. And they can do it convincingly through both their verbal and nonverbal communications. Studies show that when people are asked to play a role, such as being an introvert or extravert, they are able to convince onlookers that they actually have those characteristics, regardless of whether they really do (Lippa, 1976; Pontari & Schlenker, 2000; Toris & DePaulo, 1984). In her review of the literature on self-presentation and nonverbal behavior, DePaulo (1992) concluded that,

> Virtually every study . . . [of nonverbal posing skill] has shown that people can successfully make clear to others, using only nonverbal cues, the internal state that they are actually experiencing and that they can also convey to others the impression that they are experiencing a particular internal state when in fact they are not. . . . Furthermore, when people are deliberately trying to convey an impression of a state that they are not really experiencing, their nonverbal behaviors convey that state to others even more clearly and effectively than when they really are experiencing the state but are not trying purposefully to communicate it to others." (p. 219)

DePaulo's (1992) review indicates that when people fake personality dispositions and other personal information, they present an exaggerated version of what such an individual would actually do. For example, extraverts speak faster than introverts, so when faking extraversion, people speak even more rapidly than an actual extravert would. The resulting caricature is usually convincing to onlookers.

In general, onlookers' skill at detecting deception is poor and exceeds chance by only a slight amount (DePaulo, 1992, 1994;

DePaulo, Stone, & Lassiter, 1985; Ekman & O'Sullivan, 1991). Even in close relationships such as marriage, unless trust has been shaken in some other way, partners are poor at detecting when they are being deceived (McCormack & Levine, 1990). Yet deception can be detected, often under conditions that are most disadvantageous for the deceiver. DePaulo, LeMay, and Epstein (1991) describe a motivational impairment effect in which people's attempts to deceive are most likely to go awry on those occasions when deception is most beneficial. People who are highly motivated to get away with deception are also most likely to be seen as deceptive by onlookers *if* they also doubt their ability to convince the audience (DePaulo, 1992; DePaulo et al., 1991). Under these conditions, deceivers are more likely to experience social anxiety, and behavioral signs of anxiety are likely to tip off observers. People who are confident of their social skills, however, do not seem to exhibit motivational impairment (DePaulo, 1992; DePaulo et al., 1991).

There are virtually no data on how long people can successfully maintain a deception about themselves. It is one thing to fake information for an hour and another to try to keep it up for days or longer. People may have difficulty maintaining long-term deceptions in part because potentially contradictory information needs to be monitored and suppressed, and, over time, contradictions may slip through as the actors' attention is focused elsewhere. Furthermore, faking may be too effortful and unenjoyable to maintain for long periods. For example, introverts prefer more introspective activities and may not enjoy "faking" being outgoing, even if they can get away with it for limited periods of time.

Reasons for Deceptive Effectiveness

People's effectiveness at convincing others of the genuineness of their self-presentations stems from both actors' skills and audiences' predilections. On the actors' side of the equation, skills at deception are socialized and rewarded in everyday life. Although parents condemn deceit in principle, children are socialized to suppress some feelings and be deceptive about others as part of learning how to be a polite, well-mannered individual. For example, children learn to smile and act happy even when they receive an unwelcome present or to compliment Aunt Sue's new hairstyle even though they think it is hideous. The ability to deceive may be an important component of social power and social acceptance. Keating and Heltman (1994) found that people who are rated as more dominant by peers also were better at deception, and this was true for both children and adult men (but not for women). Furthermore, this effect held over and above communication skill generally; more dominant individuals seemed to be uniquely talented in their ability to disguise the truth in ways not dependent only on their overall communication ability. Similarly, people who score high in Machiavellianism, who are highly effective at bargaining and negotiation, are also effective liars who appear honest even while manipulating others, especially when the stakes are high (Schlenker, 1980; Wilson, Near, & Miller, 1996). Yet those high in Machiavellianism are not socially effective on all dimensions, because their selfish, manipulative style can create problems in long-term relationships (Wilson et al., 1996), and they exhibit such signs of psychopathy as narcissism, anxiety, and lack of remorse (McHoskey, Worzel, & Szyarto, 1998).

DePaulo and her colleagues (DePaulo, Kashy, Kirkendol, Wyer, & Epstein, 1996; Kashy & DePaulo, 1996) found that people lie relatively frequently during their everyday interactions (e.g., college students remembered telling about two lies per day). Most of these lies were self-centered and designed to advance or protect personal interests. However, many of the lies were other-centered in that they were designed to help or protect others, and people said they did not regard their lies as serious, nor did they worry about being caught (DePaulo et al., 1996). Further, people who tell more lies tend to be more sociable and more concerned with self-presentation, again suggesting that lying often serves to improve social functioning (Kashy & DePaulo, 1996). Lies of omission and commission are used to sooth the feelings of those we like when the truth might otherwise hurt (DePaulo & Bell, 1996). This is one reason that people's impressions of how others view them are usually self-flattering versions of how those others actually do view them. The paradox is that deceit, which is condemnable in principle, plays an important role in maintaining harmony and soothing tensions in everyday life.

On the audience's side of the equation, audiences usually give actors the benefit of the doubt and assume that their self-presentations are authentic. This tendency is consistent with the correspondence bias and with the operation of social norms favoring considerateness. The correspondence bias (Jones, 1990) describes the tendency of people to attribute the behaviors of others to corresponding internal states—for example, if others act extraverted, it is because they are extraverted. The correspondence bias is even more pronounced when perceivers are cognitively busy rather than able to focus their full attention on the actor's behavior (Gilbert, Krull, & Pelham, 1988). The more hectic the occasion, the more likely audiences are to accept the self-presentations of others at face value. Goffman (1959) noted that people are predisposed to honor the claims of others and assume truthfulness, at least publicly. Doing so makes interactions flow more smoothly and reduces the tension associated with visible suspicion. Even when people detect contradictory information, they often let it slide unless it is important to their goals during interaction.

When Are People More Effective at Self-Presentation?

People differ in their self-presentation skills, including their expressiveness (DePaulo, 1992) and acting ability (M. Snyder, 1987). Going beyond these interpersonal abilities, though, people's interpersonal orientations can have a pronounced impact on how effective they are at self-presentation. Self-presentations seem to be effective when people are motivated to make a desired impression on an audience and are relatively confident they will be able to do so. This combination—the motivation to impress and self-presentation confidence—seems to provide the optimal environment for effectively communicating to others and influencing them to form the preferred impression. If either component is lacking, as when the motivation to impress the audi-

ence is low or self-presentation doubts are high, self-presentation effectiveness seems to suffer (see Schlenker et al., 1996).

One extreme is marked by cases in which people are highly motivated to impress an audience and have doubts about their ability to do so. These conditions produce high social anxiety (Leary, 1983; Leary & Kowalski, 1995; Schlenker & Leary, 1982b, 1985). Social anxiety is associated with negative affect, negative self-preoccupation, the appearance of nervousness, physical and psychological withdrawal from the situation, and self-protective presentational strategies (e.g., minimal social participation, low self-disclosure, innocuous social behaviors such as smiling and nodding). The result is an inferior performance that usually fails to make a good impression.

The other extreme is marked by cases in which the motivation to create a desired impression on an immediate audience is very low, which can occur when the audience is seen as insignificant (e.g., a servant) or the actor is overly confident that the audience has already formed the desired impression and will not change it (e.g., a spouse). These conditions produce suboptimal monitoring of self-presentation activities and audience feedback (see Schlenker et al., 1996). For example, the actor may misread the situation, fail to notice negative audience feedback, be inconsistent in matching verbal and nonverbal activities, and seem preoccupied with other goals. Marriage counselors are often confronted with complaints that, "My spouse is no longer the person I married." Seemingly secure in the other's regard, one has allowed one's own appearance and manner to deviate dramatically from the desirable behavior once exhibited during courtship. Similarly, coaches of athletic teams often warn their players about overconfidence lest they take a game for granted and fail to monitor and control their efforts effectively.

In between these extremes is the optimal situation, in which people assign reasonably high priority to how the immediate audience regards them and feel confident that they can create the desired impression. Under these conditions, people seem most effective in marshaling their verbal and nonverbal activities to create the impression they desire and can do so regardless of whether that impression is an accurate or deceptive portrayal of self (Schlenker et al., 1996).

Protecting Identity: Self-Presentations in Predicaments

Despite their best intentions, people sometimes find themselves in predicaments that threaten their desired identities. Problems may arise because of accidents, mistakes, or some other unintended faux pas, because of failures to accomplish important tasks, or because of intentional behavior that comes to the attention of audiences and jeopardizes desired appearances, as in cases in which people appear to lie or cheat. When these predicament-creating events occur, people engage in remedial activities designed to protect their identities (see Leary, 1995; Rosenfeld et al., 1995; Schlenker, 1980, 1982). These activities fall into three broad categories: accountability avoidance strategies, accounting strategies, and apology strategies (Schlenker, Weigold, & Doherty, 1991).

Accountability Avoidance Strategies

These strategies are designed to put off, avoid, or escape from tasks, situations, and audiences that threaten desired identities. People avoid tasks that produce embarrassment and will even sacrifice money to do so (B. R. Brown, 1970; Miller, 1996); they avoid social situations they expect will produce anxiety and prematurely leave those that elicit anxiety (Leary, 1995); and they conceal embarrassing or out-of-character information (Leary, 1995; Schlenker, 1980). These activities allow people to avoid or escape from an evaluative reckoning in which their behavior may be judged and found wanting by others.

The behaviors of people high in social anxiety illustrate common but pervasive avoidance strategies. Highly anxious people tend to have fewer social contacts and, when in social situations, tend to engage in behavior that avoids the evaluative spotlight (see Leary & Kowalski, 1995; Schlenker & Leary, 1985). When they are socially anxious, people initiate fewer conversations, speak less frequently, avoid eye contact, do not speak freely, and disclose less informa-

tion about themselves; the information they do reveal is usually uncontroversial and undiagnostic.

Even when people can escape from immediate audiences, they still must account to themselves and deal with inner audiences. After predicaments, these inner audiences can be potentially harsh judges, sometimes even harsher than real audiences (Tangney, Miller, Flicker, & Barlow, 1996), and self-focused attention becomes an unpleasant state that people try to terminate (Hull & Young, 1983). People can escape from aversive self-evaluation by turning to alcohol, drugs, physical exercise, meditation, television, shopping, and other activities that reduce self-consciousness (see Schlenker et al., 1991).

Actors also can try to escape accountability by denying the evaluators' legitimacy as judges. People may assert, "You have no right to judge me," and refuse to offer an explanation. They thereby try to disqualify the audience as someone to whom they might be accountable.

Accounting Strategies

When facing predicaments, people construct accounts that provide self-serving explanations. These accounts attempt to reconcile the event with the prescriptions for conduct that appear to have been violated. Accounts include (1) defenses of innocence, which assert that a violation did not occur (e.g., an accused murderer proclaims, "It was a suicide, not a murder") or that the actor was in no way involved with the violation, (2) excuses, which claim that the individual was not as responsible for the event as it might otherwise appear (e.g., claiming the consequences were unforeseeable or caused by factors beyond personal control), and (3) justifications, which claim that the event was not as negative as it might otherwise appear to be or was actually positive because the actor was working toward a valued, superordinate goal.

Accounts can be highly effective in accomplishing their objectives of minimizing the negative personal and interpersonal ramifications of predicaments (see Leary, 1995; Rosenfeld et al., 1995; Schlenker, 1980, 1982; Schlenker et al., 2001; Snyder & Higgins, 1988; Weiner, Figueroa-Munoz,

& Kakihara, 1991). Snyder and Higgins (1988) reviewed an extensive literature showing that excuses can protect self-esteem, reduce negative affect and depression, lead to better task performance, and produce better physical health. Excuses and justifications also have been shown to reduce interpersonal condemnation, even for criminal acts, provided they appear to be sincere (see Rosenfeld et al., 1995; Schlenker et al., 2001).

However, excuses also have the potential to backfire and create problems for the actor (Higgins & Snyder, 1989; Schlenker et al., 2001). These problems can include appearing to be dishonest, self-absorbed to the detriment of others, and ineffectual at accomplishing appropriate tasks. Justifications can backfire, too, because they tend to be more confrontational than excuses (Gonzalez, Pederson, Manning, & Wetter, 1990). With excuses, actors acknowledge that the relevant norms and rules apply to them but simply plead diminished responsibility. With justifications, actors often assert that the norms and rules that might seem to apply are superseded by other, more important ones. An extreme example is the terrorist who asserts that placing a bomb in a shopping area is an act to promote freedom and justice, not to murder innocents.

Coverage of the extensive literature on accounts is beyond the scope of this chapter. Interested readers are referred elsewhere (McLaughlin, Cody, & Read, 1992; Rosenfeld et al., 1995; Schlenker, 1980, 1982; Schlenker et al., 1991, 2001; Snyder & Higgins, 1988; Snyder, Higgins, & Stucky, 1983; Tedeschi & Riess, 1981).

Apologies

Apologies admit blameworthiness and regret. By accepting blame and expressing remorse, actors affirm the value of the rules that were violated and extend a promise of better future behavior (Goffman, 1971; Schlenker, 1980). Apologies thus split the self into two parts: a bad self that misbehaved and a good self that has learned a lesson and will behave more properly in the future. If the apology seems sincere and seems to fit the magnitude of the transgression (e.g., larger transgressions should be followed by greater remorse), the actor no longer seems to require rehabilitative punishment. After transgressions, people do offer apologies and, as the predicament increases in magnitude, include more apology elements, including statements of apologetic intent, expressions of remorse, offers of restitution, self-castigating comments, and requests for forgiveness (Schlenker & Darby, 1981).

If they seem sincere and fitted to the transgression, apologies produce less negative reactions toward transgressors, including more forgiveness, less blame, less punishment, less negative evaluations of the transgressors' character, less negative interpretations of the transgressors' motives, and a lower perceived likelihood that the offending behavior will be repeated (Darby & Schlenker, 1982, 1989; Gold & Weiner, 2000; Ohbuchi, Kameda, & Agarie, 1989; Scher & Darley, 1997; Schwartz, Kane, Joseph, & Tedeschi, 1978; Weiner, Graham, Peter, & Zmuidinas, 1991).

Working Together to Maintain Desired Identities

People are not on their own when it comes to constructing and protecting desired identities. People often work as teams, as in the cases of a husband and wife who act in concert to project their family image, or the employer and employee who coordinate activities to create the appropriate business image (Goffman, 1959). When people perform as a team, their identities are linked. The self-presentation of one has direct implications for the identity of the other.

Even when not part of a team, people still help one another construct and protect their identities. Goffman (1967) described two interaction rules that he considered to be moral duties: the *rule of self-respect*, by which people have a duty to "be" who they claim to be and try to maintain that "face" if confronted by inconsistencies, and the *rule of considerateness*, by which people have the duty to respect the "faces" of others. People are expected to exhibit civility, politeness, and consideration for one another's identities. For example, people help one another maintain face, whether it is by seeming not to notice another person's faux pas or by making a witty remark that deflects the spotlight from someone else's embarrassing moment without making the embarrassed party look bad. Even kindergarten children seem to take into account the possible effects of their behavior on both their own faces and the faces of classmates (Hatch, 1987).

According to politeness theory (Brown & Levinson, 1987), when accounting for their own conduct, people must consider both their own face needs and the face needs of others, particularly anyone who might be harmed by the act or the explanation. Folkes (1982) found that when people reject another person, as when they refuse a request for a date, they usually provide excuses that emphasize a reason for the rejection that is not threatening for the recipient, such as by claiming illness or another commitment rather than a lack of interest. DePaulo and colleagues (1996) found that people often said they told lies in order to save another person's feelings.

Social norms prescribe politeness to others. There are often reasons to go beyond politeness, however, and to provide significant help to others by enhancing or protecting their identities. As shall be seen, such help can accomplish both selfish and selfless goals.

Bolstering the Identities of Others: Helping Self by Boosting Others

People often try to bolster the identities of others in order to accomplish their own personal, often selfish goals. Research on ingratiation showed that people will flatter others, agree with their opinions, imitate their behaviors, and do favors for them in order to make themselves liked and to receive such rewards as better performance appraisals from supervisors (Jones & Wortman, 1973; Wayne & Kacmar, 1991). People also will praise or help others with whom they are associated and thereby bask in the reflected glory of these desirable individuals (J. D. Brown, Collins, & Schmidt, 1988; Cialdini et al., 1990; Tesser, 1988). In organizational settings, good citizenship is valued and rewarded, and people often present themselves as "good soldiers" who act selflessly on behalf of their organization. These self-presentations of being good organizational citizens seem to be motivated at least in part by self-serving, identity-boosting goals (Bolino, 1999).

Helping can also be a useful self-presentation strategy because of how it affects perceptions of the recipient's success. Gilbert and Silvera (1996) found that overhelping can be used to spoil another person's identity by causing onlookers to attribute the other's success to the help. They found that overhelping is most likely to occur when people believe their aid will be ineffective but that other onlookers will regard it as facilitative. Similarly, people who are in competition with others and who are concerned that they will lose will give performance advantages to those others, such as by playing facilitating background music while they and the others work on the task (Shepperd & Arkin, 1991). The others' success can thereby be discounted as due to the help rather than to superior relative ability.

As these lines of research show, people often receive identity support and assistance from others. However, what sometimes appears to be support is actually anything but helpful to the recipient, as in the case of overhelping as a means of spoiling identity or flattery designed to mislead another person into providing benefits. To the extent that identity support is guided primarily by the provider's selfish interpersonal goals, without regard to the welfare of the other, the recipient's benefits may be illusory, because the provider may not believe the compliments or be willing to provide more support in the future in the absence of personal profit.

Bolstering the Identities of Others: Social Support, Social Concern

The traditional view of impression management as selfish, often exploitative activity seems to have obscured its other, socially beneficial side. Using impression management to provide support for the desired identities of others is a valued, highly rewarding form of help. In everyday life, people will put in a good word for their friends to help them get the job or date they want, to help them feel good about their prospects when tackling challenging tasks, and to provide reassurance in the face of identity-threatening events. Social support that provides validation for desired identity images has been related to the psychological well-being of the recipient, because it provides a buffer against stress, reduces negative affect and depression, and enhances positive affect and self-esteem (see J. D. Brown, 1998; Schlenker & Britt, 1999, 2001). Identity support is especially valuable in close relationships, in which people's satisfaction is directly related to the extent to which their partners see them in more positive, idealized ways than they see themselves (Murray, Holmes, & Griffin, 1996a, 1996b). The social support literature has focused on the recipient of the support, however, and not on how such support is provided.

Schlenker and Britt (1999, 2001) proposed that people will strategically enhance the identities of others by using beneficial impression management. Furthermore, these helpful activities are often guided by a concern for the others' social well-being, especially family and friends whose welfare is important. In support, Schlenker and Britt (1999, Experiment 1) found that participants strategically shifted their descriptions of same-sex friends in order to help their friends make a good impression on an attractive member of the opposite sex. If an attractive, opposite-sex individual preferred extraverted others as ideal dates, participants described their friends as highly extraverted, whereas if that other preferred introverted others as ideal dates, participants described their friends as introverted. Just as people's own self-presentations shift to conform to the role expectations of attractive others (Zanna & Pack, 1975), so do their descriptions of their friends. Further, if their friends found the opposite-sex individual to be quite unattractive, participants described their friends opposite to the preferences of the other—describing their friends as extraverted to the unattractive other who preferred introverts, and as introverted to the unattractive other who preferred extraverts—as if to assert, "My friend is not your type." They thus helped their friends avoid unwanted entanglements. These effects were obtained even though participants believed that their friends would not learn of their assistance. Thus people's descriptions of their friends seemed to be strategic and goal-oriented in character because they covaried with the apparent social interests of their friends in relation to the

audience and its preferences. Pontari and Schlenker (2001) extended these results and found that members of dating couples helped one another make a good impression on a third party who their partners thought was attractive, provided that third party was of the same sex as their partners. People were not helpful when describing their romantic partners to someone of the sex opposite to their partners'.

In two other studies, participants described same-sex friends to an evaluator who was supposedly testing their friends' cognitive abilities (Schlenker & Britt, 1999, 2001). They believed that their friends either had a high social need to make a good impression, because the friends supposedly would go through a face-to-face interview with the evaluator and receive feedback, or that they did not have a need to make a good impression, because the friends would not be interviewed or receive evaluative feedback. Participants described their friends as having greater cognitive ability when their friends had to go through the evaluative interview than when they did not. Further, beneficial impression management was greater by participants who scored higher on a personality measure of empathy and by those who expressed greater caring for their friends (Schlenker & Britt, 2001). These results show that strategic impression management, in the form of bolstering the desired identity images of a friend, covaries with the social needs of the friend and is greater under conditions in which people are more concerned with the friend's welfare (i.e., those more empathic and more caring toward the friend).

Research on beneficial impression management broadens our understanding of how people strategically control information in everyday life. Impression management is not motivated strictly by selfish, manipulative goals. Just like any other social activity, impression management can be guided by a variety of goals, some of which are socially beneficial. Indeed, people's own welfare depends in large measure on procuring the good will of others. To do so, people must imagine and anticipate the expectations and preferences of others and be willing to engage in mutually beneficial activities that take the predilections of audiences into account.

Conclusions

Self-presentation is a fundamental feature of social life. Symbolic interactionists noted that people cannot interact until they define who each one will be and what they are doing together (McCall & Simmons, 1978). Similarly, Abelson (1976, p. 42) proposed that "cognitively mediated social behavior depends on the occurrence of two processes: (a) the selection of a particular script to represent the given situation and (b) the taking of a participant role within that script." Taking a participant role means selecting a particular identity and then constructing and protecting that identity for audiences. Because people's identities are directly tied to the regard and treatment they receive in social life, people make those selections with care. They construct and protect desired identity images through self-presentation.

The self-presentation literature, as illustrated by the topics in this chapter, has remarkable breadth and depth. Self-presentation involves cognitively effortful, controlled activities, as well as unconscious, automatic behaviors. Self-presentation involves manipulative, selfish activities designed to exploit others, as well as socially beneficial behaviors that help others construct and protect their desired identities. Self-presentation involves deceptions about oneself, as well as sincere portrayals of how one thinks one really is. Self-presentation involves making a desired impression on an immediate audience, as well as conducting oneself in ways that are appreciated, at least in the mind's eye, by significant, imagined audiences (e.g., a deceased parent). Research on self-presentation has come a long way from the "early days" of the 1960s. In one of the first popular uses of the term in the social psychology literature, Jones (1964) described self-presentation as one of four ingratiation tactics, along with flattery, opinion conformity, and favor doing, that were illicit activities designed to increase one's liking by powerful others. This restricted use, which focused on the manipulative, illicit side of self-presentation and on the single-minded goal of being liked, is still the way some researchers think of the term. Today, though, research on self-presentation covers far more. Self-presentation has

emerged as an important and fundamental concept in social psychology.

References

Abelson, R. P. (1976). Script processing in attitude formation and decision making. In J. S. Carroll & J. W. Payne (Eds.), *Cognition and social behavior* (pp. 33–45). Hillsdale, NJ: Erlbaum.

Aloise-Young, P. A. (1993). The development of self-presentation: Self-promotion in 6- to 10-year-old children. *Social Cognition, 11,* 201–222.

Baldwin, M. W. (1992). Relational schemas and the processing of social information. *Psychological Bulletin, 112,* 461–484.

Baldwin, M. W., Carrell, S. E., & Lopez, D. F. (1990). Priming relational schemas: My advisor and the pope are watching me from the back of my mind. *Journal of Experimental Social Psychology, 26,* 435–454.

Baldwin, M. W., & Holmes, J. G. (1987). Salient private audiences and awareness of the self. *Journal of Personality and Social Psychology, 52,* 1087–1098.

Banerjee, R., & Yuill, N. (1999). Children's explanations for self-presentational behavior. *European Journal of Social Psychology, 29,* 105–111.

Bargh, J. A. (1989). Conditional automaticity: Varieties of automatic influence in social perception and cognition. In J. S. Uleman & J. A. Bargh (Eds.), *Unintended thought* (pp. 3–51). New York: Guilford Press.

Bargh, J. A. (1996). Automaticity in social psychology. In E. T. Higgins & A. W. Kruglanski (Eds.), *Social psychology: Handbook of basic principles* (pp. 169–183). New York: Guilford Press.

Baron, R. A., Fortin, S. P., Frei, R. L., Hauver, L. A., & Shack, M. L. (1990). Reducing organizational conflict: The potential role of inducing positive affect. *International Journal of Conflict Management, 1,* 133–152.

Baumeister, R. F. (1982). A self-presentational view of social phenomena. *Psychological Bulletin, 91,* 3–26.

Baumeister, R. F., Hamilton, J. C., & Tice, D. M. (1985). Public versus private expectancy of success: Confidence booster or performance pressure? *Journal of Personality and Social Psychology, 48,* 1447–1457.

Baumeister, R. F., Hutton, D. G., & Tice, D. M. (1989). Cognitive processes during deliberate self-presentation: How self-presenters alter and misinterpret the behavior of their interaction partners. *Journal of Experimental Social Psychology, 25,* 59–78.

Baumeister, R. F., & Jones, E. E. (1978). When self-presentation is constrained by the target's knowledge: Consistency and compensation. *Journal of Personality and Social Psychology, 36,* 608–618.

Baumeister, R. F., & Ilko, S. A. (1995). Shallow gratitude: Public and private acknowledgment of external help in accounts of success. *Basic and Applied Social Psychology, 16,* 191–209.

Baumeister, R. F., & Newman, L. S. (1994). How stories make sense of personal experiences: Motives that shape autobiographical narratives. *Personality and Social Psychology Bulletin, 20,* 676–690.

Baumgardner, A. H., & Brownlee, E. A. (1987). Strategic failure in social interaction: Evidence for expectancy disconfirmation processes. *Journal of Personality and Social Psychology, 52,* 525–535.

Bennett, M., & Yeeles, C. (1990a). Children's understanding of the self-presentational strategies of ingratiation and self-promotion. *European Journal of Social Psychology, 20,* 455–461.

Bennett, M., & Yeeles, C. (1990b). Children's understanding of showing off. *Journal of Social Psychology, 130,* 591–596.

Bolino, M. C. (1999). Citizenship and impression management: Good soldiers or good actors? *Academy of Management Review, 24,* 82–98.

Bozeman, D. P., & Kacmar, K. M. (1997). A cybernetic model of impression management processes in organizations. *Organizational Behavior and Human Decision Processes, 69,* 9–30.

Brissett, D., & Edgley, C. (Eds.). (1990). *Life as theater: A dramaturgical sourcebook* (2nd ed.). Hawthorne, NY: Aldine De Gruyter.

Brodt, S. E., & Zimbardo, P. G. (1981). Modifying shyness-related social behavior through symptom misattribution. *Journal of Personality and Social Psychology, 41,* 437–449.

Brown, B. R. (1970). Face-saving following experimentally induced embarrassment. *Journal of Experimental Social Psychology, 6,* 255–271.

Brown, J. D. (1998). *The self.* New York: McGraw-Hill.

Brown, J. D., Collins, R. L., & Schmidt, G. W. (1988). Self-esteem and direct versus indirect forms of self-enhancement. *Journal of Personality and Social Psychology, 55,* 445–453.

Brown, P., & Levinson, S. C. (1987). *Politeness: Some universals in language use.* Cambridge, UK: Cambridge University Press.

Buss, A. H., & Briggs, S. R. (1984). Drama and the self in social interaction. *Journal of Personality and Social Psychology, 47,* 1310–1324.

Carnegie, D. (1940). *How to win friends and influence people.* New York: Pocket Books.

Carver, C. S., & Scheier, M. F. (1982). Control theory: A useful conceptual framework for personality-social, clinical, and health psychology. *Psychological Bulletin, 92,* 111–135.

Carver, C. S., & Scheier, M. F. (1985). Aspects of self and the control of behavior. In B. R. Schlenker (Ed.), *The self and social life* (pp. 146–174). New York: McGraw-Hill.

Cascio, W. F. (1975). Accuracy of verifiable biographical information blank responses. *Journal of Applied Psychology, 60,* 767–769.

Chartrand, T. L., & Bargh, J. A. (1999). The chameleon effect: The perception–behavior link and social interaction. *Journal of Personality and Social Psychology, 76,* 893–910.

Cheek, J. M. (1982). Aggregation, moderator variables, and the validity of personality tests: A peer-rating study. *Journal of Personality and Social Psychology, 43,* 1254–1269.

Cheek, J. M. (1989). Identity orientations and self-interpretation. In D. M. Buss & N. Cantor (Eds.), *Personality psychology: Recent trends and emerging directions* (pp. 275–285). New York: Springer-Verlag.

Cheek, J. M., & Hogan, R. (1983). Self-concepts, self-presentations, and moral judgments. In J. Suls & A. G.

Greenwald (Eds.), *Psychological perspectives on the self* (Vol. 2, pp. 249–273). Hillsdale, NJ: Erlbaum.

Chen, S., & Anderson, S. M. (1999). Relationships from the past in the present: Significant-other representations and transference in interpersonal life. In M. P. Zanna (Ed.), *Advances in experimental social psychology* (Vol. 31, pp. 123–190). San Diego, CA: Academic Press.

Cialdini, R. B., Finch, J. F., & De Nicholas, M. E. (1990). Strategic self-presentation: The indirect route. In M. J. Cody & M. L. McLaughlin (Eds.), *The psychology of tactical communication* (pp. 194–206). Clevedon, UK: Multilingual Matters.

Cooley, C. H. (1902). *Human nature and the social order.* New York: Scribner's.

Darby, B. W., & Schlenker, B. R. (1982). Children's reactions to apologies. *Journal of Personality and Social Psychology, 43,* 742–753.

Darby, B. W., & Schlenker, B. R. (1989). Children's reactions to transgressions: Effects of the actor's apology, reputation, and remorse. *British Journal of Social Psychology, 28,* 353–364.

DePaulo, B. M. (1992). Nonverbal behavior and self-presentation. *Psychological Bulletin, 111,* 203–243.

DePaulo, B. M. (1994). Spotting lies: Can humans learn to do better? *Current Directions in Psychological Science, 3,* 83–86.

DePaulo, B. M., & Bell, K. L. (1996). Truth and investment: Lies are told to those who care. *Journal of Personality and Social Psychology, 71,* 703–716.

DePaulo, B. M., Kashy, D. A., Kirkendol, S. E., Wyer, M. M., & Epstein, J. A. (1996). Lying in everyday life. *Journal of Personality and Social Psychology, 70,* 979–995.

DePaulo, B. M., LeMay, C. S., & Epstein, J. A. (1991). Effects of importance of success and expectations for success on effectiveness at deceiving. *Personality and Social Psychology Bulletin, 17,* 14–24.

DePaulo, B. M., Stone, J. I., & Lassiter, G. D. (1985). Deceiving and detecting deceit. In B. R. Schlenker (Ed.), *The self and social life* (pp. 323–370). New York: McGraw-Hill.

Doherty, K., Van Wagenen, T. J., & Schlenker, B. R. (1991, August). *Imagined audiences influence self-identifications.* Paper presented at the annual meeting of the American Psychological Association, San Francisco.

Ekman, P., & O'Sullivan, M. (1991). Who can catch a liar? *American Psychologist, 46,* 913–920.

Emler, N., & Reicher, S. (1995). *Adolescence and delinquency: The collective management of reputation.* Cambridge, MA: Blackwell.

Fandt, P. M., & Ferris, G. R. (1990). The management of information and impressions: When employees behave opportunistically. *Organizational Behavior and Human Decision Processes, 45,* 140–158.

Fenigstein, A., Scheier, M. F., & Buss, A. H. (1979). Public and private self-consciousness: Assessment and theory. *Journal of Consulting and Clinical Psychology, 43,* 522–527.

Fleming, J. H., Darley, J. M., Hilton, J. L., & Kojetin, B. A. (1990). Multiple audience problem: A strategic communication perspective on social perception. *Journal of Personality and Social Psychology, 58,* 593–609.

Folkes, V. S. (1982). Communicating the causes of social rejection. *Journal of Experimental Social Psychology, 18,* 235–252.

Friedlander, M. L., & Schwartz, G. S. (1985). Toward a theory of strategic self-presentation in counseling and psychotherapy. *Journal of Consulting Psychology, 32,* 483–501.

Gangestad, S. W., & Snyder, M. (2000). Self-monitoring: Appraisal and reappraisal. *Psychological Bulletin, 126,* 530–555.

Gergen, K. J. (1965). Interaction goals and personalistic feedback as factors affecting the presentation of self. *Journal of Personality and Social Psychology, 1,* 413–424.

Gergen, K. J., & Gergen, M. M. (1988). Narrative and the self as relationship. In L. Berkowitz (Ed.), *Advances in experimental social psychology* (Vol. 21, pp. 17–56). New York: Academic Press.

Gibson, B., & Sachau, D. (2000). Sandbagging as a self-presentational strategy: Claiming to be less than you are. *Personality and Social Psychology Bulletin, 26,* 56–70.

Gilbert, D. T., Krull, D. S., & Pelham, B. W. (1988). Of thoughts unspoken: Social inference and the self-regulation of behavior. *Journal of Personality and Social Psychology, 55,* 685–694.

Gilbert, D. T., & Silvera, D. H. (1996). Overhelping. *Journal of Personality and Social Psychology, 70,* 678–690.

Godfrey, D. K., Jones, E. E., & Lord, C. G. (1986). Self-promotion is not ingratiating. *Journal of Personality and Social Psychology, 50,* 106–115.

Goffman, E. (1959). *The presentation of self in everyday life.* Garden City, NY: Doubleday.

Goffman, E. (1967). *Interaction ritual.* Garden City, NY: Doubleday.

Goffman, E. (1971). *Relations in public.* New York: Basic Books.

Gold, G. J., & Weiner, B. (2000). Remorse, confession, group identity, and expectancies about repeating a transgression. *Basic and Applied Social Psychology, 22,* 291–300.

Gonzales, M. H., Pederson, J. H., Manning, D. J., & Wetter, D. W. (1990). Pardon my gaffe: Effects of sex, status, and consequence severity on accounts. *Journal of Personality and Social Psychology, 58,* 610–621.

Gould, S., & Penley, L. E. (1984). Career strategies and salary progression: A study of their relationships in a municipal bureaucracy. *Organizational Behavior and Human Decision Processes, 34,* 244–265.

Greenwald, A. G., & Breckler, S. J. (1985). To whom is the self presented? In B. R. Schlenker (Ed.), *The self and social life* (pp. 126–145). New York: McGraw-Hill.

Hardin, C. D., & Higgins, E. T. (1996). Shared reality: How social verification makes the subjective objective. In R. M. Sorrentino & E. T. Higgins (Eds.), *Handbook of motivation and cognition: Vol. 3. The interpersonal context* (pp. 28–84). New York: Guilford Press.

Hatch, J. A. (1987). Impression management in kindergarten classrooms: An analysis of children's face-work in peer interactions. *Anthropology and Education Quarterly, 18,* 100–115.

Higgins, E. T. (1992). Achieving "shared reality" in the communication game: A social action that creates meaning. *Journal of Language and Social Psychology, 11,* 107–131.

Higgins, R. L., & Snyder, C. R. (1989). Excuses gone awry: An analysis of self-defeating excuses. In R. C. Curtis (Ed.), *Self-defeating behaviors: Experimental research, clinical impressions, and practical implications* (pp. 99–130). New York: Plenum Press.

Hogan, R., & Cheek, J. M. (1983). Identity, authenticity, and maturity. In T. R. Sarbin & K. E. Scheibe (Eds.), *Studies in social identity* (pp. 339–357). New York: Praeger.

Holtgraves, T., & Srull, T. K. (1989). The effects of positive self-descriptions on impressions: General principles and individual differences. *Personality and Social Psychology Bulletin, 15,* 452–462.

Hoyle, R. H., Kernis, M. H., Leary, M. R., & Baldwin, M. W. (1999). *Selfhood: Identity, esteem, regulation.* Boulder, CO: Westview Press.

Hull, J. G., & Young, R. D. (1983). Self-consciousness, self-esteem, and success–failure as determinants of alcohol consumption. *Journal of Personality and Social Psychology, 44,* 1097–1109.

James, B., & Collins, D. (1997). Self-presentational sources of competitive stress during performance. *Journal of Sport and Exercise Psychology, 19,* 17–35.

James, W. J. (1890). *Principles of psychology.* New York: Holt.

Jones, E. E. (1964). *Ingratiation.* New York: Appleton-Century-Crofts.

Jones, E. E. (1990). *Interpersonal perception.* New York: Freeman.

Jones, E. E., & Pittman, T. S. (1982). Toward a general theory of strategic self-presentation. In J. Suls (Ed.), *Psychological perspectives on the self* (Vol. 1, pp. 231–262). Hillsdale, NJ: Erlbaum.

Jones, E. E., Rhodewalt, F., Berglas, S., & Skelton, J. A. (1981). Effects of strategic self-presentation on subsequent self-esteem. *Journal of Personality and Social Psychology, 41,* 407–421.

Jones, E. E., & Wortman, C. (1973). *Ingratiation: An attributional approach.* Morristown, NJ: General Learning Press.

Judge, T. A., & Bretz, R. D. (1994). Political influence behavior and career success. *Journal of Management, 20,* 43–65.

Kacmar, K. M., Delery, J. E., & Ferris, G. R. (1992). Differential effectiveness of applicant impression management tactics on employment interview decisions. *Journal of Applied Social Psychology, 22,* 1250–1272.

Kashy, D. A., & DePaulo, B. M. (1996). Who lies? *Journal of Personality and Social Psychology, 70,* 1037–1051.

Keating, C. F., & Heltman, K. R. (1994). Dominance and deception in children and adults: Are leaders the best misleaders? *Personality and Social Psychology Bulletin, 20,* 312–321.

Kelly, A. E. (2000). Helping construct desirable identities: A self-presentational view of psychotherapy. *Psychological Bulletin, 126,* 475–494.

Kowalski, R. M., & Leary, M. R. (1990). Strategic self-presentation and the avoidance of aversive events: Antecedents and consequences of self-enhancement and self-depreciation. *Journal of Experimental Social Psychology, 26,* 322–336.

Leary, M. R. (1983). *Understanding social anxiety: Social, personality, and clinical perspectives.* Beverly Hills, CA: Sage.

Leary, M. R. (1986). The impact of interactional impediments on social anxiety and self-presentation. *Journal of Experimental Social Psychology, 22,* 122–135.

Leary, M. R. (1992). Self-presentational processes in exercise and sport. *Journal of Sport and Exercise Psychology, 14,* 339–351.

Leary, M. R. (1995). *Self-presentation: Impression management and interpersonal behavior.* Madison, WI: Brown & Benchmark.

Leary, M. R., & Baumeister, R. F. (2000). The nature and function of self-esteem: Sociometer theory. In M. Zanna (Ed.), *Advances in experimental social psychology* (Vol. 32, pp. 1–62). San Diego, CA: Academic Press.

Leary, M. R., & Kowalski, R. M. (1990). Impression management: A literature review and two-component model. *Psychological Bulletin, 107,* 34–47.

Leary, M. R., & Kowalski, R. M. (1995). *Social anxiety.* New York: Guilford Press.

Leary, M. R., Nezlek, J. B., Downs, D., Radford-Davenport, J., Martin, J., & McMullen, A. (1994). Self-presentation in everyday interactions: Effects of target familiarity and gender composition. *Journal of Personality and Social Psychology, 67,* 664–673.

Leary, M. R., Tchividjian, L. R., & Kraxberger, B. E. (1994). Self-presentation can be hazardous to your health: Impression management and health risk. *Health Psychology, 13,* 461–470.

Lippa, R. (1976). Expressive control, expressive consistency, and the correspondence between expressive behavior and personality. *Journal of Personality, 44,* 541–559.

Lockwood, P., & Kunda, Z. (2000). Outstanding role models: Do they inspire or demoralize us? In A. Tesser, R. B. Felson, & J. M. Suls (Eds.), *Psychological perspectives on self and identity: The interpersonal context* (pp. 147–171). Washington, DC: American Psychological Association.

Martin, K. A., & Leary, M. R. (1999). Would you drink after a stranger? The influence of self-presentational motives on willingness to take a health risk. *Personality and Social Psychology Bulletin, 25,* 1092–1100.

McCall, G. J., & Simmons, J. F. (1978). *Identities and interactions* (2nd ed.). New York: Free Press.

McCormack, S. A., & Levine, T. R. (1990). When lovers become leery: The relationship between suspiciousness and accuracy in detecting deception. *Communication Monographs, 57,* 219–230.

McGraw, K. M. (1991). Managing blame: An experimental test of the effects of political accounts. *American Political Science Review, 85,* 1133–1157.

McHoskey, J. W., Worzel, W., & Szyarto, C. (1998). Machiavellianism and psychopathy. *Journal of Personality and Social Psychology, 74,* 192–210.

McKillop, K. J., Jr., Berzonsky, M. D., & Schlenker, B. R. (1992). The impact of self-presentations on self-beliefs: Effects of social identity and self-presentational context. *Journal of Personality, 60,* 789–808.

McLaughlin, M. L., Cody, M. J., & Read, S. J. (Eds.). (1992). *Explaining one's self to others: Reason-giving in a social context.* Hillsdale, NJ: Erlbaum.

Mead, G. H. (1934). *Mind, self, and society.* Chicago: University of Chicago Press.

Miller, R. S. (1996). *Embarrassment: Poise and peril in everyday life.* New York: Guilford Press.

Murray, S. L., Holmes, J. G., & Griffin, D. W. (1996a). The benefits of positive illusions: Idealization and the construction of satisfaction in close relationships. *Journal of Personality and Social Psychology, 70,* 79–98.

Murray, S. L., Holmes, J. G., & Griffin, D. W. (1996b). The self-fulfilling nature of positive illusions in romantic relationships: Love is not blind, but prescient. *Journal of Personality and Social Psychology, 71,* 1155–1180.

Nowak, A., Szamrej, J., & Latané, B. (1990). From private attitude to public opinion: A dynamic theory of social impact. *Psychological Review, 97,* 362–376.

Ohbuchi, K., Kameda, M., & Agarie, N. (1989). Apology as aggression control: Its role in mediating appraisal of and response to harm. *Journal of Personality and Social Psychology, 56,* 219–227.

Paulhus, D. L. (1988, August). *Automatic and controlled self-presentation.* Paper presented at the meeting of the American Psychological Association, Atlanta, GA.

Paulhus, D. L. (1991). Measurement and control of response bias. In J. P. Robinson, P. R. Shaver, & L. S. Wrightsman (Eds.), *Measures of personality and social psychological attitudes* (pp. 17–59). San Diego, CA: Academic Press.

Paulhus, D. L. (1993). Bypassing the will: The automatization of affirmations. In D. M. Wegener & J. W. Pennebaker (Eds.), *Handbook of mental control* (pp. 573–587). Englewood Cliffs, NJ: Prentice-Hall.

Paulhus, D. L., Graf, P., & van Selst, M. (1989). Attentional load increases the positivity of self-presentation. *Social Cognition, 7,* 389–400.

Paulhus, D. L., & Levitt, K. (1987). Desirable responding triggered by affect: Automatic egotism? *Journal of Personality and Social Psychology, 52,* 245–259.

Pontari, B. A., & Schlenker, B. R. (2000). The influence of cognitive load on self-presentation: Can cognitive busyness help as well as harm social performance? *Journal of Personality and Social Psychology, 78,* 1092–1108.

Pontari, B. A., & Schlenker, B. R. (2001). *Beneficial impression management in dating couples.* Manuscript submitted for publication, University of Florida.

Rhodewalt, F., & Agustsdottir, S. (1986). The effects of self-presentation on the phenomenal self. *Journal of Personality and Social Psychology, 50,* 47–55.

Rosenfeld, P., Giacalone, R. A., & Riordan, C. A. (1995). *Impression management in organizations.* New York: Routledge.

Scher, S. J., & Darley, J. M. (1997). How effective are the things people say to apologize? Effects of the realization of the apology speech act. *Journal of Psycholinguistic Research, 26,* 127–140.

Schlenker, B. R. (1975). Self-presentation: Managing the impression of consistency when reality interferes with self-enhancement. *Journal of Personality and Social Psychology, 32,* 1030–1037.

Schlenker, B. R. (1980). *Impression management: The self-concept, social identity, and interpersonal relations.* Monterey, CA: Brooks/Cole.

Schlenker, B. R. (1982). Translating actions into attitudes: An identity-analytic approach to the explanation of social conduct. In L. Berkowitz (Ed.), *Advances in experimental social psychology* (Vol. 15, pp. 193–247). New York: Academic Press.

Schlenker, B. R. (1985). Identity and self-identification. In B. R. Schlenker (Ed.), *The self and social life* (pp. 65–99). New York: McGraw-Hill.

Schlenker, B. R. (1986). Self-identification: Toward an integration of the private and public self. In R. Baumeister

(Ed.), *Public self and private self* (pp. 21–62). New York: Springer-Verlag.

Schlenker, B. R., & Britt, T. W. (1999). Beneficial impression management: Strategically controlling information to help friends. *Journal of Personality and Social Psychology, 76,* 559–573.

Schlenker, B. R., & Britt, T. W. (2001). Strategically controlling information to help friends: Effects of empathy and friendship strength on beneficial impression management. *Journal of Experimental Social Psychology, 37,* 357–372.

Schlenker, B. R., Britt, T. W., & Pennington, J. (1996). Impression regulation and management: Highlights of a theory of self-identification. In R. M. Sorrentino & E. T. Higgins (Eds.), *Handbook of motivation and cognition: Vol. 3. The interpersonal context* (pp. 118–147). New York: Guilford Press.

Schlenker, B. R., & Darby, B. W. (1981). The use of apologies in social predicaments. *Social Psychology Quarterly, 44,* 271–278.

Schlenker, B. R., Dlugolecki, D. W., & Doherty, K. J. (1994). The impact of self-presentations on self-appraisals and behaviors: The power of public commitment. *Personality and Social Psychology Bulletin, 20,* 20–33.

Schlenker, B. R., & Leary, M. R. (1982a). Audiences' reactions to self-enhancing, self-denigrating, and accurate self-presentations. *Journal of Experimental Social Psychology, 18,* 89–104.

Schlenker, B. R., & Leary, M. R. (1982b). Social anxiety and self-presentation: A conceptualization and model. *Psychological Bulletin, 92,* 641–669.

Schlenker, B. R. & Leary, M. R. (1985). Social anxiety and communication about the self. *Journal of Language and Social Psychology, 4,* 171–193.

Schlenker, B. R., & Pontari, B. A. (2000). The strategic control of information: Impression management and self-presentation in daily life. In A. Tesser, R. Felson, & J. Suls (Eds.), *Perspectives on self and identity* (pp. 199–232). Washington, DC: American Psychological Association.

Schlenker, B. R., Pontari, B. A., & Christopher, A. N. (2001). Excuses and character: Personal and social implications of excuses. *Personality and Social Psychology Review, 5,* 15–32.

Schlenker, B. R., & Trudeau, J. V. (1990). The impact of self-presentations on private self-beliefs: Effects of prior self-beliefs and misattribution. *Journal of Personality and Social Psychology, 58,* 22–32.

Schlenker, B. R., & Weigold, M. F. (1989). Goals and the self-identification process. In L. Pervin (Ed.), *Goals concepts in personality and social psychology* (pp. 243–290). Hillsdale, NJ: Erlbaum.

Schlenker, B. R., & Weigold, M. F. (1990). Self-consciousness and self-presentation: Being autonomous versus appearing autonomous. *Journal of Personality and Social Psychology, 59,* 820–828.

Schlenker, B. R., & Weigold, M. F. (1992). Interpersonal processes involving impression regulation and management. *Annual Review of Psychology, 43,* 133–168.

Schlenker, B. R., Weigold, M. F., & Doherty, K. (1991). Coping with accountability: Self-identification and evaluative reckonings. In C. R. Snyder & D. R. Forsyth (Eds.), *Handbook of social and clinical psychology* (pp. 96–115). New York: Pergamon.

Schuetz, A., Richter, K., Koehler, M., & Schiepek, G. (1997). Self-presentation in client–therapist interaction: A single case study. *Journal of Social and Clinical Psychology, 16,* 440–462.

Schwartz, G. S., Kane, T. R., Joseph, J. M., & Tedeschi, J. T. (1978). The effects of post-transgression remorse on perceived aggression, attributions of intent, and level of punishment. *British Journal of Social and Clinical Psychology, 17,* 293–297.

Shepperd, J. A., & Arkin, R. M. (1991). Behavioral other-enhancement: Strategically obscuring the link between performance and evaluation. *Journal of Personality and Social Psychology, 60,* 79–88.

Shepperd, J. A., & Socherman, R. E. (1997). On the manipulative behavior of low Machiavellians: Feigning incompetence to "sandbag" an opponent. *Journal of Personality and Social Psychology, 72,* 1448–1459.

Singer, J. A., & Salovey, P. (1993). *The remembered self: Emotion and memory in personality.* New York: Free Press.

Snyder, C. R., & Higgins, R. L. (1988). Excuses: Their effective role in the negotiation of reality. *Psychological Bulletin, 104,* 23–25.

Snyder, C. R., Higgins, R. L., & Stucky, R. J. (1983). *Excuses: Masquerades in search of grace.* New York: Wiley.

Snyder, M. (1987). *Public appearances/private realities: The psychology of self-monitoring.* San Francisco: Freeman.

Stevens, C. K., & Kristof, A. L. (1995). Making the right impression: A field study of applicant impression management during job interviews. *Journal of Applied Psychology, 80,* 587–606.

Swann, W. B., Jr. (1983). Self-verification: Bringing social reality into harmony with the self. In J. Suls & A. G. Greenwald (Eds.), *Psychological perspectives on the self* (Vol. 2, pp. 33–66). Hillsdale, NJ: Erlbaum.

Swann, W. B., Jr., Stein-Seroussi, A., & Giesler, R. B. (1992). Why people self-verify. *Journal of Personality and Social Psychology, 62,* 392–401.

Tangney, J. P., Miller, R. S., Flicker, L., & Barlow, D. H. (1996). Are shame, guilt, and embarrassment distinct emotions? *Journal of Personality and Social Psychology, 70,* 1256–1269.

Tedeschi, J. T. (Ed.). (1981). *Impression management: Theory and social psychological research.* New York: Academic Press.

Tedeschi, J. T., & Norman, N. (1985). Social power, self-presentation, and the self. In B. R. Schlenker (Ed.), *The self in social life* (pp. 293–321). New York: McGraw-Hill.

Tedeschi, J. T., & Riess, M. (1981). Predicaments and verbal tactics of impression management. In C. Antaki (Ed.), *Ordinary language explanations of social behavior* (pp. 271–309). London: Academic Press.

Tesser, A. (1988). Toward a self-evaluation maintenance model of social behavior. In L. Berkowitz (Ed.), *Advances in experimental social psychology* (Vol. 21, pp. 181–227). New York: Academic Press.

Tetlock, P. E., & Manstead, A. S. R. (1985). Impression management versus intrapsychic explanations in social psychology: A useful dichotomy? *Psychological Review, 92,* 59–77.

Tice, D. M. (1992). Self-concept change and self-presentation: The looking glass self is also a magnifying glass. *Journal of Personality and Social Psychology, 63,* 435–451.

Tice, D. M., Butler, J. L., Muraven, M. B., & Stillwell, A. M. (1995). When modesty prevails: Differential favorability of self-presentation to friends and strangers. *Journal of Personality and Social Psychology, 69,* 1120–1138.

Toris, C., & DePaulo, B. M. (1984). Effects of actual deception and suspiciousness of deception on interpersonal perceptions. *Journal of Personality and Social Psychology, 47,* 1063–1073.

Vonk, R. (1998). The slime effect: Suspicion and dislike of likeable behavior toward superiors. *Journal of Personality and Social Psychology, 74,* 849–864.

Wayne, S. J., & Kacmar, K. M. (1991). The effects of impression management on the performance appraisal process. *Organizational Behavior and Human Decision Processes, 48,* 70–88.

Wayne, S. J., Kacmar, K. M., & Ferris, G. R. (1995).

Coworkers response to others' ingratiation attempts. *Journal of Managerial Issues, 7,* 277–289.

Weiner, B., Figueroa-Munoz, A., & Kakihara, C. (1991). The goals of excuses and communication strategies related to causal perceptions. *Personality and Social Psychology Bulletin, 17,* 4–13.

Weiner, B., Graham, S., Peter, O., & Zmuidinas, M. (1991). Public confession and forgiveness. *Journal of Personality, 59,* 281–312.

Wilson, D. S., Near, D., & Miller, R. R. (1996). Machiavellianism: A synthesis of the evolutionary and psychological literatures. *Psychological Bulletin, 119,* 285–299.

Wooten, D. B., & Reed, A., II. (2000). A conceptual overview of the self-presentational concerns and response tendencies of focus group participants. *Journal of Consumer Psychology, 9,* 141–153.

Zanna, M. P., & Pack, S. J. (1975). On the self-fulfilling nature of apparent sex differences in behavior. *Journal of Experimental Social Psychology, 11,* 583–591.

26

Interpersonal Self-Regulation: Lessons from the Study of Narcissism

FREDERICK RHODEWALT
DEBORAH L. SORROW

It has been over a century since Havelock Ellis (1898) introduced the term "Narcissus-like" into the vernacular of clinical psychology, and Freud's seminal essay (1914/1953) on early development and narcissistic investment in the self is now over three quarters of a century old. The ensuing years have produced a voluminous clinical literature on narcissism. As Pulver (1970) observed, the concept of narcissism is one of the most important contributions of psychoanalysis; however, it is also one of the most confusing. In this chapter, we describe a social cognitive self-regulatory process model of narcissism (Morf & Rhodewalt, 2001a, 2001b; Rhodewalt, 1993, 2001) and present supporting evidence. It is our contention that much of the confusion concerning narcissism is reduced when it is viewed in terms of a set of coherent cognitive, motivational, and interpersonal self-regulatory processes rather than as a "trait-like" behavioral syndrome (Morf & Rhodewalt, 2001a). We also suggest that our process model of narcissism has the potential to inform basic research on the self and interpersonal behav-

ior. Elsewhere (Rhodewalt, 2001), we have compared our approach to the metaphor of the "isotope" technique in medical diagnosis. In medicine, radioactive material is injected into the patient's body and then tracked in order to determine how specific bodily systems are functioning. In research on the social construction and maintenance of the self, individual differences in narcissism serve as indicators of ego involvement, reactivity to social feedback, and sensitivity to social context. We suggest that narcissism (as well as many other social-cognitive individual differences), therefore, can be used by self-researchers in the same way that radioactive isotopes are used by physicians—to examine functioning of specific psychological systems.

We begin with a brief overview of the clinical perspective on narcissism and then describe the model that has guided and been shaped by our research. This is followed by a review of recent research produced in our and others' laboratories. We conclude by suggesting additional hypotheses and highlighting directions for future research.

The Clinical Perspective on Narcissism: Pathological Self-Love

For most of its history, the discussion of narcissism has taken place in the psychodynamic arena, and the focus has been on the developmental antecedents of adult pathology.[1] Although the debate has been lively, it has failed to generate a systematic and coherent research agenda. This situation is attributable, in part, to the fact that until recently the field has been unable to agree on a definition of the construct. Nonetheless, a brief overview of the psychoanalytic perspective is in order because it has so richly stimulated our model.

Freud (1914/1953) described two forms of narcissism: primary and secondary. He proposed that infants start life with an undifferentiated ego–id, which he termed "autoeroticism." When the ego begins to differentiate from the id, libido attaches to the ego. This phase, known as primary narcissism, is characterized by an "overvaluation of the ego" (Westen, 1990, p. 185). As development continues, some libido detaches from the ego and attaches to external objects, resulting in object love. Under certain pathological circumstances, libido detaches from these objects and reattaches to the ego, creating a phase of secondary narcissism (Chessick, 1987).

Freud's theory of narcissism has been expanded on and modified by Hans Kohut and Otto Kernberg, the two most influential theorists in the area. Kohut (1971) defines narcissism as "the libidinal investment in the self" (p. 243) and proposes that healthy adult narcissism is transformed into such beneficial phenomena as humor, art, wisdom, empathy, and acceptance of one's own mortality. He suggests that it also provides individuals with a healthy enjoyment of their own activities, adaptive disappointment at failure, and a sense of direction and goal orientedness.

Although Kohut embraced Freud's ideas of the normality and beneficial nature of some forms of narcissism, Kohut (1971) proposed a different view of its development. He suggested that narcissistic development was independent of the development of object love; pathological narcissism results from a developmental arrest of this normal system. The child's self develops and gains maturity through interactions with others (primarily the mother) that provide the child with opportunities to be mirrored (gain affirmation, approval, and enhancement) and to idealize (identify with perfect and omnipotent others). Empathic parents contribute to the healthy development of the self in two ways. First, they provide mirroring that fosters a more realistic sense of self by allowing the child to see his or her own imperfections reflected during interactions with the parent. Second, parents reveal limitations in themselves, thus disappointing the child. In order to deal with this disappointment, the child internalizes the idealized image, gaining a personal set of ideals and values. Things run awry when the parent is unempathic and fails to provide appropriate mirroring and idealization opportunities. The resulting arrested development leaves children trapped in an infantile way of relating to the world, in which they seem to expect the world to fulfill all their needs and desires. However, this apparent grandiosity and invulnerability masks a core of emptiness and isolation. Narcissists cannot satisfy their own needs or maintain their senses of self without external support; thus, they are overly dependent on other individuals to fulfill their needs for mirroring (Kohut, 1971).

Kernberg (1976) paints a portrait of the narcissist as fragile and defensive. In his view, as toddlers move from primary narcissism to object love, they may take a pathological turn if they fail to differentiate themselves from their mothers because of maternal rejection or abandonment of the child. Kernberg contends that narcissism arises from the child's reaction to a cold and unempathic mother. This "emotionally hungry" child is enraged by his parents and comes to view them as even more depriving. Narcissism in this view is a *defense* reflecting the child's attempt to take refuge in some aspect of the self that his parents valued. This defense results in a grandiose sense of self. Perceived weaknesses in the self are "split" off into a separate hidden self. The child becomes frustrated and reverts to his or her earlier narcissism. Pathological narcissism is therefore a fixation, a distortion of a normal developmental period, not simply the halting of a normal process (Manfield, 1992). Because of this distortion of normal infantile narcissism, the individual is unable to differentiate his actual self-representations, ideal self-representations, and ideal object representations, and his lack of self-knowledge causes him to depend on others for his sense of self (Raskin & Terry, 1988). Although they differ in many respects, Kernberg and Kohut both describe individuals with a childhood history of unsatisfactory social relationships who, as adults, possess *self-concepts* incorporating grandiose views of the self that embody a conflicted psychological dependence on others.

One may argue that this clinical debate, although stimulating and lively, has impeded the field's ability to arrive at a consensual definition of the disorder, which, in turn, has retarded the development of systematic research programs. This circumstance appears to have been remedied by the inclusion of narcissism as a diagnostic category in the 1980 edition of the *Diagnostic and Statistical Manual of Mental Disorders* (American Psychiatric Association, 1980 [DSM-III], 1987 [DSM-III-R]). According to the most recent edition, DSM-IV-TR (American Psychiatric Association, 2000), narcissism involves a pervasive pattern of grandiosity, self-importance, and perceived uniqueness. Narcissists are preoccupied with fantasies of unlimited success, wealth, beauty, and power. They are exhibitionistic and require attention and admiration from others while responding to criticism or threat to self-esteem with feelings of rage, shame, or humiliation. In addition, there is a set of characteristics that collectively contribute to interpersonal difficulties. For example, narcissists display entitlement and expect special treatment from others without the need to reciprocate. They also are exploitative of others. They tend to have relationships that oscillate between idealization and devaluation. Finally, narcissists are either unable or unwilling to empathize with others. According to the DSM-IV, in narcissism, "self-esteem is almost invariably very fragile; the person may be preoccupied with how well he or she is doing and how well he or she is regarded by others. . . . In response to criticism, he or she may react with rage, shame, or humiliation" (p. 350). The picture of narcissism that emerges is one of an individual who is invested in re-

ceiving, if not creating, attention, positive regard, and admiration from others and who experiences intense emotions to such input.

Although there is agreement about narcissism's defining characteristics, discussion continues about how these characteristics combine. Are there healthy versus pathological narcissists, as suggested by some (cf. Wink, 1991), or do narcissists possess both overt (perhaps healthy) and covert (perhaps unhealthy) characteristics, as suggested by others (cf. Akhtar & Thompson, 1982)? We return to these issues later in describing our model and supporting research. However, we believe that headway can be gained in understanding the dynamics of narcissism by focusing on its core components. In this respect, we concur with Westen's (1990) conclusion that narcissism should be strictly defined as "a cognitive-affective preoccupation with the self, where 'cognitive preoccupation' refers to a focus of attention on the self; 'affective preoccupation' refers to a preoccupation with one's own needs, wishes, goals, ambitions, glory, superiority, or perfection; and 'self' refers to the whole person, including one's subjective experience, actions, body" (p. 227).

Another benefit of the publication of the DSM diagnostic criteria is the development of a number of "face valid" narcissism scales. Among these scales, the Narcissistic Personality Inventory (NPI; Raskin & Hall, 1979; see Emmons, 1987; Raskin & Terry, 1988; Rhodewalt & Morf, 1995) has received the most research attention and is the one used almost exclusively in our research. Raskin and Hall (1979) based the NPI on DSM criteria for narcissistic personality disorder. Factor analyses of the NPI (Emmons, 1984, 1987) indicate that it consists of four moderately correlated factors: Leadership/Authority, Self-Absorption/Self-Admiration, Superiority/Arrogance, and Exploitiveness/Entitlement.[2] Prifitera and Ryan (1984) reported that narcissistic and nonnarcissistic psychiatric patients could be distinguished on the basis of their NPI scores, suggesting that the scale does indeed capture pathological narcissism. NPI scores in the less extreme range are thought to reflect narcissism as a personality trait, albeit a multifaceted one.

The NPI is associated with egocentrism

and self-focus (Emmons, 1987), hostility (Rhodewalt & Morf, 1995), aggression, dominance, exhibitionism, and self-centeredness (Raskin & Terry, 1988), all of which are characteristics of pathological narcissism. However, although it is plausible to assume that the model described in this chapter characterizes both trait and pathological narcissism, the empirical support comes primarily from individuals best described as exhibiting the narcissistic personality type.

The Self-Regulatory Processing Model of Narcissism

The portrait of narcissism that arises from the clinical literature is one of paradoxes (Morf & Rhodewalt, 2001a, 2001b). How can the self simultaneously be grandiose and fragile, positive but hypersensitive to criticism? Why are narcissists so reliant on the positive regard of others but so insensitive and abusive toward those on whom they rely? We believe that by viewing narcissism within a self-regulatory processing framework, one may begin to understand the underlying coherence of the construct and, thus, begin to unravel these paradoxes. The model is very indebted to contemporary social and personality perspectives on the self (Cantor, 1990; Higgins, 1996; Mischel & Shoda, 1995), but it is also beholden to earlier psychoanalytic views on narcissistic processes, particularly those of Annie Reich (1960), who argued that the narcissistic defect is an inability of a mature ego to test reality and develop an accurate sense of self. In her view, the narcissist engages in a pathological form of self-esteem regulation wherein the narcissist must chronically perform compensatory self-inflation in order to support a megalomanic self-image.

Our model portrays narcissists as individuals who possess transient, overblown, and fragile self-images that are dependent on social validation and social context or situation. The model is dynamic and recursive in that narcissistic self-esteem regulation is shaped and guided by ongoing and changing self-concerns and social contexts. Self-concerns guide behaviors that shape social context. Social context, in turn, makes salient, intensifies, or redirects current self-concerns. Finally, we view the "narcissistic self" as sharing a similar organization and function with the "normal self." Thus the study of narcissism should inform our understanding of social self-construction and interpersonal behavior among "normal" individuals.

The model, displayed in Figure 26.1, depicts the narcissistic self as comprised of three interacting units: self-knowledge, interpersonal strategies, and intrapersonal processes. We refer to these three units collectively as the narcissistic self-system. The narcissistic self-concept incorporates both the cognitive and affective or evaluative components of the self. It contains what is known about the self, the Jamesian "me." This "cognitive self" component (Linville & Carlston, 1994) is the mental repository of autobiographical information, reflected appraisals, self-ascribed traits and competencies, and self-schemata, including possible selves, self-with-others, and undesired selves. It also contains the attendant evaluations of what is known about the self or, collectively, self-esteem. The model addresses both the valence and stability of self-esteem.

The narcissistic self-concept interconnects with the social environment through a set of self-regulatory units that include both intra- and interpersonal strategies enacted to protect or enhance positive self-views. Narcissists are active manipulators of the social feedback both at the point of its generation (interpersonal regulation) and at the point of its interpretation (intrapersonal regulation). Intrapersonal strategies include distorted interpretations of outcomes and selective recall of past events. Interpersonal regulation covers a multitude of self-presentational gambits and social manipulations, also in the service of engineering positive feedback or blunting negative feedback about the self. We have found that the model has heuristic value in terms of focusing questions and guiding research. However, it should be evident that the elements are neither discrete nor static entities but, rather, personality process units that intertwine and interact with one another. Finally, the model depicted in Figure 26.1 includes both uni- and bidirectional influences. The unidirectional relations are meant to suggest that the preponderance of influence is in one di-

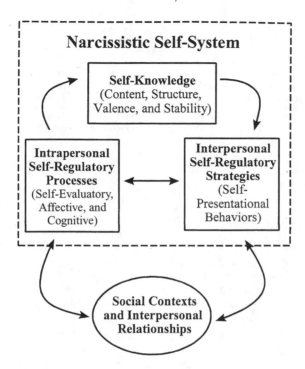

FIGURE 26.1. Self-regulatory processing model of narcissism. Data from Morf and Rhodewalt (2001a) and Rhodewalt (2001).

rection or another. Bidirectional relations indicate a more equally reciprocal and recursive set of transactions between components.

The Narcissistic Self-Concept

If narcissism at its core reflects a cognitive–affective preoccupation with the self, a central question asks, What is the nature of this self with which narcissists are so preoccupied? We have attempted to address this question by examining narcissistic self-concept content and structure through the lens of contemporary personality and social-cognitive theories and methodologies. Our research has been guided by clinical descriptions of the narcissistic self-concept, and our goal has been to characterize the self-system within the self-regulatory processing model. Most clinical observers suggest that the self-concepts of narcissists lack coherence and stability while being heavily imbued with affect. Akhtar and Thompson (1982) include in their description of the clinical features of narcissism a self-concept that is overtly

grandiose while covertly fragile and fraught with feelings of inferiority and worthlessness. They describe a narcissistic cognitive style that overtly reveals an egocentric perception of reality and covertly evidences inattention to objective aspects of events, subtle gaps in memory, and the tendency to change the meaning of reality when self-esteem is threatened. In this section, we explore these aspects of the narcissistic self-system by discussing four key questions.

Is the Narcissistic Self Positive?

The one area in which clinical observation and empirical evidence clearly agree is that narcissists project self-aggrandizing, positive views of the self. Across a number of studies using a variety of measures of self-evaluation, NPI-defined narcissism is consistently associated with high self-esteem (Emmons, 1984, 1987; Kernis & Sun, 1994; Morf & Rhodewalt, 1993; Raskin, Novacek, & Hogan, 1991; Raskin & Terry, 1988; Rhodewalt, Madrian, & Cheney, 1998; Rhodewalt & Morf, 1995, 1998;

Watson, Taylor, & Morris, 1987). For example, Rhodewalt and Morf (1995) reported that across a group of measures, NPI-defined narcissists claimed self-views that were more positive and about which they reported being more certain than did less narcissistic persons. The reader should note that these results apply only to NPI-defined narcissism and were collected in situations largely devoid of threats to the self. We return to the issue of narcissistic self-evaluations under threat in a subsequent section.

Is the Narcissistic Self Grandiose and Inflated?

One might argue that narcissists' high opinions of themselves represent an accurate reading of their accomplishments and regard from others rather than inflated, unrealistic perceptions of self. However, several studies suggest that narcissistic self-conceptions are inflated and grandiose relative to "objective" reality. For example, Rhodewalt and Eddings (2002) had men who were high and low on NPI interact with a woman via telephone for the ostensible purpose of a future date. Unknown to the men, the woman's responses were completely scripted. In essence, all men experienced the identical social interaction. Nonetheless, narcissistic men reported that the woman liked them more and thought that she would rate their personalities more positively than did less narcissistic men. Other findings indicate that narcissists overestimate their attractiveness and intelligence (Gabriel, Critelli, & Ee, 1994), their contributions to a group task (John & Robins, 1994; Robins & Beer, 2001), and their academic performance (Farwell & Wohlwend-Lloyd, 1998; Robins & Beer, 2001) relative to less narcissistic individuals. The answer is yes, narcissists' self-views are unrealistic and inflated.

The meaning of these inflated self-evaluations is less clear. At the heart of the issue is whether these positive self-evaluations reflect a true sense of high self-worth or an expression of defensiveness. In an attempt to examine this issue directly, Raskin, Novacek, and Hogan (1991) asked participants to complete measures of narcissism, self-esteem, and thought to tap defensive self-enhancement. Defensive self-enhancement had two forms: grandiosity (the need to be admired and adored) and social desirability (the need for the approval of others). Narcissism was related to grandiosity but not to social desirability. In other words, narcissists' positive self-descriptions reflect a desire to be admired but not necessarily to be liked. Raskin and colleagues note that "according to most clinical accounts, grandiosity involves two contradictory belief systems, namely an aggrandized version of the self (ideal self) and a self that corresponds to actual experience (actual self). Moreover, when threatened with failure, the grandiose person tends inconspicuously to adopt a posture consistent with his or her aggrandized self" (p. 33).

Is the Narcissistic Self "Disordered"?

Is there something about the structure or function of the narcissistic self-concept that necessitates these individuals' obsession with acquiring positive social feedback? It is possible that narcissists turn to social feedback as an on-line repository of self-knowledge because their self-concepts, although globally positive, are not as readily accessible or efficiently structured as are the self-concepts of less narcissistic individuals. This is an important question because, if such a difference were observed, it would suggest the fundamental flaw that drives the self-regulatory system. Our laboratory has conducted a number of investigations in which the goal was to uncover how the narcissistic self might be deficient.

In these investigations, we tested the notion that narcissists' self-conceptions are less accessible and less confidently held than are those of less narcissistic individuals. In short, something is lacking. According to this notion, narcissists' positive self-conceptions are poorly formed, unstable, and not as automatically accessible as they are in others. Consequently, it would follow that narcissists would be more reliant on and reactive to social and contextual feedback about their worth.

Although not exhaustive, our research on the question of deficits in narcissistic self-conceptions permits us to conclude that self-knowledge appears to be no more nor less accessible in narcissists than it is in other individuals. In a series of studies, Tschanz and Rhodewalt (2001) recorded reaction times for making me–not me judgments about trait descriptors. For example, in one study, we primed self-judgments with retrieval of either autobiographical information ("Have you behaved in a friendly way in the past month?") or social reputation information ("Does your mother think you're friendly?"). There were no effects for level of narcissism in any of these studies. Narcissists were neither faster nor slower to make unprimed self-judgments, and they were not differentially responsive to the effects of priming.

In short, we have been unable to find evidence to support the idea that narcissistic self-representations are deficient or unique. Self-knowledge appears to be as accessible among narcissists as among others. Moreover, they report being confident and certain of their self-evaluations. However, there is one potentially important qualification to these conclusions. All of these results have been generated in relatively uninvolving and nonthreatening testing situations. Given our speculation that the narcissistic self is highly context dependent and vulnerable to threat, it may be that cognitive elements of the self would be examined more sensitively across contexts and levels of threat. It may well be that the narcissistic self depicted in the clinical literature would emerge more clearly in circumstances that mirrored the clinical setting. We are currently addressing this question in our laboratory.

Our second approach has been to examine the organization of the content of narcissistic self-representations. This structural hypothesis was suggested by Robert Emmons (1987), who speculated that narcissists' self-representations may be organized such that they are low in complexity, which, in turn, accounts for the emotional lability that is a hallmark of narcissism. Emmons reported that the NPI was positively correlated with both positive and negative affect variability, consistent with his hypothesis. This hypothesis gains plausibility when one considers that differences in organization of self-knowledge have been linked to emotional reactivity (Linville, 1985). Self-complexity, an aspect of self-structure that describes the extent to which aspects of one's self-concept are differentiated, is associated with relatively stable moods compared with those with simplistic representations (Linville, 1985).

Alternatively, narcissists' self-knowledge may be more compartmentalized along positive and negative evaluative dimensions. Showers (1992a) coined the term "evaluative integration" to capture this dimension and has demonstrated that positive and negative information about the self has less emotional impact on those high in evaluative integration (low compartmentalization of good and bad self-knowledge) than on those low in evaluative integration (high compartmentalization). Showers (2000) argues that evaluative compartmentalization might be most psychologically comfortable for individuals who typically function in contexts that make accessible positive self-representations. It is only when events activate a purely negative compartment that the individual is flooded with negative evaluations and self-conceptions. Showers suggests that in such circumstances many individuals shift to a more integrated view of the self. This thinking suggests two possibilities linking narcissism, affect, and self-structure. First, narcissists may possess highly evaluatively compartmentalized self-representations. Second, they may have difficulty in shifting between compartmentalized and integrated views of the self.

We have examined the relations between self-concept structure and narcissism and, although no clear pattern that describes all narcissists has emerged, we have obtained a number of provocative findings that suggest that self-structure may moderate emotional and self-evaluative lability in some narcissists. Rhodewalt and Morf (1995, Study 1) found the predicted high NPI–low self-complexity association ($r = -.27$, $p < .05$) but have failed to replicate this association in five independent samples (Rhodewalt & Morf, 1998; Rhodewalt & Regalado, 1996; Rhodewalt et al., 1998). Likewise, we have failed to find an association between NPI-defined narcissism and low evaluative integration in three independent samples (Rhodewalt & Regalado, 1996; Rhodewalt et al., 1998). The picture is more complex, however, in that we find that evaluative integration, but not self-complexity, moderates the relation between narcissism and emotional responsiveness to social feedback. That is, although narcissism and evaluative integration are unrelated, narcissists who are also low in evaluative integration display the greatest emotional responsivity to positive and negative feedback about the self (Rhodewalt et al., 1998).

Before concluding this section, we should mention that there may be other ways in which self-concept organization is related to narcissism. Elsewhere (Rhodewalt, 2001) we have proposed that narcissists may possess selves that are highly differentiated along roles or social contexts (i.e., high self-concept differentiation; Donahue, Robins, Roberts, & John, 1993). This high differentiation might also confound the accurate assessment of self-complexity. According to Donahue and colleagues (1993), self-concept differentiation is the tendency to see oneself as possessing different traits in different social roles. Whereas high self-complexity is associated with positive outcomes and well-being, higher self-concept differentiation is related to greater intrapersonal and interpersonal distress. Self-complexity, although superficially similar to self-concept differentiation, is different in the way in which it is conceptualized and assessed. Self-concept differentiation is concerned only with an individual's sense of self in different roles, whereas self-complexity is less narrowly defined (Linville, 1985, 1987). It may be that self-complexity deals with a different level of self-structure because individuals are free to generate their own categories, thus making the measure less context dependent. There are a number of intriguing hypotheses yet to be explored; however, at present, the evidence suggests that narcissism cannot be reduced to a pathological form of underdifferentiated self-concept organization.

Is the Narcissistic Self Unstable?

As noted in the previous section, NPI-defined narcissism has been linked to emotional lability (Emmons, 1987). Is this emotional lability a general propensity to respond to events with extreme emotional reactions, or is it specific to self-related affect? Both laboratory and prospective survey studies indicate that narcissistic emotional hyperresponsiveness is specific to self-related affect, that is, self-esteem. With regard to feelings of self-worth, the narcissistic self is highly unstable (Rhodewalt et al., 1998; Rhodewalt & Morf, 1998). For

example, Rhodewalt and Morf (1998) provided participants with success and failure feedback on successive tests of intelligence. The impact of this feedback produced greater changes in the self-esteem of participants with high NPI scores than it did among participants with low NPI scores. In two daily diary studies (Rhodewalt et al., 1998), narcissists displayed greater self-esteem variability over a series of days than did less narcissistic individuals. Interestingly, in both studies, this relation was moderated by the participant's level of evaluative integration: Narcissists who were also low in evaluative integration displayed the greatest self-esteem variability. This result is compatible with Showers's (1992a, 1992b) assertion that low evaluative integration is associated with mood and self-esteem lability because external events cue self-aspects containing only positive or only negative information. This effect may be greater in narcissists because of their greater dependence on the social context for self-evaluative information.

Kernis (2002) and Rhodewalt (2001) have discussed parallels between narcissistic self-esteem instability and Kernis's research on individuals with high but unstable self-esteem. Kernis (1993) contends that high but unstable self-esteem is associated with enhanced sensitivity to evaluative events, increased concern about one's self-image, and an overreliance on social sources of evaluation. Moreover, the goal of people with high unstable self-esteem, according to Kernis, is to build more stable self-views and to enhance positive self-feelings. Thus they are especially sensitive to both positive and negative social feedback, reacting to both with more extreme affective responses than do individuals with stable self-esteem (Kernis, Cornell, Sun, Berry, & Harlow, 1993). Research also indicates that individuals with unstable high self-esteem are more hostile and angry (Kernis, Grannemann, & Barclay, 1989).

Like individuals with unstable high self-esteem, narcissists are also more likely to display antagonism toward, and a cynical mistrust of, others (Bushman & Baumeister, 1998; Rhodewalt & Morf, 1995; Ruiz, Smith, & Rhodewalt, 2001). They react to self-esteem threats by derogating the source of the threat (Morf & Rhodewalt, 1993) and devaluing the negative feedback (Kernis & Sun, 1994), while viewing positive feedback as more valid and the evaluator as more competent than do less narcissistic individuals (Kernis & Sun, 1994).

Kernis proposes that unstable self-esteem develops in individuals whose self-esteem is highly dependent on self-evaluative information from the social context. According to this view, one's self-esteem will be unstable if one encounters episodes of potentially contradictory evaluative information and if one's self-esteem is contingent on such information. Theories of narcissism also point to difficulties with interpersonal sources of evaluation and inconsistencies in the coherence of their self-concepts. Although their emphases are different, the theories of Kernberg (1976) and Kohut (1971) both argue that deficiencies in self-evaluative aspects of parent–child interactions (insufficient feedback) lay the foundation for adult narcissism. Thus narcissism and self-esteem instability may both have their origins in inconsistent or neglectful reinforcement histories that impede the development of confidently held, stable self-conceptions and require a constant vigilance for self-defining information. Kernis (2001) concludes that narcissism and unstable high self-esteem are two partially independent forms of fragile self-esteem.

The Rhodewalt and colleagues (1998) studies provide perhaps an even more illuminating finding. Not only did narcissists display greater day-to-day fluctuations in their self-esteem but also the relation between daily self-esteem and the positivity or negativity of their social interactions was significantly stronger for narcissists than it was for less narcissistic individuals. That is, narcissists' self-worth is more entrained to the quality of their most recent social interactions, whereas the self-worth of less narcissistic people is more stable and less dependent on social context.

A fascinating but perplexing aspect of narcissism is the discrepancy between the positivity of narcissists' self-conceptions and their vulnerability and reactions to perceived threat. The research described in this section has struggled with this paradox and not yet provided a complete resolution to it. One possibility is that the narcissistic self is so grounded in the ebb and flow of social interaction that it is, depending on immediate social regard, at times grandiose and at times vulnerable and threatened. That is, current self-conceptions reflect current social context. Research by Susan Andersen (Andersen & Cole, 1990; Andersen & Glassman, 1996; Andersen, Miranda, & Edwards, 2001) provides one possible explanation for how this dependency may occur. Andersen's research on transference has shown that individuals have mental representations of the significant people in their lives and that these representations are qualitatively different from individuals' representations of nonsignificant others (Andersen & Cole, 1990). When these significant-other representations are primed, it influences how individuals think of themselves by activating their mental representations of self-with-other (Hinkley & Andersen, 1996). If, as clinical theorists suggest, narcissism is a compensation for neglectful early relationships, then narcissists may possess negative self-with-other representations. The activation of these negative self-representations may help account for the instability of narcissists' self-esteem and the variability seen in their self-systems (Andersen, Miranda, & Edwards, in press).

Another way of thinking about this paradox has been suggested recently by several researchers (Brown & Bosson, 2001; Kernis, 2001; Robins, Tracy, & Shaver, 2001). Brown, Bosson, and Swann (2001) report that those with high explicit but low implicit self-esteem score higher on the NPI than people high in both types of self-esteem, and Abend, Kernis, and Hampton (2000) report that individuals with high explicit/low implicit self-esteem are more self-serving in their evaluations than are people with congruent explicit/implicit self-esteem. The prediction then would be that at a conscious level narcissists hold positive self-views; the vulnerability lies at an emotional nonverbal level. This is an interesting hypothesis, but one that requires additional research.

To summarize, the narcissistic self-concept is highly positive and inflated in that it is not closely tied to objective measures of accomplishment or social regard. Narcissists' self-concepts are similar to less narcissistic individuals' with respect to the cognitive dimensions of accessibility and structural organization. At the same time, their self-esteem is highly unstable and closely entrained to moment-to-moment perceived social regard, and this instability may be reflective of narcissists' self- and other representations or the difference in their explicit and implicit self-esteem.

Narcissism and Intra- and Interpersonal Self-Regulation

The model displayed in Figure 26.1 contains two elements that bridge narcissists' self-concepts and their social environments. In "social intelligence" terms (Cantor, 1994; Cantor & Kihlstrom, 1987), these elements contain the strategies that narcissists bring to bear on the life tasks of self-concept maintenance, protection, and enhancement. One element contains the interpersonal strategies that narcissists employ to channel their social interactions so as to elicit social feedback that sustains their self-views or meets current identity concerns. The other element is the repository of intrapersonal processes through which interpersonal feedback is embellished, distorted, or defended against. The reader will note that the two elements are reciprocally related in the model. This indicates that interpretations guide interpersonal strategy selection and that interpersonal strategies shape interpretations. It also suggests that the distinction between intra- and interpersonal processes is not always clearly defined. Often, interpersonal strategies are in the service of intrapersonal needs or share intrapersonal components.

Intra- and interpersonal self-regulatory processes are the machinery by which narcissists pursue identity goals through their social interactions. A major assumption of the model is that these self-regulatory processes are self-perpetuating in that they are only partially successful. These processes help sustain positive self-images but also fuel the vulnerabilities and interpersonal difficulties that are central to the narcissistic syndrome. The combination of intra- and interpersonal processes define the narcissistic personality in our model (Morf & Rhodewalt, 2001a).

Interpersonal Self-Regulation

Research has identified differences between narcissists and less narcissistic individuals in their use of a number of interpersonal strategies (Morf, 1994). These interpersonal strategies serve to manipulate others' impressions of, or to reduce threat to, the self. The most pervasively employed strategy is self-promotion or self-aggrandizement. To illustrate this point, Morf (1994) instructed participants who were high or low in NPI scores to interact with another individual with the goal of getting that individual to like them. Relative to participants with low NPI scores, participants with high NPI scores employed significantly more self-aggrandizing and fewer self-effacing and approval-seeking statements. Independent coders who rated audiotapes of the conversations formed more negative impressions of narcissists than of less narcissistic participants.

Further evidence of interpersonal self-esteem regulation comes from a study of narcissism and the use of self-evaluation maintenance behaviors (Morf & Rhodewalt, 1993). Self-evaluation maintenance behaviors (SEM; Tesser, 1988) involve many aspects, one of which is thinking about and relating to psychologically close others in ways that enhance or maintain positive self-evaluations. The intent of the Morf and Rhodewalt (1993) study was to explore the extent to which narcissists would engage in self-esteem-protective acts at the expense of others. Of particular interest to Morf and Rhodewalt were individuals' responses to feeling threatened by comparison with a close other. On those occasions, most individuals will do something to reduce the comparison or threat. One avenue of threat reduction is to devalue or derogate the friend on some other dimension. Morf and Rhodewalt believed that narcissists would be especially likely to engage in this form of self-evaluation maintenance because of their sense of entitlement and tendency to be exploitive of others. Threat was manipulated by having participants either slightly or substantially outperformed on an ego-relevant task. They then had the opportunity to make personality evaluations of the person who outperformed them. Cross-cutting the relative performance manipulation was a manipulation of the publicity of the personality evaluation; half of the participants believed that the evaluation was anonymous and unseen by the target, and half believed that they would have to provide their evaluations to the target in a face-to-face interaction. As expected, narcissists were more negative in their views of threatening others (compared with a nonthreatening control target). Although threatened narcissists' public evaluations of the target were not as negative as their private evaluations, the public face-to-face feedback given by narcissists was significantly more negative than the feedback offered by low-threat narcissists and high- and low-threat low narcissists in other public conditions.

The Morf (1994) and Morf and Rhodewalt (1993) findings are important because they illustrate the pathways by which narcissistic concern for the self translates into the disturbed interpersonal relationships characteristic of the narcissistic syndrome. Two additional findings support this conclusion. Rhodewalt and Morf (1998) reported that narcissists respond to threatening feedback with anger, a finding reminiscent of the "narcissistic rage" so prevalent in the clinical literature, and Bushman and Baumeister (1998) found that narcissists respond to threat with greater interpersonal aggression than do less narcissistic individuals. This anger and aggression may represent a devaluation of the source of the threatening feedback and therefore of the feedback itself. This devaluation protects the narcissistic self, but only at the expense of positive and stable interpersonal relationships.

Narcissists also engage in self-handicapping behavior more routinely than do less narcissistic people (Rhodewalt, Tragakis, & Finnerty, 2000). Self-handicaps are impediments to success created by the individual in anticipation of performing (Jones & Berglas, 1978) and serve both self-protective and self-presentational functions. The self-handicap permits one to externalize failure and claim added credit for success. However, other research has found that observers do not like self-handicappers (Rhodewalt, Sanbonmatsu, Feick, Tschanz, & Waller, 1995). Thus narcissists' propensity to engage in self-handicapping is likely to contribute to strained interpersonal relationships.

In sum, there is accumulating evidence that narcissists are actively engaged in manipulating their social interactions in an attempt to generate positive or at least nonthreatening information about the self.

However, these efforts are in the service of being admired rather than adored (Morf, Ansara, & Shia, 2000), and they have the effect of eroding the quality of the very relationships on which they are so reliant. The inevitable result is that narcissists' manipulations of their social interactions ultimately fail to accomplish the goal of positive social affirmation.

Intrapersonal Self-Regulation

Narcissists' interpersonal behaviors and related social reactions feed back on the self through a set of intrapersonal processes that include cognitive, affective, and motivational self-regulatory components. Collectively, these intrapersonal processes contribute to self-enhancing distortions of the meaning of behavioral and social feedback. This argument is supported by the clinical view of the narcissistic self-concept and cognitive style as having inflated self-regard and an egocentric perception of reality (Akhtar & Thompson, 1982).

We have already cited evidence of positive distortion in narcissistic self-evaluations (Gabriel et al, 1994; John & Robins, 1994; Rhodewalt & Eddings, 2002; Rhodewalt & Morf, 1995;). However, it has also been noted that these positive evaluations are undergirded by defensiveness, as well as genuine self-regard (Raskin et al., 1991), and that these positive self-evaluations are unstable and vulnerable to threatening social contexts (Rhodewalt et al., 1998). There is an inconsistency then between what narcissists say about themselves and the defensiveness with which they react to threatening feedback. This inconsistency may be understood by a closer examination of the processes by which narcissists understand their outcomes and the reactions they get from others.

Recent research suggests that the core narcissistic intrapersonal strategy is to make self-aggrandizing attributions for positive outcomes even when those outcomes are attributable to nonperson causes. This strategy is demonstrated most clearly in studies that provide participants with response noncontingent success feedback and then ask them to interpret the meaning of the feedback. Narcissistic participants consistently attribute such feedback to superior ability, compared with less narcissistic participants (Rhodewalt & Morf, 1998; Rhodewalt, Tragakis, & Finnerty, 2000). There is also evidence that these laboratory findings reflect a more pervasive self-aggrandizing attributional style. Using an adapted form of the Attributional Style Questionnaire (Peterson et al., 1982), Rhodewalt and Morf (1995) found that, although narcissists externalized bad outcomes no more than did others, they made more self-aggrandizing attributions for hypothetical successes than did individuals low in narcissism.

Elsewhere we have suggested that this self-aggrandizing attributional style has profound implications for narcissistic self-conceptions, affect, and interpersonal behavior (Morf & Rhodewalt, 2001a; Rhodewalt, 2001). The tendency to be self-aggrandizing is off-putting to others and should lead to negative interactions (Morf et al., 2000). It also leads narcissists to stake out claims about themselves that in all likelihood they cannot meet. Because they are so self-enhancing in their interpretations of success, failure has greater impact on their feelings of self-worth and anger than it has on the feelings of less narcissistic persons (Rhodewalt & Morf, 1998). In fact, the Rhodewalt and Morf (1998) studies demonstrated that these extreme emotional reactions to negative feedback are mediated by prior attributions for successful outcomes. For narcissists, these self-aggrandizing attributions make failure all the more threatening. These findings also highlight our earlier observation that narcissists' self-evaluations may be very different in threatening contexts than they are in neutral ones.

Exaggerated self-attributions may lead narcissists to experience rapidly alternating views of themselves as social feedback changes from moment to moment. The expression of this changing self-view is reminiscent of Kernberg's (1976) contention that narcissists frequently engage in "splitting" or dramatic shifts in self-evaluation, thereby avoiding the conflicts of dealing with their strengths and weaknesses. In our view, what appears to be splitting may be a reflection of the narcissists' use of self-attribution to maintain feelings of self-worth. However, in all likelihood, this attribution component of self-regulation contributes to self-images that are highly role or context dependent, possibly ones that are high in self-concept differentiation. Earlier in this chapter, we reported preliminary evidence suggesting that narcissists may indeed be high in self-concept differentiation (Rhodewalt & Regalado, 1996).

There are other examples of narcissistic intrapersonal self-regulation as well. Narcissists hold negative views of others, especially when those others are the source of negative feedback (Kernis & Sun, 1994; Morf & Rhodewalt, 1993). That narcissists frequently exhibit negative views of others may be viewed as the complement of their own self-aggrandizement. This contention is supported by the NPI's positive association with the Cook–Medley Hostility Scale and negative association with agreeableness on the NEO-PI (Rhodewalt & Morf, 1995). According to Costa and McCrae (1985), NEO-Agreeableness reflects a positive orientation toward other people, and Smith and Frohm (1985) provide evidence that the Cook–Medley captures a cynical mistrust of others. Taken together, these findings suggest a set of self- and person-perception-processes that lead to the construction of positive models of self and negative models of others.

Rhodewalt and Eddings (2002) provide additional evidence of intrapersonal self-esteem regulation. In response to threat, narcissists edit or distort recall of their autobiographical memories. Specifically, narcissists who were led to experience a romantic rejection recalled personal romantic histories that were more self-aggrandizing than the histories they reported 1 week prior to the rejection. More important, the greater the positive distortion in recall, the more their self-esteem was buffered from the rejection. Among less narcissistic individuals, the romantic rejection led to a recall of a more humble past and lower self-esteem. It is likely that the narcissist's defensive recall and restructuring of past events contributes to the clinical impression of a lack of coherence and continuity of the self.

Narcissism and Social Context

Much less is known about the social worlds of narcissists, and what is known is based largely on their self-reports. However, contemporary transactional views of personality (Smith & Rhodewalt, 1986) suggest that personality is reflected in choice of situations and impact on situations. Therefore, an individual's social context is greatly shaped by his or her interpersonal self-regulatory strategies. Individuals select their social contexts and interaction partners; there is evidence that narcissists select them for self-enhancement purposes. Narcissists are drawn to romantic partners who possess highly valued qualities and who are also admiring (Campbell, 1999) because this type of romantic partner is self-esteem enhancing. This same study found that narcissists do not find caring individuals particularly attractive.

Using others solely for self-esteem enhancement should take its toll on narcissists' relationships, and there is evidence to this effect. Compared with others, narcissists report having had a higher number of romantic relationships (Rhodewalt & Eddings, 2002) and having more conflictive interactions, on average, each day than do less narcissistic individuals (Rhodewalt et al., 1998). They also report romantic relationships that are characterized by extremes of emotion, jealousy, obsession, and sexual attraction (Rhodewalt & Shimoda, 2000). In sum, narcissists confess to having interpersonal relationships that are characterized by conflict, intense emotions, and instability.

There is independent evidence of the deleterious impact that narcissists inflict on their interpersonal relationships. Buss and Chiodo (1991) found that people describe their narcissistic acquaintances as acting in ways to impress others, such as bragging about their accomplishments and putting others down. Moreover, narcissists' attempts to manipulate others' impressions of them have short-term gains but long-term costs. Paulhus (1998) found that interaction partners initially found narcissists to be agreeable, competent, and entertaining, but that over repeated interactions they were viewed as arrogant and hostile. For the narcissist, behaviors that initially elicit attention and admiration ultimately result in rejection and hostility.

Narcissism, Self-Solicitation, and the Fragile Self

The model displayed in Figure 26.1 and described in this chapter characterizes narcissists as immersed in endless cycles of inter-

personal self-regulation. They attempt to use their friends to feel good about themselves. They court attention and admiration from others. They hold self-views that are positive but unstable. They are hypervigilant, seeing threat or disrespect at the slightest indication. Most important, they do this at the expense of those relationships on which they are so reliant.

Although the model lends coherence to the diverse characteristics of the syndrome, it begs the question, Why? Why can't narcissists rest on their prior accomplishments and established regard from others? Why can't they develop senses of self that are well anchored and secure? We propose that the narcissistic self is the result of a noncontingent developmental history that results in a positive but uncertain sense of self. Moreover, the self-regulatory processes described in this chapter perpetuate feelings of uncertainty and necessitate continued seeking of admiration from others—which, in turn, perpetuates continued uncertainty about the self.

Psychoanalytic theorists have described the early interpersonal experiences that they believe contribute to the development of narcissism in adulthood. Despite differences in emphasis, all point to early interactions with significant others that in some way failed to respond contingently to the thoughts, feelings, and behaviors of the child. Following from Linehan's (1993) writings on borderline personality disorder, Strauman (2001) speculates that as children, narcissists may have experienced "invalidating" environments in which their private experiences were met with neglect or, at most, muted reactions. Regardless of whether these flawed interactions led to developmental arrest or defensive self-affirming compensations, one could argue that development of the narcissistic self-system is based on response noncontingent feedback from significant others.

The adult narcissist then is concerned with maintaining and protecting a positive self-image about which he or she is not confident. Narcissists are heavily invested in producing evidence that they are who they desire to be. They do this through a set of self-regulatory strategies that collectively may be termed "self-solicitation" (Rhodewalt & Tragakis, in press). In contrast to Swann's notion of self-verification, in which individuals bring others to see them as they confidently view themselves, self-solicitation involves manipulating others to view the individual as he or she hopes to be seen. Self-verification is in the service of obtaining predictable and controllable social interactions (Swann, 1985), whereas self-solicitation is in the service of socially confirming desired self-images.

Narcissists, then, are self-solicitors who are driven by insecurely held, grandiose self-images to pursue interaction strategies that constrain others so that they provide feedback that confirms the precarious self-view. Narcissistic interpersonal self-regulation—and much of intrapersonal self-regulation—involves manipulating or constraining interpretations of the narcissist's behavior in a self-serving direction. Herein lies the rub for the narcissist. As much as they would like to believe otherwise, at some level or on some occasions they must suspect that the social feedback was not unsolicited. The narcissist's active hand in staging the social context serves as a *discounting* cue when interpreting the meaning of the social feedback with regard to the self. The strategies that are motivated by insecurity in all likelihood perpetuate that insecurity. As a consequence, narcissists must constantly appeal to their social worlds to determine if they can again solicit evidence that they are admired. And so it goes.

The analogy of the narcissist as a self-solicitor is speculative, although there are pieces of evidence that are consistent with this conjecture. Narcissists are confirmed self-handicappers. Self-handicapping is, in part, a self-presentation strategy that creates attributional ambiguity about the presence of competency or ability. This ambiguity allows the narcissist to believe that the competency or ability is preserved, but in so doing, it prevents the narcissist from knowing for certain. Another example of self-solicitation comes from research with depressed individuals who use the strategy of defensive reassurance seeking (Joiner, Katz, & Lew, 1999). These individuals ask questions such as, "Don't you love me anymore?" or "Do you think I am funny?" They do this often at the cost of damaging their relationships with others (Joiner, Metalsky, Katz, & Beach, 1999). Narcissists engage in defensive admiration seeking by implicitly—or at times explicitly—asking, "Aren't I great?" If the self-admiration seeking is successful, there is the nagging question of whether the positive response would have occurred without the solicitation. If the audience rebuffs the admiration-seeking narcissist, then the rebuff is met with hostility.

Not all available evidence is consistent with this argument. For example, narcissists claim to be more confident and certain of their positive self-views than are less narcissistic individuals (Rhodewalt & Morf, 1995). These reports may reflect a narcissistic self-aggrandizing bias rather than actual self-clarity or confidence. Nonetheless, one issue the self-soliciting view must address is the narcissist's apparent lack of insight into his or her behavior. At what level are narcissists aware of the hand they play in generating social feedback?

There is a second aspect of the self-soliciting metaphor that we find appealing. The process of self-solicitation captures the active personality process part of narcissism. It illustrates the way in which individual differences can be understood in terms of underlying cognitive, motivational, and interpersonal processes (Morf & Rhodewalt, 2001a, 2001b). Although the model and supporting research contained in this chapter has focused on the clinical construct of narcissism, it is our hope that the model may be useful to self researchers in general. Cultural observers declare that contemporary Western culture breeds narcissistic tendencies in all of us (Lasch, 1979; Wolfe, 1976). While acknowledging and, at times, celebrating the central importance of the self in the psychological world of the individual, the complexity of Western society also introduces confusion about who we are. The model proposed herein to characterize narcissism may also depict more generally the cognitive, motivational, and interpersonal processes involved in interpersonal self-regulation. An interpersonal self-regulatory process analysis of the self may prove useful in lending itself to understanding a variety of problematic self-related characteristics such as rejection sensitivity, certain eating disorders, or social anxiety, to name a few.

Acknowledgments

We wish to thank Carolyn Morf, Michael Tragakis, and Stacy Eddings for their contributions to this work.

Notes

1. An in-depth treatment of the clinical literature on narcissism is beyond the scope of this chapter, and the reader is directed to excellent overviews by Pulver (1970), Akhtar and Thompson (1982), and Cooper (1959).
2. Raskin and Terry (1988) argue for a seven-factor solution: Authority, Exhibitionism, Superiority, Entitlement, Exploitiveness, Self-Sufficiency, and Vanity. There are subtle differences in the computational approaches taken by Raskin and Terry and Emmons (1987) that may account for the slightly different factor solutions. Whether entitlement and exploitiveness are one or two factors does not appear to be a significant conceptual issue. More important is the fact that, regardless of specific factor solution, the subscales are moderately correlated. The typical range of NPI scores of participants categorized as narcissistic requires moderately high scores on all subscales. Thus the majority of high-NPI participants examined in our research score high on all facets of narcissism.

References

Abend, T., Kernis, M. H., & Hampton, C. (1999). *Discrepancies between explicit and implicit self-esteem and self-serving responses.* Manuscript submitted for publication, University of Georgia.

Akhtar, S., & Thompson, J. A. (1982). Overview: Narcissistic personality disorder. *American Journal of Psychiatry, 139,* 12–20.

American Psychiatric Association. (1980). *Diagnostic and statistical manual of mental disorders.* Washington, DC: Author.

American Psychiatric Association. (1994). *Diagnostic and statistical manual of mental disorders* (4th ed.). Washington, DC: Author.

American Psychiatric Association. (2000). *Diagnostic and statistical manual of mental disorders* (4th ed., rev.). Washington, DC: Author.

Andersen, S. M., & Cole, S. W. (1990). "Do I know you?": The role of significant others in general social perception. *Journal of Personality and Social Psychology, 59,* 384–399.

Andersen, S. M., & Glassman, N. S. (1996). Responding to significant others when they are not there: Effects on interpersonal inference, motivation, and affect. In R. M. Sorrentino & E. T. Higgins (Eds.), *Handbook of motivation and cognition* (Vol. 3, pp. 262–321). New York: Guilford Press.

Andersen, S. M., Miranda, R., & Edwards, T. (2001). When self-enhancement knows no bounds: Are past relationships with significant others at the heart of narcissism? *Psychological Inquiry, 12,* 197–202.

Brown, R. P., & Bosson, J. K. (2001). Narcissus meets Sisyphus: Self-love, self-loathing, and the never-ending pursuit of self-worth. *Psychological Inquiry, 12,* 210–213.

Brown, R. P., Bosson, J. K., & Swann, W. B., Jr. (2000). *How do I love me? Measuring self-love and self-loathing in narcissism.* Manuscript submitted for publication, University of Oklahoma.

Bushman, B., & Baumeister, R. F. (1998). Threatened egotism, narcissism, self-esteem, and direct and displaced aggression: Does self-love or self-hate lead to violence? *Journal of Personality and Social Psychology, 75,* 219–229.

Buss, D. M., & Chiodo, L. M. (1991). Narcissistic acts in everyday life. *Journal of Personality, 59,* 179–215.

Campbell, W. K. (1999). Narcissism and romantic attraction. *Journal of Personality and Social Psychology, 77,* 1254–1270.

Cantor, N. (1990). From thought to behavior: "Having" and "doing" in the study of personality and cognition. *American Psychologist, 45,* 735–750.

Cantor, N. (1994). Life task problem solving: Situational affordances and personal needs. *Personality and Social Psychology Bulletin, 20,* 235–243.

Cantor, N., & Kihlstrom, J. F. (1987). *Personality and social intelligence.* Englewood NJ: Prentice-Hall.

Chessick, R. D. (1987). Coronary artery disease as a narcissistic psychosomatic disorder: I. *Dynamic Psychotherapy, 5,* 16–29.

Cooper, A. (1959). Narcissism. In S. Arieti (Ed.), *American handbook of psychiatry* (pp. 297–316). New York: Basic Books.

Costa, P., & McCrae, R. (1985). *The NEO-PI/FFI manual supplement.* Odessa, FL: Psychological Assessment Resources.

Donahue, E. M., Robins, R. W., Roberts, B. W., & John, O. P. (1993). The divided self: Concurrent and longitudinal effects of psychological adjustment and social roles on self-concept differentiation. *Journal of Personality and Social Psychology, 64,* 834–846.

Ellis, H. (1898). Autoeroticism: A psychological study. *Alienist and Neurologist, 19,* 260–299.

Emmons, R. A. (1984). Factor analysis and construct validity of the Narcissistic Personality Inventory. *Journal of Personality and Social Psychology, 48,* 291–300.

Emmons, R. A. (1987). Narcissism: Theory and measurement. *Journal of Personality and Social Psychology, 52,* 11–17.

Farwell, L., & Wohlwend-Lloyd, R. (1998). Narcissistic processes: Optimistic expectations, favorable self-evaluations, and self-enhancing attributions. *Journal of Personality, 66,* 65–83.

Freud, S. (1953). On narcissism: An introduction. In J. Strachey (Ed. & Trans.), *The standard edition of the complete psychological works of Sigmund Freud* (Vol. 14, pp. 69–102). London: Hogarth Press. (Original work published 1914)

Gabriel, M. T., Critelli, J. W., & Ee, J. S. (1994). Narcissistic illusions in self-evaluations of intelligence and attractiveness. *Journal of Personality, 62,* 143–155.

Higgins, E. T. (1996). The "Self-Digest": Self-knowledge serving self-regulatory functions. *Journal of Personality and Social Psychology, 71,* 1062–1083.

Hinkley, K., & Andersen, S. M. (1996). The working self-concept in transference: Significant other activation and self-change. *Journal of Personality and Social Psychology, 71,* 1279–1295.

John, O. P., & Robins, R. (1994). Accuracy and bias in self-perception: Individual differences in self-enhancement and the role of narcissism. *Journal of Personality and Social Psychology, 66,* 206–219.

Joiner, T. E., Jr., Katz, J., & Lew, A. (1999). Harbingers of depressotypic reassurance seeking: Negative life events, increased anxiety, and decreased self-esteem. *Personality and Social Psychology Bulletin, 25,* 630–637.

Joiner, T. E., Jr., Metalsky, G. I., Katz, J., & Beach, S. R. H. (1999). Depression and excessive reassurance seeking. *Psychological Inquiry, 10,* 269–278.

Jones, E. E., & Berglas, S. (1978). Control of attributions about the self through self-handicapping strategies: The appeal of alcohol and the role of underachievement. *Personality and Social Psychology Bulletin, 4,* 200–206.

Kernberg, O. F. (1976). *Borderline conditions and pathological narcissism.* New York: Aronson.

Kernis, M. H. (1993). The roles of stability and level of self-esteem in psychological functioning. In R. Baumeister (Ed.), *Self-esteem: The puzzle of low self-regard* (pp. 167–182). New York: Plenum Press.

Kernis, M. H. (2001). Following the trail from narcissism to fragile self-esteem. *Psychological Inquiry, 12,* 223–225.

Kernis, M. H., Cornell, D. P., Sun, C.-R., Berry, A., & Harlow, T. (1993). There's more to self-esteem than whether it is high or low: The importance of stability of self-esteem. *Journal of Personality and Social Psychology, 65,* 1190–1204.

Kernis, M. H., Grannemann, B. D., & Barclay, L. C. (1989). Stability and level of self-esteem as predictors of anger arousal and hostility. *Journal of Personality and Social Psychology, 56,* 1013–1023.

Kernis, M. H., & Sun, C.-R. (1994). Narcissism and reactions to interpersonal feedback. *Journal of Research in Personality, 28,* 4–13.

Kohut, H. (1971). *The analysis of the self.* New York: International Universities Press.

Lasch, C. (1979). *The culture of narcissism: American life in an age of diminishing expectations.* New York: Norton.

Linehan, M. M. (1993). *Cognitive-behavioral treatment of borderline personality disorder.* NewYork: Guilford Press.

Linville, P. W. (1985). Self-complexity and affective extremity: Don't put all of your eggs in one cognitive basket. *Social Cognition, 3,* 94–120.

Linville, P. W. (1987). Self-complexity as a cognitive buffer against stress related illness and depression. *Journal of Personality and Social Psychology, 56,* 663–676.

Linville, P. W., & Carlston, D. (1994). Social cognition and the self. In P. Devine, D. L. Hamilton, & T. Ostrom (Eds.), *Social cognition: Its impact on social psychology* (pp. 143–193). San Diego, CA: Academic Press.

Manfield, P. (1992). *Split self/split object: Understanding and treating borderline, narcissistic, and schizoid disorders.* Northvale, NJ: Aronson

Mischel, W., & Shoda, Y. (1995). A cognitive–affective system theory of personality: Reconceptualizing situations, dispositions, dynamics, and invariance in personality structure. *Psychological Review, 102,* 246–268.

Morf, C. C. (1994). Interpersonal consequences of narcissists' continual effort to maintain and bolster self-esteem (Doctoral dissertation, University of Utah, 1994). *Dissertation Abstracts International, 55*(6-B), 2430.

Morf, C. C., Ansara, D., & Shia, T. (2000). *The effects of audience characteristics on narcissistic self-presentation.* Manuscript in preparation, University of Toronto.

Morf, C. C., & Rhodewalt, F. (1993). Narcissism and self-evaluation maintenance: Explorations in object relations. *Personality and Social Psychology Bulletin, 19,* 668–676.

Morf, C. C., & Rhodewalt, F. (2001a). Expanding the dynamic self-regulatory model of narcissism. *Psychological Inquiry, 12,* 243–251.

Morf, C. C., & Rhodewalt, F. (2001b). Unraveling the paradoxes of Narcissism: A dynamic self-regulatory processing model. *Psychological Inquiry, 12,* 177–196.

Paulhus, D. L. (1998). Interpersonal and intrapsychic adaptiveness of trait self-enhancement: A mixed blessing? *Journal of Personality and Social Psychology, 74,* 1197–1208.

Peterson, C., Semmel, A., Metalsky, G., Abramson, L., von Beyer, C., & Seligman, M. E. P. (1982). The Attributional Style Questionnaire. *Cognitive Therapy and Research, 6,* 287–289.

Prifitera, A., & Ryan, J. J. (1984). Validity of the Narcissistic Personality Inventory in a psychiatric sample. *Journal of Clinical Psychology, 40,* 140–142.

Pulver, S. (1970). Narcissism: The term and concept. *Journal of the American Psycho-Analytic Association, 18,* 319–341.

Raskin, R., & Hall, C. S. (1979). A narcissistic personality inventory. *Psychological Reports, 45,* 590.

Raskin, R., Novacek, J., & Hogan, R. (1991). Narcissism, self-esteem, and defensive self-enhancement. *Journal of Personality, 59,* 20–38.

Raskin, R., & Terry, H. (1988). A principal-components analysis of the Narcissistic Personality Inventory and further evidence of its construct validity. *Journal of Personality and Social Psychology, 54,* 890–902.

Reich, A. (1960). Pathologic forms of self-esteem regulation. *Psychoanalytic Study of the Child, 18,* 218–238.

Rhodewalt, F. (1993, August). Toward a model of narcissism and stress engendering behavior. In M. Scheier (Chair), *Optimism, self-representation, and health: Recent theoretical developments.* Symposium conducted at the meeting of the American Psychological Association, Toronto.

Rhodewalt, F. (2001). The social mind of the narcissist: Cognitive and motivational aspects of interpersonal self-construction. In J. P. Forgas, K. Williams, & L. Wheeler (Eds.), *The social mind: Cognitive and motivational aspects of interpersonal behavior* (pp. 177–198). New York: Cambridge University Press.

Rhodewalt, F., & Eddings, S. (2002). Narcissus reflects: Memory distortion in response to ego relevant feedback in high and low narcissistic men. *Journal of Research in Personality, 36,* 97–116.

Rhodewalt, F., Madrian, J. C., & Cheney, S. (1998). Narcissism, self-knowledge organization, and emotional reactivity: The effect of daily experiences on self-esteem and affect. *Personality and Social Psychology Bulletin, 24,* 75–87.

Rhodewalt, F., & Morf, C. C. (1995). Self and interpersonal correlates of the Narcissistic Personality Inventory: A review and new findings. *Journal of Research in Personality, 29,* 1–23.

Rhodewalt, F., & Morf, C. C. (1998). On self-aggrandizement and anger: A temporal analysis of narcissism and affective reactions to success and failure. *Journal of Personality and Social Psycholgy, 74,* 672–685.

Rhodewalt, F., & Regalado, M. (1996). [NPI-defined narcissism and the structure of the self.] Unpublished raw data, University of Utah.

Rhodewalt, F., Sanbonmatsu, D., Feick, D., Tschanz, B., & Waller, A. (1995). Self-handicapping and interpersonal trade-offs: The effects of claimed self-handicaps on observers' performance evaluations and feedback. *Personality and Social Psychology Bulletin, 21,* 1042–1050.

Rhodewalt, F., & Shimoda, V. (2000). *What's love got to do with it?: Narcissism and romantic relationships.* Manuscript in preparation.

Rhodewalt, F., & Tragakis, M. (in press). Self-handicapping and the social self: The cost and rewards of interpersonal self-construction. In J. Forgas & K. Williams (Eds.), *The interpersonal self.* Philadelphia: Psychology Press.

Rhodewalt, F., Tragakis, M., & Finnerty, J. (2000). *Narcissism and self-handicapping: Linking self-aggrandizement to behavior.* Manuscript submitted for publication.

Robins, R. W., & Beer, J. S. (2001). Positive illusions about the self: Short-term benefits and long-term costs. *Journal of Personality and Social Psychology, 80,* 340–352.

Robins, R. W., Tracy, J. L., & Shaver, P. R. (2001). Shamed into self-love: Dynamics, roots, and functions of narcissism. *Psychological Inquiry, 12,* 230–236.

Ruiz, J., Smith, T. W., & Rhodewalt, F. (2001). Distinguishing narcissism from hostility: Similarities and differences in interpersonal circumplex and five-factor correlates. *Journal of Personality Assessment, 76,* 537–555.

Showers, C. (1992a). Evaluatively integrative thinking about characteristics of the self. *Personality and Social Psychology Bulletin, 18,* 719–729.

Showers, C. (1992b). Compartmentalization of positive and negative self-knowledge: Keeping bad apples out of the bunch. *Journal of Personality and Social Psychology, 62,* 1036–1049.

Showers, C. (2000). Self-organization in emotional contexts. In J. P. Forgas (Ed.), *Feeling and thinking: The role of affect in social cognition* (pp. 283–307). New York: Cambridge University Press.

Smith, T. W., & Frohm, K. D. (1985). What's so unhealthy about hostility? Construct validity and psychosocial correlates of the Cook and Medley Ho Scale. *Health Psychology, 4,* 503–520.

Smith, T. W., & Rhodewalt, F. (1986). On states, traits, and processes: A transactional alternative to the individual difference assumptions in Type A behavior and physiological reactivity. *Journal of Research in Personality, 20,* 229–251.

Strauman, T. J. (2001). Self-regulation, affect regulation, and narcissism: Pieces of the puzzle. *Psychological Inquiry, 12,* 339–342.

Swann, W. B., Jr. (1985). The self as architect of social reality. In B. Schlenker (Ed.), *The self and social life* (pp. 100–125). New York: McGraw-Hill.

Tesser, A. (1988). Toward a self-evaluation model of social behavior. In L. Berkowitz (Ed.), *Advances in experimental social psychology* (Vol. 21, pp. 181–227). New York: Academic Press.

Tschanz, B., & Rhodewalt, F. (2001). Autobiography, reputation, and the self: On the role of evaluative valence and self-consistency of the self-relevant information. *Journal of Experimental Social Psychology, 37,* 36–48.

Watson, P. J., Taylor, D., & Morris, R. J. (1987). Narcissism, sex roles, and self-functioning. *Sex Roles, 16,* 335–350.

Westen, D. (1990). The relations among narcissism, egocentrism, self-concept, and self-esteem: Experimental, clinical, and theoretical considerations. *Psychoanalysis and Contemporary Thought, 13,* 183–239.

Wink, P. (1991). Two faces of narcissism. *Journal of Personality and Social Psychology, 61,* 590–597.

Wolfe, T. (1976). The "Me" decade and the third great awakening. In T. Wolfe, *Mauve gloves & madmen, clutter & vine, and other stories, sketches, and essays.* New York: Ferrar, Straus and Giroux.

27

Cultural Models of the Self

SUSAN E. CROSS
JONATHAN S. GORE

People define themselves using the concepts, terms, values, and ideologies provided by their cultural and social environments. The importance of the social world in the construction of the self was first articulated by Cooley (1902), Mead (1934), and Goffman (1959), but it has been lost at times in the social cognitive perspectives that have dominated research on the self in the past three decades. As the chapters in this volume reveal, much has been learned about the self as a cognitive structure, a center of motivation, and a regulator of behavior. Recently, however, investigators have returned to issues of the social and cultural origins of the self for new ideas and insights. They have realized that identity and the definition of the self depend on the cultural context. In this chapter, we describe the cultural foundations of divergent models of the self and review recent research comparing Western, independent conceptions of the self with East Asian, interdependent views of the self. We conclude the chapter with comments on how cross-cultural investigations can continue to inform research on the self and its role in behavior.

Cultural Models of the Self

Culture is a set of meanings, beliefs, and practices that guide the formation and maintenance of social institutions, the creation of social products, and the development of its members (Triandis, 1996). Key components of cultural meaning systems include beliefs about the nature of the person, what makes for an ideal person, and the person's purpose in life. Cultures vary widely in their beliefs about the nature of the person. In some cultures, children are not considered "persons" until they are several years old (Reisman, 1992). In other societies, the self may have inhabited other bodies in previous times and been reincarnated into the current body (Barth, 1997). In some American Indian societies, the self may take leave of the body and metamorphose into other forms, such as the form of a bear or an eagle (Hallowell, 1955). Hallowell, an anthropologist who was interested in the self, suggested that cultural models of the person provide individuals with psychological orientations on the self and others that direct social adaptation. He spelled out five orientations that structure the psychological environment in which the self is constituted.

First, cultural models must orient the person toward the self as a distinct entity. Using personal names, personal pronouns, and marking developmental achievements through ritual and celebration are a few of the ways in which societies acknowledge the individual as distinct from others. Although the dimensions with which distinctiveness is marked or acknowledged and the degree of distinctiveness that is believed to be optimal may vary across cultures, the first step in developing a culturally appropriate self requires recognizing one's separateness from others at some level.

Second, cultural models specify the relation of the self to others in the environment, including human others, spirit beings, animals, and inanimate beings (termed "object orientation" by Hallowell, 1955). In Japan and many other East Asian or collectivist cultures, the relation between the self and others is construed as ideally harmonious, interdependent, and interconnected. In the United States, the culturally defined relation between the self and others is construed as ideally independent, separate, with razor-sharp boundaries between the self and others (Geertz, 1975). The object orientation of some cultures may prescribe relations with nonhuman beings (such as deceased ancestors or the spirit world). In fact, relations to nonhuman others may be more important in understanding the person's goals, needs, and behavior than interpersonal relations with other humans (Hallowell, 1955).

Third, cultures provide individuals with a *spatiotemporal* orientation, in which recall of past events that are associated with the self become the foundation of self-identity and self-continuity. This orientation specifies what is to be remembered about one's past and how it influences the individual's current and future behavior. Cultures differ in the time span of recalled experiences that are viewed as self-related. In some Asian Indian cultures, individuals may recall experiences from past lives. In Ojibway groups, some persons claimed to have memories of events that occurred in utero or during early infancy (Hallowell, 1955). There also is variation in the future time perspective applied to the self, especially in the extent to which the self is believed to be immortal or eternal.

In some cultures, there is much more to this spatiotemporal orientation than one's individual history and memory. Some cultures allow for avenues by which the person may separate from self-continuity, through fugue states or culturally acceptably dissociative events. For example, a common syndrome identified in Southeast Asia is the phenomenon of "amok," in which a person (usually a male) experiences a short-term type of trance, marked by an outburst of unrestrained violence. Because the syndrome is thought to be caused by spirit possession and because the person has no memory of the event, the man is not held responsible for his behavior (Castillo, 1997). Similarly, some cultures separate the perceptions and experiences of a dream from the self, whereas other cultures interpret dream experiences as self-related. In the latter situation, the events of the dream are incorporated into the experience of the self and become part of the self-image and help direct behavior. In addition, the person may be morally responsible for behavior engaged in while dreaming. Among the Ashanti and the Kai, dreams of adultery subject the person to social sanction or punishment (Lincoln, n.d., cited in Hallowell, 1955).

Fourth, cultural models provide a *normative* orientation, specifying values, ideals, and standards toward which one should strive. In the United States, the individual, separate from social ties, obligations, and impediments, is sovereign. The maxim "To thine own self be true" dominates the understanding of how one should behave. The ideal person chooses his or her own goals and direction and recognizes his or her distinctiveness from others. In contrast, in Confucian ideology, the supreme virtue is *ren,* which means "a sensitive concern for others" (Elvin, 1985, p. 165), resulting in valuing connection to others, similarity to others, and harmony in relationships (Ho, 1995; Tu, 1994). This normative orientation establishes the grounds for self-appraisal and for the appraisal of others. In addition, it serves as the foundation for a moral order and for the understanding of one's behavior within a moral system.

By stipulating how the self is perceived in time and in relation to others and the goals and values toward which individuals should strive, cultural models of the self inevitably provide a *motivational* orientation (Hallowell, 1955). Cultural models provide motivational orientations for meeting universal needs and goals that characterize all cultures (such as the need for survival and reproduction), but the means of meeting these goals may vary across cultures. In some societies, polygamy is an acceptable means of meeting survival and reproduction needs, whereas in many other societies, monogamy is required. In a few societies, polyandry, in which one woman marries several brothers, is an acceptable route toward family survival and reproduction (Goldstein, 1987). In societies in which the person is represented as the center of relationships (Tu, 1994), social motivation will be dominant, and individuals will be "moved" by the ideals, demands, and obligations in relationships. In societies in which the individual is represented as central and relationships are peripheral and not definitive of personhood (as in individualistic cultures), individual motivation will be dominant, and persons will be "moved" by individual goals, personal wishes, and idiosyncratic ideals for self-fulfillment.

In summary, cultural models provide direction for individuals to construct socially valued and adaptive selves. There may be other important orientations or dimensions of cultural models of the self that are not included in Hallowell's list, but these five orientations provide a useful starting point for identifying dimensions of the self that may be culturally variable (see also Neisser, 1988). Thus far, psychologists have investigated few of these orientations cross-culturally, with the exception of cultural differences in the relation of the self to other humans. In the next section of this chapter, we review the research on cultural differences in perspectives on the self in relation to others and some of their consequences. At the end of the chapter we return to Hallowell's orientations as we suggest future directions for research.

Cultural Variation in the Relation between the Self and Others

The most prominent and widely researched dimensions that separate cultures' models of the person is the conception of the person as independent from others versus interdependent with others. In the United States and other societies with roots in Western European cultural traditions, the autonomous individual is viewed as separate from society and the situation. The self is the center of the person's psychological universe and is the lens through which other aspects of the world are perceived (James, 1890/1983). In this *independent* model, the person is viewed as a bounded, unique, integrated, and complete individual, who is fundamentally, morally, and legally prior to society (Geertz, 1975). The independent and self-sufficient individual enters into social relations freely and is free to leave social entanglements. In fact, social influence and obligations are potentially compromising; thus the person must be on guard to protect his or her individualism and to limit the influence of others (Markus & Kitayama, 1994). To be a culturally valued person, one must distinguish oneself from others and identify those characteristics, attributes, abilities, and ways of being that make one unique and special. These attributes become the "stuff" from which a self-concept is constructed.

This independent relation between the person and society is not assumed in collectivist cultural contexts, such as in many East Asian societies. In these cultures, the person and society are interdependent and mutually supportive. In this *interdependent* model, priority is accorded to social units and collectives such as the family, the work group, and the community rather than to the individual. The person is viewed as embedded in relationships and defined by social contexts, fundamental relationships, and social positions. Thus the person is a center of relationships; the socially valued person seeks to fit into or harmonize with relationship partners and in-groups. To be a person—to know oneself and one's place in the world—one must be a part of groups (e.g., families, work groups, and communities) and must work through them, for such is the essence of being human (Lebra, 1976; Tu, 1994). These two models of the person differ not so much in terms of the overall importance of relationships—relationships are important to humans everywhere (Baumeister & Leary, 1995)—but rather in the meanings and dynamics of relationships (Rothbaum, Pott, Azuma, Miyake, & Weisz, 2000; see also Oyserman, Coon, & Kemmelmeier, 2002).

How do cultural models get under the skin (or into the self)? Markus and Kitayama (1994; Markus, Mullally, & Kitayama, 1997) have articulated the processes whereby cultural values, beliefs, and traditions are translated into individual psychological tendencies. In their description, they integrate a focus on the broad cultural factors that influence behavior with a constructivist perspective that acknowledges that selves are constructed in particular situations, with specific actors and experiences (see Holland, Lachicotte, Skinner, & Cain, 1998). The cultural shaping of the self includes four primary levels:

1. Cultural models of the person derive first from the sociohistorical ideals and values of a society .
2. These sociohistorical ideas and values shape social customs, practices, and institutions, including linguistic practices, employment practices, and educational and legal systems.
3. These practices and institutions provide settings and situations in which individuals act and behave.
4. These experiences in everyday settings sculpt a self and shape individual psychological tendencies.

Cultural Ideals and Values Represented in Legal, Historical, and Religious Texts

The cultural shaping of the self begins with a society's core philosophical and religious heritage and traditions, which are typically expressed in valued texts and historical documents (e.g., the Bible or the Torah), legal or cultural documents (the Bill of Rights and the Declaration of Independence), and religious and national traditions (Protestantism and a tradition of mobility in the United States). These traditions and documents spell out the society's beliefs about the nature of the person, the person's relation to human and nonhuman others, normative and moral beliefs, and the other orientations described by Hallowell (1955). In Western European and North American contexts, these documents, texts, and tradi-

tions emphasize the primacy of individual rights over society's needs and the value of freedom and independence from society's demands. These values are represented in cultural products such as literature and the arts, as in Robert Frost's poem "The Road Not Taken": "Two roads diverged in a wood, and I—/I took the one less traveled by,/And that has made all the difference."

In Eastern cultural contexts, philosophical and religious traditions emphasize Buddhist ideals of empathy and self-renunciation, the Confucian ethic of proper conduct in the Five Cardinal Relationships, or Taoist beliefs that the self is one with others and with the Cosmos (Ho, 1995). These texts and the resulting religious and philosophical traditions emphasize the connectedness between persons, families, and societies and the importance of maintaining relationships. For example, the Confucian Golden Rule states, "The humane man, wishing to establish himself, seeks to establish others; wishing to be prominent himself, he helps others to be prominent" (*Analects,* as cited in Ho, 1995, pp. 133–134).

The philosophical and religious texts of the West and the East differ fundamentally in their representations of the world and the person's place in it. In Western texts and belief systems, persons are separate from the world and society and can be understood apart from the situation, context, or environment in which they are found. According to Nisbett and his colleagues (Nisbett, Peng, Choi, & Norenzayan, 2001), this view of the person is part of an *analytical* worldview, which originated in ancient Greek philosophy. The Greeks viewed the world as a collection of separable discrete objects that could be categorized in terms of their stable, universal properties. They sought abstract rules for the behavior of objects in a field and tended to ignore the environment in which the behavior occurred (Norenzayan, Choi, & Nisbett, 1999). This analytical worldview lay the foundation for modern science and Western psychology, especially a psychology of the individual.

In contrast to the analytical worldviews that characterize Western ideologies, early Confucian and Buddhist texts viewed the person and objects as continuous with and embedded in the environment. This resulted in a *holistic* worldview, in which persons and objects are understood and perceived as part of a greater whole, inseparable from the context in which they are found. Objects were viewed as part of a net of relationships, rather than in terms of discrete categories or substances. In this worldview, "anything regarded in isolation is distorted because the parts are meaningful only in their relations to the whole, like individual musical notes embedded in a melody" (Peng & Nisbett, 1999, p. 743). In this holistic perspective, the focus is on the field and the relations among elements in the field, rather than on specific objects within the field and their properties. These divergent worldviews—the analytical worldview of the Western world and the holistic worldview of the East—influence the ways in which the values, beliefs, and ideologies communicated by the texts and historical documents are played out at the second level of the cultural shaping of the self.

Core Values Produce Culture-Specific Customs, Norms, and Practices

A culture's core beliefs, values, and orientations shape cultural institutions, practices, and customs. For example, in the United States, the value of individualism is translated into a legal system that focuses on the rights of the individual. Individuals have the right to sue when others infringe on personal freedoms, and the court system in the United States makes this option relatively accessible to its citizens (Hamilton & Sanders, 1992). In contrast, in East Asia, people and court systems tend to prefer less litigious processes, such as negotiation and the use of a middleman to resolve conflicts (Leung & Fan, 1997). When a Civil Liberties Bureau was established by the American occupation forces and the Japanese Ministry of Justice after World War II, it was intended to promote individual claims against the government. Instead, it tended to be used to settle family and neighborhood disputes, promoting traditional Japanese values of maintaining social bonds rather than American values of protection of the individual (Kidder & Muller, 1991; Rosch, 1983).

The media and advertising are cultural institutions that reflect social norms and values and that also create preferences and desires. Studies of advertisements in the United States and Korea find that American advertisements typically appeal to individualism and uniqueness (Han & Shavitt, 1994). For example, one ad read, "The Internet isn't for everybody. But then again, you are not everybody" (Kim & Markus, 1999). This appeal to uniqueness in North American advertising was the foundation of a long-running promotion campaign for the Dodge Caravan that prominently displayed the single word "different." (Ironically, the Caravan was the best-selling make in its class of vehicles at the time, so buyers of a Dodge Caravan found themselves on the road with many identical vehicles.) In contrast, Korean advertisers' appeals focused on relationships with others and on conformity to group norms and social trends (Kim & Markus, 1999). One advertisement read, "Seven out of 10 people are using this product," and another emphasized following a trend with the claim, "Trend forecast for spring: Pastel colors!" Although one could certainly imagine these appeals in the United States also, the research by Kim and Markus (1999) showed that appeals to tradition and conformity to social norms were much more common in Korean ads than in North American ads.

Linguistic practices reflect and promote these cultural orientations. The grammatical rules of English highlight and foreground the actor, but in Japanese the individual is "submerged in the whole" (Ikegami, 1991, p. 290). In Japanese, the speaker will often drop the pronoun from a sentence, especially the first-person singular "I." In English, however, pronoun use is generally obligatory, especially in the first person (Kashima & Kashima, 1998). For example, the English sentence, "I cut my hair" would be translated in Japanese as "*Kami o katta*," literally "Hair cut-past" or "Cut hair" (Ikegami, 1991, p. 312). In the English version, the speaker is the primary element of the statement, whereas in the Japanese version, the speaker is an implicit element of the situation rather than the central focus. In fact, the typical American English version of this sentence highlights the speaker to an even greater degree than is at first obvious. Many North Americans describe the action of going to the hairdresser's with the statement: "I cut my hair." But who in fact did the cutting? Not the speaker, but the hairdresser. In other words, English highlights and emphasizes the agency of the person choosing to have his or her hair cut, not the actual person who did the cutting. This grammatical structure indicates that the speaker's role in initiating the action, not the hairdresser's role in carrying out the action, is what is important and should be noted. In this and other ways, the English language emphasizes the individual and individual action and control.

In Japanese, the individual is often not represented as an agent who acts but as an element in a larger whole that is shifting with time (Ikegami, 1991). One example of this comes in a comparison of the use of first-person pronouns. In Japanese, there is no simple translation of the English person pronouns "I," "me," or "mine." Instead, there are many available terms, and the situation determines which term is used. Correct usage depends on one's relationship with others in the situation, their desires, and other contextual factors (Kondo, 1990). Thus the Japanese language reflects and promotes the idea that the person is known by and understood in terms of meaningful contexts and relationships. Similarly, the Japanese language permits dropping the first-person singular pronoun (as in the "Cut-hair" example), whereas pronoun use is generally obligatory in English. As Kashima and Kashima (1998) suggest, the explicit use of first-person pronouns highlights the speaker, whereas pronoun drop reduces the prominence of the speaker and the differentiation between the speaker and the listener. Their research showed that pronoun drop was less common in cultures in which the person is conceptualized as distinct from and separate from others than in more collectivist cultures. In short, these linguistic practices of highlighting the actor as separate from or as embedded in the context reflect and reproduce the cultural beliefs and ideals concerning the nature of the person.

Settings, Episodes, and Socially Constructed Experiences

Cultural practices, customs, and institutions provide settings and situations that socialize children and adults into the norms, values,

and ideals of the society. For example, cultural ideals and customs configure parenting practices, which create "figured worlds" in which children develop (Holland et al., 1998). In the United States, a good parent–child relationship provides a "secure base" from which the child feels free to explore the world (Ainsworth, Blehar, Waters, & Wall, 1978; Bowlby, 1969). In Japan, the ideal mother–child relationship is characterized by "symbiotic harmony" (Rothbaum, Weisz, Pott, Miyake, & Morelli, 2000), in which the child is taught to be dependent on the mother and to accommodate to and to empathize with others, starting with the mother (Lebra, 1994; Weisz, Rothbaum, & Blackburn, 1984; see Rothbaum, Pott, et al., 2000, for a review of Japanese–American differences in child-rearing practices). In the United States, parents prepare children to live in a society that values individualism by having separate rooms for parents and children. In cultures that value collective, interdependent relations among people, children are prepared for the society by sleeping with their parents, grandparents, or siblings for many years. American mothers promote the development of the child's unique, independent self by recounting events in the children's lives to them, whereas Korean mothers spend about one-third the time talking about the past with their children, compared with American mothers (Mullen & Yi, 1995).

In the United States, children are encouraged to speak up, defend themselves, and protect their own rights and interests in disputes with other children. American children quickly learn that the complaint, "that's not fair," garners attention and remediation of a situation. Japanese children, in contrast, are trained to protect their relationships with others when disputes arise and to sacrifice personal interest for the greater good of interpersonal harmony. In conflict situations, Japanese children are often told to control negative emotion, to consider their behavior from the perspective of the other person, and that "to lose is to win." This reflects the cultural notion that the ideal, or mature, person is able to subordinate individual needs and goals for the good of interpersonal harmony (Lebra, 1976; Zahn-Wexler, Friedman, Cole, Mizuta, & Hiruma, 1996).

Schools also create situations in which children learn and adopt cultural values, ideals, and models. American schools and education systems reinforce the importance of the individual and stress the development of one's unique abilities and talents. Teachers are expected to tailor the educational environment to meet individual students' needs, and parents expect schools to instill in students self-reliance and self-confidence (Tobin, Wu, & Davidson, 1989). American teachers provide many opportunities for students to individuate themselves, through special tasks for high and low achievers, "show and tell," and charts of individual accomplishments (e.g., who has lost how many teeth in kindergarten classes). In Japan, in contrast, schools, especially in the early years, are expected to instill in children the ability to be productive group members and to learn to empathize with others (Lewis, 1995; Tobin et al., 1989). In Japan, students learn to work together as a group; teachers may attempt to speed up slower members of a class and to slow down more talented students so that the class moves along together. This is not viewed as a disservice to the more talented members of the class but rather as a benefit, because teachers "believe that students benefit in the long run by developing an increased sensitivity to the needs of others and a sense of security that comes from being a member of a seemingly homogenous group" (Tobin et al., 1989, pp. 25–26). Even in first grade, students end each day in a period of self-reflection and evaluation, in which they discuss as a group the ways in which they have met, or failed to meet, their goals as a class (Lewis, 1995).

Culture-Related Psychological Tendencies

As a result of participation in the social episodes and figured worlds afforded by one's cultural system, individuals develop culturally configured psychological tendencies (Markus & Kitayama, 1994). Participation in cultural practices and customs, such as sleeping with family members versus sleeping alone, working together as a group versus working alone in competition with others, and other cultural practices configure a self that seeks either to be aligned with others or independent from others and that seeks either to fit into important social environments or to stand out from them (Weisz et al., 1984). Through these and other socialization practices and customs, individuals come to find that striving for culturally approved goals is satisfying and that not achieving cultural norms and goals creates anxiety or distress (D'Andrade, 1984). Culturally patterned practices, customs, situations, and languages act as a continual priming effect, making individuals aware of some concepts and ideas frequently and forcefully (such as the importance of self-reliance, individualism, and being different in the United States versus the importance of interpersonal harmony, fitting in, and conformity in Japan) and neglecting other ideas and concepts (Lilliard, 1998). Frequent and strong activation of ideas, values, and self-views will cause them to be chronically accessible and readily available, resulting in their automatic use in perceiving the world.

Although culture provides a broad outline of the ideal or valued self (what Markus, Mullally, & Kitayama, 1997, term "selfways"), it also provides a variety of individual identities, characteristics, beliefs, attributes, preferences, wishes, needs, goals, and ways of thinking. Some of these will develop in response to particular family, school, or community environments, whereas others will be individually chosen from the "cultural supermarket" of identities (Mathews, 1996). Some cultures provide a wide array of available identities at this level (i.e., wife, mother, career person, volunteer, gardener, iconoclast, liberal, fashion plate, etc.), whereas other cultures provide relatively few choices (i.e., wife, mother, nun, prostitute). The available options at this point are generally consistent with the cultural models of the self embedded in the society's core beliefs and values; choices of identities that conflict with the culturally valued selfway may result in social sanction or reduced psychological well-being.

These processes of the cultural shaping of the self instill in a culture's members models for themselves and their relation to others that seem "natural" and "given" and that go unquestioned. In the American cultural context, this model of the self, termed the "independent self-construal" by Markus and Kitayama (1991), reflects the analytical worldview (described by Nisbett et al., 2001) in that the person is defined by stable properties, separate from his or her social context. This model of the self includes beliefs that the person has inalienable individual rights separate from and prior to society and other interpersonal commitments and that what defines a person is ultimately inside, stable, and enduring. These internal characteristics, abilities, and preferences direct behavior as the person seeks to develop, enhance, and verify them. Consequently, the person's behavior should be relatively consistent across situations and stable over time. One is motivated to protect or enhance these characteristics of the self and so one seeks out situations and relationships that allow one to express, verify, and enhance one's self-views.

In contrast, in the East Asian cultural context, models of the self reflect the holistic worldview (Nisbett et al., 2001) and include beliefs that the person is fundamentally part of a larger whole. Individuals are viewed as a "single thread in a richly textured fabric of relationships" (Kondo, 1990, p. 33). In this context, what is natural, given, or unquestioned is the person's relatedness to others and embeddedness in social contexts. Consequently, the self is not viewed as a stable, constant entity but rather is construed as "a fluid concept which changes though time and situations according to interpersonal relationships" (Hamaguchi, 1985, p. 302). This model of the self, termed the "interdependent self-construal" by Markus and Kitayama (1991), includes the belief that what defines a person is his or her social memberships, roles, and relationships; consequently, the important features of a person are "outside," and these are the features that direct and motivate behavior. One becomes a socially approved and validated person by striving for the ideal in a given situation (Kitayama, Markus, Matsumoto, & Norasakkunkit, 1997); because the ideal behavior can vary from situation to situation, or relationship to relationship, behavior may vary as well. One is motivated to approach this situation-specific ideal; thus information is sought that permits one to correct one's behavior or that allows one to better fit in to a situation.

Because social psychological theories of the self developed in a Western, individualistic cultural context, research on the self and its role and function in behavior have focused on how the self is individuated and unique, on the continued development and verification of an independent self, and on the maintenance of positive views of the self. Assumptions of the individualistic self and its consequences underlie many contemporary theories of motivation, emotion, self-esteem, and social behavior. Cross-cultural examinations of the self have shown that when the self is construed interdependently or collectively, self-related emotions, behaviors, and motivations are quite different than those observed in Western, individualistic contexts. In the following sections, we consider the topics of motivation and self-esteem in light of cultural variation in the self.

Culture and Motivation

Many aspects of motivation are universal, such as the need for survival, procreation, and human belonging. Other motivations, however, are culture specific and culturally regulated and can best be understood from inside the cultural models of the person and the self. Western psychologists seem to be much more concerned about motivation, intention, and identity than do psychologists from Eastern traditions. Although the reasons for this difference are multifaceted, some insight can be found in the nature of modern Western society. Because the societies of North America and Western Europe are ethnically and culturally diverse, there are divergent opinions of how a person should behave in a particular situation; the norms attached to particular roles and statuses in society have loosened. In many Western cultures, society no longer strictly prescribes what it means to be a married woman, a businessman, or a senior citizen. Women in their fifties give birth; grandparents give up the life of leisure to become Peace Corps volunteers; African American businessmen vocally challenge affirmative action; married couples negotiate who will work outside the home and who will care for children. In diverse, heterogeneous cultures, what one should do or be is no longer prescribed by cultural norms and expectations. Thus the individual is required to "establish internally a coherence and a continuity that will seem adequate to oneself and to others" (Camilleri & Malewska-Peyre, 1997, p. 53). As social roles and positions become less powerful in determining the individual's identity, the individual becomes more responsible for creating an identity separate from social roles, status, gender, ethnicity, and religious upbringing. Hence, in modern Western societies, identity is personally and individually constructed; persons who have not deliberately challenged and questioned the identities they were raised with (Catholic, conservative, obedient daughter, good musician, Latina) are viewed as "foreclosed" (Marcia, 1966), unenlightened, or unsophisticated. In a world in which the self is "the only or main form of reality" (Coles, 1980, p. 137), the individual who has not made an individual effort to define the self is seen as having no reality.

One consequence of the necessity to create and sustain one's own identity independent of the cultural context is that this identity must be continually verified, reexamined, updated, and defended. In the mobile Western society, in which many communities and associations are transitory or short term, individuals must continually reestablish this internal coherence and continuity as they communicate their identities to new associates and acquaintances (Camilleri & Malewska-Peyre, 1997). As a result, Western psychologists have identified a plethora of means whereby individuals protect, defend, verify, and sustain self-images. Self-affirmation, self-verification, self-enhancement, self-serving biases, self-symbolization, self-presentation, self-esteem maintenance, self-categorization, self-consistency, self-deception, self-handicapping—all are processes that Western psychologists have identified as vital for the construction, maintenance, and defense of the self-constructed identity.

In more homogenous, traditional, or Eastern cultures, identity is more closely linked to one's age, gender, status, caste, or roles; one's place in a social network is the main form of reality. Thus it is less necessary for persons to construct an internal, personal sense of identity; identities based on roles and statuses may be seldom challenged and so require little defense or scrutiny. Research comparing Icelandic and U.S. 12-year olds illustrates this difference in the attention to and importance of an internal, personal self-image (Hart & Edelstein, 1992). Iceland is very culturally homogenous; there has been little immigration for many centuries, and there is a countrywide school curriculum and set of traditional texts. Hart and Fegley (1997) report that when they asked Icelandic youths to describe themselves, using a interview technique widely used with 12-year olds in the United States, the young people often had great difficulty. They report that between 25% and 40% of the Icelandic youths found questions such as, "What are you like?" too strange to answer. Although these children were quite able to describe other people and functioned well both academically and socially, self-scrutiny and self-description were not necessary or culturally valued activities (see also Barth, 1997). Consequently, behaviors intended to defend, protect, or enhance an internal, private, self-constructed self-image may be less commonly found in homogenous cultures such as Iceland.

In a cultural context in which identity is individually selected from a wide array of cultural options, choice, personal desire, and intrinsic interest are the purest forces in motivation (Lilliard, 1998). As Bellah, Madsen, Sullivan, Swidler, and Tipton (1985) have written, in the United States "the notion of pure, undetermined choice, free of tradition, obligation, or commitment, [is] the essence of the self" (p. 152). Thus, to be an authentic person, the individual must express choices (or at least believe that he or she has expressed choices) in each and every behavior, from everyday purchases to career and relationship decisions. In fact, behaviors and goals that are constrained by external forces or social expectations are thought to be less satisfying and potent in directing behavior than are those derived purely from internal wishes and desires. In their self-determination theory of motivation, Deci and Ryan (1995; Chapter 13, this volume) argue that when individuals engage in a behavior for purely internal reasons (e.g., because it reflects their interests, wishes, and desires), they are more likely to persist at the task and to succeed in their goals. Goals that are pursued for external reasons—because of social influence or others' expectations—will not be as satisfying or successful as purely internally motivated and self-chosen goals (see also Sheldon & Elliot, 1999). Other important theories of motivation and behavior are also premised on the importance of personal choice, including reactance theory (Brehm, 1966), cognitive dissonance theory (Aronson, 1969; Festinger, 1957), and attribution theory (Morris & Peng, 1994).

In contrast, in Eastern cultural contexts, personal choice is a less important motivator of behavior. In cultures in which the self is defined by one's roles, positions, and statuses, behaving appropriately given the norms and ideals for one's roles is more important than expressing internal, private, self-selected attributes. In fact, in many cultures, there is very little discussion about why persons behave as they do; the expected behavior in a particular situation is strictly scripted, and individuals have few options for what to do in particular instances. In such situations, it is not necessary to intuit one's own or others' motivations because internal, individual differences are not predictive of behavior (Rosen, 1995). In many East Asian cultural contexts, persons and behaviors are not viewed as separable; there is no distinction between a person who acts and the actions the person performs (J. G. Miller, 1997). Consequently, understanding the person's intentions or choices is not as important as focusing on the outcome of the behavior. In Samoa, for example, only the actual outcome of persons' behavior, not their intentions, is considered in assigning blame (Lilliard, 1998).

When asked to explain others' behavior, members of collectivist cultures are more likely to focus on social and situational causes than are members of Western cultures (Choi, Nisbett, & Norenzayan, 1999; J. G. Miller, 1984). As Choi, Nisbett, and their colleagues have demonstrated, the reason is not necessarily that members of East Asian cultures ignore internal or dispositional explanations but rather that they pay more attention to and acknowledge the impact of situations on behavior. In fact, Choi and his colleagues (1999) argue that members of East Asian cultures have extensive

vocabularies for dispositions; others describe the conflict between personal desires and social responsibility that members of these cultures experience (Mathews, 1996; Oerter, Oerter, Agostiani, Kim, & Wibowo, 1996). But personal wishes, desires, and choices are not granted the priority in these cultures that they enjoy in North America. In many societies based on Confucian principles, the personal self is referred to as the "small self," and the attachment to one's family, society, and nation is the "greater self." Emblazoned on the walls of many Taiwanese schools is the admonition to "sacrifice [the] smaller self to accomplish [the] greater self" (Wu, 1994, p. 235).

This restraint or subordination of the personal or "small" self is reflected in a very different orientation toward choice in East Asian cultures compared with North American cultures. In Japan, the socially skilled person avoids directly expressing his or her choices and opinions and sidesteps choices when they are offered (captured in the Japanese term enryo; Wierzbicka, 1997). The host who offers the Japanese person too many choices creates an uncomfortable situation because it puts the person in the position of violating enryo. Instead, the good host attempts to anticipate the guest's needs and wishes and prepares accordingly (Markus & Kitayama, 1991). In the United States, offering one's guests choices may be a way of recognizing their individuality and allowing them to express their unique preferences.

Multiple studies demonstrate that choice and the psychological processes associated with the importance of choosing are less important in the motivational orientation of East Asians than is typically found in the West. Iyengar and Lepper (1999) investigated the importance of personal choice in motivation among European American children and Asian American children (from homes in which Japanese or Chinese was still the primary language). Children (ages 7 to 9) were asked to complete a set of anagram puzzles from a variety of categories (e.g., related to the family, toys, sports, food, and so forth). The experimenters manipulated who would choose the type of puzzles to be completed. In one condition, the experimenter told the children that they could pick any puzzle they wanted (personal-choice condition). In another condition, the experimenter chose the puzzle for the child (experimenter-choice condition). In the third condition, the experimenter said that the child's mother had picked which puzzle she wanted the child to do (mom-choice condition).

The Euro-American children in the personal-choice condition performed best and had the highest levels of motivation when compared with the Euro-Americans in the other conditions. The Asian American children, however, performed best and had the highest levels of motivation when they were in the mom-choice condition (Iyengar & Lepper, 1999). Although the Asian American children were more motivated in the personal-choice condition than in the experimenter-choice condition, it was clear that they most preferred that their choices were being made by a close and trusted other. The Euro-American children showed no difference between the experimenter-choice and the mom-choice conditions, because both of these conditions undermined their sense of choice. This research suggests that the assumption that autonomy and personal choice are the major contributors to high levels of motivation applies primarily to persons from Western backgrounds. As Iyengar and Lepper (1999) suggest, having choices made by a close and valued ingroup member offered the Asian American children the opportunity to promote belongingness in the relationship, which motivated high levels of performance.

Choice is a critical factor in cognitive dissonance paradigms based on the forced-choice paradigm, in which participants must choose between two options that are equally desirable. Having made a choice, participants are thought to experience postdecisional regret, resulting in dissonance reduction strategies. Such studies have not been replicated in Japan, perhaps because making choices and feeling personally responsible for those choices is not as representative of the self for Japanese, and so the possibility of making a poor choice is not as threatening to the self for Japanese as for Americans (Heine & Lehman, 1997).

For North Americans, choosing represents the establishment and fulfillment of a unique, individual self, whereas for East Asians, cases in which they are forced to choose may be construed as opportunities to demonstrate their similarity to and alignment with others. In a series of studies, Kim and Markus (1999) showed that East Asians were more likely to make choices that indicated a preference for conformity rather than uniqueness. In one study, participants were given the option of selecting a pen as compensation after completing a brief questionnaire. Participants were allowed to chose between five pens of two different colors, so that in each case, there was a majority color (3 or 4 pens) and a minority color (1 or 2 pens). Routinely, Euro-American participants selected a pen from the minority color, and East Asians selected a pen from the majority color. In other studies, Euro-American participants showed a greater preference for unique figures in an array (e.g., they preferred the diamond in a group of squares) than did Chinese American participants. Kim and Markus suggest that the participants from East Asian backgrounds revealed their desire for similarity and conformity by selecting a pen from the majority (or the majority figures), whereas the participants from Euro-American backgrounds demonstrated their preference for individuality and uniqueness by selecting one of the minority colored pens (or a minority figure). In short, for Euro-Americans, the act of choosing is an opportunity to demonstrate a sense of the self as different and unique; for the East Asians, the act of choosing is an opportunity to reinforce a sense of the self as similar to others and part of a larger group (see Bond & Smith, 1996, for a review of research on culture and conformity).

The East Asian reluctance to express one's own opinion and preferences, and choices that reflect conformity to and alignment with others, are in service to the "big self," or the self that is connected to others and society. This motivational orientation is captured in the Japanese term *wa*, which is defined as the desire for harmony within groups (Wierzbicka, 1997). In Chinese, the term *he* denotes harmony, unity, and peace with others (Gao, Ting-Toomey, & Gudykunst, 1996). Individuals are expected to promote harmony in interpersonal relationships and ingroups by behaving properly in their roles and relationships (termed "ritual propriety," or *li* in Chinese). Concern for harmony is a fundamental principle in East Asian cultural contexts and underlies much social behavior. Conflict resolution strategies that reduce animosity among the parties and that protect relationships are preferred to those that may lead to broken relationships (Leung & Fan, 1997; Markus & Lin, 1999). Negotiation and compromise are sought in business dealings rather than confrontation or litigation (Gabrenya & Hwang, 1996; Gao et al., 1996; Hamilton & Sanders, 1992). In Japanese baseball, the most important component for a successful team is *wa,* and Japanese baseball is noted for subordinating individual stardom to the team aspects of the game, such as the sacrifice bunt and the hit-and-run (Whiting, 1989). A study of Chinese in Hong Kong revealed that ratings of relationship harmony were as important as ratings of self-esteem in predicting life satisfaction; in the United States, ratings of self-esteem were much stronger than ratings of relationship harmony in predicting life satisfaction (Kwan, Bond, & Singelis, 1997).

If harmony with others in interpersonal situations is an ultimate goal in the East Asian motivational orientation, individuals may find themselves behaving quite differently in different situations. Many Western theories of motivation are based on the assumption that the self is an internal, stable structure; thus persons should behave consistently across situations (Lecky, 1945). Inconsistency denotes the lack of a stable, coherent self and is related to low self-esteem (Campbell, 1990) and poor well-being (Donahue, Robins, Roberts, & John, 1993; Sheldon, Ryan, Rawsthorne, & Ilardi, 1997). The consistency motive, particularly self-consistency, is central to many Western theories of motivation (Aronson, 1969; Swann, 1990; Swann, Rentfrow, & Guinn, Chapter 18, this volume) and personality (Pervin, 1990).

The importance of transituational consistency is notably absent in East Asian cultural contexts. Instead, East Asian philosophies explicitly recognize inconsistency in the notion of *yin* and *yang,* which are opposing but integrated forces in the world (Peng & Nisbett, 1999). These philosophical traditions view all elements of nature and being as interrelated; thus they acknowledge contradiction and complexity of causes. Har-

mony is obtained through the balance of contradictory forces or by finding the "middle way" between two extremes (Nisbett et al., 2001). Balancing the opposing forces of *yin* and *yang* provides coherence and integrity (Kitayama & Markus, 1999). Chinese proverbs, such as, "Fortune and misfortune are the twisted strands of a rope," reflect the belief that good luck and bad luck are experienced by all and that something good arises from the interplay of contradictory forces. Consequently, East Asians are much more tolerant of inconsistency, ambiguity, and contradiction than are North Americans (see Nisbett et al., 2001, for a review of Chinese dialectics).

The East Asian holistic worldview contrasts with the Western stance that contradictions must be resolved by the rejection of one of the elements of the contradiction. According to Peng and Nisbett (1999), the Western analytic worldview is based on the Aristotelian system of formal logic. In particular, the law of noncontradiction states that "it is impossible for the same thing to be both true and false at the same time" (Peng & Nisbett, 1999, p. 744). A statement is either true or false, and contradiction must be resolved. In research comparing Chinese and American responses to social situations that involved contradiction, Peng and Nisbett (1999, study 3) showed that Chinese participants tended to consider the situations from both sides and to attempt to reconcile the contradictory positions through compromise. For example, when asked to respond to a mother–daughter conflict over values, the Chinese participants were more likely to respond with statements such as, "both the mother and daughter have failed to understand each other." North Americans, in contrast, tended to view the situations from a one-sided perspective, finding fault in one position and siding with the presumably "right" position (as indicated by statements such as "the mother has to recognize the daughter's right to her own values").

In another series of studies, Choi and Nisbett (2000) hypothesized that when individuals hold a holistic view of the world that permits contradiction and inconsistency, they are less likely to experience surprise at unexpected events. "[If] one notices a host of factors and believes them to be potentially involved in complex interactions, any outcome may seem to be understandable *after the fact* because post hoc explanations may be relatively easy to generate" (Choi & Nisbett, 2000, p. 891; italics in original). Thus these individuals will be less surprised at unexpected outcomes of events. As expected, Korean participants in their studies showed greater hindsight bias after unexpected events, indicating that they "knew it all along."

This tolerance for contradiction and acceptance of opposing forces in the world may be one factor explaining the repeated finding that East Asians use more negative terms to describe themselves than do North Americans. Kanagawa, Cross, and Markus (2001), using an open-ended task in which participants respond to the question, "Who am I?" 20 times (Kuhn & McPartland, 1954), found that Japanese students included nearly twice as many negative statements in their self-descriptions as did American students. So whereas Americans will tend to distort, minimize, and ignore negative aspects of the self, Japanese are willing to acknowledge them, perhaps because internal harmony is viewed as the reconciliation of diverse and opposing forces rather than the elimination of contradiction and negativity.

Kanagawa and her colleagues (2001) also examined the hypothesis that if a Japanese person's behavior is more dependent on situational cues and norms than a Euro-American's behavior, then this variability will be reflected in the spontaneous self-concept. The participants in their study were assigned to one of four conditions for the "Who am I?" task: (1) seated alone in a research cubicle, (2) in a large group, (3) alone with a faculty member, or (4) in pairs with a peer. Americans tended to describe themselves in trait terms across all the situations to a much greater degree than did the Japanese students, emphasizing the importance to the Americans of abstract, context-free, internal attributes for self-definition. The Japanese students used a greater variety of types of statements to describe themselves than did Americans and were more likely to use situation-specific, behavioral self-descriptions (e.g., "I bought a T-shirt yesterday"; see also Rhee, Uleman, Lee, & Roman, 1995).

More important, the frequencies of the types of self-descriptions reported by the American students varied very little across the four conditions, but for the Japanese, the conditions substantially influenced the types of self-views reported. For example, the Japanese students were more likely to describe themselves in terms of their abilities when alone than in the other situations. The frequency of negative statements about the self also depended on the situation for the Japanese, but not for the Americans. The Japanese students were most negative about themselves when they were seated with a faculty member, consistent with norms of modesty and self-effacement in situations with higher status others. They were least negative in their self-descriptions when describing themselves while alone in a cubicle. These findings suggest that the power of the situation to activate different self-views is stronger in East Asian cultural contexts than in Western cultural contexts, which will result in greater variation in actual behavior.

We regret that space does not allow us to extensively review other motivational consequences of differences in cultural models of the self, but several lines of research deserve at least brief mention. For example, variation in the self influences perceptions of and desire for control. Euro-Americans tend to seek direct or primary control over their environments, whereas East Asians tend to seek to adjust to their environments and to display indirect, or secondary, means of control (Morling, 2000; Sastry & Ross, 1998; Weisz et al., 1984). Judgments of efficacy also depend on the nature of the self, and investigators have begun to pursue how a sense of collective efficacy influences individual behavior (Earley, 1993). East Asian views of the world as ever changing are reflected in Dweck and her colleagues' research into entity versus incremental implicit theories of the person (Chiu, Dweck, Tong, & Fu, 1997; Chiu, Hong, & Dweck, 1997). Others have begun to investigate the relations between self-regulatory focus and variation in self-construals (Aaker & Lee, 2001; Lee, Aaker, & Gardner, 2000). An examination of other theories of motivation, such as self-determination theory (Deci & Ryan, 1995), through the lens of interdependent models of the self will prove helpful in the development of concepts, theories, and models of motivation that can be generalized beyond Euro-American cultural borders.

Culture and Self-Regard

Cultural models of the self define the basis of self-esteem. At the most basic level, self-esteem has been defined as an attitude toward or an evaluation of oneself (Coopersmith, 1967; Rosenberg, 1965). Any evaluation requires a standard against which the object is measured. In general, the cultural ideal or model will be the primary standard against which individuals evaluate themselves (although certainly individuals will idiosyncratically elaborate on this standard; Solomon, Greenberg, & Pyszczynski, 1991). (Because the term "self-esteem" is so strongly associated with positive views of the self, we use other terms, such as "self-regard" or "self-worth," to refer to evaluations of the self as an appropriate member of society.) Thus, in the United States, the primary standard for evaluating the self is how well one meets the cultural norm of independence, autonomy, and uniqueness. In East Asian cultural contexts, the primary standard for evaluating the self is how well one meets the cultural norms of fitting into important groups, behaving appropriately in social situations, and maintaining harmony in relationships. Both the independent and the interdependent models of the self involve socially relevant dimensions (e.g., "I am special and different from others" versus "I am similar to and in harmony with others"), but the relation of the self to others varies in these two models.

Individual inferences and perceptions of how well one meets the standard and feedback from others about one's standing relative to the standard are two components of self-regard. The relative importance of these two sources of self-regard will likely vary in individualistic versus collectivistic cultural contexts. Personal inferences and evaluations will be a more important source of self-regard in Western, individualistic cultural contexts than in Eastern, interdependent cultural contexts. This orientation toward personal evaluations of worth is evident in research on cognitive and motivational processes that promote positive evaluations of the self. Examples of self-enhancing strategies include making overly positive judgments of the self (Alicke, 1985), framing self-defining traits more positively than other traits (Dunning & Hayes, 1996), and taking credit for successes while attributing failure to situational factors (Greenberg, Pyszczynski, & Solomon, 1982; see Brown, 1998, for a review). When faced with negative information about the self, individuals can self-affirm by accessing positive information that cancels out the negative feedback (Steele, 1988) or can compare themselves with others who have performed more poorly, making their own performances look better in comparison (Gibbons & Gerrard, 1991; Tesser, 1988).

Each of these self-enhancing strategies exemplifies the American perspective on self-regard: One should feel good about oneself no matter what, even if this requires distorting the information one receives so that it becomes more positive. In this cultural context, it is not enough to do one's best; one must excel and win to claim positive feelings for the self. Some theorists have argued that these self-enhancing strategies and biases are crucial for well-being and adaptation (Taylor & Brown, 1988), and others have argued that many social ills (e.g., crime, violence, teen pregnancy, poverty) are a consequence of low self-esteem (California Task Force to Promote Self-Esteem, 1990, as cited in Baumeister, 1993). In other words, positive self-regard is the hallmark of being a socially valued person in the Western, independent model of the self.

A Square Peg in a Round Hole: Applying Western Views of Self-Esteem to Eastern Cultures

Cross-cultural research consistently shows that members of collective societies are lower in self-esteem (as measured by scales developed in the West) than members of individualist societies (e.g., Bond & Cheung, 1983; Tafarodi, Lang, & Smith, 1999). In fact, distributions of scores on the Rosenberg Self-Esteem Scale (Rosenberg, 1965) within Eastern cultures show that the actual midpoint of the scores is closer to the theoretical midpoint than it is when the scale is used in Western cultures (Diener & Diener, 1995). The tendency for scores to be clustered at the high end of the distribution (as is repeatedly found in North America; Heine & Lehman, 1999) is not apparent among participants from collectivist cultures. When viewed through the lens of the Western model of the self, these findings seem to point to lower levels of self-esteem among East Asians than among Westerners. From the Western perspective, individuals with low self-esteem are viewed as deficient in resources, confused, conflicted, self-protective, and fragile (Baumeister, 1993). Is this a fair characterization of members of East Asian cultures? If, as suggested previously, self-regard is a function of fitting into the culturally approved model of the person, then East Asian responses to Western measures of self-esteem must be considered in light of the interdependent model of the self.

In the interdependent self-construal, maintaining harmony and connectedness with others is central to viewing oneself as fitting into the cultural model of the person. In these cultural contexts, the self is defined in terms of social roles, statuses, and group memberships, and the expectations of persons in these positions are socially defined and agreed on. Members of East Asian cultures are encouraged to strive toward culturally shared prototypes of the ideal person in regard to their social roles (Kitayama et al., 1997; Markus & Kitayama, 1998). Confucianism describes proper behavior in the Five Cardinal Relations (the *Wu Lun*): relations between emperor and minister, father and son, husband and wife, brothers, and friends (Gabrenya & Hwang, 1996). These cardinal relations, especially the relation between fathers and sons, form the basis of the beliefs and norms for proper behavior in interpersonal relationships (termed *li*, or "ritual propriety"; Freeman & Habermann, 1996; Ho, 1995). East Asians are encouraged to compare themselves against these ideals and to identify the ways in which they fall short of the ideals (Heine, Lehman, Markus, & Kitayama, 1999; Kitayama et al., 1997). Viewing oneself in a critical manner maintains the attitude that one must work hard to make up for one's shortcomings (Stevenson, 1995) and serves to continue improvement and movement toward the ideal. For example, pride is valued in Western culture as self-recognition of personal achievement, whereas pride in Eastern cultures is viewed as a sign of arrogance and as failure to acknowledge the contributions of others (Stipek, 1998). Indeed, in some East Asian contexts, pride or egoism is viewed as a source of suffering (Sinha & Sinha, 1997).

This self-critical orientation is developed through East Asian socialization and parenting practices. From an early age, Japanese children are encouraged to dwell on their inadequacies and shortcomings, a concept called *hansei suru* (Heine et al., 1999). Kindergarten children end each day by reflecting on their failings that day and how they can do better in the future (Lewis, 1995). In a study comparing everyday stories about a child's past among Americans and Chinese in Taiwan, P. J. Miller, Fung, and Mintz (1996) found that the Chinese mothers' stories about their toddlers were more likely to be characterized by a critical description of the child's transgressions than were the American mothers' stories. In contrast, the American mothers were more likely to recount stories about the child that were affirming and that protected the child's positive self-evaluations.

Most of the research on self-regard has found that members of collectivist cultures will employ strategies for self-effacement to express their desire for harmony and to demonstrate relatedness to others. For example, East Asians are higher in self-criticism (Heine & Lehman, 1997; Kitayama et al., 1997) and lower in unrealistic optimism (Heine & Lehman, 1995) than members of Western cultures. They are more likely than Westerners to discount the accuracy of a test that gives positive feedback and are more attentive to information that they are doing worse than others in a group (Heine, Takata, & Lehman, 2000). Japanese tend to view everyday situations as opportunities for self-criticism and criticism from others (Kitayama et al., 1997) and view themselves as further from their ideal than samples from Western cultures (Heine & Lehman, 1999). Heine and Lehman (1999) also found that self–ideal discrepancies were less strongly associated with depression and poor well-being among the Japanese in their study than among European Canadians. In North America, these discrepancies are evidence of failure, and so threaten the individual's view of himself or herself as competent and successful. In Japan, such discrepancies are common and may be viewed as admissions that one can improve and will continue to strive toward the ideal, and so reflect the culturally valued stance toward the self.

Other research findings have shown that modest self-evaluations are not attributable to group norms alone but appear to be internalized attitudes on the part of individuals with an interdependent self-construal. Hetts, Sakuma, and Pelham (1999) had participants from the United States (European Americans and Asian Americans) and recent immigrants from Asia complete an Implicit Association Test for individual terms ("Me") and collective terms ("Us"), in association with positive words ("Good") and negative words ("Bad"). A positivity index was created by subtracting the response latency for positive words from the response latency for negative words (i.e., high scores indicated quicker responses to positive words than to negative words). Recent immigrants from Asia had higher positivity scores for the collective terms than for the individual terms and also had higher positivity scores for the collective terms than did the other samples. They also had the lowest positivity scores for the individual terms compared with the other samples. European Americans had higher positivity scores for the individual terms than the collective terms. These findings indicate that the recent East Asian immigrants implicitly favored the collective terms more than the individual terms and that the reverse was true for the European Americans. One value of research using implicit measures is that participants are less likely to provide socially desirable responses; thus these findings argue against the claim by some researchers that findings of self-effacement among East Asians are primarily due to self-presentation. They support the hypothesis that group membership is more important for self-worth than individual self-esteem for East Asians.

If East Asians view the self as defined by relationships and group memberships, do they perhaps show group-serving biases that are similar to the self-serving biases of Westerners? Recent research has shown that members of both individualist cultures and collectivist cultures view their close relationships (best friend, closest family member, and romantic partner) as more positive than those of their peers (Endo, Heine, & Lehman, 2000), but this effect is stronger among Euro-Americans than Japanese (Heine & Lehman, 1997). This suggests that a relationship-serving bias exists in both cultural contexts but that the self-enhancing bias is more limited to Western culture. The motivation behind relationship-serving biases, however, may differ between cultures. Endo and her colleagues (2000) found that the relationship bias for Japanese participants was based on viewing their relationship partners more positively than themselves ("My relationships are great because the people I have a bond with are great people"), whereas for the Euro-American participants, enhancing ingroup members was related to self-enhancement ("I'm great because my relationships are better than yours").

In order to succeed in Japanese society, individuals must gain an accurate understanding of how others view them personally and within the context of their social units (Heine et al., 1999). By being sensitive to others and taking the perspective of others' evaluations, one is more likely to establish a connection with them and reap the rewards of reciprocity (Benedict, 1942). Such give-and-take relationships are very common and exemplify the yin–yang principle of balance (Kitayama & Markus, 1999). The Japanese have a highly developed script for sympathy and support, which balances the commonplace self-criticism that occurs within the culture (Kitayama et al., 1997). For example, at the end of the workday, a common parting phrase to fellow employees before returning home is Otsukaresama ("You all must be exhausted") or Gokurosama ("You all suffered hard"; Heine et al., 1999). Cultivating the cultural ideal of self-criticism and pursuit of ideal standards will lead to approval and sympathy from others.

This give-and-take orientation to self-regard also permits one person to "give" self-regard to another person. In societies with very hierarchical relationships, such as Japan and India, when lower status persons in a relationship ask for help from a higher status person, they provide the superior with an opportunity to enhance his or her regard by performing the role of nurturing subordinates (Roland, 1991). Roland (1991) describes a situation in which a Japanese man expressed anger against his stepfather for a perceived wrong by not making the kinds of requests for help that his brothers and sisters had made. In not making these requests, and therefore not being dependent on his stepfather, he threatened his stepfather's self-regard by not allowing him to act out his position of one who gives and nurtures. In other words, opportunities to affirm the self, especially the self in important roles, may be conferred by others, making the process of cultivating and maintaining self-regard a dynamic interpersonal process.

This social component of self-regard is inferred in the East Asian notion of "face," which includes the notion of one's social image that is perceived by others (Ho, 1995). Although Westerners do consider the feelings and reputations of others in social interactions, this socially shared aspect of self-regard is not as well articulated as in East Asian cultures. East Asians have an elaborate understanding of the ways in which persons may protect the face of others or give face to others (Ting-Toomey, 1994). This concern for others' face, which may be framed as an empathic appreciation for another's social esteem, may help explain aspects of East Asian culture that seem peculiar to Westerners. Even in sports, for example, Japanese seem to prefer outcomes that permit both sides in a competition to save face. A president of the Japanese Pacific Baseball League, Shinuske Hori, claimed that ties "suit the Japanese character. That way nobody loses" (Whiting, 1989, p. 25). This contrasts with the American perspective, attributed to Vince Lombardi, the famous football coach of the Green Bay Packers: "Winning is everything . . . [and] a tie is like kissing your sister."

Researchers in North American contexts are beginning to show a renewed appreciation for social influences in self-esteem. For example, Leary, Tambor, Terdal, and Downs (1995) have shown that daily fluctuations in state self-esteem reflect the individual's perceptions of being included in or excluded from social groups (see also Luhtanen & Crocker, 1992; Sabini, Siepmann, & Stein, 2001). Approval by significant others and social groups reflects cultural norms and values, however. Persons in North American cultural contexts will garner approval and inclusion in social groups when they demonstrate self-reliance, autonomy, and superiority in valued domains. Persons in East Asian cultural contexts will garner approval and inclusion when they conform to social roles and ideals, take a critical stance toward the self, and strive for harmony in relationships. In short, consideration of cultural models of the self provides clues to the ways in which people strive to be culturally appropriate persons and can further the development of a more universal theory of self-regard.

Culture Change, Biculturalism, and the Self

In the privacy of your kitchen, you admit you cannot live without your family, your history, this ideal called "your people." You cannot divorce yourself from yourself. You know you are the hyphen in American-born. Your identity scrawls the length and breadth of the page, American-born-girl. American-born-Filipina. Because you have always had one foot planted in the Midwest, one foot floating on the islands, and your arms have stretched across the generations, barely kissing your father's province, your children's future, the dreams your mother has for you. Because you were meant for the better life, whatever that is, been told you mustn't forget where you come from, what others have done for you. . . . You do your best. You try. You struggle. And somehow, when you stand in the center of a room, and the others look on, you find yourself acting out your role. Smart American girl, beautiful Filipina, dutiful daughter. (Galang, 1996, p. 86)

Those who live in multicultural worlds perhaps most acutely recognize the cultural shaping of the self. The Filipina American in the quote gives us a glimpse of a few of the factors that influence who she is—her mother's dreams, her father's homeland, others' expectations, the roles she plays, her American birth. This struggle to create a self that bridges the new—the possibilities and opportunities of life in America—and the old—the family ties, heritage, and expectations of her Filipino family—highlights cultural influences in the construction of the self. Thus far, culture has been discussed as a fairly monolithic influence on the self. But what of the person exposed to multiple cultures, through expatriation, immigration, or conquest? What of the person, like the girl in the quote, who must straddle two cultures? Must the person choose one cultural identity over the other? Or blend the two? An examination of the consequences of moving from one culture to another or of growing up with the influences of more than one culture provides a unique approach to understanding the dynamic nature of the self. In the following sections, we briefly examine the issues of self-concept change and multiple cultural identities from the perspective of cultural models of the self.

Culture Change and the Self

Thinking of the self as a core structure that is resistant to change is a popular notion held in modern Western society, and one that is reinforced by admonitions such as, "Be true to yourself." In order to understand self-concept change, however, one must assume that the self is socially constructed and malleable (Berger, 1963). If the self is molded by culture, changes in cultural environment may affect how the self is perceived (for an example, see Oyserman & Markus, 1993). When individuals migrate to new cultures, sojourn for a period of years as a student or worker, or experience culture change for other reasons, they encounter new cultural practices, institutions, and customs, and they develop new knowledge structures and scripts for behavior. For example, an Iranian immigrant living in the United States reported, "I learned to be a lot more open with feelings in the U.S., to talk more about things that bothered me. I'm a lot less shy and more aggressive, at least at work" (Hoffman, 1990, p. 286). When newly developed knowledge structures are frequently primed in a new context, how does this affect the self? The next section attempts to answer this question with a brief review of the literature on self-concept change.

Researchers who focus on self-concept change, although few, generally agree that the key component to change comes more from other people than from oneself (Hormuth, 1990; Tice, 1992). Change is especially likely to occur when a person receives feedback that threatens one's confidence in one's self-views (Swann, 1983), and when the person expects to have future interactions with the people who provide the feedback (Tice, 1992). When individuals recognize that their previous self-views are no longer consistent with their present situation or behavior, they may experience a type of identity "crisis." Swann (1983) identified several factors that contribute to such a crisis: (1) The feedback comes from a competent source, (2) it is supported by many people, (3) it is directly relevant to an important dimension of one's self-concept, and (4) it is sufficiently, but not exaggeratedly, different from one's current self-concept. For example, an American student studying in Japan who thinks of himself as intelligent and competent may experience such a crisis when his attempts to answer questions in Japanese are met with giggles or looks of confusion or when his outspokenness is met with scowls by a teacher (who expects more deferential behaviors than Americans would expect).

According to research conducted with Western participants, self-change can occur when individuals engage in behavior that is inconsistent with their current attitudes or beliefs (Aronson, 1969; Hormuth, 1990). In a new cultural context, the opportunities to engage in behaviors that are inconsistent with one's self-views or attitudes can be quite extensive. For example, Western businesspeople living overseas may find themselves working on projects in which the group's progress is more important than their individual efforts. As a result, self-views related to group membership may be activated more readily than when they were working in the West. If group projects are engaged in with high frequency, Western businesspeople may find themselves seeking group tasks in general and displaying beliefs that such tasks are preferable to individual tasks. Over time, experiences in the new culture influence thinking so that individuals apply new characteristics to themselves (Sanitioso, Kunda, & Fong, 1990) and begin to interpret past experiences in light of current motives and beliefs (Vorauer & Ross, 1993). The businessperson in the previous example may begin to "remember" events in which group projects in America were enjoyable and stimulating and may recall events in which group activities were suggested with enthusiasm.

Engaging in inconsistent behaviors is most likely to change the self-concept when these behaviors are displayed publicly (Tice, 1992; Tice & Wallace, Chapter 5, this volume). When individuals view their behavior as inconsistent with their private beliefs, they may feel compelled to adjust their self-descriptions and beliefs, especially if they expect to interact with the observers of the behavior in the future (Tice, 1992). Such inconsistencies are very likely to occur in a new cultural context. For example, Japanese cultural contexts encourage and afford modest or self-critical self-presentations, which may feel dissonant to the person with a very independent self-construal. Over time, as a person finds himself or herself engaging in behavior so as to "fit in" with the culture, this behavior becomes routinized (Hormuth, 1990). Once a behavior becomes part of people's daily lives, they are less likely to perceive environmental control over their actions and more likely to create an internal attribution for their behavior. For example, an American woman in Pakistan may learn that covering one's face in public is a cultural norm that demonstrates a woman's humility. The American woman may not like the idea of humility, but she will most likely engage in the behavior in order to avoid strange stares while in public. Over time, this behavior becomes part of her routine, and she may begin to attribute her behavior internally. Though perhaps not as humble as the Pakistani women, she may become more humble than when she first arrived. She may recognize that humility is more valued in the new culture than in American culture, and she becomes comfortable portraying this behavior in public.

Finally, individuals will develop new knowledge structures and concepts for persons and behaviors in cultures that are quite different from their culture of origin. For example, newcomers to Japan will be frequently exposed to the concept of *wa* or harmony, and visitors to Chinese societies will be required to think about *li*, or ritual propriety. In a study of American college students, Deutsch and Mackesy (1985) found that unacquainted partners who discussed a target person later used each other's self-schemas to describe themselves. Thus culture-specific concepts that are used frequently in interactions with host nationals may eventually be used to describe the self, resulting in a changed self-concept.

In summary, engagement in new cultural contexts can result in change in the self-concept as individuals receive feedback that is discrepant with their self-views, as they adopt new ways of behaving, and as they develop knowledge structures for new ways to think about persons and behavior. Note, however, that most of this research has focused on self-concept change among members of individualistic cultures and so has presumed an independent model of the self. Much less is known about self-concept change and adaptation to new cultures for individuals who have developed an interdependent self-construal or whether the processes of self-concept change may differ depending on whether a person comes from a individualistic or a collectivist culture.

After months or years of adjusting one's behavior to fit into a new cultural environment, does the individual's self-structure transform into one aligned with the new culture's model of the self? Does the original representation of the self wither away through disuse? A growing body of research on multicultural selves has shown that people who experience multiple cultures are able to shift cultural belief systems in a way that suggests that new cultural self-representations coexist with the old cultural self-representations in memory. The following section examines this phenomenon.

The Bicultural Self

Bicultural people have internalized two cultures to the extent that both cultures are "alive" inside of them (Hong, Morris, Chiu, & Benet-Martinez, 2000). Research with immigrants shows that individuals who have spent long periods of time in a new culture come to describe themselves more consistently with the new cultural norms than do recent arrivals (McCrae, Yik, Trapnell, Bond, & Paulhus, 1998). Other studies with Asian Americans and Asian international students in the United States show that measures of the independent self-construal and the interdependent self-construal are orthogonal (Cross, 1995;

Singelis, 1994). Mounting evidence indicates that individuals with exposure to two cultures can develop separate, culturally derived self-representations and that in fact this bicultural self may be most adaptive for immigrant and minority populations (Bautista de Domanico, Crawford, & DeWolfe, 1994; Kaneshiro, 1997; Ryder, Alden, & Paulhus, 2000; Sussman, 2000; see LaFromboise, Coleman, & Gerton, 1993, for a review).

Often, bicultural people find the two cultures "taking turns" guiding their thoughts and feelings, depending on particular cues in the environment (LaFromboise et al., 1993). In essence, bicultural people have the ability to interpret social and other environmental cues using the cultural framework that fits the best. Although these people acquire more than one cultural meaning system, usually only one system guides cognition at a given time, a concept termed "frame switching" (Hong et al., 2000). This suggests that multiple internalized cultures are not necessarily blended and that absorbing a second culture does not necessitate a substitution of the old cultural meaning system. An example of a Mexican American student displays this frame-switching:

> At home with my parents and my grandparents the only acceptable language was Spanish; actually, that's all they really understood. Everything was really Mexican, but at the same time they wanted me to speak good English. . . . But at school, I felt really different because everyone was American, including me. Then I would go home in the afternoon and be Mexican again. (Padilla, 1994, p. 30)

Research exploring frame switching has found that this trend occurs for many bicultural people (Morris, Nisbett, & Peng, 1995). When shown a picture of a fish swimming in front of a group of other fish, Chinese Americans who had been primed with American symbols (e.g., the American flag) tended to state that the first fish was leading the other fish (reflecting belief in an internal cause of behavior). However, when they were primed with Chinese symbols (e.g., the Great Wall), the participants tended to state that the first fish was being chased by the other fish (reflecting belief in an external cause of behavior). In other words, the students' responses revealed the

typical patterns of attribution of the primed culture (Morris & Peng, 1994).

Response styles to questionnaires have also been observed for bilingual participants (Bond, 1983; Earle, 1969). When questionnaires in English were given to Chinese participants who were fluent in English, they responded with answers that reflected Western cultural beliefs. However, when the participants received the same questionnaires translated into Chinese, they responded with answers that reflected Eastern cultural beliefs. Thus the language of the questionnaire primed the associated cultural self-representation (see also McCrae et al., 1998).

These findings shed light on self-related experiences that are often described anecdotally but have seldom been explored empirically. Many adults bemoan the experience of slipping back into old roles when they visit family or friends whom they seldom see. In these contexts, mature, middle-aged adults sometimes find themselves engaging in the adolescent behavior they thought they had outgrown. The older brother absent-mindedly patronizes his little sister, and the little sister becomes belligerent and angry in response. After the fact, they both are puzzled at their behavior, believing that they had left behind those old selves. What explains this phenomenon? These perspectives on culture change and the bicultural self suggest that in cases like this, the old self or relational schema (Baldwin, 1997)—the "little sister" or "older brother" self, which is never accessed outside of family environments—has been activated again and is influencing behavior. This old self is not gone or forgotten, but slumbers, waiting for the situation to awaken it. Is there then no hope of escaping an old and undesired self? To the extent that the individuals involved can access new selves—the professional self, the mature, sophisticated, or well-educated adult self—they may be able to switch frames and derive direction for their behavior from a more appropriate and desirable self-view.

In summary, examination of individuals who change cultures or live within two cultural environments can shed light on more ordinary aspects of changing the self or of the multiple components of the self. A cultural perspective provides many rich opportunities for theory development and testing that can guide further research within a single culture. For example, cross-cultural research has shed light on the variety of self-construals that may exist within Western cultural contexts, and researchers have adopted concepts from cross-cultural research to further the understanding of the self in Western societies. In the next section, we briefly review some of this research.

Applying Cultural Concepts to the Self in Western Societies

By making long excursions in space and time, we may find our ordinary rules completely upset, and these great upsettings will give us a clearer view and better comprehension of such small changes as may occur nearer us, in the small corner of the world in which we are called to live and move. We shall know this corner better for the journey we have taken into distant lands where we had no concern. (Poincaré, 1908/n.d., p. 21)

Although this quote from Poincaré refers to the role of astronomy and geology in understanding the physical world, it aptly summarizes the importance of cross-cultural research for understanding group and individual differences within a society. As Poincaré suggests, investigations into distant lands provide a clearer view of one's own corner of the world. For example, cross-cultural research has informed research on U.S. ethnic groups with origins in collectivist cultures. Crocker and her colleagues (Crocker, Luhtanen, Blaine, & Broadnax, 1994) have shown that group memberships are a more important contributor to self-esteem for African Americans and Asian Americans than for European Americans. African Americans and Hispanic Americans are more likely to endorse collectivist and familial cultural values than are European Americans (Gaines et al., 1997). Ethnic identity is a function of one's sociocultural position and influences attitudes, emotion, motivation, and social behavior (Gurung & Duong, 1999; Howard, 2000; Oyserman, Harrison, & Bybee, 2001; Phinney, 1990; Sellers, Smith, Shelton, Rowley, & Chavous, 1998).

Cross-cultural studies of the self also provide insight into gender differences in Western cultural contexts. Women in Western societies have traditionally been viewed as more relational, connected, and interdependent with others than men (Bakan, 1966; Gilligan, 1982; Maccoby, 1990). Integrating the cross-cultural research on the self with research on gender differences in North America, Cross and Madson (1997) argued that many gender differences in behavior can best be understood in terms of differences in the self. They argued that women in the United States are socialized to attend to relationships and to consider the needs and wishes of others, resulting in a self-view that is defined in large part in terms of relationships with others. This view of the self is distinguished from the East Asian interdependent self-construal in that it affords primacy to dyadic relationships rather than to group memberships. In other words, American women are more likely to define themselves in terms of close relationships ("I am a mother"; "I am John's girlfriend") than in terms of important groups. As a result, they have been described as constructing a *relational* self-construal (Cross, Bacon, & Morris, 2000). American men, in contrast, have been described as being more strongly socialized than women to focus on their independence, autonomy, and separation from others (but see Baumeister & Sommer, 1997; Gabriel & Gardner, 1999, for a different perspective on this topic).

These different representations of the self are thought to underlie many observed gender differences in behavior. Women in North America are more likely than men to describe themselves in terms of relationships and to evaluate themselves on the basis of relationships with others (Boggiano & Barrett, 1991; Cross et al., 2000; McGuire & McGuire, 1982; Ogilvie & Clark, 1992; Roberts & Nolen-Hoeksema, 1994; Zuckerman, 1989). Given that individuals define themselves in terms of relationships, they should be highly motivated to attend to relationship partners and to remember information about them. In fact, women tend to be more accurate than men in their perceptions of what relationship partners are thinking and feeling (Ickes, Robertson, Tooke, & Teng, 1986) and to have better memory for relationship events than do men (Ross & Holmberg, 1992). Women also exhibit more relationship-promoting behavior than do men; they are more likely than men to self-disclose in relationships (Derlega, Durham, Gockel, & Sholis, 1981) and are more likely to elicit self-disclosure from others than are men (Shaffer, Pegalis, & Bazzini, 1996; see Cross & Madson, 1997, for a review). The processes that lead to gender differences in behavior may be more easily targeted and investigated when gender is conceptualized as a cultural phenomenon leading to variation in the self-construal.

In summary, the introduction of the concept of the interdependent self-construal into Western cultural contexts has promoted a new interest in variation in the structure of the self. Researchers have begun to move beyond gender and ethnic differences and to investigate the role of relational and collective aspects of the self more generally. Many researchers now argue that people develop all three aspects of the self (the individual, relational, and collective selves) to varying degrees (see Brewer & Gardner, 1996; Sedikides & Brewer, 2000). Exciting new work has begun to probe how these aspects of the self differentially influence psychological processes. For example, several researchers have begun to investigate the cognitive consequences of the activation of the relational or collective self in North American samples (Brewer & Gardner, 1996; Cross, Morris, & Gore, 2001; Kuhnen, Hannover, & Schubert, 2001). There is much to be learned about the interrelations among these self-aspects, the influences on their development, and the situations that prime their activation, but attention to these self-aspects holds the promise of the development of a more truly global theory of the self and its role in human behavior.

Conclusions and Future Directions

East Asian psychologists sometimes complain about the Western tendency to divide the world into sharp dichotomies: East versus West; good versus bad; science versus religion; reason versus emotion; independent versus interdependent. They state that Eastern philosophical traditions do not promote such dichotomies; instead, they view all aspects of the world as interrelated and mutually controlling (Sinha & Sinha, 1997). The contrast of the independent model of the self with the interdependent model of the self has been very helpful in theory development and research; with time, the field may move away from simple dichotomies (or trichotomies) to more complex models that represent multiple dimensions of the self. One starting point is the inclusion of more of Hallowell's (1955) orientations into theoretical models. For example, a temporal perspective on the self (i.e., whether the self is viewed as existing in the past or future) may be critical for understanding individual choices, preferences, and motivations. Work on horizontal and vertical (or egalitarian and hierarchical) aspects of individualism and collectivism has also begun to move the field forward (Singelis, Triandis, Bhawuk, & Gelfand, 1995; Triandis & Gelfand, 1998)

Recent cross-cultural research has focused on one aspect of Hallowell's (1955) object orientation—the relation of the self to other humans—but has paid little attention to relations to nonhuman others and aspects of the spirit world. Given the overwhelming proportion of North Americans who believe in a god or who practice some form of religion, it is puzzling that spirituality has been largely ignored in research on the self and identity. Non-Western psychologists and cross-cultural researchers seem to have less reluctance to consider this dimension. For example, several theorists have argued that the concepts of a spiritual self and a supernatural orientation play a central role in human behavior in India (Hsu, 1963; Roland, 1991; Shweder, Much, Mahapatra, & Park, 1997).

In many East Asian cultures, particularly those based on Buddhist or Taoist beliefs, desire, craving, lust, and ambition are viewed as the source of suffering; thus one is supposed to seek to emancipate the self from this egoism (de Silva, 1993; Sinha & Sinha, 1997). In these perspectives, the individual self is seen as illusory or unreal; the ideal state requires the transcendence of selfhood and complete identification with the forces of the cosmos (Ho, 1995; Inada, 1997). To date, Western researchers have paid little attention to this perspective on the self. Initial research into the concept of the *metaphysical self*—a view of the self as a being in unity with all life—is promising (Stroink & DeCicco, 2001), but many other

questions remain. What are the consequences of this view of the self as subordinate to a greater good or a greater god?
What is the source of self-worth or well-
being in this self-view? How is the Buddhist
nonself—the renunciation of the self—
expressed and realized, and what is the importance of the nonself for theorizing about
the self?

We regret that there is not space in this
chapter to review more of the exciting developments in cultural psychology that pertain to the self. For example, many developmental psychologists are examining the
processes that influence the nature of the
self (for example, see Crystal, Watanabe,
Weinfurt, & Wu, 1998; Han, Leichtman, &
Wang, 1998; Zahn-Waxler et al., 1996, and
volumes by Greenfield & Cocking, 1994,
and Harkness & Super, 1996). There are
also many new studies linking culture and
emotion, and the self is likely to play a central role in this linkage (e.g., Mesquita,
2001; Scherer, 1997; Suh, 2000).

We also regret that we have had to paint
East Asia with a broad stroke, often lump-
ing together members of societies that view
themselves as quite different. An elaboration of the differences among these societies
(and others not mentioned here) can further
the task of developing a more global understanding of the self. East Asian psychologists are themselves best prepared to articulate these differences and to develop
concepts and theories of behavior based on
these differences (for an example, see Hsu,
1963).

There is also much to be learned about
the models of the self that prevail in African
and Latin American cultures. Although
some investigators have begun to examine
ethnographic and psychological research
from these areas for clues to their understanding of the self (e.g., Lee,
McCauley, & Draguns, 1999; Ma &
Schoeneman, 1997; Markus et al., 1997),
the fruit of this work has yet to be borne in
substantial empirical research or theory development. Rather than generally apply the
concepts developed through East Asian–
North American contrasts, researchers
would do well to collaborate with indigenous psychologists in the identification of
fundamental properties of African or Latin
American models of the person and the self

and to develop new tools and theories for
their investigation.

It is an exciting time in the history of research on the self. The concepts, theories,
and ideas uncovered by cross-cultural investigations have initiated a revolution in the
science of the self, and this revolution has
the potential to radically transform not only
research on the self but also social and personality psychology more generally (see
Cross & Markus, 1999; Fiske, Kitayama,
Markus, & Nisbett, 1998; Markus, Kitayama, & Heiman, 1996, for reviews). We
hope this chapter will stimulate new thinking and research, with the goal of developing a more comprehensive understanding of
cultural models of the self and their role in
behavior.

References

Aaker, J. L., & Lee, A. Y. (2001). "I" seek pleasures and
"we" avoid pains: The role of self-regulatory goals in information processing and persuasion. *Journal of Consumer Research, 28,* 33–49.

Ainsworth, M. D. S., Blehar, M. C., Waters, E., & Wall, S.
(1978). *Patterns of attachment: A psychological study of
the Strange Situation.* Hillsdale, NJ: Erlbaum.

Alicke, M. D. (1985). Global self-evaluation as determined
by the desirability and controllability of trait adjectives.
Journal of Personality and Social Psychology, 49,
1621–1630.

Aronson, E. (1969). A theory of cognitive dissonance: A
current perspective. In L. Berkowitz (Ed.) *Advances in
experimental social psychology* (Vol. 4, pp. 1–34). New
York: Academic Press.

Bakan, D. (1966). *The duality of human existence.* Boston:
Beacon Press.

Baldwin, M. W. (1997). Relational schemas as a source of
if–then self-inference procedures. *Review of General
Psychology, 1,* 326–335.

Barth, F. (1997). How is the self conceptualized? Variations among cultures. In U. Neisser & D. A. Jopling
(Eds.), *The conceptual self in context: Culture, experience, self-understanding* (pp. 75–91). Cambridge, UK:
Cambridge University Press.

Baumeister, R. F. (1993). Understanding the inner nature of
low self-esteem: Uncertain, fragile, protective, and conflicted. In R. F. Baumeister (Ed.), *Self-esteem: The puzzle of low self-regard* (pp. 201–218). New York: Plenum
Press.

Baumeister, R. F., & Leary, M. R. (1995). The need to belong: Desire for interpersonal attachments as a fundamental human motivation. *Psychological Bulletin, 117,*
497–529.

Baumeister, R. F., & Sommer, K. L. (1997). What do men
want? Gender differences and two spheres of belongingness. *Psychological Bulletin, 122,* 38–44.

Bautista de Domanico, Y., Crawford, I., & De Wolfe, A. S.
(1994). Ethnic identity and self-concept in Mexican-

American adolescents: Is bicultural identity related to stress or better adjustment? *Child and Youth Care Forum, 23,* 197–206.

Bellah, R. N., Madsen, R., Sullivan, W. M., Swidler, A., & Tipton, S. M. (1985). *Habits of the heart.* New York: Harper & Row.

Benedict, R. (1942). *The chrysanthemum and the sword.* Boston: Houghton Mifflin.

Berger, P. L. (1963). *Invitation to sociology: A humanistic perspective.* Garden City, NY: Anchor.

Boggiano, A. K., & Barrett, M. (1991). Gender differences in depression in college students. *Sex Roles, 25,* 595–605.

Bond, M. H. (1983). How language variation affects intercultural differentiation of values by Hong Kong bilinguals. *Journal of Language and Social Psychology, 2,* 57–66.

Bond, M. H., & Cheung, T. (1983). College students' spontaneous self-concept: The effect of culture among respondents in Hong Kong, Japan, and the United States. *Journal of Cross-Cultural Psychology, 14,* 153–171.

Bond, R., & Smith, P. B. (1996). Culture and conformity: A meta-analysis of studies using Asch's (1952b, 1956) line judgment task. *Psychological Bulletin, 119*(1), 111–137.

Bowlby, J. (1969). *Attachment and loss: Vol. 1. Attachment.* New York: Basic Books.

Brehm, J. W. (1966). *A theory of psychological reactance.* New York: Academic Press.

Brewer, M. B., & Gardner, W. (1996). Who is this "we"? Levels of collective identity and self-representations. *Journal of Personality and Social Psychology, 71,* 83–93.

Brown, J. D. (1998). *The self.* Boston: McGraw-Hill.

Camilleri, C., & Malewska-Peyre, H. (1997). Socialization and identity strategies. In J. W. Berry, P. R. Dasen, & T. S. Saraswathi (Eds.), *Handbook of cross-cultural psychology: Basic processes and human development* (Vol. 2, pp. 41–67). Boston: Allyn & Bacon.

Campbell, J. D. (1990). Self-esteem and clarity of the self-concept. *Journal of Personality and Social Psychology, 59,* 538–549.

Castillo, R. J. (1997). *Culture and mental illness: A client-centered approach.* Pacific Grove, CA: Brooks/Cole.

Chiu, C.-Y., Dweck, C. S., Tong, J. Y. Y., & Fu, J. H. Y. (1997). Implicit theories and conceptions of morality. *Journal of Personality and Social Psychology, 73,* 923–940.

Chiu, C.-Y., Hong, Y. Y., & Dweck, C. S. (1997). Lay dispositionism and implicit theories of personality. *Journal of Personality and Social Psychology, 73,* 19–30.

Choi, I., & Nisbett, R. E. (2000). The cultural psychology of surprise: Holistic theories and recognition of contradiction. *Journal of Personality and Social Psychology, 79,* 890–905.

Choi, I., Nisbett, R. E., & Norenzayan, A. (1999). Causal attribution across cultures: Variation and universality. *Psychological Bulletin, 125,* 47–63.

Coles, R. (1980). Civility and psychology. *Daedalus, 109,* 133–141.

Cooley, C. H. (1902). *Human nature and the social order.* New York: Scribner's.

Coopersmith, S. (1967). *The antecedents of self-esteem.* San Francisco: Freeman.

Crocker, J., Luhtanen, R., Blaine, B., & Broadnax, S.

(1994). Collective self-esteem and psychological well-being among White, Black, and Asian college students. *Personality and Social Psychology Bulletin, 20,* 503–513.

Cross, S. E. (1995). Self-construals, coping, and stress in cross-cultural adaptation. *Journal of Cross-Cultural Psychology, 26,* 673–697.

Cross, S. E., Bacon, P., & Morris, M. (2000). The relational-interdependent self-construal and relationships. *Journal of Personality and Social Psychology, 78,* 791–808.

Cross, S. E., & Madson, L. (1997). Models of the self: Self-construals and gender. *Psychological Bulletin, 122,* 5–37.

Cross, S. E., & Markus, H. R. (1999). The cultural constitution of personality. In L. Pervin & O. John (Eds.), *Handbook of personality theory and research* (2nd ed., pp. 378–396). New York: Guilford Press.

Cross, S. E., Morris, M. L., & Gore, J. S. (2002). Thinking about oneself and others: The relational-interdependent self-construal and social cognition. *Journal of Personality and Social Psychology, 82,* 399–418.

Crystal, D. S., Watanabe, H., Weinfurt, K., & Wu, C. (1998). Concepts of human differences: A comparison of American, Japanese, and Chinese children and adolescents. *Developmental Psychology, 34,* 714–722.

D'Andrade, R. G. (1984). Cultural meaning systems. In R. A. Shweder & R. A. LeVine (Eds.), *Culture theory: Essays on mind, self, and emotion* (pp. 65–129). Cambridge, UK: Cambridge University Press.

Deci, E. L., & Ryan, R. M. (1995). Human autonomy: The basis for true self-esteem. In M. H. Kernis (Ed.), *Efficacy, agency, and self-esteem* (pp. 31–49). New York: Plenum Press.

Derlega, V., Durham, B., Gockel, B., & Sholis, D. (1981). Sex differences in self-disclosure: Effects of topic content, friendship, and partner's sex. *Sex Roles, 7,* 433–447.

De Silva, P. (1993). Buddhist psychology: A therapeutic perspective. In U. Kim & J. W. Berry (Eds.), *Indigenous psychologies: Research and experience in cultural context* (pp. 221–239). Newbury Park, CA: Sage.

Deutsch, F. M., & Mackesy, M. E. (1985). Friendship and the development of self-schemas: The effects of talking about others. *Personality and Social Psychology Bulletin, 11,* 399–408.

Diener, E., & Diener, M. (1995). Cross-cultural correlates of life-satisfaction and self-esteem. *Journal of Personality and Social Psychology, 68,* 653–663.

Donahue, E. M., Robins, R. W., Roberts, B. W., & John, O. P. (1993). The divided self: Concurrent and longitudinal effects of psychological adjustment and social roles on self-concept differentiation. *Journal of Personality and Social Psychology, 64,* 834–846.

Dunning, D., & Hayes, A. F. (1996). Evidence for egocentric comparison in social judgment. *Journal of Personality and Social Psychology, 71,* 213–229.

Earle, M. (1969). A cross-cultural and cross-language comparison of dogmatism scores. *Journal of Social Psychology, 79,* 19–24.

Earley, P. C. (1993). East meets West meets Mideast: Further explorations of collectivistic versus individualistic work groups. *Administrative Science Quarterly, 34,* 565–581.

Elvin, M. (1985). Between the earth and heaven: Conceptions of the self in China. In M. Carrithers, S. Collins, & S. Lukes (Eds.), *The category of the person: Anthropology, philosophy, history* (pp. 156–189). Cambridge, UK: Cambridge University press.

Endo, Y., Heine, S. J., & Lehman, D. R. (2000). Culture and positive illusions in close relationships: How my relationships are better than yours. *Personality and Social Psychology Bulletin, 26,* 1571–1586.

Festinger, L. (1957). *A theory of cognitive dissonance.* Stanford, CA: Stanford University Press.

Fiske, A. P., Kitayama, S., Markus, H. R., & Nisbett, R. E. (1998). The cultural matrix of social psychology. In D. Gilbert, S. Fiske, & G. Lindzey (Eds.), *Handbook of social psychology* (pp. 915–981). New York: McGraw-Hill.

Freeman, N. H., & Habermann, G. M. (1996). Linguistic socialization: A Chinese perspective. In M. H. Bond (Ed.), *The handbook of Chinese psychology* (pp. 79–92). Hong Kong: Oxford University Press.

Gabrenya, W. K., Jr., & Hwang, K. -K. (1996). Chinese social interaction: Harmony and hierarchy on the good earth. In M. H. Bond (Ed.), *The handbook of Chinese psychology* (pp. 309–321). Hong Kong: Oxford University Press.

Gabriel, S., & Gardner, W. L. (1999). Are there "his" and "hers" types of interdependence? The implications of gender differences in collective versus relational interdependence for affect, behavior, and cognition. *Journal of Personality and Social Psychology, 77,* 642–655.

Gaines, S. O., Jr., Marelich, W. D., Bledsoe, K. L., Steers, W. N., Henderson, M. C., Granrose, C. S., Barajas, L., Hicks, D., Lyde, M., Takahashi, Y., Yum, N., Rios, D. I., Garcia, B. F., Farris, K. R., & Page, M. S. (1997). Links between race/ethnicity and cultural values as mediated by racial/ethnic identity and moderated by gender. *Journal of Personality and Social Psychology, 72,* 1460–1476.

Galang, M. E. (1996). *Her wild American self: Short stories.* Minneapolis, MN: Coffee House Press.

Gao, G., Ting-Toomey, S., & Gudykunst, W. (1996). Chinese communication processes. In M. M. Bond (Ed.), *The handbook of Chinese psychology* (pp. 280–293). Hong Kong: Oxford University Press.

Geertz, C. (1975). On the nature of anthropological understanding. *American Scientist, 63,* 47–53.

Gibbons, F. X., & Gerrard, M. (1991). Downward comparison and coping with threat. In J. Suls & T. A. Wills (Eds.), *Social comparison: Contemporary theory and research* (pp. 317–345). Hillsdale, NJ: Erlbaum.

Gilligan, C. (1982). *In a different voice: Psychological theory and women's development.* Cambridge, MA: Harvard University Press.

Goffman, E. (1959). *The presentation of self in everyday life.* New York: Doubleday.

Goldstein, M. C. (1987). When brothers share a wife. *Natural History, 96,* 39–48.

Greenberg, J., Pyszczynski, T., & Solomon, S. (1982). The self-serving attributional bias: Beyond self-presentation. *Journal of Experimental Social Psychology, 18,* 56–67.

Greenfield, P. M., & Cocking, R. R. (1994). *Cross-cultural roots of minority child development.* Hillsdale, NJ: Erlbaum.

Gurung, R. A. R., & Duong, T. (1999). Mixing and match-

ing: Assessing the concomitants of mixed-ethnic relationships. *Journal of Social and Personal Relationships, 16,* 639–657.

Hallowell, A. I. (1955). *Culture and experience.* Philadelphia: University of Pennsylvania Press.

Hamaguchi, E. (1985). A contextual model of the Japanese: Toward a methodological innovation in Japan studies. *Journal of Japanese Studies, 11,* 289–321.

Hamilton, V. L., & Sanders, J. (1992). *Everyday justice: Responsibility and the individual in Japan and the United States.* New Haven, CT: Yale University Press.

Han, J. J., Leichtman, M. D., & Wang, Q. (1998). Autobiographical memory in Korean, Chinese, and American children. *Developmental Psychology, 34,* 701–713.

Han, S.-P., & Shavitt, S. (1994). Persuasion and culture: Advertising appeals in individualistic and collectivistic societies. *Journal of Experimental Social Psychology, 30,* 326–350.

Harkness, S., & Super, C. M. (1996). *Parents' cultural belief systems: Their origins, expressions, and consequences.* New York: Guilford Press.

Hart, D., & Edelstein, D. (1992). The relationship of self-understanding to community type, social class, and teacher-rated intellectual and social competence. *Journal of Cross-Cultural Psychology, 23,* 353–365.

Hart, D., & Fegley, S. (1997). Children's self-awareness and self-understanding in cultural context. In U. Neisser & D. A. Jopling (Eds.), *The conceptual self in context: Culture, experience, self-understanding* (pp. 128–153). New York: Cambridge University Press.

Heine, S. J., & Lehman, D. R. (1995). Cultural variation in unrealistic optimism: Does the West feel more vulnerable than the East? *Journal of Personality and Social Psychology, 68,* 595–607.

Heine, S. J., & Lehman, D. R. (1997). Culture, dissonance, and self-affirmation. *Personality and Social Psychology Bulletin, 23,* 389–400.

Heine, S. J., & Lehman, D. R. (1999). Culture, self-discrepancies, and self-satisfaction. *Personality and Social Psychology Bulletin, 25,* 915–925.

Heine, S. J., Lehman, D. R., Markus, H. R., & Kitayama, S. (1999). Is there a universal need for positive self-regard? *Psychological Review, 106,* 766–794.

Heine, S. J., Takata, T., & Lehman, D. R. (2000). Beyond self-presentation: Evidence for self-criticism among Japanese. *Personality and Social Psychology Bulletin, 26,* 71–78.

Hetts, J. J., Sakuma, M., & Pelham, B. (1999). Two roads to positive regard: Implicit and explicit self-evaluation and culture. *Journal of Experimental Social Psychology, 35,* 512–559.

Ho, D. Y. F. (1995). Selfhood and identity in Confucianism, Taoism, Buddhism, and Hinduism: Contrasts with the West. *Journal for the Theory of Social Behavior, 25,* 115–139.

Hoffman, D. M. (1990). Beyond conflict: Culture, self and intercultural learning among Iranians in the U. S. *International Journal of Intercultural Relations, 14,* 275–299.

Holland, D., Lachicotte, W. J., Skinner, D., & Cain, C. (1998). *Identity and agency in cultural worlds.* Cambridge, MA: Harvard University Press.

Hong, Y., Morris, M. W., Chiu, C., & Benet-Martinez, V. (2000). Multicultural minds: A dynamic constructivist approach to culture and cognition. *American Psychologist, 55,* 709–720.

Hormuth, S. E. (1990). *The ecology of the self: Relocation and self-concept change.* New York: Cambridge University Press.

Howard, J. A. (2000). Social psychology of identities. *Annual Review of Sociology, 26,* 367–393.

Hsu, F. L. K. (1963). *Clan, caste, and club.* Princeton, NJ: Van Nostrand.

Ickes, W., Robertston, E., Tooke, W., & Teng, G. (1986). Naturalistic social cognition: Methodology, assessment, and validation. *Journal of Personality and Social Psychology, 51,* 66–82.

Ikegami, Y. (1991). "DO-language" and "BECOME-language": Two contrasting types of linguistic representation. In Y. Ikegami (Ed.), *The empire of signs: Emiotic essays on Japanese culture* (pp. 285–326). Philadelphia: Benjamins.

Inada, K. K. (1997). Buddho-Taoist and Western metaphysics of the self. In D. Allen (Ed.), *Culture and self: Philosophical and religious perspectives, East and West* (pp. 83–93). Boulder, CO: Westview Press.

Iyengar, S. S., & Lepper, M. R. (1999). Rethinking the value of choice: A cultural perspective on intrinsic motivation. *Journal of Personality and Social Psychology, 76*(3), 349–366.

James, W. (1983). *The principles of psychology.* Cambridge, MA: Harvard University Press. (Original work published 1890)

Kanagawa, C., Cross, S. E., & Markus, H. R. (2001). "Who am I?" The cultural psychology of the conceptual self. *Personality and Social Psychology Bulletin, 27*(1), 90–103.

Kaneshiro, E. N. (1997). Multiculturalism and the model minority: Japanese-Americans' ethnic identity and psychosocial adjustment. *Dissertation Abstracts International, 57,* 6652B.

Kashima, E. S., & Kashima, Y. (1998). Culture and language: The case of cultural dimensions and personal pronoun use. *Journal of Cross-Cultural Psychology, 29*(3), 461–486.

Kidder, L. H., & Muller, S. (1991). What is "fair" in Japan? In H. Steensma & R. Vermunt (Eds.), *Social justice in human relations: Vol. 2. Societal and psychological consequences of justice and injustice* (pp. 139–154). New York: Plenum Press.

Kim, H., & Markus, H. R. (1999). Deviance or uniqueness, harmony or conformity? A cultural analysis. *Journal of Personality and Social Psychology, 77,* 785–800.

Kitayama, S., & Markus, H. R. (1999). *Yin* and *yang* of the Japanese self: The cultural psychology of personality coherence. In D. Cervone & Y. Shoda (Eds.), *The coherence of personality: Social-cognitive bases of consistency, variability, and organization* (pp. 242–302). New York: Guilford Press.

Kitayama, S., Markus, H. R., Matsumoto, H., & Norasakkunkit, V. (1997). Individual and collective processes of self-esteem management: Self-enhancement in the United States and self-depreciation in Japan. *Journal of Personality and Social Psychology, 72,* 1245–1267.

Kondo, D. (1990). *Crafting selves: Power, gender and discourses of identity in a Japanese workplace.* Chicago: University of Chicago Press.

Kuhn, M. H., & McPartland, T. S. (1954). An empirical investigation of self-attitudes. *American Sociological Review, 19,* 68–76.

Kuhnen, U., Hannover, B., & Schubert, B. (2001). The semantic–procedural interface model of the self: The role of self-knowledge for context-dependent versus context-independent modes of thinking. *Journal of Personality and Social Psychology, 80,* 397–409.

Kwan, V. S. Y., Bond, M. H., & Singelis, T. M. (1997). Pancultural explanations for life satisfaction: Adding relational harmony to self-esteem. *Journal of Personality and Social Psychology, 73,* 1038–1051.

LaFromboise, T., Coleman, H., & Gerton, J. (1993). Psychological impact of biculturalism: Evidence and theory. *Psychological Bulletin, 114,* 395–412.

Leary, M. R., Tambor, E. S., Terdal, S. K., & Downs, D. L. (1995). Self-esteem as an interpersonal social monitor: The sociometer hypothesis. *Journal of Personality and Social Psychology, 68,* 518–530.

Lebra, T. S. (1976). *Japanese patterns of behavior.* Honolulu: University of Hawaii Press.

Lebra, T. S. (1994). Mother and child in Japanese socialization: A Japan–U.S. comparison. In P. M. Greenfield & R. R. Cocking (Eds.), *Cross-cultural roots of minority child development* (pp. 259–274). Hillsdale, NJ: Erlbaum.

Lecky, P. (1945). *Self-consistency: A theory of personality.* New York: Island Press.

Lee, A. Y., Aaker, J. L., & Gardner, W. L. (2000). The pleasures and pains of distinct self-construals: The role of interdependence in regulatory focus. *Journal of Personality and Social Psychology, 78,* 1122–1134.

Lee, Y.-T., McCauley, C. R., & Draguns, J. G. (1999). *Personality and person perception across cultures.* Mahwah, NJ: Erlbaum.

Leung, K., & Fan, R. M. T. (1997). Dispute processing: An Asian perspective. In H. S. R. Kao & D. Sinha (Eds.), *Cross-cultural research and methodology series: Vol. 19. Asian perspectives on psychology* (pp. 201–217). Thousand Oaks, CA: Sage.

Lewis, C. C. (1995). *Educating hearts and minds: Reflections on Japanese preschool and elementary school.* New York: Cambridge University Press.

Lilliard, A. (1998). Ethnopsychologies: Cultural variations in theories of mind. *Psychological Bulletin, 123,* 3–32.

Luhtanen, R., & Crocker, J. (1992). A collective self-esteem scale: Self-evaluation of one's social identity. *Personality and Social Psychology Bulletin, 18,* 302–318.

Ma, V., & Schoeneman, T. J. (1997). Individualism versus collectivism: A comparison of Kenyan and American self-concepts. *Basic and Applied Social Psychology, 19,* 261–273.

Maccoby, E. (1990). Gender and relationships: A developmental account. *American Psychologist, 45,* 513–520.

Marcia, J. E. (1966). Development and validation of ego-identity status. *Journal of Personality and Social Psychology, 5,* 551–558.

Markus, H., & Kitayama, S. (1991). Culture and self: Implications for cognition, emotion, and motivation. *Psychological Review, 98,* 224–253.

Markus, H., & Kitayama, S. (1994). A collective fear of the collective: Implications for selves and theories of selves. *Personality and Social Psychology Bulletin, 20,* 568–579.

Markus, H. R., & Kitayama, S. (1998). The cultural psychology of personality. *Journal of Cross-Cultural Psychology, 29,* 63–87.

Markus, H. R., Kitayama, S., & Heiman, R. J. (1996). Culture and basic psychological principles. In E. T. Higgins & A. W. Kruglanski (Eds.), *Social psychology: Handbook of basic principles* (pp. 857–913). New York: Guilford Press.

Markus, H. R., & Lin, L. R. (1999). Conflictways: Cultural diversity in the meanings and practices of conflict. In D. A. Prentice & D. A. Miller (Eds.), *Cultural divides: Understanding and overcoming group conflict* (pp. 302–333). New York: Russell Sage Foundation.

Markus, H. R., Mullally, P. R., & Kitayama, S. (1997). Selfways: Diversity in modes of cultural participation. In U. Neisser & D. Jopling (Eds.), *The conceptual self in context* (pp. 13–61). New York: Cambridge University Press.

Mathews, G. (1996). The stuff of dreams, fading: Ikigai and "the Japanese self." *Ethos, 24,* 718–747.

McCrae, R. R., Yik, M. S. M., Trapnell, P. D., Bond, M. H., & Paulhus, D. L. (1998). Interpreting personality profiles across cultures: Bilingual, acculturation, and peer rating studies of Chinese undergraduates. *Journal of Personality and Social Psychology, 74,* 1041–1055.

McGuire, W. J., & McGuire, C. V. (1982). Significant others in self space: Sex differences and developmental trends in social self. In J. Suls (Ed.), *Psychological perspectives of the self* (Vol. 1, pp. 71–96). Hillsdale, NJ: Erlbaum.

Mead, G. H. (1934). *Mind, self, and society.* Chicago: University of Chicago Press.

Mesquita, B. (2001). Emotions in collectivist and individualist contexts. *Journal of Personality and Social Psychology, 80,* 68–74.

Miller, J. G. (1984). Culture and the development of everyday social explanation. *Journal of Personality and Social Psychology, 46,* 961–978.

Miller, J. G. (1997). Cultural conceptions of duty. In D. Monro, J. F. Schumaker, & S. C. Carr (Eds.), *Motivation and culture* (pp. 178–192). New York: Routledge.

Miller, P. J., Fung, H., & Mintz, J. (1996). Self-construction through narrative practices: A Chinese and American comparison of early socialization. *Ethos, 24,* 237–280.

Morling, B. (2000). "Taking" an aerobics class in the U. S. and "entering" an aerobics class in Japan: Primary and secondary control in a fitness context. *Asian Journal of Social Psychology, 3*(1), 73–85.

Morris, M. W., Nisbett, R. E., & Peng, K. (1995). Causal attribution across domains and cultures. In D. Sperber, D. Premack, & A. J. Premack (Eds.), *Causal cognition: A multidisciplinary debate* (pp. 577–612). Oxford, UK: Clarendon Press.

Morris, M. W., & Peng, K. (1994). Culture and cause: American and Chinese attributions for social physical events. *Journal of Personality and Social Psychology, 67,* 949–971.

Mullen, M. K., & Yi, S. (1995). The cultural context of talk about the past: Implications for the development of autobiographical memory. *Cognitive Development, 10,* 407–419.

Neisser, U. (1988). Five kinds of self-knowledge. *Philosophical Psychology, 1,* 35–59.

Nisbett, R. E., Peng, K., Choi, I., & Norenzayan, A. (2001). Culture and systems of thought: Holistic versus analytic cognition. *Psychological Review, 108,* 291–310.

Norenzayan, A., Choi, I., & Nisbett, R. E. (1999). Eastern and Western perceptions of causality for social behavior: Lay theories about personalities and social situations. In D. Prentice & D. Miller (Eds.), *Cultural divides: Understanding and overcoming group conflict* (pp. 239–272). New York: Sage.

Oerter, R., Oerter, R., Agostiani, H., Kim, H.-O., & Wibowo, S. (1996). The concept of human nature in East Asia: Etic and emic characteristics. *Culture and Psychology, 2,* 9–51.

Ogilvie, D. M., & Clark, M. D. (1992). The best and worst of it: Age and sex differences in self-discrepancy research. In R. P. Lipka & T. M. Brinthaupt (Eds.), *Self-perspectives across the life span* (pp. 186–222). Albany: State University of New York Press.

Oyserman, D., Coon, H. M., & Kemmelmeier, M. (2002). Rethinking individualism and collectivism: Evaluation of theoretical assumptions and meta-analysis. *Psychological Bulletin, 128,* 3–72.

Oyserman, D., Harrison, K., & Bybee, D. (2001). Can racial identity be promotive of academic efficacy? *International Journal of Behavior and Development, 25,* 379–385.

Oyserman, D., & Markus, H. R. (1993). The sociocultural self. In J. M. Suls (Ed.), *The self in social perspective: Vol. 4. Psychological perspectives on the self* (pp. 187–220). Hillsdale, NJ: Erlbaum.

Padilla, A. M. (1994). Bicultural development: A theoretical and empirical examination. In R. G. Malgady & O. Rodriguez (Eds.), *Theoretical and conceptual issues in Hispanic mental health* (pp. 20–51). Malabar, FL: Krieger.

Peng, K., & Nisbett, R. E. (1999). Culture, dialectics, and reasoning about contradiction. *American Psychologist, 54,* 741–754.

Pervin, L. (1990). *Handbook of personality: Theory and research.* New York: Guilford Press.

Phinney, J. (1990). Ethnic identity in adolescents and adults: Review of research. *Psychological Bulletin, 108,* 499–514.

Poincaré, H. (n.d.). *Science and method.* London: Constable. (Original work published 1908).

Reisman, P. (1992). *First find your child a good mother.* New Brunswick, NJ: Rutgers University Press.

Rhee, E., Uleman, J. S., Lee, H. K., & Roman, R. J. (1995). Spontaneous self-descriptions and ethnic identities in individualistic and collectivistic cultures. *Journal of Personality and Social Psychology, 69,* 142–152.

Roberts, T., & Nolen-Hoeksema, S. (1994). Gender comparisons in responsiveness to others' evaluations in achievement settings. *Psychology of Women Quarterly, 18,* 221–240.

Roland, A. (1991). The self in cross-civilizational perspective: An Indian–Japanese–American comparison. In R. C. Curtis (Ed.), *The relational self: Theoretical convergences in psychoanalysis and social psychology* (pp. 160–180). New York: Guilford Press.

Rosch, J. (1983). Institutionalizing mediation: The evolution of the civil liberties bureau in Japan. *Law and Society Review, 18,* 701–724.

Rosen, L. (1995). Introduction. In L. Rosen (Ed.), *Other in-*

tentions: Cultural contexts and the attribution of inner states (pp. 1–11). Santa Fe, NM: School of American Research.

Rosenberg, M. (1965). *Society and the adolescent self-image*. Princeton, NJ: Princeton University Press.

Ross, M., & Holmberg, D. (1992). Are wives' memories for events in relationships more vivid than their husbands' memories? *Journal of Social and Personal Relationships, 9,* 585–604.

Rothbaum, F., Pott, M., Azuma, H., Miyake, K., & Weisz, J. (2000). The development of close relationships in Japan and the United States: Paths of symbiotic harmony and generative tension. *Child Development, 71,* 1121–1142.

Rothbaum, R., Weisz, J., Pott, M., Miyake, K., & Morelli, G. (2000). Attachment and culture: Security in the United States and Japan. *American Psychologist, 55,* 1093–1104.

Ryder, A. G., Alden, L. E., & Paulhus, D. L. (2000). Is acculturation unidimensional or bidimensional? A head-to-head comparison of the prediction of personality, self-identity, and adjustment. *Journal of Personality and Social Psychology, 79,* 49–65.

Sabini, J., Siepmann, M., & Stein, J., (2001). The really fundamental attribution error in social psychological research. *Psychological Inquiry, 12,* 1–15.

Sanitioso, R., Kunda, Z., & Fong, G. T. (1990). Motivated recruitment of autobiographical memories. *Journal of Personality and Social Psychology, 62,* 699–707.

Sastry, J., & Ross, C. E. (1998). Asian ethnicity and the sense of personal control. *Social Psychology Quarterly, 61,* 101–120.

Scherer, K. R. (1997). The role of culture in emotion-antecedent appraisal. *Journal of Personality and Social Psychology, 73,* 902–922.

Sedikides, C., & Brewer, M. B. (2000). *Individual self, relational self, collective self.* Philadelphia: Psychology Press.

Sellers, R. M., Smith, M. A., Shelton, J. N., Rowley, S. A. J., & Chavous, T. M. (1998). Multidimensional model of racial identity: A reconceptualization of African American racial identity. *Personality and Social Psychology Review, 2,* 18–39.

Shaffer, D. R., Pegalis, L. J., & Bazzini, D. G. (1996). When boy meets girl (revisited): Gender, gender-role orientation, and prospect of future interaction as determinants of self-disclosure among same- and opposite-sex acquaintances. *Personality and Social Psychology Bulletin, 22,* 495–506.

Sheldon, K. M., & Elliot, A. J. (1999). Goal striving, need satisfaction, and longitudinal well-being: The self-concordance model. *Journal of Personality and Social Psychology, 76,* 482–497.

Sheldon, K. M., Ryan, R. M., Rawsthorne, L. J., & Ilardi, B. (1997). Trait self and true self: Cross-role variation in the Big-Five personality traits and its relations with psychological authenticity and subjective well-being. *Journal of Personality and Social Psychology, 73,* 1380–1393.

Shweder, R. A., Much, N. C., Mahapatra, M., & Park, L. (1997). The "big three" of morality (autonomy, community, divinity) and the "big three" explanations of suffering. In A. M. Brandt & P. Rozin (Eds.), *Morality and health* (pp. 119–169). New York: Routledge.

Singelis, T. M. (1994). The measurement of independent and interdependent self-construals. *Personality and Social Psychology Bulletin, 20,* 580–591.

Singelis, T. M, Triandis, H. C., Bhawuk, D., & Gelfand, M. J. (1995). Horizontal and vertical dimensions of individualism and collectivism: A theoretical and measurement refinement. *Cross-Cultural Research: The Journal of Comparative Social Science, 29,* 240–275.

Sinha, D., & Sinha, M. (1997). Orientations to psychology: Asian and Western. In H. S. R. Kao & D. Sinha (Eds.), *Asian perspectives on psychology* (pp. 25–39.). New Delhi, India: Sage.

Solomon, S., Greenberg, J., & Pyszczynski, T. (1991). A terror management theory of social behavior: The psychological functions of self-esteem and cultural worldviews. In L. Berkowitz (Ed.), *Advances in experimental social psychology* (Vol. 24, pp. 93–159). San Diego, CA: Academic Press.

Steele, C. M. (1988). The psychology of self-affirmation: Sustaining the integrity of the self. In L. Berkowitz (Ed.), *Advances in experimental social psychology* (Vol. 21, pp. 261–302). New York: Academic Press.

Stevenson, H. W. (1995). The Asian advantage: The case of mathematics. In J. J. Shields, Jr. (Ed.), *Japanese schooling: Patterns of socialization, equality, and political control* (pp. 85–95). University Park: Pennsylvania State University Press.

Stipek, D. (1998). Differences between Americans and Chinese in the circumstances evoking pride, shame, and guilt. *Journal of Cross-Cultural Psychology, 29,* 616–629.

Stroink, M. L., & DeCicco, T. L. (2001). *The metapersonal self and cultural belief systems: Implications for cognition.* Manuscript submitted for publication.

Suh, E. M. (2000). Self, the hyphen between culture and subjective well-being. In E. Diener & E. M. Suh (Eds.), *Culture and subjective well-being* (pp. 63–86). Cambridge, MA: MIT Press.

Sussman, N. M. (2000). The dynamic nature of cultural identity throughout cultural transitions: Why home is not so sweet. *Personality and Social Psychology Review, 4,* 355–373.

Swann, W. B., Jr. (1983). Self-verification: Bringing social reality into harmony with the self. In J. Suls & A. G. Greenwald (Eds.), *Social psychological perspectives on the self* (Vol. 2, pp. 33–66). Hillsdale, NJ: Erlbaum.

Swann, W. B., Jr. (1990). To be adored or to be known?: The interplay of self-enhancement and self-verification. In E. T. Higgins & R. M. Sorrentino (Eds.), *Handbook of motivation and cognition* (Vol. 2, pp. 408–448). New York: Guilford Press.

Tafarodi, R. W., Lang, J. M., & Smith, A. J. (1999). Self-esteem and the cultural trade-off: Evidence for the role of individualism–collectivism. *Journal of Cross-Cultural Psychology, 30,* 620–640.

Taylor, S., & Brown, J. (1988). Illusion and well-being: A social psychological perspective on mental health. *Psychological Bulletin, 103,* 193–210.

Tesser, A. (1988). Toward a self-evaluation maintenance model of social behavior. In L. Berkowitz (Ed.), *Advances in experimental social psychology* (Vol. 21, pp. 181–227). New York: Academic Press.

Tice, D. M. (1992). Self-concept change and self-presentations: The looking glass self is also a magnifying glass. *Journal of Personality and Social Psychology, 60,* 711–725.

Ting-Toomey, S. (Ed.). (1994). *The challenge of facework: Cross-cultural and interpersonal issues.* Albany: State University of New York Press.

Tobin, J. J., Wu, D. Y. H., & Davidson, D. H. (1989). *Preschool in three cultures: Japan, China, and the United States.* New Haven, CT: Yale University Press.

Triandis, H. C. (1996). The psychological measurement of cultural syndromes. *American Psychologist, 51,* 407–415.

Triandis, H. C., & Gelfand, M. J. (1998). Converging measurement of horizontal and vertical individualism and collectivism. *Journal of Personality and Social Psychology, 74,* 118–128.

Tu, W. (1994). Embodying the universe: A note on Confucian self-realization. In R. T. Ames, W. Dissanayake, & T. P. Kasulis (Eds.), *Self as person in Asian theory and practice* (pp. 177–186). Albany: State University of New York Press.

Vorauer, J. D., & Ross, M. (1993). Making mountains out of molehills: An informational goals analysis of self-

and social perception. *Personality and Social Psychology Bulletin, 19,* 620–632.

Weisz, J. R., Rothbaum, R. M., & Blackburn, T. C. (1984). Standing out and standing in: The psychology of control in America and Japan. *American Psychologist, 39,* 955–969.

Whiting, R. (1989). *You gotta have Wa.* New York: Macmillan.

Wierzbicka, A. (1997). *Understanding cultures through their key words: English, Russian, Polish, German, and Japanese.* New York: Oxford University Press.

Wu, D. Y. H. (1994). Self and collectivity: Socialization in Chinese preschools. In R. T. Ames, W. Dissanayake, & T. P. Kasulis (Eds.), *Self as person in Asian theory and practice* (pp. 235–250). Albany: State University of New York Press.

Zahn-Wexler, C., Friedman, R. J., Cole, P. M., Mizuta, I., & Hiruma, N. (1996). Japanese and United States preschool children's responses to conflict and distress. *Child Development, 67,* 2462–2477.

Zuckerman, D. M. (1989). Stress, self-esteem, and mental health: How does gender make a difference? *Sex Roles, 20,* 429–444.

PART VI

PHYLOGENETIC AND ONTOLOGICAL DEVELOPMENT

28

Subjectivity and Self-Recognition in Animals

ROBERT W. MITCHELL

Given the difficulties clarifying conceptions of the self in humans (see, e.g., Bermúdez, Marcel, & Eilan, 1995; Gallagher & Shear, 1999; Kolak & Martin, 1991), even after hundreds of years of philosophical thought (Levin, 1992), it may seem foolhardy to concern oneself with extrapolations of these conceptions to nonhuman animals. Yet thinking about what animals know about themselves and how they think about themselves is intriguing to many observers of animals (Griffin, 2001b), and application of notions of self to animals of various species provides intriguing similarities and contrasts (Mitchell, 1993c, 1994b). Although the self in animals arises as a recurrent topic today largely because of evidence that apes, dolphins, killer whales, and perhaps elephants recognize themselves in mirrors, there are other perspectives on the nature of animal selfhood. I begin with a brief description of the ideas of early scientists who concerned themselves with understanding self-awareness in animals. I then examine the self in animals in relation to three perspectives: subjective experience, self-recognition, and (briefly) self-evaluation.

The Darwinian Tradition

Although touched on earlier (e.g., Lamarck, 1809/1984), scientific concerns about animals' self-awareness became particularly important when Darwin proposed to examine human psychology as an outgrowth of evolutionary processes. If human beings evolved from nonhuman ancestors, some germ of recognized human qualities might be present in extant animals. Darwin (1871/1896, pp. 83–84) reasoned as follows:

> It may be freely admitted that no animal is self-conscious, if by this term it is implied, that he reflects on such points, as whence he comes or whither he will go, or what is life and death, and so forth. But how can we feel sure that an old dog with an excellent memory and some power of imagination, as shewn by his dreams, never reflects on his past pleasures or pains in the chase? And this would be a form of self-consciousness. On the other hand ... how little can the hard-worked wife of a degraded Australian savage, who uses very few abstract words, and cannot count above four, exert her self-consciousness, or reflect on the

nature of her own existence. It is generally admitted, that the higher animals possess memory, attention, association, and even some imagination and reason. If these powers, which differ much in different animals, are capable of improvement, there seems no great improbability in more complex faculties, such as the higher forms of abstraction, and self-consciousness, &c., having been evolved through the development and combination of the simpler ones.

Darwin's argument attacked the problem from both ends, animal and human: dogs have skills needed for imagining themselves in past experiences, and thus animals have faculties from which a more developed self-consciousness, of the human type, could evolve; and some humans (purportedly) can barely engage in self-reflection. Compared to a dog's self-consciousness, that of some human beings is (in this presentation) not all that distinctive or remarkable. In Darwin's view, dogs' rudimentary self-consciousness consists in having subjectively experienced images of or within an event—not unlike what people commonly experience when imagining in dreams. How the dog is imagined in the event—as a visually represented dog or as a point of view looking onto a scene—is unstated.

Romanes (1889/1975), Darwin's friend and promoter, elaborated Darwin's concerns but articulated somewhat different conceptions of self-consciousness, offering distinctions between "outward" and "inward" forms (developed from ideas of Wright, 1873/1958). Outward self-consciousness is "the practical recognition of self as an active and a feeling agent" (Romanes, 1889/1975, p. 199). The organism experiences itself perceptually as a distinct unified entity; this outward self-consciousness is a natural outgrowth of the organism's being a self-moving, sentient, goal-directed organism. The "unreflective or primary self" present in outward self-consciousness can be conceived "simply as subject of experience" (Baldwin, 1901/1960, p. 507). Outward self-consciousness supplies the locus of a self as embodied and "here" where the body is (see, e.g., Sully, 1892).

Inward self-consciousness requires a separation of self into observer and observed, thinker and thought. In its most complex form, inward self-consciousness is aware-

ness of subjectivity, which requires turning the unreflective self into an observing self that attends to its internal mental states (and is not simply at one with its own experiences, as in outward self-consciousness; Romanes, 1889/1975). Romanes believed that animals show the beginnings of inward self-consciousness in having internal images (as Darwin surmised), yet animals cannot "intentionally contemplate" these internal states: rather, they experience in their minds an "internal—though unintentional—play of ideation" (p. 196) over which they have little control (compare Lamarck, 1809/1984, p. 382). Animals recognize the significance of these ideational images (in that they respond to them in dreams, homesickness, and pining for absent friends), recognize that other organisms have mental states like their own (in that they engage in deception and pretense), and even recognize that another animal recognizes their mental states (by analogical comparison with its own); yet (for inexplicable reasons) "mental existence is . . . never *thought upon* subjectively" (Romanes, 1889/1975, p. 198). In human children (but not animals), conceptual development (assisted by language) allows for an awareness of the distinction between imagination (internal mental images) and perception, which awareness is inward self-awareness (Sully, 1892). Speech constantly impresses on the growing child the subjectivity present in his or her own, and others', activities.

In an attempt to characterize how the human sort of inward self-awareness might develop in nonhuman organisms without the aid of speech, Wright (1873/1958) posited that experience of internal imagery *simultaneously* with the perception of the object expressed in the internal imagery might lead to some initial awareness of internal states as such. For example, a dog thinking of (that is, having internal images of) her master while suddenly confronted with her master would allow the dog to consciously recognize that one is a substitute for the other. For Wright, experiential recognition of the representational nature of imagery (viewed as a re-presentation of perception) might "plant the germ of the distinctively human form of self-consciousness" (p. 77), which involves (in his view) focusing attention on mental states themselves. It is made clear later in this chapter that exactly this recognition of an identity relation between "inner" and "outer," present in the match between kinesthesis and vision, leads to the preliminary recognition of self attendant in mirror-self-recognition and generalized imitation (Guillaume, 1926/1971; Mitchell, 1993c, 1997a).

The most elaborate form of human self-consciousness, argued Hobhouse (1901), is perhaps never observed in animals—that form of self-consciousness that rules behavior and with which humans act in accord. What animals lack is a desire to live up to standards that they demarcate for themselves. Whereas animals have a conception of self that allows them to achieve goals, the "consciousness of self [in a person] is a permanent regulative force distinct from the desires or plans of action which he forms from day to day" (Hobhouse, 1901, p. 312). In this view, human-specific attributes such as morality, embarrassment, shame, and regret derive in various ways from our self-images, which themselves derived from social interaction (Cooley, 1902/1964; Guillaume, 1926/1971; Mead, 1934/1974).

In their descriptions of notions of the self, the preceding authors differentiated aspects that still engage authors today: the seeming necessity of a notion of self in perceptual experience, whether animals experience subjectivity, whether animals experience mental images of themselves, the relation between body image and self, the impact of language on self-awareness, and the presence of a self-image that guides and evaluates one's actions (see, e.g., Bermúdez et al., 1995; Mitchell, 1994b). Along these lines, I explore three aspects of self in nonhumans: self as subject of experience, self as object of awareness (as in mirror-self-recognition), and self as actor controlled by standards.

The Self as a Subject of Experience

Usually, when talking of the self, psychologists focus on "higher level" cognitive processes involving mirror-self-recognition and the reflective self-awareness discussed by Hobhouse (1901). However, many psychologists (particularly those studying infants) and philosophers are concerned with initial states of awareness of self and with demarcating the self as a subject of experience. Consequently, I focus in this first section on the nature of this potentially unreflective self present in bodily experience, conscious experience, and the first-person perspective.

The Experiencing Bodily Self

A self seems immanently present in perceptual experiences, in that these are self-specifying—perceptions place the organism as the locus of its perceptual experiences (Butterworth, 2000; Evans, 1982; Gibson, 1966; Neisser, 1988). One directly experiences the spatial extent and movement of the body via kinesthesis, tactility, and somasthesis (Brewer, 1995; Mitchell, 1994b; Sheets-Johnstone, 1990), and visual and auditory perceptions localize one as "here" in relation to them (Evans, 1982; Gibson, 1966). The fact that an animal knows where its body and body parts are at any given moment indicates a form of self-awareness based in part on tactile–kinesthetic invariants (Mitchell, 1993a; Sheets-Johnstone, 1990). These invariants offer a unity to the experience of the body itself (Merleau-Ponty, 1962/1981). The phenomenon of phantom limbs, in which people (and apparently monkeys too) experience somasthetically (but not visually) the presence of a part of the body even when it is not there (either because of a birth defect or amputation) suggests that the feeling of the body's extent is to some degree biologically preprogrammed (Butterworth, 2000; Melzack, 1989, 1992; cf. Kinsbourne, 1995). Bodily self-movement implies some form of self-knowledge in the sense that the organism experiences itself moving (Sheets-Johnstone, 1998). Tactility—feelings of movement produced in relation to contact with the world—likely evolved into kinesthesis—feelings of organized bodily movement—resulting in "a direct sensitivity to movement through internally mediated systems of corporeal awareness" (Sheets-Johnstone, 1998, p. 286). Although one may be tempted to discount the implicit knowledge of self derived from perception as irrelevant to true self-consciousness, child development researchers argue instead that the original unreflective experience of self in humans derives from perceptual experience and is the basis from which more elaborate self-consciousness develops (Butterworth, 2000; Meltzoff, 1990; Neisser, 1988).

Animals in general have knowledge of the spatial extent of their bodies (Brewer, 1995) in that they usually do not walk or fly into other objects. Simply eating requires knowledge of body and bodily changes in relation to the world (for remarkable instances of such knowledge, see descriptions of eating by echolocating bats and tongue-extending chameleons in Curio, 1976). Some perceptual modalities, such as echolocation by dolphins, seem to take into account the perceiver's presence in the environment, in that the perceiver must discount sounds from echolocation that reflect off its own body (Mitchell, 1995). Many predatory and social animals seem to know how to hide their bodies from prey, predators, and conspecifics: Coyotes ambush prey, bears stealthily follow hunters, and monkeys and apes hide from each other to enact secret copulations, attack, and obtain food (Byrne & Whiten, 1990; McMahan, 1978; Mills, 1919/1976).

A more complicated awareness of bodily appearance is present in cephalopods (octopus and squid) when they change their bodily reflectance, pattern, and color (even though they are color-blind) to make their bodies match (or be saliently different from) their background (Hanlon & Messenger, 1996; Moynihan, 1985). Although some aspects of these bodily transformations, such as color matching, are clearly automatic processes, other aspects show remarkable flexibility: In some cases, these organisms transform their bodily shapes to match seaweed, fish, or their own jets of ink sprayed defensively to avoid predators. They are "visibly aware of their appearance as well as their surrounding" (Moynihan, 1985, p. 104).

Animals may even categorize their own activities: For example, rats can learn to push specific levers following specific actions such as face washing, rearing, and walking (but not scratching) or following nonaction—being immobile (Benninger, Kendall, & Vanderwolf, 1974; Morgan & Nicholas, 1979). These findings suggest to some that rats have a representation of themselves in action—a self-representation (Benninger et al., 1974)—though an alter-

native is that the rats are using self-specifying perceptual experiences without representing themselves as such (Morgan & Nicholas, 1979).

These indications that perceptions provide specification of a self as locus and experiencer of movement support the presence of a body schema—"the body's nonconscious appropriation of habitual postures and movements, its incorporation of various significant parts of the environment into its own experiential organization" (Gallagher, 1995, p. 226). For example, human infants and baby chicks make movements to compensate for an apparent loss of balance when the walls of a room they are in begin (as a result of experimental manipulation) to move toward them, which shows awareness of their body's posture and orientation in relation to their environment—a basic comprehension of their body as a locus (Butterworth, 2000). Such responses indicate a self that is specified by perception (the "ecological self"), an initial state from which more complex notions of self derive (Butterworth, 2000; Neisser, 1988). An organism's ability for coordinated movement indicates both long-term and short-term body schemas; the long-term schema provides intuitive knowledge of the possibilities for coordination and spatial position of the body's trunk and appendages, and the short-term schemas provide information about the current content and position of these body parts and changes among them (O'Shaughnessy, 1980, 1995). Yet immediate bodily experience is not always encoded in memory. For example, 4- to 8-year-old children who were either blind or had their eyes closed lost track of which finger had been lightly touched by an experimenter when they overturned their hand, and sometimes even when their hand remained stationary (McKinney, 1964).

The self may extend beyond the body, as when animals treat others and objects as possessions (James, 1890; Lancaster & Foddy, 1988; Mitchell, 1994b). For example, canids and primates exhibit jealousy of the attention others receive (Breuggeman, 1978; Goodall, 1986; Mitchell, 1994b; Smuts, 1985), and chimpanzees and baboons experience grief following the death of another (Goodall, 1986; Smuts, 1985). Such actions suggest a concept of "mine" or that others are part of "me."

Experience of the External World and Consciousness in Relation to Self-Awareness

Normally when we have experiences, we are conscious (aware) during them—that's what makes them experiences! In this conception, to have an experience is to be conscious, which is, simultaneously, to be a subject of an experience. But there are some experiences that can occur seemingly on autopilot, during which we seem unaware of them. For example, while driving a car on a habitual route, many of us become bound up in our thoughts and drive quite appropriately without any attention to our awareness of our surroundings (we may suddenly become aware of our surroundings but have no memory of our experience of what was happening beforehand in relation to them). This bifurcation of experience (into "aware" thoughts and "unaware" perceptions) is called "dissociation" and is present in other circumstances, such as hypnosis (E. Hilgard, 1986/1991; J. Hilgard, 1970). One philosopher (Carruthers, 1992) called such experiences as driving on autopilot "nonconscious experiences" and claimed that animals have experiences that are always of the nonconscious variety. This claim raises concerns about animals having a self because, if animals are without conscious experiences, they cannot be subjects of experiences. However, Carruthers's (1992) conceptualization is problematic because dissociative (nonconscious) experiences such as those while driving occur in humans only after skill is obtained in a given area (e.g., driving a car) and indicate a split in consciousness, not its complete absence. In addition, during initial skill learning, full consciousness is present, which suggests that conscious experience is developmentally prior to dissociative experience. So, from this perspective, it seems unlikely that animals always have nonconscious experiences.

Another attempt by Carruthers (1992) to attribute only nonconscious experiences to animals is to claim that their experiences are like those of people with blindsight. In blindsight, people who have lost functioning in part of their brain report no conscious visual experiences in (part of) their visual field but are still able to respond accurately to visual stimuli from this visual field, believing all the while that they are only guessing about these stimuli (Weiskrantz, 1986, 1997). Again, as with dissociation, it is unclear whether nonconscious experiences of the sort found in blindsight can occur without the blindsighted individual having had prior conscious experiences (although it is conceivable; see Evans, 1982). Indeed, the behavior of a macaque monkey named Helen after an operation that induced essentially total blindsight in this previously sighted monkey was quite different from that of a normal monkey (Humphrey, 1974). For example, Helen seemed able to use only her body (but not other objects) as a guide for the location of food items that she knew to be present but could not see.

Ironically for Carruthers's (1992) claims, this and other evidence in monkeys of differences between normal visual experiences and those during blindsight suggests that monkeys normally enjoy conscious experiences. In one study, three macaques who had had the striate cortex of their left cerebral hemisphere removed (producing blindsight in part of their right visual field) were tested, along with a normal macaque, in a task in which they had to touch a light wherever it appeared on a screen (Cowey & Stoerig, 1995). (Destriated monkeys can learn to respond to some visual stimuli in the affected visual field.) After all four monkeys learned to respond accurately to stimuli in both visual fields, they received stimuli only in the left visual field and were also given "blank" trials with no stimulus, in which case they had to press a black rectangle to indicate stimulus absence. After all four monkeys learned this task, on every 20th trial a salient visual stimulus appeared in the right visual field. Although previously all four monkeys had touched similar stimuli in the right visual field, now only the normal monkey did; the three destriated monkeys pressed the black rectangle, indicating a blank trial. One interpretation is that the destriated monkeys were reporting their awareness of a lack of awareness of the visual stimulus in the right visual field (e.g., Baars, 2001; Griffin, 2001a), but there are alternative interpretations (Weiskrantz, 1997); perhaps the destriated monkeys might not be as attentive to the stimuli in the right visual field as they had been. Still, the fact that these monkeys had previously reported the presence of (and therefore their detection of) right-visual-field stimuli in the initial study suggests that they experienced these stimuli as different from ones in the left visual field. If, as Carruthers contended, blindsight is taken to indicate normal animal experience, then the destriated macaques could not have responded discriminatively to probes in the affected and unaffected visual fields, as the experiences would be identical; hence blindsight is not representative of normal (conscious) experience for monkeys.

Internal Mental States as One's Own

Evidence of experienced internal mental states in animals is harder to find than evidence of bodily or perceptual awareness. It is fairly well established that many vertebrate species have mental images (see, e.g., Louie & Wilson, 2001; Rilling & Neiworth, 1987; Rojas-Ramírez & Drucker-Colin, 1977; Terrace, 1984) and can distinguish among their own internal states (e.g., learning to push particular levers following particular internal feelings such as hunger and thirst; see Benninger et al., 1974). But do such internal experiential worlds indicate that animals reflect on or think about their internal states, indicating an inward-looking self (see Martin, 1995)? Or is Romanes (1889/1975) correct in thinking that animals have internal experiences but do not think about or reflect on them?

Von Uexküll (1909/1985) hypothesized that the development of the nervous system in animals eventually resulted in the creation of a "counterworld" of inner experiences, derived from perceptual experiences, which animals could to some degree experience internally, independent of concurrent perceptual experiences (a view quite in keeping with earlier sensationalist philosophies concerning human consciousness, such as Locke's [1690/1905]). Von Uexküll's ideas, much like Romanes's (1889/1975), raised the question as to how much animals could contemplate their internal worlds and use them to benefit themselves, which would suggest self-conscious appreciation of these mental states as their own. One study

(Hampton, 2001) examined this question in relation to macaques' ability to distinguish their knowledge from their lack of knowledge. In this study, two macaques (M1 and M2) had to touch an image on an interactive computer screen. Then, after a delay varying from 12.5 seconds to 4 minutes, they were presented with either one stimulus (for one-third of the trials) or two stimuli.

1. If presented with one stimulus (on the left), the monkey had to select it to proceed to a memory task, in which each corner of the screen contained an image, one of which was the previously shown image. (This is the forced-choice test.) The monkey received a peanut (a preferred food) if it touched this image but had to wait 15 seconds before the next trial if it touched another image.
2. If presented with two stimuli, selection of the leftmost also led to the memory test, but now it could be freely chosen because selection of the rightmost stimulus allowed the monkey to "opt out" of the memory test; its selection led to an image of wheat that, if touched, provided a (less preferred) monkey pellet.

The results showed that, as the delay increased, M1 was less and less accurate on forced-choice tests than on freely chosen tasks and chose more often to avoid the memory test; he consistently opted out at the 200-second delay (his longest delay). M2 performed only slightly worse on forced-choice than on freely chosen tests but still showed a steady increase in opting out as the delay increased. When, in an experimental variation, the monkeys were initially shown no image and were then presented with the two stimuli, M1 always chose to opt out, and M2 chose to opt out 60% of the time: Each acted as he had done previously under the longest delay.

One interpretation of this study is that, when given a choice, the monkeys opted out when they knew that they did not remember the original stimulus, and they chose the memory test when they knew that they did remember it. Consequently, they were aware of and could reflect on their internal states (or lack thereof) and use this contemplation to act. The implication for self-knowledge is that monkeys are able to use their awareness of their mental states to make reasonable behavioral choices in accord with those mental states, suggesting that monkeys experience their mental images as their own (and are aware that they can use their bodies to make choices based on those mental images). However, the monkeys' choices might simply show that they can engage in rule following using mental experiences without any awareness of their possession of the mental images: If an internal mental image of what seems to be the last image shown is present in awareness, they choose to take the memory test; if not, they choose to opt out. The self need not be cognized, and the mental images need not be experienced as *belonging* to the monkey (see discussion of this general topic in Campbell, 1994; Evans, 1982; Mitchell, 2000; P. F. Strawson, 1958/1964, 1959/1963, 1966). But then again, mental images and other experiences might be experienced as belonging to the self in the sense of their happening inside the body (Cassam, 1995), although how this sense of belonging would be articulated and understood by an animal is unclear. If it could be shown that animals had mental images representing themselves, the idea that at least *these* images were experienced as belonging to the self would be better supported.

Darwin's example of a dog reminiscing about its past successes in the hunt—and thus having an autobiographical memory—raises just this question in relation to a dog's "representation of . . . self in the context of the remembered event" (Kinsbourne, 1995, p. 218). There are at least two ways in which the self can be present: implicitly, as a perceiver of the hunt; and literally represented, in an image of itself in the hunt. (Note that the literal self-representation requires the presence of the implicit self to experience "seeing" the imagined event.) The questions raised for either self are how the dog knows that its mental experience is a memory (i.e., a self-relevant past experience) and how it could develop a visual image of itself.

One explanation for how an organism knows a mental image is self-relevant is that it experiences a "background of body sensation" that "anchor[s] the event to the individual's autobiography": "Background awareness of one's body (its feeling, its potential for action) puts the stamp of personal

experience on the scene. Conversely, one may imagine a scene and know that it has not been previously experienced because the background of bodily sensation is missing from the image" (Kinsbourne, 1995, p. 218). Kinsbourne's description seems an accurate analysis of how we know which character we are in our dreams, but, as this idea suggests, it need not clearly distinguish previously experienced action from imagined action—often, imagining oneself participating in a novel activity has concomitant bodily feelings (including its potential for action), and, often, remembering oneself in a scene occurs without them.

The odd thing about the second type of self-representation is that one can remember an event by putting a mental image of oneself into the event, producing an image of oneself which one has never actually seen. So, for example, a dog might have a memorial representation of a hunt in which it "sees" itself (in its visual imagination) at the center of the hunt, with forest and other animals all around. How a dog might represent itself visually in imagination is unclear, however, as dogs do not recognize themselves in mirrors (Zazzo, 1982) and thus seem incapable of developing a visual image of themselves (though see Mitchell, 1993c, for a means by which dogs might develop a visual self-image). In addition, even if the dog maintained a visual image of itself, how it would connect this image with bodily feelings needs to be explained (see the later discussion of kinesthetic–visual matching).

So in the instance of Darwin's reminiscing dog, we are left with the impression of a subject looking on an imagined scene with no clear way to relate this scene to itself or to some previously experienced reality. Unless the dog has an awareness of points of view different from its own current one (perhaps including divergent points of view within itself, distinguishing plans and hopes from memories, for example), all imagined experiences would be from the same point of view and therefore from the perspective of a self which is unaware of itself.

Can a Self Have Only One Perspective or Must It Have More?

In most, perhaps all, of the descriptions of animal selfhood presented in the previous two sections, the self is a background for conscious experience (O'Shaughnessy, 1995)—being a subject of experience is identical to being or having a self, and this self as experiencer need not be known to itself as such and/or requires no conceptualization to implicitly understand itself (James, 1890; Merleau-Ponty, 1962/1981). The self of this sort in both human and nonhuman animals might be viewed as a mere "reification" of "the perception of the interconnection of internal experience which accompanies the experience itself" (Wundt, 1894/1907, p. 250), but such perception seemingly indicates the existence of a subject of experience.

Some authors have claimed that such a subject of experience has "self-awareness" of a very limited "egocentric" type:

> To have egocentric self-awareness is not to apprehend a pure self apart from the experience, but to be acquainted with an experience in its first-personal mode of presentation, that is, from "within." . . . The subject or self referred to in *self*-awareness is . . . not something apart from or beyond the experience, but simply a feature or function of its givenness. (Zahavi, 2000, p. 64)

Similarly, Eilan (1995, pp. 341–345), borrowing from Evans (1982), situated the organism in "egocentric space" in which resulting perceptual representations are "essentially perspectival" in that the spatial contents of this space are implicitly self-relational (the cat is in front of me, the dog is to my side); interestingly, it is just such self-relational representations that were lost in the monkey Helen's blindsight (Humphrey, 1974). In Eilan's view, the subject need not think of itself as a subject with a point of view in order to be one. In these views, having an experience means having a first-person perspective, and having a first-person perspective means having a self (or, identically, a subject) that experiences this first-person perspective. Having a (first-person) perspective seems a normal part of animals' experiences (Griffin, 2001b; Merleau-Ponty, 1942/1967, 1960/1982; von Uexküll, 1909/1985; Yerkes & Yerkes, 1929).

Yet the animal's "perspective" on the world here is, implicitly, in comparison with our own, not one of many alternative points of view it uses to examine itself. The question, "What is it like to be a bat?" proposed by Nagel (1979) to promote inquiry into the nature of nonhuman experience has the implied notion, "for whom?" For a bat, presumably, its experience is not "like" anything; the experience simply is (Glover, 1981; Lycan, 1987). Whether most animals recognize that their perspective is distinctly perspectival—one of several ways of viewing the world—is not clear (Quiatt, 1997).

Self as Idea and Object

The Conceptual Basis for Self-Awareness

The notion that conscious experiences per se specify a self, subject, or "first person" perspective is reasonable. But the self so specified is implicit in consciousness and appears "purely formal, or *empty*" (Evans, 1982, p. 232) when there appears no possibility for "third person" or other points of view. A self with awareness of alternative perspectives marks an idea of the self more elaborate than (and inclusive of) the self as subject of experience and is more in line with what people usually think of when they talk of "the self." Galen Strawson (1999a, 1999b, 2000), focusing on momentary unified experience, proposed that the minimal version of self-experience requires an individual psychological event of an embodied organism that has a perspective or point of view. Having a point of view, in Strawson's view, requires recognizing that there is more than one point of view, which itself requires conceptualization of experience per se. And having a concept requires an ability to apply that concept in more than one context (e.g., beyond the self; see also Evans, 1982, p. 158).

Thus attribution of perspective to an organism implies its capacity for multiple perspectives (or at least more than one) on a given environment (P. F. Strawson, 1966), which to some seems unlikely for nonhuman animals (Bermúdez, 1995; Carruthers, 1992). Indeed, Eilan (1995, p. 255) admitted that "There is a yawning chasm between your detached representation of yourself as an object [the typical view of self-awareness] and your representationally silent occurrence as an extended . . . point of view." As a way to introduce perspective taking (that is, having the ability to take multiple points of view) into normal experience, Bermúdez (1995) posited that this ability may be a natural outgrowth of intentional action. Having an intention requires both "grasping that there are different possibilities for action open to me" and the "subject's representing himself as an agent" (p. 172). But Bermúdez admitted that distinguishing agency from some simpler form of responsiveness to environmental contingencies is not a simple task and that it seems to raise similar problems to those he attempted to solve by introducing his conceptualization.

It would be interesting to discover if animals, like humans, can envision themselves from both internal and external points of view, knowing how something looks from inside the body and how it would look if perceived from outside the body (see, e.g., Natsoulas & Dubanoski, 1964). Examples of noninstinctual feigning by animals introduce (as Romanes, 1889/1975, suggested) the possibility that they may take such opposing perspectives on their own behavior. (Mirror-self-recognition, discussed later, also raises this possibility.) Wittgenstein (1949/1992) believed intentional feigning to be problematic for understanding mind, in that the same behavior indicated different mental states, but in fact feigning supports the presence of complex mentality because the feigning entity appears to take two perspectives into account: the normative one and the deceptive one. The problem is that it is unclear whether noninstinctual feigning requires such perspective taking: It may be that an organism that (e.g.) appears to be in pain but is not is simply replicating behaviors it knows have certain consequences because it wishes to experience those consequences again, and it may have no recognition that its own "real" and "feigned" instances are different (see Mitchell, 1986, 1999). Though imperfect, the best evidence for a fuller comprehension of intentional feigning as such comes from great apes (see Byrne & Whiten, 1990; de Waal, 1982, 1986; Miles, Mitchell, & Harper, 1996; Mitchell, 1986, 1993a).

Evidence for a conceptual understanding of the self that includes multiple perspectives can be difficult to pin down (Bermúdez et al., 1995; Mitchell, 2000, 2002b; P. F.

Strawson 1958/1964). What seems necessary for having more than an implicit notion of self—having a point of view that goes beyond simply having experiences—is a conceptual structure underlying the experience to support point of view. According to Evans (1982, pp. 231–232), a perceiver must have the idea of "a persisting subject of experience, located in time and space" and must be capable of "ascribing to himself [this] property which he can conceive as being satisfied by a being not necessarily himself." In this view, an organism's perceptual awareness must be allied with a conceptual understanding that there are subjects of experience per se if that organism is to be credited with self-consciousness. Otherwise, it is unclear how the organism knows that these perceptual experiences belong to it. P. F. Strawson (1959/1963) earlier made a similar point, that ascribing states of consciousness to oneself requires knowledge of how to ascribe states of consciousness per se, and both depend on having a concept of a "person." For P. F. Strawson, the concept of a person requires the idea of an entity that is both mental and physical, psychological and bodily. Because the concept of a person is essential to self-ascription and because self-ascription requires attributing states of consciousness to one's own body, "a necessary condition of states of consciousness being ascribed at all is that they should be ascribed to the *very same things* as certain corporeal [bodily] characteristics, a certain physical situation, etc." (P. F. Strawson, 1959/1963, p. 98). As noted similarly by Evans (1982, p. 213), "our self-conscious thoughts about ourselves . . . rest upon various ways we have of gaining knowledge of ourselves as physical [i.e., corporeal] things. If there is to be a division between the mental and the physical, it is a division which is spanned by the Ideas we have of ourselves."

Kinesthetic–Visual Matching: Two Perspectives on the Bodily and Experiential Self

What ideas or concepts might an animal have that span the mental and the physical and provide the animal with a conceptual understanding of point of view? What might the minimal "concept of a person" be that would allow an organism to experience a self (or have a self-experience)? The necessary conceptualization (or at least one important one) appears to be skill at kinesthetic–visual matching (KVM): the recognition of close similarity or identity between one's experience of a body's spatial extent and movements (kinesthesis) and how that looks (vision) either for the self or another (see Guillaume, 1926/1971; Mitchell, 1993c, 1993d, 1997a, 1997b, 2000, 2002a, 2002b). As Rensch (1960, p. 343) suggested, "the evolution of the concept of self [beyond that of a body scheme] might . . . be furthered by the ability to imitate the actions of other animals, i.e. to transpose visual conceptions into locomotory conceptions of the animal's own body." KVM provides an animal with two perspectives on its behavior: one kinesthetic, the other visual. It also offers the kind of conceptual translation between—or redescription of (Cenami Spada, 1997)—mental and physical that allows an organism the possibility for "ascribing to himself a property which he can conceive as being satisfied by a being not necessarily himself" (Evans 1982, p. 232). As Wittgenstein (1953/1965, p. 98e) proposed, "Think . . . how one can imitate a man's face without seeing one's own in a mirror."

An organism with KVM skills not only could recognize that it looks like its image in a mirror and in this way become aware of its visual appearance (thereby providing a representation of the self from "over there"; Anderson, 1984, 1993) but also could understand what others are experiencing kinesthetically when their activities are similar to its own and could imitate their actions to gain further information (though it need not do so). KVM also solves the problem of self-representation as exemplified in Darwin's dog: If the dog could match between a mentally represented visual image of a dog and its own actions (which seems unlikely), it could have a visual self-representation, and it could recognize itself in a visual image of the hunt. Expressed earliest by Guillaume (1926/1971), the idea of KVM as an explanation for self-recognition and bodily–facial imitation has been repeatedly and apparently independently discovered by numerous authors (for a history, see Mitchell, 1997c, 2002b). In what follows, I focus on evidence of self-recognition in animals and the theoretical implications of this evidence for animals' understanding of themselves.

Self-Recognition and the Mark Test

The earliest reports of self-recognition in animals (Hayes, 1951, 1954; Hayes & Hayes, 1955; Hoyt, 1941) described home-reared apes—gorilla Toto and chimpanzee Viki—who both used the mirror to explore their teeth; Viki also tried to pull out loose teeth, put on lipstick, and clean her face. Two decades later, members of the same ape species provided evidence that they recognized themselves in mirrors: A gorilla (age 3–5 years) initially inspected the image in the mirror, touching the mirror, and then

> looked at the mirror with his head placed between his legs. . . . Later he stood on his hands, resting his feet on the mirror. Returning to a sitting position, he lifted one leg and looked at his reflection, inspecting the parts of him that he ordinarily could not see. He obviously recognized himself and was unafraid. (Riopelle, Nos, & Jonch, 1971, p. 88; see also Riopelle, 1970; Riopelle et al., 1976)

Four chimpanzees similarly responded to their mirror-image by

> grooming parts of the body which would otherwise be visually inaccessible without the mirror, picking bits of food from between the teeth while watching the mirror image, visually guided manipulation of anal–genital areas by means of the mirror, picking extraneous material from the nose by inspecting the reflected image, making faces at the mirror, blowing bubbles, and manipulating food wads with the lips by watching the reflection. (Gallup, 1970, p. 86)

Gallup (1970) also noticed a decline in social responding with greater exposure to the mirror, but such a decline is no longer considered an important factor in the development of self-recognition because many children and apes continue to show social behaviors (and even look behind the mirror) after it is clear that they self-recognize (Lewis & Brooks-Gunn, 1979; Miles, 1994; Povinelli, Rulf, Landau, & Bierschwale, 1993; Zazzo, 1982).

To offer further evidence that chimpanzees recognize that the image in the mirror is their own, Gallup (1970) introduced the "mark test" to animal research (a test similar to that independently introduced to child development research by Amsterdam, 1972). Gallup anaesthetized two chimpanzees with mirror experience (as well as two other chimpanzees without mirror experience) and marked an eyebrow ridge and the top of the opposite ear with a nontactile, odorless red dye. After the chimpanzees recovered from the anesthesia and were presented with a mirror, the mirror-experienced chimpanzees touched the marks; by contrast, the mirror-inexperienced chimpanzees did not respond to the marks (Gallup, 1970). One chimpanzee, after touching the mark, looked at and smelled its fingers, and similar behaviors have been noted in an orangutan (Lethmate & Dücker, 1973), a siamang (*Hylobates syndactylus*; Ujhelyi, Merker, Buk, & Geissmann, 2000), a gorilla (Swartz & Evans, 1994), and other chimpanzees (who did so "often," though no quantitative information is provided; Povinelli et al., 1993, p. 361). Oddly, the actual frequency of looking at and smelling the fingers that touched the mark is unknown, yet it is often presented as a typical chimpanzee response (e.g., Anderson & Gallup, 1997; Gallup, 1994; see discussion by Swartz & Evans, 1997).

Variations in mark test procedure and in criteria for passing the mark test are common. In some studies, video images rather than, or as well as, mirror images are used (e.g., Law & Lock, 1994; Lewis & Brooks-Gunn, 1979; Marten & Psarakos, 1995). Studies with human children avoid anesthesia, and the children are marked surreptitiously, often on the nose; mark-directed behavior begins around 18–21 months of age (later for autistic and retarded children), though earlier mark-directed behaviors have been reported (Amsterdam, 1972; Johnson, 1983; Lewis & Brooks-Gunn, 1979; see Mitchell, 1997a, for an overview). In some cases, human children who do not respond to the mark have been asked by experimenters looking only at the mirror to "wipe off the stain" (Asendorpf, Warkentin, & Baudonnière, 1996). The mark is also applied surreptitiously in many animal studies, providing evidence of self-recognition in orangutans (Lethmate & Dücker, 1973; Miles, 1994), elephants (Simonet, 2000), gorillas (Patterson & Cohn, 1994), and a

siamang (Ujhelyi et al., 2000). In some studies, sham marking is used, in which an animal is repeatedly touched, but not marked, in the area to be marked until it habituates to the touch; it is then marked (Delfour & Marten, 2001; Marten & Psarakos, 1994; Reiss & Marino, 2001; Shillito, Gallup, & Beck, 1999). Accidental markings, in which animals' faces are marked unintentionally, have also provided evidence of passing the mark test in gorillas (Parker, 1991, 1994) and gibbons (Ujhelyi et al., 2000). In studies with dolphins and killer whales, either tactile or nontactile dyes have been used, and in both cases these animals have repeatedly contorted their bodies to look via the mirror at the marked parts, indicating self-recognition (Delfour & Marten, 2001; Marten & Psarakos, 1994, 1995; Reiss & Marino, 2001).

In studies with macaque monkeys, unlike those with apes and cetaceans, the few animals showing responses to (or near) the marks have been extensively trained to respond to marks (e.g., Boccia, 1994; Howell, Kinsey, & Novak, 1994; Itakura, 1987, 1988; Thompson & Boatright-Horowitz, 1994), and none show self-exploration, suggesting to many (though not all; Itakura, 1988) that these responses are not the same sort of phenomenon shown by apes (Anderson, 1994; Gallup, 1994). Studies purporting to provide evidence of self-recognition in cotton-top tamarins (a small South American primate; Hauser, Kralik, Botto-Mahan, Garrett, & Oser, 1995) and pigeons (Epstein, Lanza, & Skinner, 1981) are not only empirically flawed but unreplicable (Anderson & Gallup, 1997; Thompson & Contie, 1994; cf. Hauser & Kralik, 1997).

Although Gallup originally conceived of the mark test as offering a more objective test of self-recognition than does mere behavioral description of acts suggestive of self-recognition, he was in fact offering another criterion that, it turns out, is just as prone to interpretation as are others (see Gallup, 1994):

> [If the] question is "What is passing?" in relation to the mark test . . . [t]he easy answer is "touching the mark on the head while using the mirror to guide the hand to the mark." However, behavior is rarely as simple as that. (Swartz, Sarauw, & Evans, 1999, p. 286)

Killer whales, for example, do not have hands to make contact with the marks, so evidence of self-recognition consists of their rubbing the marks off on the side of their tanks and returning to look at their images in the mirror (Delfour & Marten, 2001). Gorillas (as well as some chimpanzees; Thompson & Boatright-Horowitz, 1994) may respond to marks on their face that are visible in their mirror image by wiping the mark off their face when *away* from the mirror (Patterson & Cohn, 1994; Shillito et al., 1999; Swartz, Sarauw, & Evans, 1999), suggesting not only a remarkable knowledge of and memory for the location of the mark on their face even without the presence of the mirror image but also an embarrassment in the mirror context (Patterson & Cohn, 1994). Similar embarrassment is reported for some human children (Lewis & Brooks-Gunn, 1979), but for others the presence of observers can have a facilitating effect on passing the mark test: 5 of 24 children in the 12- to 17-month-old group in Johnson's (1983) study touched a surreptitiously placed mark on their nose only when their mother was also visible with them on video; none of the children in this age group touched the mark during a prior period when they were visible alone on the video.

Touching the mark is often a relative category: One must touch the mark more often while looking in the mirror than before. (Obviously, attempts should be made to avoid marking animals in areas they seem to touch spontaneously.) Most studies required, as the criterion for passing the mark test, that animals touch the area that is marked more often while looking in the mirror than when not looking in the mirror. In some studies, passing the mark test required that the observing animal touch the area more often when looking in the mirror after the mark has been applied to it than it did during a prior session in which it looked in the mirror before the mark had been applied (Lewis & Brooks-Gunn, 1979; Shillito et al., 1999). Another study compared the number of touches to the mark when the marked individual was either looking or not looking into a mirror with passing the mark test, indicated by more touches in the former than the latter condition (Lin, Bard, & Anderson, 1992). Still another study (Povinelli et al., 1993) apparently required

that the number of mark contacts (by fingers) while the animal was watching the mirror image be five or more. Of the chimpanzees who passed this criterion, compared with their mirror-monitored mark contacts, all showed equal or fewer mark contacts (by fingers) when they were not looking in an available mirror and fewer such mark contacts during the control period prior to the appearance of the mirror. Of the chimpanzees who did not pass this criterion, only two showed any mark contacts (by fingers) while looking in the mirror. Thus, one chimpanzee (Todd) who touched (by fingers) the marks on his face three times while looking at himself in the mirror was deemed not to pass the mark test. Todd never touched these marks with his fingers before the mirror was presented, but did so five times while the mirror was present but he was not looking into it (p. 362). It might very well be that Todd persisted in touching the marks after noticing them in the mirror and referred back to the mirror a few times, suggesting that he recognized the image as his own. (As noted previously in relation to gorillas, if one recognizes via the mirror that one's face is marked and where, finding the mark on one's face should not be difficult even without the aid of a mirror; thus deliberate focused touching of the mark after seeing oneself in the mirror indicates self-recognition.) The fact that tamarins touched their dyed hair on looking at their reflection in the mirror (Hauser et al., 1995) is not evidence for self-recognition without evidence that they touched their dyed hair less *before* they looked at it in the mirror (Anderson & Gallup, 1997).

The directedness with which an animal touches the mark while looking at itself in a mirror is also important as evidence of self-recognition. As noted by Swartz and Evans (1991), part of the evidence for self-recognition in chimpanzees is the attention the animal focuses on the mark when it is in front of the mirror compared with its more perfunctory mark-directed behavior when the mirror is not present. Yet a gorilla that twice touched the mark, apparently deliberately, while watching himself in the mirror but who also had more cursorily touched it twice before he was shown the mirror was still viewed as not recognizing himself because of the identity in the number of touches in the two circumstances (Shillito et al., 1999). In several studies, neither behavioral criteria nor reliability checks were provided for mark test behaviors; apparently these behaviors are viewed as rather obvious. For example, Povinelli and colleagues (1993, p. 361) distinguished touches to the mark (contact by fingers) and rubs to the mark (contact by hand but not by fingers) to differentiate "intentional" from "inadvertent" contacts but offered no evidence that these can be reliably distinguished or that the means of contact (finger vs. hand) clearly differentiated the intentionality of the contact.

Although passing the mark test suggests that the animal knows that the mirror image is of its own body, an alternative interpretation is that the organism believes that it is confronted with another organism, not itself, and that it checks to see if it has a mark at the same place as the image animal (see Mitchell, 1993c). For example, some (but not most) human children touched an area on their own faces at a particular location after observing their mothers or other children with facial marks in the same location (Johnson, 1983; Lewis & Brooks-Gunn, 1979), suggesting that passing the mark test need not indicate recognition of "self" (unless some understanding of mirrors is assumed; see Mitchell, 1993c). Povinelli and colleagues (1993, p. 370) stated that "[o]ur results show that there is no need to accept this copycat hypothesis because our subjects that passed the mark test all had 4–7 hr of visual exposure to their marked partner before the unveiling of the mirror." However, the relevance of these results to the hypothesis is unclear. Again, even if the chimpanzees had been exposed to another chimpanzee with marks on its face, they might still have viewed their own mirror image as a totally different chimpanzee, and again checked to see if there were similar marks on their own face. (Note that the mirror image would have marks on opposing locations compared with the marked conspecific the chimpanzees experienced before being presented with a mirror; all chimpanzees were marked on the right eyebrow ridge and on top of the left ear.) According to Gallup (1994), apes contrast with human children in this respect; apes groom another's face if it is marked, but not

their own (see, e.g., Lethmate & Dücker, 1973). However, as de Veer and van den Bos (1999) noted, more extensive evidence supporting this view remains to be presented. If accurate, this interspecific contrast suggests that, unlike human self-images, those of apes do not incorporate the other in quite the same way (see Mitchell, 1993c). (Note that cotton-top tamarins apparently do not touch dyed hair on their own bodies after observing another with dyed hair, and they only rarely touch the other's dyed hair [Hauser et al., 1995].)

Criteria for and Conceptual Underpinnings of Self-Recognition

The various criteria proposed for mirror-self-recognition are (1) passing the mark test, (2) self-exploration (usually manual) using the mirror to see parts otherwise not visible, (3) experimenting with "contingent" bodily and facial gestures and watching them in the mirror (also called "contingency testing"; see Parker, Mitchell, & Boccia, 1994), and (4) among linguistically skilled humans and apes, verbally identifying the image as oneself (Anderson, 1993). (The significance of mirror-directed behaviors such as bubble making by chimpanzees and cetaceans or extended staring into the eyes of the mirror animal in gibbons is unclear. This evidence should be examined further in relation to other criteria [see Delfour & Marten, 2001; Marten & Psarakos, 1994; Swartz & Evans, 1991; Ujhelyi et al., 2000].) Behavioral expression of self-conscious emotions such as embarrassment provides a non-mirror-based means by which to discern self-consciousness in human children (Lewis, Sullivan, Stanger, & Weiss, 1989), and such emotions seem present in sign-using apes (Miles, 1994; Patterson & Cohn, 1994). Indeed, as noted before, embarrassment is present in some gorillas' responses to marked mirror images in that they avoided scrutiny when removing the mark (Patterson & Cohn, 1994; Shillito et al., 1999).

Work by Swartz and Evans (1991) provided the first evidence that normal chimpanzees did not always satisfy all of the nonlinguistic mirror-based indicators of self-recognition and that some normal chimpanzees showed none of these criteria.

So far, at least some members of each ape genus—*Pan* (chimpanzee), *Gorilla* (gorilla), *Pongo* (orangutan), and *Hylobates* (siamang and gibbon)—have shown evidence of each of the nonlinguistic criteria for self-recognition, but even among chimpanzees (*Pan troglodytes*—the most studied species) sometimes only about half of those tested satisfy a given criterion (see Swartz et al., 1999; Ujhelyi et al., 2000). In addition, older chimpanzees appear to lose interest in their mirror images (Povinelli et al., 1993). Obviously, the mirror image means something different to human beings (almost all of whom self-recognize) than to other species. Bonobos (*Pan paniscus*—also called pygmy chimpanzees) have never been mark tested but show contingent bodily gestures, contingent facial gestures, and/or self-exploration (Hyatt & Hopkins, 1994; Inoue-Nakamura, 1997; Walraven, van Elsacker, & Verheyen, 1995; Westergaard & Hyatt, 1994). Gorillas tend to show contingent bodily gestures and contingent facial gestures (Shillito et al., 1999; Swartz & Evans, 1994; Swartz et al., 1999) and less frequently show self-exploration (Hoyt, 1941; Inoue-Nakamura, 1997; Law & Lock, 1994; Riopelle et al., 1971). However, two human-reared sign-using gorillas engaged in a variety of self-exploratory behaviors (Patterson & Cohn, 1994). Depending on one's criteria, two to seven gorillas have passed the mark test (Parker, 1991, 1994; Patterson & Cohn, 1994; Shillito et al., 1999; Swartz & Evans, 1994). (Gallup [1994; Shillito et al., 1999], who for many years denied that the gorilla Koko recognized herself in mirrors, now acknowledges her self-recognition but remains suspicious of accounts of other gorillas' self-recognition.) Suggested instances of self-exploration by tamarins, in which one looked at her back in the mirror and another looked through her legs at her rear end and then looked directly at it (Hauser et al., 1995), were not deemed acceptable evidence of self-exploration by other observers of these behaviors (Anderson & Gallup, 1997). Dolphins and killer whales, of course, are exempt from engaging in some forms of self-exploration by definition, as they cannot move their flippers to their mouths, and other forms of self-exploration and contingency testing are difficult to detect or interpret, so researchers of these animals have focused on the mark test (see Delfour & Marten, 2001; Marten & Psarakos, 1994, 1995; Mitchell, 1995; Reiss & Marino, 2001).

Although Anderson (1993) was willing to accept success on two out of any three pieces of evidence as criterial for self-recognition, the problem arises as to why animals might show some types of evidence but not others if all are indicative of self-recognition (Mitchell, 1993d). Exactly what each of these activities indicates for self-recognition needs to be articulated.

The most ambiguous criterion for self-recognition is labeling the self. Apparently children and great apes can learn, at an age well before they show other evidence of self-recognition, that their own name refers to both their body and the mirror image of their body (Gallup, 1975; Miles, 1994), so that self-labeling need not indicate self-recognition. On the other hand, correct use of "I" or "me" (as well as "you") implies a recognition of self from different perspectives when used by children (Brigaudiot, Morgenstern, & Nicolas, 1996; Loveland, 1984) and apes (Miles, 1994; Patterson & Cohn, 1994). Given that few apes have learned either names or pronouns for self (see Itakura, 1994), this criterion is rarely employed in conferring self-recognition on animals.

Theoretically, contingent bodily gestures and contingent facial gestures provide an animal with evidence that its own actions or movements are contingent with those of the animal in the mirror (perhaps comparable to the way turning on a light switch is contingent with the appearance of light), from which the animal could (perhaps) induce that the image is of itself in the mirror. (Indeed, an orangutan which showed only contingent bodily gestures and a gorilla which showed only contingent facial gestures both passed a mark test; Lethmate & Dücker, 1973; Swartz & Evans, 1994). Obviously something more than mere contingency is necessary to induce belief that the mirror image is of one's own body. Both contingent bodily gestures and contingent facial gestures would seem likely to lead to self-recognition if the animal could use these behaviors to recognize that the contingent image in the mirror is visually the same as itself. (Animals such as monkeys appear to have little problem recognizing that the image looks like a monkey [Anderson, 1994], though whether they know that they themselves look like a monkey is unclear.) If the animal recognized such visual similarities (e.g., its hand looks like the image in the mirror and moves in the same way as the hand of the image in the mirror), then contingent bodily gestures would tell the animal that the image animal moves *when* it does and *the way* it does. From such facts and other knowledge (such as knowledge that its hand is connected to its body and that the hand in the mirror is connected to a body), it might infer that the image is of itself (see Mitchell, 1993c).

For contingent facial gestures to lead to self-recognition, the animal would need to recognize that, when it moves its face in contorted ways, the image animal moves its face in the same way (see Parker, 1991). For most animals, recognition of similarity between their own face and that in the mirror is not possible purely through visual–visual comparison: The animal cannot visually observe its own face as such until it recognizes itself in the mirror, and, until such self-recognition occurs, the animal cannot recognize that the image in the mirror looks like its own face because it does not know what its face looks like (Mitchell, 1993c). However, many orangutans enjoy looking into their extended mouth when it is full of food and will sometimes look at their image in the mirror when engaged in such behavior (Lethmate & Dücker, 1973); consequently orangutans might be able to use visual–visual matching to detect that some of their facial behaviors are visually the same as those in the image animal.

Another means an animal might use to recognize the similarity between movements of the animal itself and the animal in the mirror is kinesthetic–visual matching (KVM). If an animal engaged in contingent bodily gestures and contingent facial gestures has KVM, it should recognize that its actions are not only contingent with those in the mirror but also look like those in the mirror, which should further support self-recognition. Such awareness of behavioral similarity between one's own actions and those of another are present outside the mirror context in children at 14 months of age: When they are being imitated by another

person, they test the imitation by changing their behavior and watching what the other does, but they do not do the same thing toward a person whose behavior is only contingent with their own (Meltzoff, 1990). Such findings indicate that they recognize themselves as the source of the other's actions and that their actions are similar to those of the other, but they can (hopefully!) retain the belief that they are different from the other person. If an animal has KVM and engages in contingent bodily gestures (particularly with parts of the body) and contingent facial gestures, it would presumably come to the conclusion that the animal in the mirror is an image of itself (Mitchell, 1993c, 1993d, 1997a, 1997b). (It could alternatively, of course, come to the conclusion that there is a remarkably adept imitator of its own behavior present in a weird alternative universe inside the mirror space.) It would be interesting to see how different species respond to mirror information that provides strikingly discrepant information between kinesthesis and vision (see, e.g., Gregory, 1997, p. 250). When six chimpanzees who passed the mark test in a regular mirror were confronted with their mirror images in mildly distorting mirrors (both concave and convex) and in a multiplying (triptych) mirror, all showed contingent bodily gestures, contingent facial gestures, and self-exploration, which suggests that these behaviors are interesting or enjoyable for chimpanzees even when they do not provide precise information about their visual self-image (Kitchen, Denton & Brent, 1996).

Theoretically, self-exploration indicates minimally that the animal recognizes that the animal image in the mirror provides information about its own body, which presumably means that the animal knows that the image in the mirror is an image of itself. It also indicates that the animal, on seeing the mirror image, desires to gain visual information from the mirror image about bodily and facial aspects it has known only tactually and kinesthetically (Mitchell, 1993d). One might posit that self-exploration indicates only being intrigued by the novelty of the experience of seeing oneself, without any desire to gain visual information about one's body. Certainly being so intrigued is part of the explanation for self-exploration. But it is unclear whether this idea fully explains self-exploration: Why would being intrigued by the new experience of seeing oneself lead so consistently to moving the body so as to see (and, in the case of apes, manually manipulate) one's rear end and/or inside one's mouth if one were not interested in gaining visual information about these areas? In some instances, the interest in gaining visual information about the self is more obvious, as when a chimpanzee and a gorilla each used a mirror to explore a broken tooth, a chimpanzee used a mirror to extract a bad tooth with pliers, and a gorilla and a bonobo each used a mirror to examine extensively inside its mouth (Calhoun & Thompson, 1988; Hayes & Hayes, 1955; Hoyt, 1941; Hyatt & Hopkins, 1994; Law & Lock, 1994).

The empirically observed relationships among contingent bodily gestures, contingent facial gestures, and self-exploration are currently under debate (see Table 28.1 for some representative definitions of these categories). In one investigation of 105 chimpanzees (Povinelli et al., 1993), the frequencies of contingent bodily gestures, contingent facial gestures, and self-exploration were somewhat correlated (with ranges from .42 to .51) in chimpanzees. Yet in this study and others, individual chimpanzees and other apes varied in which of these activities they exhibited and in the order and frequency in which they exhibited them (Lethmate & Dücker, 1973; Ujhelyi et al., 2000). For example, Lin and colleagues (1992) stated (without providing data) that they observed more contingent bodily gestures than contingent facial gestures across all age groups of chimpanzees from 2 to 5 years old, but Povinelli and colleagues (1993, Figures 2 and 3) observed about equal frequencies in the same age group (note that Povinelli's "weak" and "compelling" instances combined are somewhat comparable to those of Lin et al.'s instances of contingent bodily gestures and contingent facial gestures; see Table 28.1).

The developmental relations among contingent bodily gestures, contingent facial gestures, and self-exploration are also under debate, particularly by those studying chimpanzees. Lin and colleagues (1992) observed a slight increase in contingent bodily gestures, contingent facial gestures, and self-

exploration across 2- to 5-year-old chimpanzees, but their criteria for each behavior (see Table 28.1) are open to interpretation (Povinelli et al., 1993). Povinelli and colleagues (1993), using more exclusive criteria for these behaviors, stated (without providing data) that contingent bodily gestures and contingent facial gestures occurred prior to self-exploration for "most" chimpanzees who showed all of these behavior patterns over a 5-day (5–8 hours per day) exposure to mirrors, but they also presented descriptions of individual animals who did not show this pattern (e.g., p. 354). In addition, Povinelli and colleagues claimed that "CB [contingent bodily] and CF [contingent facial] movements can be detected in young (and old) chimpanzees that do not show SE [self-exploratory] behaviors or pass the mark test" (p. 366), but the evidence indicated that this pattern was rare. (The pattern appeared more salient in another study by Eddy, Gallup, & Povinelli, 1996.)

Although it is theoretically possible that some animals could use contingency behaviors to detect themselves in mirrors, these behaviors alone are not adequate as evidence of self-recognition in that they can occur prior to more certain indications of self-recognition (Mitchell, 1993c). Human children show evidence of contingent bodily gestures and contingent facial gestures 6 to 9 months before they pass the mark test (e.g., Lewis & Brooks-Gunn, 1979). Some macaques show contingent bodily gestures but fail to show contingent facial gestures or self-exploration (Boccia, 1994). Close observation of the sequencing of behaviors over several days of mirror exposure showed that contingent bodily gestures and contingent facial gestures preceded self-exploration in one gibbon (*Hylobates leucogenys*) and that contingent bodily gestures (but no contingent facial gestures) preceded self-exploration in another (*Hylobates gabriellae*; Ujhelyi et al., 2000).

This last study, as well as another of an orangutan by Robert (1986), suggest that contingent bodily gestures might be usefully separated into two categories: one being contingent whole body movements (developmentally earlier), the other contingent movements of body parts while the rest of the body remains still (with contingent facial gestures a special case of the latter). The

TABLE 28.1. Criteria for Contingent Body Movements, Contingent Facial Movements, and Self-Explorations in Three Studies.

Povinelli et al. (1993, pp. 350–351)	Lin, Bard, & Anderson (1992, p. 122)	Swartz & Evans (1991, p. 486)
Contingent body movements: CB	Contingent body movement	
Compelling: Animal made two or more repetitions of a bodily movement while engaged in visual exploration; this often included rapid visual alternation from the body part to the mirror. (Examples are slowly waving hand, poking fingers repetitively through the mesh, moving slowly forward and backward, moving one leg slowly while standing on the other foot.)	Movement of the head or body while the chimpanzee visually follows the movements in the mirror.	
Weak: Examples of weak bouts of CB included an animal's waving its arms in front of the mirror without looking continuously into the mirror or watching itself in the mirror while performing some nonrepetitive action.		
Contingent facial movements: CF	Contingent facial movement	Self-referred behaviors
Compelling: Animal made unusual facial contortions while it was judged to be looking at its own image.	Movement of parts of the face while the chimpanzee visually follows the movements in the mirror; novel mouth movements.	Using the mirror to investigate the effects of certain behaviors, e.g. blowing bubbles, making faces, or making noises with the mouth while looking into the mirror.
Weak: Examples of weak CF behaviors included certain instances of an animal's lip smacking, sucking on the caging wire while manipulating the lips or tongue, and alternately glancing into the mirror, as well as mild facial contortions seen in other contexts.		
Self-exploration: SE	Mirror-guided body-directed behavior	Self-directed behaviors
Compelling: Animal used fingers or hands to manipulate parts of the body otherwise not visible (e.g., facial areas and anal–genital region). Animal had to be looking into mirror and must have been judged to be looking at its own image.	Use of the mirror image to direct some action toward the chimpanzee's own body, exclusive of the face. Mirror-guided face-directed behavior	Manipulation of the body using the mirror to guide the body-directed movements.
Weak: Weak bouts of SE were recorded in cases when a chimpanzee was observed scratching its face, head, nose, or body while engaging in [visual exploration] of the mirror and in cases when a subject actively groomed a part of its body that it could see directly while it alternately glanced into the mirror.	Use of the mirror image to direct some action toward one's own face, exclusive of the marked spot (e.g., the chimpanzee watches itself scratch its face).	

Note. Criteria are direct quotes.

fact that chimpanzees can use simultaneous video images of their arm and its surroundings to move it toward a desired location (Menzel, Savage-Rumbaugh, & Lawson, 1985) indicates that they do not necessarily require an image of their whole body to recognize their body parts. Interestingly, human children at 21 months of age (around the end of the time period when most children recognize their images in mirrors) may be better able to recognize and identify parts of their own and others' faces than parts of their own and others' bodies (Lis & Venuti, 1990), suggesting that understanding of the organization of the face may precede understanding of relations among other body parts.

The empirically observed relationships between passing the mark test and the other categories (particularly self-exploration) are also controversial. Povinelli and colleagues (1993) defined positive self-recognition (SR+) as an animal's showing five or more self-exploratory behaviors, ambiguous self-recognition (SR?) as showing one to four self-exploratory behaviors, and lack of self-recognition (SR−) as showing no self-exploratory behaviors, during several days of mirror exposure. One to four months later, these researchers enacted the standard mark test (with anesthesia) on chimpanzees from all three self-recognition groups and discovered that only half of the 18 SR+ animals passed the mark test and that one each of the seven SR− and six SR? chimpanzees also did. (Note also an orangutan who passed the mark test and showed contingent bodily gestures, but not self-exploration, in Lethmate and Dücker, 1973, similarly indicating that self-exploration is not essential for passing the mark test. Oddly, Povinelli and colleagues direct the reader to SR− animals as ones who show contingent bodily [CB] gestures and contingent facial [CF] gestures without self-exploration [p. 353], but later make the claim that "no subjects that showed only CF or CB behaviors pass the [mark] test" [p. 366]. Yet one of the SR− animals passed the mark test. So either this claim is false, or this SR− animal showed *no* evidence of contingent facial gestures, contingent bodily gestures, *or* self-exploration, yet still passed the mark test.) Povinelli and colleagues took their findings to indicate that self-exploration and passing the mark

test are dissociable responses, but others have mistakenly accepted the greater likelihood of SR+ chimpanzees passing the mark test (compared to SR? or SR− chimpanzees) as evidence that "both conditions [self-exploration and passing the mark test] measure the same phenomenon" (de Veer & van den Bos, 1999, p. 461). Clearly self-exploration is neither necessary nor sufficient for passing the mark test. Why not?

One hypothesis is that passing the mark test indicates not only that the animal knows (presumably) that the mirror image is a self-image (consistent with self-exploration) but also that it has a visually based general representation of faces (which it can apply to its own face) and that it cares when there is a deviation from that representation (Mitchell, 1993c, 1993d). If chimpanzees have a general representation of chimpanzee faces per se, including their own (rather than a specific representation of their own face), the chimpanzees showing self-exploration studied by Povinelli and colleagues might not have passed the mark test because they had visual access to another chimpanzee who had similar facial marks prior to self-observation in the mirror. These chimpanzees were marked two at a time, and when they came out of anesthesia, each of the pair "had visual and auditory access to each other but were just outside each other's physical reach" (Povinelli et al., 1993, p. 361). Consequently, any general facial representation might have been amended to include odd facial marks appearing spontaneously. Under normal circumstances, without such exposure to another chimpanzee with facial marks, the mark on its own face might have provided a "glaring deviation from what the chimpanzee normally perceives about others like itself," which might have induced exploration of the mark (Mitchell, 1993d, p. 361); but with ample evidence on the face of another that such marks appear spontaneously, exploration of the mark might not always have been deemed necessary.

Another hypothesis is that chimpanzees who showed self-exploration could develop a "rich or stable representation of their physical appearance," specifically of their own facial features, which would allow these animals to pass the mark test (Povinelli et al., 1993, p. 365). Failure to pass the mark test, by contrast, occurred because some chimpanzees who had shown self-exploration forgot their self-specific facial features (remember, these chimpanzees were given a mark test 1 to 4 months after they had last observed themselves in the mirror); upon again figuring out that the image in the mirror is of itself (as evinced by self-exploration), each of these chimpanzees simply included the facial marks into its self-image. (Of course a simple way to test the "forgetting" hypothesis is to test chimpanzees with only a short delay between self-exploration and the mark test.) Evidence consistent with the self-specific facial learning hypothesis is that SR+ chimpanzees were more likely to show contingent facial gestures and pass the mark test than were SR? and SR- chimpanzees; and some apes who pass the mark test in other studies (e.g., Lethmate & Dücker, 1973) spent a long time staring at themselves in mirrors.

However, several findings suggest that chimpanzees' retention (or forgetting) of a highly specific facial representation is unlikely to be the explanation for passing (or failing) the mark test. First, the chimpanzees in the age group that showed the most self-exploration apparently showed little extensive exploration of the visual information in the mirror (they looked at it for less than 2 minutes per half hour); indeed, the age group that showed the most frequent self-exploration showed only moderate visual exploration (Povinelli et al., 1993, p. 355). In addition, it is unknown how much of this visual exploration of images in the mirror allowed for visual exploration of the face; the best estimate of time spent looking at the face is the duration of contingent facial gestures, but the average total time spent engaged in contingent facial gestures by the SR+ chimpanzees was less than 50 seconds (p. 352). (The total time they spent staring at their unmoving face was not reported.) Consequently, it is unclear whether SR+ chimpanzees observed their face long enough to gain a detailed facial representation. More likely than chimpanzees' forgetting their own distinctive facial features is that they never learned them.

Second, in human children, recognition of their own facial features (as in a photograph) occurs some time after mirror self-recognition (Bigelow, 1981). Gaining evidence of facial self-recognition outside the mirror task with nonverbal chimpanzees is difficult but necessary to obtain independent evidence of a representation of facial features (de Veer & van den Bos, 1999). One suggestive study has shown that a sign-using orangutan can associate, with the appropriate names, its own photograph and those of two chimpanzees, as well as each animal's own distinctively colored feeding bowl (Itakura, 1994).

Third, given that forgetting of information is likely to increase with the length of time since learning the information, the forgetting hypothesis would predict that chimpanzees who experienced less time between learning of their facial features and seeing their face with marks on it would be more likely to pass the mark test. However, the amount of time between mirror exposure prior to marking and mirror exposure after marking was unrelated to passing the mark test (see Povinelli et al., 1993, Table 5).

Myriad explanations for self-recognition have been offered (for review, see Mitchell, 1993d; Parker & Mitchell, 1994). Although the evidence is far from conclusive, so far it supports kinesthetic–visual matching as a necessary and perhaps sufficient condition for self-recognition, as well as for generalized skill at bodily and facial imitation and at recognizing that one is being imitated (Guillaume, 1926/1971; Mitchell, 1993c, 1993d, 1997a, 1997b, 2002a, 2002b; see also Parker, 1991). Kinesthetic–visual matching is, then, a basis for self-knowledge, which exists even before recognizing oneself in a mirror (Mitchell, 1993c). Authors who were initially skeptical of this idea (Anderson, 1993; Gallup & Povinelli, 1993) now recognize the significance of KVM for self-recognition (Anderson & Gallup, 1999), one of them even mistakenly attributing the initial presentation of the idea to himself (Povinelli, 2000, p. 332). (Note that other cross-perceptual matching skills, such as tactile–kinesthetic matching, might also serve as a basis for self-knowledge.)

A generalized capacity for bodily (including facial) imitation has so far been detected in a few great apes (a chimpanzee, a gorilla, an orangutan) and some dolphins (Bauer & Johnson, 1994; Chevalier-Skolnikoff, 1977; Custance, Whiten, & Bard, 1995; Miles et al., 1996; Parker, 1991; Tayler & Saayman, 1973), as well as in most human children studied (Asendorpf & Baudonnière, 1993; Guillaume, 1926/1971; Hart & Fegley, 1994; Meltzoff, 1990; Piaget, 1945/1962). Although some other animals perhaps provide evidence of a limited capacity for imitation (e.g., see Bugnyar & Huber, 1997; Voelkl & Huber, 2000), at present they provide no evidence of a generalized capacity for bodily and facial imitation (see Mitchell, 2002a, 2002b). The limited facial imitation observed in human and chimpanzee neonates (Bard & Russell, 1999; Meltzoff, 1990) suggests a more rudimentary matching skill (see discussion in Maratos, 1998; Mitchell, 1993c, 1997b, 2002c) on which KVM might develop (Meltzoff, 1990); claims that the facial imitation skills of human neonates indicate a generalized imitation ability (Gallup & Povinelli, 1993) seem overstated (Mitchell, 1993c, 1993d, 1997b; Užgiris, 1999).

Self-Evaluation

Many behaviors of human beings offer evidence that they try to live up to some standards or norms for their behavior (Duval & Wicklund, 1972; Rosenberg, 1988). For example, using a mirror to create a more attractive self, following moral or social codes, and trying to be consistent in one's attitudes and behaviors all suggest an agent who acts in accordance with a self-representation based on standards. Hobhouse's (1901) idea that animals lack a set of standards or norms for the self that they use to evaluate their actions seems to be relatively well accepted for even the most cognitively sophisticated animals (de Waal, 1991; Mitchell, 1993b, 1994b). However, exactly what evidence would support this conclusion is not always clear. Animals do not seem to use mirrors to make themselves more attractive to themselves or others, suggesting a lack of visual standards of attractiveness (Mitchell, 1993c), although chimpanzees do, like children (Guillaume, 1926/1971), play "dress up" in front of mirrors (Roberts & Krause, 2002). Self-conscious emotions such as pride, shame, and guilt offer evidence of standards used toward the self in language-using human

children (Lewis et al., 1989), but evidence of these in animals seems always open to debate and divergent interpretation (see Mitchell & Hamm, 1997). For example, dog owners frequently believe that their pet, having soiled on the carpet, shows shame when confronted with the evidence, but more dispassionate witnesses might disagree (see Mitchell, Thompson, & Miles, 1997). One could suggest that an animal's acting dominant toward others in relation to food or other positively valued items indicates a self-conception based on standards for its own behavior, but these "standards" do not appear particularly complex.

Without language, evidence of self-consistency in relation to standards seems impossible to determine. Nonhuman animals who use language, such as sign-using apes, evaluate their actions using terms such as "good" and "bad," which suggests awareness of some standards (Miles, 1994; Patterson & Cohn, 1994), and points to the fact that such standards are socially induced (via language), even among humans (Cooley, 1902/1964). In a sense, standards have to do with living in accord with someone's perspective on how one should live and act— and only sometimes is that perspective exclusively one's own. As H. L. Mencken wryly noted, "Conscience is the inner voice that warns us that somebody may be looking" (quoted in MacHale, 1998, p. 194). For most of us, the expected thoughts of others concerning our actions influence our evaluations of our actions, and maintaining the positive regard of others is an important constraint on our behavior. But these influences and constraints rely on language and other culturally shared behaviors and beliefs. How important the others' view is for animals remains a topic of debate (Anderson, 1993; Gallup & Povinelli, 1993; Mitchell, 1993c, 1993d).

Conclusion

From this discussion, it seems clear that if animals are conscious, they are (minimally) subjects of experience, and in this sense possess a self. This self as experiencer is unreflective, implicit, and perhaps not even represented. Even we humans retain this experiential self, which exists as part of all of our perceptions and conscious thinking. This self is possible because of perception, which (through various perceptual mechanisms) specifies the self's embodiment and location and informs it of its movements, spatial extent, position relative to the world, and appearance (among other features).

The self as an idea or object of thought makes its appearance with cross-perceptual matching, perhaps most importantly the match between kinesthesis and vision. The existence of kinesthetic–visual matching is documented in animals such as apes and dolphins by the evidence of, for example, self-recognition and generalized bodily and facial imitation skills. Kinesthetic–visual matching also allows organisms to create a visual self-representation that they can use to plan their own activities, as well as to recreate others' activities with their own bodies. Indeed, it is likely that kinesthetic–visual matching survived evolutionarily as a result of its utility in planning one's activities in imagination, learning from others via apprenticeship in extractive foraging, or both (Mitchell, 1994a; Parker, 1993; Parker & Gibson, 1979; Parker & Mitchell, 1994). Note, however, that determining the adaptive value of kinesthetic–visual matching requires knowledge of its extent across species and evolutionary contexts (Harvey & Pagel, 1991), knowledge that we are only beginning to obtain (de Veer & van den Bos, 1999).

The presence of kinesthetic–visual matching in dolphins and perhaps elephants, as well as in great and lesser apes, suggests that the search for the adaptive context for development of kinesthetic–visual matching needs to be broadened beyond primates. Although animals such as monkeys that have visual–visual matching skills do not appear to use them to match their own bodily extremities with their image in the mirror, visual–visual matching of facial movements may foster self-recognition in animals such as orangutans, who can almost simultaneously observe their own mouth both directly and in a mirror. Much work needs to be done in clarifying the criteria for self-recognition and the extent of imitative skills in self-recognizing animals. Different researchers studying the same and different species have used different criteria to decide whether or not animals recognize themselves in mirrors, and in some cases the relationship between these criteria and their significance for self-recognition needs to be articulated.

Differences between chimpanzees (the most studied nonhuman species) and humans in responses to their mirror image suggest that self-recognition may be conceptualized differently by members of these two species. For more mature humans, mirrors become a means by which to transform themselves in relation to some socially induced visual standard, whereas for chimpanzees and other animals, as for young children, the mirror is merely a means of transforming one's image in fun or to be more natural, if it is used at all (Mitchell, 1993c). Although great apes raised by humans can evaluate their actions in terms of social standards, these same species growing up among conspecifics appear to be without a means of developing such self-evaluation. However, the fact that we are only beginning to understand the extent of cultural influences in great apes (Whiten et al., 1999) means that we must maintain an open mind about their understandings of themselves.

Acknowledgments

I am grateful to editors Mark Leary and June Price Tangney for their patience and perspicacious commentaries.

References

Amsterdam, B. (1972). Mirror self-image reactions before age two. *Developmental Psychobiology, 5,* 297–305.

Anderson, J. R. (1984). Monkeys with mirrors: Some questions for primate psychology. *International Journal of Primatology, 5,* 81–98.

Anderson, J. R. (1993). To see ourselves as others see us. *New Ideas in Psychology, 11,* 339–343.

Anderson, J. R. (1994). The monkey in the mirror: A strange conspecific. In S. T. Parker, R. W. Mitchell, & M. L. Boccia (Eds.), *Self-awareness in animals and humans* (pp. 315–329). New York: Cambridge University Press.

Anderson, J. R., & Gallup, G. G., Jr. (1997). Self-recognition in *Saguinus?* A critical essay. *Animal Behaviour, 54,* 1563–1567.

Anderson, J. R., & Gallup, G. G., Jr. (1999). Self-recognition in nonhuman primates: Past and future challenges. In M. Haug & R. E. Whalen (Eds.), *Animal models of human emotion and cognition* (pp. 175–194). Washington, DC: American Psychological Association.

Asendorpf, J. B., & Baudonnière, P. M. (1993). Self-awareness and other-awareness: Mirror self-recognition and synchronic imitation among unfamiliar peers. *Developmental Psychology, 29,* 88–95.

Asendorpf, J. B., Warkentin, V., & Baudonnière, P. M. (1996). Self-awareness and other-awareness II: Mirror self-recognition, social contingency awareness, and synchronic imitation. *Developmental Psychology, 32,* 313–321.

Baars, B. J. (2001). On the difficulty of distinguishing between conscious brain functions in humans and other mammals, using objective measures. *Animal Welfare, 10*(Supp.), S31–S40.

Baldwin, J. M. (1960). *Dictionary of philosophy and psychology* (Vol. 2). Gloucester, MA: Peter Smith. (Original work published 1901)

Bard, K. A., & Russell, C. L. (1999). Evolutionary foundations of imitation: Social cognitive and developmental aspects of imitative processes in non-human primates. In J. Nadel & G. Butterworth (Eds.), *Imitation in infancy* (pp. 89–123). New York: Cambridge University Press.

Bauer, G., & Johnson, C. M. (1994). Trained motor imitation by bottlenose dolphins (*Tursiops truncatus*). *Perceptual and Motor Skills, 79,* 1307–1315.

Benninger, R. J., Kendall, S. B., & Vanderwolf, C. H. (1974). The ability of rats to discriminate their own behaviours. *Canadian Journal of Psychology, 28,* 79–91.

Bermúdez, J. L. (1995). Ecological perception and the notion of a nonconceptual point of view. In J. L. Bermúdez, A. Marcel, & N. Eilan (Eds.), *The body and the self* (pp. 153–173). Cambridge, MA: MIT Press.

Bermúdez, J. L., Marcel, A., & Eilan, N. (Eds.). (1995). *The body and the self.* Cambridge, MA: MIT Press.

Bigelow, A. E. (1981). The correspondence between self- and image-movement as a cue to self-recognition for young children. *Journal of Genetic Psychology, 139,* 11–26.

Boccia, M. L. (1994). Mirror behavior in macaques. In S. T. Parker, R. W. Mitchell, & M. L. Boccia (Eds.), *Self-awareness in animals and humans* (pp. 350–360). New York: Cambridge University Press.

Breuggeman, J. (1978). The function of adult play in free-ranging *Macaca mulatta.* In E. O. Smith (Ed.), *Social play in primates* (pp. 169–191). New York: Academic Press.

Brewer, B. (1995). Bodily awareness and the self. In J. L. Bermúdez, A. Marcel, & N. Eilan (Eds.), *The body and the self* (pp. 291–309). Cambridge, MA: MIT Press.

Brigaudiot, M., Morgenstern, A., & Nicolas, C. (1996). "Guillaume i va pas gagner, c'est d'abord maman": Genesis of the first-person pronoun. In C. E. Johnson & J. H. V. Gilbert (Eds.), *Children's language* (Vol. 9, pp. 105–116). Mahwah, NJ: Erlbaum.

Bugnyar, T., & Huber, L. (1997). Push or pull: An experimental study on imitation in marmosets. *Animal Behaviour, 54,* 817–831.

Butterworth, G. (2000). An ecological perspective on the self and its development. In D. Zahavi (Ed.), *Exploring the self* (pp. 19–38). Amsterdam: Benjamins.

Byrne, R. W., & Whiten, A. (1990). Tactical deception in primates: The 1990 database. *Primate Report, 27,* 1–101.

Calhoun, S., & Thompson, R. L. (1988). Long-term retention of self-recognition by chimpanzees. *American Journal of Primatology, 15,* 361–365.

Campbell, J. (1994). *Past, space, and self.* Cambridge, MA: MIT Press.

Carruthers, P. (1992). *The animals issue.* New York: Cambridge University Press.

Cassam, Q. (1995). Introspection and bodily self-ascription. In J. L. Bermúdez, A. Marcel, & N. Eilan (Eds.), *The body and the self* (pp. 311–336). Cambridge, MA: MIT Press.

Cenami Spada, E. (1997). Amorphism, mechanomorphism, and anthropomorphism. In R. W. Mitchell, N. S. Thompson, & H. L. Miles (Eds.), *Anthropomorphism, anecdotes, and animals* (pp. 37–49). Albany: State University of New York Press.

Chevalier-Skolnikoff, S. (1977). A Piagetian model for describing and comparing socialization in monkey, ape, and human infants. In S. Chevalier-Skolnikoff & F. E. Poirier (Eds.), *Primate biosocial development: Biological, social, and ecological determinants* (pp. 159–187). New York: Garland.

Cooley, C. H. (1964). *Human nature and the social order.* New Brunswick, NJ: Transaction Books. (Original work published 1902)

Cowey, A., & Stoerig, P. (1995). Blindsight in monkeys. *Nature, 373,* 247–249.

Curio, E. (1976). *The ethology of predation.* Berlin: Springer-Verlag.

Custance, D. M., Whiten, A., & Bard, K. A. (1995). Can young chimpanzees (*Pan troglodytes*) imitate arbitrary actions? Hayes and Hayes (1952) revisited. *Behaviour, 132,* 837–859.

Darwin, C. (1896). *Descent of man.* New York: Appleton. (Original work published 1871)

Delfour, F., & Marten, K. (2001). Mirror image processing in three marine mammal species: Killer whales (*Orcinus orca*), false killer whales (*Pseudorca crassidens*) and California sea lions (*Zalophus californianus*). *Behavioural Processes, 53,* 181–190.

de Veer, M. W., & van den Bos, R. (1999). A critical review of methodology and interpretation of mirror self-recognition research in nonhuman primates. *Animal Behaviour, 58,* 459–468.

de Waal, F. B. M. (1982). *Chimpanzee politics: Power and sex among apes.* New York: Harper & Row.

de Waal, F. B. M. (1986). Deception in the natural communication of chimpanzees. In R. W. Mitchell & N. S. Thompson (Ed.), *Deception: Perspectives on human and nonhuman deceit* (pp. 221–244). Albany: State University of New York Press.

de Waal, F. B. M. (1991). The chimpanzee's sense of social regularity and its relation to the human sense of justice. *American Behavioral Scientist, 34,* 334–349.

Duval, S., & Wicklund, R. A. (1972). *A theory of objective self-awareness.* New York: Academic Press.

Eddy, T. J., Gallup, G. G., Jr., & Povinelli, D. J. (1996). Age differences in the ability of chimpanzees to distinguish mirror-images of self from video images of others. *Journal of Comparative Psychology, 110,* 38–44.

Eilan, N. (1995). Consciousness and the self. In J. L. Bermúdez, A. Marcel, & N. Eilan (Eds.), *The body and the self* (pp. 337–357). Cambridge, MA: MIT Press.

Epstein, R., Lanza, R. P., & Skinner, B. F. (1981). "Self-awareness" in the pigeon. *Science, 212,* 695–696.

Evans, G. (1982). *The varieties of reference.* Oxford, UK: Clarendon Press.

Gallagher, S. (1995). Body schema and intentionality. In J. L. Bermúdez, A. Marcel, & N. Eilan (Eds.), *The body and the self* (pp. 225–244). Cambridge, MA: MIT Press.

Gallagher, S., & Shear, J. (Eds.). (1999). *Models of the self.* Thorverton, UK: Imprint Academic.

Gallup, G. G., Jr. (1970). Chimpanzees: Self-recognition. *Science, 167,* 86–87.

Gallup, G. G., Jr. (1975). Towards an operational definition of self-awareness. In R. H. Tuttle (Ed.), *Socioecology and psychology of primates* (pp. 309–341). Paris: Mouton.

Gallup, G. G., Jr. (1994). Self-recognition: Research strategies and experimental design. In S. T. Parker, R. W. Mitchell, & M. L. Boccia (Eds.), *Self-awareness in animals and humans* (pp. 35–50). New York: Cambridge University Press.

Gallup, G. G., Jr., & Povinelli, D. J. (1993). Mirror, mirror on the wall, which is the most heuristic theory of them all? A response to Mitchell. *New Ideas in Psychology, 11,* 295–325.

Gibson, J. J. (1966). *The senses considered as perceptual systems.* Boston: Houghton Mifflin.

Glover, J. (1981). Critical notice of Nagel's *Mortal Questions. Mind, 90,* 292–301.

Goodall, J. (1986). *The chimpanzees of Gombe: Patterns of behavior.* Cambridge, MA: Harvard University Press.

Gregory, R. (1997). *Mirrors in mind.* Oxford, UK: Freeman.

Griffin, D. R. (2001a). Animals know more than we used to think. *Proceedings of the National Academy of Sciences, 98,* 4833–4834.

Griffin, D. R. (2001b). *Animal minds: From cognition to consciousness.* Chicago: University of Chicago Press.

Guillaume, P. (1971). *Imitation in children* (2nd ed.). Chicago: University of Chicago Press. (Original work published 1926)

Hampton, R. R. (2001). Rhesus monkeys know when they remember. *Proceedings of the National Academy of Sciences, 98,* 5359–5362.

Hanlon, R. T., & Messenger, J. B. (1996). *Cephalopod behaviour.* New York: Cambridge University Press.

Hart, D., & Fegley, S. (1994). Social imitation and the emergence of a mental model of self. In S. T. Parker, R. W. Mitchell, & M. L. Boccia (Eds.), *Self-awareness in animals and humans* (pp. 149–165). New York: Cambridge University Press.

Harvey, P. H., & Pagel, M. D. (1991). *The comparative method in evolutionary biology.* Oxford, UK: Oxford University Press.

Hauser, M. D., & Kralik, J. (1997). Life beyond the mirror: A reply to Anderson and Gallup. *Animal Behaviour, 54,* 1568–1571.

Hauser, M. D., Kralik, J., Botto-Mahan, C., Garrett, M., & Oser, J. (1995). Self-recognition in primates: Phylogeny and the salience of species-typical traits. *Proceedings of the National Academy of Sciences, 92,* 10811–10814.

Hayes, C. (1951). *The ape in our house.* New York: Harper and Brothers.

Hayes, C. (1954). An ape uses our household tools. *Popular Science, 164,* 121–124, 272.

Hayes, K. J., & Hayes, C. (1955). The cultural capacity of chimpanzee. In J. A. Gavan (Ed.), *The non-human primates and human evolution* (pp. 110–125). Detroit, MI: Wayne University Press.

Hilgard, E. (1991). Dissociative phenomena and the hidden observer. In D. Kolak & R. Martin (Eds.), *Self and identity: Contemporary philosophical issues* (pp. 89–114). New York: Macmillan. (Reprinted from Hilgard, E. (1986). *Divided consciousness* [Expanded ed.]. New York: Wiley.)

Hilgard, J. (1970). *Personality and hypnosis: A study of imaginative involvement.* Chicago: University of Chicago Press.

Hobhouse, L. (1901). *Mind in evolution.* London: Macmillan.

Howell, M., Kinsey, J., & Novak, M. A. (1994). Mark-directed behavior in a rhesus monkey after controlled, reinforced exposure to mirrors. *American Journal of Primatology, 13,* 216.

Hoyt, A. M. (1941). *Toto and I: A gorilla in the family.* Philadelphia: Lippincott.

Humphrey, N. K. (1974). Vision in a monkey without striate cortex: A case study. *Perception, 3,* 241–255.

Hyatt, C. W., & Hopkins, W. D. (1994). Self-awareness in bonobos and chimpanzees: A comparative perspective. In S. T. Parker, R. W. Mitchell, & M. L. Boccia (Eds.), *Self-awareness in animals and humans* (pp. 248–253). New York: Cambridge University Press.

Inoue-Nakamura, N. (1997). Mirror self-recognition in nonhuman primates: A phylogenetic perspective. *Japanese Psychological Research, 39,* 266–275.

Itakura, S. (1987). Use of a mirror to direct their responses in Japanese monkeys (*Macaca fuscata fuscata*). *Primates, 28,* 343–352.

Itakura, S. (1988). Monkeys and mirrors: Reconsideration of self-mirror-image recognition. *Japanese Psychological Review, 31,* 538–550.

Itakura, S. (1994). Symbolic representation of possession in a chimpanzee. In S. T. Parker, R. W. Mitchell, & M. L. Boccia (Eds.), *Self-awareness in animals and humans* (pp. 241–247). New York: Cambridge University Press.

James, W. (1890). *The principles of psychology.* New York: Holt.

Johnson, D. B. (1983). Self-recognition in infants. *Infant Behavior and Development, 6,* 211–222.

Kinsbourne, M. (1995). Awareness of one's own body: An attentional theory of its nature, development, and brain basis. In J. L. Bermúdez, A. Marcel, & N. Eilan (Eds.), *The body and the self* (pp. 205–223). Cambridge, MA: MIT Press.

Kitchen, A., Denton, D., & Brent, L. (1996). Self-recognition and abstraction abilities in the common chimpanzee studied with distorting mirrors. *Proceedings of the National Academy of Sciences, 93,* 7405–7408.

Kolak, D., & Martin, R. (Eds.). (1991). *Self and identity: Contemporary philosophical issues.* New York: Macmillan.

Lamarck, J. B. (1984). *Zoological philosophy.* Chicago: University of Chicago Press. (Original work published 1809)

Lancaster, S., & Foddy, M. (1988). Self-extensions: A conceptualization. *Journal for the Theory of Social Behaviour, 18,* 77–94.

Law, L. E., & Lock, A. J. (1994). Do gorillas recognize themselves on television? In S. T. Parker, R. W. Mitchell, & M. L. Boccia (Eds.), *Self-awareness in animals and humans* (pp. 308–312). New York: Cambridge University Press.

Lethmate, J., & Dücker, G. (1973). Untersuchungen zum Selbsterkennen im Spiegel bei Orang-utans und einigen anderen Affenarten [Investigation of self-recognition in the mirror by orangutans and some other types of apes]. *Zeitschrift für Tierpsychologie, 33,* 248–269.

Levin, J. D. (1992). *Theories of the self.* Washington, DC: Hemisphere.

Lewis, M., & Brooks-Gunn, J. (1979). *Social cognition and the acquisition of self.* New York: Plenum Press.

Lewis, M., Sullivan, M., Stanger, C., & Weiss, M. (1989). Self-development and self-conscious emotions. *Child Development, 60,* 146–156.

Lin, A. C., Bard, K. A., & Anderson, J. R. (1992). Development of self-recognition in chimpanzees (*Pan troglodytes*). *Journal of Comparative Psychology, 106,* 120–127.

Lis, A., & Venuti, P. (1990). The development of body schemes in children ages 18–36 months. In L. Oppenheimer (Ed.), *The self-concept* (p. 23–30). Berlin: Springer-Verlag.

Locke, J. (1905). *An essay concerning human understanding.* Chicago: Open Court. (Original work published 1690)

Louie, K., & Wilson, M. A. (2001). Temporally structured replay of awake hippocampal ensemble activity during rapid eye movement sleep. *Neuron, 29,* 145–156.

Loveland, K. A. (1984). Learning about points of view: Spatial perspective and the acquisition of "I/you." *Journal of Child Language, 11,* 535–556.

Lycan, W. G. (1987). *Consciousness.* Cambridge, MA: MIT Press.

MacHale, D. (Ed.). (1998). *Wit.* New York: MJF Books.

Maratos, O. (1998). Neonatal, early and later imitation: Same order phenomenon? In F. Simion & G. Butterworth (Eds.), *The development of sensory, motor and cognitive capacities in early infancy: From perception to cognition* (pp. 145–160). Hove, UK: Psychology Press.

Marten, K., & Psarakos, S. (1994). Evidence of self-awareness in the bottlenose dolphin (*Tursiops truncatus*). In S. T. Parker, R. W. Mitchell, & M. L. Boccia (Eds.), *Self-awareness in animals and humans* (pp. 361–379). New York: Cambridge University Press.

Marten, K., & Psarakos, S. (1995). Using self-view television to distinguish between self-examination and social behavior in the bottlenose dolphin (*Tursiops truncatus*). *Consciousness and Cognition, 4,* 205—224.

Martin, M. G. F. (1995). Bodily awareness: A sense of ownership. In J. L. Bermúdez, A. Marcel, & N. Eilan (Eds.), *The body and the self* (pp. 267–289). Cambridge, MA: MIT Press.

McKinney, J. P. (1964). Hand schema in children. *Psychonomic Science, 1,* 99–100.

McMahan, P. (1978). Natural history of the coyote. In R. L. Hall & H. S. Sharp (Eds.), *Wolf and man: Evolution in parallel* (pp. 41–54). New York: Academic Press.

Mead, G. H. (1974). *Mind, self and society.* Chicago: University of Chicago Press. (Original work published 1934)

Meltzoff, A. N. (1990). Foundations for developing a concept of self: The role of imitation in relating self to other and the value of social mirroring, social modeling, and self practice in infancy. In D. Cicchetti & M. Beeghly (Eds.), *The self in transition: Infancy to childhood* (pp. 139–164). Chicago: University of Chicago Press.

Melzack, R. (1989). Phantom limbs, the self, and the brain. *Canadian Psychology, 30,* 1–16.

Melzack, R. (1992). Phantom limbs. *Scientific American, 266,* 120–126.

Menzel, E. W., Jr., Savage-Rumbaugh, E. S., & Lawson, J. (1985). Chimpanzee (*Pan troglodytes*) spatial problem solving with the use of mirrors and televised equivalents of mirrors. *Journal of Comparative Psychology, 99,* 211–217.

Merleau-Ponty, M. (1967). *The structure of behavior.* Boston: Beacon Press. (Original work published 1942)

Merleau-Ponty, M. (1981). *Phenomenology of perception.* London: Routledge and Kegan Paul. (Original work published 1962)

Merleau-Ponty, M. (1982). The child's relations with others. In J. M. Edie (Ed.), *The primacy of perception* (pp. 96–155). Evanston, IL: Northwestern University Press. (Reprinted in translation from Merleau-Ponty, M. [1960]. Les relations avec autrui chez l'enfant. *Cours de Sorbonne.* Paris: Centre de Documentation Universitaire.)

Miles, H. L. (1994). ME CHANTEK: The development of self-awareness in a signing orangutan. In S. T. Parker, R. W. Mitchell, & M. L. Boccia (Eds.), *Self-awareness in animals and humans* (pp. 254–272). New York: Cambridge University Press.

Miles, H. L., Mitchell, R. W., & Harper, S. (1996). Simon says: The development of imitation in an enculturated orangutan. In A. Russon, K. Bard, & S. T. Parker (Eds.), *Reaching into thought: The minds of the great apes* (pp. 278–299). Cambridge, UK: Cambridge University Press.

Mills, E. A. (1976). *The grizzly: Our greatest wild animal.* Sausalito, CA: Comstock Editions. (Original work published 1919)

Mitchell, R. W. (1986). A framework for discussing deception. In R. W. Mitchell & N. S. Thompson (Eds.), *Deception: Perspectives on human and nonhuman deceit* (pp. 3–40). Albany: State University of New York Press.

Mitchell, R. W. (1993a). Animals as liars: The human face of nonhuman duplicity. In M. Lewis & C. Saarni (Eds.), *Lying and deception in everyday life* (pp. 59–89). New York: Guilford Press.

Mitchell, R. W. (1993b). Humans, nonhumans, and personhood. In P. Singer & P. Cavalieri (Eds.), *A new equality: The great ape project* (pp. 237–247). London: Fourth Estate.

Mitchell, R. W. (1993c). Mental models of mirror-self-recognition: Two theories. *New Ideas in Psychology, 11,* 295–325.

Mitchell, R. W. (1993d). Recognizing one's self in a mirror? A reply to Gallup and Povinelli, de Lannoy, Anderson, and Byrne. *New Ideas in Psychology, 11,* 351–377.

Mitchell, R. W. (1994a). The evolution of primate cognition: Simulation, self-knowledge, and knowledge of other minds. In D. Quiatt & J. Itani (Eds.), *Hominid culture in primate perspective* (pp. 177–232). Niwot, CO: University Press of Colorado.

Mitchell, R. W. (1994b). Multiplicities of self. In S. T. Parker, R. W. Mitchell, & M. L. Boccia (Eds.), *Self-awareness in animals and humans* (pp. 81–107). New York: Cambridge University Press.

Mitchell, R. W. (1995). Evidence of dolphin self-recognition and the difficulties of interpretation. *Consciousness and Cognition, 4,* 229–234.

Mitchell, R. W. (1997a). A comparison of the self-aware-ness and kinesthetic–visual matching theories of self-recognition: Autistic children and others. *New York Academy of Sciences, 818,* 39–62.

Mitchell, R. W. (1997b). Kinesthetic–visual matching and the self-concept as explanations of mirror-self-recognition. *Journal for the Theory of Social Behavior, 27,* 101–123.

Mitchell, R. W. (1999). Deception and concealment as strategic script violation in great apes and humans. In S. T. Parker, R. W. Mitchell, & H. L. Miles (Eds.), *The mentalities of gorillas and orangutans* (pp. 295–315). Cambridge, UK: Cambridge University Press.

Mitchell, R. W. (2000). A proposal for the development of a mental vocabulary, with special reference to pretense and false belief. In K. Riggs & P. Mitchell (Eds.), *Children's reasoning and the mind* (pp. 37–65). Hove, UK: Psychology Press.

Mitchell, R. W. (2002a). Imitation as a perceptual process. In C. L. Nehaniv & K. Dautenhahn (Eds.), *Imitation in animals and artifacts* (pp. 441–469). Cambridge, MA: MIT Press.

Mitchell, R. W. (2002b). Kinesthetic–visual matching, imitation, and self-recognition. In M. Bekoff, C. Allen, & G. Burghardt (Eds.), *The cognitive animal* (pp. 345–351). Cambridge, MA: MIT Press.

Mitchell, R. W. (2002c). Review of *Imitation in Infancy. British Journal of Developmental Psychology, 20,* 150–151.

Mitchell, R. W., & Hamm, M. (1997). The interpretation of animal psychology: Anthropomorphism or behavior reading? *Behaviour, 134,* 173–204.

Mitchell, R. W., Thompson, N. S., & Miles, H. L. (Eds.). (1997). *Anthropomorphism, anecdotes, and animals.* Albany: State University of New York Press.

Morgan, M. J., & Nicholas, D. J. (1979). Discrimination between reinforced action patterns in the rat. *Learning and Motivation, 10,* 1–22.

Moynihan, M. (1985). *Communication and noncommunication in cephalopods.* Bloomington: Indiana University Press.

Nagel, T. (1979). *Mortal questions.* New York: Cambridge University Press.

Natsoulas, T., & Dubanoski, R. A. (1964). Inferring the locus and orientation of the perceiver from responses to stimulation of the skin. *American Journal of Psychology, 77,* 281–285.

Neisser, U. (1988). Five kinds of self-knowledge. *Philosophical Psychology, 1,* 37–59.

O'Shaughnessy, B. (1980). *The will: A dual aspect theory* (Vol. 1). Cambridge, UK: Cambridge University Press.

O'Shaughnessy, B. (1995). Proprioception and the body image. In J. L. Bermúdez, A. Marcel, & N. Eilan (Eds.), *The body and the self* (pp. 175–203). Cambridge, MA: MIT Press.

Parker, S. T. (1991). A developmental model for the origins of self-recognition in great apes. *Human Evolution, 6,* 435–449.

Parker, S. T. (1993). Imitation and circular reactions as evolved mechanisms for cognitive construction. *Human Development, 36,* 309–323.

Parker, S. T. (1994). Incipient mirror self-recognition in zoo gorillas and chimpanzees. In S. T. Parker, R. W. Mitchell, & M. L. Boccia (Eds.), *Self-awareness in animals and humans* (pp. 301–307). New York: Cambridge University Press.

Parker, S. T., & Gibson, K. R. (1979). A developmental model for the evolution of language and intelligence in early hominids. *Behavioral and Brain Sciences, 2,* 367–408.

Parker, S. T., & Mitchell, R. W. (1994). Evolving self-awareness. In S. T. Parker, R. W. Mitchell, & M. L. Boccia (Eds.), *Self-awareness in animals and humans* (pp. 413–428). New York: Cambridge University Press.

Parker, S. T., Mitchell, R. W., & Boccia, M. L. (Eds.). (1994). *Self-awareness in animals and humans.* New York: Cambridge University Press.

Patterson, F. G. P., & Cohn, R. H. (1994). Self-recognition and self-awareness in lowland gorillas. In S. T. Parker, R. W. Mitchell, & M. L. Boccia (Eds.), *Self-awareness in animals and humans* (pp. 273–290). New York: Cambridge University Press.

Piaget, J. (1962). *Play, dreams, and imitation in childhood.* New York: Norton. (Original work published 1945)

Povinelli, D. J. (2000). *Folk physics for apes: The chimpanzee's theory of how the world works.* Oxford, UK: Oxford University Press.

Povinelli, D. J., Rulf, A. B., Landau, K. R., & Bierschwale, D. T. (1993). Self-recognition in chimpanzees (*Pan troglodytes*): Distribution, ontogeny, and patterns of emergence. *Journal of Comparative Psychology, 107,* 347–372.

Quiatt, D. (1997). Silent partners? Observations on some systematic relations among observer perspective, theory, and behavior. In R. W. Mitchell, N. S. Thompson, & H. L. Miles (Eds.), *Anthropomorphism, anecdotes, and animals* (pp. 220–236). Albany: State University of New York Press.

Reiss, D., & Marino, L. (2001). Mirror self-recognition in the bottlenose dolphin: A case of cognitive convergence. *Proceedings of the National Academy of Sciences, 98,* 5937–5942.

Rensch, B. (1960). *Evolution above the species level.* New York: Columbia University Press.

Rilling, M. E., & Neiworth, J. J. (1987). Theoretical and methodological considerations for the study of imagery in animals. *Learning and Motivation, 18,* 57–79.

Riopelle, A. J. (1970). Growing up with Snowflake. *National Geographic, 138,* 491–503.

Riopelle, A. J., Jonch Cuspinera, A., Nos De Nicolau, R., Carbó, R. L., & Sabater Pi, J. (1976). Development and behavior of the white gorilla. In P. H. Oehser (Ed.), *National Geographic Society Research Reports 1968* (pp. 355–367). Washington, DC: National Geographic Society.

Riopelle, A. J., Nos, R., & Jonch, A. (1971). Situational determinants of dominance in captive young gorillas. *Proceedings of the Third International Congress of Primatology, 3,* 86–91.

Robert, S. (1986). Ontogeny of mirror behavior in two species of great apes. *American Journal of Primatology, 10,* 109–117.

Roberts, W. P., & Krause, M. A. (2002). Pretending culture: Social and cognitive features of pretense in apes and humans. In R. W. Mitchell (Ed.), *Pretending and imagination in animals and children* (pp. 269–279). Cambridge, UK: Cambridge University Press.

Rojas-Ramírez, J. A., & Drucker-Colin, R. R. (1977). Phylogenetic correlations between sleep and memory. In R. R. Drucker-Colín & J. L. McGaugh (Eds.), *Neurobiology of sleep and memory* (pp. 57–74). New York: Academic Press.

Romanes, G. J. (1975). *Mental evolution in man.* New York: Arno Press. (Original work published 1889)

Rosenberg, M. (1988). Self-objectification: Relevance for the species and society. *Sociological Forum, 3,* 548–565.

Sheets-Johnstone, M. (1990). The case for tactile–kinesthetic invariants. In M. Sheets-Johnstone (Ed.), *The roots of thinking* (pp. 365–386). Philadelphia: Temple University Press.

Sheets-Johnstone, M. (1998). Consciousness: A natural history. *Journal of Consciousness Studies, 5,* 260–294.

Shillito, D. J., Gallup, G. G., Jr., & Beck, B. B. (1999). Factors affecting mirror behaviour in western lowland gorillas, *Gorilla gorilla. Animal Behaviour, 57,* 999–1004.

Simonet, P. (2000). *Elephants recognize themselves* [Online]. Available: http://www.santabarbarazoo.org/zoonooz_arch/ oct2000.html#Elephants [2001, June 25].

Smuts, B. (1985). *Sex and friendship in baboons.* New York: Aldine.

Strawson, G. (1999a). "The self." In S. Gallagher & J. Shear (Eds.), *Models of the self* (pp. 1–24). Thorverton, UK: Imprint Academic.

Strawson, G. (1999b). The self and the SESMET. In S. Gallagher & J. Shear (Eds.), *Models of the self* (pp. 483–518). Thorverton, UK: Imprint Academic.

Strawson, G. (2000). The phenomenology and ontology of the self. In D. Zahavi (Ed.), *Exploring the self* (pp. 39–54). Amsterdam: Benjamins.

Strawson, P. F. (1963). *Individuals.* Garden City, NJ: Anchor Books. (Original work published 1959)

Strawson, P. F. (1964). Persons. In D. F. Gustafson (Ed.), *Essays in philosophical psychology* (pp. 377–403). New York: Anchor Books. (Reprinted from Strawson, P. F. [1958]. Persons. In H. Feigl, M. Scriven, & G. Maxwell [Eds.], *Minnesota studies in the philosophy of science, vol. II: Concepts, theories, and the mind–body problem* [pp. 330–353]. Minneapolis: University of Minnesota Press.)

Strawson, P. F. (1966). *The bounds of sense.* London: Routledge.

Sully, J. (1892). *The human mind* (Vol. 1). New York: Appleton.

Swartz, K. B., & Evans, S. (1991). Not all chimpanzees (*Pan troglodytes*) show self-recognition. *Primates, 32,* 483–496.

Swartz, K. B., & Evans, S. (1994). Social and cognitive factors in great ape mirror behavior and self-recognition. In S. T. Parker, R. W. Mitchell, & M. L. Boccia (Eds.), *Self-awareness in animals and humans* (pp. 189–206). New York: Cambridge University Press.

Swartz, K. B., & Evans, S. (1997). Anthropomorphism, anecdotes, and mirrors. In R. W. Mitchell, N. S. Thompson, & H. L. Miles (Eds.), *Anthropomorphism, anecdotes, and animals* (pp. 296–306). Albany: State University of New York Press.

Swartz, K. B., Sarauw, D., & Evans, S. (1999). Comparative aspects of mirror self-recognition in great apes. In S. T. Parker, R. W. Mitchell, & H. L. Miles (Eds.), *The mentalities of gorillas and orangutans* (pp. 283–294). Cambridge, UK: Cambridge University Press.

Tayler, C. K., & Saayman, G. S. (1973). Imitative behaviour by Indian Ocean bottlenose dolphins (*Tursiops aduncus*) in captivity. *Behaviour, 44,* 286–298.

Terrace, H. (1984). And now . . . the thinking pigeon. In G. Ferry (Ed.), *The understanding of animals* (pp. 261–271). Oxford, UK: Basil Blackwell and New Scientist.

Thompson, R. K. R., & Contie, C. L. (1994). Further reflections on mirror-usage by pigeons: Lessons from Winnie-the-Pooh and Pinocchio too. In S. T. Parker, R. W. Mitchell, & M. L. Boccia (Eds.), *Self-awareness in animals and humans* (pp. 392–409). New York: Cambridge University Press.

Thompson, R. L., & Boatright-Horowitz, S. L. (1994). The question of mirror-mediated self-recognition in apes and monkeys: Some new results and reservations. In S. T. Parker, R. W. Mitchell, & M. L. Boccia (Eds.), *Self-awareness in animals and humans* (pp. 330–349). New York: Cambridge University Press.

Ujhelyi, M., Merker, B., Buk, P., & Geissmann, T. (2000). Observations on the behavior of gibbons (*Hylobates leucogenys, H. Gabriellae,* and *H. lar*) in the presence of mirrors. *Journal of Comparative Psychology, 114,* 253–262.

Uzgiris, I. (1999). Imitation as activity: Its developmental aspects. In J. Nadel & G. Butterworth (Eds.), *Imitation in infancy* (pp. 186–206). Cambridge, UK: Cambridge University Press.

Voelkl, B., & Huber, L. (2000). True imitation in marmosets. *Animal Behaviour, 60,* 195–202.

von Uexküll, J. (1985). Environment [*Umwelt*] and inner world of animals. In G. Burghardt (Ed.), *Foundations of comparative ethology* (pp. 222–245). Stroudsburg, PA: Van Nostrand Reinhold. (Reprinted in translation from von Uexküll, J. [1909]. *Umwelt and Innenwelt der Tiere.* Berlin: Springer Verlag.)

Walraven, V., van Elsacker, L., & Verheyen, R. (1995). Reactions of a group of pygmy chimpanzees (*Pan paniscus*) to their mirror images: Evidence of self-recognition. *Primates, 36,* 145–150.

Weiskrantz, L. (1986). *Blindsight: A case study and implications.* Oxford, UK: Clarendon Press.

Weiskrantz, L. (1997). *Consciousness lost and found.* New York: Oxford University Press.

Westergaard, G. C., & Hyatt, C. W. (1994). The responses of bonobos (*Pan paniscus*) to their mirror images: Evidence of self-recognition. *Human Evolution, 9,* 273–279.

Whiten, A., Goodall, J., McGrew, W. C., Nishida, T., Reynolds, V., Sugiyama, Y., Tutin, C. E., Wrangham, R. W., & Boesch, C. (1999). Chimpanzee cultures. *Nature, 399,* 682–685.

Wittgenstein, L. (1965). *The philosophical investigations.* New York: Macmillan. (Original work published 1953)

Wittgenstein, L. (1992). *Last writings on the philosophy of psychology: Vol. 2. The inner and the outer.* Oxford, UK: Blackwell. (Original work published 1949)

Wright, C. (1958). The evolution of self-consciousness. In E. H. Madden (Ed.), *The philosophical writings of Chauncey Wright* (pp. 71–97). New York: Liberal Arts Press. (Reprinted from Wright, C. [1873].

The evolution of self-consciousness. *North American Review, 116,* 251–273.)

Wundt, W. (1907). *Lectures on human and animal psychology* (4th ed.). New York: Macmillan. (Original work published 1894)

Yerkes, R. M., & Yerkes, A. W. (1929). *The great apes.* New Haven, CT: Yale University Press.

Zahavi, D. (2000). Self and consciousness. In D. Zahavi (Ed.), *Exploring the self* (pp. 55–74). Amsterdam: Benjamins.

Zazzo, R. (1982). The person: Objective approaches. In W. W. Hartup (Ed.), *Review of child development research* (Vol. 6, pp. 247–290). Chicago: University of Chicago Press.

29

Evolution of the Symbolic Self: Issues and Prospects

CONSTANTINE SEDIKIDES
JOHN J. SKOWRONSKI

The construct of self is indispensable to psychology. Research on the self has increased threefold in the past 30 years, far exceeding the growth rate of published research in psychology as a whole (Tesser, 2000). It is astounding to realize that one out of seven recently published articles in psychology examined aspects of the self. This figure is even more impressive in light of the fact that it does not include research on the construct of "identity." The timely publication of this volume reflects this impressive growth and affirms the centrality of the construct of self (and identity) for psychology and, indeed, for all the social sciences.

The contributions in this volume document the pivotal role of the self in human functioning, both within psychology (e.g., social and personality, developmental, clinical, cognitive, comparative) and within other social science disciplines (e.g., sociology, anthropology). This chapter complements these contributions by taking an evolutionary perspective on the self. We conceptualize the self as an evolutionary adaptation. We explore ideas concerning the temporal ori-

gins of the self, the evolutionary pressures that led to the emergence of the self, and the functions of the self—functions that led to its maintenance, propagation, and continued evolution.

We begin with a word of caution: Our evolutionary accounts, both past (Sedikides & Skowronski, 1997, 2000; Skowronski & Sedikides, 1999) and present, leave us with a persistent sense of ambivalence. Because the ecological and social environment (i.e., social organization) in which our forebears lived have left very few high-definition imprints, it is difficult to grasp the magnitude of the evolutionary forces that acted on them. Unlike laboratory experimentation, in which the implications of the accumulated evidence can be clear, our struggle to understand how the self has been shaped by evolution has led us to the uncomfortable realization that the evidence is weak or even contradictory. Hence, we admit that the state of the current evidence is such that alternative accounts can be written about how, when, and why evolution has shaped the self. The challenge, then, for us and for colleagues who approach the self from the standpoint of evolutionary psychology is to rigorously police our perspectives in trying to determine those ideas that are scientifically plausible and those that are not.

Of course, we attempt to refrain from giving an utterly implausible account. We devote the first section of the chapter to definitional clarifications and to an exposition of a plausible evolutionary timeline for the species under consideration, *Homo sapiens*. In the second section, we present parts of our account as a set of unresolved issues. Throughout both sections, we discuss elements of the uncertainty that we feel in our evolutionary exposition.

Definitional Clarifications

We are concerned with the evolution of an apparently unique human characteristic, the *symbolic self*. Even here, our self-confessed uncertainty emerges: Is the symbolic self truly unique? The story of evolutionary theory is littered with examples of characteristics that were thought to be unique to humans (e.g., tool use, higher cognitive functions such as mathematics and language). In at least some cases, the motive behind these exceptions was to separate humans from the so-called "lower animals." We have no such motive. Instead, we believe that there is a fundamental continuity between related species and that one consequence of this continuity is that an attribute rarely arises *de novo,* out of nothing. Instead, evolution often proceeds by reworking, amplifying, or diminishing existing characteristics. One implication of this principle is that a researcher ought to be able to find evidence of a self in other species, especially in those species that are close to humans on the bush of evolution. Indeed, evidence suggests that some animals (e.g., chimpanzees) do possess rudimentary forms of a self-concept. However, the evidence also currently indicates that the self-concept that has emerged in humans is different from that observed in other species—both quantitatively and qualitatively (see Sedikides & Skowronski, 1997, for a more detailed discussion).

What is the human symbolic self? The symbolic self can be thought of as a dynam-

ic system with at least three important capacities (Sedikides & Skowronski, 2000). One capacity is its representational ability. The symbolic self serves as the repository for mental representations of a person's attributes, which can range from abstract (e.g., knowledge about one's own typical responses to situations) to concrete (e.g., critical and temporally located episodes in one's life; Skowronski, Betz, Thompson, & Shannon, 1991) and from negative to positive (Staats & Skowronski, 1992). Additionally, these representations can extend into the future (e.g., goals) and can be metacognitive (e.g., beliefs about how others might perceive one's behavior). In short, the representational capacity of the symbolic self stores the essential library of an individual's past and present and is the repository for an individual's aspirations.

The second capacity of the symbolic self concerns its executive or agentic function. We have proposed three classes of motives as the fundamental forces that guide this executive function (Sedikides & Skowronski, 2000): valuation (i.e., protecting and enhancing the self), learning (i.e., pursuing a relatively accurate image of the self, improving skills and abilities), and homeostasis (i.e., seeking and endorsing information that is consistent with the self). These motives have several consequences. For example, the executive function of the symbolic self can instigate information-seeking behavior (e.g., pursuing feedback that will stabilize the representational component, drawing inferences about others) or choice behavior (e.g., goal setting, attempts to control outcomes). Additionally, the symbolic self can provoke defensive responses to unfavorable feedback through such strategies as rationalization or derogation. The symbolic self can also instigate the experience of positive emotions (e.g., pride, high self-esteem) in response to favorable outcomes and the experience of negative emotions (e.g., shame, guilt, or embarrassment) in response to unfavorable outcomes. In summary, the executive and regulatory capacity of the symbolic self renders it a potent initiator, mediator, or moderator of an individual's thinking, feeling, and behaving.

In agreement with Damasio (1999), we believe that to be conscious means to have a sense of the self. Hence, the third capacity of the symbolic self is its reflexive potential. This is the organism's ability to depict itself in its ongoing relation with other objects. This reflexive potential is manifested in continuous interplay between the representational and executive functions of the symbolic self. For example, the symbolic self's reflexive potential allows the organism to modify long-term goals so that those goals are congruent with anticipated environmental changes. Furthermore, a by-product of this interplay is the working self, which consists of self-knowledge that is momentarily accessible in working memory. Situational features and situation-specific goals set by the executive system can cause the working self to vary. Thus the reflexive characteristic of the symbolic self allows the self-system to respond flexibly and dynamically to environmental contingencies by selectively activating or deactivating aspects of stored self-knowledge. However, this is not to say that the reflexive potential of the symbolic self is unlimited. Biological constraints or past learning history may cause some aspects of self-knowledge to be more easily accessed than others or to be in a chronic state of activation. Hence, an individual may show some evidence of consistency in goals or behaviors across situations despite the diverging demands that different situations might place on the self-system. Nonetheless, its reflexive potential allows the self some measure of flexibility in determining which goals will be pursued and how they will be pursued in any given situation.

Timeline for Human Evolution

We next offer a timeline for the emergence of the *Homo sapiens* species, a necessary backdrop for understanding when the symbolic self has emerged in our evolutionary ancestry. As befits our introductory remarks about uncertainty, we emphasize that this is only one of several plausible timelines that a theorist might be able to concoct from the available data. However, we also note that the timeline of human evolution that we offer is, indeed, a plausible one: In fact, it is arguably the most plausible timeline in light of the evidence collected so far (McKie, 2000).

Our timeline is straightforward. Approxi-mately 6 million years ago, one group of hominids became reproductively isolated from an alternative line of great apes that led to chimpanzees and bonobos. Between 3.8 and 5.5 million years ago, these isolated hominids evolved into several species of bipedal African apes of the genus *Australopithecus*. The principal species were *Australopithecus anamensis, Australopithecus afarensis,* and *Australopithecus africanus.* The members of these species were approximately 4 feet tall, had ape-sized brains, exhibited a vegetarian lifestyle, and lacked stone tools. In this last case, it is probably best to say that there is currently no evidence of stone tool use (e.g., shards, scraping patterns) for members of these species.

Between 2.5 and 3 million years ago, global ecological changes (i.e., a general cooling of the climate) and a decline in the amount of forested area available induced some of these early hominids to move from an arboreal lifestyle to a savannah (a mix of grasslands and trees) lifestyle. By this time, the *Australopithecines* had essentially given way to a new genus, *Homo*. Several species of *Homo* (*Homo rudolfensis, Homo habilis, Homo erectus*)—along with *Australopethicus boseii*—apparently coexisted in East Africa. Other *Homo* species thrived in South and North Africa. These early *Homo* ancestors had a larger brain and physique than the early *Australopithecines* and used stone tools.

By 1.8 million years ago, one of the East African four, *Homo erectus,* showed evidence of several lifestyle changes that were congenial to a savannah lifestyle. These changes included an omnivorous diet. In addition to consumption of fruits, insects, and greens, this diet included tubers and meat. Such a diet provides two elements that are critical to the evolution of a larger brain: the nutrients that are necessary to support the construction of an enlarged brain and the energy to run it. If the processing power conferred by larger and more complex brains granted an evolutionary advantage (as opposed to the construction of larger and more complex bodies), then individuals who were born with the means to make such enlarged brain structures should have been favored over those who could not. The physiological mechanism to accomplish this task of trait selection may have been neoteny: slowing the maturation rate of several different aspects of human development relative to the rate of growth of the brain. This larger-brained (relative to body size) *Homo erectus* was successful enough to have spread across Africa.

Between 200,000 and 300,000 years ago, as the process of speciation continued, *Homo sapiens* appeared on the scene. This species, the modern humans, had an unusual confluence of characteristics (Foley & Lahr, 1997; Klein, 1989; Stringer & McKie, 1996). The species members had large brains (nearly three times as large as the australopithecines, adjusting for differences in body size) and a relatively tall and strong physique. The species also had an array of powerful cognitive capacities, which included symbolic communicative abilities and abstract thinking. An example of this capability is that the species used purpose-built tools, and refined those tools. *Homo sapiens* also showed evidence of complex social organization, relatively sophisticated cultural practices, and a penchant for relentless networking and expansion. Current DNA and anthropological evidence indicates that this species poured out of Africa and populated much of the rest of the world. The evidence also suggests that *Homo sapiens* replaced indigenous hominid species in Europe (i.e., Neanderthals) and Asia (i.e., a population of *erectus*-like species in Java) either by displacing them (i.e., taking over their habitats) or, less frequently, obliterating them. There is currently no convincing DNA evidence supporting the notion of successful interbreeding among *Homo sapiens* and other hominid species. By roughly 30,000 years ago, *Homo sapiens* was the only *Homo* species found on earth.

When in this hypothetical timeline did the human capability for self-representation evolve? Because evolution is a continuous process, exact dates are obviously difficult to discern. Nonetheless, in our prior work (Sedikides & Skowronski, 1997), we associated the origin of a rudimentary human self-concept with the appearance of *Homo erectus* in the late Pleistocene epoch. This species had been subject to strong evolutionary pressures that accompanied the movement from the forests to the savannah grasslands. In addition, a relatively large brain, a hunting lifestyle, and a structured

social organization characterized *Homo erectus*. Furthermore, an expanded and lowered pharynx, which is a physiological necessity for complex articulate speech, had evolved by late *Homo erectus*. This development suggests that *Homo erectus* was a species for which communication was important. In our view, the combination of burgeoning cognitive capacities, the ability to produce elaborate communications, and an intricate social structure is a combination that is well suited to the evolution of a sense of self. Given the confluence of these characteristics, the late Pleistocene seemed like a reasonable bet as the period in which a rudimentary human capacity for a self-concept emerged.

However, this likely represented only the first relatively primitive glimmerings of the human ability to cognitively represent the self. If this self-representational ability did indeed enhance fitness in the environment, evolution certainly would have worked to amplify this characteristic with the passage of time. Can we identify a more recent time period during which artifacts point to the presence of the symbolic self in *Homo sapiens*? Considerable controversy surrounds such a date (Leary & Cottrell, 1999), although the issue has been addressed indirectly rather than directly. One argument is that the symbolic self was manifestly present 30,000 to 60,000 years ago, as evidenced by burials, personal adornment, and representational art (Mithen, 1996). Another argument is that the symbolic self was not present until approximately 10,000 years ago, as evidenced by a lifestyle that was characterized by delayed-return contingencies (e.g., the ability to temporally disentangle one's purposeful efforts from its intended consequences), such as dependence on agricultural subsistence (Martin, 1999). A third argument is that the symbolic self was not present until as recently as 2,800 to 3,000 years ago and coincided with such cultural innovations as religion, abstract art, philosophy, and science (Jaynes, 1976).

Our own inclination (in agreement with Leary & Cottrell, 1999) is to use the earliest of these dates, but we admit that this choice is as much a reflection of personal preference as it is a reflection of the evidence. It seems to us that the features cited by Mithen (1996), such as personal adornment, are difficult to imagine in the context of an organism without a well-evolved symbolic self. Why would an organism without a well-evolved symbolic self waste time and resources creating and wearing items that do not have any apparent function other than to convey status to conspecifics or to make the wearer feel good about him- or herself? Skeptics might reply that such "unnecessary" created or adopted adornments are found in animals that possess only a rudimentary capability for distinguishing between the self and the external world (e.g., the bowers of bower birds, the shells of hermit crabs). Male bower birds, for example, will create relatively elaborate bowers for the purpose of attracting a female mate. We recognize the validity of such counterexamples but would still argue that it is the breadth of the behaviors described by Mithen that is persuasive to us. A theorist might be able to generate specific evolutionary-based explanations (e.g., sexual selection) for specific behaviors, such as adopting adornments, but it strikes us as difficult to use such explanations when an array of behaviors that seem to have a multitude of purposes (adornment, representational art, burial) emerges—an array whose purpose can seemingly be easily understood by presupposing a sense of self.

Why Has the Symbolic Self Evolved in Humans?

Evolution does not occur in a vacuum: Existing genetic variations among species members are selected by environmental pressures. Hence, the timeline that we have proposed needs to be tied to these selection pressures. Given the timeline that we have established, what are the selection pressures that could have worked toward the evolution of the human symbolic self? In light of the fate of other related species, this is an intriguing question. For most of its evolutionary past, *Homo sapiens* cohabited with more than 20 *Homo* species. Yet, it is now the sole *Homo* species remaining. We speculate on the reasons for this curious state of affairs, beginning with a summary of the selection pressures that the species likely endured. More specifically, we review two broad classes of selection pressures: ecologi-

cal and social (Sedikides & Skowronski, 1997).

Ecological Pressures

One idea that serves to explain the emergence of the self is that the self is a natural by-product or consequence of the expansion of cognitive abilities that has characterized the evolutionary line leading to modern humans. Numerous studies suggest that the emergence of cognitive abilities (among which we include the capacity to construct a self) is related to selection pressures revolving around, and stemming from, food acquisition. For example, among frugivore (fruit-feeding) primates, the irregular distribution (both temporal and spatial) of food supplies is linked with larger brain-to-body ratios. In addition, omnivorous foragers (i.e., those that feed on both animal and vegetable substances) have the largest brain-to-body ratios among primates. Such findings are intriguing given that our evolutionary ancestors had to make a change from an arboreal (and presumably largely vegetarian) lifestyle to one that was suited to life on the savannah. The new lifestyle included an omnivorous diet and food sources that were distributed widely in time and space.

Why is difficulty in locating food associated with bigger brains? Larger brains provide the processing capacity necessary to complete the difficult and varied tasks associated with the omnivorous habit of the human ancestors. For example, enhanced memory and categorization processes facilitate locating and recognizing food sources, and heightened spatial memory and cognitive mapping facilitate effective food search. Handling, processing, and storing food can be enhanced by strengthening cognitive representation abilities and the capacity to anticipate future events.

Furthermore, the challenges associated with hunting may have added to the selection of cognitive abilities by evolution. Effective pursuit in hunting presupposes accurate perception of fast-moving prey, accurate mental orientation and rotation, rapid recognition and taxonomic memory, as well the ability to act quickly. Approaching game closely and being competent in stalking requires sophisticated planning and decision-making abilities. Finally, planning an optimal route of attack necessitates the capacity to remember the history of encounters with specific prey and the capacity to imagine how such prey might react to an attack in these new circumstances.

More important, ecological pressures associated with finding and handling food may have prompted the emergence of symbolic reasoning by the time that *Homo sapiens* emerged. Effective remembering, imagining, and planning involve symbolic reasoning: the capacity to think by manipulating images or concepts. Similar mental skills are involved in tool construction and use. For example, excellence in flint knapping (i.e., shaping the flint by breaking off pieces with quick blows) presupposes planning and imagination while working the stone, and developing optimal shapes for the flints requires knowledge about the effectiveness of different flint shapes and their potential functions in hunting.

We argue that the symbolic self evolved as an additional way to enhance responding to these food-related selection pressures. Thanks to the representational (e.g., memory for past achievements, storage of future expectations) and regulatory components of the symbolic self, in the presence of such a self humans were better able to make critical decisions, such as choosing a good hunting route or an effective food distribution strategy. Additionally, the reflexive capacity of the symbolic self allowed humans to consider long-term plans, to gauge whether these plans matched the needs of the present self, to simulate the results of alternative plans on the basis of expected utility, and to take action based on the results of those simulations (e.g., set goals). These processes led to the formation of a concept of selfhood. Humans presented this concept to others, expected others to concur with it, were inclined to believe that others did concur (a process that we term "projected appraisal"), and expected others to confirm this self-conception.

In this context, emotions become a potentially important source of feedback and subsequent motivation. Feelings of happiness result from goal attainment, and the type of match achieved between the organisms' objectives and their achievements is critical for feelings related to the private self. Self-esteem (i.e., one's evaluation of or liking for the self) or pride can be high when the match is successful. On the other hand, low self-esteem, dejection, or shame can result when the match is unsuccessful (Tangney, Burggraf, & Wagner, 1995). This function of self-relevant feelings can confer crucial evolutionary advantages. Not only can such feelings provide immediate feedback regarding the attainment of one's goals, but they can also affect subsequent goal-directed effort.

In summary, the ecological-pressures perspective offers a linear account for the evolution of the symbolic self. According to this perspective, the symbolic self (1) was derived largely from the complex interactions that hominids had with their changing habitats; (2) was a function of symbolic abilities that emerged in response to environmental demands; (3) was formed as a private self-construction; (4) was communicated to conspecifics through the mechanism of projected appraisal, thus producing the public or social self; and (5) included achievement-based self-feelings (i.e., self-esteem, pride, shame).

Social Pressures

Given that the self is actively involved in humans' social lives, consider the possibility that the social lifestyle adopted by humans played a role as a selection pressure in the continuing evolution of the self. According to this social-pressures perspective, the evolution of human cognitive abilities (and, by extension, the symbolic self) has been prompted or aided by the social habit of humans' ancestors. It is certainly the case that, from an evolutionary perspective, membership in social groups comes with both pros and cons. Among the direct benefits are improved predation (e.g., hunting efficiency, food sharing), reduction of predation risk, and cooperative defense of essential resources (e.g., food sources and mates) against rival groups. However, one other apparent consequence of group living in terrestrial primates is its relation to thinking prowess: Group size in terrestrial primates is positively associated with brain size, even controlling for lifestyle differences (e.g., diet).

One can speculate that this association

might be attributable to the cognitive demands of within-group interactions. These demands are a function of the complexity of a group's social organization and the roles, rules, and relationship patterns that exist within that organization. Humans seem to be prone to peculiarly complex patterns of interactions and social relationships. For example, consider group hierarchical status. In some animals, status is straightforward: One learns and knows one's place in the pecking order, and that status typically changes only with the death of a higher ranked member of the group. Such rigid status hierarchies do not seem to call for much cognitive firepower, aside from a bit of memory. In contrast, status hierarchies in humans do not exhibit this rigid quality. Human status hierarchies are loose and free-flowing and seem to be easily modifiable depending on circumstances, such as coalition formation and change.

This flexibility in status would have placed cognitive demands on our evolutionary forebears. Group members would have been uncertain about their relative standing and would have needed to engage in numerous cognitive tasks to discern their current status. These tasks included paying attention to the situation, decoding others' nonverbal signals, guessing their intentions, and remembering the history of past interactions with each group member. In addition, such interactions are multifaceted and governed by numerous rules. Cooperative interactions (e.g., feeding, grooming, fighting) can be based on relationship type (e.g., kinship, friendship) and on several preconditions, such as role differentiation (i.e., in terms of status or division of labor), effort coordination, conformity, loyalty, and fear of social exclusion. Likewise, competitive interactions (e.g., intrasexual competition for suitable mates) can pose several cognitive demands on the human mind, such as remembering and recognizing one's own and others' social ranks, monitoring competitors' ranks, deceiving higher ranked competitors, monitoring the sexual receptivity and fitness of potential mates, exhibiting physical and social prowess in an effort to attract potential mates, safeguarding (on the part of females) against male attempts at forced copulation, cheating, and detection of cheating.

Clearly, in such a challenging environment it is beneficial to be cognitively proficient. Such proficiency allows individuals to engage in a constant, elaborate, and ever-changing cost–benefit analysis of whether to stay in the group, form a coalition, or exit the group for the sake of joining another. In such an environment, it is easy to see how the demands of the social context acted as a selection pressure that spurred the cognitive capacities required for the construction of the symbolic self.

Additional cognitive demands (e.g., maintaining a level of alertness, defending offspring and territory, initiating hostilities at an opportune time) are placed on individuals when intergroup competition occurs. Thus, in addition to a need for the individual to function well within a group context, it makes sense that individuals would be well served if their group also functioned well. High levels of group performance might sometimes be increased by factors that enhance the coordination among group members. Hence, various mechanisms may have evolved as a way to facilitate group function via enhanced coordination. For example, researchers in developmental psychology have suggested that mimicry may be a consequence of innate imitative capabilities (Nadel & Butterworth, 1999), and recent research examining the "chameleon effect" demonstrates that people will nonconsciously mimic the behavior of others (Chartrand & Bargh, 1999). Such mimicry serves to coordinate people's actions and to promote interpersonal bonds. This principle of coordination extends to the self. Coordination can be facilitated when an individual's self-concept is in agreement with the other group members' perceptions of that individual. Coordination can also be achieved via the process of *reflected appraisal*: An individual assimilates the perceptions of others so that those perceptions become integrated into the self. Humans' linguistic capabilities are well suited to this process of reflected appraisal ("Here's what I think of you. . .").

Such appraisals can obviously have emotional consequences, so it makes sense that self-related feelings partially stem from such social feedback. In fact, some authors speculate that self-esteem has evolved as a sociometer (Leary, Tambor, Terdal, & Downs, 1995), a running gauge of others' evaluations of the self. In addition, self-esteem can serve as an important cue for the organism's ever-changing ranking in the group, thus instigating dominance or deference behavior (Barkow, 1989). Other self-feelings can also fulfill social functions. For example, embarrassment promotes the appeasement of group members after an occasional transgression (Keltner & Buswell, 1997), guilt motivates an individual to assure group members that a desirable change in his or her behavior is in the offing (Tangney, 1998), and shame can lead an individual to barricade the self from the social environment in an effort to minimize further failure and debilitating defeat and to regroup (Weisfeld & Wendorf, 2000).

Reflected appraisal is not the only mechanism available for producing similarity between self-appraisals and others' appraisals. For example, individuals might come to reflect hypothetically on how others might think about and respond to the individual's behavior via processes such as perspective taking and role taking. Using these processes, individuals can run mental simulations in which they imagine how others can and might perceive them under various circumstances. Based on such thought processes, individuals can consider others as organisms like the self, attributing intentions to them, and, more generally, attributing cognitive and affective states to them.

Group living may have molded the social construction of the self in another critical way. In a flexible and shifting social context, human functioning was aided by the ability to develop multiple self-representations: The ability to remember and consistently show the "right" self to others (i.e., the self that others have seen on previous occasions) would facilitate smooth interactions with them. In order to do this, an individual needs to remember others' perceptions of the self, to anticipate how others expect him or her to behave in different circumstances, and to improvise consistent personas in response to the demands of various social roles. These abilities are all crucial elements of self-presentation. Indeed, in a flexible social environment, self-presentational skills (e.g., deception, self-deception) can be particularly useful.

In summary, the social-pressures perspective offers a linear account of the evolution of the self. According to this perspective, the symbolic self was largely a social self that: (1) emerged out of complex social interaction processes, especially the need for perspective taking and role taking, that may have resulted in the development of a capacity for a theory of mind; (2) was facilitated by the emergence of language; (3) was shaped by others' impressions of the individual (i.e., the private self was shaped by the public self through processes such as reflected appraisal); (4) was mainly in the service of impression management; and (5) was characterized by affiliation-based self-feelings (i.e., self-esteem, guilt, embarrassment).

A Clarification

We wish to add a clarification. Our argument is that the symbolic self is a trait that was selected and distributed in the human population because of its high adaptive value. Indeed, we propose that the emergence of this adaptation is relatively unique to the hominid evolutionary past. However, many of the evolutionary pressures that we discussed (e.g., hunting, group living) would seem to be applicable to other species, such as wolves, hyenas, and tigers. Why don't these animals have a symbolic self?

The answer to our rhetorical question is that evolution works within species rather than between species. That is, natural selection does not magically conjure up adaptations from thin air. A trait must be present in the species genome before natural selection exerts its modifying influence. Thus we are assuming that somewhere during the progress of evolution a fortunate accident occurred. A mutation and/or a favorable mating produced hominid individuals with the capacity for a symbolic self, a capacity that (as far as we know) has not emerged as yet in other species. Such happy accidents often spread rapidly through a reproductively isolated population and can enable members of that population to move into new ecological niches. Certainly, this scenario of isolation, favorable mutation, then expansion seems to provide a good fit to the "out of Africa" theory that is currently the leading description of the spread of humans across the globe.

On the Relation between the Ecological and Social Self

The ecological- and social-pressures perspectives offer divergent linear accounts for the evolution of the self. It is obvious that the self-concept contains elements both of the private and public self. How did both come to be? One viewpoint is that of synergism. From this viewpoint, ecological and social pressures operated synergistically, leading to the simultaneous evolution of the ecological and social selves. A second viewpoint is that social pressures drove the evolution of the self. That is, the social or public self was primary and subsequently gave rise to the emergence of the private self through reflection, internalization, and efficacy-based self-feelings. According to a third viewpoint, the ecological self was primary. That is, the private self emerged first, and the public-self component was superimposed on this private self by means of processes such as reflected appraisal.

We believe that evolutionary reasoning and contemporary empirical findings are most consistent with this last viewpoint. To begin with, there is a conceptual problem in proposing specific social mechanisms (e.g., language, reflected appraisal) as the sole engine that drove the evolution of the self. As Tomasello (1999) put it, "invoking language as an evolutionary cause of human cognition is like invoking money as an evolutionary cause of human economic activity" (p. 94). Tomasello argues that language (and, by implication, the kinds of reflected appraisal that can result from language use) can transform the nature of the symbolic self but cannot create it. Furthermore, these mechanisms themselves must have evolved from previous capabilities, such as crude communicative attempts. In short, it is probably the case that the evolution of sophisticated communication capabilities and the social context in which humans existed worked to transform the symbolic self, expanding it from a private to a social self. However, we suspect that it was ecological pressures that were initially responsible for the evolution of the self.

Several lines of inquiry support the primacy of the private self. First, the developmental emergence of the self (in the 2nd year of life) does not necessitate a social context (Howe, 2000; Howe & Courage, 1997). Furthermore, the chronic attributes of the private self are impressively stable across situations (Bem & Allen, 1974; Markus, 1977) and across both relatively short time periods (Pelham, 1991; Pelham & Wachsmuth, 1995, Study 1) and the life course (Caspi, Bem, & Elder, 1989; McCrae & Costa, 1994). Even when private self-attributes change, they do so slowly and in a predictable order (Damon & Hart, 1986; Deutsch, Ruble, Brooks-Gunn, Flemming, & Stangor, 1988). Finally, the stability of the private self is achieved by such strategies as the vigorous disposal and discounting of threatening feedback (Campbell & Sedikides, 1999; Sedikides & Green, 2000) and the selective pursuit of confirming feedback (Greenwald, 1980; Swann, 1983).

Additional evidence suggests that the self is primarily regulated by the volume, availability, accessibility, and inescapability of private feelings and thoughts (Andersen, 1984; Andersen, Glassman, & Gold, 1998). Indeed, it is the private self, with its needs for autonomy and competence (Deci & Ryan, 2000), that regulates personal strivings (Emmons, 1989), personal projects (Little, 1983), or life tasks (Cantor, Markus, Niedenthal, & Nurius, 1986), with the social context serving as the background for individual action (Carver & Scheier, 1998; Higgins & May, 2001). The autonomy and competence needs of the private self have universal (i.e., cross-cultural) appeal (Sheldon, Elliot, Kim, & Kasser, 2001).

Even more to the point, the mechanism of projected appraisal is unusually potent and is arguably more prevalent than reflected appraisal. For example, humans form an impression of how others view them on the basis of their own self-conceptions (projected appraisal) rather than on the basis of external feedback (reflected appraisal). Furthermore, humans are not accurate in determining how specific others view them (Felson, 1993; Kenny & DePaulo, 1993), and they overestimate the consistency in the impressions that others have of them (Kenny & DePaulo, 1993). These findings imply that social feedback plays a secondary role in the formation of the self, largely involving the verification of the projected self (Schoeneman, 1981; Sedikides & Skowronski, 1995).

In summary, the evidence collected so far suggests that the private aspect of the symbolic self has evolutionary primacy and sets the stage for the subsequent evolution of the social aspect of the symbolic self. This viewpoint does not deny the obvious synergy between the two selves; the viewpoint only shifts the relative importance for the initial evolution of the symbolic self to ecological pressures. Moreover, the viewpoint has the potential to generate useful empirical queries, paleontological and otherwise. Do prehistoric artifacts point to the primacy of the ecological self? At what temporal stage do signs of social selection pressures become more definite? Also, at what time in prehistory did social selection pressures emerge as an influence on the continuing development of the symbolic self (Caporael, 1997)?

Interestingly, the point at which social pressures may have begun to have increasing impact on the development of the symbolic self may coincide with evidence pointing to the emerging influence of culture in evolution. A core argument of the social-pressures perspective is that the symbolic self had the capacity for abstract or symbolic reasoning about both the self and others. Tomasello (1999) argues that this is a key development in human evolution. That is, the ability to understand others by using a "theory of mind" derived from the self, or, as Povinelli, Bering, and Giambrone (2000) put it, a "cognitive specialization for reasoning about [others' mental] states," may be the key development that distinguishes humans from other primate species. Certainly, current evidence suggests that humans, and not other animals, whether primates (Cheney & Seyfarth, 1996; Tomasello & Call, 1997) or great apes (i.e., chimpanzees; Povinelli et al., 2000), have a theory of mind.

The evolution of a theory of mind in humans may have facilitated the influence of cultural evolution on human species. Gould (2000) argued that cultural evolution can interact with natural selection in complex ways, and Tomasello (1999) noted that cultural transmission is a moderately common evolutionary process. However, Tomasello maintained that a specific form of cultural inheritance, namely cumulative cultural evolution, is unique to *Homo sapiens*. In cumulative cultural evolution, existing artifacts and social practices (e.g., tools, linguistic symbols, social organization routines) are modified, improved, and eventually transmitted to a new generation through imitative, instructive (i.e., carried out through instruction), or collaborative learning.

How can a theory of mind be a basis for cumulative cultural evolution? A theory of mind allows the organism to gain an understanding of the meaning of various artifacts and practices. By using the self as an analogy, humans can maximize imitative, instructive, and collaborative learning and thus come to a new appreciation of the individual and social functions served by various implements and actions. Because other humans can be conceptualized as intentional beings like the self, such a theory of mind makes the meaning of such cultural achievements easier to comprehend. That is, such theories allow humans to appreciate the intent and motivation behind the creation of cultural traditions.

Importantly, this appreciation provides a direction for subsequent action: The capacity for attributions of intentions can have powerful motivational consequences. For example, such attributions can allow an understanding of the improvements in a constructed object or a procedure that need to be preserved (What does this currently do?), as well as for the type of refinements that needed to be made (How can it do it better?). Furthermore, communicative organisms such as humans are motivated to convey this understanding to others ("Let me tell you how to do this better").

The presence of a theory of mind has intriguing implications when considered in combination with other human cognitive capabilities, such as: (1) long-term forward planning and goal setting; (2) mental simulation of goal evaluation and evaluation-contingent affective states (e.g., pride or shame); and (3) awareness of own mortality. Foresight can exert a multiplicative effect on the capacity for a theory of mind. Not only are humans able to understand the present intentions, needs, and goals of conspecifics, but they may also be in a position to modify cultural gains on the basis of their estimations for anticipated optimal functions of these gains. Additionally, humans are capable of mentally simulating conspecifics' perceived relevance of various artifacts and practices in the near and distant future. Hence, one can argue that it was to the evolutionary benefit of humans to engage in deliberate and constant improvement of cultural achievements: Their young's prospects for survival and reproductive success was enhanced by such knowledge. Paraphrasing Hamilton (1964), we term this knowledge "simulated inclusive fitness."

Is an Evolutionary Psychology Research Agenda on the Symbolic Self Possible?

The final issue that we consider is whether the ideas that we have described are testable. That is, from the standpoint of empirically oriented psychologists, is it possible to have a research agenda examining the symbolic self that is grounded in these evolutionary ideas?

We believe that explanations of human behavior derived from an evolutionary psychology analysis are testable and falsifiable (Ketelaar & Ellis, 2000). According to Buss's (1995) description of the hierarchical structure of evolutionary explanations for psychological phenomena, a researcher begins with meta-theoretical assumptions, offers a middle-level theory, derives hypotheses, and then proceeds with testing specific predictions that emanate from each hypothesis.

Consider the symbolic self from this hierarchical perspective. The symbolic self is widely observed in the human population. We have conceptualized the self as an adaptation. The naturalistic fallacy notwithstanding, there is no doubt that the symbolic self (i.e., its representational, agentic, and reflexive components) currently serves vital psychological functions. We consider as a suitable middle-level hypothesis the proposal that a strong (but *not* necessarily an overinflated) symbolic self, an idea that can be termed "selfness," is positively associated with psychological health. Stated otherwise, individuals high in selfness enjoy better psychological health than those who are low in selfness. For example, the absence of self-

ness is related to such personal ailments as alienation, alcoholism, and suicide (Baumeister, 1991). Psychological health also promotes reproductive fitness: Individuals who look psychologically healthy are preferred as mates over those who look psychologically unhealthy (Buss, 1989; Symons, 1979). Hence, selfness promotes reproductive fitness.

One line of research has begun to test directly the selfness hypothesis. Gramzow, Sedikides, Panter, and Insko (2000) proposed that the representational (or structural) and executive (or regulatory) components of the self are related to psychological health. They operationalized the representational component in terms of self-complexity (number of self-attributes that are structurally independent of each other; Linville, 1985), self-discrepancies (degree to which actual self-attributes are congruent with ideal or obligatory self-attributes; Higgins, 1987), self-consistency (degree to which self-attributes are perceived to be consistent with each other; Gergen & Morse, 1967), role conflict (whether socially defined roles are perceived as conflictual; Donahue, Robins, Roberts, & John, 1993), and self-attitude ambivalence (whether the self is perceived as containing both extremely positive and extremely negative attributes; Kaplan, 1972). Furthermore, Gramzow and colleagues operationalized the executive component of the self in terms of ego strength (the ability to perceive and accept reality and to defend against anxiety and displeasure; Barron, 1953), ego control (the tendency to withhold or express impulse; Block, 1961; Funder & Block, 1989), ego resiliency (the ability to modulate one's ego control; Block, 1961; Funder & Block, 1989), and hardiness (control, or the perception of having an impact over outcomes; commitment, or the perception of meaning and purpose in one's life; and challenge, or the interpretation of life changes as challenges rather than threats; Kobasa, 1979). Finally, Gramzow and colleagues operationalized psychological health in terms of the absence of depression and agitation.

Selfness was, indeed, positively associated with psychological health. The results suggested that the regulatory component of the self is strongly related to psychological health. Additionally, with one exception, all facets of the representational component of the symbolic self were linked with psychological health. The exception was self-complexity. However, there is an explanation for this null effect. Relevant theory (Linville, 1985) predicts that self-complexity will serve as a buffer against the emotional stress that occurs in response to stressful life events, a prediction that has received empirical support elsewhere (Linville, 1987). The null effect in the Gramzow and colleagues (2000) study is likely due to participants having been stress free when completing the relevant measures.

Although the Gramzow and colleagues (2000) study was the first comprehensive attempt to examine the beneficial psychological health effects of selfness, the literature is generally consistent with the view that a strong sense of self is positively related to psychological health. For example, agency-based self-regulation in the pursuit of one's goals is related to higher satisfaction with life, greater feelings of vitality, and positive daily moods (Sheldon & Kasser, 1995). Also, a clearly articulated self is related to high subjective well-being and self-esteem and to low neuroticism (Campbell, 1990; Campbell et al., 1996). Additionally, a stable sense of self is linked to lower levels of depression (Kernis et al., 1998) and higher feelings of mastery (Waschull & Kernis, 1996). Interestingly, self-esteem stability is related to self-esteem level. In turn, higher self-esteem is related to positive affect, greater subjective well-being, reduced death anxiety, and successful coping (Leary & Baumeister, 2000).

Another important testimony to the evolutionary significance of the construct of selfness comes from the attachment literature. According to attachment theory (Bowlby, 1973, 1980), the quality of infant–caregiver interactions results in mental working models (i.e., cognitive representations of attachment figures and the self) that shape the self-concept, direct affect regulation, and organize cognition, emotion, and behavior in adolescent and adult relationships. Ainsworth, Blehar, Waters, and Wall (1978) distinguished among three attachment styles: secure (characterized by confidence in the responsiveness of attachment figures in times of need, comfort with interdependence, trust, and closeness), avoidant (characterized by insecurity in the intentions of other persons and emotional distance), and anxious-ambivalent (characterized by a desire for intimacy coupled with insecurity about others' responses to this desire and fear of rejection). Hazan and Shaver (1987) demonstrated the continuity of attachment styles from childhood to adulthood: Adults who were securely attached to their close relationships reported more secure child–caregiver interactions than adults who manifested avoidant or anxious-ambivalent attachment styles.

We argue that secure attachments constitute an operationalization of selfness. Compared with their avoidant and anxious-ambivalent counterparts, securely attached persons have a more complex, clear, and balanced self-concept (Mikulincer, 1995), have higher self-esteem, and feel special and valued by others (Bartholomew & Horowitz, 1991; Griffin & Bartholomew, 1994). More important, securely attached individuals are preferred as mates and companions over anxious-ambivalent and avoidant individuals (Chappell & Davis, 1998). Securely attached persons have high mate value.

Indeed, attachments have been conceptualized from an evolutionary psychology perspective as adaptive (i.e., serving reproductive goals) responses to caregiver environments (Belsky, 1999; Simpson, 1999). Individuals in securely attached relationships have positive and supportive interactions (Senchak & Leonard, 1992; Simpson, Rholes, & Nelligan, 1992), and they provide socialization experiences to their children that foster the belief that the world is relatively safe and that others can be trusted in the context of long-term and rewarding relationships. Also, securely attached caregivers invest in parental care and thus maximize the chances of survival and reproduction in their progeny. Unsurprisingly, securely attached caregivers are likely to have securely attached children (van IJzendoorn, 1995). As stated earlier (Chappell & Davis, 1998), securely attached persons have high mate value.

An important prospect for future research is to articulate additional predictions derived from the selfness hypothesis. Several lines of research might explore the nonsocial roots of the self. If the self developed to provide an advantage to humans' interaction with the environment, then an investigator ought to be able to find continuing evidence of that advantage. For example, one line of research might explore the fading-affect bias in autobiographical memory. This bias refers to the tendency for negative autobiographical events to lose their affective intensity more quickly as time passes than do positive events. Hence, people may continue to get a "rosy glow" when they recall positive events from their lives, but are less likely to experience a "bummed out" feeling when they think of negative events. A series of recent studies by Walker, Skowronski, Gibbons, Vogl, and Thompson (in press) found that mild, nonclinical depressives were particularly likely to experience high levels of negative affect when recalling negative autobiographical memories and hence showed a reduced fading-affect bias relative to the emotions experienced by nondepressives. One might speculate that those who are low in selfness may show a similar retention of negative affect across time. Another line of research might explore the extent to which selfness is related to effective goal setting, emotional regulation, and responsiveness to the environment. Those who are high in selfness should tend to do well in all three areas. These proficiencies may also spill over into task performance: Those who are high in selfness will perform better on any number of tasks than those who are not. The reason is that those who are high in selfness will be better able to "tune into" the environment by making better choices and more effectively regulating motivation and emotion than those who are low in selfness.

Additionally, the issue of whether selfness is related to proficiency in dealing with the social world needs to be explored. If the continuing evolution of the self was advantageous to a person's ability to manage his or her social affairs, we ought to find evidence of such advantages in current social relations. For example, selfness ought to be positively related to leadership effectiveness, relationship stability, the ability to adapt to new social situations, accuracy in social perception and social memory, accuracy in autobiographical memory, and accuracy in perceiving how one is perceived by others.

Summary and Conclusion

In our previous work (Sedikides & Skowronski, 1997, 2000; Skowronski & Sedikides, 1999), we argued that the emergence of the symbolic self in humans was an evolutionary adaptation. In this chapter, we have tried to improve on and refine our past accounts. Specifically, we: (1) refined the definition of the symbolic self, (2) updated the discussion of a plausible evolutionary timescale for the evolution of the symbolic self, (3) described some of the ecological and social pressures that may have led to the continuing evolution of the self, and (4) considered issues of primacy with respect to the environmental- versus social-pressures question. Finally, we described new data that speak to some of the issues that we raised in discussing the evolutionary origins of the symbolic self and posed new testable research questions that might be formulated as a result of considering the evolutionary origins and functions of the symbolic self.

We hope that this effort will stimulate further theoretical advances and will spur empirical forays into the functions of, and possible evolutionary origins of, selfness. After all, if the symbolic self is truly one of the few adaptations that separates humans from other animal species on the bush of evolution, how can researchers settle for anything less?

References

Ainsworth, M. D. S., Blehar, M. C., Waters, E., & Wall, S. (1978). *Patterns of attachment: A psychological study of the strange situation.* Hillsdale, NJ: Erlbaum.

Andersen, S. M. (1984). Self-knowledge and social inference: 2. The diagnosticity of cognitive/affective and behavioral data. *Journal of Personality and Social Psychology, 46,* 294–307.

Andersen, S. M., Glassman, N. S., & Gold, D. A. (1998). Mental representations of the self, significant others, and nonsignificant others: Structure and processing of private and public aspects. *Journal of Personality and Social Psychology, 75,* 845–861.

Barkow, J. H. (1989). *Darwin, sex, and status: Biological approaches to mind and culture.* Toronto, Ontario, Canada: University of Toronto Press.

Barron, F. (1953). An ego-strength scale which predicts response to psychotherapy. *Journal of Consulting Psychology, 5,* 327–333.

Bartholomew, K., & Horowitz, L. (1991). Attachment styles among young adults: A test of a four-category model. *Journal of Personality and Social Psychology,* *61,* 226–244.

Baumeister, R. F. (1991). *Escaping the self: Alcoholism, spirituality, masochism, and other flights from the burden of selfhood.* New York: Basic Books.

Belsky, J. (1999). Modern evolutionary theory and patterns of attachment. In J. Cassidy & P. R. Shaver (Eds.), *Handbook of attachment: Theory, research, and clinical applications* (pp. 141–161). New York: Guilford Press.

Bem, D. J., & Allen, A. (1974). On predicting some of the people some of the time: The search for cross-situational consistencies in behavior. *Psychological Review, 81,* 506–520.

Block, J. (1961). Ego-identity, role variability, and adjustment. *Journal of Consulting and Clinical Psychology, 25,* 392–397.

Bowlby, J. (1973). *Attachment and loss: Vol. 2. Separation, anxiety, and anger.* New York: Basic Books.

Bowlby, J. (1980). *Attachment and loss: Vol. 3. Loss, sadness and depression.* New York: Basic Books.

Buss, D. M. (1989). Sex differences in human mate preferences: Evolutionary hypotheses tested in 37 cultures. *Behavioral and Brain Sciences, 12,* 1–49.

Buss, D. M. (1995). Evolutionary psychology: A new paradigm for psychological science. *Psychological Inquiry, 6,* 1–30.

Campbell, J. D. (1990). Self-esteem and clarity of the self-concept. *Journal of Personality and Social Psychology, 59,* 538–549.

Campbell, J. D., Trapnell, P. D., Heine, S. J., Katz, I. M., Lavallee, L. F., & Lehman, D. R. (1996). Self-concept clarity: Measurement, personality correlates, and cultural boundaries. *Journal of Personality and Social Psychology, 70,* 141–156.

Campbell, W. K., & Sedikides, C. (1999). Self-threat magnifies the self-serving bias: A meta-analytic integration. *Review of General Psychology, 3,* 23–43.

Cantor, N., Markus, H., Niedenthal, P., & Nurius, P. (1986). On motivation and the self-concept. In R. M. Sorrentino & E. T. Higgins (Eds.), *Motivation and cognition: Foundations of social behavior* (pp. 96–127). New York: Guilford Press.

Caporael, L. R. (1997). The evolution of truly social cognition: The core configurations model. *Personality and Social Psychology Review, 1,* 276–298.

Carver, C. S., & Scheier, M. F. (1998). *On the self-regulation of behavior.* New York: Cambridge University Press.

Caspi, A., Bem, D. J., & Elder, G. H., Jr. (1989). Continuities and consequences of interactional styles across the life course. *Journal of Personality and Social Psychology, 57,* 375–406.

Chappell, K. D., & Davis, K. E. (1998). Attachment, partner choice, and perception of romantic partners: An experimental test of the attachment-security hypothesis. *Personal Relationships, 5,* 327–342.

Chartrand, T. L., & Bargh, J. A. (1999). The chameleon effect: The perception–behavior link and social interaction. *Journal of Personality and Social Psychology, 76,* 893–910.

Cheyney, D. L., & Seyfarth, R. M. (1996). Function and intention in the calls of non-human primates. *Proceedings of the British Academy, 88,* 59–76.

Damasio, A. (1999). *The feeling of what happens: Body and emotion in the making of consciousness.* New York: Harcourt Brace.

Damon, W., & Hart, D. (1986). Stability and change in children's self-understanding. *Social Cognition, 4,* 102–118.

Deci, E. L., & Ryan, R. M. (2000). The "what" and "why" of goal pursuits: Human needs and the self-determination of behavior. *Psychological Inquiry, 11,* 227–268.

Deutsch, F. M., Ruble, D. N., Brooks-Gunn, J., Flemming, A., & Stangor, C. (1988). Information-seeking and material self-definition during the transition to motherhood. *Journal of Personality and Social Psychology, 55,* 420–431.

Donahue, E. M., Robins, R. W., Roberts, B. W., & John, O. P. (1993). The divided self: Concurrent and longitudinal effects of psychological adjustment and social roles on self-concept differentiation. *Journal of Personality and Social Psychology, 64,* 834–846.

Emmons, R. A. (1989). The personal striving approach to personality. In L. A. Pervin (Ed.), *Goal concepts in personality and social psychology* (pp. 87–126). Hillsdale, NJ: Erlbaum.

Felson, R. B. (1993). The (somewhat) social self: How others affect self-appraisals. In J. Suls (Ed.), *Psychological perspectives on the self* (Vol. 4, pp. 1–26). Hillsdale, NJ: Erlbaum.

Foley, R., & Lahr, M. (1997). Mode 3 technologies and the evolution of modern humans. *Cambridge Archeological Journal, 7,* 3–36.

Funder, D. C., & Block, J. (1989). The role of ego-control, ego-resiliency, and IQ in delay of gratification in adolescence. *Journal of Personality and Social Psychology, 57,* 1041–1050.

Gergen, K. J., & Morse, S. J. (1967). Self-consistency: Measurement and validation. *Proceedings of the 75th Annual Convention of the American Psychological Association, 2,* 207–208.

Gould, S. J. (2000). More things in heaven and earth. In H. Rose & S. Rose (Eds.), *Alas, poor Darwin: Arguments against evolutionary psychology* (pp. 85–128). London: Random House.

Gramzow, R. H., Sedikides, C., Panter, A. T., & Insko, C. A. (2000). Aspects of self-regulation and self-structure as predictors of perceived emotional distress. *Personality and Social Psychology Bulletin, 26,* 188–206.

Greenwald, A. G. (1980). The totalitarian ego: Fabrication and revision of personal history. *American Psychologist, 35,* 603–618.

Griffin, D., & Bartholomew, K. (1994). Models of the self and other: Fundamental dimensions underlying measures of adult attachment. *Journal of Personality and Social Psychology, 67,* 430–445.

Hamilton, W. D. (1964). The genetic evolution of social behavior (Parts 1 & 2). *Journal of Theoretical Biology, 7,* 1–52.

Hazan, C., & Shaver, P. (1987). Romantic love conceptualized as an attachment process. *Journal of Personality and Social Psychology, 52,* 511–524.

Higgins, E. T. (1987). Self-discrepancy: A theory relating self and affect. *Psychological Review, 94,* 319–340.

Higgins, E. T., & May, D. (2001). Individual self-regulatory functions: It's not "we" regulation, but it's still social. In C. Sedikides & M. F. Brewer (Eds.), *Individual self, relational self, collective self* (pp. 47–67). Philadelphia: Psychology Press.

Howe, M. L. (2000). *The fate of early memories: Developmental science and the retention of childhood experiences*. Washington, DC: American Psychological Association.

Howe, M. L., & Courage, M. L. (1997). The emergence and early development of autobiographical memory. *Psychological Review, 104,* 499–523.

Jaynes, J. (1976). *The origin of consciousness in the breakdown of the bicameral mind*. Boston: Houghton Mifflin.

Kaplan, K. J. (1972). On the ambivalence–indifference problem in attitude theory and measurement: A suggested modification of the semantic differential technique. *Psychological Bulletin, 77,* 361–372.

Keltner, D., & Buswell, B. N. (1997). Embarrassment: Its distinct form and appeasement functions. *Psychological Bulletin, 122,* 250–270.

Kenny, D. A., & DePaulo, B. M. (1993). Do people know how others view them? An empirical and theoretical account. *Psychological Bulletin, 114,* 145–161.

Kernis, M. H., Whisenhunt, C. R., Waschull, S. B., Greenier, K. D., Berry, A. J., Herlocker, C. E., & Anderson, C. A. (1998). Multiple facets of self-esteem and their relations to depressive symptoms. *Personality and Social Psychology Bulletin, 24,* 657–668.

Ketelaar, T., & Ellis, B. J. (2000). Are evolutionary explanations unfalsifiable? Evolutionary psychology and the Lakatosian philosophy of science. *Psychological Inquiry, 11,* 1–21.

Klein, R. (1989). *The human career: Human biological and cultural origins*. Chicago: University of Chicago Press.

Kobasa, S. C. (1979). Stressful life events, personality, and distress: An inquiry into hardiness. *Journal of Personality and Social Psychology, 37,* 1–11.

Leary, M. R., & Baumeister, R. F. (2000). The nature and functions of self-esteem: Sociometer theory. In M. P. Zanna (Ed.), *Advances in experimental social psychology* (Vol. 32, pp. 1–62). San Diego, CA: Academic Press.

Leary, M. R., & Cottrell, C. A. (1999). Evolution of the self, the need to belong, and life in a delayed-return environment. *Psychological Inquiry, 10,* 229–232.

Leary, M. R., & Tambor, E. S., Terdal, S. K., & Downs, D. L. (1995). Self-esteem as an interpersonal monitor: The sociometer hypothesis. *Journal of Personality and Social Psychology, 68,* 518–530.

Linville, P. W. (1985). Self-complexity and affective extremity: Don't put all of your eggs in one cognitive basket. *Social Cognition, 3,* 94–120.

Linville, P. W. (1987). Self-complexity as a cognitive buffer against stress-related illness and depression. *Journal of Personality and Social Psychology, 52,* 663–676.

Little, B. R. (1983). Personal projects: A rationale and method for investigation. *Environment and Behavior, 15,* 273–309.

Markus, H. (1977). Self-schemata and processing information about the self. *Journal of Personality and Social Psychology, 35,* 63–78.

Martin, L. L. (1999). I-D compensation theory: Some implications of trying to satisfy immediate-return needs in a delayed-return culture. *Psychological Inquiry, 10,* 195–208.

McCrae, R. R., & Costa, P. T. (1994). The stability of personality: Observation and evaluations. *Current Directions in Psychological Science, 3,* 173–175.

McKie, R. (2000). *Ape man: The story of human evolution*. London: BBC Worldwide Ltd.

Mikulincer, M. (1995). Attachment style and the mental representation of the self. *Journal of Personality and Social Psychology, 69,* 1203–1215.

Mithen, S. (1996). *The prehistory of the mind: The cognitive origins of art, religion, and science*. London: Thames & Hudson.

Nadel, J., & Butterworth, G. (Eds.). (1999). *Imitation in infancy. Cambridge studies in cognitive perceptual development*. New York: Cambridge University Press.

Pelham, B. W. (1991). On confidence and consequence: The certainty and importance of self-knowledge. *Journal of Personality and Social Psychology, 60,* 518–530.

Pelham, B. W., & Wachsmuth, J. O. (1995). The waxing and waning of the social self: Assimilation and contrast in social comparison. *Journal of Personality and Social Psychology, 69,* 825–838.

Povinelli, D. J., Bering, J. M., & Giambrone, S. (2000). Toward a science of other minds: Escaping the argument by analogy. *Cognitive Science, 24,* 509–541.

Schoeneman, T. J. (1981). Reports of the sources of self-knowledge. *Journal of Personality, 49,* 284–292.

Sedikides, C., & Green, J. D. (2000). On the self-protective nature of inconsistency/negativity management: Using the person memory paradigm to examine self-referent memory. *Journal of Personality and Social Psychology, 79,* 906–922.

Sedikides, C., & Skowronski, J. J. (1995). On the sources of self-knowledge: The perceived primacy of self-reflection. *Journal of Social and Clinical Psychology, 14,* 244–270.

Sedikides, C., & Skowronski, J. J. (1997). The symbolic self in evolutionary context. *Personality and Social Psychology Review, 1,* 80–102.

Sedikides, C., & Skowronski, J. J. (2000). On the evolutionary functions of the symbolic self: The emergence of self-evaluation motives. In A. Tesser, R. Felson, & J. Suls (Eds.), *Psychological perspectives on self and identity* (pp. 91–117). Washington, DC: American Psychological Association.

Senchak, M., & Leonard, K. (1992). Attachment style and marital adjustment among newlywed couples. *Journal of Social and Personal Relationships, 9,* 51–64.

Sheldon, K. M., Elliot, A. J., Kim, Y., & Kasser, T. (2001). What is satisfying about satisfying events? Testing 10 candidate psychological needs. *Journal of Personality and Social Psychology, 80,* 325–339.

Sheldon, K. M., & Kasser, T. (1995). Coherence and congruence: Two aspects of personality integration. *Journal of Personality and Social Psychology, 68,* 531–543.

Simpson, J. A. (1999). Attachment theory in modern evolutionary perspective. In J. Cassidy & P. R. Shaver (Eds.), *Handbook of attachment: Theory, research, and clinical applications* (pp. 115–140). New York: Guilford Press.

Simpson, L., Rholes, W., & Nelligan, J. (1992). Support seeking and support giving within couples in an anxiety-provoking situation: The role of attachment styles. *Journal of Personality and Social Psychology, 62,* 434–446.

Skowronski, J. J., Betz, A. L., Thompson, C. P., & Shannon, L. (1991). Social memory in everyday life: Recall of self-events and other-events. *Journal of Personality and Social Psychology, 60,* 831–843.

Skowronski, J. J., & Sedikides, C. (1999). Evolution of the

symbolic self. In D. H. Rosen & M. C. Luebbert (Eds.), *Evolution of the psyche* (pp. 78–94). Westport, CT: Greenwood.

Staats, S., & Skowronski, J.J. (1992). Perceptions of self-affect: Now and in the future. *Social Cognition, 10,* 415–431.

Stringer, C., & McKie, R. (1996). *African exodus: The origins of modern humanity.* London: Jonathon Cape.

Swann, W. B. (1983). Self-verification: Bringing social reality into harmony with the self. In J. Suls & A. G. Greenwald (Eds.), *Psychological perspectives on the self* (Vol. 2, pp. 33–66). Hillsdale, NJ: Erlbaum.

Symons, D. (1979). *The evolution of human sexuality.* New York: Oxford University Press.

Tangney, J. P. (1998). How does guilt differ from shame? In J. Bybee (Ed.), *Guilt and children* (pp. 1–17). San Diego, CA: Academic Press.

Tangney, J. P., Burggraf, S. A., & Wagner, P. E. (1995). Shame-proneness, guilt-proneness, and psychological symptoms. In J. P. Tangney & K. W. Fischer (Eds.), *Self-conscious emotions: The psychology of shame, guilt, embarrassment, and pride* (pp. 343–367). New York: Guilford Press.

Tesser, A. (2000). On the confluence of self-esteem main-tenance mechanisms. *Personality and Social Psychology Review, 4,* 290–299.

Tomasello, M. (1999). *The cultural origins of human cognition.* Cambridge, MA: Harvard University Press.

Tomasello, M., & Call, J. (1997). *Primate cognition.* Oxford, UK: Oxford University Press.

Walker, W. R., Skowronski, J. J., Gibbons, J. A., Vogl, R. J., & Thompson, C. P. (in press). On the emotions that accompany autobiographical memory: Dysphoria disrupts the fading affect bias. *Cognition and Emotion.*

Waschull, S. B., & Kernis, M. H. (1996). Level and stability of self-esteem as predictors of children's intrinsic motivation and reasons for anger. *Personality and Social Psychology Bulletin, 22,* 4–13.

Weisfeld, G. E., & Wendorf, C. A. (2000). The involuntary defeat strategy and discrete emotions theory. In L. Sloman & P. Gilbert (Eds.), *Subordination and defeat: An evolutionary approach to mood disorders and their therapy* (pp. 121–145). Mahwah, NJ: Erlbaum.

Van IJzendoorn, M. H. (1995). Adult attachment representations, parental responsiveness, and infant attachment: A meta-analysis on the predictive validity of the Adult Attachment Interview. *Psychological Bulletin, 11,* 387–403.

30

The Development of Self-Representations during Childhood and Adolescence

SUSAN HARTER

Interest in self-processes has burgeoned in the past decade within many branches of psychology. Cognitive developmentalists, particularly those of a neo-Piagetian persuasion, have addressed normative changes in the emergence of a sense of self (e.g., Case, 1985, 1992; Fischer, 1980; Harter, 1997; Higgins, 1991). Developmentalists interested in memory processes have also described how the self is crafted through the construction of narratives that provide the basis for autobiographical memory (see Fivush, 1987; Nelson, 1986, 1993; Snow, 1990). Contemporary attachment theorists, building on the earlier efforts of Ainsworth (1973, 1974) and Bowlby (1980), have provided new insights into how interactions with caregivers come to shape the representations of self and others that young children come to construct (see Bretherton, 1991, 1992; Cassidy, 1990; Cicchetti, 1990, 1991; Cicchetti & Beeghly, 1990; Pipp, 1990; Sroufe, 1990). Clinicians within the psychodynamic tradition have also contributed to our understanding of how early socialization experiences come to shape the structure and content of self-evaluations and contribute to psychopathology (Blatt, 1995; Bleiberg, 1984; Kernberg, 1975; Kohut, 1977; Winnicott, 1965). Moreover, social and personality theorists have devoted considerable attention to those processes that produce individual differences in perceptions of self, particularly among adults (see Baumeister, 1987, 1993; Epstein, 1991; Epstein & Morling, 1995; Kernis, 1993; Kihlstrom, 1993; Leary & Downs, 1995; Markus & Wurf, 1987; Showers, 1995; Swann, 1996; Steele, 1988).

Clearly, there is a "new look" to many of these contemporary formulations. However, the field has also witnessed a return to many of the classic issues that captured the attention of historical scholars of the self. For example, new life has been breathed into James's (1890, 1892) distinction between the I-self—the self as subject, agent, knower—and the Me-self—the self as object, as known. In addition, James's analysis of the antecedents of self-esteem has now been put to an empirical test (see Harter, 1993, 1998). There has also been a resurgence of interest in the formulations of those symbol-ic interactionists, namely, Baldwin (1897), Cooley (1902), and Mead (1934), who placed heavy emphasis on how interactive processes with caregivers shape the develop-ing self.

Interest in self-processes has escalated, in part due to increasing emphasis on their functional role in development. Thus, far from being an epiphenomenon, the self has taken center stage as a dynamic actor, play-ing a variety of roles. In fact, it is commonly asserted that the very architecture of the self-theory, by evolutionary design, is ex-tremely functional across the life span. At-tachment theorists (e.g., Bretherton, 1991; Cassidy, 1990; Sroufe, 1990) have observed how working models of the self have *orga-nizational* significance, providing young children with a set of expectations that al-lows them to guide their behavior more effi-ciently. The development of self-relevant scripts also gives the toddler predictive structure; moreover, the emergence of auto-biographical memories, scaffolded by the narrative coconstruction of the self, serves to define the self and to cement social bonds (e.g., Crittenden, 1994; Fivush, 1987; Hud-son, 1990; Nelson, 1993; Snow, 1990).

For those focusing on childhood and ado-lescence, the self serves to shape goals (e.g., Dweck, 1991; Ruble & Frey, 1991) and to provide self-guides that aid in appropriate social behaviors and self-regulation (e.g., Higgins, 1991). Positive self-affects, in the form of pride, serve to foster an emotional investment in one's competencies and to en-ergize one toward further accomplishments. Negative self-conscious emotions, particu-larly guilt, have also been afforded very functional, social properties across the life span in that they provoke behaviors direct-ed toward reparation, rebonding, and the maintenance of emotional attachments (see Barrett, 1995; Tangney & Fischer, 1995). Social psychologists who address adult self-processes have also articulated a number of similar functions. Markus and colleagues (e.g., Markus & Kitayama, 1991; Markus & Nurius, 1986; Markus & Wurf, 1987; Oyserman & Markus, 1993) have focused on how the self organizes, interprets, and gives meaning to experience, regulates af-fect, and motivates action by providing in-centives, standards, plans, and scripts (see

also Carver & Scheier, 1990; Greenwald, 1980). Moreover, the construction of future possible selves (Markus & Nurius, 1986) further organizes behavior and energizes the individual to pursue selected goals. Discrep-ancies between real and ideal self-concepts can also motivate the individual to achieve his or her ideals in the service of self-improvement (Banaji & Prentice, 1994; Bandura, 1990; Oosterwegel & Oppen-heimer, 1993; Rogers, 1951).

Epstein and colleagues (e.g., Epstein, 1991; Epstein & Morling, 1995) have iden-tified four basic needs that require the con-struction of a self. The individual needs (1) to maintain a favorable sense of his or her attributes, which in turn will help (2) to maximize pleasure and minimize pain. Moreover, one needs (3) to develop and maintain a coherent picture of the world, as well as to (4) maintain relatedness with oth-ers. The first self-enhancement function has also been addressed by others (e.g., Beach & Tesser, 1995; Steele, 1988; Tesser, 1988; Tesser & Cornell, 1991). Certain social psy-chologists have emphasized more specific motives. For example, Greenberg, Pyszczyn-ski, and Solomon (1995) concur that the pursuit of positive self-esteem is a superor-dinate goal toward which humans aspire. However, they also argue that self-esteem serves as an anxiety buffer against adults' terror over their eventual death. Leary and Downs (1995) have identified a different so-cial function, namely avoidance of social ex-clusion. They argue that behaviors that maintain self-esteem decrease the likelihood that one will be ignored or rejected by other people. Clearly, across different theorists addressing different stages of development, the functions of various self-representations have surfaced as an important considera-tion. (However, as we shall see in our later treatment of the liabilities of self-develop-ment, not all investigators are as sanguine about the positive functions of self-process-es.)

Definitions of Self

Self terminology abounds: self-concept, self-image, self-esteem, self-worth, self-evalua-tions, self-perceptions, self-representations, self-schemas, self-affects, self-efficacy, and self-monitoring, to name but a few. Certain scholars of the self have argued that the plethora of terminology and contradictory definitions, both conceptual and operational, have rendered much of the literature uninterpretable (see Wylie, 1979, 1989). Given that varying conceptualizations define the landscape of the self literature, leading to potential confusion in how terms are to be interpreted, it is critical to clarify the terminology to be employed in this chapter. At the broadest level, I focus on self-representations, namely, attributes or characteristics of the self that are consciously acknowledged by the individual through language—that is, how one describes oneself. The terms "self-representations," "self-perceptions," and "self-descriptions" are used interchangeably to denote this general process. However, other representations of self are more explicitly *self-evaluative* in that they make specific reference to one's positive or negative attributes (e.g., "I am scholastically competent" or "I am not that popular"). Where the focus has been the assessment of the valence of self-representations, the term "self-evaluations" will be employed.

It has become increasingly important to the field to distinguish between self-evaluations that represent global characteristics of the individual (e.g., "I am a worthwhile person") and those that reflect the individual's sense of adequacy across particular domains, such as one's cognitive competence (e.g., "I am smart"), social competence (e.g., "I am well liked by peers"), athletic competence (e.g., "I am good at sports"), and so forth (see Bracken, 1996; Epstein, 1991; Harter, 1986b, 1997; Marsh, 1986, 1987; Rosenberg, 1979). Conceptualizations and instruments that aggregate domain-specific self-evaluations into a single score (e.g., Coopersmith, 1967) have been found wanting in that they mask the meaningful distinctions between one's sense of adequacy across domains.

With regard to terminology, global self-evaluations have typically been referred to as "self-esteem" (Rosenberg, 1979), "self-worth" (Harter, 1982, 1993), or "general self-concept" (Marsh, 1986, 1987). In each case, the focus is on the overall evaluation of one's worth or value as a person. In this chapter, I employ the terms "self-esteem"

and "self-worth" interchangeably. It is important to appreciate the fact that this general evaluation is tapped by its own set of items that explicitly ask about one's perceived worth as a person (e.g., "I feel that I am a worthwhile person"); that is, it is *not* a summary statement of self-evaluations across different domains.

Consistent with the literature, the term "self-concept" is primarily reserved for evaluative judgments of attributes within discrete domains such as cognitive competence, social acceptance, physical appearance, and so forth. Thus I make reference to "domain-specific self-evaluations." As will become evident, such a focus allows the investigator to construct a *profile* of self-evaluations across domains for individuals or for particular subgroups of interest. Moreover, the separation of global self-esteem or self-worth from domain-specific evaluations allows one to address the issue of whether evaluations in some domains are more predictive of global self-esteem than are others.

The I-Self versus the Me-Self

This chapter also builds on another distinction in the literature. The majority of scholars who have devoted thoughtful attention to the self have come to a similar conclusion: Two distinct but intimately intertwined aspects of self can be meaningfully identified—self as *subject* (the I-self) and self as *object* (the Me-self). William James (1890) introduced this distinction, defining the I-self as the actor or *knower*, whereas the Me-self was the object of one's knowledge, "an empirical aggregate of things objectively known" (p. 197). James also identified particular features or components of both the I-self and the Me-self. Components of the I-self included (1) *self-awareness*, an appreciation for one's internal states, needs, thoughts, and emotions; (2) *self-agency*, the sense of the authorship over one's thoughts and actions; (3) *self-continuity*, the sense that one remains the same person over time; and (4) *self-coherence*, a stable sense of the self as a single, coherent, bounded entity. Components of the Me-self included the "material me," the "social me," and the "spiritual me." The distinction between the I-self and the Me-self has proved amazingly viable and appears as a recurrent theme in most theoretical treatments of the self (see Dickstein, 1977; Harter, 1999; Lewis, 1991, 1994; Wylie, 1979).

Until recently, major empirical attention had been devoted to the Me-self, to the study of the self as an object of one's knowledge and evaluation, as evidenced by the myriad number of studies on self-concept and self-esteem (see Harter, 1999; Wylie, 1979). More recently, the I-self, which James himself regarded as an elusive construct, has become more prominent in accounts of self-development. As the chapters in this volume demonstrate, both the structure and content of the Me-self at any given developmental level necessarily depend on the particular I-self capabilities, namely, those cognitive processes that define the knower. Thus, the cognitive-developmental changes in I-self processes will directly influence the nature of the self-theory that the child is constructing.

Most scholars conceptualize the self as a *theory* that must be cognitively constructed. Those theorists within the tradition of adult personality and social psychology have suggested that the self-theory should possess the characteristics of any formal theory, defined as a hypothetico-deductive system. Such a personal epistemology should, therefore, meet those criteria by which any good theory is evaluated, namely, the degree to which it is parsimonious, empirically valid, internally consistent, coherently organized, testable, and useful. From a developmental perspective, however, the self-theories created by children cannot meet these criteria, given numerous cognitive limitations that have been identified in Piagetian (1960) and neo-Piagetian formulations (e.g., Case, 1992; Fischer, 1980); that is, the I-self in its role as constructor of the Me-self does not, in childhood, possess the capacities to create a hierarchically organized system of postulates that are internally consistent, coherently organized, testable, or empirically valid. In fact, it is not until late adolescence, if not early adulthood, that the abilities to construct a self-portrait that meets the criteria of a good formal theory potentially emerge. Therefore, in our developmental analysis of the self as a cognitive construction, it is essential to examine how the changing characteristics of the I-self processes that define

each developmental stage directly affect the Me-self, namely, the self-theory that is being constructed.

Antecedents and Consequences of the Self as a Cognitive and Social Construction

In examining the development of the self, this chapter focuses on the *antecedents* of self-representations, as well as on their functional *consequences*. With regard to antecedents, it becomes evident that the self is both a *cognitive* and a *social* construction, two major themes around which the material to be presented is organized. From a cognitive-developmental perspective, the construction of self-representations is inevitable. As neo-Piagetians (e.g., Case, 1992; Fischer, 1980) and self theorists (e.g., Epstein, 1973, 1981, 1991; Greenwald, 1980; Kelly, 1955; Markus, 1980; Sarbin, 1962) have forcefully argued, our species has been designed to actively create *theories* about our world and to make *meaning* of our experiences, including the construction of a theory of self. Thus the self is, first and foremost, a *cognitive construction*. The particular cognitive abilities and limitations of each developmental period (I-self processes or the self as subject) will represent the template that dictates the features of the self-portrait to be crafted (the Me-self or the self as object). As becomes evident, a cognitive-developmental analysis focuses primarily on changes in the *structure* of the self-system, namely, how self-representations are conceptually organized. As such, primary emphasis is given to processes responsible for those normative developmental changes that result in *similarities* in self-representations among individuals at a given developmental level.

Previous ontogenetic accounts highlighted major qualitative differences in the nature of self-descriptions associated with broad stages of development. Within the field of development, observers were initially struck by the most outstanding markers in the psychological landscape, namely, dramatic differences that defined the stage models of the day (e.g., Piaget, 1960). More recent treatments of self-development fill in the gaps by providing a more detailed account of the progression of substages of self-understanding. As a result, we have necessarily had to alter our views about whether the development of self-representations is best viewed as a discontinuous or continuous process. Employing frameworks of the past, self-development was viewed as largely discontinuous, with an emphasis on the saltatory nature of the conceptual leaps from one broadly defined stage to another. From this perspective, theorists highlighted the dramatic *differences* between the self-descriptions and evaluations of young children, older children, and adolescents. However, there has been a shift in emphasis that is reflected in this chapter. The development of self-representations is now viewed as more continuous, in that investigators specify more ministeps or substages that occur, including how such levels build on and transform one another.

In focusing on normative developmental changes, we see how cognitive development affects two general characteristics of the self-structure, the levels of *differentiation* and of *integration* that the individual can bring to bear on the postulates in his or her self-theory. With regard to differentiation, emerging cognitive abilities allow the individual to create self-evaluations that differ across various domains of experience. Moreover, they permit the older child to distinguish between real and ideal self-concepts, which can then be compared with one another, creating potential discrepancies that have further consequences for one's self-esteem. During adolescence, newfound cognitive capabilities support the creation of multiple selves in different relational contexts.

With regard to integration, cognitive abilities that emerge across the course of development allow the individual to construct higher order generalizations about the self in the form of trait labels (e.g., demonstrated skills in math, science, and language arts are subsumed under the self-concept of "smart"). Abilities that emerge in middle childhood also permit the individual to construct a concept of his or her worth as a person, namely, global self-esteem. Further cognitive advances in adolescence allow one to successfully intercoordinate seemingly contradictory self-attributes (e.g., "How can I be both cheerful and depressed?") into meaningful abstractions about the self (e.g.,

"I'm a moody person"). These themes are addressed in subsequent sections of this chapter.

In addition to an exploration of the cognitive developmental antecedents of the self, emphasis is placed on the self as a *social* construction. Thus attention is devoted to an examination of how socialization experiences in children's interactions with caregivers, peers, teachers, and in the wider sociocultural context will influence the particular *content* and *valence* of one's self-representations. Socialization factors as experienced by the I-self (or self as subject) will therefore affect the Me-self (or self as object). Those building on the symbolic interactionist perspective (Baldwin, 1895; Cooley, 1902; Mead, 1934), as well as those of an attachment theory persuasion, have focused on how socialization experiences with caregivers produce *individual differences* in the content of self-representations, including whether evaluations of the self are favorable or unfavorable. I examine how the reactions of significant others determine whether the child comes to view the self as competent versus incapable, as lovable versus undeserving of others' affection, as worthy of esteem versus lacking in value. Although cognitive developmentalists emphasize the fact that children are active agents in their own development, including the construction of self, those from the symbolic interactionist and attachment perspectives alert us to the fact that children are also at the mercy of the particular caregiving hand they have been dealt.

A second goal of this chapter is to examine certain consequences of these cognitive and social processes. Why, for example, should we care about self-development? I argue that self-representations and self-evaluations are of little interest unless it can be demonstrated that they have broader behavioral implications and unless there are ramifications for how individuals adapt to or cope with the developmental tasks that confront them. As observed earlier in this chapter, the self has been afforded many *positive* functions, namely, organizational, motivational, and protective (e.g., to maximize pleasure and minimize pain).

Unfortunately, as becomes evident in this chapter, self-processes do not always conform to this functional job description.

Rather, there are numerous potential negative correlates and consequences on the path to self-development. Paradoxically, some of these forks in the road are inevitable, given developmental advances; that is, emerging cognitive developmental structures not only pave the way for a more mature self-structure but also usher in the potential for a variety of negative correlates and consequences. The path to self-development, therefore, can represent a veritable minefield. As others have also pointed out, there are costs to development (Leahy, 1985), as new cognitive acquisitions provoke vulnerabilities for the self-system (Higgins, 1991). These liabilities are apparent at every level of development. Thus attention is devoted to both positive and negative outcomes that result from normative developmental acquisitions. There are also *individual differences* in the extent to which the self performs its supposed positive functions. For example, some individuals suffer from low self-esteem, leading to feelings of depressed affect, low energy, and in some cases suicidal thinking and behaviors (see Baumeister, 1993; Harter, 1999). I explore these consequences, including the multiple pathways to low self-esteem.

Overview of Specific Topics

I turn next to an analysis of how the self is both cognitively and socially constructed during childhood and adolescence. Although self-development begins at birth and proceeds through predictable stages during infancy (see Harter, 1998), this chapter focuses on those *verbal* representations of self that begin to emerge toward the end of the second year of life. Attention is devoted to cognitive developmental processes that represent I-self changes that, in turn, influence developmental differences in the nature of the Me-self, in both children and adolescents. The focus is on *normative developmental* changes that lead to similarities in the self-structure among individuals at a given developmental level. Within this framework, emphasis is placed on how cognitive developmental advances lead to more mature self-structures, while at the same time they usher in potential liabilities that may compromise the functionality of the self-system.

The focus then shifts to *individual differ-*

ences in self-*evaluative* judgments, namely, domain-specific self-concepts, as well as global self-worth or self-esteem. I explore James's (1892) theory of self-esteem in which he argues that it is a function of the relationship between one's perceived successes and one's pretensions or aspirations for success across different domains. Attention then shifts to those social sources of self-evaluation initially observed by the symbolic interactionists (Baldwin, 1897; Cooley, 1902; Mead, 1934). Child-rearing practices leading to individual differences in self-esteem are examined against a backdrop of models specifying how the opinions of others are internalized.

I then examine a broader model of the causes and consequences of self-worth that has emerged in my own work. A central assumption in my thinking is that self-processes must have meaningful *consequences* if they are to be considered worthy of study. One constellation of negative consequences associated with low self-worth (depressed affect, hopelessness, and suicidal ideation) has been central to my work. Although these efforts have resulted in a general model that has been empirically supported by group data, I have also documented the fact that there are multiple pathways to these outcomes that need to be considered in understanding how the pattern of antecedents can differ across individuals. In keeping with the theme that self-processes can go awry, leading to negative consequences, several liabilities are addressed, including the development of false-self behavior. A revision of my model is also presented, one that includes anger (in addition to depression in the original model) and violent ideation (in addition to suicidal ideation in the original model). I apply this model to the histories of recent school shooters.

High self-esteem has typically been viewed as a psychological commodity to be sought after, as a correlate of positive mental health. However, this view has recently been challenged by theorists, for example, Damon (1995) and Seligman (1993), who are critical of what they consider to be an overemphasis by educators, clinicians, and parents on promoting high self-esteem among our youth, particularly when these efforts lead to an inflated sense of esteem. Moreover, Baumeister, Smart, and Boden

(1999) have observed that certain individuals with high self-esteem who have narcissistic tendencies (including an inflated sense of self-esteem) can, in the face of threats to the ego, externalize blame and react violently to others. These arguments are reviewed. Finally, this chapter points to practical applications in considering interventions to promote realistically positive self-evaluations that serve adaptive mental health functions.

Developmental Differences in Self-Representations during Childhood and Adolescence

A central theme in this chapter is that the self is both a cognitive and a social construction. In this section, six stages of self-development are described, three in childhood and three during adolescence, focusing on both cognitive and social processes (see Table 30.1 and Table 30.2). Developmental differences in the structure, content, and valence of self-representations are highlighted. As I observed previously, it is critical to understand that developmental changes in the I-self (here viewed as cognitive processes) will affect the Me-self (namely, how one describes oneself). It is also imperative to realize that the self is constructed in the crucible of social relationships that will also affect these dimensions, particularly the content and valence of the Me-self. (See Harter, 1999, for more detailed discussion of these levels with illustrative cameo descriptions for each of the six stages.)

Toddlerhood to Early Childhood (Approximately Ages 2–4)

Theory and evidence (see Fischer, Hand, Watson, Van Parys, & Tucker, 1984; Griffin, as cited in Case, 1992; Harter, 1999; Higgins, 1991; Watson, 1990) indicate that the young child can construct very concrete cognitive representations of observable features of the self (e.g., "I know my ABCs; I can count; I can run fast; I live in a big house"). Damon and Hart (1988) label these as "categorical identifications" in that the young child understands the self only as separate, taxonomic attributes that may be physical (e.g., "I have blue eyes"), active (e.g., "I play ball"), social (e.g., "I have two

sisters"), or psychological (e.g., "I am happy"). Case (1992) has referred to this level as "interrelational," in that young children can forge rudimentary links in the form of discrete event–sequence structures that are defined in terms of physical dimensions, behavioral events, or activity. However, they cannot coordinate two such structures (see also Griffin, 1992), in part because of working memory constraints that prevent the young child from holding several features in mind simultaneously.

Fisher's (1980) formulation is very similar. He has labeled these initial structures as "single representations." Such structures are highly differentiated from one another, because the cognitive limitations at this stage render the child incapable of integrating single representations into a coherent self-portrait. One manifestation of this self-structure is the inability to acknowledge that one can possess opposing attributes, for example, "good" and "bad" or "nice" and "mean" (Fischer et al., 1984). Children also deny that they can experience two *emotions,* both same-valence feelings (e.g., mad and sad) and opposite-valence emotions (e.g., happy and sad) at the same time (Harris, 1983; Harter & Buddin, 1987), leading to unrealistic perceptions of the emotional experience of self and others.

Moreover, self-evaluations during this period are likely to be unrealistically positive, as young children have difficulty distinguishing between their desired and their actual competence, a confusion initially observed by both Freud (1952) and Piaget (1932). For contemporary cognitive developmentalists, this problem stems from another cognitive limitation of this period, namely the inability to bring social comparison information to bear meaningfully on their competencies (Frey & Ruble, 1990). The ability to use social comparison toward the goal of self-evaluation requires that the child be able to relate one concept (one's own performance) to another (someone else's performance), a skill that is not sufficiently developed in the young child.

Higgins (1991), building on the models of Case (1985), Fischer (1980), and Selman (1980), has focused more on the interaction between the child's cognitive abilities and the role of socializing agents. He has provided evidence that at Case's stage of inter-

TABLE 30.1. Normative-Developmental Changes in Self-Representations during Childhood

Age period	Salient content	Structure/ organization	Valence accuracy	Nature of comparisons	Sensitivity to others
Very early childhood	Concrete, observable characteristics; simple taxonomic attributes in the form of abilities, activities, possessions, preferences	Isolated representations; lack of coherence, coordination; all-or-none thinking	Unrealistically positive; inability to distinguish real from ideal selves	No direct comparisons	Anticipation of adult reactions (praise, criticism); rudimentary appreciation of whether one is meeting others' external standards
Early to middle childhood	Elaborated taxonomic attributes; focus on specific competencies	Rudimentary links between representations; links typically opposites; all-or-none thinking	Typically positive; inaccuracies persist	Temporal comparisons with self when younger; comparisons with age-mates to determine fairness	Recognition that others are evaluating the self; initial introjection of others' opinions; others' standards becoming self-guides in regulation of behavior
Middle to late childhood	Trait labels that focus on abilities and interpersonal characteristics; comparative assessments with peers; global evaluation of worth	Higher-order generalizations that subsume several behaviors; ability to integrate opposing attributes	Both positive and negative evaluations; greater accuracy	Social comparison for purpose of self-evaluation	Internalization of others' opinions and standards, which come to function as self-guides

TABLE 30.2. Normative-Developmental Changes in Self-Representations during Adolescence

Age period	Salient content	Structure/ organization	Valence accuracy	Nature of comparisons	Sensitivity to others
Early adolescence	Social skills, attributes that influence interactions with others or one's social appeal; differentiation of attributes according to roles	Intercoordination of trait labels into single stractions; abstractions compartmentalized; all-or-none thinking; opposites; don't detect, integrate, opposing abstractions	Positive attributes at one point in time; negative attributes at another; leads to innacurate overgeneralizations	Social comparison continues, although less overt	Compartmentalized attention to internalization of different standards and opinions of those in different relational contexts
Middle adolescence	Further differentiation of attributes associated with different roles and relational contexts	Initial links between single abstractions, often opposing attributes; cognitive conflict caused by seemingly contradictory characteristics; concern over which reflect one's true self	Simultaneous recognition of positive and negative attributes; instability leading to confusion and inaccuracies	Comparisons with significant others in different relational contexts; personal fable	Awareness that the differing standards and opinions of others represent conflicting self-guides, leading to confusion over self-evaluation and vacillation with regard to behavior; imaginary audience
Late adolescence	Normalization of different role-related attributes; reflecting personal beliefs, values, and moral standards; interest in future selves	Higher-order abstractions that meaningfully integrate single abstractions and resolve inconsistencies, conflict	More balanced, stable view of both positive and negative attributes; greater accuracy; acceptance of limitations	Social comparison diminishes as comparisons with one's own ideals increase	Selection among alternative self-guides; construction of one's own self-standards that govern personal choices; creation of one's own ideals toward which the self aspires

relational development, very young children can place themselves in the same *category* as the parent who shares their gender, which forms an initial basis for *identification* with that parent. For example, the young boy can evaluate his overt behavior with regard to the question: "Am I doing what Daddy is doing?" Attempts to match that behavior, as well as cultural ideals concerning gender-appropriate behavior, will determine which attributes become incorporated into the young child's self-definition. Thus one observes the influence of the socializing environment on the self.

Higgins (1991) has noted that at the interrelational stage, young children can also form structures that allow them to detect the fact that their behavior evokes a reaction in caregivers, which in turn causes psychological reactions in themselves. These experiences shape the self to the extent that the child chooses to engage in behaviors designed to please the parents. Stipek, Recchia, and McClintic (1992), in a laboratory study, have provided empirical evidence for this observation, demonstrating that slightly before the age of 2, children begin to anticipate adult reactions, seeking positive responses to their successes and attempting to avoid negative responses to failure. At this age, they also find that young children show rudimentary appreciation for adult standards by turning away from adults and hunching their shoulders in the face of failures (see also Kagan, 1984, who has reported similar distress reactions). Although young children are beginning to recognize that their behavior has an impact on others, their I-self cannot yet evaluate their Me-self, consistent with the first stage of Selman's (1980) developmental model of self-awareness.

Early to Middle Childhood (Approximately Ages 5–7)

At the next level, children show some abilities to intercoordinate concepts that were previously compartmentalized (Case, 1985; Fischer, 1980). For example, they can form a category or representational *set* that relates a number of their competencies (good at running, jumping, climbing) to one another. Of particular interest are the structures that Fischer (1980) labels as "representational mappings," a level that was missing in earlier de-

velopmental models. Mappings represent links that are unidirectional or nonreversible. Thus representations are linked or mapped onto one another. One very common type of mapping involves a link in the form of *opposites*. For example, in the domain of physical concepts, children can oppose up and down, taller and shorter, thinner and wider, although they cannot yet demonstrate the reversible operation required for conservation. Educational instruction, as well as television programming (e.g., *Sesame Street*), serve to facilitate the detection and utilization of such opposites.

With regard to descriptions of self and other, the ability to oppose attributes perceived as "good" and "bad" (e.g., "nice" vs. "mean," "smart" vs. "dumb") is especially salient (Fischer, Shaver, & Carnochan, 1990; Harter, 1986b; Ruble & Dweck, 1995). Given that "good" is defined as the opposite of "bad" and that the young child continues to identify self-attributes as positive, such a cognitive construction precludes the young child from acknowledging his or her negative characteristics (although *others* may be perceived as bad). Thus the child overdifferentiates good and bad. The very structure of such mappings, therefore, results in the unidimensional or all-or-none thinking that typically leads to self-descriptions that remain laden with virtuosity. (In child-rearing situations involving harsh discipline for misbehavior, or for a subset of children with very negative socialization histories involving abuse, maltreatment, or neglect, children may at times conclude that they are *all bad*, an unfortunate liability at this stage for such children. However, the underlying structure is the same, namely a mapping in the form of opposites that results in all-or-none, unidimensional thinking.) In Case's (1992) theory and its application to the self (Griffin, 1992), similar structures are posited. In fact, this stage is labelled "unidimensional" thinking. Evidence reveals that although children at this level can develop representational sets or categories for self-attributes and self-emotions, they cannot as yet integrate attributes or affects of opposing valence, for example, smart versus dumb (Harter, 1986b), nice versus mean (Fischer et al., 1984), or happy versus sad (Harter & Buddin, 1987).

Higgins (1991) has moved beyond a consideration of the structural features of self-descriptors at this age level in examining how an increasing cognitive appreciation for the perspective of *others* influences self-development. The relational structures of this level allow the child to realize that socializing agents have a particular *viewpoint* (not merely a reaction) toward them and their behavior. As Selman (1980) has observed, the improved perspective-taking skills at this age permit the child to realize that others are actively *evaluating* the self, although they have not yet internalized these evaluations sufficiently to evaluate the self independently. Nevertheless, as Higgins argues, the viewpoints of others begin to function as "self-guides" as the child comes to identify further with what they perceive socializing agents expect of the self. These self-guides function to aid children in the regulation of their behavior. The findings of Stipek and colleagues (1992) provide direct evidence that these processes begin to be observed shortly after the age of 3.

With regard to the interaction between cognitive-developmental level and the socializing environment, there are some advances with regard to the ability to utilize social comparison information, although there are also limitations. Frey and Ruble (1985, 1990), as well as Suls and Sanders (1982), have provided evidence that children first focus on *temporal* comparisons (how I am performing now, compared with when I was younger) rather than comparisons with age-mates. Such temporal comparisons are particularly gratifying given the rapid skill development at this age level, and therefore such comparisons contribute to the positive self-evaluations that typically persist at this age level. Evidence (see Ruble & Frey, 1991) now reveals that younger children do engage in certain forms of social comparison; however, it is directed toward different goals than for older children. For example, young children use such information to determine if they have received their fair share of rewards, rather than for purposes of self-evaluation.

Middle to Late Childhood
(Approximately Ages 8–11)

The major advance of this age period is the ability to coordinate self-representations that were previously differentiated or considered to be opposites. In Case's (1985, 1992) theory, this level is labeled "bidimensional" thought. In identifying similar structures, Fischer (1980) labels this stage as "representational systems." Siegler's (1991) strategy construction processes at this level also include higher order generalizations of features previously compartmentalized. These frameworks lead to the expectation, supported by findings (see Harter, 1999), that the child is capable of forming higher order concepts, namely trait labels, based on the integration of more specific behavioral features of the self. Thus the higher order generalization that one is smart integrates observations of success in both English and social studies. Similarly, the child could construct a hierarchy for the construct "dumb," coordinating perceptions of lack of ability in mathematics and in science. In the domain of social relationships, the self can be viewed as both rowdy (with close friends and with kids on the bus) and shy (around someone they don't know and with someone who is more competent). Thus concepts previously viewed as opposing can now be integrated, leading to both positive and *negative* self-evaluations.

Such bidimensional thought is applied to emotion concepts, as well, as a growing number of empirical studies indicate (Carroll & Steward, 1984; Donaldson & Westerman, 1986; Fischer et al., 1990; Gnepp, McKee, & Domanic, 1987; Harris, 1983; Harris, Olthof, & Meerum-Terwogt, 1981; Harter, 1986b; Harter & Buddin, 1987; Reissland, 1985). Thus one can develop a representational system by integrating *happy* (when one is playing sports) with *sad* (when my efforts on the team are not successful). With the emerging ability to integrate positive and negative concepts about the self, the child is much less likely to engage in the type of all-or-none thinking observed in the previous stages, in which typically only one's positive attributes were touted. As a result, self-descriptions begin to represent a more balanced presentation of one's abilities in conjunction with one's limitations, perceptions that are likely to be more veridical with others' views of the self.

For Case (1985, 1992), the emergence of these structures partially depends on experiences in which two lower order features, for example, perceptions of smartness and dumbness, are activated simultaneously or in rapid sequence. Thus events that make each of these attributes salient will foster such bidimensional structures. Moreover, Case emphasizes the general role of *practice*. Repeated exposure to such events (e.g., "On my report card I got an A in English but only a C+ in Math") should reinforce this type of intercoordination. One can imagine scenarios in which there would be little environmental support for such integration. For example, children who are severely abused typically develop negative self-perceptions that not only lead them to feel unworthy and unlovable but to experience a profound sense of inner badness, as if they were inherently "rotten to the core," as revealed in clinical observations (Briere, 1992; Harter, 1999; Herman, 1992; Terr, 1990; Westen, 1993), as well as research (Fischer & Ayoub, 1994). In abusing environments, family members typically offer and continue to reinforce negative evaluations of the child that are then incorporated into the child's self-portrait. As a result, there may be little scaffolding for the kind of self-structure that would allow the child to develop, as well as integrate, both positive and negative self-evaluations. Moreover, negative self-evaluations that become *automatized* (Siegler, 1991) are even more resistant to change.

The more balanced view of self, in which both positive and negative attributes of the self are acknowledged, is also fostered by social comparison. A number of studies conducted in the 1970s and early 1980s (reviewed in Frey & Ruble, 1990; Ruble & Frey, 1991) have presented evidence that it is not until middle childhood that one could utilize comparisons with others as a barometer of the skills and attributes of the self (see also Damon & Hart, 1988). From a cognitive developmental perspective, the ability to use social comparison information toward the goal of *self-evaluation* requires that children compare their own performance with that of another simultaneously, a skill that is not sufficiently developed at younger ages (see also Moretti & Higgins, 1990). Age stratification in school stimulates greater attention to individual differences between age-mates (Mack, 1983). The primary motive for children in this age period to utilize social comparison is for personal competence assessment. Moreover, with increasing age, children shift from more conspicuous forms of social comparison to more subtle avenues as they become more aware of the negative social consequences of overt forms, for example, being accused of boasting about their superior performance (Pomerantz, Ruble, Frey, & Greulich, 1995).

The ability to utilize social comparison information for the purpose of self-evaluation is founded on cognitive developmental advances and is supported by the socializing environment. However, it also ushers in potential liabilities, as others have cogently observed (Maccoby, 1980; Moretti & Higgins, 1990), contributing to individual differences in self-evaluation. With the emergence of the ability to rank order the performance of other students in the class, all but the most competent children will fall short. Jacobs (1983) has noted that this is a major liability for children with learning disabilities. Other research supports this observation in that learning-disabled students who were mainstreamed were found to have more negative perceptions of their scholastic competence than those in self-contained classrooms restricted only to learning-disabled students (Renick & Harter, 1988). Thus the very ability and penchant to compare the self with others makes one's self-concept vulnerable in those domains that are valued (e.g., scholastic competence, athletic prowess, and peer popularity). Moreover, to the extent that negative self-evaluations are now organized as relatively stable dispositional *traits* (rather than mere behaviors), they may be more resistant to disconfirmation.

The advances of this period also have implications for those looking-glass-self processes that require the ability to incorporate the opinions of significant others. For Higgins (1991), the newfound cognitive ability to form dispositional traits leads children to construct a more general evaluation of themselves as *persons*. This observation is consistent with my own empirical work demonstrating that the concept of global self-worth or self-esteem—namely, how much one likes oneself as a person—does not emerge until middle childhood (Harter, 1990b). Higgins has further observed that the child can now focus on the "type of person" that others desire or expect him or her to be. Further cognitive acquisitions at this age allow the child to incorporate these expectations into self-guides that become even more internalized. Thus, as Selman (1980) also notes, the child incorporates both the standards and opinions of significant others, allowing the I-self to directly evaluate the Me-self.

Early Adolescence (Approximately Ages 12–14)

During this period, the young adolescent becomes capable of thinking abstractly (Case, 1985; Fischer, 1980; Flavell, 1985; Harter, 1983; Higgins, 1991). The ability to construct abstractions can be applied to inanimate features of one's world, as well as to self and others (see Table 30.2). This cognitive advance represents further intercoordination in that now trait labels are integrated into abstractions. For example, one may construct an abstraction of the self as *intelligent* by combining such traits as *smart* and *creative*. One also may create an abstraction that oneself is an "airhead," given situations in which one feels dumb and uncreative. Similarly, one may construct abstractions that one is an extrovert (integrating the traits of being rowdy and talkative), as well as that one is an introvert in certain situations (when one is shy and quiet). With regard to emotion concepts, one can be depressed (combining *sad* and *mad*), as well as cheerful (combining *happy* and *excited*). With regard to the *content* of these abstractions, Damon and Hart (1988) report that in the self-portraits of young adolescents, interpersonal attributes and social skills that influence interactions with others or one's social appeal are typically quite salient.

From a traditional Piagetian perspective, the formal operational skills that emerge during this age period should not only usher in abstract thinking but should also equip the adolescent with the tools to construct a formal, hypothetico-deductive theory (Piaget, 1960). Such a theory, be it about physical phenomena in the universe or about psychological attributes of the self, should meet certain criteria, for example, internal consistency, and should represent an integrated nomological network of postulates

(Epstein, 1973). However, a neo-Piagetian analysis indicates that the newfound abstract representations are compartmentalized; that is, they are quite distinct from one another (Case, 1985; Fischer, 1980; Harter, 1990a; Higgins, 1991). For Fischer (1980), they are overdifferentiated from one another because the young adolescent lacks "cognitive control" over such abstractions and therefore can think about them only as isolated self-attributes. However, this inability to integrate seemingly contradictory characteristics of the self (*intelligent* vs. *airhead, extrovert* vs. *introvert, depressed* vs. *cheerful*) has the psychological advantage of sparing the adolescent conflict over opposing attributes in one's self-theory (Harter & Monsour, 1992). Increased differentiation functions as a cognitive buffer, reducing the possibility that negative attributes in one sphere may spread or generalize to another sphere (see Higgins, 1991; Linville, 1987; Simmons & Blyth, 1987).

Middle Adolescence (Approximately Ages 15–16)

During this period, further cognitive links are forged (Case, 1985; Fischer, 1980) in that the teenager can now begin to relate one abstraction to another (e.g., one can recognize that it is possible to be both intelligent and an airhead, both an extrovert and an introvert, both cheerful and depressed). Within Fischerian theory, these abstract "mappings" bear features in common with the earlier representational mappings in that such links often take the form of opposites. However, the mapping structure is an immature form of relating two abstract concepts to one another in that one cannot yet integrate such self-representations in a manner that would resolve the apparent contradiction. Thus, at the level of abstract mappings, the adolescent still does not possess the cognitive tools necessary to construct an integrated theory of self in which the postulates, namely, personal attributes, are internally consistent. Moreover, an awareness of the opposites within one's self-portrait causes considerable intrapsychic conflict, confusion, and distress (Fischer et al., 1990; Harter & Monsour, 1992; Higgins, 1991), given the inability to coordinate these seeming contradictions. Mappings also lead to instability in the self-portrait, another form of lack of cognitive control. As a result, adolescents at this stage may frequently demonstrate all-or-none thinking (Harter, 1990b), vacillating from one extreme to the other (e.g., they may view themselves as brilliant at one point in time and a total airhead at another).

A major contextual factor contributing to the contradictions experienced at this age level involves socialization pressure to develop different selves in different roles or relationships (Erikson, 1968; Grotevant & Cooper, 1986; Hill & Holmbeck, 1986; Rosenberg, 1986). Such pressures provide a backdrop for the emergence of the "conflict of the different Me's" (James, 1890). Several studies have provided evidence that the self-descriptions of adolescents vary across different roles, for example, self with parents, close friends, romantic partners, and classmates (Gecas, 1972; Griffin, Chassin, & Young, 1981; Hart, 1988; Harter & Monsour, 1992; Rosenberg, 1986). Conflicts between opposing attributes in these different relational contexts have been found to be particularly problematic for adolescents at this age, in comparison with attributes within a role (Harter, Bresnick, Bouchey, & Whitesell, 1997). Higgins (1991) describes this new vulnerability in terms of conflicting *self-guides* across different roles, as adolescents attempt to meet the incompatible expectations of parents versus peers. Such discrepancies have been found to produce confusion, uncertainty, and indecision with regard to self-regulation and self-evaluation, consistent with the findings reported previously.

The vulnerability of this period is exacerbated by the ability to reflect on one's thinking and to ponder internal events, which brings about a dramatic increase in introspection (see Broughton, 1978; Erikson, 1968; Harter, 1990b; Rosenberg, 1979). In their search for a coherent self, adolescents in this age period are often morbidly preoccupied with how they appear in the eyes of others (see also Elkind, 1967; Lapsley & Rice, 1988). Such self-consciousness includes the search for "who I am," as the adolescent seeks to establish self-boundaries and to more clearly sort out the multiple "Me's" that provide for a very crowded self-landscape. The creation of a coherent self-portrait also shifts to a larger canvas during this and the subsequent period, in which broad brushstrokes must come to define the social, occupational, religious, and political *identities* that one will assume.

Late Adolescence

The cognitive advances during this period involve the construction of higher order abstractions that represent the meaningful intercoordination of single abstractions. As such, they should provide the older adolescent with new cognitive solutions for developing a more integrated theory of self. Neo-Piagetians (see Case, 1985; Fischer, 1980) observe that developmental acquisitions at these higher levels typically require greater scaffolding by the social environment in the form of support, instruction, and so forth, in order for individuals to function at their optimal levels. If these new skills are fostered, they should aid the adolescent in integrating opposing attributes in a manner that does not produce conflict or distress. For example, one could integrate one's extraversion and introversion by constructing the higher order abstraction that one is "flexible" across different social situations. One may integrate one's tendencies to be both intelligent and an airhead under the higher order abstraction of "inconsistent." Being both cheerful and depressed could similarly be coordinated under the rubric of "moody." Such higher order abstractions provide self-labels that bring meaning and therefore legitimacy to what formerly appeared to be troublesome contradictions within the self.

Findings (Harter & Monsour, 1992; Harter et al., 1997) indicate that not only do older adolescents utilize these strategies but that they also seek to normalize inconsistency by asserting that it would be strange and undesirable to display the same attributes across different relational contexts. Higgins (1991) has described the reduction in conflict as a function of further levels of internalization. Thus adolescents come to construct their *own* standards that represent an integration of a complex array of alternative self-guides that become less tied to their social origins. These findings are consistent with those of Damon and Hart (1988), who have reported that in late adolescence the self is described in terms of an organized system of beliefs and values that include dimensions of personal choice and moral standards.

The Distinction between Global and Domain-Specific Self-Evaluations

The previous sections focused on more normative developmental processes that define changes in the structure, content, and valence of self-representations across childhood and adolescence. Emphasis now shifts to models and methods for examining *individual differences* in the valence of self-evaluations, asking the question of why some children and adolescents view the self favorably, whereas others report very unfavorable descriptions of self. In addressing this question, it is first necessary to distinguish between *global* perceptions of one's worth as a person (self-esteem or self-worth) and more *domain*-specific self-concepts (see Harter, 1999). A variety of multidimensional models have emerged in recent years, demonstrating that self-evaluations are multifaceted and that judgments will vary tremendously across domains, providing a *profile* of self-evaluations for given individuals (see Bracken, 1996; Harter, 1982, 1985, 1990b, 1993, 1999; Hattie, 1992; Marsh, 1986, 1987, 1993; Marsh & Hattie, 1996; Mullener & Laird, 1971; Oosterwegel & Oppenheimer, 1993; Shavelson & Marsh, 1986).

However, in each of these multidimensional models, the construct of global self-esteem or self-worth has also been retained. This construct is *not* assessed by aggregating the domain-specific scores but rather is tapped by its own set of items asking about how much one likes oneself overall as a person, values one's worth, and so forth. Of particular interest is the question of whether some domain-specific self-evaluations contribute more heavily to the prediction of global self-esteem than do others. From a developmental perspective, two features are noteworthy. The ability to make judgments of one's worth as a person does not emerge until middle childhood. Younger children are able to make judgments of their competence or adequacy in particular domains, although their self-evaluations are not as

clearly differentiated (Harter & Pike, 1984). However, they do not possess a conscious, verbalizable concept of their overall self-esteem. Young children do *exude* a sense of their self-esteem, and these behavioral manifestations (e.g., displays of confidence, exploration) can be reliably rated by observers (Haltiwanger, 1989; Harter, 1999).

Secondly, the number of domains that can be differentiated increases with development across the periods of early childhood, middle and late childhood, adolescence, and adulthood (see Harter, 1999, for a listing of the specific domains at each developmental period). For example, the Self-Perception Profile for Children (Harter, 1985) taps five specific domains: Scholastic Competence, Athletic Competence, Peer Likability, Physical Appearance, and Behavioral Conduct, in addition to Global Self-Worth. The Self-Perception Profile for Adolescents (Harter, 1988) adds three new domains: Close Friendship, Romantic Appeal, and Job Competence. Additional domains are included on the Self-Perception Profile for College Students (Neemann & Harter, 1987) and the Self-Perception Profile for Adults (Messer & Harter, 1989), which can be found in Harter (1999). At every developmental level, preliminary interviews and focus groups were conducted to determine the domains that the majority felt were most salient.

Another popular series of multidimensional instruments has been developed by Marsh and Hattie (1996). Their self-description questionnaires tap domains appropriate for children, adolescents, and young adults, in addition to assessing general self-concept. The Multidimensional Self-Concept Scale developed by Bracken (1992, 1996) is the most recent such measure. For a comprehensive review of these and other self-concept measures, see Keith and Bracken (1996). The Harter and Marsh scales have also been reviewed by Wylie (1989). These instruments have been developed primarily for children and adolescents in Western, industrialized countries. Elsewhere (Harter, 1999), I have cautioned against using these measures in Eastern countries such as China, Japan, and Korea, where the findings reveal that for several reasons they are not culturally appropriate. Of particular interest in countries in which the scale has excellent psychometric properties (the United States, Canada, England, France, Australia, Greece, Netherlands, Spain, Italy, Israel) are the very robust gender differences obtained. Females report significantly more negative self-perceptions in the areas of Physical Appearance and Athletic Competence (see Harter, 1999, for interpretations).

The Jamesian Discrepancy Model of Self-Esteem

The fact that an individual starting in middle childhood can make both global judgments of his/her worth as a person, as well as domain-specific self-evaluations, is very relevant to James's (1892) theory of the *antecedents* of self-esteem. James emphasized the need to consider perceptions of success in relation to pretensions, namely, aspirations or intentions to be a success across the domains of one's life. For James, the congruence or the discrepancy between these two dimensions were critical in that they represented the determinants of one's level of global self-esteem. According to this formulation, individuals do not scrutinize their every action or attribute; rather, they focus primarily on their perceived adequacy in domains in which they have aspirations to succeed. Thus the individual who perceives the self positively in domains in which he or she aspires to excel will have high self-esteem. Those who fall short of their ideals, creating a discrepancy between perceived successes and their pretensions, will experience low self-esteem.

It is critical to appreciate that, from a Jamesian perspective, inadequacy in domains deemed unimportant to the self should not adversely affect self-esteem. For example, an individual may judge the self not to be athletic. However, if athletic prowess is not an aspiration, then self-esteem will not be negatively affected. Thus the individual with high self-esteem is able to *discount* the importance of domains in which he or she is not competent, whereas the individual with low self-esteem appears unable to devalue success in domains of inadequacy.

Several years ago, both Rosenberg (1979) and Tesser and colleagues (see Tesser, 1980, 1988) provided initial documentation of this formulation among adolescents and adults, respectively. More recently (see Harter, 1990b, 1999), I have documented the utility of this model for older children, adolescents, college students, and adults in the world of work and family. I have employed several data-analytic strategies, each of which tells the same story, and have constructed actual discrepancy scores between importance ratings and competence judgments in each domain. Averaging these across domains, initially, I have determined that the larger the discrepancy, that is, the more one's importance ratings exceed one's perceived adequacy or competence, the lower one's self-worth. Across numerous studies, these correlations typically range from .55 to .72. Employing a second procedure, in which I have examined self-worth as a function of the average absolute competence/adequacy judgments for *only* those domains rated very important or sort of important, a systematic, linear relationship emerges (see Figure 30.1). Thus relatively low self-worth is reported for those acknowledging that they lack competence or adequacy in domains for which they have aspirations of success, namely, those who are unable to discount the importance of domains in which they feel inadequate. As perceived success in domains deemed important increases across groups, parallel gains in self-worth are reported. Employing this second strategy, we find that the relationship between competence in important domains and self-worth ($r = .70$) far exceeds the correlation between competence in unimportant domains and self-worth ($r = .30$), a difference that would be predicted from a Jamesian perspective.

Third, an even more direct test of the role of importance, including the discounting process, involves a comparison of the importance attached to domains in which individuals feel incompetent or inadequate, among groups with high and low self-worth. According to James (1892), although individuals with high self-worth may and do have domains in which they feel inadequate, they should be able to discount the importance of these domains. In contrast, individuals with low self-worth should give higher ratings of importance to domains in which they feel inadequate. Thus we examined importance ratings for

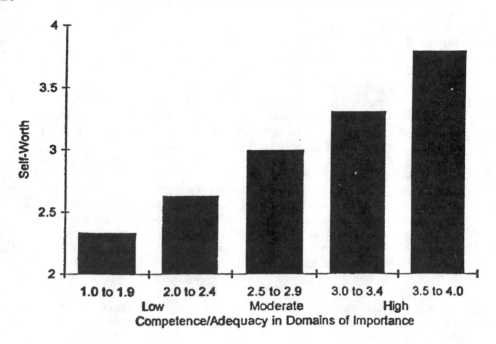

FIGURE 30.1. Self-worth as a function of level of competence/adequacy in important domains.

only those areas in which both participants with low and with high self-worth reported that they felt incompetent or inadequate. To examine the generality of this principle, we included normally achieving, learning-disabled, and behaviorally disordered groups of adolescents (Harter, Whitesell, & Junkin, 1999). We first identified individuals with high and low self-worth within each educational group. After selecting only those domains in which members of both groups indicated that they felt incompetent or inadequate, we examined the *importance ratings* attached to those domains.

Our findings directly supported the Jamesian hypothesis. Adolescents with high self-worth were better able to discount the importance of domains in which they reported weaknesses; that is, their importance scores were significantly ($p < .0001$) lower than the importance scores of the adolescents with low self-worth. Moreover, this pattern was observed across all three types of students. Thus these findings provide further confirmation for the contention that the inability to discount the importance of areas in which one reports personal limitations is a characteristic of individuals with low self-worth.

In a fourth procedure (described in detail in Harter, 1999), we wrote vignettes in which older children were presented with a situation in which a domain (the participant's own worst domain) was considered to be very important to the story child, who eventually learned that he or she was not very competent in that arena. Participants were asked to rate how important the domain was now, given the story child's inadequacy. Findings revealed a systematic pattern for children with high self-esteem to discount the importance of that domain, whereas the children with low self-esteem continued to tout the importance of domains of incompetence. (Elsewhere [Harter, 1999], I have described the clinical implications of taking importance into account in intervention efforts to enhance the self-esteem of individuals who do not value themselves as persons.)

This package of findings suggests that there may be different routes to high self-esteem. One may first evaluate one's competencies and then place importance on those domains in which they feel that they are adequate, discounting the importance of those in which they perceive limitations. Alternatively, one may first establish a hierarchy of importance and attempt to develop competencies in domains deemed most critical. Both processes could be operative across different individuals. To date, findings do not speak directly to these processes; however, this would be an important area for further research. Finally, although the different procedural approaches we have employed support James's formulation, the value of considering importance ratings in the prediction of self-esteem is controversial (see Harter, 1999; Marsh, 1986, 1993; Marsh & Hattie, 1996, for these arguments.)

Are Some Domains More Predictive of Global Self-Worth Than Others?

The answer is a resounding "yes," and the findings are highly consistent across countries in which the scales have excellent psychometric properties. Physical appearance correlates most highly with global self-worth (average *r* of .64), athletic competence consistently bears the lowest relationship (average *r* of .31), and falling in between are scholastic competence, social acceptance, and behavioral conduct (average correlations are from .45 to .48). The values are obtained normatively at every developmental level and are also obtained in other populations (learning disabled, gifted, children in Special Olympics) in which one might expect other domains to be more highly correlated, given their salience (e.g., scholastic competence for the first two groups and athletic competence for the third).

Why should appearance (one's outer self) be so highly related to global self-worth (one's inner self)? Clearly, a critical contributing factor involves the emphasis that contemporary society places on appearance at every age (see Harter, 1999, in which this literature is reviewed). Another possibility is that one's outer self is always on display for others, as well as the self, to observe. In contrast, in other domains one has more control over whether, when, and how personal adequacy will be revealed. Of particular interest is the directionality of this relationship. When asked which comes first, 60% of adolescents report that appearance comes first, that is, they are basing their self-worth on how they think they look. The remainder report the opposite directionality, namely, how much they value themselves as persons affects how attractive they think they are. The first directionality, basing one's self-worth on how one thinks one looks, is particularly pernicious for females, whose perceptions of attractiveness are significantly lower than for males. These females not only report much more negative evaluations of their looks but also lower self-worth (see Harter, 1999, for interpretations). Interventions to reverse the directionality, albeit difficult in this society, should have positive benefits.

Social Sources of Individual Differences in Self-Evaluation

As observed in the introduction, several historical scholars—James Mark Baldwin (1897), Charles Horton Cooley (1902), and George Herbert Mead (1925, 1934)—set the conceptual stage on which the drama of the self in social interaction was enacted. For these *symbolic interactionists*, the self was primarily a social construction crafted through linguistic exchanges (i.e., symbolic interactions) with others. Thus the personal self develops in the crucible of interpersonal relationships with significant others. Recently, there has been a resurgence of interest in these formulations that emphasized how interactive processes, initially with caregivers, profoundly shape the developing self (see Bretherton, 1991; Case, 1992; Cicchetti, 1990; Harter, 1998; Sroufe, 1990). These interactions represent experiences by the self as subject that in turn influence the content of the Me-self.

Of particular interest in this chapter is how the messages of approval or disapproval that caregivers communicate to the child are incorporated into the child's sense of worth as a person. Thus the focus is on those processes through which the child comes to adopt the *opinions* that significant others are perceived to hold toward the self, that is, reflected appraisals that come to define one's sense of self as a person. Each of the symbolic interactionists assumed an implicit internalization process through which the child came to adopt and eventually to own personally the initial values and opinions of significant others. Cooley (1902), in his "looking-glass-self" formulation, was perhaps most explicit in observing that significant others constituted social mirrors into which the child gazes in order to detect his or her opinions toward the self. These perceived opinions, in turn, are incorporated into the evaluation of one's worth as a person. For Mead (1925), the attitudes of different significant others toward the self were psychologically averaged across these individuals, resulting in the "generalized other," which represented their shared perspective on the self.

Although the symbolic interactionists pointed to critical processes in the normative construction of the self, they did not alert us to the fact that self-development, so dependent on social interactions, could go awry. Caregivers who provide nurturance, approval, and support that is positive will provoke the child to internalize favorable images of self. However, caregivers lacking in nurturance, encouragement, and approval, as well as socializing agents who are rejecting or punitive, will produce children with very negative self-evaluations. Liabilities also emerge for those who remain drawn like a magnet to the social mirror as a source of self-evaluation, seemingly unable to incorporate the standards and opinions of others in a personal sense of self that guides behavior.

In the previous section, evidence for James's model of the antecedents of global self-worth or esteem was presented. It was demonstrated that perceptions of competence or adequacy in domains deemed important were a powerful predictor of self-worth. However, approval from significant others represents another critical source of self-worth for the developing child and adolescent. James's explanation is not incompatible with a looking-glass-self model of self-worth; it is merely incomplete. Thus evidence for an additive model, in which both Jamesian and looking-glass-self processes combine to produce an individual's level of self-worth, is presented.

The capacities to engage in looking-glass-self processes, as well as to construct working models of self, do not emerge at one particular point in development but evolve gradually over the course of childhood. Rudimentary skills begin to appear at about 2 years of age. Stipek and colleagues (1992)

report that, toward the goal of anticipating positive parental responses and avoiding negative reactions, 2-year-olds begin to develop an appreciation for parental standards. In addition, they show some initial ability to evaluate whether they have met these standards. Thereafter, children gradually begin to internalize the standards of parents, allowing them to engage in self-evaluation independent of adults' reactions. Further contributing to looking-glass-self processes is the increasing ability throughout childhood to appreciate the parents' evaluative perspective toward the self. Through increasing perspective-taking skills, children come to recognize not only that parents have standards that they expect to be met but also that parents form an evaluative opinion about the child (Higgins, 1991; Leahy & Shirk, 1985; Oosterwegel & Oppenheimer, 1993; Selman, 1980). Through these processes, the I-self gradually becomes capable of evaluating the Me-self.

The Influence of Different Sources of Approval on Self-Worth

Based on considerable evidence (see Harter, 1999), there is a general consensus of opinion that support from significant others is a critical determinant of global self-worth or self-esteem. However, a more differentiated picture is beginning to emerge with regard to support from different sources of support—for example, parents versus peers—in either more public or more private relational contexts. From a looking-glass-self perspective, one can ask the question: "Mirror, mirror, on the wall, whose opinion is the most critical of all?"

In my own research documenting the looking-glass-self formulation, I have broadened the examination of the *sources* of approval to whom children turn. For older children and adolescents, I have identified four sources of potential support: parents, teachers, classmates, and close friends. I then created self-report items tapping the extent to which one feels that these others approve of or value the self. Through the construction of such items, I have been able to examine directly the link between the perceived regard from others and the perceived regard for the self (i.e., global self-worth).

Across numerous studies with older children and adolescents, as well as with college students and adults in the world of work and family, I have found that the correlations between perceived support from significant others and self-worth range from .50 to .65 (Harter, 1990b, 1993). As anticipated from Cooley's (1902) model, those with the lowest levels of support report the lowest self-worth, those with moderate support have moderate levels of self-worth, and those receiving the most support hold the self in the highest regard. Among the four sources of support that we have examined, we have repeatedly demonstrated that for older children and adolescents, perceived classmate and parent approval are the best predictors. Thus, Cooley's looking-glass-self model on the origins of self-worth appears to be clearly documented, with regard to the link between one's perceptions of the approval of others and one's sense of worth as a person.

That said, for Cooley's looking-glass-self processes to be most adaptive, children should come to *internalize* the attitudes of others to the extent that they are no longer directly dependent on such evaluations. In another strand of research (Harter, Stocker, & Robinson, 1996), we addressed the issue of the directionality of the link between approval and self-worth. We asked adolescents to indicate whether they consciously *endorsed* the looking-glass-self formulation ("if others approve of me then I will value myself as a person") or the opposite metatheory ("if I first value myself as a person then others will approve of me"). Findings revealed a number of liabilities for those "looking-glass-self" students who endorsed the first option. They reported lower levels of approval, more fluctuating approval, lower levels of self-esteem, and more fluctuating self-esteem. In addition, teachers blind to students' directionality orientation reported that the first group of students were more socially distractible. From all of our findings, we have concluded that during childhood, the directionality of approval and self-worth is, as Cooley (1902) argued, from approval to self-worth. However, those who come to *internalize* these initially external social evaluations such that their sense of self-worth *precedes* their perceptions of approval have the healthier psychological outcomes.

To date, we have not examined whether *others'* reports of the approval they provide predict self-worth. Interestingly, the literature suggests that the link between people's self-perceptions and how they are actually viewed by others is weak (Juhasz, 1992; Kenny, 1988; Shrauger & Schoeneman, 1979). Moreover, perceptions of support have been found to be more predictive of self-evaluations than have more objective indices of support (Berndt & Burgy, 1996; Felson, 1993; John & Robbins, 1994; Rosenberg, 1979; Shrauger & Schoeneman, 1979). Thus, as Rosenberg concluded, "We are more or less unconsciously seeing ourselves as we *think* others, who are important to us and whose opinion we trust, see us" (1979, p. 97).

An Additive Model of the Determinants of Self-Worth

Our findings reveal that both James's (1892) and Cooley's (1902) formulations, taken together, provide a powerful explanation for the level of self-worth displayed by older children and adolescents (Harter, 1987, 1990b). As can be seen in Figure 30.2, the effects of these two determinants are additive. At each level of social support (representing the average of classmate and parental approval), greater competence in domains of importance leads to higher self-worth. Similarly, at each level of competence in domains of importance, the more support one garners from classmates and parents, the higher one's self-worth. Those individuals with the lowest self-worth, therefore, are those who report both incompetence in domains of importance and the absence of supportive approval from others. Those with the highest self-worth report the highest levels of competence in domains of importance, as well as the highest level of parental and peer support.

More recently, we have become interested in the importance attached to support from different sources; that is, just as competence in domains deemed important is critical to James's formulation, by the same logic, might not support from sources judged to be important be a better predictor of self-worth than support alone? There may be very legitimate reasons why children would discount the importance of support from

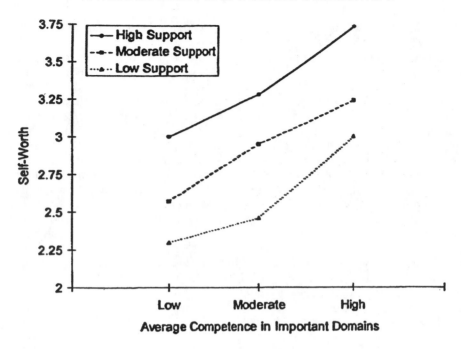

FIGURE 30.2. Additive effects of competence/adequacy in domains of importance and social support on self-worth.

particular sources, particularly if it were not forthcoming. As discussed earlier, there are a number of reasons why children may not be able to garner the support of significant others. To address this issue, we constructed items tapping the importance of approval or acceptance from each of the primary sources in our model (e.g., parents, teachers, and peers). Analogous to our data-analytic strategy in examining James's hypothesis, we have examined the correlations between support from important and from unimportant sources. The pattern of findings is quite similar. We find that support from important sources correlates much more highly with self-worth ($r = .52$) than does support from sources deemed unimportant ($r = .22$). Thus the same processes appear to be operative for both formulations in that importance of success in particular domains and the importance of support from each source both contribute to our understanding of the level of self-worth (Harter, 1999).

The Powerful Link between Self-Worth and Depression

Considerable attention has been devoted to an analysis of the determinants of self-worth in the lives of children and adolescents. Yet why should we be concerned about self-worth unless we can demonstrate that it plays a vital role in individuals' lives and can document the fact that it performs some critical function? The efforts of numerous self-worth researchers may well be misguided if self-worth reduces to an epiphenomenon that has little impact on everyday functioning.

Initially, therefore, attention was directed to the potential *mediational* role of self-worth, in an effort to identify constructs critical to the lives of individuals that self-worth might affect. What are some likely candidates? What outcomes of any significance might self-worth influence? A major candidate is one's *mood* or affect, along the dimension of cheerful to depressed. Recent theory and research has placed increasing emphasis on cognitions that give rise to or accompany depression. Cognitions involving the *self* have found particular favor. There is clear historical precedent for including negative self-evaluations as one of the constellation of symptoms experienced in depression, beginning with Freud's (1917/1968) observations of the low self-esteem displayed by adults suffering from depressive disorders. Those within the psycho-analytic tradition have continued to afford low self-esteem or low self-worth a central role in depression (Bibring, 1953; Blatt, 1974).

In my own studies, I consistently find that among older children and adolescents, self-worth is highly related to affect along a continuum of cheerful to depressed (with correlations ranging from .72 to .80). These findings are consistent with those of other investigators (Battle, 1987; Beck, 1975; Kaslow, Rehm, & Siegel, 1984). Of particular relevance to this chapter is our finding that older children and adolescents within our normative samples who report low self-worth consistently report depressed affect (Harter, 1986b, 1990b, 1993; Renouf & Harter, 1990). Among a clinical sample of inpatient adolescents with psychiatric diagnoses of depression, we have also found a powerful link between self-worth and self-reported depressed affect. Among those reporting depressed affect, 80% also report low self-worth (Harter, Marold, & Whitesell, 1992).

Although it is clear that self-worth or self-esteem is highly correlated with depressive reactions, the directionality of this link cannot be determined through conventional statistical procedures with data collected at one point in time. Moreover, other constructs, namely hopelessness about one's future (see Beck, 1987), reveal that the perceived inability to control the events in one's life is another feature associated with depression (see also Baumeister, 1990; Pfeffer, 1988; Rutter, 1986; Seligman, 1975) and strongly correlated with global self-worth and depressed affect (r's in the .70s in our data). Thus, in our model (see Figure 30.3) we have created a depression–adjustment composite that combined global self-worth, affect/mood (along a continuum of cheerful to depressed), and hope (hopeful to hopeless). We have found strong statistical support for this model in that perceptions of competence/adequacy in certain domains judged more important in the peer culture (physical appearance, likability by peers, athletic competence) are predictive of peer approval support. Conversely, perceptions of adequacy in the domains of scholastic competence and behavioral conduct, rated as more important to parents, are more predictive of parental approval. Thus, although there are direct effects of competence in domains of importance on the depression–adjustment composite, much of the

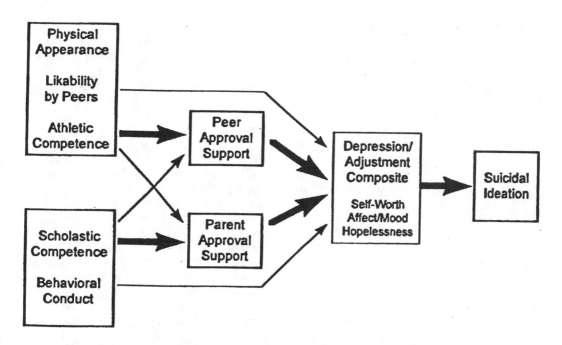

FIGURE 30.3. General model of the predictors of depression/adjustment and suicide.

effect is mediated by approval from peers and parents (Harter, 1999).

Finally, we extended our model to one potential outcome, suicidal ideation. The incidence of suicide among adolescents has tripled in recent decades, leading to efforts to identify the determinants of this major mental health threat to our youth (see Alcohol, Drug Abuse, and Mental Health Administration, 1989; Noam & Borst, 1994; Pfeffer, 1986, 1988). Several broad classes of risk factors implicated in depression and suicidal behaviors have captured the attention of researchers, including biological precursors, epidemiological correlates, and social–psychological stressors. We have been particularly committed to an examination of the third class of risk factors. Evidence to date has revealed a constellation of social–psychological correlates that are predictive of suicidal behavior, including depressed affect, poor self-concept in particular domains, real–ideal discrepancies, low self-worth, hopelessness, and lack of social support (see Baumeister, 1990; Carlson & Cantwell, 1980; Cicchetti & Schneider-Rosen, 1986; Pfeffer, 1986; Rutter, Izard, & Read, 1985).

From a developmental perspective, these particular risk factors become increasingly salient as one moves into adolescence (see Emery, 1983). Self-awareness, self-consciousness, introspectiveness, and preoccupation with one's self-image dramatically increase (see review by Harter, 1990a). Self-worth becomes more vulnerable (Rosenberg, 1986), and adolescents become more aware of the relationship between self-worth, social support, and depressed affect (Harter & Marold, 1993). With regard to the support system, the impact of peer support increases dramatically (Brown, 1990; Savin-Williams & Berndt, 1990). Although young adolescents are beginning to make bids for autonomy from their parents, they are nevertheless struggling to remain connected (Cooper, Grotevant, & Condon, 1983; Grotevant & Cooper, 1986; Steinberg, 1990); thus parent support continues to be critical.

Multiple Pathways to Self-Worth and Its Correlates

The model presented in Figure 30.3 has found considerable and robust support uti-

lizing path-analytic techniques with normative samples of older children and adolescents. However, although theoretically driven models documenting general relations among predictors and outcomes are very useful, they do not speak to the specific precursors of depressive reactions for a given individual. The inspection of the profile of scores for individuals reveals that not all youths who experience low self-worth, depressed affect, and hopelessness report perceived limitations in both predictive clusters of competence/adequacy, namely, those that are more peer salient and more parent salient. Nor do all adolescents report the lack of both peer and parental support. Thus we sought to identify empirically subgroups of adolescents who manifest different patterns of predictors, defined by the components in our model, that represented different pathways to depressive reactions (Harter & Whitesell, 1996). From several normative samples of adolescents, we first identified those who reported the constellation of low self-worth, depressed affect, and hopelessness, namely, adolescents who were experiencing self-reported depressive symptomatology. We then looked for subgroups of individuals whose scores represented different combinations of predictors. These efforts have resulted in the identification of six potential pathways to depression. These patterns of pathways differ in the number of predictors of depression. In the first pattern, all predictors in the general model are relevant.

However, other patterns represented only a subset of these predictors. For example, for some individuals, only the domains of appearance, likability, and athletic competence, coupled with peer support, were predictive of the depression–adjustment composite. For other individuals, the converse was true, in that only perceptions of inadequacy in the domains of scholastic competence and behavioral conduct, coupled with low parent support, were predictive. A complete description of these patterns is beyond the scope of this chapter. Detailed descriptions of these patterns, coupled with clinical examples, are presented in Harter (1999). However, the point of these analyses is to demonstrate that the general model does not necessarily apply to all individuals low or high on the depression–adjustment composite; and for the purposes of intervention, one needs to identify the specific predictors for a given individual.

Extension of the Model in Light of the Profiles of the School Shooters

In the past 5 years we have witnessed tragedy in the schools, as white adolescent males from suburban areas have randomly shot at their classmates, killing anywhere from 2 to 12 of them. An examination of the 11 major school shootings between 1996 and 2001, as reported in the media, reveals commonalities that we have found interesting in light of our model. Many of these youth felt incompetent in the domains that our model identifies, and all experienced not only lack of peer approval but active rejection and humiliation. Some had histories of poor scholastic competence and behavioral conduct, and some experienced parental rejection or neglect. Many were reported to have low self-esteem, and some had been diagnosed as depressed, with suicidal intentions. All were obviously violent at the time of the shooting event, although few had histories of violence. Based on these observations, we expanded our model to include *anger* as an affect (in addition to depressed affect in the original model) and *violent* ideation, as well as suicidal ideation (in the original model). Preliminary findings (Low & Harter, 2001a) have revealed that the model fits well with these additions and that, not surprisingly, given the literature on the comorbidity of internalizing and externalizing symptoms (Achenbach & Edelbrock, 1983; Curran, 1987; Deffenbacher & Swaim, 1999; Gispert, Davis, Marsh, & Wheeler, 1987; Khan, 1987; Renouf & Harter, 1990; Rutter, 1987), violent and suicidal ideation correlate ($r = .55$). Adolescents also responded to vignettes (see Harter, 1999) in which we simulated the kinds of events that the actual school shooters experienced (e.g., teased or bullied by teens, spurned by a romantic interest, put down by a teacher). Participants then were asked to report their levels of humiliation, feelings of unfairness, anger at the perpetrator, blame of the perpetrator, depression, difficulty of getting the event out of their minds, as well as the type of response that this

would provoke in them (from passivity to active violent ideation). Somewhat surprisingly, humiliation has received little attention in the literature on emotion, in general, and the adolescent literature, in particular, despite the fact that adolescence is a time of heightened sensitivity to the reactions of others, self-consciousness, and general vulnerability. The closest construct is the shame–anger reaction in which being publicly shamed leads to acts of revenge (see Tangney & Dearing, in press). Thus there is a need to further examine links between shame and humiliation, including similarities and differences, research that I have begun with college students.

Findings from our adolescent study (Harter, 2001; Low & Harter, 2001b) revealed that for the sample as a whole, humiliation and perceptions of unfairness were highly related to anger at and blame of the perpetrator, as well as to the difficulty of getting the event out of one's mind. Analyses of nonviolent versus violent ideators further revealed that the two groups differed significantly on many of these variables. These included anger at the perpetrator, blaming of the perpetrator, difficulty of getting the event out of one's mind, and how often such an event had actually happened to them, with the violent ideators reporting higher levels on each. Moreover, on the variables included in our general model, violent ideators reported significantly greater aggression, lower self-worth, greater depressed affect, more hopelessness, and greater suicidal ideation. Thus we are developing a more comprehensive formulation on how our expanded model may reveal psychosocial processes predictive of violence. One eventual goal is to develop a measure that may be of help in identifying youth at risk for both suicidal and violent ideation.

Liabilities Associated with Exceedingly High Self-Esteem for Some Individuals

Throughout this chapter, high self-esteem has been presented as a psychological commodity to be sought after or fostered as an index of positive mental health. However, as Baumeister and colleagues (1999) have cogently argued, there would appear to be liabilities for a subset of individuals with exceedingly high self-esteem. They observe that individuals with high self-esteem who also have *narcissistic* tendencies (including an inflated sense of self), *low empathy* for others, but high *sensitivity* to potential negative evaluations of others can, in the face of threats to the ego, externalize blame and react *violently* toward others. In support of this formulation, Baumeister and colleagues draw on descriptions of (1) how psychopaths with favorable opinions of themselves commit violence, (2) how many murderers tend to have an inflated sense of self, (3) how rapists have a sense of male superiority, (4) how in many cases of domestic violence, an abusive husband's sense of superiority, status, or esteem is threatened, and (5) how many delinquent youth who are narcissistic, who feel entitled, and who externalize blame often engage in violent behavior. However, there has been no systematic research to examine their model directly or to identify the subset of individuals with high self-esteem who are at risk for violence, particularly during the period of adolescence. These authors conclude that we need careful studies of the way in which ego threats lead to violence and that in such studies we not only need to examine self-esteem but to include measures that directly tap *narcissism*, as well (Baumeister et al., 1999).

Recently my colleagues and I sought, in a pilot effort, to see if we could identify such a subgroup (Harter, 1999). A data set designed for a somewhat different set of research hypotheses consisted of (1) global self-esteem scores, (2) need for approval items, and (3) a cluster of empathy items, which are some of the predictive factors in Baumeister and colleagues' (1999) formulation. We also used a measure of threat to the ego, which tapped responses to a vignette in which a same-sex, same-age story character was teased and publicly put down for the way he or she looked and dressed and then shoved and subjected to additional loud, insulting comments when he or she tried to get away. After reading the vignette, the participant was asked to put himself or herself in the position of the victim and report on his or her level of (1) humiliation, (2) anger at the perpetrator, (3) blame of the perpetrator, and (4) violent ideation, namely

how much he or she would think about seriously harming the perpetrator, on a 4-point scale. We identified two groups of participants with extremely high self-esteem (3.75 to 4.00 on a 4-point scale, mean of 3.9 for each group), one group ($N = 9$) that was also *low* on *empathy* (2.7) and *high* on *need for approval* (3.5; both also 4-point scales), and a second group ($N = 14$) who reported high levels of empathy (3.5) and low need for approval (2.3).

Despite the small numbers, we found large and highly significant differences for the two groups in the predicted direction for (1) humiliation (3.6 vs. 2.7), (2) anger at the perpetrator (4.0 vs. 3.4), (3) blame of the perpetrator (3.9 vs. 3.1), and (4) desire to seriously harm the perpetrator (3.5 vs. 1.3). Thus, exceedingly high self-esteem, associated with lack of empathy and high need for approval, does appear to be associated with blaming and violent ideation in the face of threats to one's self-esteem (Harter, 1999).

Baumeister and colleagues (1999) contend that those with very low self-esteem and depression are not as likely to show the pattern of anger, blame, and harm. However, the literature on the comorbidity of depressed affect and anger, of clinical diagnoses of depression and conduct-disordered behavior, and of self- and other-reported internalizing and externalizing symptoms would argue otherwise (see Achenbach & Edelbrock, 1983; Curran, 1987; Deffenbacher & Swaim, 1999; Renouf & Harter, 1990; Rutter, 1987). We identified a subset of *low self-esteem* and *affectively depressed* (self-reported) adolescents with high levels of humiliation (3.39), anger (3.63), and blame (3.64) who also indicated that they would plan to seriously harm the perpetrator (3.5) (Harter, 2001). Moreover, consistent with the literature on comorbidity, they were also relatively suicidal. Thus it would appear that there are individuals at both ends of the self-esteem–affect spectrum who are at risk for violence.

Is the Construct of Self-Esteem in Trouble?

Baumeister and colleagues (1999) have raised a red flag in terms of certain liabilities associated with high self-esteem among a subset of particular individuals. Moreover, not all theorists would support the type of model that I have developed, in which self-worth or personal esteem plays a central role. There are those who would question the importance of self-esteem, contending that the focus on perceptions of global worth has been misguided. For example, Damon (1995) and Seligman (1993) have been critical of what they consider to be an overemphasis by educators and clinicians on promoting high self-esteem among our youth or among depressed individuals, particularly when these efforts lead to an inflated sense of esteem. Damon views such efforts as not only misguided but also possibly detrimental, arguing that they divert educators from teaching skills and deprive students of the thrill of actual accomplishment. It is Damon's contention that self-esteem has become an overrated commodity and that the effusive praise that parents or teachers heap on children to make them feel good is often met with suspicion by children; moreover, it interferes with the goal of building specific skills in the service of genuine achievement. In a similar vein, Seligman argues that self-esteem is merely an epiphenomenon, a reflection of whether one's commerce with the world is going well or badly, with little explanatory power in and of itself. He contends that if it becomes a focal point in treatment, it will distract clinicians from identifying the more specific causes of psychological problems such as depression.

At one level, global self-esteem or self-worth would appear to have little explanatory power because, as a mediator, it has been causally implicated in so many different child and adolescent problem behaviors, including depression and suicide, eating disorders, antisocial behaviors, and delinquency (most recently, gang membership), as well as teen pregnancy (see Mecca, Smelser, & Vasconcellos, 1989, who review evidence on the links between self-esteem and these problem behaviors). Thus we do not now understand what specific forces lead one individual with low self-worth to terminate his or her own life, whereas another, with an eating disorder, will put his or her life at risk. Still another may terminate someone *else's* life (as in gang shootings or random school violence), and yet another, through pregnancy, will create a *new* life. Knowing

that a child or adolescent has low self-esteem or self-worth, therefore, will not allow us to predict which *particular* outcome will ensue.

However, it is very important to emphasize that, in our zeal for parsimonious explanatory models, we must not ignore the fact that the *phenomenological* self-theory as experienced by children, adolescents, and adults is not necessarily parsimonious. Self-evaluations, including global self-worth, are very salient constructs in one's working model of self and, as such, can wield powerful influences on affect and behavior. Thus the challenge is to develop models that identify the specific antecedents of different outcomes while preserving the critical role of self-representations as phenomenological mediators. This perspective, although not embraced by all theorists in the field, can serve as a framework for intervention strategies to instill realistic and positive self-evaluations (see Harter, 1999, for intervention strategies based on both the cognitive and social processes that underlie the construction of the self).

Conclusions and Future Directions

Clear developmental advances and limitations profoundly influence the structure, content, and valence of the self-representations of children and adolescence, as this six-stage formulation has indicated. Cognitive developmental factors (the I-self) play heavily into how the self can be crafted at each level (the Me-self). In addition, there are individual differences at each developmental level with regard to how favorably children and adolescents evaluate themselves, differences that are dependent on how competent or adequate one feels in domains of importance (initially from James), as well as on the reactions of critical socializing agents (parents, peers, and additional significant others), as initially articulated in the theories of symbolic interactionists and later by attachment theorists.

There are clearly many new directions in which self-processes could be examined. The developmental sequence described has not really been documented through appropriate longitudinal methodologies that would be more compelling. The directionality of the links between particular self-concept domains and sources of approval and global self-worth requires further study. My own findings reveal that those individuals who base their self-worth on their appearance, as well as on approval from others, fare worse on a variety of outcomes. Those who seem to have internalized positive feelings of worth that they feel precede evaluations of appearance or approval report much better correlates and outcomes, although this internalization process has not been directly examined. Another new direction involves the construct of "relational self-worth" (Harter, Waters, & Whitesell, 1998). We have determined that in addition to global self-worth, older children and adolescents develop relationship-specific evaluations of their worth as persons (e.g., with parents, close friends, classmates) that are highly related to the support they receive within that particular relationship. However, these processes have yet to be investigated. Finally, there is a need to study correlates and outcomes other than depression and violence, as well as to examine situations in which high self-esteem is a liability at different developmental levels.

Troublesome is the fact that the developmental literature has not been integrated with the burgeoning literature in the field of adult social psychology that has also identified numerous processes relevant to self-esteem, in particular. Such topics include self-enhancement strategies (Baumeister, 1993), self-verification (Swann, 1996), self-stability (Kernis, 1993), self-complexity (Linville, 1987; Showers, 1995)—the list goes on. What we need, it seems, is some convergence in which developmental considerations are respected by adult social psychologists and whereby developmental psychologists think about the ontogenetic origins of the processes that have been documented by social psychologists in adults and at what ages and stages these might emerge and why. Our fields (developmental approaches and adult psychological processes) have been for too long discrete areas of inquiry. Merely applying the adult psychological processes (and measures) to children and adolescents is not sufficient. Rather, it seems that we need some thoughtful coordination, a priori, of how what we know about developmental processes might

lead to differences with age in light of these adult conceptualizations. Let us work together toward these goals.

References

Achenbach, T. M., & Edelbrock, C. S. (1983). *Manual for the Child Behavior Checklist and Revised Child Behavior Profile.* Burlington: University of Vermont.

Ainsworth, M. (1973). The development of infant–mother attachment. In B. Caldwell & H. Ricciuto (Eds.), *Review of child development research* (Vol. 3, pp. 1–94). Chicago: University of Chicago Press.

Ainsworth, M. (1974). Infant–mother attachment and social development: Socialization as a product of reciprocal responsiveness to signals. In M. Richards (Ed.), *The integration of the child into the social world* (pp. 99–135). Cambridge, UK: Cambridge University Press.

Alcohol, Drug Abuse, and Mental Health Administration. (1989). *Report of the Secretary's Task Force on Youth Suicide* (DHHS Publication No. ADM 89–1621). Washington, DC: U.S. Government Printing Office.

Baldwin, J. M. (1895). *Mental development of the child and the race: Methods and processes.* New York: Macmillan.

Baldwin, J. M. (1897). *Social and ethical interpretations in mental development: A study in social psychology.* New York: Macmillan.

Banaji, M. R., & Prentice, D. A. (1994). The self in social contexts. *Annual Review of Psychology, 45,* 297–325.

Bandura, A. (1990). Conclusion: Reflections on nonability determinants of competence. In R. J. Sternberg & J. Kolligian, Jr. (Eds.), *Competence considered* (pp. 316–352). New Haven, CT: Yale University Press.

Barrett, K. C. (1995). A functionalist approach to shame and guilt. In J. P. Tangney & K. W. Fischer (Eds.), *Self-conscious emotions: The psychology of shame, guilt, embarrassment, and pride* (pp. 25–63). New York: Guilford Press.

Battle, J. (1987). Relationship between self-esteem and depression among children. *Psychological Reports, 60,* 1187–1190.

Baumeister, R. F. (1987). How the self became a problem: A psychological review of historical research. *Journal of Personality and Social Psychology, 52,* 163–176.

Baumeister, R. F. (1990). Suicide as escape from self. *Psychological Review, 97,* 90–113.

Baumeister, R. F. (1993). Understanding the inner nature of low self-esteem: Uncertain, fragile, protective, and conflicted. In R. F. Baumeister (Ed.), *Self-esteem: The puzzle of low self-regard* (pp. 201–218). New York: Plenum Press.

Baumeister, R. F., Smart, L., & Boden, J. M. (1999). Relation of threatened egotism to violence and aggression: The dark side of high self-esteem. In R. Baumeister (Ed.), *The self in social psychology* (pp. 288–314). New York: Psychology Press.

Beach, S. R. H., & Tesser, A. (1995). Self-esteem and the extended self-evaluation maintenance model: The self in social context. In M. H. Kernis (Ed.), *Efficacy, agency, and self-esteem* (pp. 145–168). New York: Plenum Press.

Beck, A. T. (1975). *Depression: Causes and treatments.* Philadelphia: University of Pennsylvania Press.

Beck. A. T. (1987, May). *Hopelessness as a prediction of ultimate suicide.* Paper presented at the joint meetings of the American Association of Suicidology and the International Association for Suicide Prevention, San Francisco, CA.

Berndt, T. J., & Burgy, L. (1996). The social self-concept. In B. A. Bracken (Ed.), *Handbook of self-concept* (pp. 171–209). New York: Wiley.

Bibring, E. (1953). The mechanism of depression. In P. Greenacre (Ed.), *Affective disorders: Psychoanalytic contribution to their study* (pp. 13–48). New York: International Universities Press.

Blatt, S. J. (1974). Levels of object representation in anaclitic and introjective depression. *Psychoanalytic Study of the Child, 29,* 107–157.

Blatt, S. J. (1995). Representational structures in psychopathology. In D. Cicchetti & S. Toth (Eds.), *Rochester Symposium on Developmental Psychopathology: Emotion, cognition, and representation* (Vol. 6, pp. 1–34). Rochester, NY: University of Rochester Press.

Bleiberg, E. (1984). Narcissistic disorders in children. *Bulletin of the Menninger Clinic, 48,* 501–517.

Bowlby, J. (1980). *Attachment and loss: Vol. 3. Loss, sadness, and depression.* New York: Basic Books.

Bracken, B. (1992). *Multidimensional Self-Concept Scale.* Austin, TX: PRO-ED.

Bracken, B. (1996). Clinical applications of a context-dependent multi-dimensional model of self-concept. In B. Bracken (Ed.), *Handbook of self-concept* (pp. 463–505). New York: Wiley.

Bretherton, I. (1991). Pouring new wine into old bottles: The social self as internal working model. In M. R. Gunnar & L. A. Sroufe (Eds.), *Self processes and development: The Minnesota Symposium on Child Development* (Vol. 23, pp. 1–41). Hillsdale, NJ: Erlbaum.

Bretherton, I. (1992). The origins of attachment theory: John Bowlby and Mary Ainsworth. *Developmental Psychology, 28,* 759–775.

Briere, J. (1992). *Child abuse trauma: Theory and treatment of the lasting effects.* Newbury Park, CA: Sage.

Broughton, J. (1978). The development of the concepts of self, mind, reality, and knowledge. In W. Damon (Ed.), *Social cognition* (pp. 75–100). San Francisco: Jossey-Bass.

Brown, B. B. (1990). Peer groups and peer cultures. In S. S. Feldman & G. Elliot (Eds.), *At the threshold: The developing adolescent* (pp. 171–196). Cambridge, MA: Harvard University Press.

Carlson, G. A., & Cantwell, D. P. (1980). Unmasking masked depression in children and adolescents. *American Journal of Psychiatry, 137,* 443–449.

Carroll, J. J., & Steward, M. S. (1984). The role of cognitive development in children's understandings of their own feelings. *Child Development, 55,* 1486–1492.

Carver, C. S., & Scheier, M. F. (1990). Origins and functions of positive and negative affect: A control-process. *Psychological Review, 97,* 19–35.

Case, R. (1985). *Intellectual development: Birth to adulthood.* New York: Academic Press.

Case, R. (1992). *The mind's staircase.* Hillsdale, NJ: Erlbaum.

Cassidy, J. (1990). Theoretical and methodological considerations in the study of attachment and the self in young children. In M. T. Greenberg, D. Cicchetti, & E. M. Cummings (Eds.), *Attachment in the preschool years: Theory, research, and intervention* (pp. 87–120). Chicago: University of Chicago Press.

Cicchetti, D. (1990). The organization and coherence of socioemotional, cognitive, and representational development: Illustrations through a developmental psychopathology perspective on Down syndrome and child maltreatment. In R. Thompson (Ed.), *Nebraska Symposium on Motivation: Vol. 36. Socioemotional development* (pp. 266–375). Lincoln: University of Nebraska Press.

Cicchetti, D. (1991). Fractures in the crystal: Developmental psychopathology and the emergence of self. *Developmental Review, 11,* 271–287.

Cicchetti, D., & Beeghly, M. (1990). Perspectives on the study of the self in transition. In D. Cicchetti & M. Beeghly (Eds.), *The self in transition: Infancy to childhood* (pp. 1–15). Chicago: University of Chicago Press.

Cicchetti, D., & Schneider-Rosen, K. (1986). An organizational approach to childhood depression. In M. Rutter, C. E. Izard, & P. B. Read (Eds.), *Depression in young people: Developmental and clinical perspectives* (pp. 71–134). New York: Guilford Press.

Cooley, C. H. (1902). *Human nature and the social order.* New York: Scribner's.

Cooper, C. R., Grotevant, H. D., & Condon, S. M. (1983). Individuality and connectedness both foster adolescent identity formation and role taking skills. In H. D. Grotevant & C. R. Cooper (Eds.), *Adolescent development in the family: New directions for child development* (pp. 43–59). San Francisco: Jossey-Bass.

Coopersmith, S. (1967). *The antecedents of self-esteem.* San Francisco: Freeman.

Crittenden, P. M. (1994). Peering into the black box: An exploratory treatise on the development of self in young children. In D. Cicchetti & S. L. Toth (Eds.), *Rochester Symposium on Developmental Psychopathology: Vol. 5. Disorders and dysfunctions of the self* (pp. 79–148). Rochester, NY: University of Rochester Press.

Curran, D. K. (1987). *Adolescent suicidal behavior.* Washington, DC: Hemisphere.

Damon, W. (1995). *Greater expectations: Overcoming the culture of indulgence in America's homes and schools.* New York: Free Press.

Damon, W., & Hart, D. (1988). *Self-understanding in childhood and adolescence.* New York: Cambridge University Press.

Deffenbacher, J. L., & Swaim, R. C. (1999). Anger expression in Mexican American and White non-Hispanic adolescents. *Journal of Counseling Psychology, 46,* 61–69.

Dickstein, E. (1977). Self and self-esteem: Theoretical foundations and their implications for research. *Human Development, 20,* 129–140.

Donaldson, S. K., & Westerman, M. A. (1986). Development of children's understanding of ambivalence and causal theories of emotion. *Developmental Psychology, 22,* 655–662.

Dweck, C. S. (1991). Self-theories and goals: Their role in motivation, personality and development. In R. Dienstbier (Ed.), *Nebraska Symposium on Motivation: Vol. 38. Perspectives on motivation* (pp. 199–235). Lincoln: University of Nebraska Press.

Elkind, D. (1967). Egocentrism in adolescence. *Child Development, 38,* 1025–1034.

Emery, P. E. (1983). Adolescent depression and suicide. *Adolescence, 18,* 245–258.

Epstein, S. (1973). The self-concept revisited or a theory of a theory. *American Psychologist, 28,* 405–416.

Epstein, S. (1981). The unity principle versus the reality and pleasure principles, or the tale of the scorpion and the frog. In M. D. Lynch, A. A. Norem-Hebeisen, & K. Gergen (Eds.), *Self-concept: Advances in theory and research* (pp. 82–110). Cambridge, MA: Ballinger.

Epstein, S. (1991). Cognitive–experiential self theory: Implications for developmental psychology. In M. R. Gunnar & L. A. Sroufe (Eds.), *The Minnesota Symposia on Child Development: Vol. 23. Self processes and development* (pp. 111–137). Hillsdale, NJ: Erlbaum.

Epstein, S., & Morling, B. (1995). Is the self motivated to do more than enhance and/or verify itself? In M. H. Kernis (Ed.), *Efficacy, agency, and self-esteem* (pp. 9–26). New York: Plenum Press.

Erikson, E. H. (1968). *Identity, youth, and crisis.* New York: Norton.

Felson, R. B. (1993). The (somewhat) social self: How others affect self-appraisals. In J. Suls (Ed.), *Psychological perspectives on the self* (Vol. 4, pp. 1–26). Hillsdale, NJ: Erlbaum.

Fischer, K. W. (1980). A theory of cognitive development: The control and construction of hierarchies of skills. *Psychological Review, 87,* 477–531.

Fischer, K. W., & Ayoub, C. (1994). Affective splitting and dissociation in normal and maltreated children: Developmental pathways for self in relationships. In D. Cicchetti & S. Toth (Eds.), *Rochester Symposium on Developmental Psychopathology: Vol. 5. Disorders and dysfunctions of the self* (pp. 149–222). Rochester, NY: University of Rochester Press.

Fischer, K. W., Hand, H. H., Watson, M. W., Van Parys, M., & Tucker, J. (1984). Putting the child into socialization: The development of social categories in preschool children. In L. Katz (Ed.), *Current topics in early childhood education* (Vol. 5, pp. 27–72). Norwood, NJ: Ablex.

Fischer, K. W., Shaver, P., & Carnochan, P. (1990). How emotions develop and how they organize development. *Cognition and Emotion, 4,* 81–127.

Fivush, R. (1987). Scripts and categories: Interrelationships in development. In U. Neisser (Ed.), *Concepts and conceptual development: Ecological and intellectual factors in categorization* (pp. 233–251). Cambridge, UK: Cambridge University Press.

Flavell, J. H. (1985). *Cognitive development* (2nd ed.). Englewood Cliffs, NJ: Prentice-Hall.

Freud, S. (1952). *A general introduction to psychoanalysis.* New York: Washington Square Press.

Freud, S. (1968). Mourning and melancholia. In J. Strachey (Ed. & Trans.), *The standard edition of the complete psychological works of Sigmund Freud* (Vol. 14, pp. 237–260). London: Hogarth Press. (Original work published 1917)

Frey, K. S., & Ruble, D. N. (1985). What children say when the teacher is not around: Conflicting goals in so-

cial comparison and performance assessment in the classroom. *Journal of Personality and Social Psychology, 48,* 550–562.

Frey, K. S., & Ruble, D. N. (1990). Strategies for comparative evaluation: Maintaining a sense of competence across the life span. In R. J. Sternberg & J. Kolligian, Jr. (Eds.), *Competence considered* (pp. 167–189). New Haven, CT: Yale University Press.

Gecas, V. (1972). Parental behavior and contextual variations in adolescent self-esteem. *Sociometry, 36,* 332–345.

Gispert, M., Davis, M. C., Marsh, L., & Wheeler, K. (1987). Predictive factors in repeated suicide attempts by adolescents. *Hospital and Community Psychology, 38,* 390–393.

Gnepp, J., McKee, E., & Domanic, J. A. (1987). Children's use of situational information to infer emotion: Understanding emotionally equivocal situations. *Developmental Psychology, 23,* 114–123.

Greenberg, J., Pyszczynski, T., & Solomon, S. (1995). Toward a dual-motive depth psychology of self and social behavior. In M. H. Kernis (Ed.), *Efficacy, agency, and self-esteem* (pp. 73–101). New York: Plenum Press.

Greenwald, A. G. (1980). The totalitarian ego: Fabrication and revision of personal history. *American Psychologist, 7,* 603–618.

Griffin, N., Chassin, L., & Young, R. D. (1981). Measurement of global self-concept versus multiple role-specific self-concepts in adolescents. *Adolescence, 16,* 49–56.

Griffin, S. (1992). Structural analysis of the development of their inner world: A neo-structural analysis of the development of intrapersonal intelligence. In R. Case (Ed.), *The mind's staircase* (pp. 189–206). Hillsdale, NJ: Erlbaum.

Grotevant, H. D., & Cooper, C. R. (1986). Individuation in family relationships. *Human Development, 29,* 83–100.

Haltiwanger, J. (1989, April). *Behavioral referents of presented self-esteem in young children.* Paper presented at the meeting of the Society for Research in Child Development, Kansas City, MO.

Harris, P. L. (1983). What children know about the situations that provoke emotion. In M. Lewis & C. Saarni (Eds.), *The socialization of affect* (pp. 162–185). New York: Plenum Press.

Harris, P. L., Olthof, T., & Meerum-Terwogt, M. (1981). Children's knowledge of emotion. *Journal of Child Psychology and Psychiatry, 45,* 247–261.

Hart, D. (1988). The adolescent self-concept in social context. In D. K. Lapsley & F. C. Power (Eds.), *Self, ego, and identity* (pp. 71–90). New York: Springer-Verlag.

Harter, S. (1982). The perceived competence scale for children. *Child Development, 53,* 87–97.

Harter, S. (1983). Developmental perspectives on the self-system. In P. Mussen (Series Ed.) & E. M. Hetherington (Vol. Ed.), *Handbook of child psychology: Vol. 4. Socialization, personality, and social development* (4th ed., pp. 275–385). New York: Wiley.

Harter, S. (1985). *The Self-Perception Profile for Children.* Unpublished manual, University of Denver, Denver, CO.

Harter, S. (1986a). Cognitive-developmental processes in the integration of concepts about emotions and the self. *Social Cognition, 4,* 119–151.

Harter, S. (1986b). Processes underlying the construction, maintenance, and enhancement of the self-concept in children. In J. Suls & A. G. Greenwald (Eds.), *Psychological perspectives on the self* (Vol. 3, pp. 137–181). Hillsdale, NJ: Erlbaum.

Harter, S. (1987). The determinants and mediational role of global self-worth in children. In N. Eisenberg (Ed.), *Contemporary issues in developmental psychology* (pp. 219–242). New York: Wiley.

Harter, S. (1988). *The Self-Perception Profile for Adolescents.* Unpublished manual, University of Denver, Denver, CO.

Harter, S. (1990a). Adolescent self and identity development. In S. S. Feldman & G. R. Elliot (Eds.), *At the threshold: The developing adolescent* (pp. 352–387). Cambridge, MA: Harvard University Press.

Harter, S. (1990b). Causes, correlates and the functional role of global self-worth: A life-span perspective. In R. Sternberg & J. Kolligian, Jr. (Eds.), *Competence considered* (pp. 67–98). New Haven, CT: Yale University Press.

Harter, S. (1993). Causes and consequences of low self-esteem in children and adolescents. In R. F. Baumeister (Ed.), *Self-esteem: The puzzle of low self-regard* (pp. 87–116). New York: Plenum Press.

Harter, S. (1997). The personal self in social context: Barriers to authenticity. In R. D. Ashmore & L. Jussim (Eds.), *Self and identity: Fundamental issues* (pp. 81–105). New York: Oxford University Press.

Harter, S. (1998). The development of self-representations. In W. Damon (Series Ed.) & N. Eisenberg (Vol. Ed.), *Handbook of child psychology: Vol. 3. Social, emotional, and personality development* (5th ed., pp. 553–617). New York: Wiley.

Harter, S. (1999). *The construction of the self.* New York: Guilford Press.

Harter, S. (2001, April). *What have we learned from Columbine: The role of the self-system in school violence.* Paper presented at Society for Research in Child Development, Minnesota.

Harter, S., Bresnick, S., Bouchey, H. A., & Whitesell, N. R. (1997). The development of multiple role-related selves during adolescence. *Development and Psychopathology, 9,* 835–854.

Harter, S. & Buddin, B. J. (1987). Children's understanding of the simultaneity of two emotions: A five-stage developmental acquisition sequence. *Developmental Psychology, 23,* 388–399.

Harter, S., & Marold, D. B. (1993). The directionality of the link between self-esteem and affect: Beyond causal modeling. In D. Cicchetti & S. L. Toth (Eds.), *Rochester Symposium on Developmental Psychopathology: Vol. 5. Disorders and dysfunctions of the self* (pp. 333–370). Rochester, NY: University of Rochester Press.

Harter, S., Marold, D. B., & Whitesell, N. R. (1992). A model of psychosocial risk factors leading to suicidal ideation in young adolescents. *Development and Psychopathology, 4,* 167–188.

Harter, S., & Monsour, A. (1992). Developmental analysis of conflict caused by opposing attributes in the adolescent self-portrait. *Developmental Psychology, 28,* 251–260.

Harter, S., & Pike, R. (1984). The pictorial scale of perceived competence and social acceptance for young children. *Child Development, 55,* 1969–1982.

Harter, S., Stocker, C., & Robinson, N. S. (1996). The perceived directionality of the link between approval and self-worth: The liabilities of a looking glass self orientation among young adolescents. *Journal of Research on Adolescence, 6,* 285–308.

Harter, S., Waters, P., & Whitesell, N. R. (1998). Relational self-worth: Differences in perceived worth as a person across interpersonal contexts. *Child Development, 69,* 756–766.

Harter, S., & Whitesell, N. R. (1996). Multiple pathways to self-reported depression and adjustment among adolescents. *Development and Psychopathology, 9,* 835–854.

Harter, S., Whitesell, N. R., & Junkin, L. J. (1999). Similarities and differences in domain-specific and global self-evaluations of learning disabled, behaviorally-disordered, and normally achieving adolescents. *American Educational Research Journal, 35,* 653–680.

Hattie, J. (1992). *Self-concept.* Hillsdale, NJ: Erlbaum.

Herman, J. (1992). *Trauma and recovery.* New York: Basic Books.

Higgins, E. T. (1991). Development of self-regulatory and self-evaluative processes: Costs, benefits, and tradeoff. In M. R. Gunnar & L. A. Sroufe (Eds.), *The Minnesota Symposia on Child Development: Vol. 23. Self processes and development* (pp. 125–166). Hillsdale, NJ: Erlbaum.

Hill, J. P., & Holmbeck, G. N. (1986). Attachment and autonomy during adolescence. In G. J. Whitehurst (Ed.), *Annals of child development* (Vol. 3, pp. 145–189). Greenwich, CT: JAI Press.

Hudson, J. A. (1990). The emergence of autobiographical memory in mother–child conversation. In R. Fivush & J. A. Hudson (Eds.), *Knowing and remembering in young children* (pp. 166–196). New York: Cambridge University Press.

Jacobs, D. H. (1983). Learning problems, self-esteem, and delinquency. In J. E. Mack & S. L. Ablon (Eds.), *The development and sustenance of self-esteem in childhood* (pp. 209–222). New York: International Universities Press.

James, W. (1890). *Principles of psychology.* New York: Holt.

James, W. (1892). *Psychology: The briefer course.* New York: Holt.

John, O. P., & Robbins, R. W. (1994). Accuracy and bias in self-perception: Individual differences in self-enhancement and the role of narcissism. *Journal of Personality and Social Psychology, 66,* 206–219.

Juhasz, A. M. (1992). Significant others in self-esteem development: Methods and problems in measurement. In T. M. Brinthaupt & R. P. Lipka (Eds.), *The self: Definitional and methodological issues* (pp. 204–235). Albany: State University of New York Press.

Kagan, J. (1984). *The nature of the child.* New York: Basic Books.

Kaslow, N. J., Rehm, L. P., & Siegel, A. W. (1984). Social-cognitive and cognitive correlates of depression in children. *Journal of Abnormal Child Psychology, 12,* 605–620.

Keith, L. K., & Bracken, B. A. (1996). Self-concept instrumentation: An historical and evaluative review. In B. A.

Bracken (Ed.), *Handbook of self-concept* (pp. 91–170). New York: Wiley.

Kelly, G. A. (1955). *The psychology of personal constructs.* New York: Norton.

Kenny, D. (1988). Interpersonal perception: A social relations analysis. *Journal of Social and Personal Relationships, 5,* 247–261.

Kernberg, O. F. (1975). *Borderline conditions and pathological narcissism.* New York: Aronson.

Kernis, M. H. (1993). The roles of stability and level of self-esteem in psychological functioning. In R. F. Baumeister (Ed.), *Self-esteem: The puzzle of low self-regard* (pp. 167–180). New York: Plenum Press.

Khan, A. U. (1987). Heterogeneity of suicidal adolescents. *Journal of the American Academy of Child and Adolescent Psychiatry, 26,* 92–96.

Kihlstrom, J. F. (1993). What does the self look like? In T. K. Srull & R. S. Wyer, Jr. (Eds.), *Advances in social cognition: Vol. 5. The mental representation of trait and autobiographical knowledge about the self* (pp. 79–90). Hillsdale, NJ: Erlbaum.

Kohut, H. (1977). *The restoration of the self.* New York: International Universities Press.

Lapsley, D. K., & Rice, K. (1988). The "new look" at the imaginary audience and personal fable: Toward a general model of adolescent ego development. In D. K. Lapsley & F. C. Power (Eds.), *Self, ego, and identity: Integrative approaches* (pp. 109–129). New York: Springer-Verlag.

Leahy, R. L. (1985). The costs of development: Clinical implications. In R. L. Leahy (Ed.), *The development of the self* (pp. 267–294). New York: Academic Press.

Leahy, R. L., & Shirk, S. R. (1985). Social cognition and the development of the self. In R. L. Leahy (Ed.), *The development of the self* (pp. 123–150). New York: Academic Press.

Leary, M. R., & Downs, D. L. (1995). Interpersonal functions of the self-esteem motive: The self-esteem system as a sociometer. In M. H. Kernis (Ed.), *Efficacy, agency, and self-esteem* (pp. 123–140). New York: Plenum Press.

Lewis, M. (1991). Ways of knowing: Objective self-awareness or consciousness. *Developmental Review, 11,* 231–243.

Lewis, M. (1994). Myself and me. In S. T. Parker, R. W. Mitchell, & M. L. Boccia (Eds.), *Self-awareness in animals and humans: Developmental perspectives* (pp. 20–34). New York: Cambridge University Press.

Linville, P. W. (1987). Self-complexity as a cognitive buffer against stress-related illness and depression. *Journal of Personality and Social Psychology, 52,* 663–676.

Low, S., & Harter, S. (2001a). *Extension of a model of the determinants and correlates of self-esteem, depression, and suicidal ideation to aggression and violent ideation.* Unpublished manuscript, University of Denver.

Low, S., & Harter, S. (2001b). *Young adolescents' reactions to potentially humiliating events that have emerged in the media reports of the school shooters: Affective, cognitive, and behavior dimensions.* Unpublished manuscript, University of Denver.

Maccoby, E. (1980). *Social development.* New York: Wiley.

Mack, J. E. (1983). Self-esteem and its development: An overview. In J. E. Mack & S. L. Ablong (Eds.), *The de-velopment and sustaining of self-esteem* (pp. 1–44). New York: International Universities Press.

Markus, H. (1980). The self in thought and memory. In D. M. Wegner & R. R. Vallacher (Eds.), *The self in social psychology* (pp. 42–69). New York: Oxford University Press.

Markus, H., & Nurius, P. (1986). Possible selves. *American Psychologist, 41,* 954–969.

Markus, H., & Wurf, E. (1987). The dynamic self-concept: A social psychological perspective. *Annual Review of Psychology, 38,* 299–337.

Markus, H. R., & Kitayama, S. (1991). Culture and the self: Implications for cognition, emotion, and motivation. *Psychological Review, 98,* 224–253.

Marsh, H. W. (1986). Global self-esteem: Its relation to specific facets of self-concept and their importance. *Journal of Personality and Social Psychology, 51,* 1224–1236.

Marsh, H. W. (1987). The hierarchical structure of self-concept and the application of hierarchical confirmatory factor analysis. *Journal of Educational Measurement, 24,* 17–19.

Marsh, H. W. (1993). Academic self-concept: Theory, measurement, and research. In J. Suls (Ed.), *Psychological perspectives on the self* (Vol. 4, pp. 59–98). Hillsdale, NJ: Erlbaum.

Marsh, H. W., & Hattie, J. (1996). Theoretical perspectives on the structure of self-concept. In B. A. Bracken (Ed.), *Handbook of self-concept* (pp. 38–90). New York: Wiley.

Mead, G. H. (1925). The genesis of the self and social control. *International Journal of Ethics, 35,* 251–273.

Mead, G. H. (1934). *Mind, self, and society from the standpoint of a social behaviorist.* Chicago: University of Chicago Press.

Mecca, A. M., Smelser, N. J., & Vasconcellos, J. (Eds.). (1989). *The social importance of self-esteem.* Berkeley: University of California Press.

Messer, B., & Harter, S. (1989). *The Self-Perception Profile for Adults.* Unpublished manual, University of Denver, Denver, CO.

Moretti, M. M., & Higgins, E. T. (1990). The development of self-esteem vulnerabilities: Social and cognitive factors in developmental psychopathology. In R. J. Sternberg & J. Kolligian, Jr. (Eds.), *Competence considered* (pp. 286–314). New Haven, CT: Yale University Press.

Mullener, N., & Laird, J. D. (1971). Some developmental changes in the organization of self-evaluations. *Developmental Psychology, 5,* 233–236.

Neeman, J., & Harter, S. (1987). *The Self-Perception Profile for College Students.* Unpublished manual, University of Denver, Denver, CO.

Nelson, K. (1986). *Event knowledge: Structure and function in development.* Hillsdale, NJ: Erlbaum.

Nelson, K. (1993). Events, narratives, memory: What develops? In C. A. Nelson (Ed.), *Minnesota Symposium on Child Psychology: Vol. 26. Memory and affect* (pp. 1–24). Hillsdale, NJ: Erlbaum.

Noam, G. G., & Borst, S. (Eds.). (1994). *Children, youth, and suicide: Developmental perspectives.* San Francisco: Jossey-Bass.

Oosterwegel, A., & Oppenheimer, L. (1993). *The self-system: Developmental changes between and within self-concepts.* Hillsdale, NJ: Erlbaum.

Oyserman, D., & Markus, H. R. (1993). The sociocultural self. In J. Suls (Ed.), *Psychological perspectives on the self* (Vol. 7, pp. 187–220). Hillsdale, NJ: Erlbaum.

Pfeffer, C. R. (1986). *The suicidal child.* New York: Guilford Press.

Pfeffer, C. R. (1988). Risk factors associated with youth suicide. *Psychiatric Annals, 18,* 652–656.

Piaget, J. (1932). *The moral judgment of the child.* New York: Harcourt, Brace & World.

Piaget, J. (1960). *The psychology of intelligence.* Patterson, NJ: Littlefield-Adams.

Pipp, S. (1990). Sensorimotor and representational internal representational working models of self, other, and relationship: Mechanisms of connection and separation. In D. Cicchetti & M. Beeghly (Eds.), *The self in transition: Infancy to childhood* (pp. 243–264). Chicago: University of Chicago Press.

Pomerantz, E. V., & Ruble, D. N., Frey, K. S., & Greulich, F. (1995). Meeting goals and confronting conflict: Children's changing perceptions of social comparison. *Child Development, 66,* 723–738.

Reissland, N. (1985). The development of concepts of simultaneity in children's understanding of emotions. *Journal of Child Psychology and Psychiatry, 26,* 811–824.

Renick, M. J., & Harter, S. (1988). *The Self-Perception Profile for Learning Disabled Students.* Unpublished manual, University of Denver, Denver, CO.

Renouf, A. G., & Harter, S. (1990). Low self-worth and anger as components of the depressive experience in young adolescents. *Development and Psychopathology, 2,* 293–310.

Rogers, C. R. (1951). *Client-centered therapy.* Boston: Houghton Mifflin.

Rosenberg, M. (1979). *Conceiving the self.* New York: Basic Books.

Rosenberg, M. (1986). Self-concept from middle childhood through adolescence. In J. Suls & A. G. Greenwald (Eds.), *Psychological perspective on the self* (Vol. 3, pp. 107–135). Hillsdale, NJ:Erlbaum.

Ruble, D. N., & Dweck, C. (1995). Self-conceptions, person conception, and their development. In N. Eisenberg (Ed.), *Review of personality and social psychology: Vol. 15. Development and social psychology: The interface* (pp. 109–139). Thousand Oaks, CA: Sage.

Ruble, D. N., & Frey, K. S. (1991). Changing patterns of comparative behavior as skills are acquired: A functional model of self-evaluation. In J. Suls & T. A. Wills (Eds.), *Social comparison: Contemporary theory and research* (pp. 70–112). Hillsdale, NJ: Erlbaum.

Rutter, M. (1986). The developmental psychopathology of depression: Issues and perspectives. In M. Rutter, C. E. Izard, & P. B. Read (Eds.), *Depression in young people: Developmental and clinical perspectives* (pp. 3–32). New York: Guilford Press.

Rutter, M. (1987). Psychosocial resilience and protective mechanisms. *American Journal of Orthopsychiatry, 57,* 316–331.

Rutter, M., Izard, C. E., & Read, P. B. (Eds.). (1986). *Depression in young people: Developmental and clinical perspectives.* New York: Guilford Press.

Sarbin, T. R. (1962). A preface to a psychological analysis of the self. *Psychological Review, 59,* 11–22.

Savin-Williams, R. C., & Berndt, T. J. (1990). Friend and peer relations. In S. S. Feldman & G. Elliot (Eds.), *At the threshold: The developing adolescent* (pp. 277–307). Cambridge, MA: Harvard University Press.

Seligman, M. E. P. (1975). *Helplessness: On depression, development, and death.* San Francisco: Freeman.

Seligman, M. E. P. (1993). *What you can change and what you can't.* New York: Fawcett Columbine.

Selman, R. L. (1980). *The growth of interpersonal understanding.* New York: Academic Press.

Shavelson, R. J., & Marsh, H. W. (1986). On the structure of self-concept. In R. Schwarzer (Ed.), *Anxiety and cognition* (pp. 305–330). Hillsdale, NJ: Erlbaum.

Showers, C. (1995). The evaluative organization of self-knowledge: Origins, process, and implications for self-esteem. In M. H. Kernis (Ed.), *Efficacy, agency, and self-esteem* (pp. 101–122). New York: Plenum Press.

Shrauger, J. S., & Schoeneman, T. J. (1979). Symbolic interactionist view of self-concept: Through the looking glass darkly. *Psychological Bulletin, 86,* 549–573.

Siegler, R. S. (1991). *Children's thinking* (2nd ed.). Englewood Cliffs, NJ: Prentice-Hall.

Simmons, R. G., & Blyth, D. A. (1987). *Moving into adolescence: The impact of pubertal change and school context.* New York: Aldine de Gruyter.

Snow, K. (1990). Building memories: The ontogeny of autobiography. In D. Cicchetti & M. Beeghly (Eds.), *The self in transition: Infancy to childhood* (pp. 213–242). Chicago: University of Chicago Press.

Sroufe, L. A. (1990). An organizational perspective on the self. In D. Cicchetti & M. Beeghly (Eds.), *The self in transition: Infancy to childhood* (pp. 281–308). Chicago: University of Chicago Press.

Steele, C. M. (1988). The psychology of self-affirmation: Sustaining the integrity of the self. In L. Berkowitz (Ed.), *Advances in experimental social psychology* (Vol. 21, pp. 261–302). San Diego, CA: Academic Press.

Steinberg, L. (1990). Interdependency in the family: Autonomy, conflict, and harmony in the parent-adolescent relationship. In S. Feldman & G. Elliot (Eds.), *At the threshold: The developing adolescent* (pp. 255–276). Cambridge, MA: Harvard University Press.

Stipek, D., Recchia, S., & McClintic, S. (1992). Self-evaluation in young children. *Monographs of the Society for Research in Child Development, 57,* 1–84.

Suls, J., & Sanders, G. (1982). Self-evaluation via social comparison: A developmental analysis. In L. Wheeler (Ed.), *Review of personality and social psychology* (Vol. 3, pp. 67–89). Beverly Hills, CA: Sage.

Swann, W. B., Jr. (1996). *Self-traps.* New York: Freeman.

Tangney, J. P., & Dearing, R. L. (in press). *Shame and guilt.* New York: Guilford Press.

Tangney, J. P., & Fischer, K. W. (Eds.). (1995). *Self-conscious emotions: The psychology of shame, guilt, embarrassment, and pride.* New York: Guilford Press.

Terr, L. (1990). *Too scared to cry.* New York: Basic Books.

Tesser, A. (1980). Self-esteem maintenance in family dynamics. *Journal of Personality and Social Psychology, 39,* 77–91.

Tesser, A. (1988). Toward a self-evaluation maintenance model of social behavior. In L. Berkowitz (Ed.), *Advances in experimental social psychology* (Vol. 21, pp. 181–227). New York: Academic Press.

Tesser, A., & Cornell, D. (1991). On the confluence of self

processes. *Journal of Experimental Social Psychology, 27,* 501–526.

Watson, M. (1990). Aspects of self development as reflected in children's role playing. In D. Cicchetti & M. Beeghly (Eds.), *The self in transition: Infancy to childhood* (pp. 281–307). Chicago: University of Chicago Press.

Westen, D. (1993). The impact of sexual abuse on self structure. In D. Cicchetti & S. Toth (Eds.), *Rochester Symposium on Developmental, Psychopathology: Vol. 5.*

Disorders and dysfunctions of the self (pp. 223–250). Rochester, NY: University of Rochester Press.

Winnicott, D. W. (1965). *The maturational processes and the facilitating environment.* New York: International Universities Press.

Wylie, R. C. (1979). *The self concept: Theory and research on selected topics* (Vol. 2). Lincoln: University of Nebraska Press.

Wylie, R. C. (1989). *Measures of self-concept.* Lincoln: University of Nebraska Press.

31

Disturbances of Self and Identity in Personality Disorders

DREW WESTEN
AMY KEGLEY HEIM

Mr. B could fill a room with his presence. A promising artist whose promise was not materializing rapidly enough for his taste, he came to psychotherapy bitter, angry, and depressed at his life circumstances. His field was not an easy one in which to gain prominence, and he felt grossly underappreciated. "I'm a god," he once said with utter earnestness, but no one seemed to acknowledge his apotheosis. He wavered between this kind of exalted view of himself and a despondent, secret fear that perhaps he was not who he thought he was. In fact, he was typically most grandiose when he was most threatened—when passed over in some way, when he failed to receive expected praise, and so forth. His ideal self—who he wanted (and in this case, thoroughly expected) to be—was as unrealistic as his conscious views of himself. He would have been satisfied with nothing but greatness, and when he feared that he might not be recognized, he became filled with a sense of helpless, impotent rage.

Mr. B is a prototypic example of a narcissistic personality disorder—someone who is grandiose, dismissing and devaluing of others, envious, lacking in the capacity to put himself in another person's mind and empathize with the other's feelings, and prone to responding to failure or criticism with rage and humiliation. Patients with personality disorders provide a useful vantage point on the self and identity, because many personality disorders include disturbances in self and identity at their core, and understanding what happens when self and identity go awry can provide insight into their normal structure and function, just as understanding memory deficits in amnesic patients can provide insight into the structure and function of memory.

We begin this chapter by briefly examining the multiple meanings of self, which we later apply to personality disorders. Next we consider some methodological issues of particular relevance to studying aspects of self in individuals for whom lack of self-knowledge may be diagnostic. We then turn to the clinical, theoretical, and empirical literature on disturbances in self and identity in personality disorders. We conclude by examining the data on the etiology of those disturbances.

Domains of Self and Identity

Despite the considerable prominence enjoyed by "the self" in psychological theory and research over the past 20 years, in many respects the self is a construct characterized by identity confusion. Definitions of self range from "the entire person from a psychological perspective" (McCrae & Costa, 1982) to "what one 'takes oneself to be'" (Markus & Cross, 1990). Theorists often use self-related terms interchangeably, such as self and identity, or self and self-concept.

Here we briefly outline a set of distinctions among "self-relevant" terms that reflect an effort to integrate social psychological views of self with views of self that emerged independently from clinical observation (Westen, 1985, 1992). These two vantage points on the self have much to offer one another because of their complementary strengths and weaknesses. Social psychological research has profitably applied and adapted concepts and methods from cognitive science to the domain of self, and social psychologists routinely use methods that are replicable and allow causal inference—hallmarks of cumulative science that have often been absent from clinical treatments of the self. The clinical setting, in contrast, allows access to people's views of self over months or years and permits exploration of the complex, highly idiosyncratic associative networks that constitute self-experience in its naturalistic setting—networks that influence the way people feel, behave, and experience themselves in highly self-relevant, emotion-laden situations.

The value of clinical concepts and data is likely to become more apparent as researchers increasingly view the self-concept as having *attitude-like* properties—that is, as representations that are associated with affective and behavioral propensities. Many of the characteristics now understood to vary among attitudes—such as the extent to which they are implicit or explicit; their complexity and integration; their affective valence, intensity, and ambivalence; and so forth—have been central to clinical (particularly psychodynamic) descriptions of the self. Indeed, research and clinical observation are converging on a set of propositions about the self that would have been controversial just a decade ago. For example, self-representations have both conscious and unconscious (explicit and implicit) aspects, and, like attitudes toward other objects, explicit views of self may be very different (and sometimes opposite) from implicit views. Further, it is now clear that many if not most aspects of the self-concept are affect laden and are associated with multiple and often contradictory (ambivalent, or, more accurately, multivalent) affective evaluations that are differentially activated under different circumstances.

For the purposes of this chapter, we offer the following (telegraphic) distinctions among several phenomena related to self, beginning with the "self" itself. Although psychologists have used the term to refer to a variety of phenomena, we would likely do well to hyphenate virtually every structure or process for which we would like to reserve the word "self," such as self-esteem, self-reflection, or self-knowledge. If, for example, we use the terms "self" and "self-concept" interchangeably, as frequently occurs in the literature, we confront a logical inconsistency: If our self-concept is our concept of our self, then our self-concept is, by definition, our concept of our self-concept (because self and self-concept are synonymous). This is surely not what we mean by the self-concept (although people's self-concepts may include their understanding of the way they see themselves—something absent in many patients with personality disorders who have trouble taking their own mental processes as objects of thought and hence distinguishing who they are from who they think they are). Logically, the only coherent (if psychologically unsatisfying) use of the term is the colloquial definition of self as *the person*—body, mental contents, attributes, and the like. This is what we mean when we say, "He was only thinking of him*self*," or "She has a negative view of her*self*" (Westen, 1992, 1994a).

It follows that *self-schemas* or *self-representations* are mental representations of the self or person, which can be implicit or explicit. Contemporary thinking about the nature of mental representations may be useful in rethinking what we mean by self-schemas or self-representations (for a review, see Smith, 1998). From a connectionist point of view, a representation is not a static entity but a *potential for reactivation* of a network of units (metaphorically or literally interpreted as neurons) that have been previously activated together. Thus the particular "shape" of a person's representations of self at any given time (Sandler & Rosenblatt, 1962) will reflect the confluence of *chronically* activated networks (potentials for reactivation of well-worn ways of viewing the self) and *recently* activated networks (thoughts, perceptions, etc.). Current and recent experiences will activate and inhibit particular views and experiences of self— that is, they will make some views of self more likely to influence thought, feeling, and behavior. A connectionist model of self would suggest that people have multiple networks representing different aspects of self active outside of awareness at any given time, which collaborate and conflict in ways that produce an explicit self-representation.

A clinically informed connectionist model would add that networks that are active but that do not find conscious representation (whether because they simply do not reach the requisite level of activation or because they are actively inhibited from consciousness) may nonetheless play a substantial role in shaping people's feelings and actions. Further, virtually no representation of self is free of emotional entailments (although some representations, of course, have less of an affective "charge" than others). If I behave aggressively toward someone and interpret my act as assertive or as hostile, I will have two very different feelings about myself. Thus, if we were to integrate a connectionist account with a similarly dynamic view of affect regulation, we might suggest that a person's explicit representations of self at any given time are likely to reflect two simultaneous constraint satisfaction processes: one designed to settle on a representation based on goodness of fit to the data, and the other designed to settle on a representation that maximizes positive and minimizes negative affect (Westen, 1994b, 1998, 1999).

The extent to which a representation of self is distorted by emotional constraints (in a moderately positive direction, as in most people; in a strongly positive direction, as in narcissists; or in a negative direction, as in many depressed and personality-disordered individuals with depressive dynamics) should depend on the extent to which cognitive and emotional constraints are strong or weak (that is, on whether the situation is clear or ambiguous enough to allow multiple attributions and whether different equilibrated solutions would produce weak or strong emotional responses). The degree to which the person's representation of self "fits the facts" should also depend on personality variables such as the individual's tolerance for negative affects of different kinds, ability to regulate self-esteem, and so forth. In this view, "self-enhancement" is a shorthand for an equilibration process by which people regulate emotions such as shame, guilt, anxiety, and pride in the context of cognitive constraints on self-representation that leave enough room for alternative attributions and, hence, for motivated cognition.

Aside from actual self-representations of this sort, people also have a multitude of *desired, feared,* and *ideal* self-representations associated with various affects (Higgins, 1990; Strauman, 1996; Westen, 1985, 1994b). Clinical experience suggests that these representations may also be either implicit or explicit. For example, many people have strong fears of becoming like a parent with whom they have attempted to disidentify (see McWilliams, 1998), and they may become guilty or angry when their behavior resembles that of the parent, even though they may not be consciously aware of why they are feeling what they are feeling and what provoked it. Reducing a discrepancy between wished-for, feared, or ideal self-representations and their corresponding actual self-representations leads to various positive and negative affect states (e.g., guilt, shame, anxiety, embarrassment, pride). Thus people are motivated to change their actual self-representations to increase their correspondence with desired or ideal self-representations and to maximize their discrepancy from feared representations. They can do this by changing who they are (e.g., behaving differently), altering their actual self-representations, or changing their desires, wishes, or ideals for themselves.

When we ask research participants to describe themselves, we typically call on them to access prototypic, explicit representations, which are what we usually mean by the global term, "self-concept." The same is usually true when we ask them about their *self-esteem,* or affective valuation of the self. People tend to have a general "level" of self-esteem to which they gravitate, which is usually loosely congruent with their prototypic self-concept. Self-esteem, in this sense, is the affective component of the person's prototypic attitude toward the self. Even at the level of explicit prototypes, however, people have specific views of themselves (e.g., of their abilities in different domains), which are associated with different affective evaluations (Harter, 1996).

In everyday life, on-line constructions of self and associated feelings reflect in part the activation of particular affect-laden "potentials" (chronically activated networks), as well as discrepancies between actual, feared, desired, and wished-for self-representations. As a result, people experience fluctuations in self-esteem, as different twists of the neural kaleidoscope lead to novel but nonrandom patterns of self-experience. Of particular relevance in this regard are relationship schemas, or *self-with-other representations,* that are often involved in the activation of specific views of self (Baldwin, 1992; Ogilvie & Ashmore, 1991). For a patient with a narcissistic personality disorder such as Mr. B, a perceived slight or criticism, a representation of self with critical or dismissing other, is likely to activate networks that represent a *shamed or humiliated self,* with the attendant affect (which may or may not attain conscious expression). (On the activation of states of mind that include representations and affects, see Horowitz, 1998).

Thus far, we have described a number of ways in which the person can take the self as object—that is, we have focused on *representations of self.* As James (1890/1918) observed, however, the self as object is not isomorphic with a person's subjective sense of self, or self as subject. This *sense of self* includes (1) a sense of continuity of experience (sense of self as having continuity of consciousness and memory over time); (2) a sense of agency (sense of self as an active agent of one's actions); and (3) an experiential sense of self as thinker and feeler of one's own thoughts (Westen, 1992). The sense of self is rarely an object of reflection and has received little empirical attention, although it is central to many psychological views of self and can become disrupted in

certain forms of psychopathology and by certain nonnormative experiences, such as sexual abuse (Westen, 1994a).

Identity is probably the broadest self-related concept, and it shares many aspects of Markus's "dynamic self-concept" (Markus & Wurf, 1987). Most definitions of identity derive at least in part from Erikson (1963, 1968), who emphasized that identity is both a highly personal construction, developed through the integration of various identifications and disidentifications with significant others and reference groups, and a social construction, developed through internalization of roles and reflected appraisals of others. Important components of identity include (1) a sense of personal sameness or continuity over time and across situations, (2) a sense of inner agency, (3) a commitment to certain self-representations as self-defining, (4) a commitment to certain roles as self-defining, (5) acknowledgement of one's role commitments and views of self by significant others, (6) a commitment to a set of core values and ideal self-standards, and (7) and commitment to a worldview that gives life meaning (Wilkinson-Ryan & Westen, 2000).

To summarize, we should be careful when using the term "self" that we all have the same processes in mind when using the same word. Some of the more psychologically meaningful uses of the term may be better denoted by more specific terms, notably "self-representation" (implicit and explicit views of self), "self-esteem" (feelings about the self), "sense of self" (experience of continuity, consciousness, and agency), and "identity" (commitment to aspects of self as defining and meaningful over time).

Assessing Domains of Self and Identity

Equally important as definitional clarity is the question of how to operationalize these constructs. The traditional way of measuring self-relevant thoughts and feelings is via self-report. For example, the most widely used self-esteem scale, the Rosenberg Self-Esteem Scale (SES; Rosenberg, 1965), consists of 10 items that tap the individual's feelings of general self-worth (e.g., "All in all, I am inclined to feel I am a failure"). Other measures, such as the Tennessee Self-

Concept Scale (TSCS; Roid & Fitts, 1994), assess numerous specific domains of self-esteem, such as feelings about the social self and physical self. Other instruments assess highly specific domains of self-esteem (for a review, see Byrne, 1996), such as the Sexual Self-Esteem Scale (Gaynor & Underwood, 1995) and the Body Esteem Scale (BES; Franzio & Shields, 1984).

From a clinical point of view, self-report instruments such as these can be very useful in tapping explicit, but not implicit, self-esteem (Westen, 1985, 1991, 1992), a problem that has recently prompted development of implicit measures that we suspect are likely to revolutionize the literatures on self and self-esteem (Devos & Banaji, Chapter 8, this volume). Traditional self-report measures rely on a set of largely implicit assumptions that are problematic: (1) that conscious and unconscious views of self are similar; (2) that the representations activated when people are asked to describe explicit, prototypic aspects of self are the same representations activated in everyday life that guide relevant thought, feeling, and behavior; (3) that people have the expertise and knowledge to report on dimensions of self that may be subtle; and (4) that defensive and self-presentation biases are either minimal or can be detected using self-report scales designed to detect bias. For example, if Mr. B, described at the beginning of this chapter, were to complete the Rosenberg Self-Esteem Scale, he would almost certainly strongly endorse many items indicative of high self-esteem. Multiple sources of narrative and behavioral data suggested, however, that Mr. B was at times filled with self-doubt, feelings of inferiority, and abject despair about himself—feelings that were only consciously accessible to him in fleeting moments under very specific circumstances. Even if an occasional item "caught" some of these feelings, his score would be difficult to distinguish from that of someone with moderately high self-esteem who rated every item a solid 4 out of 5, as opposed to mostly 5s with an occasional 1 or 2.

An increasing body of data suggests that the kind of defensive inflation of explicit views of self characteristic of people such as Mr. B can be measured reliably using observational methods such as narrative interviews or observation of behavior in groups and that this kind of defensive distortion of self-representations comes at considerable cost to the individual (not to mention those around him or her). For example, Shedler, Mayman, and Manis (1993) found that individuals who scored high on a self-report measure of positive mental health but low on a clinician-based assessment of the same construct (assessed from participants' earliest memories) showed higher levels of coronary reactivity than both individuals with genuinely good mental health and those who acknowledged their distress (e.g., anxiety). Colvin and Block (1994) have shown that individuals described by neutral observers of their behavior as narcissistic suffer in multiple ways interpersonally that are not revealed by their self-reports.

Similarly, Robins and Beer (2001) found that self-enhancement of personal abilities can have short-term benefits but that people who rely on substantial self-enhancement ultimately experience less well-being and show worse adaptation than people who perceive themselves more accurately. In a longitudinal study, along with completing questionnaire measures of variables such as narcissism and self-esteem, college freshmen rated their expected academic performance in college. The researchers then collected data regarding their actual performance annually until graduation. The investigators operationalized academic self-enhancement by computing the discrepancy between prior academic performance (as measured by high school GPA and SAT scores) and self-reported performance. Students who self-enhanced early in their academic careers were more likely to disengage from academics over time, as reality failed to support their inflated expectations, and were more likely to drop out of school.

In general, self-report instruments have difficulty teasing apart genuine self-esteem and associated representations of self from impression management and self-deception (Farnham, Greenwald, & Banaji, 1999). Thus, in recent years, several researchers have developed methods for assessing implicit aspects of self-concept (e.g., Aidman, 1999; Bosson, Swann, & Pennebaker, 2000; Greenwald & Farnham, 2000; Pelham & Hetts, 1999). For example, Greenwald and Farnham (2000) have adapted the Implicit Associations Test (IAT; Greenwald,

McGhee, & Schwartz, 1998) to measure implicit self-esteem and self-concept. The procedure rests on the premise that the strength of association between pairs of concepts and attributes (e.g., self–good, other–bad) is reflected in response latency.

Researchers have developed other methods of accessing implicit aspects of self as well. Ogilvie and Ashmore (1991) developed a way of measuring self-with-other representations that samples people's explicit self-representations but avoids asking them to make generalizations about patterns in the way they represent themselves across relationships. Participants rate themselves on a set of dimensions across numerous relationships of their choosing (such as relationships with a sibling, boss, parent, etc.). A hierarchical-classes analysis reduces the data to a small set of clusters of prominent self-with-other themes, that is, ways the person describes self with others that appear to cut across a subset of relationships. Although this method does not, strictly speaking, measure implicit representations, it *aggregates* data within participants in ways that capture implicit themes or personal constructs.

Westen and colleagues (Westen & Cohen, 1993; Westen & Muderrisoglu, 2001; Westen & Shedler, 1999a, 1999b) have been approaching the measurement of aspects of self through narrative methods. Their method is predicated on the view that the representations of self that influence thought, feeling, and behavior in everyday life, like many other personality processes, are less likely to be revealed in participants' answers to direct questions about themselves of the format, "Are you the kind of person who . . ." than in their narrative descriptions of their lives (and particularly of emotionally meaningful interpersonal interactions). The assumptions underlying this method rest on clinical observation and on research showing that this is, in fact, the way clinicians of all theoretical persuasions assess personality (Westen & Arkowitz-Westen, 1998), as well as on the burgeoning literature in cognitive neuroscience on the pervasive role of implicit processes in thought, feeling, and behavior.

In this view, by virtue of the "architecture" of cognition, emotion, and motivation, people cannot be expected to report what is implicit, even if their reports are not substantially biased by motives for self-presentation or self-esteem maintenance. Nor should we expect that people without expertise in personality assessment—namely, participants themselves—should be uniformly the best observers of personality, particularly in cases such as personality disorders, in which lack of self-insight is diagnostic. In fact, self-report questionnaires and structured interviews have produced poor validity coefficients in diagnosing personality disorders such as narcissistic, paranoid, and passive–aggressive (Perry, 1992). (In fact, passive–aggressive personality disorder was deleted from the latest edition of the DSM (American Psychiatric Association, 1994), in part because it could not be measured reliably by asking people to describe themselves.) In contrast, recent data suggest that narrative-based assessment of patients' personality pathology produces correlations between the treating clinician and a pair of independent interviewers in the range of $r = .80$ (Westen & Muderrisoglu, 2001).

In describing these methods that rely less on self-report, we do not mean to offer the simple view that self-reports are bad and other forms of measurement are good. Whether self-reports provide valid data about aspects of self depends on the way they are used. When used to assess people's explicit, prototypic views of self, well-constructed self-report instruments produce valid data. To the extent that the aim is not simply to know about people's generalizations about themselves, however, the use of self-report methods can become problematic. If the aim is to understand self-representations as they manifest in daily life (and, presumably, as they affect thought, feeling, and behavior), we might do well to rely less on participants to aggregate their views over time, essentially providing their explicit theories about themselves. At the very least, we might do well to ask them to describe what they are thinking and feeling in situations relevant to the domain of interest and to aggregate these descriptions over time ourselves. Perhaps most important, when used to assess people's self-representations without qualifying by level of consciousness (implicit or explicit), as has been the norm in psychological research on aspects of self,

self-reports are likely to produce misleading data for a substantial subset of individuals for whom discrepancies between implicit and explicit views are as psychologically interesting as their convergence (Westen, 1998).

Measurement of identity is another field that has seen substantial progress in recent years. Based on Erikson's theory, Marcia (1966, 1980) devised a semistructured interview to assess adolescents' and adults' levels of commitment and exploration with regard to occupational choices and ideological concerns. Using the data from these interviews, individuals can be reliably classified into four identity statuses, which represent different levels of identity resolution: identity achievement, moratorium, foreclosure, and identity diffusion.

Identity achievement in Marcia's system represents the most mature level of identity development. Individuals with this status have explored and subsequently made commitments to various occupational and ideological choices. Moratorium is often a stage on the way to identity development, although it may also represent a permanent state of instability. In moratorium, the individual explores various identity issues without making any firm commitments. Individuals with a foreclosed status have prematurely settled on occupations and beliefs that others have prescribed for them, without undertaking a period of exploration or questioning. Individuals with this status typically express black-and-white views and lean toward an authoritarian stance to the world. Identity diffusion, the status most relevant to personality pathology, is not unusual in normal adolescence and early adulthood. It describes those individuals who have not determined an ideological or occupational direction and who may be characterized by social isolation, withdrawal, and a lack of a sense of continuity over time. In a broader sense, identity diffusion is Erikson's term for the failure to achieve an integrated sense of self. Identity diffusion typically involves phenomena such as a subjective sense of incoherence, inability to commit to roles, and repeated shifts in ideology. Marcia's (1980) identity statuses have generated considerable research over the past 20 years, documenting the relationship between identity status and a range of

theoretically related variables, such as personality (e.g., security-seeking; Kroger, 1995); attitudes (e.g., AIDS attitudes; Moore & Barling, 1991); object relations (Marcia, 1994); and level of integrative complexity (Slugoski, Marcia, & Koopman, 1984).

To summarize, assessment of aspects of self and identity is less straightforward than it might appear and less straightforward than has typically been the case, although exciting new methodological developments promise to change the way researchers measure and understand self-related processes. Of particular importance is the development of methods of assessing implicit self-representations and implicit aspects of self-esteem, which are especially important to address in research with clinical populations, such as in patients with personality disorders. Self-reports are likely to be appropriate for some purposes and not for others; for this reason, they should not be the default in assessment. Self-reports are most likely to be valid when (1) processes being reported are available to introspection, such as behaviors and conscious phenomenology; (2) processes being reported do not require training, expertise, or norms (e.g., "I have high self-esteem" relative to whom?) that lay observers may not have; (3) domains being assessed do not have implications for self-esteem and hence are less likely to elicit defensive biases; and (4) domains being assessed are only minimally relevant with respect to social desirability, so that self-presentation biases are less likely to be engaged.

Self and Identity in Personality Disorders

Issues of self play a role in many forms of psychopathology. People who are depressed tend to have negative views of self. Individuals with schizophrenia often have difficulty representing key aspects of self at all and distinguishing the most basic attributes of self (thoughts, feelings, etc.) from those of others. This is perhaps most apparent in auditory hallucinations, in which individuals with schizophrenia may mistake their own psychological processes for someone else's voice. The most blatant form of identity disturbance is found in dissociative identity disorder (DID; APA, 1994), formerly called multiple personality disorder. In DID, the patient's identity consists of two or more partial identities, sometimes called part-selves or alters, that are "split off" and carry out different functions. In this disorder, usually the result of extreme sexual and/or physical abuse in childhood (Lewis & Yeager, 1994), the person may have no awareness of actions carried out in one state while in another. What distinguishes DID is not only the fragmented identity in the Eriksonian sense but also profound deficits in the *sense of self*—particularly the subjective experience of self as agent and as continuous through time.

Profound disturbances in aspects of self also distinguish many forms of personality disorder. For example, McWilliams (1994) describes the self-representations of the "paranoid self" as involving a polar opposition between an "impotent, humiliated, and despised" self-image and an "omnipotent, vindicated, triumphant one" (p. 214). Individuals with paranoid personality disorder frequently maintain self-esteem through attempts to thwart authority figures or institutions. Success in defying authority provides a sense of vindication and temporary feelings of safety and moral righteousness.

What Are Personality Disorders?

Personality disturbances have captured the attention of observers for much of recorded history, beginning at least with Hippocrates' and Galen's efforts to link character styles to biological variables (an approach recently brought back into currency by Cloninger; Cloninger, Svrakic, Bayon, & Przybeck, 1999). Modern interest in personality pathology emerged in the 19th century when Prichard (1835) coined the term "moral insanity" to describe deviant behavior patterns in individuals whose reasoning processes, unlike those of patients with psychosis, remained intact. (This distinction remains the basis of the "insanity defense," which is predicated on a view of people as either capable or incapable of moral decision making based on the intactness of their cognition.)

The concept of *personality disorder* emerged in the 1930s and 1940s in the psychoanalytic literature, as clinicians and the-

orists discovered a class of patients whose problems seemed to lie less in circumscribed symptoms (such as phobias or obsessive–compulsive thoughts and rituals) than in their enduring ways of thinking, understanding themselves and others, regulating their impulses and feelings, and interacting with other people (Kernberg, 1975; Reich, 1933). Coupled with similar observations in the early to mid-20th century by descriptive psychiatrists of patients who seemed to have enduring melancholic traits or peculiarities of thinking that did not quite cross the threshold for psychosis, the concept of personality disorder found its way into the official *Diagnostic and Statistical Manual of Mental Disorders (DSM)*.

In the original version of the manual (APA, 1952), the disorders presently termed personality disorders (PDs) were grouped under headings such as "personality pattern disturbance" and "personality trait disturbance." The major impetus to research on PDs came with the publication of DSM-III (APA, 1980), which introduced a multiaxial system of diagnosis, including a separate "axis" devoted primarily to PDs. The current edition of the DSM (DSM-IV; APA, 1994) defines a personality disorder as "an enduring pattern of inner experience and behavior that deviates markedly from the expectations of the individual's culture, is pervasive and inflexible, has an onset in adolescence or early adulthood, is stable over time, and leads to distress or impairment" (p. 629). The PDs include 10 disorders, grouped into three thematic clusters based loosely on factor-analytic research. The odd or eccentric cluster (cluster A) includes schizotypal, schizoid, and paranoid PDs. The three disorders share social peculiarity and withdrawal, with varying degrees and types of cognitive disturbance. The dramatic, emotional, or erratic cluster (cluster B) includes histrionic, borderline, narcissistic, and antisocial PDs. These PDs share features such as self-centeredness, impulsivity, and difficulty empathizing with others' experience. The anxious or fearful cluster (cluster C) includes obsessive–compulsive, avoidant, and dependent PDs. These disorders (particularly obsessive–compulsive) are less easily characterized by a single set of shared features, although one central thread is anxiety (warded off in obsessive–compulsive individuals, expressing itself strongly in social situations in avoidant individuals, and tied to fears of separation and independence in dependent patients).

To illustrate the diagnosis of the personality disorders, we use the example of narcissistic personality disorder, an example of which opened this chapter. Narcissistic personality disorder (NPD) is characterized by a "pervasive pattern of grandiosity (in fantasy or behavior), need for admiration, and lack of empathy, beginning by early adulthood and present in a variety of contexts" (APA, 1994, p. 661). NPD has nine criteria, of which five are necessary to make the diagnosis: (1) has a grandiose sense of self-importance; (2) is preoccupied with fantasies of unlimited success, power, brilliance, beauty, or ideal love; (3) believes that he or she is "special" and unique and can only be understood by, or should associate with, other special or high-status people (or institutions); (4) requires excessive admiration; (5) has a sense of entitlement; (6) is interpersonally exploitative; (7) lacks empathy, is unwilling to recognize or identify with the feelings and needs of others; (8) is often envious of others or believes that others are envious of him or her; and (9) shows arrogant, haughty behaviors or attitudes (p. 661).

The DSM-IV classification is not flawless, and although substantially influenced by empirical research, particularly since the inception of DSM-III, it continues to face numerous challenges. For example, many researchers have argued that a dimensional system would more accurately describe individuals with personality pathology than the current categorical system, and the 10 diagnoses included in the manual are highly overlapping (Clark, Livesley, & Morey, 1997; Oldham et al., 1992; Westen & Shedler, 2000; Widiger, 1993). Nonetheless, the DSM-IV provides a rough map of the terrain of personality disturbance that represents a significant advance over the babble of personality descriptions that existed before some effort to standardize categories and criteria.

Pathology of Self in Personality Disorders

The clinical literature offers a wealth of phenomenological and theoretical descriptions of pathology of self in patients with PDs, although empirical literature has only more recently begun to emerge. The disorders that have received the most attention are borderline and narcissistic. This makes considerable sense, given the central role of self-pathology in both disorders: the identity confusion characteristic of borderline patients and the grandiosity characteristic of narcissistic patients. We review, as well, the empirical findings on other disorders for which data are available.

Self and Identity in Borderline Pathology

Kernberg (1976, 1984) has provided the most extensive theoretical and phenomenological description of borderline pathology. Kernberg focuses on what he calls borderline personality *organization* (BPO), which he locates on a continuum between psychotic and neurotic (by which he means relatively high-functioning) forms of personality structure. Patients with borderline personality organization lack the overt disturbances in self and reality testing characteristic of psychotic patients. However, they lack the capacity to regulate impulses and emotion and to understand the self and others in ways that allow healthier people to love and to work successfully. While similar in many respects to the DSM-IV diagnosis of borderline personality disorder (BPD), BPO is a broader construct that encompasses a number of DSM-IV PDs in addition to BPD. For Kernberg, patients with paranoid, schizoid, schizotypal, and antisocial personality disorders typically function at a borderline level, as do many patients with histrionic and dependent personality disorders.

In Kernberg's conceptualization, pathology of self is a hallmark of borderline pathology. People with more adaptive forms of personality organization can integrate contradictory representations of the self and others and can represent themselves as essentially the same person across time and situations, even though they recognize that they may behave differently at different times. In contrast, patients with BPO suffer from a lack of integration of self-representations, for which Kernberg (1984) uses Erikson's term, "identity diffusion" (Clarkin, Kernberg, & Somavia, 1998; Kernberg, 1984). As outlined by Kernberg (1975,

1984) and elaborated by Akhtar (1984, 1992), the identity diffusion seen in patients with BPO consists of six basic clinical features. The first involves contradictory character traits that produce representations of self that are difficult to integrate. The patient may evidence gross contradictions in behavior (e.g., behaving alternately in ways that are prudish and promiscuous), perceptions of self (e.g., seeing the self as a complete success or a total failure), or vocational interests. These contradictions make it difficult for the patient and others to get a clear picture of the person as an integrated person. The second feature is the temporal discontinuity of the self, whereby the patient lacks a sense of the self as continuous through time. The sense of "a life lived in pieces" captures this experience (Pfeiffer, 1974). Third is a lack of authenticity, manifest in a chameleon-like identity in which the person changes who she is and perceives herself to be depending on who she is with—a phenomenon first described by Deutsch (1942) as the "as-if" personality. (We use the female pronoun here and the male pronoun later in describing narcissistic personality disorder as a convenience, reflecting the differential rates of the two disorders in men and women.) Fourth are feelings of emptiness and emotional numbing that lead to feelings of inner deadness and fears of being alone (because aloneness becomes nothingness if the self can only be defined in relation to significant others). A fifth feature is gender dysphoria, manifest in opposite-gender behaviors and confusion regarding choice of sexual partner and the gender to which one belongs. The sixth feature is an inordinate ethnic and moral relativism, which involves a lack of stable values and cultural or ethnic affiliation. Similar to the chameleon-like quality of the inauthentic self described previously, the patient's beliefs and values may change along with those of members of her social group. Akhtar (1992) added a seventh clinical feature often observed in patients with identity diffusion: disturbances in body image, seen particularly in borderline patients with bulimia.

Focusing more specifically on borderline personality *disorder* as defined in DSM-III and DSM-IV, Westen and Cohen (1993) summarized the most central components of identity disturbance believed to characterize BPD as taken from the extant theoretical, clinical, and empirical literatures. Their description resembles Kernberg's (1975) and Akhtar's (1984) descriptions of BPO in many respects. It includes the following features: (1) a lack of consistently invested goals, values, ideals, and relationships; (2) a tendency to make temporary hyperinvestments in roles, value systems, worldviews, and relationships that ultimately break down and lead to a sense of emptiness and meaninglessness; (3) gross inconsistencies in behavior over time and across situations that lead to a relatively accurate perception of the self as lacking coherence; (4) difficulty integrating multiple representations of the self at any given time; (5) a lack of a coherent life narrative or sense of continuity over time; and (6) a lack of continuity of relationships that results in the loss of shared memories that contribute to a coherent sense of self over time. In terms of the distinctions with which we began, most of these disturbances are disturbances in the sense of self (the subjective experience of agency and continuity over time) and identity, although borderline patients are also prone to particular representations of self (e.g., self as globally bad or loathsome; Westen et al., 1992) and self-with-other paradigms (e.g., abandoned self–rejecting other, victimized self–victimizing other; Nigg, Lohr, Westen, Gold, & Silk, 1992). In addition, as emphasized by Kernberg (1984) and supported by subsequent research (Baker, Silk, Westen, Nigg, & Lohr, 1992), borderline patients tend to "split" their representations of self and others into good and bad and to have difficulty forming coherent, integrated representations that incorporate both positive and negative features in ways that capture the realities of human personality.

Empirical research on identity disturbance in borderline personality disorder is sparse. Taylor (1995) points out that the DSM criterion that captures identity disturbance has proved one of the least reliable criteria among the PDs, stemming largely from the vagueness of the item ("identity disturbance: markedly and persistently unstable self-image or sense of self" [DSM-IV, APA, 1994, p. 654]) and its nonspecificity to BPD. In an effort to refine the concept of identity disturbance empirically, Wilkinson-Ryan and Westen (2000) developed a 36-item identity-disturbance instrument for clinician report, based on clinical, theoretical, and empirical descriptions of identity disturbance. Their aims were (1) to use factor analysis to identify whether identity disturbance is a unitary construct; (2) to examine the relation between aspects of identity disturbance and BPD; and (3) to assess the extent to which borderline pathology independently contributes to variance in identity diffusion, holding constant a history of sexual abuse. The role of sexual abuse is of significance because between 50% and 75% of patients with BPD report a history of sexual abuse (see Zanarini, 1997) and because sexual abuse is known to disrupt multiple aspects of self, leading to dissociation (and, in extreme cases, dissociative identity disorder).

Using a practice research network approach, in which researchers quantify descriptions of patients provided by a random sample of clinicians using psychometric instruments designed for clinician report, Wilkinson-Ryan and Westen (2000) found identity disturbance to be a multidimensional construct consisting of four factors: role absorption (tendency to define the self based on a single role or label, such as "adult child of an alcoholic"), painful incoherence (the patient's subjective distress and concern about lack of coherence), inconsistency (objective inconsistency of behavior, which the patient typically does not find troubling), and lack of commitment (to roles, values, and long-term relationships). Three of the four factors distinguished borderline patients from other patients in the sample, including those with other PDs, with painful incoherence most associated with BPD. The lack of commitment factor did not distinguish between patients with BPD and patients with other forms of pathology, casting doubt on its specificity as a diagnostic criterion, despite its centrality in the clinical construct. Although all factors also correlated with a history of sexual abuse, regression analysis showed that BPD diagnosis continued to predict identity disturbance on all four dimensions when sexual abuse history was held constant. Sexual abuse history contributed independently to only one identity disturbance factor, painful

incoherence, suggesting that the identity disturbance seen in borderline patients is *sui generis* and does not appear to be a consequence of abuse history.

Self and Identity in Narcissistic Personality Disorder

Although many of Kernberg's major contributions have been in the understanding of borderline phenomena, his theories of narcissistic disturbance contributed substantially to the development of the diagnosis of NPD in DSM-III, just as they did to the borderline diagnosis. According to Kernberg (1984), whereas borderline patients lack an integrated identity, narcissistic patients are developmentally more advanced, in that they have been able to develop a consistent view of themselves. A core feature of their pathology, however, lies in the view of self that they need to construct to maintain self-esteem, namely one that is grossly inflated. According to Kernberg, not only are the conscious self-representations of narcissistic patients inflated but so also are the representations that constitute their ideal self. Actual and ideal self, in his view, exist in dynamic relation to one another: One reason that narcissistic patients must maintain such an idealized view of self is that they have a correspondingly grandiose view of who they should and must be, divergence from which leads to tremendous feelings of shame, failure, and humiliation.

The concept of a grandiose self is central to the theory of Heinz Kohut, one of the other major theorists of narcissistic personality pathology, whose ideas, like those of Kernberg, contributed to the DSM diagnosis of NPD (Goldstein, 1985). Like many other theorists, Kohut's (1971, 1977) use of the term "self" is inconsistent, sometimes used to refer to all of personality and at other times limited to self-representations. His main contribution, however, was his attempt to describe the self as a core structure at the heart of personality (hence the term "self psychology," which refers to the theoretical system he developed within psychoanalysis).

The Kohutian self in this distinctive sense is the nucleus of a person's central ambitions and ideals and the talents and skills used to actualize them (Kohut, 1971; Wolf,

1988). It develops through two pathways, or what Kohut calls "poles" of the self, which provide the basis for self-esteem. The first is what he calls the *grandiose self*—an idealized representation of self that emerges in children through empathic mirroring by their parents ("mommy, watch!") and provides the nucleus for later ambitions and strivings. The second he calls the *idealized parent imago*—an idealized representation of the parents, which provides the foundation for ideals and standards for the self. Parental mirroring allows the child to experience himself as reflected in the eyes of a loving and admiring parent; idealizing a parent or parents allows the child to identify with and become like an idealized other. In the absence of adequate experiences with parents who can mirror the child and serve as appropriate targets of idealization (for example, when the parents are self-involved or abusive), the child's self-structure cannot develop, preventing the achievement of cohesion, vigor, and normal self-esteem (which Kohut describes as "healthy narcissism"). As a result, the child develops a disorder of the self, of which pathological narcissism is a prototypic example.

Most research on NPD of relevance to self has examined the diagnostic efficiency of various diagnostic criteria. The results of these studies generally support the centrality of grandiose representations and grandiose fantasies as defining features of narcissistic patients (Gunderson, Ronningstam, & Smith, 1995). In two studies not limited to DSM criteria, Westen and Shedler (1999a; Shedler & Westen, 1998) used a personality pathology Q-sort with a large national sample of patients with PDs to examine the psychological characteristics of patients diagnosed with different PDs. Both studies produced similar findings; we describe here the larger study ($N = 530$) with the most recent version of the Q-sort (Westen & Shedler, 1999a). The following items related to self were among the 20 most highly ranked (i.e., highly descriptive) items out of the 200 items in the instrument in an aggregate description of patients diagnosed by their treating clinicians with NPD: has an exaggerated sense of self-importance; tends to feel mistreated, misunderstood, or victimized; and expects self to be "perfect" (an item that supports Kernberg's view of the

narcissistic patient's exaggerated ideal self). When the investigators ignored clinicians' DSM-IV diagnoses and instead derived diagnostic prototypes empirically using Q-factor analysis (a clustering technique), the narcissistic cluster that emerged included the following items among those most descriptive: has fantasies of unlimited success, power, beauty, talent, brilliance, and so forth; has an exaggerated sense of self-importance; expects self to be "perfect"; tends to feel false or fraudulent; and has a disturbed or distorted body image (sees self as unattractive, grotesque, disgusting, etc.; Westen & Shedler, 1999b). Interestingly, this empirically derived prototype included not only the manifestly grandiose self-representations, fantasied self-representations, and ideal self-representations of narcissistic patients but also some of their underlying fears about themselves, such as feelings of fraudulence and unattractiveness. We are unaware of self-report studies similarly finding such fears to be characteristic of the explicit prototypic views of self reported by narcissistic patients. The discrepancy between self- and observer reports corroborates theoretical assertions that implicit and explicit representations may be very different in narcissistic patients (e.g., Westen, 1990), with the latter primarily reflecting overt grandiosity and the former reflecting both grandiose ideal self-representations and dreaded devalued (feared) representations of self.

Other Research on Self and Identity Disturbance in Personality Disorders

Empirical literature relating to self in other personality disorders is limited. Two recent studies have linked self-esteem to PD diagnosis or PD traits (Sinha & Watson, 1997; Watson, 1998). These studies found that low self-esteem was a significant predictor of 7 of 11 PD diagnoses and showed the strongest association with borderline personality disorder, avoidant personality disorder, dependent personality disorder, and obsessive–compulsive personality disorder. The link to self-esteem makes sense in light of depressive and self-doubting dynamics seen clinically in patients with many PDs, particularly those found in these studies to have low self-esteem.

Research using Benjamin's (1974, 1996a, 1996b) Structural Analysis of Social Behavior (SASB) is also relevant to issues of self in PDs. The SASB is a three-dimensional circumplex model with three surfaces that provides a sophisticated method of assessing complex interpersonal and intrapersonal processes. Of particular relevance is one surface of the SASB, called the "introject circumplex," which captures the way an individual treats him- or herself. It is so named because of the assumption that internalized (introjected) treatment by significant others shapes the self-concept and associated ways of "interacting" with oneself, a view amply supported by research (Benjamin, 1974, 1996a). One axis of the introject circumplex represents the attachment dimension (in this case, attachment to self), with end points of self-love and self-hate. Although systematic work with samples of patients with PDs remains to be done, Benjamin has recently offered an extensive application of the SASB to the study and treatment of PDs (1993, 1996a, 1996b), and research on the introject surface is likely to provide useful information on self-esteem and self-abuse in patients with PD.

Etiology of Self Pathology in Personality Disorders

As with most forms of psychopathology, prime etiological variables include genetic influences, environmental events, and gene–environment interactions and transactions. Here we provide a brief overview of three areas of research of relevance to the etiology of PDs that have particular implications for the origins of self-disturbance: behavior genetics, attachment, and trauma.

Behavior Genetics

The vast majority of behavior-genetic studies of personality have focused on normal personality traits, such as those that make up the Five-Factor Model (Widiger & Trull, 1992) and Eysenck's (1967, 1981) three-factor model (extraversion, neuroticism, and psychoticism). These studies have generally shown moderate to large heritability for a range of personality traits, from 30% to 60% (Livesley, Jang, Jackson, & Vernon,

1993; Plomin & Caspi, 1999). The most frequently studied traits, extraversion and neuroticism, have produced heritability estimates of 54% to 74%, and of 42% to 64%, respectively (Eysenck, 1990). When measures other than self-report are used, heritability estimates decrease somewhat but remain within the moderate range (e.g., Plomin & Caspi, 1999).

Compared to research on normal personality traits, studies of the heritability of PDs have been rare (see Nigg & Goldsmith, 1994). The most common design has been family studies, in which researchers begin with the PD proband and then assess other family members. The major limitation of this method is that familial aggregation of disorders can support either genetic or environmental causes. Hence, twin and adoption studies tend to provide more definitive data.

A number of family, twin, and adoption studies have focused on the genetic basis of PDs, although the majority of these studies have examined only a subset of the DSM PDs, particularly schizotypal, antisocial, and borderline personality disorders. These disorders appear to reflect a continuum of heritability, with schizotypal most strongly linked to genetic influences, antisocial linked both to environmental and genetic variables, and borderline showing the smallest estimates of heritability.

Research on the heritability of schizotypal personality disorder provides the clearest evidence of a genetic component to a personality disorder. (Schizotypal personality disorder is defined by criteria such as odd beliefs or magical thinking, unusual perceptual experiences, odd thinking and speech, suspiciousness, inappropriate or constricted affect, and behavior or appearance that is odd or eccentric.) Early observers of schizophrenia (e.g., Bleuler, 1911/1950; Kraepelin, 1896/1919) often noted peculiarities in language and behavior among the relatives of their schizophrenic patients. Bleuler called this presentation "latent schizophrenia" and considered it to be a less severe and more widespread form of schizophrenia. Further research into the constellation of symptoms characteristic of relatives of schizophrenic patients ultimately resulted in the creation of the DSM diagnosis of schizotypal personality disorder (SPD; Spitzer, Endicott, & Gibbon, 1979). A genetic relationship between schizophrenia and SPD is now well established (Kendler & Walsh, 1995; Lenzenweger, 1998). For example, using data from the Roscommon Family Study, Kendler and his colleagues (e.g., Kendler et al., 1993; Kendler, McGuire, Gruenberg, & Walsh, 1995; Kendler & Walsh, 1995) found a significant familial relationship between SPD and schizophrenia. Torgersen (1984) found that 33% (7 of 21) of identical co-twins had SPD, whereas only 4% (1 of 23) of fraternal co-twins shared the diagnosis.

Antisocial personality disorder, in contrast, appears to have both genetic and environmental roots, as documented in adoption studies (Cadoret, Yates, Troughton, Woodworth, & Stewart, 1995). An adult adoptee whose biological parent had an arrest record for antisocial behavior is four times more likely to have problems with aggressive behavior than a person without a biological vulnerability. At the same time, a person whose *adoptive* parent had antisocial personality disorder is more than three times more likely to develop the disorder, regardless of biological history.

In contrast to schizotypal and antisocial personality disorders, research on the behavioral genetics of BPD has yielded much less evidence of heritability. Modest degrees of familiality have emerged in several studies (e.g., Reich, 1989); however, the bulk of the evidence does not support genetic explanations (Dahl, 1993; Nigg & Goldsmith, 1994). For example, Torgerson (1984), in the only twin study on borderline PD, failed to find evidence for the genetic transmission of the disorder, although the sample was relatively small. However, some authors (e.g., Nigg & Goldsmith, 1994; Widiger & Allen, 1994) have suggested that the personality trait neuroticism, which is highly heritable, is at the core of many borderline features (e.g., negative affect and sensitivity to stress). Further, other components of BPD have shown substantial heritability, including one of particular importance for our present purposes—problems with identity (Livesley et al., 1993).

Although behavioral genetic data are proving increasingly important in understanding the etiology of personality disorders (e.g., Livesley, Jang, & Vernon, 1998),

their relevance to aspects of self remains unclear. With some notable exceptions, studies have not examined self-representations, sense of self, identity, or other related constructs. Nevertheless, to the extent that one can take personality self-descriptions as a mixture of relatively accurate descriptions of personality and as self-representations ("theories" of the self; Epstein, 1973), they are likely to provide at least indirect data on the heritability of some aspects of self. Further, because traits such as neuroticism are likely to be accompanied by particular kinds of self-representations (e.g., negative views of self), then aspects of self can be presumed, like other personality traits, to range in heritability, with most showing moderate heritability.

Attachment

An environmental variable that has proven robust as a predictor of various forms of personality pathology is attachment history. Bowlby (1969, 1973) defined attachment as a behavioral system designed to provide proximity to attachment figures, who ensure the protection and hence the survival of offspring. The balance between proximity, which is essential for survival, and distance, which is necessary over time for exploration, is achieved behaviorally and is regulated by an "internal organization" that includes representations of the self and attachment figures. According to Bowlby, the major determinant of the quality of the child's attachment is the caregiver's ability to respect the child's desire for a secure base while facilitating his or her exploratory behaviors and remaining available to offer the child love and care when needed (Bowlby, 1977). Provided these conditions are met, the child is likely to develop a secure attachment characterized by "a representational model of himself as being both able to help himself and as worthy of being helped" (1977, p. 206). Subsequent research has supported the central role of maternal sensitivity or attunement in the development of secure "internal working models" of relationships in infancy (e.g., De Wolff & van IJzendoorn, 1997).

Ainsworth, Blehar, Waters, and Wall (1978) devised the Strange Situation to identify the attachment patterns of infants.

This method involves brief separations of caregiver and infant and observation of the infant's reactions, particularly during reunion periods. Two-thirds of infants show secure attachment, meaning that they show distress when separated and pleasure on reunion. Insecure infants exhibit either resistant-ambivalent or avoidant attachment styles. Resistant-ambivalent infants experience their caregiver as unable consistently to meet their needs, resulting in considerable separation anxiety, a reluctance to explore their surroundings because of preoccupation with the caregiver, and alternations between clinging and resistant behavior. In contrast, infants experiencing repeated rejection by their caregivers when seeking to have their needs met tend to develop an avoidant style. As a result, they typically deny their need for love and emotional support and adopt an outwardly self-sufficient style; in the Strange Situation such infants will show little outward concern regarding the coming and going of the caregiver. More recently, a fourth type of attachment has been identified as disorganized (Main & Solomon, 1990). The disorganized pattern usually results from chronic neglect or abuse (Cicchetti, Toth, & Lynch, 1995) and is indicated by confused and disoriented behavior when the infant reunites with the caregiver. The child may appear frightened in the caregiver's presence and be very difficult to soothe.

A quantum leap forward in linking infant attachment to later outcomes came with the development of the Adult Attachment Interview (AAI; George, Kaplan, & Main, 1985), which was devised to assess the attachment status of adults through an analysis of narrative accounts of important attachment relationships during childhood. The AAI yields four primary attachment classifications that closely parallel the infant attachment styles: autonomous (secure), dismissing (avoidant), preoccupied (resistant), and unresolved (disorganized).

Given the extent to which many PDs are disorders of attachment at core (e.g., the social distancing of schizoid and avoidant patients; the detachment of antisocial patients; the unstable, disorganized attachments of patients with BPD), attachment history and attachment status are of obvious relevance to the development of PDs and of related

disturbances of self (see, e.g., Nakash-Eisikovits, Dutra, & Westen, in press). For example, Rosenstein and Horowitz (1996) assessed the attachment status of adolescent inpatients and found strong associations between a dismissing attachment style and the presence of conduct disorder, substance abuse, narcissistic personality disorder, antisocial personality disorder, and self-reported narcissistic, antisocial and paranoid traits. In contrast, adolescents with a more preoccupied attachment style were more likely to have a mood disorder, obsessive–compulsive personality disorder, histrionic personality disorder, borderline personality disorder, or schizotypal personality disorder, and self-reported avoidant, anxious, and dysthymic traits. Other research suggests that adult patients with BPD (Fonagy et al., 1996) and adults who were hospitalized as adolescents for severe personality pathology (Allen, Hauser, & Borman-Spurrell, 1996), are likely to be classified as "unresolved" using the AAI. These individuals tend to have incoherent internal working models of both self and others.

Fonagy and colleagues have studied severe personality disorders, primarily BPD, from an attachment perspective, focusing on the development of what they call *mentalization* (e.g., Fonagy, Target, & Gergely, 2000). Mentalization involves the capacity to understand one's own and others' mental states, such as thoughts, wishes, beliefs, and feelings. A hallmark of mentalization is the ability to attribute beliefs, desires, and other mental states to others that are based neither on one's own beliefs and desires nor on simple physical realities. In other words, it refers to the capacity to imagine another person's mental experience, which is crucial in understanding and predicting their actions. Development of this capacity depends on the responses of caregivers, who both make inferences about and help clarify the contents of the child's mind and allow the child to explore the mind of the caregiver. This process provides the child with reflected appraisals of self, while simultaneously providing important information about the mental states of other people. Secure attachment to the caregiver should both reflect and facilitate this process.

Fonagy and colleagues (1996) have operationalized mentalizing capacity as assessed from AAI narratives and have used these data to study the relation between parents' mentalization ability and the attachment status of their children. Compared with low-mentalizing parents, parents scoring in the higher range of mentalizing capacity were three to four times more likely to have securely attached children (Fonagy, Steele, Moran, Steele, & Higgitt, 1991). Painful and traumatic experiences can lead people to shut down their internal worlds, a reaction already apparent by the preschool years in maltreated children (Cicchetti, 1991). Thus parents who are low in mentalizing may be transmitting this characteristic directly to their infants through social learning processes or by reproducing in their behavior some of the same parenting practices (such as abuse or neglect) that led them as children to close their minds to their own and others' mental states.

Fonagy's research on mentalizing dovetails with research on the understanding of social causality in adult and adolescent patients with BPD. Borderline patients show significantly lower levels of understanding of causality in the social world than patients with other psychiatric disorders (e.g., major depression), as assessed from narratives such as early memories (similar to the AAI) and Thematic Apperception Test stories (e.g., Westen, Ludolph, Misle, Ruffins, & Block, 1990). Thus the stories they tell show less attention to people's internal states, less coherence, and more unexplained or peculiar transitions.

Research on mentalizing is relevant to questions about self and identity because the complexity and depth of representations of others tend to correlate highly with the complexity and depth of representations of self (Bornstein & O'Neill, 1992; Leigh, Westen, Barends, & Mendel, 1992; Levy, Blatt, & Shaver, 1998). Thus children who learn to avoid thinking about other minds—either because of their own maltreatment or because they have learned to avoid thinking about mental states from their parents, who themselves were maltreated—are unlikely to form complex, multifaceted representations of self. They are also less likely to have the kind of comforting, comfortable, and appropriately mirroring interactions with caregivers that help children develop positive self-esteem and to internalize methods of self-soothing and self-regulation that help people regulate their self-esteem.

Trauma

Attachment and trauma tend to be strongly associated, or at least interdependent (Allen, Coyne, & Huntoon, 1998; van der Kolk, 1987). The presence of trauma often suggests a problematic attachment history, whereas problematic attachment, particularly disorganized or unresolved attachment status, usually signals the presence of prior trauma. As with problematic attachment, traumatic experiences may have profound effects on multiple aspects of self and identity, depending on the type of trauma (e.g., physical and sexual abuse, combat experiences, assault, motor vehicle accidents) and variables such as severity and frequency of the trauma and the age of the victim at the time of the traumatic event or events.

Physical and sexual abuse of children are among the most common forms of childhood trauma. Childhood trauma, particularly sexual abuse, may have profound effects on the development of self and identity in survivors. For example, dissociation in many sexual abuse survivors disrupts the organization of self-representations and the continuous sense of selfhood over time and across situations, contributing to an impaired sense of identity (Davies & Frawley, 1994; Westen, 1994a).

Self-esteem also suffers, as children often blame themselves for the abuse out of a desire to avoid having to regard the world (and/or an attachment figure who abuses them) as malevolent and unsafe. Numerous studies of both clinical and nonclinical samples of survivors of child sexual abuse have identified self-esteem as a key area affected by the abuse experience (Bolger, Patterson, & Kupersmidt, 1998; Brayden, Deitrich-MacLean, Dietrich, & Sherrod, 1995; Kendall-Tackett, Williams, & Finkelhor, 1993; Romano & DeLuca, 2001). Finkelhor and Browne (1985) developed a model of sexual abuse-related trauma that proposed four dynamics that account for the effects of the trauma, including stigmatization, betrayal by a trusted person, powerlessness, and traumatic sexualization (which refers to the child's sexuality having been shaped in a developmentally inappropriate way as a result of the abuse). Although all four have implications for the development of self and identity, the dynamics of stigmatization and powerlessness may have the most impact on the victim's self-esteem.

Sexual abuse survivors also frequently experience feelings of self-blame, either internalized from being blamed by significant others or internally generated as a way to attain a sense of control over the future and a hope of redeeming the self by changing or atoning in some way. Recent studies (Coffey, Leitenberg, Henning, Turner, & Bennett, 1996; Hazzard, Celano, Gould, Lawry, & Webb, 1995; Liem & Boudewyn, 1999) find that self-blame for abuse in both children and adults who were sexually abused as children is a strong predictor of current psychological distress, such that individuals with high scores on measures of self-blame also show elevations on measures such as the Brief Symptom Inventory (Derogatis & Melisaratos, 1983) and the Beck Depression Inventory (Beck, Ward, Mendelson, Mock, & Erbaugh, 1961).

The effects of early abuse on aspects of self can be seen as early as these dimensions of self can be measured. In self-recognition studies, maltreated toddlers frequently display neutral or negative affect on recognition of themselves in the mirror, suggesting feelings of shame or badness (Cicchetti, 1991). From an attachment perspective, childhood sexual abuse is likely to have a substantial impact on internal working models of self and relationships, particularly when the abuser was an attachment figure or when attachment figures either did not protect the child or did not respond in protective and nonblaming ways following disclosure.

Research has demonstrated clear links between trauma and the development of personality disorders, most notably borderline and antisocial personality disorder, although links to specific aspects of self and identity are yet to be studied. Childhood trauma, particularly sexual abuse, has been linked to BPD in a number of studies (Herman & van der Kolk, 1989; Westen et al., 1990; Zanarini, 1997). Although early trauma is likely to have particularly profound effects on the development of a sense of self

and identity through its impact on subsequent development, later traumatic events also affect functioning in these domains. For example, self-related disturbances have been observed in combat veterans from the Vietnam War (Brende, 1982, 1983). During war, some soldiers dissociate, particularly when committing or observing atrocities, and the requisites of war often encourage the loss of a sense of personal agency. Some of these experiences later persist as symptoms of posttraumatic stress and related disorders. Experiences of adult rape can also affect the sense of personal agency and can reduce self-esteem through feelings of self-blame (Ullman, 1997).

Using data from the Children in the Community Study, a community-based, prospective longitudinal study conducted in upstate New York beginning in the 1970s, several studies have provided evidence for a link between child abuse and neglect and later development of PDs. Participants with a documented history of maltreatment in childhood were more than four times more likely to have received a PD diagnosis during early adulthood than their nonabused peers, and different types of maltreatment (e.g., neglect, sexual abuse, physical abuse) showed differential relationships with Axis II PDs (Johnson, Cohen, Brown, Smailes, & Bernstein, 1999). A history of neglect was associated with greater risk of symptoms of antisocial, borderline, narcissistic, avoidant, passive–aggressive, and schizotypal personality disorder. Sexual abuse history was associated with a higher incidence of symptoms of borderline, histrionic, and depressive personality disorder. Physical abuse history was associated with increased risk for symptoms of antisocial, borderline, dependent, depressive, passive–aggressive, and schizoid personality disorder.

To summarize, if research on the etiology of PDs is in its infancy, research on the etiology of self pathology in PDs is probably best described as embryonic. Data on behavioral genetics and attachment relationships provide suggestive evidence for the influence of both biology and early experience on the subsequent development of self-related pathology in personality disorders. Children who are temperamentally high on negative affect (neuroticism) are likely to be more vulnerable to negative self-evaluation, and children with disrupted or abusive attachment relationships tend to have difficulty forming complex and accurate representations of their own minds, which may inhibit identity formation and make self-regulation through self-reflection more difficult. Data on the influence of traumatic experiences such as sexual abuse provide more direct evidence of a link between childhood experience and self-related pathology, with pervasive impact of trauma on domains such as self-esteem. Adolescent and adult experiences (such as rape) no doubt can substantially influence domains of self as well, although at least theoretically, the impact of such experiences should generally be less pervasive and more readily treatable, particularly for individuals without a prior traumatic history.

Conclusion

As we have suggested throughout this chapter, personality disorders provide a potentially important vantage point for studying self and identity, but much of the empirical landscape remains to be developed. Clinical observation points to a number of phenomena that can substantially enrich our understanding of the normal development and functioning of aspects of self, such as:

1. Dissociation, which has implications for the sense of agency and continuity at the core of the sense of self
2. Contradictory or alternating self-representations, as seen in BPD, which have implications for the organization of self-representations and the way people gain control over the activation of representations
3. Grandiose and unrealistic actual and ideal self-representations, as seen in NPD, which have implications for theories of possible selves and mental health (e.g., the extent to which positive illusions may have a curvilinear relation with mental health)
4. Substantial divergences between implicit and explicit self-esteem and implicit and explicit self-representations, as seen in narcissistic and antisocial personality disorders, which have implications for the understanding of attitudinal aspects

of self-representation and for the role of affect regulation and self-esteem regulation in personality
5. Difficulty maintaining commitment to values, standards, and roles, as in BPD, which has implications for the understanding of how people normally establish and maintain identity.

Collaborations between social and clinical psychologists are likely to prove particularly useful, allowing researchers to apply methods and concepts from each subdiscipline to the samples and phenomena that have traditionally been defined as the terrain of the other, to test the limits of each approach, and to forge integrations between them.

Acknowledgments

Preparation of this chapter was supported in part by Grant Nos. MH59685 and MH60892 from the National Institute of Mental Health to Drew Westen.

References

Aidman, E. V. (1999). Measuring individual differences in implicit self-concept: Initial validation of the Self-Apperception Test. *Personality and Individual Differences, 27,* 211–228.

Ainsworth, M., Blehar, M., Waters, E., & Wall, S. (1978). *Patterns of attachment: A psychological study of the Strange Situation.* Hillsdale, NJ: Erlbaum.

Akhtar, S. (1984). The syndrome of identity diffusion. *American Journal of Psychiatry, 141*(11), 1381–1385.

Akhtar, S. (1992). *Broken structures: Severe personality disorders and their treatment.* Northvale, NJ: Aronson.

Allen, J., Coyne, L., & Huntoon, J. (1998). Complex posttraumatic stress disorder in women from a psychometric perspective. *Journal of Personality Assessment, 70*(2), 277–298.

Allen, J., Hauser, S., & Borman-Spurrell, E. (1996). Attachment theory as a framework for understanding sequelae of severe adolescent psychopathology: An 11-year follow-up study. *Journal of Consulting and Clinical Psychology, 64*(2), 254–263.

American Psychiatric Association. (1952). *Diagnostic and statistical manual of mental disorders.* Washington, DC: Author.

American Psychiatric Association. (1994). *Diagnostic and statistical manual of mental disorders* (4th ed.). Washington, DC: Author.

Baker, L., Silk, K., Westen, D., Nigg, J., & Lohr, N. (1992). Malevolence, splitting, and parental ratings by borderlines, *Journal of Nervous and Mental Disease, 180,* 258–264.

Baldwin, M. (1992). Relational schemas and the processing

of social information. *Psychological Bulletin, 112*(3), 461–484.

Beck, A., Ward, C., Mendelson, M., Mock, J., & Erbaugh, J. (1961). An inventory for measuring depression. *Archives of General Psychiatry, 4,* 561–571.

Benjamin, L. S. (1974). Structural analysis of social behavior. *Psychological Review, 81,* 392–425.

Benjamin, L. S. (1996a). *Interpersonal diagnosis and treatment of personality disorders* (2nd ed.). New York: Guilford Press.

Benjamin, L. S. (1996b). An interpersonal theory of personality disorders. In J. F. Clarkin & M. Lenzenweger (Eds.), *Major theories of personality disorder* (pp. 141–220). New York: Guilford Press.

Bleuler, E. (1950). *Dementia praecox or the group of schizophrenias.* New York: International Universities Press. (Original work published 1911)

Bolger, K., Patterson, C., & Kupersmidt, J. (1998). Peer relationships and self-esteem among children who have been maltreated. *Child Development, 69*(4), 1171–1197.

Bornstein, R., & O'Neill, R. (1992). Parental perceptions and psychopathology. *Journal of Nervous and Mental Disease, 180*(8), 475–483.

Bosson, J. K., Swann, W. B., & Pennebaker, J. W. (2000). Stalking the perfect measure of implicit self-esteem: The blind men and the elephant revisited? *Journal of Personality and Social Psychology, 79,* 631–643.

Bowlby, J. (1969). *Attachment and loss: Vol. 1. Attachment.* New York: Basic Books.

Bowlby, J. (1973). *Attachment and loss: Vol. 2. Separation, anxiety, and anger.* New York: Basic Books.

Bowlby, J. (1977). The making and breaking of affectional bonds: I. Aetiology and psychopathology in the light of attachment theory. *British Journal of Psychiatry, 130,* 201–210.

Brayden, R., Deitrich-MacLean, G., Dietrich, M., & Sherrod, K. (1995). Evidence for specific effects of childhood sexual abuse on mental well-being and physical self-esteem. *Child Abuse and Neglect, 19*(10), 1255–1262.

Brende, J. (1982). Electrodermal responses in post-traumatic syndromes: A pilot study of cerebral hemisphere functioning in Vietnam veterans. *Journal of Nervous and Mental Disease, 170*(6), 352–361.

Brende, J. (1993). A psychodynamic view of character pathology in Vietnam combat veterans. *Bulletin of the Menninger Clinic, 47*(3), 193–216.

Byrne, B. (1996). *Measuring self-concept across the lifespan: Issues and instrumentation.* Washington, DC: American Psychological Association.

Cadoret, R., Yates, W., Troughton, E., Woodworth, G., & Stewart, M. (1995). Genetic-environmental interaction in the genesis of aggressivity and conduct disorders. *Archives of General Psychiatry, 52*(11), 916–924.

Cicchetti, D. (1991). Fractures in the crystal: Developmental psychopathology and the emergence of self. *Developmental Review, 11,* 271–287.

Cicchetti, D., Toth, S., & Lynch, M. (1995). Bowlby's dream comes full circle: The application of attachment theory to risk and psychopathology. *Advances in Clinical Child Psychology, 17,* 1–75.

Clark, L., Livesley, W., & Morey, L. (1997). Personality disorder assessment: The challenge of construct validity. *Journal of Personality Disorders, 11*(3), 205–231.

Clarkin, J., Kernberg, O., & Somavia, J. (1998). Assessment of the patient with borderline personality disorder for psychodynamic treatment. In J. Barron (Ed.), *Making diagnosis meaningful: Enhancing, evaluation and treatment of psychological disorders* (pp. 299–318). Washington, DC: American Psychological Association.

Cloninger, C. R., Svrakic, D., Bayon, C., & Przybeck, T. (1999). Measurement of psychopathology as variants of personality. In C. R. Cloninger (Ed.), *Personality and psychopathology* (pp. 33–65). Washington, DC: American Psychiatric Press.

Coffey, P. Leitenberg, H., Henning, K., Turner, T., & Bennett, R. (1996). Mediators of the long-term impact of child sexual abuse: Perceived stigma, betrayal, powerlessness, and self-blame. *Child Abuse and Neglect, 20*(5), 447–455.

Colvin, C., & Block, J. (1994). Do positive illusions foster mental health? An examination of the Taylor and Brown formulation. *Psychological Bulletin, 116*(1), 3–20.

Davies, J. M., & Frawley, M. G. (1994). *Treating the adult survivor of childhood sexual abuse: A psychoanalytic perspective.* New York: Basic Books.

Derogatis, L., & Melisaratos, N. (1983). The Brief Symptom Inventory: An introductory report. *Psychological Medicine, 13,* 595–605.

Deutsch, H. (1942). Some forms of emotional disturbance and their relationship to schizophrenia. *Psychoanalytic Quarterly, 11,* 301–321.

De Wolff, M., & van IJzendoorn, M. (1997). Sensitivity and attachment: A meta-analysis on parental antecedents of infant attachment. *Child Development, 68*(4), 571–591.

Epstein, S. (1973). The self-concept revisited, or a theory of a theory. *American Psychologist, 28,* 404–416.

Epstein, S. (1990). Cognitive–experiential self-theory. In L. A. Pervin (Ed.), *Handbook of personality: Theory and research* (pp. 165–192). New York: Guilford Press Press.

Erikson, E. (1963). *Childhood and society* (2nd ed.). New York: Norton.

Erikson, E. (1968). *Identity: Youth and crisis.* New York: Norton.

Eysenck, H. (1967). *The biological basis of personality.* Springfield, IL: Charles C. Thomas.

Eysenck, H. (1981). *A model for personality.* New York: Springer-Verlag.

Eysenck, H. (1990). Genetic and environmental contributions to individual differences: Three major dimensions of personality. *Journal of Personality, 58,* 245–261.

Farnham, S., Greenwald, A., & Banaji, M. (1999). Implicit self-esteem. In D. Abrams & M. Hogg (Eds.), *Social identity and social cognition* (pp. 230–248). Cambridge, MA: Blackwell.

Finkelhor, D., & Browne, A. (1985). The traumatic impact of child sexual abuse: A conceptualization. *American Journal of Orthopsychiatry, 55,* 530–541.

Fonagy, P., Leigh, T., Steele, M., Steele, H., Kennedy, R., Mattoon, G., Target, M., & Gerber, A. (1996). The relation of attachment status, psychiatric classification, and response to psychotherapy. *Journal of Clinical and Consulting Psychology, 64*(1), 22–31.

Fonagy, P., Steele, H., Moran, G., Steele, M., & Higgitt, A. (1991). The capacity for understanding mental states: The reflective self in parent and child and its significance for security of attachment. *Infant Mental Health Journal, 13,* 200–217.

Fonagy, P., Target, M., & Gergely, G. (2000). Attachment and borderline personality disorder: A theory and some evidence. *Psychiatric Clinics of North America, 23*(1), 103–122.

Franzio, S., & Shields, S. (1984). The Body Esteem Scale: Multidimensional structure and sex differences in a college population. *Journal of Personality Assessment, 48,* 173–178.

Gaynor, P., & Underwood, J. (1995). Conceptualizing and measuring sexual self-esteem. In P. E. Shrout & S. T. Fiske (Eds.). *Personality research, methods, and theory: A festschrift honoring Donald W. Fiske* (pp. 333–347). Hillsdale, NJ: Erlbaum.

George, C., Kaplan, N., & Main, M. (1985). *An adult attachment interview: Interview protocol.* Unpublished manuscript, Department of Psychology, University of California, Berkeley.

Goldstein, W. (1985). DSM-III and the narcissistic personality. *American Journal of Psychotherapy, 39*(1), 4–16.

Greenwald, A., & Farnham, S. (2000). Using the Implicit Association Test to measure self-esteem and self-concept. *Journal of Personality and Social Psychology, 79*(6), 1022–1038.

Greenwald, A. G., McGhee, D. E., & Schwartz, J. L. K. (1998). Measuring individual differences in implicit cognition: The Implicit Association Test. *Journal of Personality and Social Psychology, 74,* 1464–1480.

Gunderson, J. G., Ronningstam, E., & Smith, L. E. (1995). Narcissistic personality disorders. In W. J. Livesley (Ed.), *The DSM-IV personality disorders* (pp. 201–212). New York: Guilford Press.

Harter, S. (1996). Historical roots of contemporary issues involving self-concept. In B. Bracken (Ed.), *Handbook of self-concept: Developmental, social, and clinical considerations* (pp. 1–37). New York: Wiley.

Hazzard, A., Celano, M., Gould, J., Lawry, S., & Webb, C. (1995). Predicting symptomatology and self-blame among child sex abuse victims. *Child Abuse and Neglect, 19*(6), 707–714.

Herman, J., & van der Kolk, B. (1989). Childhood trauma in borderline personality disorder. *American Journal of Psychiatry, 146,* 490–495.

Higgins, E. T. (1990). Personality, social psychology, and person-situation relations: Standards and knowledge activation as a common language. In L. Pervin (Ed.), *Handbook of personality: Theory and research* (pp. 301–338). New York: Guilford Press.

Horowitz, M. (1998). *Cognitive psychodynamics: From conflict to character.* New York: Wiley.

James, W. (1918). *Principles of psychology.* New York: Holt. (Original work published 1890)

Johnson, J., Cohen, P., Brown, J., Smailes, E., & Bernstein, D. (1999). Childhood maltreatment increases risk for personality disorders during early adulthood. *Archives of General Psychiatry, 56,* 600–606.

Kendall-Tackett, K., Williams, L., & Finkelhor, D. (1993). Impact of sexual abuse on children: A review and synthesis of recent empirical studies. *Psychological Bulletin, 113*(1), 164–180.

Kendler, K. S., McGuire, M., Gruenberg, A. M., O'Hare, A., Spellman, M., & Walsh, D. (1993). The Roscommon Family Study: 3. Schizophrenia-related personality dis-

order in relatives. *Archives of General Psychiatry, 50,* 781–788.

Kendler, K. S., McGuire, M., Gruenberg, A. M., & Walsh, D. (1995). Schizotypal symptoms and signs in the Roscommon Family Study. *Archives of General Psychiatry, 52,* 296–303.

Kendler, K. S. & Walsh, D. (1995). Schizotypal personality disorder in parents and the risk for schizophrenia in siblings. *Schizophrenia Bulletin, 21*(1), 47–52.

Kernberg, O. (1975). *Borderline conditions and pathological narcissism.* New York: Aronson.

Kernberg, O. (1976). *Object relations theory and clinical psychoanalysis.* New York: Aronson.

Kernberg, O. (1984). *Severe personality disorders.* New Haven, CT: Yale University Press.

Kohut, H. (1971). *The analysis of the self.* New York: International Universities Press.

Kohut, H. (1977). *The restoration of the self.* Madison, CT: International Universities Press.

Kraepelin, E. (1919). *Dementia praecox and paraphrenia.* Chicago: Chicago Medical Book. (Original work published 1896)

Kroger, J. (1995). The differentiation of "firm" and "developmental" foreclosure identity statuses: A longitudinal study. *Journal of Adolescent Research, 10*(3), 317–337.

Leigh, J., Westen, D., Barends, A., & Mendel, M. (1992). Assessing complexity of representations of people from TAT and interview data. *Journal of Personality, 60,* 809–837.

Lenzenweger, M. F. (1998). Schizotypy and schizotypic psychopathology. In M. F. Lenzenweger & R. H. Dworkin (Eds.), *Origins and development of schizophrenia: Advances in experimental psychopathology* (pp. 93–122). Washington, DC: American Psychological Association.

Levy, K., Blatt, S., & Shaver, P. (1998). Attachment styles and parental representations. *Journal of Personality and Social Psychology, 74*(2), 407–419.

Lewis, D., & Yeager, C. (1994). Abuse, dissociative phenomena and childhood multiple personality disorder. *Child and Adolescent Psychiatric Clinics of North America, 3*(4), 729–743.

Liem, J., & Boudewyn, A. (1999). Contextualizing the effects of childhood sexual abuse on adult self- and social functioning: An attachment theory perspective. *Child Abuse and Neglect, 23*(11), 1141–1157.

Livesley, W., Jang, K., Jackson, D., & Vernon, P. (1993). Genetic contributions to dimensions of personality disorder. *American Journal of Psychiatry, 150*(12), 1826–1831.

Livesley, W., Jang, K., Jackson, D., & Vernon, P. (1998). Phenotypic and genetic structure of traits delineating personality disorder. *Archives of General Psychiatry, 55*(10), 941–948.

Livesley, W. J., Jang, K. L., & Vernon, P. A. (1998). Phenotypic and genetic structure of traits delineating personality disorder. *Archives of General Psychiatry, 55,* 941–948.

Main, M., & Solomon, J. (1990). Procedures for identifying infants as disorganized/disoriented during the Ainsworth Strange Situation. In M. T. Greenberg, D. Cicchetti, & E. M. Cummings (Eds.), *Attachment in the preschool years* (pp. 121–160). Chicago: University of Chicago Press.

Marcia, J. (1966). Development and validation of ego identity status. *Journal of Personality and Social Psychology, 3,* 551–558.

Marcia, J. (1980). Identity in adolescence. In J. Adelson (Ed.), *Handbook of adolescent psychology* (pp. 159–187). New York: Wiley.

Marcia, J. (1994). Ego identity and object relations. In J. Masling & R. Bornstein (Eds.), *Empirical studies of psychoanalytic theories: Vol. 5. Empirical perspectives on object relations theory.* (pp. 59–103). Washington, DC: American Psychological Association.

Markus, H., & Cross, S. (1990). The interpersonal self. In L. A. Pervin (Ed.), *Handbook of personality: Theory and research* (pp. 576–608). New York: Guilford Press.

Markus, H., & Wurf, E. (1987). The dynamic self-concept: A social psychological perspective. *Annual Review of Psychology, 38,* 299–337.

McCrae, R., & Costa, P. (1982). *Emerging lives, enduring dispositions: Personality in adulthood.* Boston: Little, Brown.

McWilliams, N. (1994). *Psychoanalytic diagnosis: Understanding personality structure in the clinical process.* New York: Guilford Press.

McWilliams, N. (1998). Relationship, subjectivity, and inference in diagnosis. In J. Barron (Ed.), *Making diagnosis meaningful* (pp. 197–226). Washington, DC: American Psychological Association Press.

Moore, S., & Barling, N. (1991). Developmental status and AIDS attitudes in adolescence. *Journal of Genetic Psychology, 152*(1), 5–16.

Nakash-Eisikovits, O., Dutra, L., & Westen, D. (in press). The relationship between attachment patterns and personality pathology in adolescents. *Journal of the American Academy of Child and Adolescent Psychiatry.*

Nigg, J., & Goldsmith, H. (1994). Genetics of personality disorders: Perspectives from personality and psychopathology research. *Psychological Bulletin, 115*(3), 346–380.

Nigg, J., Lohr, N. E., Westen, D., Gold, L., & Silk, K. R. (1992). Malevolent object representations in borderline personality disorder and major depression. *Journal of Abnormal Psychology, 101,* 61–67.

Ogilvie, D. M., & Ashmore, R. D. (1991). Self-with-other representation as a unit of analysis in self-concept research. In R. C. Curtis (Ed.), *The relational self: Theoretical convergences in psychoanalysis and social psychology* (pp. 282–314). New York: Guilford Press.

Oldham, J., Skodol, A., Kellman, H., Hyler, S., Rosnick, L., & Davies, M. (1992). Diagnosis of DSM-III-R personality disorders by two semistructured interviews: Patterns of comorbidity. *American Journal of Psychiatry, 149,* 213–220.

Pelham, B., & Hetts, J. (1999). Implicit and explicit personal and social identity: Towards a more complete understanding of the social self. In T. Tyler, R. Kramer, & O. John (Eds.), *The psychology of the social self* (pp. 115–143). Mahwah, NJ: Erlbaum.

Perry, J. C. (1992). Problems and considerations in the valid assessment of personality disorders. *American Journal of Psychiatry, 149,* 1645–1653.

Pfeiffer, E. (1974). Borderline states. *Diseases of the Nervous System, 35,* 212–219.

Plomin, R., & Caspi, A. (1999). Behavioral genetics and personality. In A. L. Pervin (Ed.), *Handbook of person-*

ality: Theory and research (pp. 251–276). New York: Guilford Press.

Prichard, J. (1835). *A treatise on insanity.* London: Sherwood, Gilbert & Piper.

Reich, J. H. (1989). Familiality of DSM-III dramatic and anxious personality clusters. *Journal of Nervous and Mental Disease, 177,* 96–100.

Reich, W. (1933). *Character analysis.* New York: Farrar, Straus, and Giroux.

Robins, R., & Beer, J. (2001). Positive illusions about the self: Short-term benefits and long-term costs. *Journal of Personality and Social Psychology, 80*(2), 340–352.

Roid, G., & Fitts, W. (1994). *Tennessee Self-Concept Scale (TSCS).* Los Angeles, CA: Western Psychological Services.

Romano, E., & DeLuca, R. (2001). Male sexual abuse: A review of effects, abuse characteristics, and links with later psychological functioning. *Aggression and Violent Behavior, 6*(1), 55–78.

Rosenberg, M. (1965). *Society and the adolescent self-image.* Princeton, NJ: Princeton University Press.

Rosenstein, D., & Horowitz, H. (1996). Adolescent attachment and psychopathology. *Journal of Consulting and Clinical Psychology, 64*(2), 244–253.

Sandler, J., & Rosenblatt, B. (1962). The concept of the representational world. *Psychoanalytic Study of the Child, 17,* 128–145.

Shedler, J., Mayman, M., & Manis, M. (1993). The *illusion* of mental health. *American Psychologist, 48,* 1117–1131.

Shedler, J., & Westen, D. (1998). Refining the measurement of Axis II: A Q-sort procedure for assessing personality pathology. *Assessment, 5,* 335–355.

Sinha, B., & Watson, D. (1997). Psychosocial predictors of personality disorder traits in a non-clinical sample. *Personality and Individual Differences, 22*(4), 527–537.

Slugoski, B., Marcia, J., & Koopman, R. (1984). Cognitive and social interactional characteristics of ego identity statuses in college males. *Journal of Personality and Social Psychology, 47*(3), 646–661.

Smith, E. R. (1998). Mental representation and memory. In D. T. Gilbert, S. T. Fiske, & G. Lindzey (Eds.), *Handbook of social psychology, Vol. 1* (pp. 391–445). New York: McGraw-Hill.

Spitzer, R. L., Endicott, J., & Gibbon, M. (1979). Crossing the border into borderline personality and borderline schizophrenia. *Archives of General Psychiatry, 36,* 17–24.

Strauman, T. (1996). Stability within the self: A longitudinal study of the structural implications of self-discrepancy theory. *Journal of Personality and Social Psychology, 71*(6), 1142–1153.

Taylor, S. (1995). Commentary on borderline personality disorder. In W. J. Livesley (Ed.), *The DSM-IV personality disorders* (pp. 165–172). New York: Guilford Press.

Torgersen, S. (1984). Genetic and nosological aspects of schizotypal and borderline personality disorders. *Archives of General Psychiatry, 41,* 546–554.

Ullman, S. (1997). Attributions, world assumptions, and recovery from sexual assault. *Journal of Child Sexual Abuse, 6*(1), 1–19.

van der Kolk, B. A. (1987). The separation cry and the trauma response: Developmental issues in the psychobiology of attachment and separation. In B. A. van der Kolk (Ed.), *Psychological trauma* (pp. 31–62). Washington,

DC: American Psychiatric Press.

Watson, D. (1998). The relationship of self-esteem, locus of control, and dimensional models to personality disorders. *Journal of Social Behavior and Personality, 13*(3), 399–420.

Westen, D. (1985). *Self and society: Narcissism, collectivism, and the development of morals.* New York: Cambridge University Press.

Westen, D. (1990). The relations among narcissism, egocentrism, self-concept, and self-esteem. *Psychoanalysis and Contemporary Thought, 13,* 185–241.

Westen, D. (1991). Cultural, emotional, and unconscious aspects of self. In R. C. Curtis (Ed.), *The relational self: Theoretical convergences in psychoanalysis and social psychology* (pp. 181–210). New York: Guilford Press.

Westen, D. (1992). The cognitive self and the psychoanalytic self: Can we put our selves together? *Psychological Inquiry, 3*(1), 1–13.

Westen, D. (1994a). The impact of sexual abuse on aspects of self. In D. Cicchetti & S. Toth (Eds.), *Rochester Symposium on Developmental Psychopathology* (Vol. 5, pp. 641–667). Rochester, NY: University of Rochester Press.

Westen, D. (1994b). Toward an integrative model of affect regulation: Applications to social-psychological research. *Journal of Personality, 62,* 641–647.

Westen, D. (1998). The scientific legacy of Sigmund Freud: Toward a psychodynamically informed psychological science. *Psychological Bulletin, 124,* 333–371.

Westen, D. (1999). Psychodynamic theory and technique in relation to research on cognition and emotion: Mutual implications. In T. Dalgleish & M. Power (Eds.), *Handbook of cognition and emotion* (pp. 727–746). New York: Wiley.

Westen, D., & Arkowitz-Westen, L. (1998). Limitations of Axis II in diagnosing personality pathology in clinical practice. *American Journal of Psychiatry, 155,* 1767–1771.

Westen, D., & Cohen, R. P. (1993). The self in borderline personality disorder: A psychodynamic perspective. In Z. V. Segal & S. J. Blatt (Eds.), *The self in emotional distress: Cognitive and psychodynamic perspectives* (pp. 334–360). New York: Guilford Press.

Westen, D., Ludolph, P., Misle, B., Ruffins, S., & Block,

M. J. (1990). Physical and sexual abuse in adolescent girls with borderline personality disorder. *American Journal of Orthopsychiatry, 60,* 55–66.

Westen, D., Moses, M. J., Silk, K. R., Lohr, N. E., Cohen, R., & Segal, H. (1992). Quality of depressive experience in borderline personality disorder and major depression: When depression is not just depression. *Journal of Personality Disorders, 6,* 382–393.

Westen, D., & Muderrisoglu, S. (2001). *Reliability and validity of personality disorder assessment using a systematic clinical interview.* Unpublished manuscript, Boston University.

Westen, D., & Shedler, J. (1999a). Revising and assessing Axis II, Part I: Developing a clinically and empirically valid assessment method. *American Journal of Psychiatry, 156,* 258–272.

Westen, D., & Shedler, J. (1999b). Revising and assessing Axis II, Part II: Toward an empirically based and clinically useful classification of personality disorders. *American Journal of Psychiatry, 156,* 273–285.

Westen, D., & Shedler, J. (2000). A prototype matching approach to personality disorders: Toward DSM-V. *Journal of Personality Disorders, 14,* 109–126.

Widiger, T. (1993). Validation strategies for the personality disorders. *Journal of Personality Disorders* (Suppl.), 34–43.

Widiger, T., & Allen, F. (1994). Toward a dimensional model for the personality disorders. In P. Costa & T. Widiger (Eds.), *Personality disorders and the five-factor model of personality* (pp. 19–39). Washington, DC: American Psychological Association.

Widiger, T., & Trull, T. (1992). Personality and psychopathology: An application of the five-factor model. *Journal of Personality, 60,* 363–393.

Wilkinson-Ryan, T., & Westen, D. (2000). Identity disturbance in borderline personality disorder: An empirical investigation. *American Journal of Psychiatry, 157*(4), 528–541.

Wolf, E. S. (1988). *Treating the self: Elements of clinical self psychology.* New York: Guilford Press.

Zanarini, M. (Ed.). (1997). *Role of sexual abuse in the etiology of borderline personality disorder.* Washington, DC: American Psychiatric Press.

PART VII

EPILOGUE

32

The Next Generation of Self Research

JUNE PRICE TANGNEY
MARK R. LEARY

Questions about the nature of the self have captured the attention of philosophers for centuries and of behavioral scientists since the latter part of the 19th century. After the seminal speculative writings of James, Cooley, Baldwin, Mead, and others, the "first generation" of empirical research on the self that emerged in the middle of the 20th century focused primarily on self-esteem. Various methods were developed to assess individual differences in level of self-esteem and efforts made to determine the causes, correlates, and consequences of high versus low self-regard. At this time, self-esteem was conceptualized as a fairly stable attribute and was seen largely in the province of personality psychology.

This volume summarizes what may be viewed as the *second generation* of self research, which started in the 1980s. At that time, researchers' conceptualizations of the self became markedly more rich and differentiated, owing to a confluence of factors (see Leary & Tangney, Chapter 1, this volume; Mischel & Morf, Chapter 2, this volume). Perhaps most important, researchers from a range of subdisciplines began to investigate properties and mechanisms of the self, each from their unique vantage point. No longer solely the domain of personality psychology, theory and research on the self began to pop up across the behavioral and social sciences. In mainstream social psychology, work involving social cognition, attitudes, group processes, social influence, and interpersonal relationships began to explore self-processes. Basic research on motivation and emotion also began to draw on self-related constructs (such as self-efficacy, identity, self-enhancement, self-verification, self-discrepancy, and self-conscious emotions), and clinical research on affective and personality disorders often traced these difficulties to problems with self and identity. Myriad lines of research in developmental psychology likewise incorporated the self, and, of course, personality psychology continued to investigate individual differences in self-related attributes, not just trait self-esteem but also self-consciousness, self-monitoring, and identity orientation, among others. In addition, sociologists, who had long embraced the importance of the self for understanding the link between the individual and the social order (Cooley, 1902), devoted increasing attention to self and identity (Stets & Burke, Chapter 7, this volume). In this second generation of self research, researchers moved beyond a focus on self-esteem to a wide array of constructs and processes that involve the human capacity for self-awareness.

In editing this *Handbook,* we were struck by how well developed these emerging lines of self research have become and by the degree of integration that is emerging across many of the domains. Over the past few years, the self has coalesced into an exciting, vital, definable field, rich now and even more promising for the future. In this closing chapter, we offer some final thoughts, underscoring four overarching and nearly inescapable themes that recur across multiple chapters in this *Handbook*—evolutionary processes, self-esteem, development, and culture—and speculating on what might be in store for the third generation of empirical research on the self in the 21st century.

Why Did the Self Evolve?

Answers to many basic questions about the self may lie in understanding the self's functions for the individual. What does the self do? Paralleling a trend across the behavioral sciences, self researchers have recently begun to explore the self from an evolutionary perspective. In reviewing archeological, historical, and anthropological evidence, psychologists have grappled with two distinct sets of questions. One set of questions concerns the evolutionary functions of the self. Why is it helpful to have a self? How were human beings selected for "selfness"? What is it about the self that enhances one's chances for survival, or more to the point, increases one's inclusive fitness? In short, what evolutionary pressures and developments brought about the modern self? A second set of related questions concerns at what point during human evolution the self emerged. In this volume, Mitchell (Chapter 28) discussed evidence regarding the presence of a self in nonhuman animals. Mitchell suggests that, although rudiments of self-awareness may be seen among certain nonhuman primates, no other animals possess the capacity for self-awareness and self-representation possessed by human be-

ings. When in the course of human history do we find evidence that people could think consciously about themselves? Sedikides and Skowronski (Chapter 29) address the important question of when and why the human self evolved, and the evolution of the self is also addressed, at least in passing, by Brewer (Chapter 24), Baumeister and Vohs (Chapter 10), Tesser (Chapter 14), Pyszczynski, Greenberg, and Goldenberg (Chapter 16), and Leary and MacDonald (Chapter 20).

We found these ideas about the origins of the self so intriguing that we couldn't resist adding a few thoughts into the mix. Without wading into controversies regarding the point at which self-awareness first appeared among human beings or the nature of the evolutionary pressures that fostered self-awareness in the distant prehistoric past, we believe it is also worth considering more recent developments that may have provided fertile ground for an ever more elaborated and differentiated sense of self. In our view, a cultural event critical to the development of the modern self was the shift from hunting and gathering to sedentary farming that occurred approximately 10,000 years ago (see Martin, 1999). The advent of agriculture and, for the first time, sedentary communities allowed people to specialize, opening the door to more differentiated identities. Once groups of human beings began cultivating food, it was possible for one person to produce enough food to feed multiple individuals, thereby freeing people up to do more than just hunting, gathering, and scavenging for their next meal. Some individuals could now specialize as toolmakers, clothesmakers, builders, farmers, merchants, and so on. Thus people's identities became increasingly differentiated, both in terms of their self-perceptions ("I'm the person who makes the tools") and in terms of how others viewed them ("She's the group's main toolmaker"). The shift from hunting–gathering to agriculture was also likely critical to the development of the self in a second respect. The shift from nomadic to sedentary existence allowed people to accrue more personal possessions because people were no longer limited to what they could carry on their backs. For the first time, they made relatively permanent homes filled with personal objects, creating both a sense of ownership and a unique space that likely fostered a sense of individual identity and self.

Regarding the functional advantages of the self, one key factor may be motivation toward mastery and excellence that a sense of self helps to confer. In the world of the hunter–gatherer, the primary motives likely stemmed from points rather low on the hierarchy of needs—food to satisfy hunger, social acceptance for protection and support, sex to satisfy lust, shelter and clothing in service of safety and comfort. Once these basic needs were satisfied (as after a good meal), motivation presumably decreased. But as people developed a sense of self—an identity as a toolmaker, for instance—they were able to become invested in their work, think about how their work was viewed by others, take pride in their accomplishments, and strive toward excellence. In short, the ability to self-reflect permitted the pursuit of long-term personal goals that were no longer tied to an immediate reinforcement. The ultimate result would be a better product (a better tool, house, crop, boot), which would certainly confer an advantage in the struggle to survive and reproduce.

And then, of course, there are questions about the future of the self. Is the human self still evolving? Has the self reached a stable point, or will it continue to grow and differentiate in new directions? Certainly, our identities continue to become increasingly complex, not least owing to advances in communication technology, the explosive growth in information, the World Wide Web, the dizzying array of choices we face each day, the diversity of our communities, our transience, and our Palm Pilots (Gergen, 1991). The question is whether changes in the *content* of human identities, moving into the 21st century, will have implications for the basic cognitive–affective *processes* that underlie them. What are the evolutionary pressures, if any, operating on the self?

Throughout most of human history, self and identity have been shaped by two sets of interacting forces—natural selection and contextual influences based on changes in the social, cultural, and physical environment. In modern, industrialized societies, in which success in procreation is more a matter of choice than inclusive fitness, evolutionary pressures that selectively favored adaptive change are much different than they have been throughout human history, if they exist at all. Much more influential than in the past are our social, cultural, and technological environments—the effects of which are not necessarily positive. The ultimate question for self psychologists working from a sociobiological perspective is: In what direction will our new self lead?

What's the Deal with Self-Esteem?

One of the ironies in the study of self and identity is that, although the first generation of self research focused primarily on self-esteem and the second generation has explored it in even greater depth, we still lack consensus regarding what self-esteem is and what it does. Researchers remain divided on fundamental questions such as why people have self-esteem and even whether high self-esteem is desirable. Such questions are not only important theoretically to several specific areas of investigation but also have extensive applied implications. Entire philosophies and methods of parenting and teaching have been developed to enhance children's self-esteem. Are these approaches something that researchers would recommend, or should efforts to enhance children's self-esteem be discouraged?

Part of the ambiguity and the dearth of definitive answers stem from inconsistencies in what researchers mean when they refer to "self-esteem." Among other things, it is critical to distinguish between *level* of self-esteem and the *basis* for self-esteem. Many of the apparently negative "effects" of high self-esteem appear to derive from particular strategies of defending and protecting self-esteem (Baumeister et al, 1996; Crocker & Park, Chapter 15, this volume; Rhodewalt & Sorrow, Chapter 26, this volume; Tesser, Chapter 14, this volume) or from the basis for constructing self-esteem (Dweck, Higgins, & Grant-Pillow, Chapter 12, this volume; Pyszczynski, Greenberg, & Goldenberg, Chapter 16, this volume; Ryan & Deci, Chapter 13, this volume) rather than from simply whether the person's self-esteem is high or low (Kernis & Goldman,

Chapter 6, this volume). Problems arise when one's self-esteem is undeserved, based on inappropriate factors, or maintained in ways that are personally or socially maladaptive.

In this context, it may be useful to reexamine the notion of "inflated" self-esteem. Discussions of the negative effects of high self-esteem often incorporate the notion that some people have "inflated" self-esteem—that their self-esteem is too high, higher than it should be. It is worth asking, then, What does it mean to say that someone has inflated self-esteem? Who are these people with more self-esteem than they deserve? If we consider representative items from Rosenberg's (1965) self-esteem scale, the most widely used measure of trait self-esteem, we find that respondents rate the accuracy of statements such as, "I feel that I'm a person of worth, at least on a equal plane with others," "I feel I have a number of good qualities," "On the whole, I'm satisfied with myself," and "I take a positive attitude toward myself." Only one of the 10 items involves any hint of social comparison ("I'm able to do things as well as most other people"). Thus high scores on the Rosenberg denote high self-esteem, a sense of self-worth, but not necessarily an inflated, grandiose self-image.[1]

What does it mean, then, for a person's self-esteem to be too high? Is the suggestion here that the average college freshman, unemployed person, or mentally retarded individual *shouldn't* on the whole take a positive attitude toward themselves? Self-esteem researchers seem to hold one of two opinions on this question. Some would argue that, with the exception of an extreme and minute portion of the population (serial child molesters, Hannibal Lechter, Osama bin Laden), it is difficult to argue that anyone's score on Rosenberg's scale is higher than it "should" be. People are entitled to feel good about themselves, assuming that they are not evil and unrepentant reprobates. The other view is that some people ought not, in fact, have high self-esteem because the conditions that the self-esteem system evolved to monitor are not present. For example, dominance theory (Barkow, 1980) suggests that self-esteem evolved to monitor one's relative dominance, and sociometer theory (Leary & Downs, 1995) links self-

esteem to being socially valued and accepted by other people. From these perspectives, self-esteem is "too" high when it is not commensurate with the person's true degree of dominance or acceptance, respectively. In effect, the person is receiving inaccurate information about his or her social standing, which can lead to interpersonal miscalculations and other kinds of maladaptive behavior. Like many disagreements among self researchers, this one stems from fundamental differences in how self-related constructs are conceptualized.

More generally, our understanding of the causes and consequences of level of self-esteem would be enhanced by greater precision in our use of terms. As many of the chapters in this volume emphasize, terms such as self-concept, self-esteem level, self-esteem stability, self-esteem maintenance, self-efficacy, self-regulation, and narcissism each represent distinct constructs that offer a unique contribution to our understanding of the self. Yet these terms are often used inconsistently, resulting in confusion and undermining communication across areas.

A case in point involves the distinction between narcissism and high self-esteem. In conceptualizing narcissism, social psychologists tend to focus on grandiosity, an exaggerated sense of self-importance, and an overestimation of one's abilities. But there is much more to the concept of narcissism. Clinical theorists, drawing on a long history of "object relations," typically use the term "narcissism" to refer to a distinctly pathological form of self-focus and fluctuating self-regard that stems from fundamental defects in the self-system (e.g., Kohut, 1971). The narcissist is not simply an impervious, overconfident, conceited jerk, but rather someone with a damaged sense of self. Attempts to shore up this damaged self-image with unrealistic fantasies of grandiosity inevitably alternate with a grinding sense of emptiness and self-loathing. Other hallmarks of narcissism include a pervasive self-focus, a corresponding inability to focus on and empathize with others, a painful vulnerability to criticism and rejection, and a history of shallow and chaotic relationships. People with high self-esteem do not typically fit this profile. Yet much of the theory surrounding the "dark side" of self-esteem (e.g., Baumeister et al., 1996) entails descriptions more akin to narcissism than high self-esteem.

Developmental Questions about the Self: Much Fertile Ground Awaits

Harter (Chapter 30, this volume) emphasized how much rich territory remains unexplored at the interface between developmental psychology and what have historically been "adult" social psychological approaches to the self. At first glance, broad questions about the development of the self (e.g., How does [some aspect of the self] develop?) are misleadingly simple, masking several distinct types of developmental questions. This is not merely a matter of measuring self-esteem in children and adults to see if they differ. For example, developmental researchers interested in self-esteem could examine not only developmental changes in level of self-esteem but also developmental changes in the composition of self-esteem (e.g., Is social self-esteem more closely linked to global self-esteem in adolescence compared with middle adulthood?) and developmental changes in the implications of self-esteem (e.g., Is self-esteem more important to resilience in the face of failure at earlier than later stages of development?)

In most areas of self research, four distinct types of developmental questions can be examined. The first two questions concern normative developmental changes: First, are there developmental changes in the *level* of a given self-related construct across the lifespan? For example, is the self of a 6-year-old as complex as the self of a 60-year-old? Are there developmental differences in the degree to which people engage in self-evaluation maintenance strategies? Are adolescents more inclined to engage in social comparisons, relative to younger children or adults?

The second set of questions involves developmental changes in the *quality* of a given self-related construct across the lifespan. For example, does the nature or organization of the self change with age (e.g., are there age-related changes in degree of compartmentalization)? Are children inclined to engage in different kinds of self-evaluation maintenance strategies than their parents? Do the elderly make different types of so-cial comparisons, relative to younger individuals?

The third and fourth kinds of developmental questions focus on individual differences. Compared with children, adolescents as a group may have more complex selves, make more and different types of social comparisons, and so on. But *within* a given age group, substantial individual differences exist along these dimensions. The third developmental question is, Where do these differences come from? What do we know about the developmental roots of individual differences in these self-attributes or self-processes? For example, what biological, cognitive, and early environmental factors foster the development of more versus less complex selves? Are certain cultural or family socialization contexts associated with the development of specific types of self-evaluation maintenance strategies or with the propensity to engage in social comparisons?

Fourth and finally, we may ask whether developmental changes exist in the implications of those individual differences: Are some individual differences more critical— more adaptive or maladaptive—at certain life stages than at other life stages? For example, do self-complexity and compartmentalization have different implications for psychological adjustment and resilience under stress for adolescents versus adults? Can self-complexity be a liability at certain critical phases of development? Are certain self-evaluation maintenance strategies effective in maintaining self-esteem among children but less so among adults? Does the relationship between upward social comparison and life satisfaction shift with increasing age?

These are just a sampling of the kinds of questions that can be examined at the intersection of developmental and self psychology. As illustrated in Table 32.1, each of these four basic developmental questions can be posed in reference to most, if not all, of the self-related attributes and processes described in this volume. The X's denote areas in which at least some empirical research has been conducted. In most cases, the empirical research is still in its infancy, and much work remains in these domains. But what we find striking about Table 32.1 is that most boxes represent virgin territory, yet to be addressed in the research literature. We hope that this volume will encour-

TABLE 32.1. Blueprint for Developmental Research on the Self

Self-attribute or process	Developmental changes in level	Developmental changes in quality	Etiology of individual differences	Developmental changes in the implications of individual differences
Cognitive aspects of the self (memory, information processing)				
Stability/variability in the self				
Organization of the self (complexity, compartmentalization)			×	
Implicit aspects of the self				
Self-awareness	×			
Self-control and self-regulation	×		×	
Goals and the self (mastery vs. performance, promotion vs. prevention)			×	
Self-efficacy				
Self-determination				
Trait self-esteem	×	×		
Self-esteem maintenance	×		×	
Self-verification				
Social comparison				
Self-relevant emotions	×		×	
Self in person perception and social judgment				
The self in relationships			×	
Social identity				×
Self-presentation		×		
Sociocultural aspects of self				
Disorders of the self				

Note. × denotes areas in which some empirical research has been conducted.

age social and personality psychologists to consider developmental issues in the context of their research. Similarly, we hope that developmental researchers incorporate into their own research many of the rich ideas and methods summarized in this volume.

Culture and Self

A repeating theme across many of the chapters is the intimate link between self and culture. It seems critical to consider cultural context when considering the nature, meaning, and functions of certain self-attributes.

As emphasized by Cross and Gore (Chapter 27, this volume; see also Markus & Kitayama, 1991), culture plays a pivotal role in the construction of self-beliefs and identity. As a result, there are likely fundamental differences in the nature of the self-related phenomena in qualitatively distinct cultures.

As with developmental aspects of the self, questions about cultural differences in the self may, at first glance, appear deceptively simple (e.g., How does [some aspect of the self] differ across cultures?). Here, too, four distinct types of questions about self and culture can be posed, paralleling the developmental questions just discussed.

The first two questions again concern differences in level or quality—in this instance, differences across cultural groups. First, are there cultural differences in the *level* of a given self-related construct? We might ask, for example, whether people from different cultures vary in level of self-esteem, self-consciousness, mastery motives, or death anxiety. Are there cultural differences in the degree of overlap between self and others that underlies intimacy?

Second, are there cultural differences in the *quality* of a given self-related construct? For example, does the relative importance of self-esteem in specific domains vary as a function of culture (e.g., Is social self-esteem more closely linked to global self-esteem in interdependent vs. independent cultures)? Are there cultural differences in the kinds of contexts that give rise to mastery motives or to death anxiety? Are there cultural differences in the degree of intimacy across distinct types of relationships (e.g., romantic partner, family member, acquaintance in the community), or in overlap between self and other people (Aron, Chapter 22, this volume)?

The third and fourth questions focus on individual differences (most often involving interaction or moderator effects). Although cultures may differ in mean level of an attribute, substantial individual differences exist within each cultural group, differences that may have culturally specific antecedents and consequences. Are there cultural differences in the etiology or developmental roots of individual differences in certain self-attributes or self-processes? For example, are there cultural differences in the types of parenting styles that give rise to high self-esteem or an emphasis on mastery versus performance goals? Are there cultural differences in the types of early experiences that foster a lifelong vulnerability to death anxiety or the capacity engage in close intimate relationships?

Finally, we can address questions regarding cultural differences in the implications of those individual differences. We may ask, for example, whether high self-esteem and the pursuit of mastery versus performance goals are more adaptive in independent versus interdependent cultural contexts. Can high self-esteem and a mastery orientation be a liability in some contexts but not in others? Does the relationship between death anxiety and creativity differ across cultures? Does the relationship between psychological adjustment and relationship intimacy, or overlap between self and other, vary as a function of interdependence of culture?

Again, these are just a sample of the kinds of questions about self and culture that can be examined. As in Table 32.1, regarding developmental aspects of the self, each of these four basic questions about culture can be posed in reference to most, if not all, of the self-related attributes and processes described in this volume. (We did not construct a parallel table to show areas of self research as they relate to culture because the vast majority of the cells in such a table would be empty due to the dearth of relevant research.) In recent years, self researchers have begun to make some inroads into this extensive territory, mostly with regard to the first question concerning mean differences across cultures. But most of the existing research focuses on only two cultures—Japanese and North American—and the other three questions about the link between self and culture have barely been addressed. In the coming years, we will surely learn more about the self around the globe.

Conclusions

In reading our colleagues' exceptional contributions to this *Handbook of Self and Identity,* we were impressed by the degree of integration already evident across the chapters. Researchers examining diverse functions and aspects of the self have not only staked out important new territory but are also remarkably well informed about each others' work. Each line of research presented in the foregoing chapters has been enriched both theoretically and methodologically by a consideration of related constructs and mechanisms. In this closing chapter, we have offered some final thoughts about what the future may hold for research on the self, focusing on evolutionary processes, self-esteem, development, and culture. More generally, however, we anticipate rapid growth and progress as researchers take the level of integration up a step further, integrating the "midlevel" theories presented here. What is needed next is a new level of self-theory that focuses on processes that bridge the breadth of phenomena linked to the uniquely human capacity for self-awareness. Many of the contributions in this volume (most notably Chapter 2) have made an important step in this direction, perhaps marking the beginning of the third generation of research on the self.

Note

1. The Janis–Field Feelings of Inadequacy scale (1959), another measure of self-esteem used widely in social and personality psychology, similarly eschews items evaluating self-worth in terms of comparison with others. Only one item involves direct social comparison ("How often do you feel inferior to most of the people you know?"). The Janis–Field suffers from other problems, however. Most notably, only a minority of items (6) seem to directly assess feelings of self-worth. The majority of items (17) assess some form of anxiety—primarily social or performance anxiety (see also Church, Truss, & Velicer, 1980).

References

Barkow, J. (1980). Prestige and self-esteem: A biosocial interpretation. In D. R. Omark, F. F. Strayer, & D. G. Freedman (Eds.), *Dominance relations: An ethological view of social conflict and social interaction* (pp. 319–332). New York: Garland STPM Press.

Baumeister, R. F., Smart, L., & Boden, J. M. (1996). Relation of threatened egotism to violence and aggression: The dark side of high self-esteem. *Psychological Review, 103,* 5–33.

Church, M. A, Truss, C. V., & Velicer, W. F. (1980). Structure of the Janis-Field Feelings of Inadequacy Scale. *Perceptual and Motor Skills, 50,* 935–939.

Cooley, C. H. (1902). *Human nature and the social order.* New York: Scribner's.

Gergen, K. J. (1991). *The saturated self.* New York: Basic Books.

Janis, I. L., & Field, P. B. (1959). A behavioral assessment of persuasibility: Consistency of individual differences. In C. I. Hovland & I. L. Janis (Eds.), *Personality and persuasibility* (pp. 29–54). New Haven, CT: Yale University Press.

Kohut, H. (1971). *The analysis of the self.* New York: International Universities Press.

Leary, M. R., & Downs, D. L. (1995). Interpersonal functions of the self-esteem motive: The self-esteem system as a sociometer. In M. Kernis (Ed.), *Efficacy, agency, and self-esteem* (pp. 123–144). New York: Plenum Press.

Markus, H. R., & Kitayama, S. (1991). Culture and the self: Implications for cognition, emotion, and motivation. *Psychological Review, 98,* 224–253.

Martin, L. (1999). I–D compensation theory: Some implications of trying to satisfy immediate-return needs in a delayed-return culture. *Psychological Inquiry, 10,* 195–208.

Rosenberg, M. (1965). *Society and the adolescent self-image.* Princeton, NJ: Princeton University Press.

Author Index

Subject Index

Page numbers followed by *f* indicate figure, *n* indicate note, and *t* indicate table.

691